Free Student Aid.

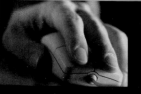

Log on.

Tune in.

Succeed.

Research Navigator™ is a great media resource that can help you succeed in your personal health course. Offering three exclusive online databases of credible and reliable source material, Research Navigator™ includes EBSCO's Content Select Academic Journal Database, The New York Times Search by Subject Archive, and "Best of the Web" Link Library. Research Navigator™ can help you make the most of your research time.

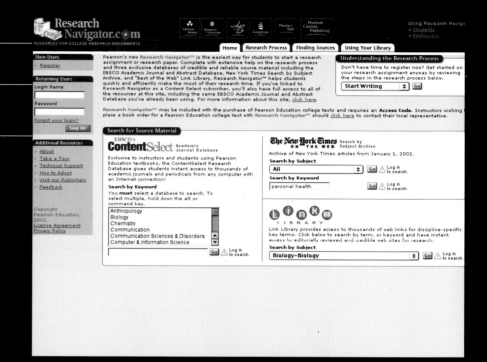

What your system needs to use these media resources:

WINDOWS™
266 MHz minimum CPU
Windows 98, NT, 2000, ME, XP
64 MB RAM installed
800 X 600 screen resolution, thousands of colors
56K Internet connection
Browser: Internet Explorer 5.0 and higher;
   Netscape 4.7, 7.0
Plug-Ins: Adobe Acrobat Reader

MACINTOSH™
266 MHz minimum CPU
OS 9.2 or higher
64 MB RAM available
800 x 600 screen resolution, thousands of colors
56K Internet connection
Browser: Internet Explorer 5.0 and higher;
   Netscape 4.7, 7.0
Plug-Ins: Adobe Acrobat Reader

Got technical questions?

For technical support, please visit www.aw.com/techsupport and complete the appropriate online form. You can also call our tech support hotline at 800-6-Pro-Desk (800-677-6337) Monday-Friday, 8 a.m. to 5 p.m. CST.

Here's your personal ticket to success:

How to log on to Research Navigator™:

1. Go to www.aw.com/donatelle.
2. Click the cover of *Donatelle, Access to Health, 8th Edition.*
3. Click the Research Navigator™ link located on the left side of the website.
4. Click on the "Register" button located under the "New User" sectin on the left side of the Research Navigator™ home-page.
5. Scratch off the foil below to reveal your pre-assigned access code.
6. Enter your access code exactly as it appears below.

7. Complete the online registration form to create your own personal Log In Name and Password.
8. Once your personal Log In Name and Password are confirmed by email, you can either go back to www.aw.com/donatelle and click Research Navigator™ or go to www.research navigator.com and type in yoru new Log In Name and Password under "Returning Users" and click "Log In."

Your Access Code is:

Record your new login name and password on the back of this card.

Cut out this card and keep it handy. It's your ticket to valuable information.

Important: Please read the License Agreement, located on the launch screen before using ResearchNavigator. By using the web site, you indicate that you have read, understood, and accepted the terms of this agreement.

Access
to Health

Access to Health

EIGHTH EDITION

Rebecca J. Donatelle, Ph.D.
Oregon State University

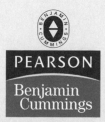

PEARSON

Benjamin
Cummings

San Francisco   Boston   New York
Cape Town   Hong Kong   London   Madrid   Mexico City
Montreal   Munich   Paris   Singapore   Sydney   Tokyo   Toronto

Publisher: Daryl Fox
Acquisitions Editor: Deirdre McGill
Development Manager: Claire Brassert
Project Editor: Susan Malloy
Assistant Editor: Christina Pierson
Cover Designer: Yvo Riezebos
Photo Researcher: Brian Donnelly, Cypress Integrated Systems
Manufacturing Buyer: Stacey Weinberger
Project Coordination: Elm Street Publishing Services, Inc.
Production Editor: Steven Anderson
Composition: Thompson Type
Cover Printer: Phoenix Color
Printer and Binder: Courier Kendallville

Cover Photo: © Nicholas Wilton/Images.com, Inc.

Credits can be found on page C-1 and C-2.

ISBN 0-8053-5564-2

Library of Congress Cataloging-in-Publication Data
    Donatelle, Rebecca J., 1950–
Access to health / Rebecca J. Donatelle.—8th ed.
        p. cm.
    Includes bibliographical references and index.
    ISBN 0-8053-5564-2 (alk. paper)
    1. Health. I. Title.

RA776.D66 2004
613—dc21

                                        2003043784

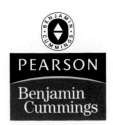

About the Author

Rebecca J. Donatelle is a teacher and mentor for undergraduate and graduate students in the Department of Public Health at Oregon State University. Although her main emphasis is in the area of Public Health Promotion and Health Education, she teaches a wide range of students from many disciplines on the Oregon State campus. Donatelle is an Associate Professor in Public Health and is the Coordinator of Public Health Promotion and Education Programs in the College of Health and Human Sciences. She has a Ph.D. in Community Health/Health Education, a Master of Science degree in Health Education, and a Bachelor of Science degree with majors in both Health/Physical Education and English. She is also a Certified Health Education Specialist.

Among the courses that she teaches are Principles of Health Behaviors, Stress and Health, Violence and Public Health, Epidemiology and Control of Chronic Diseases, and Introduction to Human Disease (Communicable). Recently, she has developed a new course on Complementary and Alternative Medicine.

In addition to her teaching responsibilities, Donatelle is an active researcher in the area of health behaviors, and she has been the principal investigator on a number of randomized, controlled trials focusing on motivating behavior change, the use of social support in facilitating behavior change, and the use of community supports to assist individuals in changing high-risk behaviors. Currently, she is working with pregnant women who smoke in an effort to get them to reduce or stop smoking during pregnancy and beyond. She has also conducted extensive research in the area of decision making and factors influencing the use of alternative and traditional health care providers for treatment of low back pain; illness and sick role behaviors; women's decisions about treatment for breast cancer and cardiac rehabilitation; and stress in health and disease.

Donatelle has received the Leadership Award, an Outstanding Teacher Award, and a Robert Wood Johnson Foundation Presidential Award for Promising New Research in the Smoke-Free Families National Initiative. She has been an active member of several state and national committees and task forces and continues to work to reduce risk for high risk populations, particularly women and older adults. In addition to *Access to Health,* Donatelle is the author of *Health: The Basics, Fitness for Health,* and *AIDS and STIs in a Global Society,* and she has written several chapters and manuscripts for various health-related books and journals.

Preface

At no time in human history have so many people been concerned about health. Newspaper headlines frequently proclaim that a new disease or environmental threat is on the rise. TV news shows employ medical doctors, health promotion specialists, dietary specialists, natural healers, and other professionals to cover the latest health breakthroughs and threats. We hear a constant litany of health do's and don'ts, stressing care in how we treat our bodies, minds, and spirits; however, these recommendations often seem confusing or contradictory. We worry about what illnesses we might catch from others; about environmental threats to health; about whether the foods we eat, the neighborhoods we live in, and the genes that we inherit pose health risks that require constant monitoring.

We face a number of challenges to our health that might have seemed unimaginable to our ancestors. Killer diseases that defy antibiotics, mysterious maladies that sap energy and restrict quality of life, harmful drugs that can lead to addiction, a health care system that excludes more and more people, and an increasingly degraded environment arc all causes for a great concern. Knowing how best to respond to these challenges, and which individual and societal resources should be enlisted in order to reduce risks to health and promote health, is the responsibility of each individual.

Juxtaposed against the threats to health are positive developments: new insights into specific health problems, new strategies for reducing risks, and new policies and programs designed to help us be healthier. Protective measures to promote well-being include the decision recently enacted in Corvallis, Oregon, to ban smoking in all public places (all bars, restaurants, etc.); mandate the use of seat belts and bicycle helmets; insurance coverage for mammograms; and labels that accurately describe the contents of food products. Public health programs encourage safer sex through condom use, ensure that children get adequate nutrition, and require immunization of all children in the United States. These developments indicate that people are working hard to make a difference.

As a consumer, making the best choices to ensure health is challenging, at best. Navigating the ever-changing sea of information about health may frustrate even the most knowledgeable among us. Today's health consumers face an astounding array of advertisements for health products and services, news flashes about diseases and cures, conventional and alternative treatments to choose from, and often contradictory information. To make matters worse, unproven products are advertised alongside those that are scientifically validated. Many nutrition supplements, such as herbs and nutritional compounds, are not regulated for consumer protection. Overworked health professionals may be pressed for time to explain health issues and reassure patients. Some health organizations target worried consumers and play on their vulnerabilities and desires (promising quick fixes for those who want to lose weight, be sexy, or add years to life). Needless to say, consumers need strategies for dealing with health concerns.

For health educators, preparing a new generation of students to be savvy consumers, armed with accurate information for making wise health decisions, is a formidable task. Writing an introductory health text for this population of students, in a field where information changes moment by moment, can be extremely challenging. Clearly, no *one* text can answer all of a student's questions, give solid advice about all possible topics, or even attempt to cover the vast spectrum of hotly debated health issues. After more than 30 years of teaching public health students and students from a wide array of health and nonhealth disciplines, we hope to provide the most accurate and up-to-date information about issues and topics that are most relevant to today's students. We strive to take students beyond what they were taught in high school and provide thought-provoking, scientifically valid information representing the culmination of years of research, rather than single-source, often spurious results of unsubstantiated research. We want to teach students how to evaluate information and process it in a systematic, reasoned way as they endeavor to make informed decisions about health. We believe that by challenging students to think about and discuss controversial health topics, they will become the citizens that future generations can rely on to develop sound policies, programs, and key health services.

This opportunity to assist a new generation of students to become future agents for change in the area of health is something we take seriously. Although issues of individual decision making and lifestyle are key features of *Access to Health*, we believe that individual health is also strongly influenced by public health actions and policy. Thus, we also focus on policies, programs, and services that *promote health and prevent premature disease and disability*. In addition, we are mindful of disparities in health and the underlying reasons for difference in risks based on race, ethnicity, age, gender, geographic region, and other factors. Recognizing that many of today's health problems know no national or international boundaries, we challenge students to think globally as they consider health risks and seek creative solutions to health problems. By reading, questioning, gaining greater understanding of the factors that contribute to individual and societal health, and contemplating possible actions that may reduce risk, *Access to Health* prepares students for their own development as well as possible futures in the field.

As we prepared this text, we spent countless hours talking with students, interacting with them in classes, and testing what "works" and what "does not work" in today's introductory health classes. Even more time was spent talking with course instructors, surveying selected features and finding out how instructors assess whether such features benefit students. As always, we invited comments and suggestions on how to make this the ***best*** edition of *Access to Health* yet and the foremost personal health text on the market today.

We are pleased with the overwhelming success that *Access to Health* has enjoyed through its many revisions and changes, and we are gratified that many of you have continued to use this text. We hope that this edition once again meets the high standards we have previously established and that its rich foundation of scientifically valid and current citations, its wealth of technological tools and resources, and its thought-provoking exercises will continue to stimulate students to share our enthusiasm for health and to actively engage in health promotion and disease prevention.

New to This Edition

As in our previous editions, we are committed to a tradition of excellence with the eighth edition of *Access to Health*. As such, this text maintains many features that it has become known for, while also focusing on exciting new health trends. The eighth edition has been updated, line by line, so that all facts and figures reflect cutting-edge research. This careful attention to detail ensures that students will be getting the latest information about health topics as this text goes to press. As is the tradition with *Access to Health,* we include "hot" areas of interest for today's students. We maintain the heart and focus of *Access to Health,* but offer readers something new and different, which we hope will help them gain greater insights into the controversies, issues, and realities of today's health marketplace. The most noteworthy changes include the following:

- **New opportunities for self-assessment and behavior change.** The revision and replacement of many Assess Yourself boxes ensure that they ask the questions that are relevant to students' lives. For example, students have the opportunity to consider how tattoos and piercing, safer sex, and the use of club drugs affect their overall health assessment in Chapter 1, and sources of stress specific to college students are assessed in the new Assess Yourself box in Chapter 3. The new Behavior Change Contracts encourage students to follow through with the changes suggested by the results of these self-assessments.

- **Increased coverage of the mind-body connection and spirituality,** plus the role of spirituality and emotional health in overall health status. New figures summarizing major themes of spirituality, new information on mental health problems and anxiety disorders, and a new table on the signs and symptoms of depression as well as information on other factors important to one's overall mental health are included. Groundbreaking material on self-inflicted cutting behaviors is designed to prompt student thinking and discussion about an emerging problem among adolescents and young adults.

- **Expanded and updated coverage on violence, terrorism, and bioterrorism in Chapter 4** designed to increase student awareness of the tremendous toll that violence takes in America and throughout the world and the potential threats of these forms of violence on future generations. New facts and figures are included on trends in crime, economic implications of crime, and the emotional and physical burden of violent crime among selected populations. Date rape, stranger rape, and marital rape are all discussed in terms of factors that contribute to these crimes, the impact on those affected by rape, and related societal issues.

- **Significant expansion in the areas of personal fitness, strength and conditioning, and newer forms of fitness regimens,** including information on Pilates, yoga, tai chi, and the role of strength and conditioning in increased metabolic rates and weight loss. We also cover a unique, often ignored, area: exercise programs for overweight, obese, and/or very out-of-shape individuals. Information on factors to consider when buying exercise equipment and fitness club memberships should be of interest to students of all ages.

- **A significant revision and expansion of our groundbreaking chapter on Complementary and Alternative Medicine.** Although we were the first to offer a full chapter devoted to this topic, keeping up with trends in research and verifying new information requires considerable thought, research, and effort. Not only did we reorganize this chapter to be more user friendly, we substantially increased content and research-based information in response to reviewer comments and suggestions. Students are encouraged, via thought-provoking exercises and skills development, to be critical consumers, ask key questions, and seek scientifically defensible facts from reliable resources as they consider various CAM products and services, as well as more traditional medical remedies.

- **Major updates, revisions, and additions in the areas of nutrition and weight management,** including new guidelines on organic foods, the importance of soy and flax in healthy diets, the roles of antioxidants, lycopene, omega-3, and omega-6 fats in a healthy diet, new vegetarian Food Guide Pyramid guidelines, the use of food as medicine, and other topics that are of interest to today's adults. Because new information about nutrition and diet surfaces daily, we tried to find the most reputable sources and summarize those areas that students seem to have the most questions about. In addition, the growing epidemic of obesity in America today provided impetus for significant updating and expansion of our sections on weight control and eating behaviors.

- **Expanded coverage of environmental issues and concerns** including our roles and responsibilities for environmental health, conservation, and protection of the environment. We added new information on the Air Quality Index, potential risks from prolonged exposure to cell phones, and dangers from molds and other environmental health risks at home and outdoors. Comparisons in consumption patterns between Americans and persons in other nations is designed to stimulate discussion and critical thinking.
- **New and expanded coverage of infectious and chronic diseases** such as diabetes, West Nile Virus, resistant bacterial diseases, pathogens related to bioterrorism threats, hepatitis A, B, and C, tuberculosis, and the growing global burden of disease from HIV/AIDS is presented. In addition, new statistics on cancer and heart disease and new guidelines for blood pressure monitoring are included.
- **Continued focus on diversity and the importance of recognizing differences** in health statistics, health risks, and other health-related factors based on gender, race, ethnicity, age, socioeconomic status, sexual orientation, relationship status, culture, country of origin, and other sociodemographic factors.
- **New coverage of topics relevant to college-aged populations.** Whether the topic is information on new contraceptives such as NuvaRing, Lunelle, Ortho Evra, and Mirena; water and health; abuse of OxyContin; skin cancer; the connection between stress and health; or a vast array of other topics, we have tried to focus on areas of relevance to a new generation of healthy-savvy students. In many instances, we have updated facts and figures as we go to press and hope that you will find these data to be interesting and important. If you have topics that you would like to see included or expanded upon, please feel free to email the author at *Becky.Donatelle@orst.edu*.

Maintaining a Standard of Excellence

With every edition, the challenge for the author and specific chapter authors has been to make the book "better" than before, and to provide information and material that surpass the competition at every level. As such, we have painstakingly considered our reviewer feedback from the previous edition and strengthened and improved pedagogical standards.

- Chapter 1 establishes both the individual and social context of health and disease and the importance of health to society as a whole, a dual approach used throughout the text. In order to assist students in their efforts to achieve health, we provide a foundation for sound decision making based on well-established theories of health behavior. Decision making through critical thinking and awareness continues to form the cornerstone of each chapter. This is shown in pedagogical tools such as the "What Do You Think?" opening scenarios that include reflective

questions and the "Taking Charge" section that introduces students to how they might best use a particular chapter in building their own positive health behaviors.

- The roles of the community, health policies, and health services in disease prevention and health promotion are integrated throughout the text. The public health approach is often ignored in health texts in favor of individual action only. We believe that optimum health changes will occur only in environments that are conducive to change, in which individuals can maximize resources to make long-term behavior changes. This underlying philosophy concerning the capacity for change is incorporated throughout the text and highlighted in the Checklist for Change at the closing section of each chapter.
- Within a strong pedagogical framework, the importance of building health skills is emphasized and integrated consistently throughout the text. Readers will learn specific applications in every chapter through the Assess Yourself, Skills for Behavior Change, and Taking Charge sections.

Special Features

Each chapter in *Access to Health* includes the following special feature boxes designed to help students think about healthy behavior skills as well as how to apply the concepts in everyday life:

- **Assess Yourself** boxes provide quick, general indicators of personal health status in various areas, which students may consider when initiating behavior change.
- **New Horizons in Health** boxes present information on "hot interest" topics. These include late-breaking information or high-interest pieces that should be singled out for special emphasis.
- **Health Ethics: Conflict and Controversy** boxes provide a forum for discussing controversial issues and the relative ethics of these topics.
- **Reality Check** boxes focus attention on potential risks and health and safety issues by providing the most current facts and statistics. Their main purpose is to inform students about risks and lead them to recognize their own potential health problems.
- **Skills for Behavior Change** boxes focus on practical strategies that students can use to improve health or reduce their risks from negative health behaviors.
- **Women's Health/Men's Health** boxes include newsworthy health-related topics focusing on health, research, and treatment issues related to gender. In addition, pending legislation and policies affecting men's and women's health are explored.
- **Health in a Diverse World** boxes promote acceptance of diversity on college campuses and beyond and strategies for adapting to an increasingly diverse world. They also encourage understanding of domestic and international perspectives on health.

Learning Aids

Chapter Objectives   Each chapter is introduced with a set of objectives tied to the major sections of the chapter. The objectives serve as a helpful tool when learning and reviewing key concepts of the chapter.

What Do You Think? Scenarios   These scenarios are designed to prompt discussions that are relevant to the chapter and that apply to students' experiences.

What Do You Think? Questions   Groups of questions appear throughout each chapter to encourage students to think critically as they read the text.

Running Glossary of Key Terms   To emphasize and support understanding of the meaning of terms, these terms are bold-faced in the text and defined in the margin next to where they are first introduced. Key terms are also listed in alphabetical order at the end of the text.

Taking Charge   At the end of each chapter, Taking Charge wraps up the chapter contents with a focus on application by the student. Included is a Checklist for Change to help students assess their personal health attitudes and habits and their community's health status, with recommendations on how to make changes for both. In addition, the following features are included: Summary, Questions for Discussion and Reflection, Application Exercises, and Further Reading. These features follow up on the chapter's objectives, content, and concepts as well as expand on the scenarios and class discussions. New to Taking Charge is Accessing Your Health on the Internet. This section provides descriptions of relevant online resources, including sites from organizations such as the World Health Organization (WHO), Centers for Disease Control and Prevention (CDC), and the Mayo Clinic. These links and hundreds more can be found on the Companion Website for *Access,* described in more detail later.

   In addition, two appendixes give practical information in an easy format. **Appendix A** concerns first aid, describing procedures that may prevent injury and save lives. **Appendix B** gives nutritional information about a broad array of foods. Students can evaluate current eating behaviors and plan for improved nutrition.

For Students *and* Instructors

MyHealthClass   An online standard course management system (built on the CourseCompass™ platform) loaded with valuable free student and instructor resources.

   MyHealthClass features preloaded content—all described in detail below—gathered together at one convenient Internet address: www.myhealthclass.com. Included on the site are a Behavior Change Log Book and Wellness Journal, Health on the Net, Take Charge of Your Health! Worksheets, and links to StudentBody101.com and the Companion Website. In addition, MyHealthClass offers access to Research Navigator™, eThemes of the Times, and the computerized test bank.

Student Supplements

Behavior Change Log Book and Wellness Journal   This assessment tool helps students track daily activity and nutritional intake to create a long-term nutrition and fitness plan. It also includes topics for journal-based activities and behavior change contracts.

Take Charge of Your Health! Self-Assessment Workbook with Review and Practice Tests   Includes self-assessment activities for each chapter, worksheets, and review/practice tests.

Health on the Net   An excellent enhancement to interactive student learning, this catalog of Internet resources provides tips for researching online, course-specific URLs, and MLA and APA guidelines.

StudentBody101.com   This dynamic website, accessed at www.studentbody101.com, focuses on alcohol, drugs, stress, fitness, tobacco, and sexuality and facilitates active learning by posting current journal articles, self-assessments, online discussions, and behavior change tips. It is accredited by Health on the Net.

Study Guide for StudentBody101.com   This supplement guides students through the StudentBody101 website and ensures that each student gets the most out of the site.

Companion Website   This website, designed for easy navigation and not password protected, can be accessed at www.aw.com/donatelle. It offers a range of activities including self-assessments, practice quizzes, open-ended critical thinking questions, weblinks, and audio and video clips. Online flashcards allow students to quiz themselves on key terms from the text. Also included is eThemes of the Times, a site containing 30 *New York Times* articles reporting on the latest health news and research.

Research Navigator™   A six-month subscription to this online resource (free with all new copies of the text) offers extensive help on the research process and three databases of credible and reliable source material: EBSCO's Content Select™ Academic Journal Database, *New York Times* Search by Subject Archive, and "Best of the Web" Link Library.

Instructor Supplements

Discovery Health Channel Health and Wellness Lecture Launcher Videos   Created in partnership between Discovery Health Channel and Benjamin Cummings, these VHS tapes feature quick lecture-launcher clips on topics from nutrition to stress management to substance abuse. There are 24 clips in all in this two-volume set, each five to ten minutes in length. Additional videos are available from the Benjamin Cummings Video Series and from Films for the Humanities to qualified adopters.

Instructor's Resource Manual with Media Guide   This resource provides individual and classroom activities, chapter objectives, outlines, and Companion Website resources to reinforce chapter concepts and develop effective student learning. It also offers ideas for incorporating the Discovery Health Channel videos into the course.

Instructor's Resource Binder   This three-ring binder accommodates all of the printed supplements for *Access to Health*.

Printed Test Bank and Computerized Test Bank   The test bank includes multiple-choice, short-answer, true/false, matching, and essay questions for each chapter. The cross-platform Test Bank CD-ROM allows you to create tests, edit questions, and add your own material to existing exams. It includes the entire printed Test Bank.

PowerPoint® Presentation CD-ROM   This cross-platform CD-ROM is a lecture resource containing figures and tables from the book as well as customizable lecture outlines.

Transparency Acetates   The figures and tables are also available in full color for lecture presentations.

Take Charge of Your Health! Worksheets   A sampling of 45 self assessments from the *Take Charge!* workbook that is available separately from the workbook.

Instructor's Guide for StudentBody101.com   Tips for using the online resource of StudentBody101 are featured in this guide, with ideas for conducting discussions, assigning writing activities, and more.

Course Management   WebCT and Blackboard are also available; consult your Benjamin Cummings sales representative for details.

Acknowledgments

After writing eight editions of *Access to Health*, I can only marvel at the dedication and professionalism of the many fine publishing experts who have helped make such a text successful. With each subsequent edition of *Access*, their skills in dealing with the complexities and considerations of the publication process have become more apparent. From the excellent, hands-on initial efforts of Joe Heider and Ted Bolen of Prentice Hall during my "early apprentice" days as an author, to the continued professionalism of Suzy Spivey, Joe Burns, Mary Kriener, Max Chuck, and others at Allyn and Bacon, I have been extremely fortunate in having a steady stream of fine publishing teams to help me create the foundations of a text that was responsive to students, creative in approach, and reflective of the most important health trends of the times.

Having had such an outstanding group of prior publishing teams, I was initially concerned to learn that *Access to Health* was transferred to another publisher. These concerns were quickly allayed as I met with Acquisitions Editor Deirdre McGill, Publisher Daryl Fox, and the outstanding group of editorial staff from Benjamin Cummings who would work with me on subsequent editions of the text. Although I wouldn't have thought it was possible to beat past publishing efforts, I must honestly say that my experiences with Benjamin Cummings have been the best of my publishing years, and remarkably—it just keeps getting better! From the wonderful guidance, thoughtful suggestions, and patient prodding demonstrated by Susan Teahan, my initial project editor with *Health: The Basics*, to the superb effort, expertise, and guidance shown by Susan Malloy in this edition of *Access to Health* and related supplements, I have been extremely impressed by the high level of skill that the Benjamin Cummings editorial staff exhibits. These two women have been wonderful to work with and many thanks are due each of them for the ways in which they make an author's work come to fruition. I have worked with many others over the years and these two are among the absolute finest in their field. In addition, I would like to acknowledge the wonderful editorial assistance provided by Developmental Editor Alice E. Fugate, who did an outstanding job in a short time frame to merge some of the newest features of *Health: The Basics* with content from *Access to Health* and in suggesting revisions and modifications based on reviewer comments and market demands. This was a huge and complicated task and Alice did a remarkable job. Although these women were key contributors to the finished work, there were many other people who worked on this revision of *Access to Health*.

In particular, I would like to thank my Production Editor, Becky Dodson, for her invaluable assistance in final book development and refinement, and Christina Pierson, Assistant Editor, for preparing the manuscript and overseeing the complete supplements package. I would also like to thank the Benjamin Cummings marketing and sales force, particularly Marketing Manager Sandra Lindelof, who spent countless hours making sure that *Access to Health* got into instructors' hands. Part of the success of any book depends on the efforts of those who work diligently to make sure that the strengths of the book are outlined and that instructors are able to make good decisions about what their students will be reading. In keeping with my overall experiences with Benjamin Cummings, the sales staff and editorial staff are among the best of the best. I am very lucky to have them working with me on this project and want to extend a special thanks to all of them!

In addition, many colleagues, students, and staff members have provided the feedback, reviews, extra time and assistance, and encouragement that have helped me meet the demands of rigorous publishing deadlines over the years. With each edition of the book, your assistance has made the vision for *Access to Health* a reality. Rather than just creating an upscale version of a high school text, we have worked diligently to provide a text that is "alive" for readers. With each edition, we would not have developed a book like this one without the outstanding contributions of several key people. Whether acting as reviewers, generating new ideas, providing expert commentary, or writing chapters, each of these professionals has added his or her skills to our collective endeavor.

Contributors to the Eighth Edition

Dr. Patricia Ketcham (Oregon State University): Chapter 7, Reproductive Choices: Making Responsible Decisions; Chapter 11, Addictions and Addictive Behavior: Threats to Wellness; Chapter 12, Drinking Responsibly: A Lifestyle Challenge on Campus; Chapter 13, Tobacco and Caffeine: Daily Pleasures, Daily Challenges; Chapter 14, Illicit Drugs: Use, Misuse, and Abuse; Chapter 22, Consumerism: Selecting Health Care Products and Services; and Appendix A, Injury Prevention and Emergency Care.

Donna Champeau (Oregon State University): Chapter 6, Sexuality: Choices in Sexual Behavior; Chapter 20, Dying and Death: The Final Transition.

Reviewers for the Eighth Edition

Clearly, *Access to Health* continues to be an evolving "work in progress." With each new edition, we have built on the combined expertise of many colleagues throughout the country who are dedicated to the education and behavioral changes of students. We thank the many reviewers of the past seven editions of *Access to Health* who have made such valuable contributions. For the eighth edition, reviewers who have helped us continue this tradition of excellence include Jan Adair, Minnesota State University; Barbara Anton, Minnesota State University; Jeremy Barnes, Southeast Missouri State University; Jill Black, Cleveland State University; Kim Clark, California State University San Bernadino; Craig Elder, Southeast Missouri State University; Rebecca Leas, Clarion University; Irene O'Boyle, Central Michigan University; Miguel Perez, California State University Fresno; and Pat Rada-Sidinger, Colorado Mountain College.

We have also had invaluable feedback from the colleagues who attended our Health Summits: Thanks to Daniel Adame, Emory University; Fran Babich, Butte College; Elizabeth Barrington, San Diego Mesa College; Christine Beyer, Kennesaw State University; Larry Bryant, Georgia Southern University; Donna Cobb, University of Central Oklahoma; Sandy Collins, Los Angeles Southwest College; Trey Cone, University of Central Oklahoma; Shae Donham, Northeastern State University; Linda Glatte, San Diego State University; Kathy Hixon, Northeastern State University; Jane Hoffmeyer, Georgia Perimeter University; Amy Howton, Kennesaw State University; Erica Jackson, Auburn University; Bushra Jonna, Grossmont College; Raeann Koerner, Ventura College; Teri McFarland, Palomar College; James Noto, San Diego State University; Rusty Pippin, Baylor University; Jan Riggs, Los Angeles Southwest College; Teresa Snow, Georgia Institute of Technology; J Stelzer, Valdosta State University; Matt Wilson, Georgia Southern University; Debbie Wulff, Grossmont College, and to the Health and Physical Education Department at Utah Valley State College, especially its chair, Vance Hillman.

Brief Contents

Contents

Chapter 6
Sexuality: Choices in Sexual Behavior   152

Chapter 7
Reproductive Choices: Making Responsible Decisions   174

Appendixes

Feature Boxes

Assess Yourself

Health Ethics: Conflict and Controversy

Health in a Diverse World

New Horizons in Health

Reality Check

Skills for Behavior Change

Women's Health/Men's Health

Access to Health

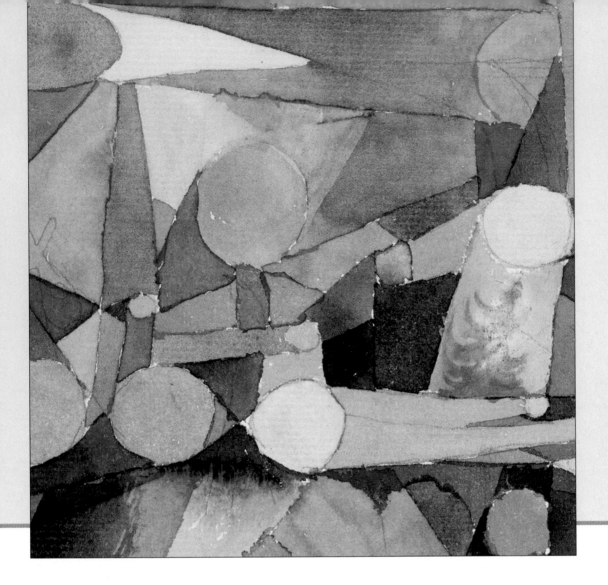

Objectives

* Discuss health in terms of historical perspectives, multidimensional elements, and the importance of a health-promoting lifestyle in preventing premature disease and disability.

* Discuss the health status of Americans, the factors that contribute to health, and the importance of *Healthy People 2010* and the Agency for Health Care, Research, and Quality (AHRQ) guidelines in establishing national goals for promoting health.

* Evaluate the role of gender in health status, health research, and health training.

* Discuss the health challenges faced by people of various racial and cultural backgrounds.

* Explain the importance of understanding our differences and developing a global perspective on population health.

* Provide a rationale for focusing on risk behaviors as a means of influencing health status.

* Evaluate sources of health information, particularly the Internet, to determine reliability.

* Examine how predisposing factors, beliefs, attitudes, and significant others affect a person's behavior changes.

* Survey behavior-change techniques, and learn how to apply them to personal situations.

* Apply decision-making techniques to your own lifestyle.

Promoting Healthy Behavior Change

What do you think?

In 2001, the leading cause of death for Americans ages 15–24 was unintentional injury, followed by homicide/legal intervention, and suicide. Americans aged 25–44 were also most likely to die from unintentional injuries, but other leading causes of death included cancer and heart disease.

Why might unintentional injury be prevalent among these two age groups? ✳ *What types of unintentional injuries might be typical for each group?* ✳ *Why might homicide and legal intervention rates be higher in younger Americans?* ✳ *What policies or programs might reduce these death rates?*

Bev reads on the Internet that bananas coming into the United States from South America have been contaminated with a particularly virulent strain of bacteria that affects the nervous system. She quickly e-mails all of her friends, telling them to stop eating bananas! Later, she finds out that this was all a hoax and there is no truth to the rumor. Not only is she embarrassed, she gets numerous e-mail replies telling her that she is easily duped. She also gets a letter from a large grocery chain, threatening a lawsuit for spreading rumors that may hurt business.

Have you ever been victimized by believing health claims that you've seen on the Internet? ✳ *What can you do to ensure that you are not unknowingly spreading false or misleading information?* ✳ *As a consumer, how can you find out if such claims are worthy of consideration?*

Concerned about your health? You are not alone. At no time in U.S. history have so many individuals, government agencies, educational systems, community groups, businesses, and health care organizations been so concerned about health or so vocal in their attempts to influence daily health habits. Billboards graphically display the dangers of drinking and driving and the impact of cigarette smoke, even on people who don't smoke. Television ads warn of the dangers of unsafe sexual activity and illegal drugs while touting the miraculous benefits of an endless arsenal of prescription medicines designed to "fix" everything from arthritis and high cholesterol to panic attacks and depression. Even the president held a special press conference in 2002 to warn U.S. citizens that over half of us are overweight and unfit, and the health of the country is in jeopardy due to epidemic rates of obesity, diabetes, and other lifestyle-related maladies. On a daily basis, you are challenged to "Just do it, but don't overdo it"; "Be all you can be, but be yourself"; "Drink your milk, but maybe you should consider soy"; "Eat cruciferous vegetables, but buy organic" —and if you want to look and feel good, exercise, exercise, exercise, but not to the point of being obsessed!

Although conflicting health claims abound, research that would provide a clear message about their authenticity is scarce or written in technical language that is hard for the typical person to interpret. Many people are confused about what they should and should not do. Sound familiar? We often assume that the government and the medical profession will protect us, only to find out later that what we've been told is true, may in fact be false. As an example, for the past three decades doctors have advised women who've gone through menopause to take hormone replacement therapy as protection against heart disease and stroke. Research appeared to support this recommendation. In 2002, however, the findings of a more carefully controlled clinical trial dealt women a considerable blow: Not only does hormone replacement therapy *not* protect against heart disease, stroke, and blood clots, it actually seems to increase the risk for these diseases![1]

In this case, health researchers, practitioners, and others on whom we rely appear to have based long-standing prevention and treatment regimens on faulty premises. How many other health recommendations are false or misleading? Our best scientists often struggle to determine which research is valid and which provides only a preliminary indicator of hazards or benefits. How can the average person figure out what is accurate and what is bogus?

Suffice it to say, answering these questions is not an easy task. It is fairly easy to see why individuals struggle so hard to "get it right" when it comes to making health decisions that may affect them or those they care about. It should also come as no surprise that in spite of all of the emphasis on health in society today and all of our collective resources aimed at prevention, intervention, and treatment, the health status of Americans continues to be plagued by old problems (see the New Horizons in Health box on "America's Mixed Health Bag: Improvements, Disparities, and Continuing Problems").

Why is being healthy so challenging for so many of us? What can we do to overcome these challenges, make better decisions about our behaviors, and become wiser, more responsible health consumers? There are no easy answers, because health is influenced by a myriad of factors—some that we can control and some that we can't. But the good news is that many people have found the skills and motivation to look objectively at where they are, plan carefully, and make decisions that improve their life and health. They have learned how to use the technological and community resources that are at their disposal in ways that are likely to enhance rather than diminish their health. Perhaps more importantly, they have found their own unique ways to make behavior changes that are long term. Have you ever wondered how one of your friends managed to lose weight and is now out kayaking and running in triathlons, when you can't seem to lose an ounce, and the latest trip up the stairs leaves you panting for breath? Or why another friend seems to thrive under pressure, while it makes you break down into a screaming fit or tears? Why do so many good health intentions remain only intentions, without progressing to the action phase?

This text is not designed to provide a foolproof recipe for achieving health or to answer all of your questions. It *is* designed to provide fundamental knowledge about health topics, to help you utilize personal and community resources to create your own health profile, and to challenge you to think more carefully before making decisions that affect your health or the health of others. It shows how policies, programs, media, culture, and ethnic, gender, and socioeconomic status influence health, directly and indirectly, both in the United States and around the world.

It is our hope that you will gain appreciation for the many achievements that we've made in health and the many challenges that lie ahead. Additionally, it is our hope that you will begin to look at global health not in an ethnocentric way, in which you are only able to appreciate those who look and talk like you and have habits and customs like yours, but rather in a more inclusive way.

Health decisions should be based on the best available research and should be consistent with who you are, your values and beliefs, and who you want to become. Although your health is not always totally within your control, certain behavior choices will affect you positively today and reduce future health risks. For those risk factors that are beyond your control, you must learn to react, adapt, respond appropriately, and use a reasoned, rather than purely emotional, rationale for your choices. By making informed, rational decisions, you will improve both the quality and the length of your own life and have a positive influence on those around you. (See the Reality Check box for tips on using the Internet to gather useful information.)

America's Mixed Health Bag: Improvements, Disparities, and Continuing Problems

Our national preoccupation with health should make it easier to get healthy, stay healthy, and live a long and productive life. However, while we are doing better in some areas, we still have a long way to go in others. A national survey of trends in health behaviors from 1991–2000, known as the Behavioral Risk Factor Surveillance System, indicates that Americans are buckling up (seat belts) but chugging down (alcohol) more than ever, that they are fatter and less fit than at any time in our nation's history, and that they are getting their cancer screening tests, but still smoking too much. Specific findings in this research are that:

- Binge drinking, particularly among college-aged adults, increased in one-third of all states and declined in only three states. Increases concentrated in the South and Midwest, where Wisconsin had the highest amount of binge drinking in 1999 (19.6 percent, compared with 16.4 percent in 1991). Illinois had the greatest increase during the study, jumping from 7.3 percent to 13.9 percent.
- Most states reported increases in seat belt use, mammograms, adult vaccinations, and screening for cervical cancer.
- Levels of physical inactivity rose in 3 of 48 states and declined in 11 states.
- Cholesterol screening increased in 13 of 47 states and decreased in 5 states.
- Obesity rose in *all* states. Well over half of all Americans are either overweight or obese.
- Smoking increased in 14 of 47 states. It declined in only one state, Minnesota.

Another national report, summarizing trends in racial and ethnic-specific health indicators in the United States as part of *Healthy People 2000,* indicates that although we are doing better as a population, there are still great disparities in our overall health status. According to Surgeon General David Satcher, "Americans of all ages and in every racial and ethnic group have better health today . . . but until all groups are equally protected, our work isn't done." Here are key points from this report:

- All racial and ethnic groups experienced improvements in rates for 10 key health indicators: prenatal care, infant mortality, teen births, death rates for heart disease, homicide, motor vehicle crashes, work-related injuries, tuberculosis rates, syphilis rates, and air quality.
- Five more health indicators—total death rate and death rates for stroke, lung cancer, breast cancer, and suicide—improved in all groups *except* American Indians and Alaska Natives.
- The percent of children living in poverty improved for all groups *except* Asian or Pacific Islanders.
- Percent of low birthweight infants improved only among African American and non-Hispanic groups.

Still other findings from recent years highlight America's ongoing health concerns:

- Sales of red meat, butter, and other high-fat foods, once on the decline, are seeing an unprecedented rise.
- Salad bars, low-fat grilled items, and portion control are on the decline, as consumers opt for super-sized burgers and monster meals at popular restaurant chains.
- Cigarette smoking among our nation's young has declined, but certain groups—particularly young women—continue to smoke at high rates.
- Depression, mental health problems, certain infectious diseases, and other preventable ailments are on the rise.

- The diabetes rate among young adults is skyrocketing—up over 30 percent in the past decade.
- Increasing numbers of Americans lack access to basic health care.

As our population becomes more diverse—with growing numbers of Hispanics, Asians, and African Americans as well as other racial and ethnic minorities and persons who live in the United States illegally—poverty continues to be the single greatest barrier to health care, creating a burgeoning population of underserved or unserved individuals. One of the greatest lessons is that we need to tailor interventions and prevention activities to the unique needs of diverse groups.

Sources: D. Nelson et al., "State Trends in Health Risk Factors and Receipt of Clinical Preventive Services Among Adults During the 1990s," *Journal of the American Medical Association* 287 (20) (May 22/29,2002); National Center for Health Statistics, "Healthy People 2000, Trends in Racial and Ethnic-Specific Rates for Health Status Indicators: United States, 1990–1998. Statistical Note No. 23.16 pp. (PHS) 2002." (see http://www.cdc.gov/nchs/releases/02news/healthimpr.htm); J. Seidell, "Dietary Fat and Obesity: An Epidemiological Perspective," *American Journal of Clinical Nutrition* 67 (1998): 546–552; U.S. Department of Health and Human Services, Centers for Disease Control and Prevention (2002) (see http://www.cdc.gov); National Institute for Mental Health (2002) (see http://www.nimh.nih.gov); National Center for Health Statistics (2000) (see http://www.cdc.gov/nchs/search/search.htm); Agency for Healthcare Research and Quality (2002) (see http://www.ahcpr.gov).

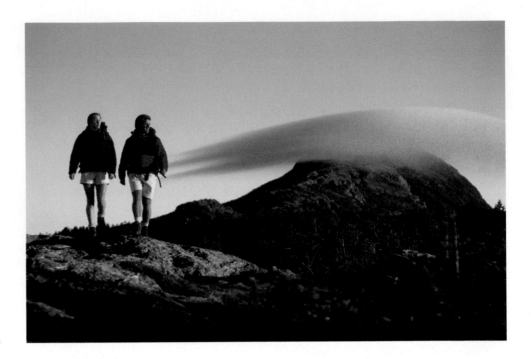

Today, health and wellness mean taking a positive, proactive attitude toward life and living it to its fullest.

Putting Your Health in Perspective

Although we use the term **health** almost unconsciously, few people understand the broad scope of the word or what it really means. For some, *health* simply means the antithesis of sickness. To others, it means being in good physical shape and able to resist illness. Still others use terms like **wellness,** or *well-being,* to include a wide array of factors that seem to lead to positive health status. Why all of these variations? In part, the differences are due to an increasingly enlightened way of viewing health that has taken shape over time. In addition, as our collective understanding of illness has improved, so has our ability to understand the many nuances of health. Our progress to current understandings about health has evolved over centuries, and we have a long way to go in achieving a truly comprehensive view of this complex subject.

Health   The ever-changing process of achieving individual potential in the physical, social, emotional, mental, spiritual, and environmental dimensions.

Wellness   The achievement of the highest level of health possible in each of several dimensions.

Medical Model   A model in which health status was focused primarily on the individual and a biological or diseased organ perspective.

Ecological or Public Health Model   A model in which diseases and other negative health events are viewed as a result of an individual's interaction with his/her social and physical environment.

Health: Yesterday and Today

Prior to the 1800s, if you weren't sick, you were not only regarded as lucky, but also healthy. When deadly epidemics such as bubonic plague, pneumonic plague, influenza, tuberculosis, and cholera killed millions of people, survivors were believed to be of hearty, healthy stock, and congratulated themselves on their good fortune. Poor health was often associated with poor hygiene and unsanitary conditions, and certain stigmas were attached to households that harbored any of these illnesses. Not until the late 1800s and early 1900s did researchers slowly begin to discover that victims of these epidemics were not simply unhealthy or dirty. Rather, they were victims of environmental factors (microorganisms found in contaminated water, air, and human waste) that made them sick and over which they often had little control. Public health officials moved swiftly to address these problems, and as a result, the term *health* became synonymous with *good hygiene.* Colleges offered courses in health and hygiene, the predecessors of the course you are in today.

Throughout the years, perceptions of health were dominated by the **Medical Model,** in which health status focused primarily on the individual and a biological or diseased organ perspective. The surest way to bring about improved health was to cure or *treat* disease. Health and health status were primarily considered to be a result of something that happened to a person due to poor behavior, contact with a pathogen, or other negative influence on the body. Restoring health via medicines or therapy was the main goal of this model, and government resources focused on initiatives that led to treatment of disease as a means of intervention. Even today, there are those who believe that it is cheaper to give someone a medicine to control a disease than it would be to prevent the disease from developing in the first place.

Consumer Beware: Hoaxes, Rumors, and Other Perils of the Internet

Looking for reliable health information on the Internet? Wondering if that e-mail warning of a deadly pathogen in your hamburger is fact or fiction? Dazed by searching for a topic, only to be confronted with 300,000 websites in your search results? Each year more than 100 million people seek health information on the Internet. Many of them end up frazzled, confused, and—worst of all—misinformed.

Clearly, not all health websites are created equal. Where should you start? Here are some tips to point you in the right direction:

✔ Websites sponsored by an official government agency, a university or college, or a hospital/medical center typically offer accurate, up-to-date information about a wide range of health topics. Government sites are easily identified by their .gov extensions (for example, the National Institute of Mental Health is http://www.nimh.nih.gov); college and university sites typically have .edu extensions (Johns Hopkins University is http://www.jhu.edu). Hospitals often have an .org extension (Mayo Clinic: http://www.mayohealth.org), although some of these may not be so readily identifiable. Major philanthropic foundations, such as the Robert Wood Johnson Foundation, the Legacy Foundation, the Kellogg Foundation, and others, often provide information about selected health topics.

✔ Links associated with well-established, professionally peer-reviewed journals such as the *New England Journal of Medicine* (http://www.nejm.org/) or the *Journal of the American Medical Association (JAMA)* (http://www.amaassn.org/) are good sources. While some of these sites require a fee for access, often you can locate basic abstracts and information, such as a weekly table of contents that can help you conduct a search. Other times, you can pay a basic fee for a certain number of hours of unlimited searching.

✔ For consumer news and updates on health-related hoaxes, consult the Centers for Disease Control and Prevention. The CDC provides consumer alerts on topics such as buying antibiotics online and e-mail health hoaxes. A sampler of recent e-mail scares: anthrax in the mail, poisonous perfume samples in the mail, underarm deodorants causing breast cancer, and transmission of HIV by contact with unused feminine (sanitary) pads. If you receive an e-mail warning about a health topic, check the hoax and rumor site at the CDC (http://www.cdc.gov/hoax_rumors.htm) before giving it credibility.

✔ Use discretion, and don't believe everything you read. Cross-check information against reliable sources to see if facts and figures are consistent. Quackery runs rampant on the Internet, particularly on sites that are trying to sell you a quick fix for a health problem. Just because a source claims to be a physician or an expert does not mean that this is true. When in doubt, check with your own medical doctor, health education professor, or state health division website. There are many government and education-based sites that are independently sponsored and reliable. The following is just a sample. Others are provided in each chapter as we cover specific topics:

1. Adam: www.adam.com
2. Intelihealth: www.intelihealth.com
3. Dr. Koop.com: www.drkoop.com
4. Web MD: http://my.webmd.com
5. Drug Infonet: www.druginfonet.com
6. Health AtoZ.com: www.healthatoz.com

In 2001, it became easier to determine whether a website is reliable. The American Accreditation Healthcare Commission (http://www.urac.org) has devised 50 criteria that health sites must meet to win its "seal of approval." A rating scale and visible seal will tell you at a glance whether a site meets these rigorous standards. In addition to policing the accuracy of health claims, this accreditation will evaluate health information and provide a forum for reporting misinformation, privacy violations, and other complaints.

Source: Laura Landro, "Health Journal: Online Groups Step Up Attempts to Enforce Standards," *The Wall Street Journal,* July 20, 2001, p. B1.

Around 1900, health professionals began to focus on an **Ecological** or **Public Health Model** of health. Under this model, diseases and other negative health events are viewed more as a result of an individual's interaction with his/her social and physical environment. Thus, polluted air and water, hazardous work conditions, negative influences in the home and social environment, abuse of drugs and alcohol, stress unsafe behavior, diet, sedentary lifestyle, and cost, quality, and access to health care all are viewed as potent forces affecting one's health status. If factors in the external environment and individual behaviors affect health risk, it seems logical that to prevent negative health outcomes, we must work to diminish these threats. Under the Ecological or Public Health Model, prevention and intervention strategies become elevated to their proper place in improving the health of individuals and entire populations.

In the late 1940s, progressive thinkers in public health began to be more proactive in pushing for programs and policies that took an ecological approach to prevention. At an international conference in 1947 focusing on global health issues, the World Health Organization (WHO) took the landmark step of trying to clarify what *health* truly meant:

"Health is the state of complete physical, mental, and social well-being, not just the absence of disease or infirmity."[2] For the first time, the concept of health came to be officially defined as more than the absence of disease.

Not until the 1960s and 1970s, however, did the definition of health began to more closely mirror the comprehensive ecological model that public health professionals had been advocating for decades. Scientists argued that health was much more than the absence of disease; in fact, their definition included the physical, social, and mental elements of life, as well as environmental, spiritual, emotional, and intellectual dimensions. To be truly healthy, a person must be capable of functioning at an optimal level in each of these areas, as well as interacting with others and the greater environment, in a productive and spiritually healthy manner. In addition, public health leaders argued that it wasn't just length of life or the number of disease-free years that mattered, but rather living life to the fullest and reaching your potential for a happy, healthy, and productive life. Today, *quality of life* is recognized as being as important as years of life.

Investigation into the environment as the primary cause of diseases has continued for decades and the medical model still persists in some cultures, particularly those that are ravaged by outbreaks of disease and seemingly insurmountable poverty and poor social conditions. Today, however, more people understand that it is often a broken "system" that causes major diseases to spread unchecked. See the "Achievements in Public Health" section of this chapter for a graphic indication of how public health has worked to improve health status. As a classic example, consider life expectancy. In the early 1900s the average life expectancy in America was only 47 years, largely because of the vast numbers of individuals who died before age 5 from childhood diseases. Public health improvements in sanitation and the development of vaccines and antibiotics have added many years to the average life span since then.

Today, because most childhood diseases are preventable or curable and because massive public health efforts are aimed at reducing the spread of infectious diseases, average life expectancy for Americans is 76.9 years with many people living well into their 80s and 90s and more. According to **mortality** (death rate) statistics, people are now living longer than at any previous time in our history. **Morbidity** (illness) rates also indicate that people less frequently contract the common infectious diseases that devastated previous generations. Longer life and less frequent disease are not proof that people are indeed *healthier,* however.

Mortality   Death rate.

Morbidity   Illness rate.

Activities of daily living (ADLs)   Performance of tasks of everyday living, such as bathing and walking up the stairs.

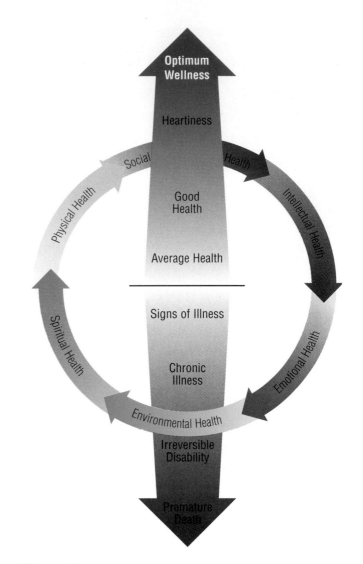

Figure 1.1
The Dimensions of the Health and Wellness Continuum

The Evolution toward Wellness

René Dubos, biologist and philosopher, aptly summarized the thinking of his contemporaries by defining *health* as "a quality of life, involving social, emotional, mental, spiritual, and biological fitness on the part of the individual, which results from adaptations to the environment."[3] The concept of *adaptability,* or the ability to successfully cope with life's ups and downs, became a key element of the overall health definition. Eventually the term *wellness* became popular and not only included the previously mentioned elements, but also implied that there were levels of health in each category. To achieve *high-level wellness,* a person would move progressively higher on a continuum of positive health indicators. Those who fail to achieve these levels may move to the illness side of the continuum. Today, the terms *health* and *wellness* are often used interchangeably to mean the dynamic, ever-changing process of trying to achieve one's potential in each of several interrelated dimensions. These dimensions typically include those presented in Figure 1.1.

- *Physical health.* This dimension includes characteristics such as body size and shape, sensory acuity and responsiveness, susceptibility to disease and disorders, body functioning, physical fitness, and recuperative abilities. Newer definitions of physical health also include our ability to perform normal **activities of daily living** (ADLs), or those tasks that are necessary to normal existence in today's society. Being able to get out of bed in the morning, being able to bend over to tie your shoes, or other daily tasks are examples of ADLs.
- *Intellectual health.* This dimension refers to the ability to think clearly, reason objectively, analyze critically, and use "brainpower" effectively to meet life's challenges. It means learning from successes and mistakes and making sound, responsible decisions that take into consideration all aspects of a situation.
- *Social health.* This dimension refers to the ability to have satisfying interpersonal relationships: interactions with others, adaptations to various social situations, and daily behaviors.
- *Emotional health.* This dimension refers to the feeling component—to be able to express emotions when appropriate, to control them when not, and to avoid expressing them in an inappropriate manner. Feelings of self-esteem, self-confidence, self-efficacy, trust, love, and many other emotional reactions and responses are all part of emotional health.
- *Environmental health.* This dimension refers to an appreciation of the external environment and the role individuals play in preserving, protecting, and improving environmental conditions.
- *Spiritual health.* This dimension may involve a belief in a supreme being or a specified way of living prescribed by a particular religion. Spiritual health also includes the feeling of unity with the environment—a feeling of oneness with others and with nature—and a guiding sense of meaning or value in life. It also may include the ability to understand and express one's purpose in life; to feel a part of a greater spectrum of existence; to experience love, joy, pain, sorrow, peace, contentment, and wonder over life's experiences; and to care about and respect all living things.

A *well* individual might display the following characteristics:

- A realistic sense of self, including personal capabilities and limitations.
- An appreciation of all living things, no matter how ugly or beautiful, how unique or different, or how great or small.
- A willingness to understand imperfection, to forgive others' mistakes, and to grow from personal mistakes or shortcomings.
- The ability to laugh, cry, and genuinely "feel" emotions without getting lost in emotional upsets.
- The ability to function at a reasonable level physiologically.
- The ability to maintain and support healthy relationships with family, friends, intimate partners, and strangers.
- An appreciation for one's role in preserving and protecting the environment.

- A sense of satisfaction with life and an appreciation for the stages of the life experience.
- A zest for living, coupled with a curiosity about what each new encounter, each new day will bring.
- A respect for self, as well as a respect for others.
- A realistic perspective about life's challenges and the skills to cope with life's stresses and challenges.
- A balance in all things.

Many people believe that wellness can best be achieved by adopting a *holistic* approach, in which a person emphasizes the integration of and balance among mind, body, and spirit. Achieving wellness means attaining the optimum level of wellness for a given person's unique set of limitations and strengths. A physically disabled person may be functioning at his or her optimum level of performance; enjoy satisfying interpersonal relationships; work to maintain emotional, spiritual, and intellectual health; and have a strong interest in environmental concerns. In contrast, those who spend hours lifting weights to perfect the size and shape of each muscle but pay little attention to nutrition may *look* healthy but may not maintain a healthy balance in all areas of health. Although we often consider physical attractiveness and other external trappings in measuring the overall health of a person, appearance and physical performance indicators are actually only two signs of physical health, indicating little about the other dimensions. Complete the appraisal in the Assess Yourself box to gain perspective on your own level of wellness in each dimension.

> **What do you think?**
> *René Dubos, a renowned bacteriologist who developed many key philosophies about health, is credited with saying, "Measure your health by your sympathy with morning and spring."*
> ❋ *What do you think Dubos meant by this statement?* ❋ *Discuss how well your own health measures up when weighed against this criterion.*

New Directions for Health

In response to the many indications that Americans were not as healthy as they should be, in 1990 the U.S. Surgeon General proposed a national plan for promoting health among individuals and groups. Known as *Healthy People 2000,* the plan outlined a series of long-term objectives.[4] Critics of this plan complained that it was just a large wish list, that it needed some unifying plan to help bring about the outlined changes, and that there was little financial support to ensure that the objectives could be achieved. Although many communities worked toward these goals and the plan helped solidify plans for many regions of the country, as a nation we still had a long way to go by the new millennium.

How Healthy Are You?

Although we all recognize the importance of being healthy, it can be a challenge to sort out which behaviors are most likely to cause problems or which ones pose the greatest risk. Even when we recognize our unique risks and know what to do, it isn't always easy to stay motivated enough to maintain a specific set of health behaviors. Before you decide where to start, it is important to take a careful look at your health status right now. Think carefully about where you believe that you are today in each of the dimensions of health. Circle the number in each category that you think *best* describes you. Rate your health status in each of the following dimensions by circling the number on the line that comes closest to describing the way you are most of the time.

	POOR HEALTH		AVERAGE HEALTH		EXCELLENT HEALTH
Physical health	1	2	3	4	5
Social health	1	2	3	4	5
Emotional health	1	2	3	4	5
Environmental health	1	2	3	4	5
Spiritual health	1	2	3	4	5
Intellectual health	1	2	3	4	5

After completing the above section, how would you rate your *overall* health?_____

Which area(s), if any, do you think you should you work on improving? _____

If we were to ask your closest friends how healthy they think you are, which area(s) do you think they would say you need to work on and improve?_____

By completing the following assessment, you will have a clearer picture of health areas in which you excel and those that could use varying degrees of work. Taking this assessment will also help you to reflect on various components of health that you may not have thought much about.
  Use the results from this assessment as a guide and as a way to begin analyzing potential areas for improvement and/or maintenance. Answer each question, then total your score for each section and fill it in on the Personal Checklist at the end of the assessment for a general sense of your health profile. Think about the behaviors that influenced your score in each category. Would you like to change any of them? Choose the area that you'd like to improve, then complete the Behavior Change Contract at the end of this book. Use the contract to think through and implement a behavior change over the course of this class.
  Each of the categories in this questionnaire is an important aspect of the total dimensions of health, but this is not a substitute for the advice of a qualified health care provider. Consider scheduling a thorough physical examination by a licensed physician or setting up an appointment with a mental health counselor at your school if you think you need help making a behavior change.
  For each of the following, indicate how often you think the statements describe you.

PHYSICAL HEALTH

	Never	Rarely	Some of the Time	Usually or Always
1. I am happy with my body size and weight.	1	2	3	4
2. I engage in vigorous exercises such as brisk walking, jogging, swimming, or running for at least 30 minutes per day, 3–4 times per week.	1	2	3	4
3. I do exercises designed to strengthen my muscles and increase endurance at least 2 times per week.	1	2	3	4
4. I do stretching, limbering up, and balance exercises such as yoga, pilates, or tai chi to increase my body awareness and control and increase my overall physical health.	1	2	3	4
5. I feel good about the condition of my body and would be able to respond to most demands placed upon it.	1	2	3	4
6. I get at least 7–8 hours of sleep each night.	1	2	3	4

	Never	Rarely	Some of the Time	Usually or Always
7. I try to add moderate activity to each day, such as taking the stairs instead of the elevator and walking whenever I can instead of riding.	1	2	3	4
8. My immune system is strong and my body heals itself quickly when I get sick or injured.	1	2	3	4
9. I have lots of energy and can get through the day without being overly tired.	1	2	3	4
10. I listen to my body; when there is something wrong, I try to make adjustments to heal it or seek professional advice.	1	2	3	4

SOCIAL HEALTH

	Never	Rarely	Some of the Time	Usually or Always
1. When I meet people, I feel good about the impression I make on them.	1	2	3	4
2. I am open, honest, and get along well with other people.	1	2	3	4
3. I participate in a wide variety of social activities and enjoy being with people who are different than I.	1	2	3	4
4. I try to be a "better person" and work on behaviors that have caused problems in my interactions with others.	1	2	3	4
5. I get along well with the members of my family.	1	2	3	4
6. I am a good listener.	1	2	3	4
7. I am open and accessible to a loving and responsible relationship.	1	2	3	4
8. I have someone I can talk to about my private feelings.	1	2	3	4
9. I consider the feelings of others and do not act in hurtful or selfish ways.	1	2	3	4
10. I try to see the good in my friends and do whatever I can to support them and help them feel good about themselves.	1	2	3	4

EMOTIONAL HEALTH

	Never	Rarely	Some of the Time	Usually or Always
1. I find it easy to laugh, cry, and show emotions like love, fear, and anger and try to express these in positive, constructive ways.	1	2	3	4
2. I avoid using alcohol or other drugs as a means of helping me forget my problems.	1	2	3	4
3. When viewing a particularly challenging situation, I tend to view the glass as "half full" rather than "half empty" and perceive problems as opportunities for growth.	1	2	3	4
4. When I am angry, I try to let others know in nonconfrontational and nonhurtful ways, trying to resolve issues rather than stewing about them.	1	2	3	4
5. I try not to worry unnecessarily and try to talk about my feelings, fears, and concerns rather than letting them become chronic issues.	1	2	3	4
6. I recognize when I am stressed and take steps to relax through exercise, quiet time, or other calming activities.	1	2	3	4

(continued on page 12)

	Never	Rarely	Some of the Time	Usually or Always
7. I feel good about myself and believe others like me for who I am.	1	2	3	4
8. I try not to be too critical and/or judgmental of others and to understand differences or quirks that I may note in others.	1	2	3	4
9. I am flexible and adapt or adjust to change in a positive way.	1	2	3	4
10. My friends regard me as a stable, emotionally well-adjusted person whom they trust and rely on for support.	1	2	3	4

ENVIRONMENTAL HEALTH

	Never	Rarely	Some of the Time	Usually or Always
1. I am concerned about environmental pollution and actively try to preserve and protect natural resources.	1	2	3	4
2. I buy recycled paper and purchase biodegradable detergents and cleaning agents whenever possible.	1	2	3	4
3. I recycle my garbage, purchase refillable containers when possible, and try to minimize the amount of paper and plastics that I use.	1	2	3	4
4. I try to wear my clothes for longer periods between washing to reduce water consumption and the amount of detergents in our water sources.	1	2	3	4
5. I vote for pro-environment candidates in elections.	1	2	3	4
6. I write my elected leaders about environmental concerns.	1	2	3	4
7. I turn down the heat and wear warmer clothes at home in winter and use the air conditioner only when necessary or at higher temperatures in summer.	1	2	3	4
8. I am aware of lead pipes in my living area, chemicals in my carpet, and other potential hazards and try to reduce my exposure whenever possible.	1	2	3	4
9. I use both sides of the paper when taking class notes or doing assignments.	1	2	3	4
10. I try not to leave the faucet running too long when I brush my teeth, shave, or shower.	1	2	3	4

SPIRITUAL HEALTH

	Never	Rarely	Some of the Time	Usually or Always
1. I believe life is a precious gift that should be nurtured.	1	2	3	4
2. I take time to enjoy nature and the beauty around me.	1	2	3	4
3. I take time alone to think about what's important in life—who I am, what I value, where I fit in, and where I'm going.	1	2	3	4
4. I have faith in a greater power, be it a God-like force, nature, or the connectedness of all living things.	1	2	3	4
5. I engage in acts of caring and goodwill without expecting something in return.	1	2	3	4
6. I feel sorrow for those who are suffering and try to help them through difficult times.	1	2	3	4
7. I look forward to each day as an opportunity for further growth and challenge.	1	2	3	4

	Never	Rarely	Some of the Time	Usually or Always
8. I work for peace in my interpersonal relationships, in my community, and in the world at large.	1	2	3	4
9. I have a great love and respect for all living things, and regard animals, etc., as important links in a vital living chain.	1	2	3	4
10. I go for the gusto and experience life to the fullest.	1	2	3	4

INTELLECTUAL HEALTH

	Never	Rarely	Some of the Time	Usually or Always
1. I carefully consider my options and possible consequences as I make choices in life.	1	2	3	4
2. I learn from my mistakes and try to act differently the next time.	1	2	3	4
3. I follow directions or recommended guidelines, avoid risks, and act in ways likely to keep myself and others safe.	1	2	3	4
4. I consider myself to be a wise health consumer and check reliable information sources before making decisions.	1	2	3	4
5. I am alert and ready to respond to life's challenges in ways that reflect thought and sound judgment.	1	2	3	4
6. I have at least one hobby, learning activity, or personal growth activity that I make time for each week; something that improves me as a person.	1	2	3	4
7. I actively learn all I can about products and services before making decisions.	1	2	3	4
8. I manage my time well rather than let time manage me.	1	2	3	4
9. My friends and family trust my judgment.	1	2	3	4
10. I think about my self-talk (the things I tell myself) and then examine the evidence to see if my perceptions and feelings are sound.	1	2	3	4

Although each of these six dimensions of health is important, there are some factors that don't readily fit one dimension. As college students, you face some unique risks that others may not have. For this reason, we have added an additional section to this self-assessment that focuses on personal health promotion and disease prevention. Answer these questions and add your results to the Personal Checklist in the following section.

PERSONAL HEALTH PROMOTION/DISEASE PREVENTION

	Never	Rarely	Some of the Time	Usually or Always
1. I know the warning signs of common sexually transmitted infections, such as genital warts (HPV), chlamydia, and herpes, and read new information about these diseases as a way of protecting myself.	1	2	3	4
2. If I were to be sexually active, I would use protection such as latex condoms, dental dams, and other means of reducing my risk of sexually transmitted infections.	1	2	3	4
3. I find ways other than binge drinking when at parties or during happy hours to loosen up and have a good time.	1	2	3	4
4. When I have more than 1 or 2 drinks, I ask someone who is not drinking to drive me and my friends home.	1	2	3	4
5. I have eaten too much in the last month and have forced myself to vomit to avoid gaining weight.	4	3	2	1

(continued on page 14)

	Never	Rarely	Some of the Time	Usually or Always
6. I have several piercings and have found that I enjoy the rush that comes with each piercing event.	4	3	2	1
7. If I were to have a tattoo or piercing, I would go to a reputable person who follows strict standards of sterilization and precautions against blood-borne disease transmission.	1	2	3	4
8. I engage in extreme sports and find that I enjoy the highs that come with risking bodily harm through physical performance.	4	3	2	1
9. I am careful not to mix alcohol or other drugs with prescription and over-the-counter drugs.	1	2	3	4
10. I practice monthly breast/testicle self-examinations.	1	2	3	4

PERSONAL CHECKLIST

Now, total your scores in each of the health dimensions and compare them to what would be considered optimal scores. Which areas do you need to work on? How does your score compare with how you rated yourself in the first part of the questionnaire?

	Ideal Score	Your Score
Physical health	40	_____
Social health	40	_____
Emotional health	40	_____
Environmental health	40	_____
Spiritual health	40	_____
Intellectual health	40	_____
Personal health promotion/disease prevention	40	_____

What Your Scores in Each Category Mean

Scores of 35–40: Outstanding! Your answers show that you are aware of the importance of these behaviors in your overall health. More important, you are putting your knowledge to work for you by practicing good health habits that should reduce your overall risks. Although you received a very high score on this part of the test, you may want to consider areas where your scores could be improved.

Scores of 30–34: Your health practices in these areas are very good, but there is room for improvement. Look again at the items you answered that scored one or two points. What changes could you make to improve your score? Even a small change in behavior can help you achieve better health.

Scores of 20–29: Your health risks are showing! Find information about the risks you are facing and why it is important to change these behaviors. Perhaps you need help in deciding how to make the changes you desire. Assistance is available from this book, your professor, and student health services at your school. Consider making a change by filling out the Behavior Change Contract at the end of this book.

Scores below 20: You may be taking unnecessary risks with your health. Perhaps you are not aware of the risks and what to do about them. Identify each risk area and make a mental note as you read the associated chapter in the book. Whenever possible, seek additional resources, either on your campus or through your local community health resources, and make a serious commitment to behavior change. If any area is causing you to be less than functional in your class work or personal life, seek professional help. In this book you will find the information you need to help you improve your scores and your health. Remember that these scores are only indicators, not diagnostic tools.

Healthy People 2010 and Other Initiatives

A new plan, *Healthy People 2010*, takes the Healthy People 2000 initiative to the next level. *Healthy People 2010* is a nationwide program with two broad goals: (1) eliminate health disparities, and (2) increase the life span and quality of life. The plan includes 28 focus areas, each representing a public health priority such as nutrition, tobacco use, substance abuse, access to quality health services, and common health conditions, for example, heart disease and diabetes. Under these focus areas are a list of Leading Health Indicators (LHIs) that spell out specific health issues (see Table 1.1).

For each focus area, the plan presents specific objectives for the nation to achieve during the next decade. For instance, nutrition data show that only 42 percent of Americans aged 20 and older are at their healthy weight; the goal is to raise that number to 60 percent. In the focus area of physical activity and fitness, 40 percent of Americans ages 18 and older do not engage in any leisure-time physical activity. The objective is to reduce this number to 20 percent by 2010.[5]

Although the Healthy People documents provide a blueprint for health planning in the next decade, other programs and agencies also offer recommendations for improving the health of Americans. In the public sector, the *Agency for Health Care, Research, and Quality* (AHRQ) offers additional direction for national health care efforts through its *AHRQ Guidelines,* a set of objectives for health care providers to meet in specific areas of practice. Other government agencies and research centers also address specific health co-cerns. An example is *Best Practices for Comprehensive Tobacco Control Programs,* which recommends budgets and treatment guidelines to curb smoking.[6]

A New Focus on Health Promotion

The objectives of *Healthy People 2010* have prompted action to promote health and prevent premature disability through social, environmental, policy-related, and community-based programming, In addition, a new emphasis on assisting individuals in their pursuit of specific behavior changes is emerging. Changing behavior without help is not easy, however.

Table 1.1
What Is *Healthy People 2010*?

Overarching Goals

1. Increase quality and years of healthy life
2. Eliminate health disparities

Focus Areas

1. Access to quality health services
2. Arthritis, osteoporosis, and chronic back conditions
3. Cancer
4. Chronic kidney disease
5. Diabetes
6. Disability and secondary conditions
7. Educational and community-based programs
8. Environmental health
9. Family planning
10. Food safety
11. Health communication
12. Heart disease and stroke
13. HIV
14. Immunization and infectious diseases
15. Injury and violence prevention
16. Maternal, infant, and child health
17. Medical product safety
18. Mental health and mental disorders
19. Nutrition and overweight
20. Occupational safety and health
21. Oral health
22. Physical activity and fitness
23. Public health infrastructure
24. Respiratory disease
25. Sexually transmitted disease
26. Substance abuse
27. Tobacco use
28. Vision and hearing

Leading Health Indicators

1. Physical activity
2. Overweight and obesity
3. Tobacco use
4. Substance abuse
5. Responsible sexual behavior
6. Mental health
7. Injury and violence
8. Environmental quality
9. Immunization
10. Access to health care

Source: Office of Disease Prevention and Health Promotion, U.S. Department of Health and Human Services. 2000. (see www.health.gov/healthypeople/About/hpfact.htm).

The term **health promotion** describes the educational, organizational, procedural, environmental, social, and financial supports that help individuals and groups reduce negative health behaviors and promote positive change.

Health promotion programs identify healthy people who are engaging in **risk behaviors**, or behaviors that increase susceptibility to negative health outcomes, and motivate them to change their actions. Effective stop-smoking programs, for instance, don't simply say "Just do it." Instead, they provide information about risk behaviors and possible consequences to smokers and their sidestream smoke victims (educational supports); they encourage smokers to participate in smoking cessation classes and allow time off for worker attendance, or they set up buddy systems of social supports to help them (organizational supports); they establish rules governing smokers' behaviors and supporting their decisions to change, such as banning smoking in the workplace and removing cigarettes from vending machines (environmental supports); and they provide monetary incentives to motivate people to participate (financial supports).[7]

Health promotion programs also encourage those with sound health habits to maintain them. By attempting to modify behaviors, increase skills, change attitudes, increase knowledge, influence values, and improve health decision making, health promotion goes well beyond the simple information campaign. By basing programs and services in communities, organizations, schools, and other places where most people spend their time, health promotion increases the likelihood of long-term success on the road to health and wellness.

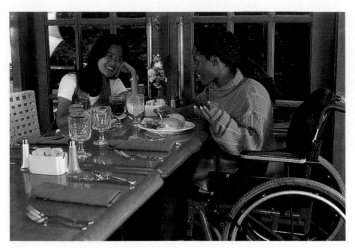

The motivation to improve quality of life within the framework of one's own unique capabilities is crucial to achieving health and wellness.

Whether we use the term *health* or *wellness,* we are talking about a person's overall responses to the challenges of living. Occasional dips into the ice cream bucket and other dietary slips, failures to exercise every day, flare-ups of anger, and other deviations from optimal behavior should not be viewed as major failures. Actually, the ability to recognize that each of us is an imperfect being, attempting to adapt in an imperfect world, signals individual well-being.

We must also remember to be tolerant of others. Rather than be warriors against pleasure in our zeal to change the health behaviors of others, we need to be supportive, understanding, and nonjudgmental. *Health bashing*—intolerance or negative feelings, words, or actions aimed at people who fail to meet our own expectations of health—may indicate our own deficiencies in the psychological, social, and/or spiritual dimensions of the health continuum.

Disease Prevention

Most health promotion initiatives include the term **disease prevention**. What does it really mean? Historically, the health literature describes three types of prevention: primary, secondary, and tertiary.

In a general sense, *prevention* means taking positive actions *now* to avoid becoming sick *later.* Getting immunized against diseases such as polio, deciding not to smoke cigarettes, and practicing safer sex constitute **primary prevention**—actions designed to reduce risk and avoid health problems before they start. **Secondary prevention** (also referred to as **intervention**) involves recognizing health risks or early problems and taking action (intervening) to stop the behavior before it leads to actual illness. Getting a young smoker to quit or reduce the number of cigarettes smoked is an example of secondary prevention. The third type of prevention, **tertiary prevention,** involves treatment and/or rehabilitation after the person is already sick. Typically, tertiary prevention is practiced by licensed health care professionals operating under the medical model of health.

Health promotion   Combined educational, organizational, policy, financial, and environmental supports to help people reduce negative health behaviors and promote positive change.

Risk behaviors   Behaviors that increase susceptibility to negative health outcomes.

Disease prevention   Actions or behaviors designed to keep people from getting sick.

Primary prevention   Actions designed to stop problems before they start.

Secondary prevention (intervention)   Intervention early in the development of a health problem.

Incidence   The number of new cases.

Prevalence   The number of existing cases.

Tertiary prevention   Treatment and/or rehabilitation efforts.

Certified Health Education Specialists (CHES) Academically trained health educators who have passed a national competency examination for prevention and intervention programming.

In the United States, two of every three deaths and one of every three hospitalizations are linked to preventable lifestyle behaviors, such as tobacco use, sedentary lifestyle, alcohol consumption, and overeating. This means that primary and secondary prevention offer our best hope for reducing the **incidence** (number of new cases) and **prevalence** (number of existing cases) of disease and disability.

It is clear that we need to move from a mind-set of tertiary prevention to focus on earlier intervention designed to remove barriers and help individuals succeed in their behavior change strategies. Health educators in U.S. schools and communities offer an affordable and effective delivery of prevention and intervention programs. **Certified Health Education Specialists (CHESs)** make up a trained cadre of public health workers with special credentials and competencies to plan, implement, and evaluate prevention programs that offer scientifically sound, behaviorally based methods to help individuals and communities increase the likelihood of success. As a nation that historically spends little on prevention (less than 5 percent of our total national funding for health goes to prevention), however, such a shift has been and will continue to be difficult.

Achievements in Public Health

To those of us in the field of public health, the saying "we've come a long way, baby" accurately reflects the health achievements of the past 100 years. According to the Centers for Disease Control and Prevention (CDC), here are the ten greatest public health achievements of the twentieth century:

1. *Vaccinations.* Vaccinations have eradicated smallpox, eliminated poliomyelitis, and significantly controlled a number of infectious diseases, including measles, rubella, tetanus, diphtheria, and *Haemophilus influenzae* Type B, all of which claimed the lives of large numbers of people in the early 1900s.
2. *Motor vehicle safety.* Improvements in motor vehicle safety have resulted from engineering efforts to make both vehicles and highways safer and from successful efforts to change personal behavior, such as the use of safety belts, child safety seats, and motorcycle helmets, and the avoidance of drinking and driving.
3. *Workplace safety.* Work-related health risks common at the beginning of the last century are now under better control or completely eliminated. Since 1980, the rate of fatal occupational injuries has fallen by 40 percent.
4. *Control of infectious diseases.* Clean water and improved sanitation have greatly reduced the development and transmission of infectious diseases since 1900. In addition, antimicrobial therapy, such as the discovery of and treatment with antibiotics, has greatly reduced the risk of contracting diseases such as tuberculosis and sexually transmitted infections.
5. *Cardiovascular disease (CVD) and stroke deaths.* Efforts to educate the public on how to modify health risk factors, such as quitting smoking and controlling high blood pressure, coupled with improved access to early detection and better treatment, have reduced rates of CVD and stroke.
6. *Safe and healthy foods.* Since 1900, technology for eradicating microbial contaminants from foods has improved dramatically. In addition, identification of essential micronutrients and establishment of food-fortification programs have almost eliminated major nutritional deficiency diseases such as rickets, goiter, and pellagra.
7. *Maternal and infant care.* Better hygiene and nutrition, improved availability of antibiotics, greater access to health care, and technological advances in medicine have greatly reduced the risks to infants and mothers. Since 1900, infant mortality has decreased by 90 percent, and maternal mortality has declined by 99 percent.
8. *Family planning.* Access to family planning and contraceptive services has altered social and economic roles of women. Family planning has provided health benefits that have reduced the number of infant, child, and maternal deaths; increased opportunities for preconception counseling and screening; and increased the use of barrier contraceptives to prevent unwanted pregnancies and sexually transmissible infections.
9. *Fluoridated drinking water.* Fluoridation of drinking water began in 1945 and by 1999 reached an estimated 144 million persons in the United States. Fluoridation safely and inexpensively prevents tooth decay, regardless of socioeconomic status or access to health care. It has played an important role in reducing tooth decay in children and tooth loss in adults.
10. *Recognition of tobacco as a health hazard.* Public antismoking campaigns have changed social norms to prevent initiation of tobacco use, promote cessation of use, and reduce exposure to environmental tobacco smoke. Since the 1964 Surgeon General's report on the health risks of smoking, millions of smoking-related health problems have been prevented and many lives have been saved.[8]

While past achievements are indeed remarkable, they also raise questions about where we're going in the new century. Will the future of our health rest solely in the hands of researchers, technological wizardry, and pharmaceutical houses? What roles will public health practitioners and the health care system play? What will our own role be in health promotion and disease prevention in the twenty-first century? Interviews with leading experts in health-related fields offer some clues.

- *New drugs.* By 2010, experts predict a new arsenal of medicines for diseases such as Alzheimer's and multiple sclerosis, which defy treatment today. Genetically targeted drugs will home in on certain conditions, and new, slow-release vaccinations will control diseases such as diabetes.
- *Cancer.* By the year 2015, cancer deaths are expected to drop by 21 percent, with 13 percent fewer people ever getting cancer. Although many of our cancer-producing behaviors, such as smoking, will persist, we will have better methods of genetic screening for risk, targeted vaccines that control certain cancers, and less invasive treatments. Cancer treatment will be less debilitating.

- *Bacteria and infectious diseases.* Infectious diseases are the number one cause of death worldwide, with emergent resurgent diseases on the increase. By 2010, a new strain of antibiotics will provide an improved prognosis for resistant diseases, but an as yet undiscovered virus could have the potential to wipe out over one-third of the world's population.
- *Spirituality.* Spirituality training will become a common element of traditional medical training. Insurers will reimburse it, and medical schools will teach alternative medicine.
- *Heart disease.* As baby boomers age, heart disease will increase, but better diagnostic tests will exist and better drug treatment will be developed, including proteins that create small arteries when main arteries are blocked.
- *Colds and flu.* Although there won't be a cure for the cold in 2010, new vaccines will cut the cost of inoculating a child in a developing country from $100 to 10 cents, and drugs will provide great relief for many. A pandemic flu also is projected, however.
- *Foods.* By 2010, we'll have more "medical" foods that combine supplements, micronutrient additives, and medicines to boost food content, protect against disease, and bolster the immune system.
- *Aging.* By 2010, advances in medicine will include a "Methuselah" gene, which currently doubles or triples life span in roundworms; calorie-restricted meals that increase longevity; and proteins that might halt the brain declines found in Alzheimer's disease.[9]

While we've come a long way, the possibilities for health and well-being in the future defy the imagination. Living longer, living more disease-free years, and injecting more quality into the extra years of life will be major goals of the future. The more we learn about the remarkable resilience of the human body and spirit, and the more technology stretches our imagination and enlarges our possibilities, the more likely that the twenty-first century will rival the twentieth for major health-related achievements.

> **What do you think?**
> *What do you consider the greatest achievements in public health in the twentieth century?*
> ✳ *Do you think we will become more reliant on technology for better health in the future?* ✳ *Why or why not?*

Preparing for Better Health in the Twenty-First Century

Although we've made dramatic improvements in many health areas, there are challenges ahead. To make additional strides, people must have a sense of both individual and social responsibility. Although it is important that each of us

---

HEALTH IN A DIVERSE WORLD

Global Health Challenges in the New Century

THE GLOBAL IMPACT OF HEALTH DISPARITIES

With all of our health concerns in the United States, it is often easy to overlook health-related issues and problems in other regions of the world. However, as we move to a global economy and travel to the most remote areas of the world becomes possible, we are likely to see dramatic developments in global health. In nonindustrialized countries, where four-fifths of the planet's population live, noncommunicable diseases such as depression and heart disease are fast replacing the traditional enemies of infectious disease and malnutrition as the leading causes of disability and premature death. Consider the following:

- Worldwide, premature deaths—defined as occurring before age 50—will be cut in half by the year 2025. While this is positive, it also increases the likelihood of costly chronic diseases.
- Global life expectancy is projected to reach 73 years by 2025. Many thousands of people born at the end of the twentieth century will live through the twenty-first century to see the advent of the twenty-second. For example, France is projected to have 150,000 centenarians by the year 2050, compared to 200 in 1950.
- Some gaps in health between rich and poor countries are at least as wide as they were half a century ago and are becoming wider still. While people in most countries are living longer and enjoy improved access to health care, life expectancy in other nations is actually decreasing. Between 1976 and 1995, 16 countries with a combined population of 300 million experienced such decreases. Many were in Africa.
- Over one-third of the global population lacks access to essential drugs; an average of only 50 percent of patients take their prescriptions correctly, and up to 75 percent of antibiotics are prescribed inappropriately, leading to a growing threat of antimicrobial resistance.
- In 1998 the global population was 5.8 billion; by 2025 it will reach 8 billion. Although women will bear fewer babies—an average of 2.3 compared to 2.9 in 1995 and 5.0 in 1955—the world has never been so densely populated nor suffered such a strain on natural resources. However, the under-20 population will be only 32 percent

work to preserve and protect our own health, it is also important to become actively engaged in the health of our communities, our nation, and the global population. The mark of a truly healthy person is whether the individual focuses beyond the "me" aspects of human existence, and becomes equally concerned with the "we" aspects of health, as well as having a sense of responsibility about the greater environment that we live in.

Focusing on Global Health Issues

Everyone's health is profoundly affected by economic, social, behavioral, scientific, and technological factors. The world economy has become increasingly interconnected and globalized; every day, 2 million people worldwide move across national borders. Global commerce and communication have benefited people in virtually every country while creating a remarkable degree of mutual interdependence.[10] In addition to their undoubted advantages, however, these changes also bring health risks that cannot be addressed by one country alone. Some obvious examples include infectious diseases, contaminated foodstuffs, terrorism, and illegal or banned toxic substances.[11]

Each of us must do our part to improve our own health, protect the health of others, and work for social justice in related health areas. This requires taking the time to understand the vast differences in health status across various social groups and actively promoting community actions that erase disparities (see the Health in a Diverse World box).

HEALTH IN A DIVERSE WORLD

of the total in 2025, compared to 40 percent in 2002.

- Mental and behavioral disorders are common today worldwide, affecting more than 25 percent of all people at some time during their lives. It was estimated that in 1990, mental and neurological disorders accounted for 10 percent of the total Disability Adjusted Life Years (DALYs) lost to all diseases and injuries. This was 12 percent in 2000 and is projected to be 15 percent of the growing disease burden in 2020. Common disorders which can cause severe disability include depression, substance use disorders, schizophrenia, epilepsy, Alzheimer's disease, mental retardation, and disorders of childhood and adolescence.
- By the year 2020, tobacco use (a major risk factor for lung cancer, emphysema, and asthma) is expected to kill more people than any single disease, surpassing even the HIV epidemic.

Severe, persistent poverty also contributes to huge disparities in health status. Many people of the world have insufficient resources to care for basic sustenance needs. War, infectious diseases, contaminated water and air, and solid waste pollution deplete the strength of those who are struggling to survive. Poor access to health care and necessary medicines, shortages of food, and depression often plague individuals as they face daily challenges for survival.

CHANGING RISKS IN THE FUTURE

According to a new body of research compiled by researchers at the Harvard School of Public Health and the World Health Organization (WHO) and colleagues throughout the world, the Global Burden of Disease, a projection ranking major threats to health, indicates massive shifts in health threats. Using a unique new method of rating, researchers attempted to assess the impact of risk on years of healthy life lost, a roundabout way of building quality of life into an age-old formula that looks at risk only in terms of death rates. Thus, a risk factor that causes you to be disabled or function at less than optimal capacity is shown to have an immediate impact even though you may not die from it. Using this new formula, the following comparisons in rank order of disease burden for the 15 leading causes were computed. This is an approximate listing of comprehensive health risks for the global population.

1990	2020 PROJECTIONS
1. Lower respiratory infections	1. Ischemic heart disease
2. Diarrheal diseases	2. Unipolar major depression*
3. Perinatal conditions	3. Road traffic accidents
4. Unipolar major depression	4. Cerebrovascular diseases
5. Ischemic heart disease	5. Chronic obstructive pulmonary disease
6. Cerebrovascular disease	6. Lower respiratory infections
7. Tuberculosis	7. Tuberculosis
8. Measles	8. War
9. Road traffic accidents	9. Diarrheal diseases
10. Congenital abnormalities	10. HIV disease
11. Malaria	11. Perinatal conditions
12. Chronic obstructive pulmonary disease	12. Violence
13. Falls	13. Congenital abnormalities
14. Iron-deficiency anemia	14. Self-inflicted injuries
15. Protein-energy malnutrition	15. Trachea, bronchus, and lung cancers

Among females and in developing countries, unipolar major depression is projected to become the leading cause of disease burden.
Sources: The World Health Report, "Mental Health: New Understanding, New Hope," (2001) (see http://www.who.int/whr/2001/main/en/chapter2/index.htm); C. Murray and D. Lopez, Global Health in the 21st Century (2001) (see http://healthlink.mcw.edu/article/977858884.html); *The Global Burden of Disease: Summary* (Cambridge, MA: Harvard University Press, 1996).

What do you think?
What implications do developments in global health have for people living in the United States today? ✻ What international programs, policies, and/or services might help control the world's health problems in the next decade? ✻ Are there actions that individuals can take to help?

Focusing on Your Health

In this country, we tend to focus on the leading causes of death rather than those factors that threaten the lives or futures of young Americans. A 20-year-old typically does not view death as an imminent threat; thus, the motivation for behavior change is not as great as it perhaps should be. It is important to consider how your current actions affect you right now *and* in the future. Also, think about how your actions may affect others and the global environment. For example, do you have days when you're tired all the time or disinterested in what is going on around you? Or perhaps you are a bit dissatisfied with yourself, your friends, your career choices, or other things in your life. In contrast, you probably also have days when you wake up full of energy, when you look forward to the next fun event, and when you later fall into bed exhausted, yet excited about the next day. Some of the time, you probably hear about the latest environmental threat or a catastrophe in another region of the world and "tune in" with great interest. Other times, you can hardly take time to worry about yourself, let alone others. What is the difference between the "blah" version of you and the "actively engaged" version? To a great extent, it probably depends on what you eat, the amount of exercise and sleep you get, the excitement you feel in meeting challenges and being rewarded, and whether you take time to refresh the spiritual side of your life. It also depends on how much time you've taken to inform yourself about community and global health problems. In short, your investment in healthy behaviors contributes to how well you live each day.

By focusing on health behaviors that energize and refresh you, you can become actively engaged in life. If you skip that early morning walk because you can't drag yourself out of bed, if you don't socialize because you are worried about how "fat" you look or think you "don't have anything to wear," if you find that your interactions with others cause stress, it may be time to reexamine your health status. What are your current health risks? Future health risks? What can you do to improve your current situation? While ADLs are performance-based measures typically used to assess func-

Women's Health Initiative (WHI) National study of postmenopausal women, in conjunction with the NIH mandate for equal research priorities for women's health issues.

tioning in the later years of life, perhaps we need to focus on them much earlier. In addition, rather than rating ourselves based on what everyone else is doing, we need to consider potential differences based on race, socioeconomic opportunity, gender, age, and other variables. It takes effort and judgment to achieve our personal best.

What do you think?
Based on the wellness dimensions discussed here, what are some of your strengths in each dimension? ✻ What are some of your deficiencies? ✻ What one or two things can you do to enhance your strong areas? ✻ To improve on your weaknesses?

Gender Differences and Health Status

You don't have to be a health expert to know that there are physiological differences between men and women. Although much of male and female anatomy is identical, major differences exist in susceptibility to disease and other health factors. Many disorders—osteoporosis, multiple sclerosis, and Alzheimer's disease, for example—are far more common in women than in men. Finally, although women live longer than men, they don't necessarily enjoy a better quality of life.[12]

Much of the current interest in exploring women's health came after 1990, when a highly publicized government study raised concern about the uneven numbers of women included in clinical trial research conducted by the National Institutes of Health (NIH). The NIH established the Office of Research on Women's Health (ORWH) in 1990 to oversee the representation of women in NIH studies. According to Vivian Pinn, ORWH's director, "For too long, medicine has viewed women as 'abnormal men' when considering health problems."[13]

Researchers have historically excluded women of childbearing age from clinical trials of many new drugs. One reason has been a concern about whether a medication might harm a fetus; another has been that women's menstrual cycles can influence the effects of a drug. Of course, men and women do vary physiologically, so the elimination of women from many studies means that the results from these studies cannot be applied to women directly. According to social psychologist Carol Tavris, "If you want to know the effects of Drug X and you throw women out of your study because the menstrual cycle affects their responses to medication, you cannot then extrapolate from your study of men to women, precisely because the menstrual cycle affects their responses to medication."[14] To address these concerns, the government has specified that equal amounts of money and time must be spent on men's and women's health research.[15] The National Heart, Blood, and Lung Institute is conducting the **Women's Health Initiative (WHI)**. This 15-year, $625

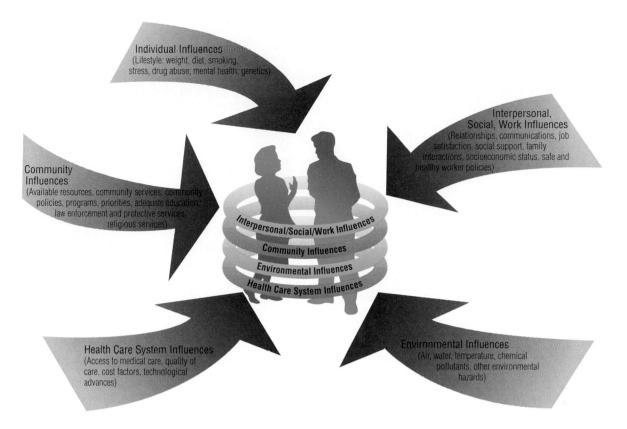

Figure 1.2
Factors That Influence Health Status

million study focuses on the leading causes of death and disease in more than 160,000 postmenopausal women. WHI researchers hope to find out how a healthful lifestyle and increased medical attention can help prevent women's cancers, heart disease, and osteoporosis.[16] The breakthrough discoveries about hormone replacement therapy, mentioned earlier in this chapter, are part of the WHI.

> **What do you think?**
> *Do you think there are true disparities between men's and women's health status?* ✳ *What are some indicators or examples?* ✳ *Can you think of programs, policies, or individual actions that would reduce such disparities?*

Improving Your Health

Table 1.2 on page 22 summarizes the leading causes of death in the United States, by age. Note that Americans aged 15–24 are most likely to die from unintentional injuries, followed by homicide/legal intervention and suicide. Unintentional injuries are also the major killer in the next age group, 25–34, followed by suicide and homicide.

Individual behavior is a major determinant of good health, but heredity, access to health care, and the environ-

ment can also influence health status (see Figure 1.2). When these factors are considered together and form the basis of a person's lifestyle choices, the net effect on health can be great.

Benefits of Healthy Behaviors

Although mounting evidence indicates that there are significant benefits to being healthy, many people find it difficult to become and remain healthy. Most experts believe that several key behaviors will help us live longer, such as:

- Getting a good night's sleep (minimum of seven hours).
- Maintaining healthy eating habits.
- Managing weight.
- Participating in physical recreational activities.
- Avoiding tobacco products.
- Practicing safer sex.
- Limiting intake of alcohol.
- Scheduling regular self-exams and medical checkups.

Several other actions may not add "years to your life"—but they can add significant "life to your years." They include:

- Controlling the real and imaginary stressors in life.
- Forming and maintaining meaningful relationships with family and friends.
- Making time for yourself.
- Participating in at least one fun activity each day.

Table 1.2
Leading Causes of Death in the United States by Age (Years)

Rank	All Ages	1–4	5–9	10–14	15–24	25–34	35–44	45–54	55–64	65+
1.	Diseases of heart 725,192	Unintentional injuries 1,898	Unintentional injuries 1,459	Unintentional injuries 1,632	Unintentional injuries 13,656	Unintentional injuries 11,890	Malignant neoplasms 16,732	Malignant neoplasms 46,681	Malignant neoplasms 89,067	Diseases of heart 607,265
2.	Malignant neoplasms 549,838	Congenital anomalies 549	Malignant neoplasms 509	Malignant neoplasms 503	Homicide and legal intervention 4,998	Suicide 5,106	Unintentional injuries 15,231	Diseases of heart 34,994	Diseases of heart 64,167	Malignant neoplasms 390,122
3.	Cerebrovascular diseases 167,366	Malignant neoplasms 418	Congenital anomalies 207	Homicide and legal intervention 246	Suicide 3,901	Homicide 4,231	Diseases of heart 13,600	Unintentional injuries 11,639	Chronic lower respiratory 11,297	Cerebrovascular diseases 148,599
4.	Chronic lower respiratory diseases 124,181	Homicide and legal intervention 376	Homicide and legal intervention 186	Suicide 242	Malignant neoplasms 1,724	Malignant neoplasms 4,005	Suicide 6,466	Chronic liver disease cirrhosis 6,368	Cerebrovascular diseases 9,652	Chronic lower respiratory diseases 108,112
5.	Unintentional injuries 67,860	Diseases of heart 183	Diseases of heart 116	Congenital anomalies 221	Diseases of heart 1,069	Diseases of heart 3,066	Human immunodeficiency 6,232	Cerebrovascular diseases 5,563	Diabetes mellitus 9,097	Pneumonia and influenza 57,282
6.	Diabetes mellitus 68,399	Pneumonia and influenza 130	In situ and benign neoplasms 64	Diseases of heart 161	Congenital anomalies 434	Human immunodeficiency virus infection 2,729	Chronic liver diseases and cirrhosis 3,302	Suicide 5,081	Unintentional injuries 7,285	Diabetes mellitus 51,843
7.	Pneumonia and influenza 63,730	Conditions of perinatal period 92	Chronic lower respiratory diseases 49	Chronic lower respiratory diseases 90	Chronic lower respiratory diseases 209	Diabetes mellitus 582	Homicide and legal intervention 3,206	Diabetes mellitus 4,735	Chronic liver diseases and cirrhosis 5,637	Alzheimer's disease 44,020
8.	Alzheimer's disease 44,536	Septicemia 87	Septicemia 47	Influenza and pneumonia 47	Human immunodeficiency virus infection 198	Cerebrovascular diseases 580	Cerebrovascular diseases 2,574	Human immunodeficiency infection 3,907	Suicide 2,896	Unintentional injuries 32,219
9.	Nephritis, nephrotic syndrome, and nephrosis 35,525	In situ and benign neoplasms 63	Influenza and pneumonia 46	Cerebrovascular diseases 39	Cerebrovascular diseases 182	Congenital anomalies 465	Diabetes mellitus 1,942	Chronic lower respiratory diseases 3,110	Nephritis, nephrotic syndrome, and nephrosis 2,864	Nephritis, nephrotic syndrome, and nephrosis 29,938
10.	Septicemia 30,680	Chronic lower respiratory disease 54	Human immunodeficiency virus infection 38	In situ and benign neoplasms 37	Influenza and pneumonia 179	Liver disease 407	Influenza and pneumonia 1,063	Influenza and pneumonia 1,697	Septicemia 2,714	Septicemia 24,626

Source: "10 Leading Causes of Death, United States, 2001, All Races, Both Sexes," National Center for Injury Prevention and Control, Centers for Disease Control and Prevention, Data from National Center for Health Statistics Vital Statistic System (see http://www.cdc.gov//ncipc/pub-res/research_agenda/chart.htm).

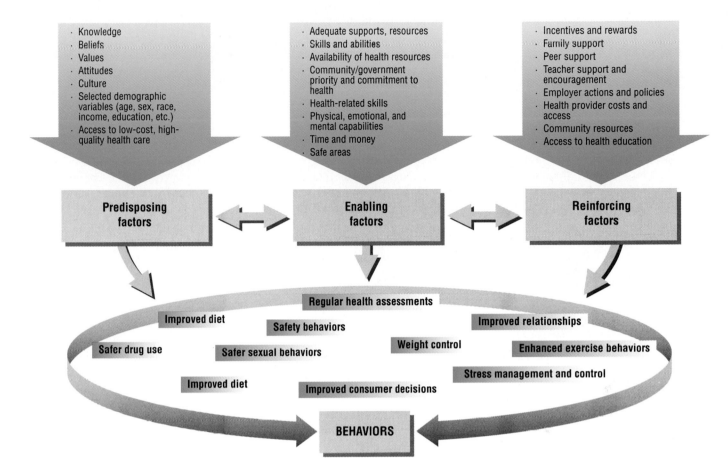

Figure 1.3
Factors That Influence Behavior-Change Decisions

- Respecting the environment and the people in it.
- Considering alternatives when making decisions and assessing how actions affect others.
- Valuing each day and making the best of opportunities.
- Viewing mistakes as opportunities to learn and grow.
- Being as kind to yourself as to others.
- Understanding the health care system and using it wisely.

Though it's easy to list things that one should do, change is not always easy. All of us, no matter where we are on the health/wellness continuum, have to start somewhere. All people have faced personal and external challenges to their attempts to change health behaviors—some have not done so well, some have been extremely successful, and some have made only small changes that add up to significant improvements in how they feel and how they live. The key is to identify the behaviors most in need of change, determine goals and the actions necessary to achieve them, set up a plan of action, and get started. But first, it is important to take a look at factors that contribute to current patterns of behavior.

Changing Your Health Behaviors

Mark Twain said that "habit is habit, and not to be flung out the window by anyone, but coaxed downstairs a step at a time." The chances of successfully changing negative habits improve when you identify a key behavior that you want to change and develop a plan for gradual change that allows you time to unlearn negative patterns and substitute positive ones. Many experts advocate dissecting a given health behavior into smaller parts and working on them one at a time in "baby steps" (see the Skills for Behavior Change box).

First, identify what is most important to you or what causes you the greatest immediate and long-term risks. For example, if you are concerned about your weight, assess your eating patterns and decide where you can make changes that you can live with. Too many of us decide on New Year's Day that we are going to lose weight, exercise more, find more friends, and essentially reinvent ourselves overnight! Is it any wonder that we don't keep most of these resolutions?

Factors That Influence Behavior Change

Figure 1.3 identifies major factors that influence behavior and behavior-change decisions. They can be divided into three general categories: predisposing, enabling, and reinforcing.

Predisposing Factors Our life experiences, knowledge, cultural and ethnic inheritance, and current beliefs and values are all *predisposing factors* influencing behavior and behavior

Staging for Change

On any given morning, many of us get out of bed and resolve to change a given behavior today. Whether it be losing weight, drinking less, exercising more, being nicer to others, managing time better, or some other change, we start out with enthusiasm and high expectations. Within a short time, however, a vast majority of people return to doing whatever it was they thought they shouldn't be doing.

Why do so many good intentions fail? According to Dr. James Prochaska, psychologist and head of the Health Promotion Partnership at the University of Rhode Island, and Dr. Carlos DiClimente, it's because we are going about things in the wrong way. According to Prochaska and DiClimente, fewer than 20 percent of us are really prepared to take action. Yet, health professionals continue to exhort us to "Just Do It! And do it now!" After considerable research, Prochaska and DiClimente believe that behavior changes usually do not succeed if they start with the change itself. Instead, we must go through a series of "stages" to adequately prepare ourselves for that eventual change. Our chances of keeping those New Year's resolutions will be greatly enhanced if we have proper reinforcement and help during each of the following stages:

1. *Precontemplation*. People in the precontemplation stage have no current intention of changing. They may have tried to change a behavior before and given up, or they may be in denial and unaware of any problem. People in this stage don't have to worry about failure and have no intention of taking any actions.
Strategies for Change: Although a very touchy area, sometimes a few frank, yet kind words from friends may be enough to make precontemplators take a closer look at themselves. This is not to say that you should become a "warrior against pleasure" or tell people what to do when they haven't asked for advice. Recommended readings or tactful suggestions, however, can be useful.

2. *Contemplation*. In this phase, people recognize that they have a problem and begin to contemplate the need to change. Acknowledgment usually results from increased awareness, often due to feedback from family and friends or access to information. Despite this acknowledgment, people can languish in this stage for years, realizing that they have a problem but lacking the time or energy to make the change.
Strategies for Change: Often, contemplators need a little push to get them started. This may come in the form of helping them set up a change plan (e.g., an exercise routine), buying a helpful gift (i.e., a low-fat cookbook), sharing articles about a particular problem, or inviting them to go with you to hear a speaker on a related topic. People often need skill building or time to think about a course of action. Your assistance can help them move off the point of indecision.

3. *Preparation*. Most people at this point are close to taking action. They've thought about what they might do and may even have come up with a plan. Rather than thinking about why they can't begin, they have started to focus on what they can do.
Strategies for Change: Follow a few standard guidelines: Set realistic goals (large and small), take small steps toward change, change only a couple of things at once, reward small milestones, and seek support from friends. Identify those factors that have enabled success or served as a barrier to success in the past, and modify them where possible. Complete a Behavior Change Contract to help you commit to making these changes.

4. *Action*. In the action stage, people begin to follow their action plans. Those who have prepared for change, thought about alternatives, engaged social support, and made a plan of action are more ready for action than those who have given it little thought. Unfortunately, too many people start behavior change here rather than going through the first three stages. Without a plan, without enlisting the help of others, or without a realistic goal, failure is likely.
Strategies for Change: Publicly stating the desire to change helps ensure success. Encourage friends who are making a change to share their plans with you. Offer to help, and try to remove potential obstacles. Social support and the buddy system can motivate even the most reluctant person.

5. *Maintenance*. Maintenance requires vigilance, attention to detail, and long-term commitment. Many people reach their goals, only to relax and slip back into the undesired behavior. In this stage, it is important to be aware of the potential for relapses and develop strategies for dealing with such challenges. Common causes of relapse include overconfidence, daily temptations, stress or emotional distractions, and self-deprecation.
Strategies for Change: During maintenance, continue taking the same actions that led to success in the first place. Find fun and creative ways to maintain positive behaviors. This is where a willing and caring support group can be vital. Knowing where on your campus to turn for help when you don't have a close support network is also helpful.

6. *Termination*. By this point, the behavior is so ingrained that the current level of vigilance may be unnecessary. The new behavior has become an essential part of daily living. Can you think of someone you know who has made a major behavior change that has now become an essential part of that person's life?

change. Factors that may predispose us to certain conditions include age, sex, race, income, family background, educational background, and access to health care. For example, if your parents smoked, you are 90 percent more likely to start smoking than someone whose parents didn't. If your peers smoke, you are 80 percent more likely to smoke than someone whose friends don't.

Enabling Factors Skills and abilities; physical, emotional, and mental capabilities; and resources and accessible facilities that make health decisions more convenient or difficult are *enabling factors*. Positive enablers encourage you to carry through on your intentions. Negative enablers work against your intentions to change. For example, if you would like to join a local fitness center but discover that the closest one is four miles away and the membership fee is $500, those negative enablers may convince you to stay home. On the other hand, if your school's fitness center is two blocks away, stays open until midnight, and offers a special student membership, those positive enablers will probably convince you to join. Identifying positive and negative enabling factors and devising alternative plans when the negative factors outweigh the positive are part of planning for behavior change.

Reinforcing Factors *Reinforcing factors* include the presence or absence of support, encouragement, or discouragement that significant people in your life bring to a situation. For example, if you decide to stop smoking and your family and friends continue smoking in your presence, you may be tempted to start smoking again. In other words, your smoking behavior was reinforced. If, however, you are overweight and you lose a few pounds and all your friends tell you how terrific you look, your positive behavior will be reinforced and you will be more likely to continue your weight-loss plan.

The manner in which you reward or punish yourself also plays a role. Accepting small failures and concentrating on your successes can foster further achievements. Berating yourself because you binged on ice cream or argued with a friend may create an internal environment in which failure becomes almost inevitable. Telling yourself that you're worth the extra time and effort and giving yourself a pat on the back for small accomplishments are often overlooked factors in positive behavior change.

Motivation

Wanting to change is a prerequisite of the change process, but there is much more to the process than motivation. Motivation must be combined with common sense, commitment, and a realistic understanding of how best to move from point A to point B.[17] *Readiness* is the state of being that precedes behavior change. People who are ready to change possess the knowledge, attitudes, skills, and internal and external resources that make change a likely reality. For someone to be

ready for change, certain basic steps and adjustments in thinking must occur. The Skills for Behavior Change box describes the *Stages of Change* model of health behavior change.

Some of us need a little boost before we are able to change our behaviors. Rewards, or incentives for successfully reaching goals that we set, are effective ways to keep ourselves on track. Several studies have pointed out that those who set up a system of rewards for behavioral change are often successful. For example, allow yourself something that you really enjoy after losing 5 pounds, rather than depriving yourself until you lose all 30 of the pounds that you want to lose.[18]

> **What do you think?**
> *If you were trying to adopt a healthy new behavior, for example, starting to exercise 30 minutes per day, who could you ask to support you? * What factors could make this change difficult? * Why do you think you weren't successful in doing it before? * What skills will you need to succeed? * How ready are you?*

Beliefs and Attitudes

We often assume that when rational people realize there is a risk in what they are doing, they will act to reduce that risk. But this is not necessarily true. Consider the number of health professionals who smoke, consume junk food, and act in other unhealthy ways. They surely know better, but their "knowing" is disconnected from their "doing." Why is this so? Two strong influences on behavior are beliefs and attitudes.

A **belief** is an appraisal of the relationship between some object, action, or idea (for example, smoking) and some attribute of that object, action, or idea (for example, smoking is expensive, dirty, and causes cancer—or it is relaxing). Beliefs may develop from direct experience (perhaps you have trouble breathing after smoking for several years) or from secondhand experience or knowledge conveyed by other people (maybe you watched your grandfather, a long-time smoker, die of lung cancer).[19] An **attitude** is a relatively stable set of beliefs, feelings, and behavioral tendencies in relation to something or someone.

Belief Appraisal of the relationship between some object, action, or idea and some attribute of that object, action, or idea.

Attitude Relatively stable set of beliefs, feelings, and behavioral tendencies in relation to something or someone.

Do Beliefs and Attitudes Influence Behavior? It seems logical to conclude that your beliefs will influence your behavior. If you believe (make the appraisal) that taking drugs (an action) is harmful (attribute of that action), you will not use drugs. If you believe that drinking and driving are incompatible, you will never drink and drive. Or will you?

Psychologists studying the relationship between beliefs and health behaviors have determined that although beliefs may subtly influence behavior, they may not actually cause people to change behavior. In 1966 psychologist I. Rosenstock developed a classic theory, the **Health Belief Model (HBM),** to show when beliefs affect behavior change.[20] Although many other models attempt to explain the influence of beliefs on behaviors, the HBM remains one of the most widely accepted. It holds that several factors must support a belief before change is likely:

- *Perceived seriousness of the health problem.* How severe would the medical and social consequences be if the health problem was to develop or be left untreated? The more serious the perceived effects, the more likely that action will be taken.
- *Perceived susceptibility to the health problem.* Next, what is the likelihood of developing the health problem? People who perceive themselves at high risk are more likely to take preventive action.
- *Cues to action.* Those who are reminded or alerted about a potential health problem are more likely to take action.

Three other factors are linked to perceived risk for health problems: *demographic variables,* including age, gender, race, and ethnic background; *sociopsychological variables,* including personality traits, social class, and social pressure; and *structural variables,* including knowledge about or prior contact with the health problem.

The Health Belief Model is followed many times every day. Take, for example, smokers. Older smokers are likely to know other smokers who have developed serious heart or lung problems as a result of smoking. They are thus more likely to perceive tobacco as a threat to their health than a teenager who has just begun smoking. The greater the perceived threat of health problems caused by smoking, the greater the chance a person will quit. However, many chronic smokers know the risks yet continue to smoke. Why do they fail to take actions to avoid further harm? According to Rosenstock, some people do not believe that they will be affected by a severe problem—they act as if they believe they have some kind of immunity—and are unlikely to change their behaviors. In some cases, they may think that even if they get cancer or have a heart attack, the health care system will cure them. They also may feel that the immediate pleasure outweighs the long-range cost.

Intentions to Change

Our attitudes tend to reflect our emotional responses to situations and also tend to follow from our beliefs. According to the **Theory of Reasoned Action,** our behaviors result from

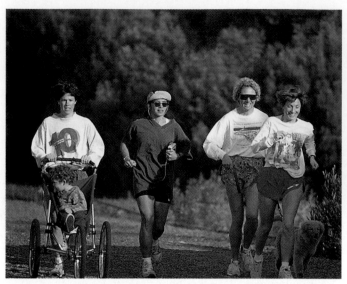

The support and encouragement of friends who have similar goals and interests will strengthen your commitment to develop and maintain positive health behaviors.

our intentions to perform actions. An intention is a product of our attitude toward an action and our beliefs about what others may want us to do.[21] A behavioral intention, then, is a written or stated commitment to perform an action.

In brief, the more consistent and powerful your attitudes about an action and the more you are influenced by others to take that action, the greater will be your stated intention to do so. The more you verbalize your commitment to change, the more likely you are to succeed.

Significant Others as Change Agents

Many of us are highly influenced by the approval or disapproval (real or imagined) of close friends, loved ones, and the social and cultural groups to which they belong. Such influences can support healthy behavior, or they can interfere with even the best intentions.

Your Family From the time of your birth, your parents have given you strong cues about which actions are socially acceptable and which are not. Brushing your teeth, bathing, wearing deodorant, and chewing food with your mouth closed are probably all behaviors that your family instilled in you long ago. Your family culture influenced your food choices, your religious beliefs, your political beliefs, and all your other values and actions. If you deviated from your family's norms, your mother or father probably let you know fairly quickly. Good family units share a dedication to the healthful development of all family members, unconditional trust, and a commitment to work out difficulties.

When the loving family unit does not exist, when it does not provide for basic human needs, or when dysfunctional, irresponsible individuals try to build a family under the influence of drugs or alcohol, it becomes difficult for a child to learn positive health behaviors. Healthy behaviors get their start in healthy homes; unhealthy homes breed unhealthy habits. Healthy families provide the foundation for a clear and necessary understanding of what is right and wrong, what is positive and negative. Without this fundamental grounding, many young people have great difficulties.[22]

Your Social Bonds Like family, personal environments also mold behaviors. If you deviated from the actions expected in your hometown, you probably suffered strange looks, ostracism by some high school cliques, and other negative social reactions. The more you value the opinions of other people, the more likely you are to change a behavior that offends them. If you couldn't care less what they think, you probably brush off their negative reactions or suggested changes. How often have you told yourself, "I don't care what so-and-so thinks. I'll do what I darn well please"? Although most of us have thought or said these words, often we care too much about what even the insignificant people in our lives think. In general, the lower your level of self-esteem and self-efficacy, the higher the chances that others will influence your actions.

Sometimes, the influence of others can be a powerful social support for positive behavior changes.[23] At other times, we are influenced to drink too much, party too hard, eat too much, or engage in some other negative action because we don't want to be left out or criticized. Understanding the subtle and not-so-subtle ways in which other people influence our actions is an important step toward changing our behaviors.

Choosing a Behavior-Change Strategy

Once you have analyzed all the factors that influence what you do, you must decide which behavior-change technique will work best for you. Options include shaping, visualization, modeling, controlling the situation, reinforcement, and changing self-talk.

Shaping

Regardless of how motivated you are, some behaviors are almost impossible to change immediately. To reach your goal, you may need to take a number of individual steps, each designed to change one small piece of the larger behavior. This process is known as **shaping**.

For example, suppose that you have not exercised for a while. You decide that you want to get into shape and your goal is to be able to jog three to four miles every other day. You realize that you'd face a near-death experience if you tried to run even just a few blocks in your current condition. So you decide to start slowly and build up to your desired fitness level gradually. During week 1, you will walk for one hour every other day at a slow, relaxed pace. During week 2,

you will walk for the same amount of time but will speed up your pace and cover slightly more ground. During week 3, you will speed up even more and will try to go even farther. You will continue taking such steps until you reach your goal.

Whatever the desired behavior change, all shaping involves the following items:

- Starting slowly and trying not to cause undue stress during the early stages of the program.
- Keeping the steps small and achievable.
- Being flexible and ready to change if the original plan proves uncomfortable.
- Refusing to skip steps or to move to the next step until the previous step has been mastered.

Behaviors don't develop overnight, so they won't change overnight.

Visualization

Mental practice and rehearsal can help change unhealthy behaviors into healthy ones. Athletes and others use a technique known as **imagined rehearsal** to reach their goals. By visualizing their planned action ahead of time, they will be prepared when they put themselves to the test.

For example, suppose you want to ask someone out on a date. Imagine the setting (walking together to class) for the action. Then practice exactly what you're going to say ("Mary, there's a great concert this Sunday and I was wondering if . . .") in your mind and out loud. Mentally anticipate different responses ("Oh, I'd love to, but I'm busy that evening") and what you will say in reaction ("How about if I call you sometime this week?"). Careful mental and verbal rehearsal (you could even try out your scenario on a good friend) will greatly improve the likelihood of success.

Modeling

Modeling, or learning behaviors through careful observation of other people, is one of the most effective strategies for changing behavior. For example, suppose that you have

---

Health Belief Model (HBM)   Model for explaining how beliefs may influence behaviors.

Theory of Reasoned Action   Model for explaining the importance of our intentions in determining behaviors.

Shaping   Using a series of small steps to get to a particular goal gradually.

Imagined rehearsal   Practicing, through mental imagery, to become better able to perform an event in actuality.

Modeling   Learning specific behaviors by watching others perform them.

trouble talking to people you don't know very well. One of the easiest ways to improve your communication skills is to select friends whose "gift of gab" you envy. Observe their social skills. Do they talk more or listen more? How do people respond to them? Why are they such good communicators? If you carefully observe behaviors you admire and isolate their components, you can model the steps of your behavior-change strategy on a proven success.

Controlling the Situation

Sometimes, the right setting or the right group of people will positively influence your behaviors. Many situations and occasions trigger certain actions. For example, in libraries, houses of worship, and museums, most people talk softly. Few people laugh at funerals. The term **situational inducement** refers to an attempt to influence a behavior by using situations and occasions to control it.

For example, you may be more apt to stop smoking if you work in a smoke-free office, a positive situational inducement. But a smoke-filled bar, a negative situational inducement, may tempt you to resume. Careful consideration of which settings will help and which will hurt your effort to change, and your decision to seek the first and avoid the second, will improve your chances for change.

Reinforcement

A **positive reinforcement** seeks to increase the likelihood that a behavior will occur by presenting something positive as a reward for it. Each of us is motivated by different reinforcers. Although a special T-shirt may be a positive reinforcer for young adults entering a race, it would not be for a 40-year-old runner who dislikes message-bearing T-shirts.

Most positive reinforcers can be classified under five headings: consumable, activity, manipulative, possessional, and social.

- *Consumable reinforcers* are delicious edibles such as candy, cookies, or gourmet meals.
- *Activity reinforcers* are opportunities to watch TV, go on a vacation, go swimming, or do something else enjoyable.
- *Manipulative reinforcers* are incentives such as lower rent in exchange for mowing the lawn or the promise of a better grade for doing an extra-credit project.
- *Possessional reinforcers* are tangible rewards such as a new TV or sports car.
- *Social reinforcers* are signs of appreciation, approval, or love, such as loving looks, affectionate hugs, and praise.

Situational inducement   Attempt to influence a behavior through situations and occasions that are structured to exert control over that behavior.

Positive reinforcement   Presenting something positive following a behavior that is being reinforced.

When choosing reinforcers, determine what would motivate you to act in a particular way. Research has shown that people can be motivated to change their behaviors, such as not smoking during pregnancy or abstaining from cocaine, if they set themselves up on a *token economy* system, whereby they earn tokens or points that can be exchanged for meaningful rewards such as financial incentives.[24] The difficulty often lies in determining *which* incentive will be most effective. Your reinforcers may initially come from others (extrinsic rewards), but as you see positive changes in yourself, you will begin to reward and reinforce yourself (intrinsic rewards). Keep in mind that reinforcers should immediately follow a behavior, but beware of overkill. If you reward yourself with a movie on the VCR every time you go jogging, this reinforcer will soon lose its power. It would be better to give yourself this reward after, say, a full week of adherence to your jogging program.

What do you think?

What consumable reinforcers (food or drink) would be a healthy reward for your new behavior? ⁕ If you could choose one activity reinforcer to reward yourself after one day of success in your new behavior, what would it be? ⁕ If you could obtain something (possessional reinforcer) after you reach your goal, what would it be? ⁕ If you maintain your behavior for one week, what type of social reinforcer would you like to receive from your friends?

Changing Self-Talk

Self-talk, or the way you think and talk to yourself, can also play a role in modifying health-related behaviors. Here are some cognitive procedures for changing self-talk.

Rational-Emotive Therapy   This form of cognitive therapy or self-directed behavior change is based on the premise that there is a close connection between what people say to themselves and how they feel. According to psychologist Albert Ellis, most everyday emotional problems and related behaviors stem from irrational statements that people make to themselves when events in their lives are different from what they would like them to be.[25]

For example, suppose that after doing poorly on an exam, you say to yourself, "I can't believe I flunked that easy exam. I'm so stupid." By changing this irrational, "catastrophic" self-talk into rational, positive statements about what is really going on, you can increase the likelihood that positive behaviors will occur. Positive self-talk might be phrased as follows: "I really didn't study enough for that exam, and I'm not surprised I didn't do very well. I'm certainly not stupid. I just need to prepare better for the next test." Such self-talk will help you to recover quickly from disappointment and take positive steps to correct the situation.

Meichenbaum's Self-Instructional Methods In Meichenbaum's behavioral therapies, clients are encouraged to give themselves "self-instructions" ("Slow down, don't rush") and "positive affirmations" ("My speech is going fine—I'm almost done!") instead of self-defeating thoughts ("I'm talking too fast—my speech is terrible") whenever a situation seems to be getting out of control. Behavioral psychologist Donald Meichenbaum is perhaps best known for a process known as stress inoculation, which subjects clients to extreme stressors in a laboratory environment. Before a stressful event (e.g., going to the doctor), clients practice individual coping skills (e.g., deep-breathing exercises) and self-instructions (e.g., "I'm feel better once I know what's causing my pain"). Meichenbaum demonstrated that clients who practiced coping techniques and self-instruction were less likely to resort to negative behaviors in stressful situations.

Blocking/Thought Stopping By purposefully blocking or stopping negative thoughts, a person can concentrate on taking positive steps toward behavior change. For example, suppose you are preoccupied with your ex-partner, who has recently deserted you for someone else. You consciously stop thinking about the situation and force yourself to think about something more pleasant (e.g., dinner tomorrow with your best friend). By refusing to dwell on negative images and forcing yourself to focus elsewhere, you can save wasted energy, time, and emotional resources and move on to positive change.

Changing Your Behavior

Many strategies have proved effective in making behavior changes. Before you begin this process, take stock of what has contributed to maintaining the behavior.

Self-Assessment: Antecedents and Consequences

Behaviors, thoughts, and feelings always occur in a context—the situation. Situations can be divided into two components: the events that come before and after. *Antecedents* are the setting events for a behavior; they cue or stimulate a person to act in certain ways. Antecedents can be physical events, thoughts, emotions, or the actions of other people. *Consequences*—the results of behavior—affect whether a person will repeat a behavior.[26] Consequences can also consist of physical events, thoughts, emotions, or the actions of other people.

Suppose you are shy and must give a speech in front of a large class. The antecedents include walking into the class, feeling frightened, wondering if you are capable of doing a good job, and being unable to remember a word of your speech. If the consequences are negative—if your classmates laugh and you get a low grade—your terror about speaking in public will be reinforced, and you will continue to dread this kind of event. In contrast, if you receive positive feedback from the class and instructor, you may actually learn to like speaking in public.

Learning to recognize the antecedents of a behavior and acting to modify them is one method of changing behavior (see the Reality Check box on page 30). A diary noting your undesirable behaviors and identifying the settings in which they occur can be a useful tool. Figure 1.4 identifies several factors that can make behavior change more difficult.

Analyzing Personal Behavior

Successful behavior change requires determining what you want to change. All too often we berate ourselves by using generalities: "I'm lousy to my friends; I need to be a better person." Determining the specific behavior you would like to change—in contrast to the general problem—will allow you to set clear goals. What are you doing that makes you a lousy friend? Are you gossiping or lying about your friends? Have you been a "taker" rather than a "giver"? Or are you really a good friend most of the time?

Let's say the problem is gossiping. You can now analyze this behavior by examining the following components:

- *Frequency.* How often are you gossiping—all the time, or only once in a while?
- *Duration.* How long have you been doing this?
- *Seriousness.* Is your gossiping just idle chatter, or are you really trying to injure the other person? What are the consequences for you? For your friend? For your friendship?
- *Basis for problem behavior.* Is your gossip based on facts, perceptions of facts, or deliberate embellishment of the truth?
- *Antecedents.* What kinds of situations trigger your gossiping? Do some settings or people bring out the gossip in you more than others? What triggers your feelings of dislike for or irritation toward your friends? Why are you talking behind their backs?

Decision Making: Choices for Change

Choosing among alternatives isn't easy, particularly when friends, family, media influences, and pleasurable options tempt you. "Just saying no" is usually easier said than done. However, if you are trying to fit in, be liked, or satisfy other emotional needs, decision making will become even more difficult. That's why anticipating what might occur in a given setting and thinking through all possible safe alternatives is important as you implement behavior change.

For example, knowing that you are likely to be offered a drink when you go to a party, what kind of response could you make that would be okay in your social group? If someone is flirting with you and the situation takes on a distinct sexual overtone, what might you do to prevent the situation from turning bad? Advance preparation will help you stick to your behavior plan.

Evaluating Personal Risk

A simple glance at newspaper headlines or a session watching the evening news can easily make your hair stand on end. Anthrax, West Nile virus, polluted water, diabetes, HIV, and a host of other health risks seem to be stalking us. Making sense of these potential threats is often challenging and requires an understanding of the concept of *risk*. Essentially, risk implies that there is some chance that something bad may happen to you. The question is when it is likely to happen. Is it inevitable? Is it something you can prevent through changes in your own behavior? Should you believe what you read?

Clearly, each of us is born with a *genetic propensity* toward certain risks. Diseases like diabetes, sickle-cell disease, and hypercholesterolemia are among a long list of diseases that appear to have distinct genetic links. If your grandparents and parents had one of these conditions, chances are increased that you will also have that disease.

Another factor that increases your risk is age, or relative longevity. If you live long enough, you will be likely to develop certain conditions, such as arthritis, certain memory-sapping dementias, several of the cardiovascular diseases, and various forms of cancer. For example, although you may hear that a woman has a 1 in 8 chance of contracting breast cancer, in truth, that is a woman's risk in the later years of her life. The risk is much lower for women in their 20s and 30s. A quick look at the leading causes of death by age (Table 1.2) indicates which risks are greatest by age.

Other factors that increase your risk include the environment that you live in, your exposure to toxic chemicals, your socioeconomic status, your race, your level of education, and lifestyle behaviors. These and a host of other factors, either individually or collectively, can spell health or disease risk for each of us.

QUESTIONS TO ASK

While we can read information that tells us that we are at risk, many of us are left wondering what we can do to reduce our risk or whether we should believe all of the hype to begin with. Although there are many reputable sources of information available, the best place to start is by checking information from government agencies and databases, institutions of higher education resources, or top-ranked peer-reviewed journals. Such journals require that a panel of professional experts review the scientific merits of a study and resultant health claims and determine whether the claims are valid and/or reliable. There are several additional things that you can do to ensure that you are getting the most accurate information available.

1. *Cross-check the information from two or three of the above sources.* Are they basically saying the same thing? Is conflicting information being given? If there is conflicting information, you'll need to continue your search and confirm information with additional sources.
2. *Is the source reliable?* Just because a magazine is published and in your library doesn't mean that it uses good science in making health claims. Even in your doctor's office, you may find trade magazines that publish articles written by people who may be good writers but lack sufficient expertise to make the claims that they are making, or people who are paying for space to advertise and have a vested interest in making a claim, even though it may be false.
3. *What are the credentials of the authors?* Just because someone has a Ph.D., M.D., or other set of initials behind his or her name doesn't mean that he or she is an expert. For example, a Ph.D. in counseling may decide to write about a particular health activity, even though he may not have all of the facts. An M.D. with little background in the area may decide to write an article about teen pregnancy. Look for information on the specific background of the authors. What are their degrees in? Where are they working now? Have

they published related research in peer-reviewed journals? Those working, teaching, or doing research in the area that they are writing about have more credibility than those who are not in the field.
4. *Where does the research come from?* Who paid for the research? Was it a drug company, business, or service provider who may have a vested interest in a particular outcome?
5. *What research methods were used?* Was it part of a randomized, controlled trial that is representative of the people being studied and about whom the claims are being made? Taking a course in research methods and basic statistics while in college will help you assess the merits of a particular study. In general, studies that include randomized, controlled samples that are applicable to populations are the most reliable. However, be careful not to make decisions about risk based on the results of only one study that hits the nightly news. Factors to consider when you judge information from scientific studies include:

LESS RELIABLE

Small number of subjects
Unpublished
Not repeated
Nonhuman subjects
Results not related to
   group in question
   (e.g., men vs. women)
No limitations mentioned
Not compared to other research
Author credentials unclear

MORE RELIABLE

Larger number of subjects
Published in peer-reviewed journal
Results verified in multiple studies
Human subjects
Results related to group in question
   (men vs. women)
Limitations discussed
Compared to other research
Author credentials clear

6. *If the source is one of thousands on the Internet, how can you know which ones to believe?* Start with sites from the government (such as the CDC and National Center for Health Statistics), professional health organizations, health-related foundations, and higher education/university–based sites. Reports and journals from agencies such as the American Heart Association, the American Cancer Society, and the National Cancer Institute also provide accurate information.

7. *How does this risk compare to others?* While you may very well be afraid of being killed in an airplane crash, statistically your risk is much smaller than that of being killed while driving your car to campus each day. Keeping your risk in perspective is an important factor in being able to rationally cope with life's challenges.

8. *Is the risk real?* Sometimes health risks are sensationalized or played up in the media because of their shock value rather than because they are real risks for you. For example, you may hear a lot about a murder in your area (although chances are low that you would be a victim) and not hear much at all about the fact that a sexually transmitted disease is raging through the campus community. You might be led to worry about a small risk that appears to be big and to ignore big risks that appear to be small.

9. *Look carefully at what the numbers really mean.* If rates are listed as 1 in 100, remember that this is the same as 1 percent, or 10 in 1,000, or 10,000 out of 1 million. Normally health risks are listed per 100,000 people.

Remember that when you consider risks you should look at your risk at a particular point in time, whether you are looking at it today or in 30 years. Then, consider what science tells you is the best course of action for reducing risk. Also, consider these questions:

✔ What actions are best for me? Which are most compatible with my current situation? How much time/effort am I really willing to invest? What sacrifices will I have to make for a given result?
✔ Where can I find information that will help me make a better decision?

KNOW YOUR "RISK" TERMINOLOGY

Once you've evaluated whether there is a real risk for you, you should also familiarize yourself with the risk terminology that is typically used in reporting epidemiological data.

Risk-specific attack rate is the number of persons who became ill who reported the risk behavior divided by the total number of people who reported the risk behavior. For example, if 150 students went to a dormitory picnic, all ate warm potato salad, and 30 got sick, there would be 30 cases and 120 noncases for an attack rate of 25 percent.

Relative risk is the attack rate among those exposed to the risk factor divided by the attack rate in those who were not exposed. If those who ate potato salad were no more likely to become ill than those who did not, the attack rates would be equal and the relative risk would be 1. If those who ate potato salad were more likely to become ill than those who did not, this ratio would be *greater than* 1 and potato salad would be a risk factor for illness.

Overall, knowing what the terms mean, assessing the reliability and validity of the source, and keeping abreast of new studies/information will help you have a better understanding of what the threats to your health are and what you can do to reduce risk. Careful study of the information found in the following chapters should provide the necessary foundation for risk reduction.

Sources: Health Insight, "A Consumer's Guide to Taking Charge of Health Information" (August 2002) (see http://www.healthinsight. harvard.edu/guide.html). K E. Nelson, C. Williams, and N. Graham, *Infectious Disease Epidemiology: Theory and Practice* (Aspen Publishers, 2001), pp. 140–142.

Remember that things typically don't "just happen." By staying alert to potential problems, being aware of your alternatives, maintaining a good sense of your own values, and sticking to your beliefs under pressure, you can gain control over many situations in your life.

Setting Realistic Goals

Changing behavior is not easy, but sometimes we make it even harder by setting unrealistic and unattainable goals. To start making positive changes, ask yourself these questions.

● *What do I want?* What is your ultimate goal—to lose weight? Exercise more? Reduce stress? Have a lasting relationship? Whatever it is, you need a clear picture of the eventual target outcome.
● *Which change is the greatest priority at this time?* Often people decide to change several things all at once. Suppose that you are gaining unwanted weight. Rather than saying, "I need to eat less, start jogging, and really get in shape," you need to be specific about your current behavior. Are you eating too many sweets? Too many foods high in fat? Perhaps a realistic goal, therefore, would be, "I am going to try to eat

OBSTACLE	STRATEGY
Stress (intrinsic and extrinsic)	Identify potential sources of stress, and find constructive ways to lower stress level.
Social pressures to repeat old habits	Enlist the support of friends. Identify specifics of these pressures.
Not expecting mistakes, perfectionist, hypercritical	Accept that slips are inevitable, but maintain control. Acknowledge that humans are imperfect beings.
Self-blame for poor coping or a weak personality	Blame pressures from the environment or lack of skills, rather than innate weakness.
Lack of effort, lack of motivation	Assess effort and make sure it is adequate. Provide rewards for successes.
Faulty beliefs, low self-efficacy	Develop new skills, focus on successes, and plan ahead for difficult situations. Change self-talk.

Figure 1.4

Obstacles to Behavior Change. Psychologists offer a number of explanations for why you may fail in your efforts to change your behavior and strategies for overcoming these obstacles.

Source: From *Self-Directed Behavior: Self-Modification for Personal Adjustment,* by D. L. Watson and R. G. Tharp, Copyright 1997, 1993, 1989, 1985, 1981, 1977, 1972 Brooks/Cole Publishing Company, Pacific Grove, CA 93950, a division of Thomson Publishing Inc. Reprinted by permission of the publisher.

less fat during dinner every day." Choose the behavior that constitutes your greatest problem, and tackle that first. You can always work on something else later. Take small steps, experiment with alternatives, and find the best way to meet your unique goals.

- *Why is this important to me?* Think through why you want to change. Are you doing it because of your health? To look better? To win someone else's approval? Usually, doing things because it's right for you rather than to win others' approval is a sound strategy. If you are doing it for someone else, what happens when that other person isn't around?
- *What are the potential positive outcomes?* What do you hope to accomplish with this change?
- *What health-promoting programs and services can help me get started?* Nearly all campuses and communities have programs and services designed to support positive behavior change. It may mean buying a self-help book, speaking to a counselor, or enrolling in an aerobics class at the local fitness center.

- *Are there family or friends whose help I can enlist?* Social support is one of your most powerful allies. Getting a friend to walk with you on a regular basis, asking your partner to help you stop smoking by quitting at the same time, and making a commitment with a friend to never let each other drive if you've had something to drink—these are all examples of how people can help each other make positive changes.

What do you think?

Why is it sometimes hard to make decisions? ✳ *What factors influence your decision making?* ✳ *Select one behavior that you want to change and refer to the Behavior Change Contract at the end of this book.* ✳ *Using the goal-setting strategies discussed here, outline a plan for change.*

Managing Behavior Change

Behavior change can be a challenge. Recognize that you are a unique individual, with your own emotional makeup, physical characteristics, and values and beliefs. Finding the right behavior-change strategy involves perseverance, introspection, planning, and motivation. Regardless of the model or the strategies employed, each person has a unique road to follow. Each chapter in this book describes specific activities and choices that will enable you to adopt and maintain healthy behaviors.

Checklist for Change

Making Personal Choices

☐ Are you ready to make this change? Are you in a healthy emotional state? Are you doing it for yourself or to please someone else?

☐ Have you completed a personal health history to assess your risks from various sources?

☐ Do you have an action plan with short- and long-term goals? Have you set priorities?

☐ Assess your personal resources. Where can you go for support and advice?

☐ Have you planned alternative actions in case you run into obstacles or begin to sabotage yourself?

☐ List several reinforcers and supports that will keep you motivated along the way.

☐ Establish a set of guidelines for success. Will you set small goals to achieve at selected intervals, or will you consider yourself successful only if you meet your ultimate goal?

Making Community Choices

☐ Have you taken time to become educated about issues and concerns affecting others in your community?

☐ Have you prioritized actions to take to help change community behaviors? Do you have a particular goal?

☐ Do you analyze what is happening in your school, community, state, and nation by reading about issues, actively discussing problems and possible solutions, and developing personal opinions?

☐ Do you listen carefully to what your elected officials say and take constructive action if you disagree with them?

☐ Do you vote for officials whose policies, rhetoric, and past histories indicate that they support improvements in the environment, education, and health care for all people?

☐ Do you volunteer at least once every term to help others who are less fortunate?

☐ Do you purchase products and services from companies that have proven records of supporting the health and well-being of others through their organizational practices?

Summary

✳ Health encompasses the whole dynamic process of fulfilling one's individual potential in the physical, social, emotional, spiritual, intellectual, and environmental dimensions of life. Wellness means achieving the highest level of health possible along several dimensions.

✳ Although the average American life span has increased over the past century, we need to increase the span of quality life. The programs *Healthy People 2000* and *2010* and documents such as the *AHRQ Guidelines* have established a set of national objectives for achieving longer life and quality of life for all Americans through health promotion and disease prevention.

✳ Gender continues to play a major role in health status and care. Women live longer but have more medical problems than do men. The recent inclusion of women in medical research and training attempts to close the gap in health care.

✳ For the U.S. population as a whole, the leading causes of death are heart disease, cancer, and stroke. But in the 15- to 24-year-old age group, the leading causes are unintentional injuries, homicide/legal intervention, and suicide. Many of the risks associated with heart disease, cancer, and stroke can be reduced through lifestyle changes. Many of the risks associated with accidents, homicide, and suicide can be reduced through preventive measures.

✳ Worldwide commerce and travel are bringing dramatic changes in global health. In nonindustrialized countries, noncommunicable diseases such as depression and heart disease are replacing infectious disease and malnutrition as leading causes of disability and death.

✳ Several factors contribute to a person's health status, and a number of them are within our control. Beliefs and attitudes, intentions to change, support from significant others, and readiness to change are factors over which individuals have some degree of control. Access to health care, genetic predisposition, health policies that support positive choices, and other factors are all potential reinforcing, predisposing, and enabling factors that may influence health decisions.

* Applying behavior-change techniques, such as shaping, visualizing, modeling, controlling the situation, and rein-forcing, and changing self-talk help people succeed in making behavior changes.

* Decision making has several key components. Each person must explore his or her own problems, the reasons for making change, and the expected outcomes. The next step is to plan a course of action best suited to individual needs.

Questions for Discussion and Reflection

1. How are the terms *health* and *wellness* similar? What, if any, are important distinctions between these terms? What is health promotion? Disease prevention? What does it really mean to be healthy? Considering the various dimensions of health, describe someone that you believe to have many of these characteristics.

2. How healthy are Americans today? Are we doing better or worse in terms of health status in America? Who is not doing better in an era when health is the "buzz" and everyone seems to be interested in improving health? What factors influence today's disparities in health?

3. What are some of the major global health problems today? Why is it increasingly important that we consider individual, community, U.S., and global health when we consider the health of populations?

4. What are some of the major differences in the way males and females are treated in the health care system? Why do you think these differences exist? Why are people treated differently based on race, sexual orientation, religion, marital status, and age?

5. What are the leading causes of death across different ages and races? What are the leading causes of death for people ages 15 to 24? Why are these statistics so different? Explain why it is important to look at these statistics by age rather than just in total. What lifestyle changes can you make to lower your risks for contracting major diseases?

6. What major differences exist between the leading causes of death for Americans and for people in other regions of the world?

7. What is the Health Belief Model? The Theory of Reasoned Action? How may each of these models be working when a young woman decides to smoke her first cigarette? Her last cigarette?

8. Explain the predisposing, reinforcing, and enabling factors that might influence a young welfare mother as she decides whether to sell drugs to support her children.

9. Using the Stages of Change model, discuss what you might do (in stages) to help a friend stop smoking. Why is it important that a person be ready to change before trying to change?

Application Exercises

Reread the What Do You Think? scenarios at the beginning of the chapter and answer the following questions.

1. What can you do to ensure that you are getting the most accurate and reliable health information upon which to make your health decisions? How can you protect yourself from false or misleading information on the Internet?

2. From what you learned in this chapter, why are young people at high risk for accidents, homicide, and suicide? Why do these risks decline with age?

Accessing Your Health on the Internet

Visit the following Internet sites to explore further topics and issues related to personal health. To visit an organization's website, go to the Companion Website for *Access to Health, Eighth Edition* at www.aw.com/donatelle, click on the book image, and select "Accessing Your Health on the Internet" from the navigation menu on the left.

1. *National Center for Health Statistics.* Outstanding place to start for information about health status in the United States. Links to key documents such as *Health United States* (published annually), national survey information, and information on mortality by age, race,

gender, geographic location, and other important data. Includes comprehensive information provided by the Centers for Disease Control and Prevention (CDC) as well as easy links to at least ten of the major health resources currently being utilized for policy and decision making about health in the United States.

2. *CDC Wonder.* Clearinghouse for comprehensive information from the CDC, including special reports, guidelines, and access to national health data.

3. *National Health Information Center.* An excellent resource for consumer information about health.

4. **Web MD.** Reputable and comprehensive overview of various diseases and conditions. Written for the public in an easy-to-understand format with links to more in-depth information.

5. **Mayo Clinic.** Another reliable resource for specific information about health topics, diseases, and treatment options. Easy to navigate and consumer friendly.

Further Reading

Olpin, M., and D. Gotthoffer. *Health on the Net 2002*. Boston: Allyn & Bacon, 2002.

This easy-to-use resource makes the vast potential of the Internet easily accessible to health students.

Robins, Alexander, and Abby Wilner. *Quarterlife Crisis: The Unique Challenges of Life in Your 20s*. J. P. Tarcher Paperbacks, 2001.

Overview of challenges facing young adults in America today.

U.S. Department of Health and Human Services. *Healthy People 2010: National Health Promotion and Disease Prevention Objectives for the Year 2010*. Washington, DC: Government Printing Office, 1998.

This plan contains the Surgeon General's long-range goals for improving the life span for all Americans by three years and improving access to health for all Americans, regardless of sex, race, socioeconomic status, and other variables.

U.S. Department of Health and Human Services. *Health United States: 2002*. Centers for Disease Control and Prevention. Washington, DC: Government Printing Office, 2002.

Provides an up-to-date overview of U.S. health statistics, risk factors, and trends

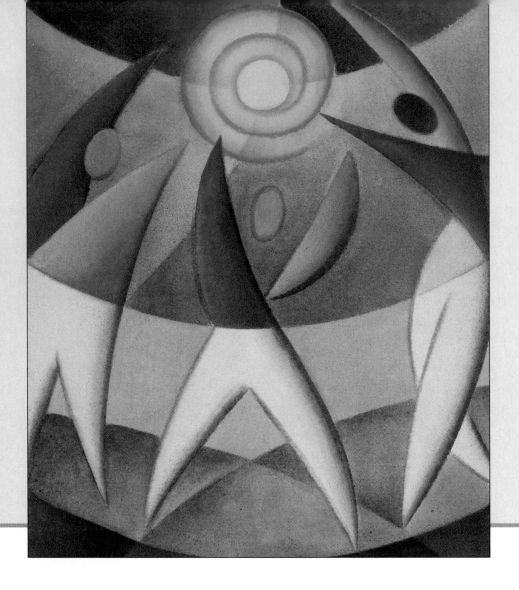

Objectives

* Define psychosocial health in terms of its mental, emotional, and social components, and identify the basic elements shared by psychosocially healthy people.

* Identify the internal and external factors influencing psychosocial health, and consider how each may affect you.

* Discuss the positive steps can take to enhance psychosocial health.

* Discuss the dimension of spirituality and the role that it plays in health and wellness.

* Discuss the mind–body connection and how emotions (including optimism and happiness) influence health status.

* Identify and describe common psychosocial problems of adulthood, and explain their causes, methods of prevention, and available treatments.

* Describe different types of anxiety disorders and their key risk factors.

* Illustrate the warning signs of suicide and actions that can be taken to help a suicidal individual.

* Identify the different types of health professionals, popular types of therapy, and strategies for selecting a good therapist.

2 Psychosocial Health

Being Mentally, Emotionally, Socially, and Spiritually Well

What do you think?

Amy is a 20-year-old junior majoring in health education. She is chronically tired and often blasts her friends with verbal outbursts when she is angry. She is cynical and hostile to others when she is stressed. She often feels like crying, but the tears never come. Amy can't sleep well, and she is gaining weight. Even her closest friends are getting fed up with her, and rarely invite her out.

If you were Amy's friend, what would you do to help her? ✳ *Do you know anyone with some of these same symptoms?* ✳ *What might cause them?* ✳ *What campus programs and services might be helpful?* ✳ *Why is it difficult to confront someone like this?*

Martin is a sophomore majoring in public health at a large university. He is outgoing, warm, and popular. Recently, he was selected to represent his group in a class and deliver a five-minute overview of his state's environmental policies. That morning, Martin felt nauseated and dizzy and had a slight, dull headache. As class time approached, his heart rate increased and his face grew flushed. By the time the instructor called on him to deliver the report, Martin was visibly shaken; his hands trembled, he was perspiring profusely, and he felt so weak that he could barely get out of his seat. He excused himself, went to the bathroom, and vomited, then left the building, feeling abject embarrassment.

Have you ever experienced anything like Martin's predicament? ✳ *What did you do?* ✳ *How would you describe Martin's problem?* ✳ *What services on campus might help him cope with this type of situation?* ✳ *As a friend, what might you have said to Martin after class?*

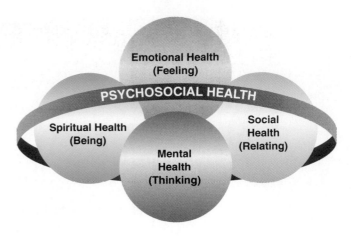

Figure 2.1
Psychosocial Health. Psychosocial health is a complex interaction of mental, emotional, social, and spiritual health.

ave there been days when you felt mentally and physically exhausted? Were you so tired that you found it hard to stay awake long enough to study or go out with friends? In contrast, have there been other days when you felt energized from the moment you woke up in the morning? Although you were busy all day, you may have felt too awake to even think about going to bed.

Your experience illustrates the close link between psychosocial and physical health. Although often overlooked during the pursuit of a fit and firm body, a fit mind can be equally important in determining not only the number of years we live, but also the quality of those years. Like Amy and Martin, all of us go through times when life seems difficult. Whatever the cause for the "lows" in our lives, they have the power to sap energy, drain emotions, and break the spirit. Over the long haul, they can even shorten life expectancy.

However, human beings possess a resiliency that enables us to cope, adapt, and thrive, regardless of life's challenges. How we feel and think about ourselves, those around us, and our environment can tell us a lot about our psychosocial health and whether we are healthy emotionally, spiritually, and mentally. Increasingly, health professionals recognize that having a solid social network, being emotionally and mentally healthy, and acknowledging and developing spiritual capacity can put life into years, as well as add years to life.

Defining Psychosocial Health

Psychosocial health encompasses the mental, emotional, social, and spiritual dimensions of health (see Figure 2.1). It is the result of a complex interaction between a person's history and conscious and unconscious thoughts about and interpretations of the past. Psychosocially healthy people are emotionally, mentally, socially, intellectually, and spiritually resilient. Despite occasional slips, they respond to challenges, disappointments, joys, frustrations, and pain in appropriate ways most of the time. Most authorities identify several basic elements shared by psychosocially healthy people.[1]

• They feel good about themselves. Psychosocially healthy people are not typically overwhelmed by fear, love, anger, jealousy, guilt, or worry. They know who they are and have

a realistic sense of their capabilities. They respect themselves even though they realize they aren't perfect.
• They feel comfortable with other people. Healthy people enjoy satisfying and lasting personal relationships and do not take advantage of others, nor do they allow others to take advantage of them. They can give love, consider others' interests, respect personal differences, and feel responsible for their fellow human beings.
• They control tension and anxiety. They recognize the underlying causes and symptoms of stress and anxiety in their lives and consciously work to avoid irrational thoughts, unnecessary aggression, hostility, excessive excuse making, and blaming others for their problems.
• They meet the demands of life. They try to solve problems as they arise, accept responsibility, and plan ahead. Acknowledging that change is inevitable, they welcome new experiences.
• They curb hate and guilt by acknowledging and combating their tendencies to respond with hate, anger, thoughtlessness, selfishness, vengeful acts, or feelings of inadequacy. Rather than knocking others aside to get ahead, they reach out to help others—even those they don't particularly care for.
• They maintain a positive outlook by approaching each day with a presumption that things will go well. They block out most negative and cynical thoughts and give the good things in life star billing. They look to the future with enthusiasm rather than dread.
• They enrich the lives of others because they recognize that there are others whose needs are greater than their own.
• They cherish the things that make them smile. Reminders of good experiences brighten their day. Fun is an integral part of their lives. So is making time for themselves.
• They value diversity. Psychosocially healthy people do not feel threatened by people who are of a different race, gender, religion, sexual orientation, ethnicity, or political party. They appreciate creativity in others as well as in themselves.
• They appreciate nature. They take the time to enjoy their surroundings and are conscious of their place in the universe.

Psychosocial health   The mental, emotional, social, and spiritual dimensions of health.

Mental health   The "thinking" part of psychosocial health, includes your values, attitudes, and beliefs.

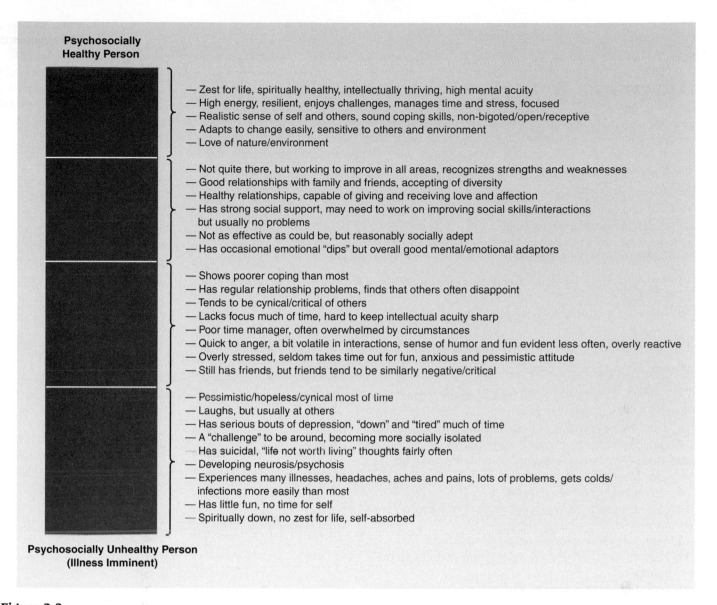

Psychosocially Healthy Person

— Zest for life, spiritually healthy, intellectually thriving, high mental acuity
— High energy, resilient, enjoys challenges, manages time and stress, focused
— Realistic sense of self and others, sound coping skills, non-bigoted/open/receptive
— Adapts to change easily, sensitive to others and environment
— Love of nature/environment

— Not quite there, but working to improve in all areas, recognizes strengths and weaknesses
— Good relationships with family and friends, accepting of diversity
— Healthy relationships, capable of giving and receiving love and affection
— Has strong social support, may need to work on improving social skills/interactions but usually no problems
— Not as effective as could be, but reasonably socially adept
— Has occasional emotional "dips" but overall good mental/emotional adaptors

— Shows poorer coping than most
— Has regular relationship problems, finds that others often disappoint
— Tends to be cynical/critical of others
— Lacks focus much of time, hard to keep intellectual acuity sharp
— Poor time manager, often overwhelmed by circumstances
— Quick to anger, a bit volatile in interactions, sense of humor and fun evident less often, overly reactive
— Overly stressed, seldom takes time out for fun, anxious and pessimistic attitude
— Still has friends, but friends tend to be similarly negative/critical

— Pessimistic/hopeless/cynical most of time
— Laughs, but usually at others
— Has serious bouts of depression, "down" and "tired" much of time
— A "challenge" to be around, becoming more socially isolated
— Has suicidal, "life not worth living" thoughts fairly often
— Developing neurosis/psychosis
— Experiences many illnesses, headaches, aches and pains, lots of problems, gets colds/infections more easily than most
— Has little fun, no time for self
— Spiritually down, no zest for life, self-absorbed

Psychosocially Unhealthy Person
(Illness Imminent)

Figure 2.2
Psychosocially Healthy Individuals versus Psychosocially Unhealthy Individuals

Of course, no one ever achieves perfection. Attaining psychosocial health and wellness involves many complex processes (see Figure 2.2). This chapter will help you understand not only what it means to be psychosocially well, but also why we may run into problems. Learning how to assess your own health and to help yourself or seek help from others are important parts of psychosocial health (see the Assess Yourself box).

What do you think?

Which psychosocial qualities do you value the most in your friends? ✳ *Do you think that you are strong in these areas yourself?* ✳ *Explain your answer.*

Mental Health: The Thinking You

The term **mental health** is often used to describe the "thinking" part of psychosocial health. As a thinking being, you have the ability to reason, interpret, and remember events from a unique perspective; to sense, perceive, and evaluate what is happening; and to solve problems. In short, you are intellectually able to sort through the clutter of events, contradictory messages, and uncertainties of a situation and attach meaning (either positive or negative) to it (people often refer to this subset of mental health as intellectual health). Your values, attitudes, and beliefs about your body, your family, your relationships, and life in general are usually—at least in part—a reflection of your mental health.

A mentally healthy person is likely to respond in a positive way even when things do not go as expected. For example, a mentally healthy student who receives a D on an exam

Assessing Your Psychosocial Health

Being psychosocially healthy requires both introspection and the willingness to work on areas that need improvement. Begin by completing the following assessment scale. When you've finished, ask someone who is very close to you to take the same test and respond with their perceptions of you. Carefully assess areas where your responses differ from those of your friend or family member. Which areas need some work? Which are in good shape?

1 = never describes me
2 = describes me infrequently
3 = describes me fairly frequently
4 = describes me most of the time
5 = describes me all of the time

1. My actions and interactions indicate that I am confident in my abilities.	1	2	3	4	5
2. I am quick to blame others for things that go wrong in my life.	1	2	3	4	5
3. I am spontaneous and like to have fun with others.	1	2	3	4	5
4. I am able to give love and affection to others and show my feelings.	1	2	3	4	5
5. I am able to receive love and signs of affection from others without feeling uneasy.	1	2	3	4	5
6. I am generally positive and upbeat about things in my life.	1	2	3	4	5
7. I am cynical and tend to be critical of others.	1	2	3	4	5
8. I have a large group of people whom I consider to be good friends.	1	2	3	4	5
9. I make time for others in my life.	1	2	3	4	5
10. I take time each day for myself for quiet introspection, having fun, or just doing nothing.	1	2	3	4	5
11. I am compulsive and competitive in my actions.	1	2	3	4	5
12. I handle stress well and am seldom upset or stressed out by others.	1	2	3	4	5
13. I try to look for the good in everyone and every situation before finding fault.	1	2	3	4	5
14. I am comfortable meeting new people and interact well in social settings.	1	2	3	4	5
15. I would rather stay in and watch TV or read than go out with friends or interact with others.	1	2	3	4	5
16. I am flexible and can adapt to most situations, even if I don't like them.	1	2	3	4	5
17. Nature, the environment, and other living things are important aspects of my life.	1	2	3	4	5
18. I think before responding to my emotions.	1	2	3	4	5
19. I am selfish and tend to think of my own needs before those of others.	1	2	3	4	5
20. I am consciously trying to be a "better person."	1	2	3	4	5
21. I like to plan ahead and set realistic goals for myself and others.	1	2	3	4	5
22. I accept others for who they are.	1	2	3	4	5
23. I value diversity and respect others' rights, regardless of culture, race, sexual orientation, religion, or other differences.	1	2	3	4	5
24. I try to live each day as if it might be my last.	1	2	3	4	5

25. I have a great deal of energy and appreciate the little things in life.	1	2	3	4	5
26. I cope with stress in appropriate ways.	1	2	3	4	5
27. I get enough sleep each day and seldom feel tired.	1	2	3	4	5
28. I have healthy relationships with my family.	1	2	3	4	5
29. I am confident that I can do most things if I put my mind to them.	1	2	3	4	5
30. I respect others' opinions and believe that others should be free to express their opinions, even when they differ from my own.	1	2	3	4	5

Look at items 2, 7, 11, 15, and 19. Add up your score for these five items and divide by 5. Is your average for these items above or below 3? Did you score a 5 on any of these items? Do you need to work on any of these areas?

Now look at your scores for the remaining items. (There should be 25 items.) Total these scores and divide by 25. Is your average above or below 3? On which items did you score a 5? Obviously you're doing well in these areas. Now remove these items from this grouping of 25 (scores of 5), and add up your scores for the remaining items. Then divide your total by the number of items included. Now what is your average?

Do the same for the scores completed by your friend or family member. How do your scores compare? Which ones, if any, are different, and how do they differ? Which areas do you think you need to work on? What actions can you take now to improve your ratings in these areas? Use the Behavior Change Contract to make a positive change.

may be disappointed but will try to assess why she did poorly. Did she study enough? Did she attend class and ask questions about the things she didn't understand? Even though the test result may be important to her, she will find constructive ways to deal with her frustration: talk to the instructor, devote more time to studying before the next exam, or hire a tutor. In contrast, a mentally unhealthy person may take a distorted view and respond irrationally. She may believe that her instructor is out to get her or that other students cheated on the exam. She may allow her low grade to provoke a major crisis in her life. She may spend the next 24 hours getting wasted, decide to quit school, try to get back at her instructor, or even blame her roommate for preventing her from studying.

When a person's mental health begins to deteriorate, he or she may experience sharp declines in rational thinking ability and increasingly distorted perceptions. The person may become cynical and distrustful, experience volatile mood swings, or choose to be isolated from others. These negative reactions may even threaten the life and health of others. People who show such extreme behavior are classified as having mental illnesses, discussed later in this chapter.

Emotional Health: The Feeling You

The term **emotional health** is often used interchangeably with mental health. Although the two are closely intertwined, emotional health more accurately refers to the "feeling," or subjective, side of psychosocial health. **Emotions** are intensified feelings or complex patterns of feelings that we experience on

a minute-by-minute, day-to-day basis. Love, hate, frustration, anxiety, and joy are only a few of the many emotions we feel. Typically, emotions are described as the interplay of four components: physiological arousal, feelings, cognitive (thought) processes, and behavioral reactions. Each time you are put in a stressful situation, you react physiologically while your mind tries to sort things out. You consciously or unconsciously react based on how rationally you interpret the situation.

According to psychologist Richard Lazarus, there are four basic types of emotions: (1) emotions resulting from harm, loss, or threats; (2) emotions resulting from benefits; (3) borderline emotions, such as hope and compassion; and (4) more complex emotions, such as grief, disappointment, bewilderment, and curiosity.[2] Each of us may experience any of these feelings in any combination at any time. As rational beings, it is our responsibility to evaluate our individual emotional responses, the environmental causes of them, and the appropriateness of our actions.

Emotionally healthy people are usually able to respond in an appropriate manner to upsetting events. When they feel threatened, they are not likely to react in an extreme fashion, behave inconsistently, or adopt an offensive attack mode.

Emotional health The "feeling" part of psychosocial health, includes your emotional reactions to life.

Emotions Intensified feelings or complex patterns of feelings we constantly experience.

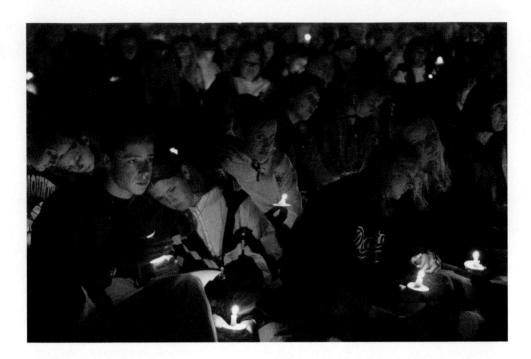

Rituals such as memorial services can be an important component of spiritual health.

Even when their feelings are trampled upon or they suffer agonizing pain because of a lost love, they keep their emotions in check. Emotionally unhealthy people are much more likely to let their feelings overpower them. They may be highly volatile and prone to unpredictable emotional outbursts and inappropriate, sometimes frightening responses to events. An ex-boyfriend who is so jealous of your new relationship that he hits you and pushes you around in front of your friends is showing an extremely unhealthy and dangerous emotional reaction. Such violent responses have become a problem of epidemic proportions in the United States (see Chapter 4).

Emotional health also affects social health. Someone feeling hostile, withdrawn, or moody may become socially isolated. People in the midst of emotional turmoil may be grumpy, irritable, or overly quiet; they may cry easily or demonstrate other disturbing emotional responses. Since they are not much fun to be around, their friends may avoid them at the very time they are most in need of emotional support. Social isolation is just one of the many potential negative consequences of unstable emotional responses.

For students, a more immediate concern is how emotional trauma or turmoil can impact academic performance. Have you ever tried to study for an exam after a fight with a close friend or family member? Emotional turmoil may seriously affect your ability to think, reason, and act rationally. Many otherwise rational, mentally healthy people do ridiculous things when they are going through a major emotional upset. Mental functioning and emotional responses are indeed intricately connected.

Social Health: Interactions with Others

Social health is the part of psychosocial health dealing with interactions with others and the ability to adapt to social situations. Socially healthy individuals have a wide range of interactions with family, friends, and acquaintances. They are able to listen, express themselves, form healthy relationships, act in socially acceptable and responsible ways, and find the best fit for themselves in society. See the Women's Health/Men's Health box and Chapter 5 for information.

Numerous studies have documented the importance of social life in achieving and maintaining health, and two aspects of social health have proven to be particularly important.[3]

- Presence of strong social bonds. **Social bonds**, or social linkages, reflect the general degree and nature of our interpersonal contacts and interactions. Social bonds serve six major functions: providing (1) intimacy, (2) feelings of belonging to or integration with a group, (3) opportunities for giving or receiving nurturance, (4) reassurance of one's worth, (5) assistance and guidance, and (6) advice. People who are more "connected" to others manage stress more effectively and are much more resilient when bombarded by life's crises.
- Presence of key social supports. **Social supports** refer to relationships that bring positive benefits to the individual. Social supports can be either expressive (emotional support, encouragement) or structural (housing, money). Families provide both structural and expressive support to children.

Social bonds Degree and nature of interpersonal contacts.

Social supports Structural and functional aspects of social interactions.

Prejudice A negative evaluation of an entire group of people that is typically based on unfavorable and often wrong ideas about the group.

Strategies for Resolving Conflict

Commander Dee Norton of the U.S. Coast Guard tells this story: A senior male officer instructed a female officer to perform a task. After listening to him describe what he wanted, the subordinate suggested a different approach that she had used successfully in her previous unit. Her boss angrily accused her of being insubordinate, because to him a good officer was a team player who obeyed orders without question. His reaction astonished and upset the junior officer, who thought he would appreciate a helpful suggestion.

Stereotyped gender roles have often taught men to value authority, confidence, and a hierarchical chain of command. Women, on the other hand, have often been encouraged to be good listeners and work cooperatively. These life lessons translate into different patterns of relating to others. Men tend to initiate interactions, speak more often, interrupt more frequently, and "hold the floor" for longer periods of time. Women tend to solicit input, ask more questions, negotiate relationships, and share power with others.

Depending on the situation, both approaches have value. Assertiveness and conviction are effective for conveying information and making rapid decisions, especially in formal hierarchies. A collaborative style is valuable for promoting cooperation and building consensus. But, as Norton's example shows, when these communication styles clash, they can lead to misunderstanding and conflict.

You can't avoid conflict; indeed, you'll face it throughout your life. Instead, learn to handle tensions constructively as they arise—people with good conflict resolution skills enjoy greater self-efficacy and stronger social bonds. Gemma Summers, a mediator and author based in Sydney, Australia, offers this four-step strategy for conflict resolution:

1. *Take your own side.* Before you bring up the issue that's upsetting you, know what you want to achieve. Make sure you can articulate what's bothering you and how you'd like to resolve it (rehearse ahead of time if necessary). Have a positive outcome in mind.
2. *Take the other side.* Listen to what the other side says, but go beyond that—try to understand as well. What's really bothering them? Perhaps you can work out a solution that will make everyone happy. Express empathy for their position.
3. *Take the neutral side.* It may not be easy, but try to see the big picture.

Place the conflict in context. Which of you has more to lose? Does the outcome really matter to you? If you feel yourself becoming emotional, go back to step 1 and focus again on the outcome that you want to achieve.

4. *Make up.* If at all possible, end your discussion on a positive note. Remember that conflict resolution is a process and one session may not be enough. Set the stage for further discussion by keeping those lines of communication open.

While Summers originally developed these guidelines for women, she notes that men find them helpful, too. The basic principles of conflict resolution transcend gender.

Sources: Michelle Conlin, "She's Gotta Have 'It,'" *Business Week*, July 22, 2002, p. 88; John Dagge, "War and Peace in the Office," *Sun Herald*, July 21, 2002, p. 2; CDR Dee Norton, "Gender and Communication—Finding Common Ground," U.S. Coast Guard, *The Leadership News*, Spring 1998 (see www.uscg.mil/hq/g-w/g-wt/g-wtl/gender.htm); and G. Summers, *How to Get What You Want Without Losing It: A Woman's Guide to Resolving Conflict* (see www.goforgoals.com.au/book.htm).

Adults need to develop their own social supports. Psychosocially healthy people create a network of friends and family with whom they can give and receive support.

Social health also reflects the way we react to others. In its most extreme forms, a lack of social health may be represented by aggressive acts of prejudice and bias toward other individuals or groups. **Prejudice** is a negative evaluation of an entire group of people that is typically based on unfavorable (and often wrong) ideas about the group. In its most obvious manifestations, prejudice is reflected in acts of discrimination against others, in overt acts of hate and bias, and in purposeful intent to harm individuals or groups.

Spiritual Health

Although mental and emotional health are key factors in overall psychosocial functioning, it is possible to be mentally and emotionally healthy and still not achieve optimal well-being. What is missing? For many people, that difficult-to-describe element that gives zest to life is the spiritual dimension. For a complete discussion of spiritual health, see the section later in this chapter and in Chapter 3.

What do you think?

What do social and emotional health mean to you? ✳ *What are your strengths and weaknesses in these areas?* ✳ *What can you do to enhance your strengths?* ✳ *What can you do to protect yourself from social health difficulties?* ✳ *From problems with emotional health?*

External Factors That Influence Psychosocial Health

Our psychosocial health is based on our expectations and how we perceive life experiences. While some experiences are under our control, others are not. External influences are those factors in life that we do not control, such as who raised us and the physical environment in which we live.

The Family   Families have a significant influence on psychosocial development. Children raised in healthy, nurturing, happy families are more likely to become well-adjusted, productive adults. Children raised in **dysfunctional families** —which show characteristics such as violence, distrust, anger, dietary deprivation, drug abuse, parental discord, sexual, physical, or emotional abuse—may have a harder time adapting to life. In dysfunctional families, love, security, and unconditional trust are so lacking that children often become confused and psychologically bruised. Yet not all people raised in dysfunctional families become psychosocially unhealthy, and not all people from healthy environments are well adjusted. Obviously, more factors are involved in our "process of becoming" than just our family.

The Wider Environment   While isolated negative events may do little damage to psychosocial health, persistent stressors, uncertainties, and threats can cause significant problems. Children raised in environments where crime is rampant and daily safety is in question, for example, run an increased risk of psychosocial problems. Drugs, crime, violent acts, school failure, unemployment, and a host of other bad things can happen to good people. But it is believed that certain protective factors, such as having a positive role model in the midst of chaos, may help children from even the worst environments remain healthy and well adjusted.

Another important influence is access to health services and programs designed to enhance psychosocial health. Going to a support group or seeing a trained therapist can be a crucial first step. Individuals from poor socioeconomic environments who cannot afford such services often find it difficult to secure help in improving their psychosocial health.

Social Supports and Social Bonds   Although often overlooked, a stable, loving support network of family and friends is key to psychosocial health. Social supports and the social bonds that come from close relationships help us get through even the most difficult times. Having those with whom we can talk, share thoughts, and practice good and bad behaviors without fear of losing their love is an essential part of growth.

Internal Factors That Influence Psychosocial Health

Many internal factors also work to shape a person's development. These factors include hereditary traits, hormonal functioning, physical health status (including neurological functioning), physical fitness, and certain elements of mental and emotional health.

Self-Efficacy   During our formative years, successes and failures in school, athletics, friendships, intimate relationships, our jobs, and every other aspect of life subtly shape our beliefs about our own personal worth and abilities. These beliefs in turn become internal influences on our psychosocial health.

Psychologist Albert Bandura used the term **self-efficacy** to describe a person's belief about whether he or she can successfully engage in and execute a specific behavior. Prior success in academics, athletics, or social interactions will lead to expectations of success in the future. In general, the more self-efficacious a person is and the more positive past experiences have been, the more likely this person will be to keep trying to execute a specific behavior successfully. Self-efficacious people are more likely to feel a sense of **personal control** over situations, that their own internal resources allow them to control events. On the other hand, someone with low self-efficacy may give up easily or never even try to change a behavior. Always being the last chosen to play basketball or long-term difficulty with making friends may make failure seem inevitable.

Learned Helplessness versus Learned Optimism   Psychologist Martin Seligman has proposed that people who continually experience failure may develop a pattern of responding known as **learned helplessness** in which they give up and fail to take any action to help themselves. Seligman ascribes this in part to society's tendency toward "victimology," blaming one's problems on other people and circumstances. While viewing ourselves as victims may make us feel better temporarily, it does not address the underlying causes of a problem. Ultimately, it erodes self-efficacy and fosters learned helplessness by making us feel that we cannot do anything to improve the situation.[4]

Countering this is Seligman's principle of *learned optimism:* Just as we learn to be helpless, so can we teach

---

Dysfunctional families   Families in which there is violence; physical, emotional, or sexual abuse; parental discord; or other negative family interactions.

Self-efficacy   Belief in one's own ability to perform a task successfully.

Personal control   Belief that one's own internal resources can control a situation.

Learned helplessness   Pattern of responding to situations by giving up because of repeated failure in the past.

Self-esteem   Sense of self-respect or self-confidence.

ourselves to be optimistic. His research provides growing evidence for the central place of mental health in overall positive development.[5] In one study, university freshmen who had been identified as pessimistic on the basis of a questionnaire were randomly assigned to an experimental group or a control group. The experimental group attended a 16-hour workshop in which they practiced social and study skills and learned to dispute chronic negative thoughts. The control group did not participate. Eighteen months later, 15 percent of the control group members were experiencing severe anxiety and 32 percent were suffering from moderate to severe depression. In contrast, only 7 percent of workshop participants suffered from anxiety and 22 percent from depression. Seligman concluded that even relatively brief interventions, such as this workshop, can produce measurable improvements in coping skills.[6]

Personality   Your personality is the unique mix of characteristics that distinguish you from others. Hereditary, environmental, cultural, and experiential factors influence how each person develops. Personality determines how we react to the challenges of life, interpret our feelings, and resolve conflicts.

Most of the recent schools of psychosocial theory promote the idea that we have the power not only to understand our behavior but also to actively change it and thus mold our own personalities. Yet although much has been written about the importance of a healthy personality, there is little consensus on what that concept really means. In general, however, people who possess the following traits often appear to be psychosocially healthy:[7]

- *Extroversion*, the ability to adapt to a social situation and demonstrate assertiveness as well as power or interpersonal involvement.
- *Agreeableness*, the ability to conform, be likable, and demonstrate friendly compliance as well as love.
- *Openness to experience*, the ability to demonstrate curiosity and independence (also referred to as *inquiring intellect*).
- *Emotional stability*, the ability to maintain social control.
- *Conscientiousness*, the qualities of being dependable, demonstrating self-control, and discipline and having a need to achieve.[8]

Life Span and Maturity   Our personalities are not static. Rather, they change as we move through the stages of our lives. Our temperaments also change as we grow, as is illustrated by the extreme emotions experienced by many people in early adolescence. Most of us learn to control our emotions as we advance toward adulthood.

The college years mark a critical transition period for young adults as they move away from families and establish themselves as independent adults. For most, this step toward maturity entails changing the nature of the relationship to parents. Managing personal finances, career strategies, and interpersonal communication are among the developmental tasks college students must accomplish. Older students often have to balance the responsibilities of family, career, and school.

The transition to independence will be easier for those who have successfully accomplished earlier developmental tasks such as learning how to solve problems, make and evaluate decisions, define and adhere to personal values, and establish both casual and intimate relationships. People who have not fulfilled these earlier tasks may find their lives interrupted by recurrent "crises" left over from earlier stages. For example, if they did not learn to trust others in childhood, they may have difficulty establishing intimate relationships as adults.

> **What do you think?**
> *Over which external factors does an individual have the most control?* ✴ *Which factors had the greatest impact on making you who you are today?*

Enhancing Psychosocial Health

Attaining self-fulfillment is a lifelong, conscious process that involves building self-esteem, understanding and controlling emotions, and learning to solve problems and make decisions. The Skills for Behavior Change box can provide ideas for improving your psychosocial health. In addition to the advice in this chapter, see Chapter 3 for tips on effective stress reduction, relaxation techniques, and other tools for enhancing your psychosocial health.

Developing and Maintaining Self-Esteem and Self-Efficacy

Self-esteem refers to one's sense of self-respect or self-worth. It can be defined as how one evaluates oneself and values one's own personal worth as an individual. People with high self-esteem tend to feel good about themselves and have a positive outlook on life. People with low self-esteem often do not like themselves, constantly demean themselves, and doubt their ability to succeed.

Our self-esteem is a result of the relationships we have with our parents and family during our formative years, our friends as we grow older, our significant others as we form intimate relationships, and with our teachers, coworkers, and others throughout our lives. If we felt loved and valued as children, our self-esteem enables us to believe that we are inherently "lovable individuals."

Find a Support Group   The best way to maintain self-esteem is through a support group—peers who share your values. The prime prerequisite for a support group is that it makes you feel good about yourself and forces you to take an honest look at your actions and choices. Although the idea of finding a support group seems to imply establishing a wholly new group, remember that old ties are often the strongest.

Tips for Building Self-Esteem

How can you build self-esteem? There are many things you can do in your day-to-day life that, when practiced regularly and added to other actions, can have a significant impact on the way you feel about yourself.

SQUELCH THAT INNER CRITIC

We are often our own worst enemies. We harp at ourselves continually about how we look and how we should have behaved in certain situations. Begin squelching that inner voice now:

- Examine your faults with a "mirror" rather than a magnifying glass. Instead of saying, "I'm stupid and I'll never get through this class," say, "I didn't do so well on this last test, but I'm going to do better. I'm doing great in another class."
- View your "mistakes" as opportunities to know yourself better or as growth experiences that will teach you to do things differently next time. If you find that you made careless mistakes on a test because you rushed through it, allow more time on your next test to double-check your work.
- The next time someone compliments you, respond positively. Say thank you rather than mumbling a protest.

FOCUS ON THE POSITIVE

Don't wallow in self-pity. Although no one is upbeat all the time, you can do a great deal to shorten the interlude between positive thoughts:

- Don't sulk. When upset, allow yourself 15 minutes to worry, then force yourself to do or think of something else.
- Don't compare yourself with others. Concentrate on improving your own performance.
- Give yourself time to feel good. When you reach an objective, allow time for fun before starting another project.
- Spend time with a friend who cares about you and isn't afraid to let you know it. Friends are crucial to positive self-esteem, say experts, because they make up your "psychic family"—an important source of support and objectivity.
- Count your blessings. Make a list of the people, events, and things in your life for which you are grateful. Include your own accomplishments. Whenever you feel cheated by life, look at this list.

Keeping in contact with old friends and important family members can provide a foundation of unconditional love that will help you through the many life transitions ahead. Try to be a support for others, too. Join a discussion, political action, or recreational group. Write more postcards and "thinking of you" notes to people who matter. This will build both your own self-esteem and that of your friends.

Complete Required Tasks   Develop a history of success by completing required tasks well. You are less likely to succeed in your studies if you leave term papers until the last minute or fail to ask about points that are confusing to you. Most college campuses provide study groups and learning centers that offer tips for managing time, understanding assignments, dealing with professors, and preparing for tests. Poor grades, or grades that do not meet expectations, are major contributors to emotional distress among college students.

Form Realistic Expectations   Set realistic expectations for yourself. If you expect perfect grades, a steady stream of Saturday-night dates and soap-opera romances, and the perfect job, you may be setting yourself up for failure. Assess your current resources and the direction in which you are heading. Set small, incremental goals that are possible to meet.

Make Time for You   Taking time to enjoy yourself is another way to boost self-esteem and psychosocial health. Viewing each new activity as something to look forward to and an opportunity to have fun is an important part of keeping the excitement in your life. Wake up focusing on the fun things you have to look forward to each day, and try to make this anticipation a natural part of your day.

Maintain Physical Health   Regular exercise fosters a sense of well-being. Nourishing meals can help you avoid the weight gain experienced by many college students. (See Chapter 9 for information on nutrition and Chapter 10 for more on the importance of exercise).

Examine Problems and Seek Help when Necessary   Sometimes you can handle life's problems alone; at other times you may need assistance. Recognize your strengths, act appropriately, and know when to seek help from friends, support groups, family, or professionals.

Sleep: The Great Restorer

Sleep serves at least two biological purposes in the body: conservation of energy so that we are rested and ready to perform during high-performance daylight hours, and restoration so that neurotransmitters that have been depleted during waking hours can be replenished. This process clears the brain of daily minutiae to prepare for a new day. Getting enough sleep to feel ready to meet daily challenges is a key factor in physical and psychosocial health.

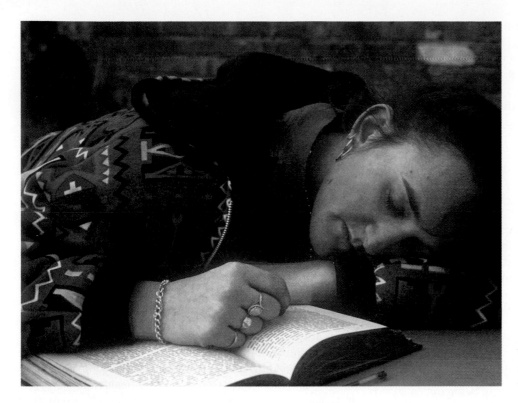

Without adequate sleep, a person may have a hard time facing the challenges of college life.

All of us can identify with that tired, listless feeling caused by sleep deprivation during periods of high stress. Either we can't find enough hours in the day for sleep, or once we get into bed, we can't fall asleep or stay asleep. **Insomnia** —difficulty in falling asleep quickly, frequent arousals during sleep, or early morning awakening—is a common complaint among 20 to 40 percent of Americans. Insomnia is more common among women than among men, and its prevalence is correlated with age and low socioeconomic status.

Some people have difficulty getting a good night's rest due to other sleep disorders. An increasingly common condition is **sleep apnea**, which is characterized by periodic episodes when breathing stops completely for 10 seconds or longer at a time.[9] Typically caused by upper respiratory tract problems in which weak muscle tone allows part of the airway to collapse, sleep apnea results in poor air exchange. This in turn raises blood pressure and lowers blood oxygen levels. Sleep apnea can pose a serious health risk.

How much sleep do we need? This depends on many factors. There is a genetically based need for sleep, different for each species. Sleep duration is also controlled by *circadian rhythms*, which are linked to the hormone *melatonin*. People may also control sleep patterns by staying up late, drinking coffee, getting lots of physical exercise, eating a heavy meal, or using alarm clocks. Most people follow characteristic stages of sleep, ranging from *Wakefulness* to *Drowsiness* to *Light Sleep* moving to *Deeper Sleep*. The most important period of sleep, known as the time of *rapid eye movement*, or *REM*, sleep, is essential to feeling rested and refreshed. In REM heart rate increases, respiration speeds up and dreaming tends to occur. If we miss REM sleep, we are left feeling groggy and sleep deprived.

Though many people turn to over-the-counter sleeping pills, barbiturates, or tranquilizers to get some sleep, the following methods for conquering sleeplessness are more effective and less risky:[10]

- Establish a consistent sleep schedule. Go to bed and get up at about the same time every day.
- Evaluate your sleep environment and change anything that could be keeping you awake. If it's noise, wear earplugs. If it's light, try room-darkening shades.
- Exercise regularly; it's hard to feel drowsy if you have been sedentary all day. Don't exercise right before bedtime, however, because activity speeds up your metabolism and makes it harder to go to sleep.
- Limit caffeine and alcohol. Caffeine can linger in your body for up to 12 hours and cause insomnia. While alcohol may make you drowsy at first, it interferes with the normal sleep-wake cycle and can make you wake up early.
- Avoid eating a heavy meal, particularly at bedtime. Don't drink large amounts of liquid before bed.
- If you're unable to get to sleep in 30 minutes, get up and do something else for awhile. Read, play solitaire, or try other relaxing activities, and return to bed when you feel drowsy.

Insomnia Difficulty in falling asleep or staying asleep.

Sleep apnea Disorder in which a person has numerous episodes of breathing stoppage during a normal night's sleep.

- If you nap, do so only during the afternoon when circadian rhythms make you especially sleepy. Don't let naps interfere with your normal sleep schedule.
- Establish a relaxing nighttime ritual that puts you in the mood to sleep. Take a warm shower, relax in a comfortable chair, don your favorite robe. Doing this consistently will cue your mind and body that it's time to wind down.[11]

Spirituality: An Inner Quest for Well-Being

Most of us have heard from others or recognized in our own lives the importance of a spiritual dimension; this might range from a tree-hugging zest for nature to a great love for a God-like deity. Philosophers and humanists have discussed spirituality, religious crusaders have promoted spirituality throughout the world, and today, researchers extol the virtues of spirituality for everything from saving interpersonal relationships to reducing stress. But what, exactly, does **spirituality** mean? Most experts agree that spiritual health refers to a belief in some unifying force that gives purpose or meaning to life, or a sense of belonging to a scheme of being that is greater than the purely physical or personal dimensions of existence. For some, this unifying force is nature; for others, it is a feeling of connection to other people; for others still, the unifying force is a god or some other spiritual symbol. Dr. N. Lee Smith, internist and associate professor of medicine at the University of Utah, defines spiritual health in the following ways:

- The quality of existence in which one is at peace with oneself and in good standing with the environment.
- A sense of empowerment and personal control that includes feeling heard and valued, and feeling in control over one's responses (but not necessarily in control of one's environment).
- A sense of connectedness to one's deepest self, to other people, and to all regarded as good.
- A sense of meaning and purpose, which provides a sense of mission by finding meaning and wisdom in the here and now.
- Enjoying the process of growth and having a vision of one's potential.
- Having hope, which translates into positive expectations.[12]

On a day-to-day basis, many of us focus on acquiring material possessions and satisfying basic human needs. But there comes a point when we discover that material possessions do not automatically bring happiness or a sense of self-worth. This realization may be triggered by a crisis. A failed relationship, a terrible accident, the death of a close friend or family member, or other loss often prompts a search for meaning, for the answer to the proverbial question "Is that all there is?" Whatever the reason, this search brings new opportunities for understanding ourselves.

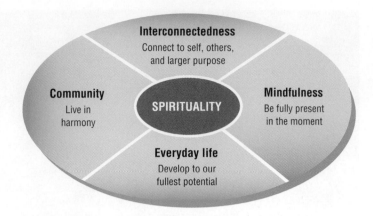

Figure 2.3
Four Major Themes of Spirituality

As we develop into spiritually healthy beings, we begin to recognize our identity as unique individuals. We reach a better appreciation of our strengths and shortcomings and our place in the universe. By developing an understanding of spirituality and how it is interwoven intricately into our existence, we embrace its power to improve health and our overall perspective on life. In turn, we may begin to notice more, feel more, and experience more of life. Perhaps most important, we gain an appreciation for the here-and-now, rather than living for aspirations that we may never achieve.

In its purest sense, spirituality addresses four main themes: *interconnectedness*, the practice of *mindfulness*, spirituality as a part of everyday life, and living in harmony with the community (see Figure 2.3).

- Interconnectedness. The concept of **interconnectedness** includes connectedness to self, to others, and to a larger meaning or purpose. Connecting with oneself involves exploring feelings, taking time to consider how you feel in a given situation, assessing your reactions to people and experiences, and taking mental notes when things or people cause you to lose equilibrium. It also involves considering your values and achieving congruence between what you consider important (your goals) and what you can do to achieve your goals without compromising your values. You may choose to connect with people in a physical, emotional, social, occupational, intellectual, or spiritual way.
- Practice of mindfulness. **Mindfulness** refers to the ability to be fully present in the moment. Mindfulness has been described as a way of nurturing greater awareness, clarity, and acceptance of present-moment reality or a form of inner "flow"—a holistic sensation felt when a person is totally involved in the moment.[13] You can achieve this inner flow through an almost infinite range of opportunities for enjoyment and pleasure, either through the use of physical and sensory skills ranging from athletics to music to yoga, or through the development of symbolic skills in areas such as poetry, philosophy, or mathematics.[14] The psychologist Abraham Maslow referred to these moments as peak

experiences, during which a person feels integrated, synergistic, and at one with the world.

• Spirituality as a part of daily life. Spirituality is embodied in the ability to discover and articulate our own basic purpose in life; to learn how to experience love, joy, peace, and fulfillment; and to help ourselves and others achieve their full potential.[15] This ongoing process of growth fosters three convictions: faith, hope, and love. **Faith** is the belief that helps us realize our purpose in life; **hope** is the belief that allows us to look confidently and courageously to the future; and **love** involves accepting, affirming, and respecting self and others regardless of who they are. Love also encompasses caring for and cherishing our environment. Rather than setting these three convictions as a goal to attain in the future, we should accept them as part of life's ongoing journey at all times.[16]

• Living in harmony with community. Our values are an extension of our beliefs about the world and attitude toward life. They are formed over time through a series of life experiences, and they are reflected in our hopes, dreams, desires, goals, and ambitions.[17] Though most people have some idea of what is important to them, many spend life largely unaware of how their values impact themselves or those around them until a life-altering event shakes up their usual perspective on life.

Spirituality: A Key to Health and Wellness Although many experts affirm the importance of spirituality in achieving health and wellness, the specific impact of this dimension remains elusive. Some researchers describe the spiritual dimension as a factor of well-being, which is achieved when four basic needs are satisfied:[18]

1. The need for having.
2. The need for relating.
3. The need for being.
4. The need for *transcendence*, or that sense of well-being that is experienced when a person finds purpose and meaning in life; nonphysical in nature, it can best be described as spiritual.

A Spiritual Resurgence Over recent decades, studies show that most Americans want spirituality in their lives, although not necessarily in the form of religion. Many find spiritual fulfillment in music, poetry, literature, art, nature, and intimate relationships.[19] Researcher Wade Clark Roof, of the University of California at Santa Barbara, found that in the 1960s and 1970s, baby boomers abandoned organized religion in large numbers: 84 percent of Jews, 69 percent of mainline Protestants, 61 percent of conservative Protestants, and 67 percent of Catholics.[20] Many dropped out of formal religious practice not because they lost interest in spirituality, but because they felt organized religion was not meeting their needs.

Today, however, we are seeing a return to formal religious participation and an increased concern for spiritual growth and development. National polls show that 9 out of 10 Americans believe in God and consider religion and/or spirituality to be important in their lives.[21] Many religious groups have spawned new philosophies that are more inclusive and often influenced by new-age ideas. An estimated 32 million baby boomers have turned to Eastern practices, new-age philosophies, 12-step programs, Greek mythology, shamanic practices, massage, yoga, and a host of other traditions and practices (see the New Horizons in Health box).[22]

For some, spirituality means a "quest for self and self-lessness"—a form of therapy and respite from a sometimes challenging personal environment. This quest for a "life force," which helps people deeply experience the moments of their lives rather than just live through them, has received much scholarly and popular attention. Self-help books that focus on spirituality consistently top the best-seller lists. Television programs promote the virtues of a spiritual or natural existence. Writers and psychologists such as William James, Gordon Allport, Erich Fromm, Viktor Frankl, Abraham Maslow, and Rollo May have made spirituality a major focus of their work.

Spiritual health courses have emerged as offshoots of public health and medical school training. For example, the Harvard Medical School of Continuing Education offers a course called "Spirituality and Healing in Medicine," which brings together scholars and medical professionals from around the world to discuss the role of spirituality in treating illness and chronic pain. Self-help workshops focusing on spiritual elements of health are popular throughout the world.

The Mind–Body Connection

Can negative emotions make a person physically sick? Can positive feelings help us stay well? Researchers are exploring the interaction between emotions and health, especially in conditions of uncontrolled, persistent stress. According to

---

Spirituality A form of well-being in which a person acknowledges the need for having, relating, being, and transcendence in the quest for meaning and purpose in life.

Interconnectedness A web of connections, including our relationship to ourselves, to others, and to a larger meaning or purpose in life.

Mindfulness Awareness and acceptance of the reality of the present moment.

Faith Belief that helps each person realize a unique purpose in life.

Hope Belief that establishes confidence and courage in facing the future.

Love Acceptance, affirmation, and respect for the self and others.

News from the World of Faith, Spirituality, and Healing Research

Dozens of studies are examining the effects of religion and spirituality on mental and physical health. Several of them provide interesting preliminary results:

- **Mental health**. A review of articles published in the *American Journal of Psychiatry* and the *Archives of General Psychiatry* during a 10-year period found that 80 percent showed a positive correlation between spirituality and better mental health.
- **Stress.** The Alameda County Study, which tracks nearly 7,000 Californians, showed that West Coast worshippers who participate in church-sponsored activities are markedly less stressed over finances, health, and other daily concerns than nonreligious types.
- **Blood pressure.** Elderly people in a Duke University study who attended religious services, prayed, or read the Bible regularly had lower blood pressure than their nonpracticing peers.
- **Recovery.** In another Duke University study, devout patients recovering from surgery spent an average of 11 days in the hospital, compared with nonreligious patients who spent 25 days.
- **Mortality.** Research on 1,931 older adults indicates that those who attend religious services regularly have a lower mortality rate.
- **Immunity.** Research on 1,700 adults found that those who attend religious services are less likely to have elevated levels of interleukin-6, an immune substance prevalent in people with chronic diseases.
- **Lifestyle.** A recent review of several studies suggests that spirituality is linked with low suicide rates, less alcohol and drug abuse, less criminal behavior, fewer divorces, and higher marital satisfaction.
- **Depression.** A Duke University study of 577 men and women hospitalized for physical illness showed that the more patients used positive coping strategies (seeking spiritual support from friends and religious leaders, praying, meditating, etc.), the lower the level of their depressive symptoms and the higher their quality of life.

After reviewing a number of studies like these, researchers at Georgetown University School of Medicine concluded that at least 80 percent of them point to a positive link between spiritual and physical well-being. People who consider themselves spiritual tend to recover more quickly from illness, live longer, and enjoy better health throughout their lives.

Sources: "Spirituality and Chronic Pain," MayoClinic.com, February 4 2002 (see http://www.mayoclinic.com/findinformation/conditioncenters/invoke.cfm?objectid=67A79059-32B9-4A7D-AA413F254B235FD1); Susan S. Larson, Oskar Pfister Address at the American Psychiatric Association, May 22, 2002., International Center for the Integration of Health & Spirituality (see http://www.nihr.org/abouticihs/introscarp.asp); D. N. Elkins, "Spirituality," *Psychology Today*, Sept. 1999, v.32, Issue 5, p. 44. Reprinted with permission from Psychology Today Magazine, Copyright © 1999 Sussex Publishers, Inc; *Journal of Gerontology: Psychological Sciences*, 1998.

one theory, the brain of an emotionally overwrought person sends signals to the adrenal glands, which respond by secreting cortisol and epinephrine (adrenaline), the hormones that activate the body's stress response. These chemicals are also known to suppress immune functioning, possibly causing subtle immune changes. What remains to be shown is whether these changes affect overall health, and if so, how.

Happiness: A Key to Well-Being

Although we can list the actions that we should perform to become physically healthy, such as eating the right foods, getting enough rest, exercising, and so on, it is less clear how to achieve that "feeling-good state" that researchers call

Subjective well-being (SWB) Feeling characterized by satisfaction with present life, relative presence of positive emotions, and relative absence of negative emotions.

subjective well-being (SWB). This refers to that uplifting feeling of inner peace and wonder that we call "happiness." After completing a major study, psychologists David Myers and Ed Deiner noted that people experience happiness in many different ways, based on age, culture, gender, and so on.[23] In spite of differences, however, SWB is defined by three central components:[24]

- Satisfaction with present life. People who are high in SWB tend to like their work and are satisfied with their current personal relationships. They are sociable, outgoing, and willing to open up to others. They also like themselves and enjoy good health and self-esteem.
- Relative presence of positive emotions. People high in SWB more frequently feel pleasant emotions, mainly because they evaluate the world around them in a generally positive way. They have an optimistic outlook, and they expect success in what they undertake.
- Relative absence of negative emotions. Individuals with a strong sense of subjective well-being experience fewer and less severe episodes of negative emotions such as anxiety, depression, and anger.

What do you think?

How do you rate on each of the components of subjective well-being? ✱ What factors influence your SWB? ✱ How has it changed over the course of your life?

Myths and Misperceptions about Happiness

Do you have to be happy all of the time to achieve subjective well-being? Of course not. Everyone experiences disappointments, unhappiness, and times when life seems unfair. However, people with SWB are typically resilient, able to look on the positive side and get themselves back on track fairly quickly, and less likely to fall into deep despair over setbacks. Several other myths about happiness are worth noting:[25]

- There is no "happiest age." Age is not a predictor of SWB. Most age groups exhibit similar levels of life satisfaction, although the things that bring joy often change with age.
- Happiness has no "gender gap." Although women are more likely than men to suffer from anxiety and depression, and men are more at risk for alcoholism and personality disorders, equal numbers of men and women report being fairly satisfied with life.
- There are minimal racial differences in happiness. For example, African Americans and European Americans report nearly the same levels of happiness, and African Americans are slightly less vulnerable to depression. Despite racism and discrimination, members of disadvantaged minority groups generally seem to "think optimistically" by making realistic self-comparisons and attributing problems less to themselves than to unfair circumstances.
- Money does not buy happiness. Wealthier societies report greater well-being. However, once the basic necessities of food, shelter, and safety are provided, there is a very weak correlation between income and happiness. Having no money is a cause of misery, but wealth itself does not guarantee happiness.

Fortunately, humans are remarkably resourceful creatures. We respond to great loss or a traumatic event, such as the death of a loved one, with an initial period of grief, mourning, and abject rage. Yet, with time and the support of loving family and friends, we pick ourselves up, brush off the bad times, and manage to find satisfaction and peace. Typically, humans learn from suffering and emerge even stronger and more ready to deal with the next crisis. Most find some measure of happiness after the initial shock and pain of loss. Those who are otherwise healthy, in good physical condition, and part of a strong social support network can adapt and cope effectively.

Does Laughter Enhance Health?

Remember the last time you laughed so hard that you cried? Remember how relaxed you felt afterward? Scientists are just beginning to understand the role of humor in our lives and health:

- Stressed-out people with a strong sense of humor become less depressed and anxious than those whose sense of humor is less well developed.
- Students who use humor as a coping mechanism report that it predisposes them to experiencing a positive mood.
- In a study of depressed and suicidal senior citizens, patients who recovered were the ones who demonstrated a sense of humor.
- Telling a joke, particularly one that involves a shared experience, increases our sense of belonging and social cohesion.

Laughter helps us in many ways. People like to be around others who are fun loving and laugh easily. Learning to laugh puts more joy into everyday experiences and increases the likelihood that fun-loving people will keep company with us.

Psychologist Barbara Fredrickson argues that positive emotions such as joy, interest, and contentment serve valuable life functions. Joy is associated with playfulness and creativity. Interest encourages us to explore our world, enhancing knowledge and cognitive ability. Contentment allows us to savor and integrate experiences, an important step to achieving mindfulness and insight. By building our physical, social, and mental resources, these positive feelings empower us to cope more effectively with life's challenges. While the actual emotions may be transient, their effects can be permanent and provide lifelong enrichment.[26]

Laughter also seems to have positive physiological effects. A number of researchers, such as Lee Berk, M.D., and Stanley Tan, M.D., have noted that laughter sharpens our immune systems by activating T-cells and natural killer cells and increasing production of immunity-boosting interferon.[27] It also reduces levels of the stress hormone cortisol.

In one experiment, Fredrickson monitored the cardiovascular responses of human subjects who suffered fear and anxiety induced by an unsettling film clip. Some of them then viewed a humorous film clip, while others did not. Those who watched the humorous film returned more quickly to their baseline cardiovascular state, indicating that laughter may counteract some of the physical effects of negative emotions.[28]

In another study, 50 women with advanced breast cancer who were randomly assigned to a weekly support group lived an average of 18 months longer than 36 cancer patients not in the support group. The implication of this finding is that the women in the support group cheered each other on and this allowed them to sleep and eat better, which promoted their survival. Other researchers have found that a fighting spirit and the determination to survive are vital adjuncts to standard cancer therapy.[29]

Relaxation therapies such as meditation and yoga offer the chance to "practice" self-initiated contentment, thus providing practical skills for dealing with day-to-day stress. These therapies have proved to be effective treatments for physical ailments such as headaches, chronic pain, and high blood pressure.[30]

While positive emotions appear to benefit physical health, evidence is accumulating that negative emotions can impair it. Studies of widowed and divorced people reveal below-normal immune-system functioning and higher rates of illness and death than among married people. Other studies have shown unusually high rates of cancer among depressed people.[31]

Some researchers believe that certain psychosocial behaviors actually make people vulnerable to illness. Psychologist Lydia Temoshok studied people with malignant melanoma (a potentially deadly skin cancer) and found that 75 percent shared common traits. They tended to be unfailingly pleasant, repress their negative feelings and emotions, and make extraordinary attempts to accommodate others. She hypothesized that this "Type C" personality signals emotional repression, which may suppress the immune system.[32]

Do these studies provide conclusive evidence of a mind–body connection? Not necessarily, because they do not account for other factors known to be relevant to health. For example, some researchers suggest that people who are divorced, widowed, or depressed are more likely to drink and smoke, use drugs, eat and sleep poorly, and be sedentary—all of which may affect the immune system. In fact, the immune system changes measured in studies of the mind–body connection are relatively small. The health consequences of such minute changes are difficult to gauge because the body can tolerate a certain amount of reduced immune function without contracting illness. The exact amount it is able to tolerate and under what circumstances are still in question.[33]

A large body of evidence points to an association between the emotions and physical health, although we still have much to learn about this relationship. Does an emotional state trigger negative behaviors that lead to decreased immune functioning? Or do emotions directly affect health by stimulating the production of hormones that tax the immune system? In the meantime, however, it appears that happiness and an optimistic mind-set don't just feel good—they are also good for you.

When Psychosocial Health Deteriorates

Sometimes circumstances overwhelm us to such a degree that we need outside assistance to help us get back on track toward healthful living.

Depression: The Full-Scale Tumble

In a recent meeting of the American Psychological Association, the organization's president remarked, "Depression has been called the common cold of psychological disturbances, which underscores its prevalence, but trivializes its impact."[34] According to experts, major depression is, in fact, one of the most common psychiatric disorders in the United States, affecting over 15 million Americans. Many of them are misdiagnosed, underdiagnosed, and not receiving treatment, despite its availability.[35]

It is normal to feel blue or depressed in response to certain experiences, such as the death of a loved one, divorce, loss of a job, or an unhappy ending to a long-term relationship. However, people with **major depressive disorder** experience a form of **chronic mood disorder** that involves, on a day-to-day basis, extreme and persistent sadness, despair, and hopelessness. People with this disorder typically feel discouraged by life and circumstances and experience feelings of intense guilt and worthlessness. Usually they show some impairment of social and occupational functioning, although their behavior is not necessarily bizarre. Approximately 15 percent of them eventually attempt suicide or succeed in committing suicide.[36]

According to the National Institutes of Mental Health (NIMH), women experience depression at nearly two times the rate of men: Between 8–11 percent of men and 19–23 percent of women become depressed. About 6 percent of women and 3 percent of men have experienced episodes severe enough to require hospitalization.[37]

There are a few exceptions to these findings, however. Among Jews, males are equally as likely as females to have major depressive episodes.[38] In recent years, there has also been a noteworthy increase in depression among children, the elderly, and adolescents, particularly adolescent girls, and perhaps in Native American and homosexual young people as well.[39] Writers, composers, and entertainers also seem to have higher than expected rates of major depression, and people experiencing chronic, unrelenting pain have the highest rates of any group.[40]

Depression can strike at any age, but the first episode usually occurs before age 40. (See Table 2.1, which lists common symptoms.) Some people experience one bout of depression and never have problems again, but others suffer recurrences throughout their lives. Stressful life events are often catalysts for these recurrences.

Risks for Depression Major depressive disorders are caused by interaction between biology, learned behavioral responses, and cognitive factors. Chemical and genetic processes may predispose people to depression, and irrational ideas and beliefs can guide them to negative coping behaviors.[41] Some people, because of genetic history, environment, situational triggers and stressors, poor behavioral skills, and brain–body chemistry, may be particularly vulnerable.

Facts and Fallacies about Depression Although it is one of the fastest-growing problems in U.S. culture, depression remains one of the most misunderstood mental disorders. Myths and misperceptions about the disease abound:[42]

• *True depression is not a natural reaction to crisis and loss.* It is a pervasive and systemic biological problem. Symptoms may come and go, and their severity will fluctuate, but they do not simply go away. Crisis and loss can lead an already

Table 2.1
Are You Depressed ?

Sadness and despair are the main symptoms of depression. Other common signs include:

- Loss of motivation or interest in pleasurable activities.
- Preoccupation with failures and inadequacies; concern over what others are thinking.
- Difficulty concentrating; indecisiveness; memory lapses.
- Loss of sex drive or interest in close interactions with others.
- Fatigue and loss of energy; slow reactions.
- Sleeping too much or too little; insomnia.
- Feeling agitated, worthless, or hopeless.
- Withdrawal from friends and family.
- Diminished or increased appetite.
- Recurring thoughts that life isn't worth living, thoughts of death or suicide.
- Significant weight loss or weight gain.

Some depressed people mask their symptoms with a forced, upbeat sense of humor or high energy levels. Communication may cease or seem frantic.

depressed person over the edge to suicide or other problems, but crisis and loss do not inevitably result in depression.

- *People will not snap out of depression by using a little willpower.* Telling a depressed person to "snap out of it" is like telling a diabetic to produce more insulin. Medical intervention in the form of antidepressant drugs and therapy is often necessary for recovery. Understanding the seriousness of the disease and supporting people in their attempts to recover are key elements.

- *Frequent crying is not a hallmark of depression.* Some people who are depressed bear their burdens in silence, or may even be the life of the party. Some depressed individuals don't cry at all. Rather, biochemists theorize that crying may actually ward off depression by releasing chemicals that the body produces as a positive response to stress.

- *Depression is not "all in the mind."* Depression isn't a disease of weak-willed, powerless people. In fact, research suggests that depressive illnesses originate with an inherited chemical imbalance in the brain. In addition, some physiological conditions, such as thyroid disorders, multiple sclerosis, chronic fatigue syndrome, and certain cancers have depressive side effects. Certain medications also are known to prompt depressive like symptoms.

- *It is not true that only in-depth psychotherapy can cure long-term clinical depression.* No single psychotherapy method works for all cases of depression.

Depression and Gender   For reasons that are not well understood, two-thirds of all people suffering from depression are women. Researchers have proposed biological, psychological, and social explanations for this fact. Women appear to be at greater risk for depression during times when their hor-

mone levels change significantly, such as the premenstrual phase of the menstrual cycle, following the birth of a child, and at onset of menopause. Men's hormone levels appear to remain more stable throughout life. Some researchers theorize that women are inherently more at risk for depression, yet evidence to support this theory is inconsistent or contrary.

Although adolescent and adult females have been found to experience depression at twice the rate of males, the college population seems to represent a notable exception, with equal rates experienced by males and females. Why? Several theories have been suggested:[43]

- The social institutions of the college campus provide more egalitarian roles for men and women.
- College women experience fewer negative events than do high school females. Males in college report more negative events than they experienced in high school.
- College women report smaller and more supportive social networks.

Depression is often preceded by a stressful event. Some psychologists therefore theorize that women might be under

Major depressive disorder   Severe depression that entails chronic mood disorder, physical effects such as sleep disturbance and exhaustion, and mental effects such as the inability to concentrate.

Chronic mood disorder   Experience of persistent sadness, despair, and hopelessness.

more stress than men and thus more prone to become depressed. However, women do not report more stressful events than men.

Finally, researchers have observed gender differences in coping strategies, or the response to certain events or stimuli, and have proposed that some women's strategies make them more vulnerable to depression. Presented with "a list of things people do when depressed," college students were asked to indicate how likely they were to engage in each behavior. Men were more likely to assert that "I avoid thinking of reasons why I am depressed," "I do something physical," or "I play sports." Women were more likely to answer "I try to determine why I am depressed," "I talk to other people about my feelings," and "I cry to relieve the tension." In other words, the men tried to distract themselves from a depressed mood whereas the women focused on it. If focusing obsessively on negative feelings intensifies these feelings, women who do this may predispose themselves to depression. This hypothesis has not been directly tested, but some supporting evidence suggests its validity.[44]

Treating Depression The best treatment involves determining the person's type and degree of depression and its possible causes. Both psychotherapeutic and pharmacological modes of treatment are recommended for clinical (severe and prolonged) depression. Drugs often relieve the symptoms of depression, such as loss of sleep or appetite, while psychotherapy can be equally helpful by improving the ability to function (see Table 2.2).[45]

In some cases, psychotherapy alone may be the most successful treatment. The two most common psychotherapeutic therapies for depression are cognitive and interpersonal therapy.

Cognitive therapy aims to help a patient look at life rationally and correct habitually pessimistic thought patterns. It focuses on the here and now rather than analyzing a patient's past. To pull a person out of depression, cognitive therapists usually need 6 to 18 months of weekly sessions comprising reasoning and behavioral exercises.

Interpersonal therapy, sometimes combined with cognitive therapy, also addresses the present but focuses on correcting chronic relationship problems. Interpersonal therapists focus on patients' relationships with their families and other people.

Antidepressant drugs relieve symptoms in nearly 80 percent of people with chronic depression. Several types of the medications known as *tricyclics* are available and work by preventing excessive absorption of mood-altering neurotransmitters. Tricyclics can take six weeks to three months to become effective. Newer antidepressant drugs, called *tetracyclics*, work in one or two weeks.

In recent years, words like Zoloft and Prozac have become such a common part of our vocabulary that it doesn't seem at all unusual to know someone who is taking an antidepressant. This could lead one to think that antidepressants can be taken like aspirin. However, countless emergency

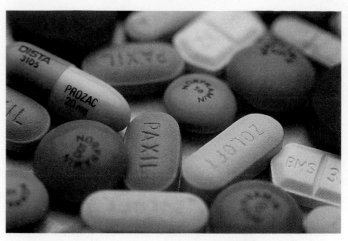

In addition to prescription antidepressant drugs, a number of related natural supplements are sold over the counter. One such supplement, melatonin, has grown in popularity in recent years.

room visits occur when people misuse antidepressants, try to quit by going "cold turkey," or suffer reactions to the drugs. The potency and dosage of each vary greatly.

Antidepressants should be prescribed only after a thorough psychological and physiological examination. If your doctor suggests an antidepressant, ask these questions first:

- What biological indicators are you using to determine whether I really need this drug? (Beware of the health professional who gives you a five-minute exam, asks you if you are feeling down or blue, and prescribes an antidepressant to fix your problems.)
- What is the action of this drug? What will it do, and when will I start to feel the benefits?
- What is your rationale for selecting this antidepressant over others?
- What are the side effects of using this drug?
- How long can I be on this medication without significant risk to my health?
- What happens if I stop taking it?
- How will you follow up or monitor the levels of this drug in my body? How often will I need to be checked?

Electroconvulsive therapy (ECT) is another treatment for depression. A patient given ECT is sedated under light general anesthesia, and electric current is applied to the patient's temples for five seconds at a time for 15 or 20 minutes. Between 10 and 20 percent of people with depression who do not respond to drug therapy are responsive to ECT. However, because it carries a risk of permanent memory loss, some therapists do not recommend ECT under any circumstances.

Clinics have been established in large metropolitan areas to offer group support for depressed people. Some clinics treat all types of depressed people; others restrict themselves to specific groups, such as widows, adolescents, or families and friends of people with depression.

Table 2.2
Drug Treatments for Depression

ANTIDEPRESSANT CLASS	INDICATIONS/CONTRAINDICATIONS	SIDE EFFECTS
TRICYCLICS (TCAs) Desipramine (Norpramin) Nortriptyline (Pamelor) Imipramine (Trofranil) Amitriptyline (Elavil) Protriptyline (Vivactil) Doxepin (Sinequan)	Due to their sedating effects, TCAs are useful for patients with insomnia. They may pose a risk for individuals with cardiovascular disease such as arrhythmias.	Most common: dry mouth, constipation. Others: weight gain, dizziness caused by a drop in blood pressure on sitting or standing up (orthostatic hypotension), changes in sexual desire, difficulty urinating, increased sweating, and sedation. TCAs can be lethal in overdose.
SELECTIVE SEROTONIN REUPTAKE INHIBITORS (SSRIs) Fluoxetine (Prozac) Sertraline (Zoloft) Paroxetine (Paxil) Fluvoxamine (Luvox) Serzone	SSRIs are generally the first-line choice because they have fewer side effects than other antidpressants, do not require blood monitoring, and are safe in overdose. Newer versions have fewer side effects.	Insomnia, agitation, sexual dysfunction, occasional nausea or heartburn, headache, occasional drowsiness, dizziness, tremor, diarrhea/constipation, and dry mouth (rare).
MONOAMINE OXIDASE INHIBITORS (MAOIs) Isocarboxazid (Marplan) Tranylcypromine (Parnate) Phenelzine (Nardil)	MAOIs can cause severe and sudden rise in blood pressure if ingested with certain drugs (e.g., over-the-counter cold preparations, diet pills, and amphetamines) or foods containing tyramine (e.g., red wines, aged cheeses). They interact with epinephrine in some topical anesthetics and are not advised with other antidepressants.	Agitation, insomnia, sexual dysfunction, disturbed appetite, faintness (like orthostatic hypotension). Weight gain is most prominent with MAOIs.
BUPROPION (WELLBUTRIN)	This drug doesn't interact significantly with other drugs. At high doses it can cause seizures in some people, most commonly those who have seizure disorders, anorexia, or bulimia. It has been used experimentally to counteract sexual side effects of SSRIs.	Agitation, insomnia, sedation, blurred vision, dizziness, headache/migraine, dry mouth, tremor, appetite loss, weight loss, excessive sweating, rapid heartbeat, constipation, rashes.
TRAZODONE (DESYREL)	Trazodone is often used with another antidepressant to alleviate insomnia induced by the initial drug.	Drowsiness, faintness, nausea, and vomiting.
MAPROTILINE (LUDIOMIL)	This drug is used to treat agitation and anxiety associated with depression but is not advised for people with seizure disorders. It is somewhat risky for patients with cardiovascular disease.	Similar to those of TCAs.
SEROTONIN AND NOREPINEPHRINE REUPTAKE INHIBITORS (SNRIs) Venlafaxine (Effexor)	SNRIs work something like a combination of an SSRI and a TCA and are useful for patients who don't respond to other antidepressants.	Similar to those of SSRIs.
NEFAZODONE (SERZONE)	This drug shouldn't be taken with the non-sedating antihistamines terfenadine (Seldane) and astemizone (Hismanal).	Headache, dry mouth, nausea, drowsiness, faintness, constipation.

Source: Table of antidepressant drugs in "Antidepressants," excerpted by permission from the December 1995 issue of *Harvard Women's Health Watch,* Vol. 3, No. 4, p. 3 © 1995, President and Fellows of Harvard College; Mark Nichols, "The Quest for a New Cure: New Drugs and Therapies Join the Battle against Depression," *Maclean's,* December 1, 1997, Vol. 110, No 48; pp. 60–63.

Anxiety Disorders: Facing Your Fears

On a recent trip to a professional conference, Marilyn Erickson (fictitious name) boarded a connecting flight at O'Hare International Airport, only to find that her husband John, a professor at a major university, was missing. Marilyn got off the plane and searched frantically throughout the airport for him. Finally, long after the plane had departed, she found him sitting on a bench outside the terminal; he was vomiting, dizzy, and distraught over the mere thought of boarding

REALITY CHECK

Cutting through the Pain

What is self-injury? Self-injury is an attempt to alter a mood state by inflicting physical harm on the body. This may include cutting (with razors, glass, knives, etc.), burning, hitting the body with an object or fists, or not allowing wounds to heal. People discover that hurting themselves brings relief from distress and turn to it as a primary coping mechanism.

Why does self-injury make some people feel better? Many factors or a combination of factors seem to be involved, including a biologic predisposition, a need to reduce tension, and a lack of experience in dealing with strong emotions. Some studies suggest that when people who self-injure feel emotionally overwhelmed, performing self-injury brings their levels of psychological and physiological tension and arousal back to a bearable level almost immediately. Simply stated, when they feel a strong uncomfortable emotion and don't know how to handle it, hurting themselves reduces the emotional discomfort quickly and calms them down.

Who is most likely to self-injure? The typical person in therapy for self-injury is a female, who is single, intelligent, well-educated, and from a middle- to upper-middle-class family. She usually started self-injuring in middle to late adolescence. Often (but not always) she has a background of physical, emotional, and/or sexual abuse or has experienced chaotic family conditions. Eating disorders are also often coreported. However, focusing only on those receiving therapeutic treatment for self-injury may vastly underreport the number of males and minorities who self-injure. One report estimates that males may account for as many as 40 percent of self-injurers, but their injuries are overlooked as a product of "macho outbursts" such as fighting or sports injuries.

How common is this behavior? It is difficult to accurately estimate the number of people who self-injure because it is sometimes difficult to distinguish self-injurious behavior from suicide attempts. In some studies, no attempt is made to distinguish between the two behaviors. And, as the injuries are often purposely hidden, reports from hospitals, police, or social service agencies underreport the occurrence. In the general population of the United States estimates of individuals engaging in self-injury range from 14 to 600 persons per 100,000 annually (.014–0.6 percent). The rates are higher in adolescents and young adults; estimates in the general college student population range from 1.8–12 percent.

Is treatment available? Treatments currently being explored range from talk therapy to teaching problem-solving skills to medications that help relieve underlying depression and anxiety that may contribute to the self-injury. What all of the treatments have in common is the aim to end the feelings that prompt the behavior, not just stop the behavior itself.

Are there signs and symptoms? Signs include scars or current cuts or abrasions and flimsy excuses for these wounds. A young woman may wear long sleeves and pants in warm weather to hide her wounds. Difficulty handling anger, social withdrawal, sensitivity to rejection, or body alienation may also be symptoms of self-injury.

What do you do if a loved one self-injures?

✔ Educate yourself; read the books or websites listed at the end of this chapter.

✔ Don't avoid the subject of self-injury; let her know that you're willing to talk.

✔ Let your friend know you understand that self-injury is helping her to cope with strong negative emotions.

✔ Be available; it may be helpful to provide distractions when she is tempted to self-injure.

✔ Show concern for the injuries. The injuries need to be treated to prevent scarring and infection.

—Susan Dobie, Oregon State University

Sources: T. M. Edwards, "What Cutters Feel," *Time,* November 9, 1998; A. R. Favazza, *Bodies under Siege: Self-Mutilation and Body Modification in Culture and Psychiatry* (Baltimore, MD: Johns Hopkins University Press, 1996); D. Martinson, "Self-Injury: A quick guide to the basics," (1988) (see www.palace.net/~llama/psych/guide.html); K. L. Suyemoto and X. Kountz, "Self-Mutilation," (2000) *The Prevention Researcher,* 7 (4): 1–4.

For Further Information: K. Conterio, and W. Lader, *Bodily Harm: The Breakthrough Healing Program for Self-Injurers* (New York: Hyperion, 1998).

S. Levenkron, *Cutting: Understanding and Overcoming Self-Mutilation* (New York: W.W. Norton and Company, 1998).

Secret Shame: Self-Injury Information and Support (see www.crystal.palace.net/~llama/selfinjury).

Self-Abuse: Self-Injury, Cutting, Self-Harm, Self-Abuse, and Body Mutilation (see www.selfabuse.com).

the plane. When Marilyn suggested catching another flight, he trembled violently and refused to budge from his bench. They returned to their home on the West Coast on a bus and missed their scheduled conference appearance.

Professor Erickson suffered from one of several **anxiety disorders**, known as a panic attack, a little-understood yet common psychological problem. Consider John Madden, former head coach of the Oakland Raiders and a true "man's man" who has outfitted his own bus and drives every weekend across the country to serve as commentator on NFL football games. What's the reason behind this exhausting driving schedule? Madden is terrified of getting on a plane.

Anxiety disorders are the number one mental health problem in the United States, affecting over 19 million people of ages 18–54 each year, or about 13 percent of all adults.[46] Some sources place the true number as high as 25 percent. Anxiety is also a leading mental health problem among adolescents, affecting 13 million youngsters ages 9–17. In just two years, the number of "hits" on the website of the Anxiety Disorders Association of America soared from 500,000 to over 21.6 million.[47] Costs associated with an overly anxious populace are growing rapidly; conservative estimates cite nearly $50 billion a year spent in doctors' bills and workplace losses in America. According to a study by the World Health Organization, the odds of developing an anxiety disorder have doubled in the past four decades.[48] These numbers don't begin to address the human costs incurred when a person is too fearful to leave the house or talk to anyone outside the immediate family. Anxiety-related ailments include generalized anxiety disorder, panic disorder, specific phobias, and social phobias.

Generalized Anxiety Disorder One common form of anxiety disorder, **generalized anxiety disorder (GAD),** is severe enough to significantly interfere with daily life. Generally, the person with this disorder is a consummate "worrier" who develops a debilitating level of anxiety. Often multiple sources of worry exist, and it is hard to pinpoint the root cause of the anxiety. A diagnosis of GAD depends on showing at least three of the following symptoms for more days than not during a period of six months.[49]

1. Restlessness or feeling keyed up or on edge.
2. Being easily fatigued.
3. Difficulty concentrating or mind going blank.
4. Irritability.
5. Muscle tension.
6. Sleep disturbances (difficulty falling or staying asleep or restless sleep)

Often GAD runs in families and is readily treatable with benzodiazepines such as Librium, Valium, and Xanax, which calm the person for short periods. More effective long-term treatments are achieved through individual therapy.

Panic Disorder *Panic attacks* are a form of **panic disorder** characterized by sudden bursts of disabling terror. The panic may be "free-floating anxiety" that has no connection with

the person's present experience. During a panic attack, at least four of the following symptoms develop abruptly and reach a peak within 10 minutes:[50]

- Palpitations, pounding of the heart, or accelerated heart rate.
- Sweating.
- Trembling or shaking.
- Sensations of shortness of breath, smothering, or choking.
- Chest pain or discomfort.
- Nausea or abdominal distress.
- Feeling dizzy, unsteady, light-headed, or faint.
- Derealization (feeling of unreality) or depersonalization (being detached from oneself).
- Fear of losing control or going crazy.
- Fear of dying.
- Paresthesias (numbness or tingling sensations).
- Chills or hot flashes.

Specific Phobias In contrast with panic disorders, **phobias,** or phobic disorders, involve a persistent and irrational fear of a specific object, activity, or situation, often out of proportion to the circumstances. About 13 percent of Americans suffer from phobias, such as fear of spiders, snakes, public speaking, and so on. Social phobias are perhaps the most common phobic response.[51]

Social Phobias A **social phobia** is an anxiety disorder characterized by the persistent fear and avoidance of social situations. Essentially, the person dreads these situations for fear of being humiliated, embarrassed, or even looked at.[52] These disorders vary in scope. Some cause difficulty only in specific situations, such as getting up in front of the class to give a report. In more extreme cases, a person avoids all contact with others.

Sources of Anxiety Disorders Because these disorders vary in complexity and degree, scientists have yet to find clear reasons why one person develops them and another doesn't. The following factors are often cited as possible causes.

Anxiety disorders Disorders characterized by persistent feelings of threat and anxiousness in coping with everyday problems.

Generalized anxiety disorder (GAD) A constant sense of worry that may cause restlessness, difficulty in concentrating, and tension.

Panic disorder Severe anxiety disorder in which a particular situation, often for unknown reasons, causes terror and panic attacks.

Phobia A deep and persistent fear of a specific object, activity, or situation that results in a compelling desire to avoid the source of the fear.

Social phobia A phobia characterized by fear and avoidance of social situations.

- *Biology.* Some scientists trace the origin of anxiety to the brain and brain functioning. Using sophisticated positron emission tomography scans (PET scans), scientists can analyze areas of the brain that react during anxiety-producing events. Families appear to display similar brain and physiological reactivity, so we may inherit our tendencies toward anxiety disorders.

- *Environment.* Anxiety may also be a learned response. Though genetic tendencies may exist, experiencing a repeated pattern of reaction to certain situations programs the brain to respond in a certain way. For example, monkeys separated from their mothers at an early age are more fearful, and their stress hormones fire more readily, than those that stayed with their mothers. If your mother (or father) screamed whenever a large spider loped into view, or if other anxiety-raising events occurred frequently, you might be predisposed to react with anxiety to similar events later in your life. Animals also experience such anxieties—perhaps from being around their edgy owners.

- *Social and Cultural Roles.* Because men and women are taught to assume different roles in society (such as man as protector, woman as victim), women may find it more acceptable to scream, shake, pass out, and otherwise express extreme anxiety. Men, on the other hand, have learned to "stuff" such anxieties rather than act upon them; thus culture and social roles may also be a factor in risks for anxiety.

Although anxiety disorders have become widely recognized in our society, newer forms of psychological disorders have begun to emerge. See the Reality Check box for information about one area of growing concern—self-mutilation.

Seasonal Affective Disorder (SAD)

An estimated 6 percent of Americans suffer from **seasonal affective disorder (SAD)**, a type of depression, and an additional 14 percent experience a milder form of the disorder known as the winter blues. SAD strikes during the winter months and is associated with reduced exposure to sunlight. People with SAD suffer from irritability, apathy, carbohydrate craving and weight gain, increases in sleep time, and general sadness. Researchers believe that SAD is caused by a malfunction in the hypothalamus, the gland responsible for regulating responses to external stimuli. Stress may also play a role.

Certain factors seem to put people at risk for SAD. Women are four times more likely to suffer from it than men. Although SAD can occur at any age, people aged 20 to 40 appear to be most vulnerable. Certain families appear to be at risk. And residents of northern states, where there are fewer hours of sunlight during the winter, are more at risk than those living in the South. An estimated 10 percent of the population in Maine, Minnesota, and Wisconsin experience SAD, compared to fewer than 2 percent of those in Florida and New Mexico.

Therapies for SAD are simple but effective. The most beneficial is light therapy, which exposes patients to lamps that simulate sunlight. Eighty percent of patients experience relief from their symptoms within four days of treatment. Other treatments for SAD include diet change (eating more complex carbohydrates), increased exercise, stress management techniques, sleep restriction (limiting the number of hours slept in a 24-hour period), psychotherapy, and antidepressants.

Schizophrenia

Perhaps the most frightening of all mental disorders is **schizophrenia**, which affects about 1 percent of the U.S. population. Schizophrenia is characterized by alterations of the senses (including auditory and visual hallucinations); the inability to sort out incoming stimuli and to make appropriate responses; an altered sense of self; and radical changes in emotions, movements, and behaviors. Victims of this disease often cannot function in society.

For decades, scientists believed that schizophrenia was an environmentally provoked form of madness. They blamed abnormal family interactions or early childhood traumas. Since the mid-1980s, however, magnetic resonance imaging (MRI) and positron emission tomography (PET) have allowed us to study brain function more closely, and scientists have recognized that schizophrenia is a biological disease of the brain. The brain damage occurs very early in life, possibly as early as the second trimester of fetal development. However, symptoms most commonly appear in late adolescence.

At present, schizophrenia is treatable but not curable. Treatments usually include some combination of hospitalization, medication, and supportive psychotherapy. Supportive psychotherapy, as opposed to psychoanalysis, can help the patient acquire skills for living in society.

Even though environmental theories of the causes of schizophrenia have been discarded in favor of biological theories, a stigma remains attached to the disease. Families of people with schizophrenia often experience anger and guilt associated with misunderstandings about the causes of the disease. They often need help in the form of information, family counseling, and advice on how to meet the schizophrenic person's needs for shelter, medical care, vocational training, and social interaction.

Gender Issues in Psychosocial Health

Unfortunately, gender bias can get in the way of correct diagnosis of psychosocial disorders. In one study, for instance, 175 mental health professionals, of both genders, were asked

---

Seasonal affective disorder (SAD) A type of depression that occurs in the winter months, when sunlight levels are low.

Schizophrenia A mental illness with biological origins that is characterized by irrational behavior, severe alterations of the senses (hallucinations), and, often, an inability to function in society.

to diagnose a patient based upon a summarized case history. Some of the professionals were told that the patient was male, others that the patient was female. The gender of the patient made a substantial difference in the diagnosis (though the gender of the clinician did not). When subjects thought the patient was female, they were more likely to diagnose hysterical personality, a "female disorder." When they believed the patient to be male, the more likely diagnosis was antisocial personality, a "male disorder."

PMS: Physical or Mental Disorder?   A major controversy is the inclusion of a "provisional" diagnosis for premenstrual syndrome (PMS) in the American Psychiatric Association's Diagnostic and Statistical Manual of Mental Disorders (fourth edition; known as DSM-IV). The provisional inclusion, in an appendix to DSM-IV, signals that PMS merits further study and may be included as an approved diagnosis in future editions of the DSM. In other words, PMS could be considered a mental disorder in the future.

PMS is characterized by depression, irritability, and other symptoms of increased stress typically occurring just prior to menstruation and lasting for a day or two. A more severe case of PMS is known as *premenstrual dysphoric disorder*, or *PMDD*. Whereas PMS is somewhat disruptive and uncomfortable, it does not interfere with daily functions; PMDD does. To be diagnosed with PMDD, a woman must have at least five symptoms of PMS for a week to 10 days, with at least one symptom being serious enough to interfere with her ability to function at work or at home. In these more severe cases, antidepressants may be prescribed. The point of contention lies in whether administering this treatment indicates that PMDD is viewed as a mental disorder rather than a physical problem.[53] Is it legitimate to attach a label indicating dysfunction and disorder to symptoms experienced only once or twice a month? Further controversy stems from the possible use (or misuse) of the diagnostic label to justify exclusion of women from certain desirable jobs.

Suicide: Giving Up on Life

Each year there are over 35,000 reported suicides in the United States. Experts estimate that there may actually be closer to 100,000 cases, due to the difficulty in determining many causes of suspicious deaths. More lives are lost to suicide than to any other single cause except cardiovascular disease and cancer. Suicide often results from poor coping skills, lack of social support, lack of self-esteem, and the inability to see one's way out of a bad situation. Factors contributing to suicide risks are common risks in many regions of the world. The Health in a Diverse World box provides key indicators of this.

Suicide: A Neglected Problem among Diverse Populations

One of the most underrated public health problems facing Americans today, suicide accounts for more than 30,000 preventable deaths each year, nearly 10,000 more than deaths from homicide. It touches all ages, races, and social groups and is on the rise in many segments of the population.

- Recent reports from the Centers for Disease Control showed the rate of suicides among black teens ages 10 to 19 increased 114 percent between 1980 and 1995.
- For every successful suicide, another 17 are attempted.

- Elderly men use the most violent means of suicide and are the most likely to be successful.
- After age 75, suicide rates are three times the national average, and after age 80, six times the national average.
- Males outnumber females five to one in completed suicides, while females are two times more likely to attempt suicide, often by using less lethal means such as drugs or alcohol. Native Americans have a higher suicide rate than whites of all ages.
- Teen suicides often occur in clusters, particularly when friends or prominent national figures, such as rock stars, commit suicide.
- Rates of suicide are considerably higher in western states, followed by the South, Northeast, and Midwest. The rate in New Jersey in 1998 was 6.4 per 100,000, while it was 21 per 100,000 in Nevada and Alaska.

- People who have never been married are twice as likely to commit suicide as currently married people. The highest rates of all occur among the divorced or widowed.
- Young gay or bisexual males are more likely to attempt suicide than heterosexual men are, but more heterosexual men successfully complete the attempt.
- Suicide rates are highest in German-speaking countries, Switzerland, Scandinavia, Eastern Europe, and Japan, and lowest in Greece, Italy, and Spain.

Sources: S. K. Goldsmith, T. C. Pellmar, A. M. Kleinman, and W. E. Bunney, editors, *Reducing Suicide: A National Imperative* (Washington, DC: National Academy Press, 2002); S. Stapleton,"The Surgeon General Calls for Suicide Prevention," 1998, *American Medical News* 41, p. 9; and "Suicide among Black Youth, 1980–1995," *Journal of the American Medical Association,* 279, p. 1431.

College students are more likely than the general population to attempt suicide; suicide is the third leading cause of death in people between the ages of 15 and 24. In fact, this age group now accounts for nearly 20 percent of all suicides.[54] The pressures, joys, disappointments, challenges, and changes of the college environment are believed to be in part responsible for these rates. However, young adults who choose not to go to college but who are searching for direction in careers, relationships, and other life goals are also at risk.

Risk factors for suicide include a family history of suicide, previous suicide attempts, excessive drug and alcohol use, prolonged depression, financial difficulties, serious illness in the suicide contemplator or in his or her loved ones, and loss of a loved one through death or rejection. Societal pressures often serve as a catalyst.

In most cases, suicide does not occur unpredictably. In fact, between 75 and 80 percent of people who commit suicide give a warning of their intentions.

Warning Signs of Suicide

Common signs of possible suicide include:[55]

- Recent loss and a seeming inability to let go of grief.
- Change in personality—sadness, withdrawal, irritability, anxiety, tiredness, indecisiveness, apathy.
- Change in behavior—inability to concentrate, loss of interest in classes.
- Diminished sexual interest—impotence, menstrual abnormalities.
- Expressions of self-hatred.
- Change in sleep patterns.
- Change in eating habits.
- A direct statement about committing suicide, such as "I might as well end it all."
- An indirect statement, such as "You won't have to worry about me anymore."
- "Final preparations," such as writing a will, repairing poor relationships with family or friends, giving away prized possessions, or writing revealing letters.
- A preoccupation with themes of death.
- A sudden and unexplained demonstration of happiness following a period of depression.
- Marked changes in personal appearance.
- Excessive risk taking and an "I don't care what happens to me" attitude.

Taking Action to Prevent Suicide

Most people who attempt suicide really want to live, but see death as the only way out of an intolerable situation. Crisis counselors and suicide hotlines may help temporarily, but the best way to prevent suicide is to get rid of conditions that may precipitate attempts, including alcoholism, drug abuse, loneliness, isolation, and access to guns.

If someone you know threatens suicide or displays any warning signs, take the following actions:

- Monitor the warning signals. Try to keep an eye on the person involved, or see that there is someone around the person as much as possible.
- Take any threats seriously. Don't just brush them off.
- Let the person know how much you care about him or her. State that you are there if he or she needs help.
- Listen. Try not to discredit or be shocked by what the person says. Empathize, sympathize, and keep the person talking. Talk about stressors and listen to the responses.
- Ask directly, "Are you thinking of hurting or killing yourself?"
- Do not belittle the person's feelings or say that he or she doesn't really mean it or couldn't succeed at suicide. To some people, these comments offer the challenge of proving you wrong.
- Help the person think about alternatives. Be ready to offer choices. Offer to go for help with the person. Call your local suicide hotline and use all available community and campus resources. Recommend a counselor or other person to talk to.
- Remember that your relationships with others involve responsibilities. If you need to stay with the person, take the person to a health care facility, or provide support, give of yourself and your time.
- Tell your friend's spouse, partner, parents, brothers and sisters, or counselor. Do not keep your suspicions to yourself. Don't let a suicidal friend talk you into keeping your discussions confidential. If your friend succeeds in a suicide attempt, you will have to live with the consequences.

> **What do you think?**
>
> *If your roommate showed some of the warning signs of suicide, what action would you take?* ✳ *Whom would you contact first?* ✳ *Where on campus might your friend get help?* ✳ *What if someone in class whom you hardly know gave some of the warning signs?* ✳ *What would you then do?*

Seeking Professional Help

A physical ailment will readily send most of us to the nearest health professional, but many Americans feel that seeking professional help for psychosocial problems is an admission of personal failure. We tend to ignore psychosocial problems until they pose a serious threat to our well-being—and even then, we may refuse to ask for the help we need. However, an increasing number of Americans are turning to mental health professionals, and nearly one in five seeks such help. Researchers cite breakdowns in support systems, high societal expectations of the individual, and dysfunctional families as the three major reasons why more people are asking for assistance than ever before.

You should consider seeking help if:

- You think you need help.
- You experience wild mood swings.

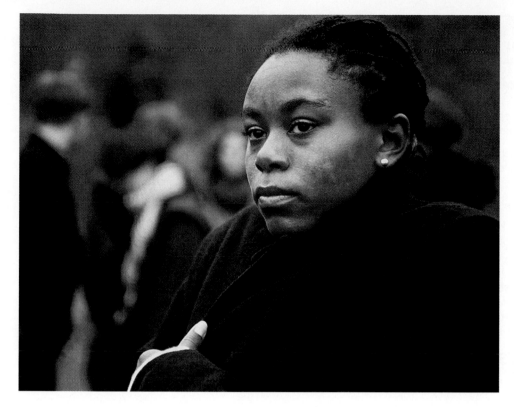

When experiencing problems such as depression or anxiety, it is unwise to try to "go it alone." A qualified, caring therapist can help.

- A problem is interfering with your daily life.
- Your fears or feelings of guilt frequently distract your attention.
- You begin to withdraw from others.
- You have hallucinations.
- You feel that life is not worth living.
- You feel inadequate or worthless.
- Your emotional responses are inappropriate to various situations.
- Your daily life seems to be nothing but repeated crises.
- You feel you can't "get your act together."
- You are considering suicide.
- You turn to drugs or alcohol to escape from your problems.
- You feel out of control.

Getting Evaluated for Treatment

If you are considering treatment for a psychosocial problem, schedule a complete evaluation first. Start with your campus health center. Consult a credentialed health professional for a thorough examination, which should include three parts:

- A physical checkup, which will rule out thyroid disorders, viral infections, and anemia—all of which can result in depressive like symptoms—and a neurological check of coordination, reflexes, and balance, to rule out brain disorders.
- A psychiatric history, which will attempt to trace the course of the apparent disorder, genetic or family factors, and any past treatments.
- A mental status examination, which will assess thoughts, speaking processes, and memory, as well as an in-depth interview with tests for other psychiatric symptoms.[56]

Once physical factors have been ruled out, you may decide to consult a professional who specializes in psychosocial health.

Mental Health Professionals

Several types of mental health professionals, or providers, are available to help you. Remember, the most important criterion is not how many degrees this person has, but whether you feel you can work together.

Psychiatrist A **psychiatrist** is a medical doctor. After obtaining an M.D. degree, a psychiatrist spends up to 12 years studying psychosocial health and disease. As a licensed physician, a psychiatrist can prescribe medications for various mental or emotional problems and may have admitting privileges at a local hospital. Some psychiatrists are affiliated with hospitals, while others are in private practice.

Psychologist A **psychologist** usually has a Ph.D. degree in counseling or clinical psychology. In addition, many states require licensure. Psychologists are trained in various types of therapy, including behavior and insight therapy. Most can

Psychiatrist A licensed physician who specializes in treating mental and emotional disorders.

Psychologist A person with a Ph.D. degree and training in psychology.

Table 2.3
Traditional Forms of Psychotherapy: Assumptions, Goals, and Methods

TYPE OF THERAPY	BASIC ASSUMPTIONS	GOALS AND METHODS
Psychoanalysis	Behavior is motivated by intrapsychic conflict and biological urges.	Discover the sources of conflict and resolve them through insight.
Psychodynamic therapy	Behavior is motivated by both unconscious forces and interpersonal experiences.	Understand and improve interpersonal skills by modifying the client's inappropriate schemas about interpersonal relationships.
Humanistic and Gestalt therapy	People are good and have innate worth.	Use techniques to enhance personal awareness and feelings of self-worth to promote personal growth and self-actualization and to enhance clients' awareness of bodily sensations and feelings.
Behavior and cognitive-behavior therapy	Behavior is largely controlled by environmental contingencies, people's perception of them, or a combination.	Change maladaptive behavior and thinking patterns by manipulating environmental variables, restructuring thinking patterns, and correcting faulty thinking or irrational beliefs.
Family/couples therapy	Problems in relationships entail everybody involved in them.	Analyze relationship patterns and other's roles in order to discover how interactions influence problems in individual functioning.

Source: Adapted from Neil R. Carlson and William Buskist, *Psychology: The Science of Behavior*, 5th ed., p. 629. Copyright ©1997 Allyn & Bacon. Reprinted by permission.

conduct both individual and group counseling sessions. Psychologists may also be trained in certain specialties, such as family counseling or sexual counseling.

Psychoanalyst A **psychoanalyst** is a psychiatrist or psychologist having special training in psychoanalysis. Psychoanalysis is a type of therapy that helps patients remember early traumas that have blocked personal growth. Facing these traumas helps them resolve conflicts and begin to lead more productive lives.

Clinical/Psychiatric Social Worker A **social worker** has at least a master's degree in social work (M.S.W.) and two years of experience in a clinical setting. Many states require an ex-

amination for accreditation. Some social workers work in clinical settings, whereas others have private practices.

Counselor A **counselor** often has a master's degree in counseling, psychology, educational psychology, or related human service. Professional societies recommend at least two years of graduate coursework or supervised practice as a minimal requirement. Many counselors are trained to do individual and group therapy. They often specialize in one type of counseling, such as family, marital, relationship, children, drug, divorce, behavioral, or personal counseling.

Psychiatric Nurse Specialist Although all registered nurses can work in psychiatric settings, some continue their education and specialize in psychiatric practice. The **psychiatric nurse specialist** can be certified by the American Nursing Association in adult, child, or adolescent psychiatric nursing.

Many different types of counseling exist, ranging from individual therapy, which involves one-on-one work between therapist and client, to group therapy, in which two or more clients meet with a therapist to discuss problems. Table 2.3 identifies traditional forms of psychotherapy.

Choosing a Therapist

Remember that in most states, anyone can use the title *therapist* or *counselor*. Choose carefully. Get recommendations for therapists through your doctor or someone you trust.

Psychoanalyst A psychiatrist or psychologist having special training in psychoanalysis.

Social worker A person with an M.S.W. degree and clinical training.

Counselor A person having a variety of academic and experiential training who deals with the treatment of emotional problems.

Psychiatric nurse specialist A registered nurse specializing in psychiatric practice.

A qualified mental health professional should be willing to answer all of your questions during an initial consultation. If he or she is unwilling, move on to the next one on your list. Fundamental questions to ask include:

- Will the therapist permit an interview before treatment begins? It is important that you find a therapist with whom you can communicate comfortably. By conducting an initial interview, you will get a sense of whether or not the therapist will be a good fit for you.
- Do you like the therapist as a person? Is this the type of person you would choose as a friend? Look beyond credentials to find someone who shows a genuine interest in you. If you sense that the therapist is watching the clock or easily distracted, look elsewhere. You should be the focal point of the entire session.
- Does the therapist demonstrate professionalism? The therapist should follow a basic code of ethics. This includes winning your trust and setting boundaries in your relationship. If your therapist is frequently late, suggests social interactions outside your therapy sessions, talks continually about himself or herself, has questionable billing practices, or doesn't want to release you from therapy, you should be concerned. These are all unprofessional behaviors.
- Will the therapist help you set your own goals? A good therapist should evaluate your general situation and help you set small goals to work on between sessions. A professional should not tell you how to help yourself, but help you discover your goals.[57]

What to Expect in Therapy

The first trip to a therapist can be extremely difficult. Most of us have misconceptions about what therapy is and about what it can do. That first visit is a verbal and mental sizing up between you and the therapist. You may not accomplish much in that first hour. If you decide that this professional is not for you, you will at least have learned how to present your problem and what qualities you need in a therapist.

1. Before meeting, briefly explain your needs. Ask what the fee is. Arrive on time. Wear comfortable clothing. Expect to spend about an hour during your first visit.
2. The therapist will want to take down your history and details about the problems that have brought you to therapy. Answer as honestly as possible. Many will ask how you feel about aspects of your life. Do not be embarrassed to acknowledge your feelings.
3. Therapists are not mind readers. They cannot tell what you are thinking. It is therefore critical to the success of your treatment that you trust this person enough to be open and honest.
4. Do not expect the therapist to tell you what to do or how to behave. The responsibility for improved behavior lies with you.
5. Find out if you can set your own therapeutic goals and timetables. Also, find out if, later in therapy, your therapist will allow you to determine what is and is not helping you. If, after your first visit (or even after several visits), you feel you cannot work with this person, say so. You have the right to find a therapist with whom you feel comfortable.

> ## What do you think?
>
> *Have you ever thought about seeing a therapist? ✳ What made you decide to go or not go? ✳ If you were to consult a therapist, what factors would you take into consideration in picking one who is "right" for you?*

Taking Charge

2

Managing Your Psychosocial Health

Psychosocial health is a complex concept. Achieving optimal psychosocial health requires careful introspection and planned action. Look at life as a constant process of discovery, and remember that even the most difficult times can provide opportunities for learning and growth. Remembering the following points and acting upon them whenever possible will help you along the way.

Checklist for Change

Making Personal Choices

☐ Consider life a constant process of discovery.

☐ Accept yourself as the best that you are able to be right now.

☐ Remember that nobody is perfect.

☐ Remember that the most difficult times in life occur during transitions and can be opportunities for growth even when they are painful.

☐ Be open to other perspectives.

☐ Recognize the sources of your own anxiety and act to reduce them.

☐ Ask for help when you need it; discuss your problems with others.

☐ Try to find joy and happiness in both the little and big things in life.

☐ Nurture your friendships.

☐ Become sensitive to and aware of your own body's signals. Take care of yourself.

- □ Find a meaning for your life and work toward achieving your goals.
- □ Develop strategies to get through problem situations.
- □ Remain open to emotional experiences—give yourself to today rather than always reserving yourself for tomorrow.
- □ Even when you fail, be proud of yourself for trying.
- □ Keep your sense of humor—learn to laugh at yourself.
- □ Never quit trying to grow, to experience, to love, and to live life to its fullest.

Summary

* Psychosocial health is a complex phenomenon involving mental, emotional, social, and spiritual health.
* Many factors influence psychosocial health, including life experiences, family, the environment, other people, self-esteem, self-efficacy, and personality. Some of these are modifiable; others are not.
* Developing self-esteem and self-efficacy and getting enough sleep are key to enhancing psychosocial health.
* Many people believe spirituality is important to wellness. Though the exact reasons have not been established, many studies show a connection.
* Happiness is a key factor in determining overall reaction to life's challenges. The mind—body connection is an important link in overall health and well-being.

* Indicators of deteriorating psychosocial health include depression. Identifying depression is the first step in treating this disorder.
* Common psychosocial problems include anxiety disorders, phobias, panic disorders, seasonal affective disorder, and schizophrenia.
* Suicide is a result of negative psychosocial reactions to life. People intending to commit suicide often give warning signs of their intentions. Such people can often be helped.
* Mental health professionals include psychiatrists, psychoanalysts, psychologists, clinical/psychiatric social workers, counselors, and psychiatric nurse specialists. A great variety of therapy methods exist, including group and individual therapy. It is wise to carefully interview a therapist before beginning treatment.

Questions for Discussion and Reflection

1. What is psychosocial health? What indicates that people are or aren't psychosocially healthy? Why might the college environment provide a real challenge to your psychosocial health?
2. Discuss the factors that influence your overall level of psychosocial health. What factors can you change? Which ones may be more difficult to change?
3. What steps could you take today to improve your psychosocial health? Which steps require long-term effort?
4. What are four main themes of spirituality, and how are they expressed in daily life?
5. Why is laughter therapeutic? How can humor help you better achieve wellness?
6. What factors appear to contribute to psychosocial difficulties and illnesses? Which of the common psychosocial illnesses is likely to affect people in your age group?

7. What are the warning signs of suicide? Of depression? Why is depression so pervasive among young Americans today? Why are some groups more vulnerable to suicide and depression than are others? What would you do if you heard a friend in the cafeteria say to no one in particular that he was going to "do the world a favor and end it all"?
8. Discuss the different types of health professionals and therapies. If you felt depressed about breaking off a long-term relationship, which professional and therapy do you think would be most beneficial? Explain your answer. What services are provided by your student health center? What fees are charged to students?
9. What psychosocial areas do you need to work on? Which are most important to you, and why? What actions can you take today?

Application Exercises

Reread the What Do You Think? scenarios at the beginning of the chapter and answer the following questions.

1. How psychosocially healthy are each of the individuals described in the scenarios presented in the chapter opener?
2. What factors may have contributed to Amy's behavior? Why might her friends be hesitant about reaching out to help her?

3. What factors may have contributed to Martin's panic attack? What would you do if someone you knew suffered from this disorder?
4. What services on your campus would be available to help these students improve their psychosocial health? What community services are available to nonstudents who have limited incomes?
5. As a friend, what could you do to help each of them?

Accessing Your Health on the Internet

Visit the following Internet sites to explore further topics and issues related to personal health. To visit an organization's website, go to the Companion Website for *Access to Health, Eighth Edition* at www.aw.com/donatelle, click on the book image, and select "Accessing Your Health on the Internet" from the navigation menu on the left.

1. *MEDWEB.* This site provides an extensive list of sites and resources for many aspects of mental health information.
2. *Mental Health Net.* Provides information for mental health practitioners as well as those whom they serve. Includes many mental health links.

3. *American Psychological Association.* Includes APA newsletters; links to other sites; information on books, journals, and employment; and public, practical, and educational materials.
4. *Other reliable sites* include those of the National Institute of Mental Health, the American Psychiatric Association, and the National Mental Health Association.

Further Reading

Dalai Lama and H. C. Cutler. *The Art of Happiness: A Handbook for Living.* New York: Riverhead, 1998.

Explores the reasons why so many people are unhappy and offers strategies for becoming happy. Through a series of interviews, the authors explore questions of meaning, motives, and the interconnectedness of life.

Julie Norem, Ph.D. *The Positive Power of Negative Thinking.* New York: Basic Books, 2002.

Explores reasons for negative thinking and mechanisms for changing the way you think. Self tests and analysis for helping you retrain your thinking processes.

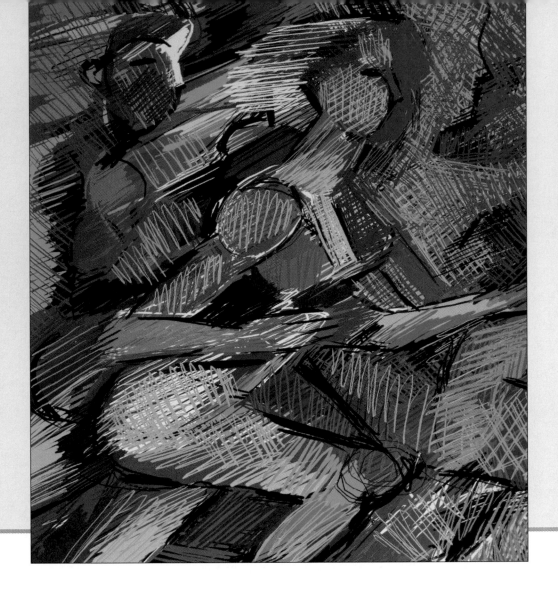

Objectives

* Define stress, and examine the potential impact of stress on health, relationships, and success in college.

* Explain the three phases of the general adaptation syndrome, and describe what happens physiologically when we experience a real or perceived threat.

* Examine the health risks that may occur with chronic stress.

* Discuss psychosocial, environmental, and self-imposed sources of stress. Examine ways in which you might reduce risks from these stressors or inoculate yourself against stressful situations.

* Examine the special stressors that affect college students and strategies for reducing risk.

* Explore techniques for coping with unavoidable stress, reducing exposure to stress, and making optimum use of positive stressors to promote growth and enrich life experiences.

* Examine the role of spirituality in enhancing life and the ability to deal with stress.

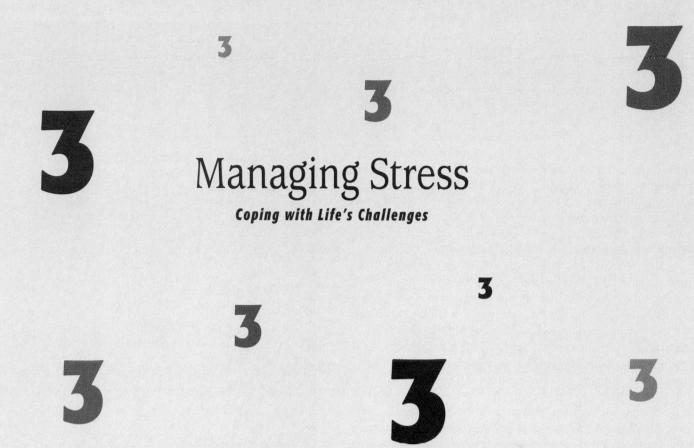

Managing Stress

Coping with Life's Challenges

What do you think?

Desirée has just set off from northern Wisconsin for her freshman year at a university in Oregon. She moves into a dorm full of strangers; many come from different cultures, and their life experiences differ from hers. She struggles to do her homework in the noise and commotion of dorm life and to keep up with seemingly endless assignments. She longs for her family and old friends, cries easily, and often stays in bed, avoiding class. By midterm, she is failing three classes and doesn't seem to care.

Beth arrives from Los Angeles to attend the same university. She lives in an active sorority, and her first week of classes is a riot—partying, meeting new people, staying up all night, and skipping class. Although she misses her friends in L.A., she is excited about her social life. She feels "wired" and has a few drinks to calm herself before studying and to help her sleep. Although she dreams of becoming an engineer, by midterm she has a GPA of 2.2.

James is another freshman at the same university. He married right after high school and has a wife and an infant daughter to support while he attends college. When the first football game takes place, he longs to be with the other students, having a good time. Instead, he goes to his part-time job and then home to study. He often feels angry and resents staying home to watch his daughter; he also finds it difficult to concentrate on his studies. By midterm, he is getting A's and B's in his classes, but he is tired and has lost interest in things that he used to enjoy.

What stressors affect each individual? ✳ How have past experiences, and choices and current situations contributed to their stress? ✳ Which student will find it most difficult to deal with stress? ✳ Why? ✳ What campus services and supports could help these students? ✳ How did your freshman experience compare to these, and how did you cope with the challenges you faced?

oud music. Relationship problems. Too much to do. Not enough time. The excitement of a new relationship. Financial worries. Stress! You can't get away from it; there's no place to hide. Seemingly, stress is an inevitable part of modern life. Whether it seems frightening or invigorating, we all experience its effect.

Often, stress is insidious, and we don't even notice things that affect us. As we sleep it encroaches on our psyche through noise or incessant worries over things that need to be done. While we work at the computer, stress may interfere in the form of noise from next door, strain on our eyes, and tension in our backs. The exact toll stress exacts from us during a lifetime of stress overload is unknown, but it is much more than an annoyance. Rather, it is a significant health hazard that can rob the body of needed nutrients, damage the cardiovascular system, raise blood pressure, and dampen the immune system's defenses, leaving us vulnerable to infections and a host of diseases. In addition, it can drain our emotional reserves, contribute to depression, anxiety, and irritability, and cause social interactions to be punctuated with hostility and anger. Stress is a major concern in the United States, and it appears to be getting worse: One-third of U.S. workers report an increase in job-related stress over the past year.[1] Although much has been written about stress, we are only beginning to understand the multifaceted nature of the stress response and its tremendous potential for harm or benefit.

What Is Stress?

Often, we think of stress as an externally imposed factor that threatens or makes a demand on our minds and bodies. But for most of us, stress usually results from an internal state of emotional tension that occurs in response to the various demands of living. Most current definitions state that **stress** is the mental and physical response of our bodies to the changes and challenges in our lives. Inherent in these definitions is the idea that we sometimes take ourselves and our lives too seriously; that we should loosen up, worry less, and gain greater control over our minds as well as our bodies.

A **stressor** is any physical, social, or psychological event or condition that causes the body to adjust to a specific situation. Stressors may be tangible, such as an angry parent or a disgruntled roommate, or intangible, such as the mixed emotions associated with meeting your significant other's parents for the first time. **Adjustment** is the attempt to cope with a given situation. **Strain** is the wear and tear the body and mind sustain during the adjustment process.

Stress and strain are associated with most daily activities. Generally, positive stress, or stress that presents the opportunity for personal growth and satisfaction, is called **eustress**. Getting married, starting school, beginning a career, developing new friendships, and learning a new physical skill all give rise to eustress. **Distress,** or negative stress,

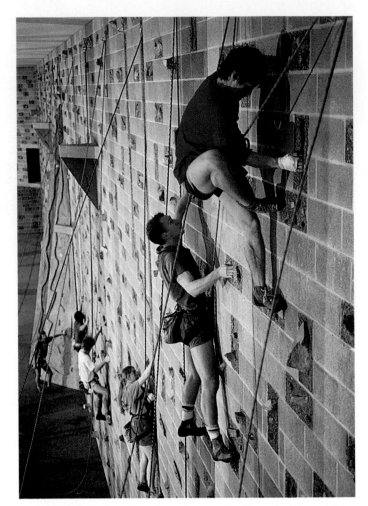

Many people enjoy the adrenaline rush of a strenuous and challenging workout.

is caused by those events, such as financial problems, the death of a loved one, academic difficulties, and the breakup of a relationship, that result in debilitative stress and strain.

In many cases, we cannot prevent the occurrence of distress: like eustress, it is a part of life. However, we can train ourselves to recognize the events that cause distress and to anticipate the reactions we have to them. We can learn to practice prestress coping skills and to develop poststress management techniques.

The Body's Response to Stress

Whenever we're surprised by a sudden stressor, such as someone swerving into our lane of traffic, the adrenal glands jump into action. These two almond-sized glands sitting atop the kidneys secrete adrenaline and other hormones into the bloodstream. As a result, the heart speeds up, breathing rate increases, blood pressure elevates, and the flow of blood to the muscles increases with a rapid release of blood sugars into the bloodstream. This sudden burst of energy and strength is believed to provide the extra edge that has helped generations of humans survive during adversity. Known as

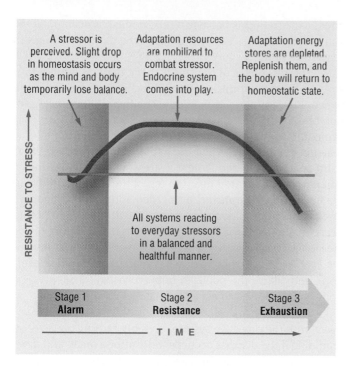

Figure 3.1
The General Adaptation Syndrome

the **fight-or-flight response,** this physiological reaction is believed to be one of our most basic, innate survival instincts. It is a point at which our bodies go on the alert either to fight or to escape.

The General Adaptation Syndrome (GAS)

What has just been described in very general terms is a complicated physiological response to stress in which our bodies move from **homeostasis,** a level of functioning in which systems operate smoothly and maintain equilibrium, to one of crisis, in which the body attempts to return to homeostasis. This adjustment is referred to as an **adaptive response.** First characterized by Hans Selye in 1936, this internal fight to restore balance when upset is known as the **general adaptation syndrome (GAS)** (see Figure 3.1), which has three distinct phases: alarm, resistance, and exhaustion.[2]

Alarm Phase When exposed to a stressor, whether real or perceived, the fight-or-flight response kicks into gear. Stress hormones flow into the body, and it prepares to do battle with whatever is causing the upset. The subconscious perceptions and appraisal of the stressor stimulate the areas in the brain responsible for emotions. Emotional stimulation, in turn, starts the physical reactions that we associate with stress (see Figure 3.2). This entire process takes only a few seconds.

Suppose that you are walking to your car after a late-night class on a dimly lit campus. As you pass a particularly dark area, you hear someone cough behind you and sense that this person is fairly close. You walk faster, only to hear

the quickened footsteps of the other person. Your senses become increasingly alert, your breathing quickens, your heart races, and you begin to perspire. The stranger is getting closer and closer. In desperation you stop, clutching your book bag in your hands, determined to use force if necessary to protect yourself. You turn around quickly and let out a blood-curdling yell. To your surprise, the only person you see is Mrs. Fletcher, a woman in your class, who has been trying to stay close to you out of her own anxiety about walking alone in the dark. She screams and jumps back off the street, only to trip and fall. You look at her in startled embarrassment, help her to her feet, and nervously laugh about your reaction. You have just experienced the *alarm* phase of GAS.

When the mind perceives a stressor (either real or imaginary), such as a potential attacker, the *cerebral cortex,* the region of the brain that interprets the nature of an event, is called to attention. If the cerebral cortex perceives a threat, it triggers an **autonomic nervous system (ANS)** response that prepares the body for action. The ANS is the portion of the central nervous system that regulates bodily functions that we do not normally consciously control, such as heart function, breathing, and glandular function. When we are stressed, the activity rate of all these bodily functions increases dramatically to give us the physical strength to protect ourselves or to mobilize internal forces.

Stress Mental and physical responses to change.

Stressor A physical, social, or psychological event or condition that requires an adjustment.

Adjustment The attempt to cope with a given situation.

Strain The wear and tear sustained by the body and mind in adjusting to or resisting a stressor.

Eustress Stress that presents opportunities for personal growth.

Distress Stress that can have a negative effect on health.

Fight-or-flight response Physiological arousal response in which the body prepares to combat a real or perceived threat.

Homeostasis A balanced physical state in which all the body's systems function smoothly.

Adaptive response Form of adjustment in which the body attempts to restore homeostasis.

General adaptation syndrome (GAS) The pattern followed in the physiological response to stress, consisting of the alarm, resistance, and exhaustion phases.

Autonomic nervous system (ANS) The portion of the central nervous system that regulates bodily functions that a person does not normally consciously control.

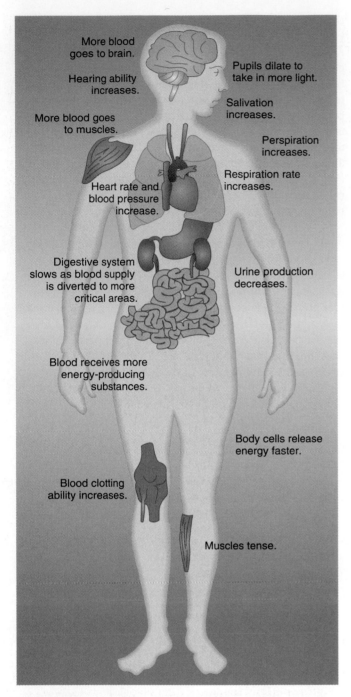

Figure 3.2
The General Adaptation Syndrome: Alarm Phase

Labels on figure:
More blood goes to brain.

Hearing ability increases.

Pupils dilate to take in more light.

More blood goes to muscles.

Salivation increases.

Perspiration increases.

Respiration rate increases.

Heart rate and blood pressure increase.

Digestive system slows as blood supply is diverted to more critical areas.

Urine production decreases.

Blood receives more energy-producing substances.

Body cells release energy faster.

Blood clotting ability increases.

Muscles tense.

The ANS has two branches: sympathetic and parasympathetic. The **sympathetic nervous system** energizes the body for either fight or flight by signaling the release of several stress hormones that speed the heart rate, increase the breathing rate, and trigger many other stress responses. The **parasympathetic nervous system** functions to slow all the systems stimulated by the stress response. Thus, the parasympathetic branch of the ANS serves as a system of checks and balances on the sympathetic branch. In a healthy person, these two branches work together in a balance that controls the negative effects of stress. However, long-term stress can strain this balance, and chronic physical problems can occur as stress reactions become the dominant forces in a person's body.

The responses of the sympathetic nervous system to stress involve a complex series of biochemical exchanges between different parts of the body. The **hypothalamus,** a section of the brain, functions as the control center of the sympathetic nervous system and determines the overall reaction to stressors. When the hypothalamus perceives that extra energy is needed to fight a stressor, it stimulates the adrenal glands, located near the top of the kidneys, to release the hormone **epinephrine,** also called adrenaline. Epinephrine causes more blood to be pumped with each beat of the heart, dilates the bronchioles (air sacs in the lungs) to increase oxygen intake, increases the breathing rate, stimulates the liver to release more glucose (which fuels muscular exertion), and dilates the pupils to improve visual sensitivity. The body is then poised to act immediately.

As epinephrine secretion increases, blood is diverted away from the digestive system, possibly causing nausea and cramping if the distress occurs shortly after a meal, and drying of nasal and salivary tissues, producing dry mouth. The alarm phase also provides for longer-term reaction to stress. The hypothalamus triggers the pituitary gland, which in turn releases another powerful hormone, **adrenocorticotrophic hormone (ACTH).** ACTH signals the adrenal glands to release **cortisol,** a hormone that makes stored nutrients more readily available to meet energy demands. Finally, other parts of the brain and body release endorphins, the body's naturally occurring opiates, which relieve pain that may be caused by a stressor.

Resistance Phase The resistance phase of the GAS begins almost immediately after the alarm phase starts. In this stage, the body has reacted to the stressor and adjusted in a way that allows the system to return to homeostasis. As the sympathetic nervous system energizes the body via the hormonal action of epinephrine, norepinephrine, cortisol, and other hormones, the parasympathetic nervous system helps control these energy levels and return the body to a normal level of functioning.

Exhaustion Phase In the exhaustion phase of the GAS, the physical and emotional energy used to fight a stressor have been depleted. The toll it takes on the body depends on the type of stress or the period of time spent under stress. Short-term stress probably would not deplete all of a person's energy reserves, but chronic stress experienced over a period of time can create continuous states of alarm and resistance, resulting in total depletion of energy and susceptibility to illness. The key to warding off the effects of stress lies in what many researchers refer to as *adaptation energy stores*, the physical and mental foundations of our ability to cope with stress.

Two levels of adaptation energy stores exist: deep and superficial. We apparently have little control over deep stores, as their size appears to be preset by heredity. Superficial adaptation energy stores, however, are renewable and

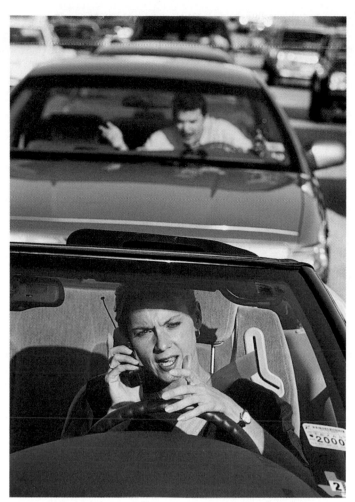

Two snapshots of stress: One driver juggles freeway driving and a phone call, while the other expresses "road rage." Both drivers may be heading for stress-related health problems.

balance between work and relaxation, practicing good nutritional habits, setting realistic goals, and maintaining supportive relationships.

What do you think?

What are your greatest sources of stress right now? ✳ *On a scale of 1–10, with 10 being the highest level, how stressed are you?* ✳ *Have you noticed any symptoms of stress?* ✳ *How can you reduce your stress?*

Stress and Your Health

Although much has been written about the negative effects of stress, researchers have only recently begun to untangle the complex web of physical and emotional interactions that actually cause the body to break down over time. Stress is often described as a "disease of prolonged arousal" that leads to other negative health effects. Nearly all systems of the body become potential targets for this onslaught, and the long-term effects may be devastating.

Much of the initial impetus for studying the health effects of stress came from indirect observations. Cardiologists in the Framingham Heart Study and other research projects noted that highly stressed individuals seemed to experience significantly greater risks for cardiovascular disease (CVD) and hypertension.[3] Monkeys exposed to high levels of unpredictable stressors in studies showed significantly increased levels of disease and mortality.[4] In a landmark study,

present the first line of defense against stress, as they are tapped into initially as the body fights stress. Only when superficial stores are exhausted does the body tap into the deep energy stores. As our adaptation energy stores are depleted, we tire more quickly and require more rest. Without this replenishing sleep, the alarm and resistance phases eventually will limit our ability to rebound properly.

As the body adjusts to chronic unresolved stress, the adrenal glands continue to release cortisol, which remains in the bloodstream for longer periods of time due to slower metabolic responsiveness. Over time, without relief, cortisol can reduce **immunocompetence,** or the ability of the immune system to respond to various onslaughts. Blood pressure can remain dangerously elevated, and our body systems become unable to respond with the same vigor they once did. The net effect? Greater chance of minor illnesses at one end of the continuum; greater risk of life-threatening disease at the other end.

Stress management, therefore, depends on the ability to replenish superficial stores and conserve deep stores. Besides getting adequate amounts of rest, adaptation energy stores can be replenished by aerobic exercise, finding a

Sympathetic nervous system Branch of the autonomic nervous system responsible for stress arousal.

Parasympathetic nervous system Part of the autonomic nervous system responsible for slowing systems stimulated by the stress response.

Hypothalamus A section of the brain that controls the sympathetic nervous system and directs the stress response.

Epinephrine Also called adrenaline, a hormone that stimulates body systems in response to stress.

Adrenocorticotrophic hormone (ACTH) A pituitary hormone that stimulates the adrenal glands to secrete cortisol.

Cortisol Hormone released by the adrenal glands that makes stored nutrients more readily available to meet energy demands.

Immunocompetence The ability of the immune system to respond to assaults

M. D. Jeremko observed that chronic stress activation can result in headaches, asthma, hypertension, ulcers, lower back pain, and other medical conditions, a finding substantiated by a meta-analysis of over one hundred similar studies. [5] A Harvard study concluded that mental health was the most important predictor of physical health.[6] While the battle over the legitimacy of these observations continues to be waged in research labs across the country, the theory that chronic stress increases susceptibility to certain ailments has gained credibility.

Stress and CVD Risks

Since Friedman and Rosenman's classic study of Type A and Type B personalities and heart disease in the late 1960s and early 1970s (discussed later in this chapter), researchers have tried to definitively link personality, emotions, and a host of other variables to heart disease.[7] It is generally assumed that too much stress contributes to, (1) increased plaque buildup in the arteries due to elevations in cholesterol level, (2) hardening of the arteries, (3) alterations in heart rhythms, (4) increased blood pressure, and (5) difficulties in cardiovascular system responsiveness due to all of the above. (For more information about CVD risks, see Chapter 15.)

Stress and Impaired Immunity

A new area of scientific investigation known as **psychoneuroimmunology (PNI)** analyzes the intricate relationship between the mind's response to stress and the ability of the immune system to function effectively. A recent article in the *Journal of the American Medical Association (JAMA)* reviews the research linking stress to adverse health consequences.[8] Among the findings: Too much stress, over a long period, can negatively regulate various aspects of the cellular immune response. In particular, stress disrupts bidirectional communication networks between the nervous, endocrine, and immune systems. When these networks fail, messenger systems that regulate hormones, blood cell formation, and a host of other health-regulating systems begin to falter or send faulty information.[9]

During prolonged stress, elevated levels of adrenal hormones destroy or reduce the ability of the white blood cells, known as natural killer T-cells, to aid the immune response. When killer T-cells are suppressed and other regulating systems aren't working correctly, illness may occur. Several key studies link stress with infectious diseases:

• Mice that are forced to live in crowded cages prior to and after infection with tuberculosis have much poorer outcomes than mice in less crowded situations. Social disruption in mice also seems to trigger outbreaks of herpes viruses.[10]

Psychoneuroimmunology (PNI) Science of the interaction between the mind and the immune system.

• Caregivers of Alzheimer's patients were vaccinated against the flu but still had a much greater chance of getting the flu or becoming ill than non-caregivers who received the same vaccine.[11]
• People with self-reported high stress levels were much more likely to develop upper respiratory infections than those who reported lower levels of stress.
• Certain changes in lifestyle may increase resistance to infectious diseases. These changes include broadening one's social involvement (e.g., joining social or spiritual groups, having a confidant, spending time with supportive friends) and maintaining healthful practices such as proper diet, exercise, and sleep.[12]
• Students' disease-fighting mechanisms are weaker during high-stress times, such as exam weeks and days when they are upset. In one experiment, a stressful event increased the severity of symptoms in a group of volunteers who were knowingly infected with a cold virus. In another, 47 percent of subjects living high-stress lives developed colds after a virus was dropped into their noses, but only 27 percent of those living relatively stress-free lives caught these colds.[13]

Though strong indicators support the hypothesis of a relationship between high stress and increased risk for disease, we are only beginning to understand this link. Some research indicates that such a relationship does not exist and that other factors such as genetics and environmental stimuli may be involved. Although these studies have pointed to the role of a positive attitude, control of stress and other psychological factors in susceptibility to disease and overall recovery, controversy over the mechanisms and benefits of stress reduction in health remains.[14]

Stress and the Mind

Stress may be one of the single greatest contributors to mental disability and emotional dysfunction in the United States. Whether it be from lost work productivity, difficulties in relationships, abuse of drugs and other substances, displaced anger and aggressive behavior, or a host of other problems, stress overload does much more than cause the heart rate to soar. Evidence suggests a strong relationship between stress and the potential for negative mental health reactions. Consider the following:[15]

• Numerous researchers have demonstrated that stressors, that interact with low self-esteem and/or maladaptive coping styles, are predictors of depression and anxiety.
• Depression and drug abuse are highly correlated with excessive exposure to stress.
• Among college students, low self-esteem or depression and concerns about stress and health were identified as unresolved problems for 35 percent and 20 percent of the respondents, respectively.
• Mature coping styles predict happiness, occupational and social success, enjoyment, and absence of addictions.
• Persons with high nervous tension have increased risk for mental illness, suicide, and coronary heart disease.

- A recent national study of Americans ages 15 to 54 found that almost half will suffer a mental and addictive disorder during their lifetime. Many of these disorders are believed to be stress related.
- Mental illness is on the increase in almost all segments of U.S. society.

Sources of Stress

Both eustress and distress have many sources. These sources include psychosocial factors, such as changes, hassles, pressure, inconsistent goals and objectives, conflict, overload, and burnout; environmental stressors, such as natural and human-made disasters; and self-imposed stress.

Psychosocial Sources of Stress

Psychosocial stress refers to the factors in our daily lives that cause stress (see the Assess Yourself box). Interactions with others, the subtle and not-so-subtle expectations we and others have of ourselves, and the social conditions we live in force us to readjust continually.

Change Any time there is change in your normal daily routine, whether good or bad, you will experience stress. The more changes you experience and the more adjustments you must make, the greater the stress effects may be. In 1967, Drs. Thomas Holmes and Richard Rahe analyzed the social readjustments experienced by over 5,000 patients, noting which events seemed to occur just prior to disease onset.[16] They determined that certain events (both positive and negative) were predictive of increased risk for illness. They called their scale for predicting stress overload and the likelihood of illness the Social Readjustment Rating Scale (SRRS).[17] The SRRS has since served as the model for scales for certain groups, including college-age students, as shown in Table 3.1. Although many other factors must be considered, in general, the more of these stressors you experience, the more you need to change your behaviors or situation before problems occur.

Hassles While Holmes and Rahe focused on major stressors, psychologists such as Richard Lazarus have focused on petty annoyances and frustrations, collectively referred to as *hassles*.[18] Minor hassles—losing your keys, slipping and falling in front of everyone as you walk to your seat in a new class, finding that you went through a whole afternoon with a big chunk of spinach stuck in your front teeth—seem unimportant, but their cumulative effects may be harmful in the long run.

Pressure Pressure occurs when we feel forced to speed up, intensify, or shift the direction of our behavior to meet a higher standard of performance.[19] Pressures can be based on our personal goals and expectations, concern about what others think, or outside influences. Among the most significant outside influences are society's demands that we compete and be all that we can be. The forces that push us to compete for the best grades, nicest cars, most attractive significant others, and highest-paying jobs create significant pressure to be the personification of American success.

Inconsistent Goals and Behaviors For many of us, negative stress effects are magnified when there is a disparity between our goals (what we value or hope to obtain in life) and our behaviors (actions that may or may not lead to those goals). For instance, you may want good grades, and your family may expect them. But if you party and procrastinate

---

Table 3.1
Chronic Stressors for College Students

Here are several chronic stressors often experienced by college students. Each has the potential to cause serious health problems, particularly if experienced on a fairly regular basis (i.e., at least two or three times per week for the past month).

1. Roommate conflict	13. Uncertainty over the right major	25. Conflict with parents
2. Homesickness	14. Missing distant friends	26. Academic performance
3. Friend conflict	15. Family illness	27. Overweight
4. Writing major papers	16. Loneliness	28. Don't fit in; no friends
5. Dieting	17. Job pressures	29. Living/housing situations
6. Money/financial problems	18. Lack of privacy	30. Tuition bills/book costs
7. Long-distance relationship	19. Friends with problems	31. Health problems/not feeling well
8. Juggling school and job	20. Parental problems/family problems	32. Difficult class or instructor
9. Time management	21. Not enough sex/intimacy	33. Unsure of job future
10. Noisy dorm or apartment	22. Behind in schoolwork	34. Not enough sleep
11. No car or car not working	23. Problem with lover	35. Problem with drugs/alcohol
12 Underweight	24. Not enough exercise	

Source: Adapted from L. Towbes and L. Cohen, "Chronic Stress in the Lives of College Students: Scale Development and Prospective Predictions of Distress." *Journal of Youth and Adolescence* 25, no. 2 (1996): 202–203. By permission of Plenum Publishers and the authors.

How Stressed Are You?

Each of us reacts differently to life's little challenges. Faced with a long line at the bookstore, most of us will get agitated and anxious for a few seconds before we start grumbling, or shrug and move on. But for others—the one in five of us whom researchers call *hot reactors*—such incidents are part of a daily health assault. These individuals may get very angry outwardly, or they may appear calm and collected. It is what is going on under the surface that is what affects health. Surges in blood pressure, increases in heart rate, nausea, sweating, and a host of other hot reactor indicators may occur. Completing the following assessment will help you think about the nature and extent of stress in your life and how you might be likely to respond to daily stressors. Although this survey is just an indicator of what stress levels might be, it should help you focus on areas that you may need to work on to reduce stress.

Part One: What Is Stressing You Out?

For each statement, indicate how often the following stressful situations or feelings are a part of your daily life.

	1 = Never	2 = Rarely	3 = Sometimes	4 = Often	5 = All the time
1. I find that there are not enough hours in the day to finish everything I have to do.	1	2	3	4	5
2. I am nervous/anxious about how I am performing in my classes.	1	2	3	4	5
3. People don't seem to notice whether I do a good job or not.	1	2	3	4	5
4. I am tired and feel like I don't have the energy to do everything that I need to get done.	1	2	3	4	5
5. I am irritable and seem to be easily bothered by things that people do.	1	2	3	4	5
6. I worry about what is happening in my family (health of a loved one, financial problems, relationship problems).	1	2	3	4	5
7. I'm worried about my finances and having enough money to pay my bills.	1	2	3	4	5
8. I don't have enough time for fun.	1	2	3	4	5
9. I am unhappy with my body (weight, fitness level, etc.).	1	2	3	4	5
10. My family and friends count on me to help them with their problems.	1	2	3	4	5
11. I am concerned about my current relationship or lack of a relationship.	1	2	3	4	5
12. I am impatient/intolerant of the weaknesses of others.	1	2	3	4	5
13. My house/apartment is a mess and I'm embarrassed to have others see it.	1	2	3	4	5
14. I worry about whether I'll get a job and be able to support myself after graduation.	1	2	3	4	5
15. I worry that people don't like me or think that I'm not someone that they'd like to be friends with.	1	2	3	4	5

Your Total Score: _____

61–75: Your stress level is probably quite high. Prioritize the areas where you scored 5's, and list two or three things for each area that you could do to reduce your stress level. Note any increase in headaches, backaches, or insomnia; that's your body telling you to lighten your load. Plan at least one fun thing to do for yourself each day. Make yourself more of a daily priority.

46–60: Your stress level is moderate. Look at those areas that are 5's and pick out two or three that you would like to change now. Make a list of things you can do to help yourself reduce stress levels today. Practice at least one stress management technique each day. Make more time for yourself. Use the Behavior Change Contract to plan how you will reduce stress.

30–45: You seem to have a lower level of stress—this is good. However, there are still areas that you could work on. Think about what these are and list things you could do now to reduce stress.

Less than 30: You seem to be doing a great job. Whatever your problems, stress isn't one of them. Even when stressful events do occur—and they will—your health probably won't suffer.

Remember, each of us has "stress slips" along the way. Think about your reactions to situations like those above. Whenever possible, make conscious choices to reduce stress.

Part Two: How Do You Respond to Stress?

Respond to each of the following stressful events with a rating of how likely you are to react to it.

  1 = I would never respond like this.
  2 = I would occasionally respond like this.
  3 = I would respond like this a lot of the time.
  4 = I would almost always/always respond like this.

Scenario #1:
You've been waiting 20 minutes for a table in a crowded restaurant, and the hostess seats a group that arrived after you.

a. You feel your anger rise as your face gets hot and your heart beats faster.	1	2	3	4
b. You yell, "Hey! I was here first!" in an irritated voice to the hostess.	1	2	3	4
c. You angrily confront the people who are being seated in front of you and tell them you were there first.	1	2	3	4
d. You say, "Excuse me" in a polite voice and inform the other group and/or the hostess that you were there first.	1	2	3	4
e. You note it, but don't react. It's no big deal and the hostess obviously didn't notice the order of arrival.	1	2	3	4

Scenario #2:
You get to a movie theater early so that you and a friend can get great seats. You strategically pick a seat that will give you a good view. Then, although the theater is nearly empty, a very large, very tall man plops himself in the seat directly in front of you. Try as you might, you cannot see the screen.

a. You say in a very loud voice: "Dang it, there's a whole theater and he has to sit right in front of us!"	1	2	3	4
b. You yell directly at the man, saying, "Can't you go sit somewhere else? I can't see!"	1	2	3	4
c. You tap the man on the shoulder and say, "Excuse me. I wonder if you could slide down a seat. I can't see."	1	2	3	4
d. You calmly nudge your friend and decide to get up and move.	1	2	3	4
e. You aren't bothered by the person in front of you; this is just part of going to the movies and no big deal.	1	2	3	4

Multiple Scenarios

a. Your sister calls out of the blue and starts to tell you how much you mean to her. Uncomfortable, you change the subject without expressing what you feel.	1	2	3	4
b. You come home to find the kitchen looking like a disaster area and your spouse/roommate lounging in front of the TV. You tense up and can't seem to shake your anger, but you decide not to bring it up.	1	2	3	4
c. Faced with a public speaking event, you get keyed up and lose sleep for a day or more, worrying about how you'll do.	1	2	3	4

(continued on page 76)

d. Your boyfriend/girlfriend/partner is seen out with another person and appears to be acting quite "close" to the person. You are a trusting person and decide not to worry about it. If your significant other has anything to tell you, you know that he/she will talk to you.

1	2	3	4

e. You aren't able to study as much as you'd like for an exam, yet you think that you really "nailed" the exam after you have taken it. When you get it back, you find that you actually did horribly. You make an appointment to talk with the professor and determine what you can do to improve on the next exam. You acknowledge that you are responsible for the low grade this time, but vow to do better next time. You are disappointed, but don't let it bother you.

1	2	3	4

Analyzing This Section:

Look carefully at each of these scenarios. Obviously, none of us is perfect and we sometimes react in ways that we later regret. The key here is to assess how you react the majority of the time.

If stressful events occur and you are able to remain calm, not experience increases in heart rate or blood pressure, and avoid outward displays or inner signs of anxiety, anger, or frustration, you are probably a cool reactor, someone who tends to roll with the punches when a situation is out of your control. This is usually indicative of a good level of coping and overall, this type of person will suffer fewer health consequences when stressed. The key here is that you really are not stressed and really are calm and unworried about the situation.

If you are the type who frets and stews about a stressor, can't sleep, or tends to react by hostile confrontation, anger, or other negative physiological overreactions, you probably are a hot reactor, someone who responds to mildly stressful situations with a "fight-or-flight" adrenaline rush that drives up blood pressure and can lead to heart rhythm disturbances, accelerated clotting, and damaged blood vessel linings. Some hot reactors can seem cool as a cucumber on the outside, but inside their bodies are silently killing them. They may be on edge or jumpy or unable to sleep, even though most people would never suspect that they are in trouble. Before you honk or make obscene gestures at the guy who cuts you off in rush hour traffic, remember that getting angry can destroy thousands of heart muscle cells within minutes. Robert S. Eliot, author of *From Stress to Strength,* says hot reactors have no choice but to calm themselves down with rational thought. Look at ways to change your perceptions and cope more effectively. Ponder the fact that the only thing you'll hasten by reacting is a decline in health. "You have to stop trying to change the world," Eliot advises, "and learn to change your response to it."

throughout the term, your behaviors are inconsistent with your goals, and significant stress in the form of guilt, last-minute frenzy before exams, and disappointing grades may result. On the other hand, if you want to dig in and work and are committed to getting good grades, this may eliminate much of your negative stress. Thwarted goals can lead to frustration, and frustration has been shown to be a significant disrupter of homeostasis.

Determining whether behaviors are consistent with goals is an essential component of maintaining balance in life. If we consciously strive to attain our goals in a direct manner, we greatly improve our chances of success.

Conflict   Conflict occurs when we are forced to make difficult decisions concerning two or more competing motives, behaviors, or impulses or when we are forced to face incompatible demands, opportunities, needs, or goals.[20] What if your best friends all choose to smoke marijuana and you don't want to smoke but fear rejection? Conflict often occurs as our values are tested. College students who are away from home for the first time often face conflict between parental values and their own set of developing beliefs.

Overload   Excessive time pressure, too much responsibility, high expectations of yourself and those around you, and lack of support can lead to **overload,** a state of being overburdened. Have you ever felt you had so many responsibilities that you couldn't possibly begin to fulfill them all? Have you longed for a weekend when you could just take time out with friends and not feel guilty? These feelings are symptoms of overload. Students suffering from overload may experience anxiety about tests, poor self-concept, a desire to drop classes or drop out of school, and other problems. In severe cases, in which they are unable to see any solutions to their problems, students may suffer from depression or turn to substance abuse.

Burnout People who regularly suffer from overload, frustration, and disappointment may eventually experience **burnout,** a state of physical and mental exhaustion caused by excessive stress. People involved in the "helping professions," such as teaching, social work, drug counseling, nursing, and psychology, experience high levels of burnout, as do people such as police officers and air-traffic controllers who work in high-pressure, dangerous jobs.

Other Forms of Psychosocial Stress Other forms of psychosocial stress include problems with overcrowding, discrimination, and socioeconomic difficulties such as unemployment and poverty. People of different ages or ethnic backgrounds may face a disproportionately heavy impact from these sources of stress. In addition to all of these we face increasing threats from technological stressors. For more information see the New Horizons in Health Box.

What do you think?

Think about the changes that you have made during the past couple of years. Which of them would you regard as positive? ❋ Negative? How did you react to these changes initially? ❋ Did your reactions change later? ❋ What are the biggest and most important changes that students must make as they enter colleges and universities, and what can they do to cope with unexpected changes?

Stress and "Isms"

Today's racially and ethnically diverse group of students, faculty members, and staff enriches everyone's educational experience yet also challenges everyone to deal with differences. Students come to the campus from vastly different contexts and life experiences. Often, those who act, speak, dress, or appear "different" face additional pressures that do not affect students considered more "typical." Students perceived as "different" may become victims of subtle and not-so-subtle forms of bigotry, insensitivity, harassment, or hostility. Race, ethnicity, religious affiliation, age, sexual orientation, or other *"isms"*—different viewpoints and backgrounds—may hang like a dark cloud over these students.[21]

Evidence of the health effects of excessive stress abound in the general population. Black Americans suffer higher rates of hypertension, CVD, and most forms of cancer than their white counterparts do. Gay men and lesbians have higher rates of suicide and are more likely to become victims of violent acts. Although poverty and socioeconomic status have been blamed for much of the spike in hypertension rates for African Americans and other marginalized groups, this chronic, physically debilitating stress may reflect real and perceived status in society more than actual poverty. Feeling that they occupy a position of low status, either due

to living conditions, financial security, or job status, can be a source of stress. The problem is exacerbated for those who are socially disadvantaged early in life and grow up without a nurturing environment. Many believe that stressors for ethnic minority students may contribute to a wide range of difficulties on Colleges campuses.[22]

Imagine what it would be like to come to campus and find yourself isolated, lacking friends, and ridiculed on the basis of who you are or how you look. Even worse, consider the fate of students such as Matthew Shepard, the young student in Wyoming who was brutally murdered for being gay, or countless other students who have been victimized because of race, nationality, or religious affiliation. They must deal with hidden fears, suffering, and difficulties caused by intolerant factions on campus in addition to "making the grade" in classes. (Chapter 4 focuses on violence and its incidence and prevalence on campus.)

Environmental Stress

Environmental stress results from events occurring in the physical environment as opposed to social surroundings. Environmental stressors include natural disasters, such as floods and hurricanes, and industrial disasters, such as chemical spills and explosions. Often as damaging as one-time disasters are **background distressors,** such as noise, air, and water pollution, although we may be unaware of them, and their effects may not become apparent for decades. As with other distressors, our bodies respond to environmental distressors with the general adaptation syndrome. People who cannot escape background distressors may exist in a constant resistance phase, which can contribute to the development of stress-related disorders.

Self-Imposed Stress

Self-Concept and Stress The **cognitive stress system** is the psychological system that governs our responses to stressors.[23] The cognitive stress system helps us recognize stressors; evaluate them on the basis of self-concept, past experiences, and emotions; and make decisions regarding how to cope with them.

Overload A condition in which a person feels overly pressured by demands.

Burnout Physical and mental exhaustion caused by excessive stress.

Background distressors Environmental stressors of which people are often unaware.

Cognitive stress system The psychological system that governs emotional responses to stress.

Taming Technostress

Telephones that ring constantly; VCRs that you can't program; e-mail lists that grow on your desktop like an out-of-control fungus; laptop computers that somehow end up in your luggage when you go on vacation; electronic organizers that beep during dinner or at the movies; voice message systems that don't allow you to talk to a live person; busy signals as you try to get on the Internet; and slow, slow, slow downloading of information. Can you feel your heart rate speeding up just thinking about these situations?

If you are like millions of other people today, you find that technology is often a daily terrorizer that raises your blood pressure, frustrates you, and prevents you from ever really "getting away from it all." In short, you may unknowingly be a victim of stressors that previous generations only dreamed (or had nightmares) about. Known as *technostress,* this problem is defined as "personal stress generated by reliance on technological devices, . . . a panicky feeling when they fail, and a state of near-constant stimulation, or being perpetually 'plugged in.'" When technostress grabs you, it may interact with other forms of stress to create a synergistic, never-ending form of stimulation that keeps your stress response reverberating all day.

Part of the problem, ironically, is that technology enables us to be so productive. Because it encourages polyphasic activity, or "multitasking," people are forced to juggle multiple thoughts and actions at the same time, such as driving while talking on cell phones or checking handheld devices for appointments. There is clear evidence that such multitasking contributes to auto accidents and other harmful consequences. What is less clear is what happens to someone who never takes downtime and is always plugged in.

What are the symptoms of technology overload? It evokes typical stress responses by increasing heart rate and blood pressure and causing irritability and memory disturbances. Over time, many stressed-out people lose the ability to relax and find that they feel nervous and anxious when they are supposed to be having fun. Headaches, stomach and digestive problems, skin irritations, more colds than usual, difficulty in wound healing, lack of sleep, ulcers, and a host of other problems may result. A study conducted by Yale University indicates that chronic stress may even thicken the waistline; increased secretions of cortisol caused even slender women to store more fat in the abdomen.

Tips for Fighting Technostress

- Exercise. Get away from any form of technology. Quiet walks or runs away from the blare of music and the sound of machines (typical in fitness centers) are best. Try to find a place that has few people and little noise—that usually means outdoors.
- Become aware of what you are doing. Log the time you spend on e-mail, voice mail, and so on. Set up a schedule to limit your use of technology. For example, limit all e-mail responses to two to three lines. Spend no more than a half-hour per day answering e-mails.
- Set up strict rules for when you can log on, and don't log on at other times.
- Give yourself more time for everything you do. If you are surfing the web for resources for a term paper, start early rather than the night before the paper is due.
- Manage the telephone—don't let it manage you. Rather than interrupting what you're doing to answer, screen calls with an answering machine. Get rid of call waiting, which forces you to juggle multiple calls, and subscribe to a voice-mail service that takes messages when you're on the phone.
- Set "time out" periods. During these times, don't answer the phone, listen to the stereo, or turn on the computer or TV. Switch off e-mail notification systems so you aren't beeped during these periods.

- Take regular breaks. Even when working, get up, walk around, stretch, do deep breathing, or get a glass of water every hour or so.
- If you are working on the computer, look away from the screen and focus on something far away every 30 minutes or so. Stretch your shoulders and neck periodically as you work. Playing soft background music can help you relax.
- Resist the urge to buy the newest and fastest technology. Such purchases not only cause financial stress but also add to stress levels due to the typical glitches that occur when installing and adjusting to new software.
- Do not take laptops, handheld devices, or other technological gadgets on vacation. If you must take a cell phone for emergencies, turn it and your voice messaging system off, and use the phone only in true emergencies.
- Back up materials on your computer at regular intervals. Writing a term paper only to lose it during a power outage will send you into hyperstress very quickly.

Sources: "Taming Technostress" from *TechnoStress: Coping with Technology@Work@Home@Play* by Dr. Larry D. Rosen and Dr. Michelle M. Weil. Copyright © 1997. Material used by permission of John Wiley & Sons, Inc.; Yale University, "Stress May Cause Excess Abdominal Fat in Otherwise Slender Women, Study Conducted at Yale Shows," *ScienceDaily Magazine,* November 23, 2000 (see http://www.sciencedaily.com /print/2000/11/001120072314.htm); "Are You a Slave to the Telephone?" MayoClinic.com, November 1, 2000 (see http://www.mayoclinic.com).

Sensory organs serve as input channels for information reaching the brain. From that point on, attention to the problem, memory, reasoning processes, and problem solving are organized in various parts of the brain. This occurs before we act on the stressor. Because learning and memory involve the changing of various proteins in brain neurons, the emotions experienced during the stress response also "tickle" the memory storage neurons and contribute to responses. Behaviorally, we will respond to the stressor in ways consistent with our memories of similar situations.

Self-esteem is closely related to the emotions engendered by past experiences. Low self-esteem can lead to helpless anger. People suffering helpless anger have usually learned that they are wrong to feel anger, so instead of expressing it in healthy ways they turn it inward. They may "swallow" their rage in food, alcohol, or other drugs, or act in other self-destructive ways. Donna Shalala, former U.S. Secretary of Health and Human Services, has instituted a program called "Girl Power," designed to improve the self-esteem of young women between the ages of 9 and 14, a time when low self-esteem is thought to trigger a host of negative health behaviors.

Research indicates that self-esteem significantly affects various disease processes. People with low self-esteem create a self-imposed distressor that can depress the immune system and increase the symptoms of diseases such as acquired immune deficiency syndrome (AIDS), herpes, multiple sclerosis, and Epstein-Barr syndrome.

Personality Types and Hardiness

A person's personality may contribute to the kind and degree of self-imposed stress he or she experiences. The coronary disease–prone personality was first described in 1974 by physicians Meyer Friedman and Ray Rosenman.[24] They identified two stress-related personality types: Type A and Type B. Type A personalities are hard-driving, competitive, anxious, time-driven, impatient, angry, and perfectionistic. Type B personalities are relaxed and noncompetitive. According to Rosenman and Friedman, people with Type A characteristics are more prone to heart attacks than their Type B counterparts.

Researchers today believe that more needs to be discovered about personality types before we can say that all Type A's have greater risks for heart disease. First of all, most people are not one personality type all the time. Second, many other unexplained variables must be explored, such as why some Type A people seem to thrive in stress-filled environments. Sometimes labeled Type C personalities (not to be confused with the cancer-prone Type C discussed in Chapter 2), these individuals appear to succeed more often than Type B personalities. They enjoy good overall health even while displaying Type A patterns of behavior.

Critics argue that these attempts to base ill health on personal behavioral patterns are crude. For example, researchers at Duke University contend that the Type A personality may be more complex than previously described. They have identified a "toxic core" in some Type A personalities.

People who have this toxic core are angry, distrustful of others, and have above-average levels of cynicism. People who are angry and hostile often have below-average levels of social support and other increased risks for ill health. It may be this toxic core rather than the hard-driving nature of the Type A personality that makes people more vulnerable to self-imposed stress.[25]

According to psychologist Susanne Kobasa, **psychological hardiness** may negate self-imposed stress associated with Type A behavior. Psychologically hardy people are characterized by *control, commitment,* and *challenge.*[26] People with a sense of control are able to accept responsibility for their behaviors and change behaviors that they discover to be debilitating. People with a sense of commitment have good self-esteem and understand their purpose in life. People with a sense of challenge see changes in life as stimulating opportunities for personal growth.

Since some Type A behavior is "learned," it can be modified. Some Type A people are able to slow down and become more tolerant, patient, and better humored. Unfortunately, many people do not decide to modify their Type A habits until after they become ill or suffer a heart attack. Prevention of heart and circulatory disorders resulting from stress entails recognizing and changing dangerous behaviors before damage is done.

Self-Efficacy and Control

Whether people cope successfully with stressful situations often depends on their level of self-efficacy, their level of situational control or belief in their skills and performance abilities.[27] If people have been successful in mastering similar problems in the past, they will be more likely to believe in their own effectiveness. Similarly, people who have repeatedly tried and failed may lack confidence in their abilities to deal with life's problems. In some cases, this insecurity may prevent them from trying to cope.

In addition, people who believe they lack control in a situation may become easily frustrated and give up. Those who feel they have no personal control tend to have an *external locus of control* and a low level of self-efficacy. People who are confident their behavior will influence the outcome tend to have an *internal locus of control.* Individuals who feel that they have limited control over their lives often have higher levels of stress. As Americans recoiled from the terrorist attack of September 11, 2001, many felt that society was "out of control." The resulting post-traumatic stress is discussed in the Health in a Diverse World box.

> **Psychological hardiness** A personality trait characterized by control, commitment, and challenge

Post-Traumatic Stress: The Aftermath of Terror

For many of us, the vivid images of the planes hitting the World Trade Center Towers on September 11, 2001, will be etched in our memory for the rest of our lives. Anger, horror, frustration, and a host of other emotions brought tears, stomach upset, and other bodily ills to those of us who sat helplessly watching the events following the attack. As horrible as this experience was for those who sat watching, the real trauma for those who lost loved ones, coworkers, and friends may have only begun.

Post-traumatic stress disorder (PTSD) is an acute stress disorder with extreme anxiety and behavioral disturbances that develops within the first hours or days after a traumatic event. Typically, persons suffering from PTSD have been soldiers returning from witnessing the atrocities of war, particularly those who saw friends killed or mangled or who experienced terrible suffering and pain themselves. Many of these soldiers continued to suffer from these experiences for decades afterward.

Other extreme traumatic events include rape or other severe physical attacks, near-death experiences in accidents, witnessing a murder or death, street crime or assault, being caught in a natural disaster, or being a victim of terrorist attacks such as the Oklahoma City bombing in the mid 1990s. Typical symptoms of PTSD include the following:

- *Dissociation*, or perceived detachment of the mind from the emotional state or even the body. In dissociation, the person may have a sense of the world as a dreamlike or unreal place and have poor memory of the events—a form of *dissociative amnesia*.
- *Acute anxiety* or nervousness, in which the person is hyperaroused, may cry easily or experience mood swings, and may experience flashbacks, nightmares, and recurrent thoughts or visual images. The sufferer may sense vague uneasiness or feel like the event is happening again and again. Some may experience intense physiological reactions, such as shaking or nausea when something reminds them of the events. In some cases, they may have difficulty returning to areas that remind them of the trauma. For example, persons experiencing PTSD related to the Pentagon and World Trade Center attacks may be unable to work in tall buildings, have difficulty getting on a plane, or feel acutely afraid when they hear planes flying overhead.
- *Persistent stress symptoms:* Sufferers may have two or more of these symptoms:
  - Difficulty falling or staying asleep.
  - Irritability or outbursts of anger or other emotions.
  - Difficulty concentrating.
  - Hypervigilance.
  - Exaggerated startle response.

If these symptoms last more than one month, post-traumatic stress disorder may be diagnosed, either as an *acute form* (less than three months in duration), or a *chronic form* (longer than three months).

A *delayed onset* form of PTSD may appear months after the event. In most people, symptoms disappear within six months.

Although exact figures for this illness may never be known, the National Institutes of Health indicates that as many as 5 to 8 percent of the American public may have chronic forms of post-traumatic stress, with the prevalence among women being almost twice that among men. Victims of rape and torture as well as concentration camp survivors have historically been among those most likely to have problems.

Therapies designed to help trauma victims recover are increasingly effective as our knowledge about this disorder grows. Schools, communities, and workplaces now routinely bring in crisis experts immediately after an event to help survivors talk through their feelings and gain support from others. A supportive family, employer, and friends and access to professional counseling are important in the recovery process. New generations of anti-anxiety drugs can help individuals who have difficulties. Sleep aids and other options are also available to ease short-term symptoms.

Sources: Posttraumatic Stress Disorder Society (see http://www.mentalhealth.com/dis1/p21-an06.html); *Mental Health: A Report to the Surgeon General* (see http://www.surgeongeneral.gov/library/mentalhealth/chapter4/sec2.html).

Stress and the College Student

College students experience numerous distressors, including changes related to being away from home for the first time, pressure to make friends in a new and sometimes intimidating setting, the feeling of anonymity imposed by large classes, and test-taking anxiety (see the Skills for Behavior Change box).

College students may be especially vulnerable because they are in a period of transition, facing several key developmental tasks: (1) achieving emotional independence from family; (2) choosing and preparing for a career; (3) preparing for a relationship, commitment, and/or family life; and (4) developing an ethical system. These tasks require that the college student develop new social roles and modify old ones, changes that can result in role strain, a major aspect of chronic stress.

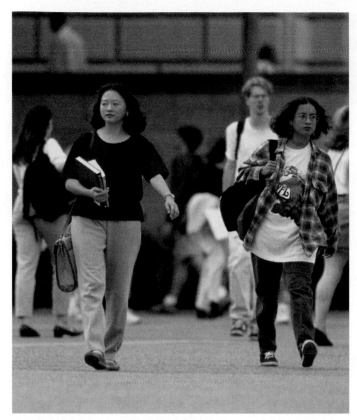

College can be a stressful time for students, whether they are young people choosing a career path or older adults returning to school to change directions later in life.

In a large study of chronic stressors, male and female college students differed significantly in the things they perceived to be significant stressors.[28] Women indicated that (1) trying to diet, (2) being overweight, (3) having an overload of schoolwork, and (4) gaining weight were among their most frequent stressors. Men, on the other hand, tended to list the following items as major stressors: (1) being underweight, (2) problems relating to commuting to school, (3) not having someone to date, (4) not enough sex, (5) being behind in schoolwork, (6) not enough friends, and (7) concerns about drug or alcohol use.[29]

Most colleges offer stress management workshops through health centers or student counseling departments. You should not ignore the symptoms of stress overload. If you experience one or more of the following symptoms, act promptly to reduce their impact:

- Difficulty keeping up with classes or difficulty concentrating on and finishing tasks.
- Frequent clashes with close friends, family, or intimate partners about trivial issues such as personal habits, appearance, and housekeeping.
- Persistent hostile or angry feelings; increased frustration with minor annoyances.
- Increased boredom and fatigue; a general sense of "the blahs."
- Disinterest in social activities or tendency to avoid others.

- Increased use of alcohol or other drugs.
- Sleep disturbances, problems with eating.
- Difficulty in maintaining an intimate relationship.
- Disinterest in sexual relationships or inability to participate in satisfactory sexual relationships.
- Frequent headaches, backaches, muscle aches, or tightness in the stomach.
- Problems making decisions; increased procrastination.
- Frequent indigestion, diarrhea, or urination.
- Frequent colds and infections.
- Tendency to be intolerant of minor differences of opinion.
- Hunger and cravings or tendency to overeat or to eat while thinking of other things.
- Inability to listen or tendency to jump from subject to subject in conversation.
- Stuttering or other speech difficulties.
- Becoming prone to accidents.

Managing Your Stress

In addition to creating stressful situations, college gives you the opportunity to evaluate and change how you manage stress. Stress can be challenging or debilitating, depending upon how we view it. The most effective way to avoid problems is to learn a number of skills known collectively as *stress management*.

Building Skills for Stress Reduction

Dealing with stress involves assessing all aspects of a stressor, examining your response and how you can change it, and learning to cope with it. Often we cannot change the requirements at our college, assignments in class, or unexpected distressors. Inevitably, we will be stuck in classes that bore us and for which we find no application in real life. We feel powerless when a loved one dies. Although the facts cannot be changed, we can change our reactions to these distressors.

Assessing Your Stressors After recognizing a stressor, evaluate it. Can you alter the circumstances to reduce the amount of distress you are experiencing, or must you change your behavior and reactions to reduce stress levels? For example, if five term papers for five different courses are due during the semester, your professors are unlikely to drop such requirements. You can, however, change your behavior by beginning the papers early and spacing them over time to avoid last-minute stress.

Changing Your Responses Changing your responses requires practice and emotional control. If your roommate is habitually messy and this causes you stress, you can choose among several responses. You can express your anger by yelling, you can pick up the mess and leave a nasty note, or you can defuse the situation with humor. The first reaction

Overcoming Test-Taking Anxiety

Doing well on a test is an ability needed far beyond college. Many careers require special exams. Tests are a fact of life in government, insurance, medicine, and other fields. And stress is a fact of tests!

But there are things you can do to get the upper hand on your anxiety. Here are some helpful hints to try on your next exam.

Before the Exam

1. Manage your time. Plan to start studying a week before your test (longer if it's a career exam). The more advance studying, the less anxiety you will feel. The final night should be limited to review. Arrive at the test a half-hour early for a final run-through. You will find that this will ease your anxiety and increase your confidence.

2. Build your test-taking self-esteem. First, take a three-by-five-inch card and write down the three reasons you will pass the exam. Carry the card with you and look at it whenever you study. Second, when you get the test, write your three reasons on the test or on a piece of scrap paper. Positive affirmations such as this will help you succeed.

3. Get adequate sleep. You need to be alert, so get a little extra sleep for a few nights before your exam.

4. Eat a balanced meal before the exam. Sugar doesn't give you energy—in fact, it tires you. Avoid rich or heavy foods (they'll make you sleepy) as well as foods that might upset your stomach. You want to feel your best.

5. Take a moderate amount of caffeine an hour before the test. Research shows that caffeine promotes alertness, motor performance, and the capacity for work, as well as decreases fatigue. A cup of coffee, tea, or a cola drink is sufficient. Be aware, though, that some people shouldn't use caffeine. Avoid it if it makes you feel shaky or if you do not regularly consume it. Test day is not the day to find our how your body reacts to caffeine.

During the Test

1. Use time management during the test. If you have 60 minutes to answer 30 multiple-choice questions, you might decide to spend the first 45 minutes taking the test (1 1/2 minutes per question) and 15 minutes reviewing your answers (30 seconds per question). Hold yourself to this schedule. After 15 minutes, you should have completed the first 10 questions. If you don't know an answer or the question is taking too long, skip it and move on. Since you allotted yourself time at the end to review, you will be able to go back.

Test makers usually allow sufficient time to complete and review a test. However, if you feel that you are a slow reader and need more time, talk to your teacher or test administrator before the exam.

2. Slow down. When you open your test book, always write RTFQ (Read the Full Question) at the top. Make sure you understand the question before answering.

3. Stay on track. If you begin to get anxious, reread your three reasons for success.

---

that comes to mind is not always the best. Stop before reacting to gain the time you need to find an appropriate response. Ask yourself, "What is to be gained from my response?"

Many people change their responses to potentially stressful events through *cognitive coping strategies*. These strategies help them prepare for stressors through gradual exposure to increasingly higher stress levels.

Stress inoculation Newer stress management technique in which a person consciously tries to prepare ahead of time for potential stressors.

Downshifting Conscious attempt to simplify life in an effort to reduce the stresses and strains of modern living.

Learning to Cope Everyone copes with stress in different ways. Some people drink or take drugs, others seek help from counselors, and still others try to forget about it or engage in positive activities such as exercise. **Stress inoculation,** one of the newer coping techniques, helps people prepare for stressful events ahead of time. For example, suppose you are petrified over speaking in front of a class. Practicing in front of friends or in front of a video camera are strategies that may inoculate and prevent your freezing up on the day of the presentation. Some health experts compare stress inoculation to a vaccine given to protect against a disease. Regardless of how you cope with a situation, your conscious effort to deal with it is an important step in stress management.

Downshifting More and more people recognize that today's lifestyle is hectic and pressure-packed, and much of their stress comes from trying to keep up. Many also question whether "having it all" is worth it. In recent years, a number of top executives have said "enough" and have voluntarily left high-paying jobs to lead a simpler life. While you may argue that it is easy to lead a simple life with a large bank account, the truth is that people of all walks of life are taking a step back and simplifying their lives. They are following a trend known as **downshifting.** Moving from a large urban area to the country or to small towns, buying a smaller house, exchanging the expensive SUV for a run-of-the-mill four-door sedan, and a host of other changes in lifestyle typify this move. Some dedicated downshifters have given up television, microwaves, phones, and even computers.

This trend toward simplicity was promoted by Henry David Thoreau in the nineteenth century, but for years it has been seen as an eccentric battle against machines or part of a back-to-nature movement. In recent years, however, the idea has become more mainstream. Large numbers of people indicate that they would give up their current lifestyles for a return to simpler times and as many are already trying to do so. In fact, consultants who once coached clients on getting ahead now run programs that teach them how to be satisfied with less. Self-help books, newsletters, and networking groups all pitch the simpler life.

Downshifting involves a fundamental shift in values and honest introspection about what is important in life. When considering any form of downshifting or perhaps even starting your career this way, it's important to move slowly and consider the following:

- *Determine your ultimate goal.* What is most important to you, and what will you need to reach that goal? What can you do without? Where do you want to live?
- *Make a short-term and long-term plan for simplifying your life.* Set up your plan in doable steps, and work slowly toward each. Begin saying no to requests for your time, and determine those people with whom it is important for you to spend time.
- *Complete a financial inventory.* How much money will you need to do the things you want to do? Pay off credit cards and eliminate existing debt, or consider debt consolidation. Get used to paying with cash. If you don't have the cash, don't buy. Will you rent or buy a home? With what kind of car could you get by?
- *Plan for health care costs.* Make sure that you budget for health insurance and basic preventive health services. This should be a top priority.
- *Select the right career.* Look for work that you enjoy and that isn't necessarily driven by salary. Can you be happy taking a lower-paying job that is less stressful and allows you the opportunity to have a life?
- *Consider options for saving money.* Downshifting doesn't mean you renounce money; it means you choose not to let money dictate your life. It's still important to save. If you're just getting started, you need to prepare for emergencies and for future plans. Avoid compulsive buying, and consider living with others to share the costs.

- *Clear out/clean out.* A cluttered life can be distressing. Take an inventory of material items and get rid of things you haven't worn or used in the last year. Donate items to charity groups. Clean as you go, and get rid of the frills.

Managing Emotional Responses

Have you ever gotten all worked up about something only to find that your perceptions were totally wrong? We often get upset not by realities but by our faulty perceptions. For example, suppose you found out that everyone except you is invited to a party. You might easily begin to wonder why you were excluded. Does someone dislike you? Have you offended someone? Such thoughts are typical. However, the reality of the situation may have absolutely nothing to do with your being liked or disliked. Perhaps you were sent an invitation and it didn't get to you.

Stress management requires that you examine your *self-talk* and your emotional responses to interactions with others. With any emotional response to a distressor, you are responsible for the emotion and the behaviors elicited by the emotion. Learning to tell the difference between normal emotions and those based on irrational beliefs can help you either stop the emotion or express it in a healthy and appropriate way.

Learning to Laugh and Cry Have you noticed that you feel better after a good laugh or cry? It isn't your imagination. Laughter and crying stimulate the heart and temporarily rev up many body systems. Heart rate and blood pressure then decrease significantly, allowing the body to relax.

Fighting the Anger Urge

Although much has been said about how hotheaded, short-fused people are at risk for health problems, recent research provides even more compelling reasons to "chill out." Stress hormones released during anger may constrict blood vessels in the heart or actually promote clot formation, which can cause a heart attack.

Anger results when differences occur between our wants, desires, and dreams and what we actually "get" in life. People who spend all their emotional energy in a quest for justice or grow frustrated over events that seem impossible to change can become driven by anger. Because anger triggers the fight-or-flight reaction, these people operate with the stress response turned on long after it should have dissipated.

Angry individuals typically display cynicism, a brooding, hypercritical view of their world. Like angry people, cynical individuals keep fight-or-flight reactions reverberating through their bodies indefinitely. Often labeled as "hostile," these chronically stressed folks frequently have weakened immune responses and increased risk of disease. Counseling designed to determine the underlying cause of anger and deal with related issues can be effective. See Figure 3.3 for strategies to control and redirect anger.

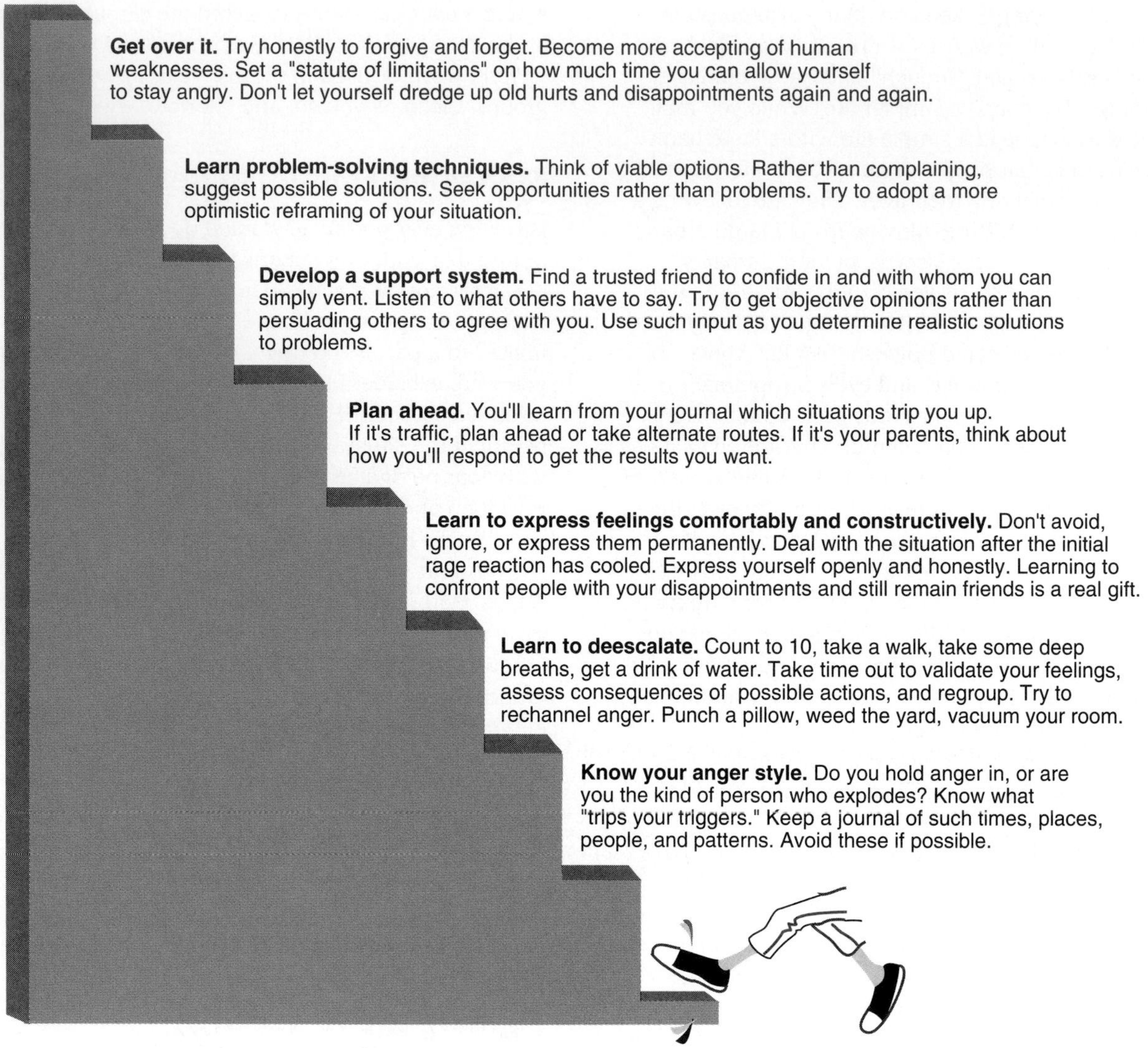

Get over it. Try honestly to forgive and forget. Become more accepting of human weaknesses. Set a "statute of limitations" on how much time you can allow yourself to stay angry. Don't let yourself dredge up old hurts and disappointments again and again.

Learn problem-solving techniques. Think of viable options. Rather than complaining, suggest possible solutions. Seek opportunities rather than problems. Try to adopt a more optimistic reframing of your situation.

Develop a support system. Find a trusted friend to confide in and with whom you can simply vent. Listen to what others have to say. Try to get objective opinions rather than persuading others to agree with you. Use such input as you determine realistic solutions to problems.

Plan ahead. You'll learn from your journal which situations trip you up. If it's traffic, plan ahead or take alternate routes. If it's your parents, think about how you'll respond to get the results you want.

Learn to express feelings comfortably and constructively. Don't avoid, ignore, or express them permanently. Deal with the situation after the initial rage reaction has cooled. Express yourself openly and honestly. Learning to confront people with your disappointments and still remain friends is a real gift.

Learn to deescalate. Count to 10, take a walk, take some deep breaths, get a drink of water. Take time out to validate your feelings, assess consequences of possible actions, and regroup. Try to rechannel anger. Punch a pillow, weed the yard, vacuum your room.

Know your anger style. Do you hold anger in, or are you the kind of person who explodes? Know what "trips your triggers." Keep a journal of such times, places, people, and patterns. Avoid these if possible.

Figure 3.3
Steps in Anger Control

Source: Adapted from Brian L. Seaward. 1999. *Managing Stress,* Jones and Barlett. pp. 97–99.

Taking Mental Action

Stress management calls for mental action in two areas. First, positive self-esteem, which can help you cope with stressful situations, comes from learned habits. Successful stress management involves mentally developing and practicing self-esteem skills.

Second, because you can't always anticipate what the next distressor will be, you need to develop the mental skills necessary to manage your reactions to stresses after they have occurred. The ability to think about and react quickly to stress comes with time, practice, experience with a variety of stressful situations, and patience.

Changing the Way You Think Once you realize that some of your thoughts may be irrational or overreactive, make a conscious effort to adjust your thinking, reframe or change the way you've been thinking, and focus on more positive patterns. Here are specific actions you can take to develop these mental skills:

• *Worry constructively.* Don't waste time and energy worrying about things you can't change or events that may never happen.

• *Look at life as being fluid.* If you accept that change is a natural part of living and growing, the jolt of changes may become less stressful.

• *Consider alternatives.* Remember that there is seldom only one appropriate action. Anticipating options will help you plan for change and adjust more rapidly.

• *Moderate expectations.* Aim high, but be realistic about your circumstances and motivation.

- *Weed out trivia.* Cardiologist Robert Eliot offers two rules for coping with life's challenges: (1) "Don't sweat the small stuff," and (2) remember that "it's all small stuff."[30]
- *Don't rush into action.* Think before you act.

Taking Physical Action

Physical activities can complement the emotional and mental strategies of stress management.

Exercise Exercise reduces stress by raising levels of endorphins—mood-elevating, pain-killing hormones—in the bloodstream. As a result, exercise increases energy, reduces hostility, and improves mental alertness.

Most of us have relieved stress by engaging in aggressive physical activity: chopping wood when we are angry is one example. Exercise performed as an immediate response can help alleviate stress symptoms. However, a regular exercise program yields even more substantial benefits. Try to engage in at least 25 minutes of aerobic exercise three or four times a week. But even simply walking up stairs, parking farther away from your destination, or standing rather than sitting helps to conserve and replenish your adaptive energy stores. Although it may not improve your aerobic capacity, a quiet walk alone or with friends can refresh your mind and calm your stress response. Plan walking breaks with friends. Stretch after prolonged periods of study at your desk. A short period of physical exercise may provide the break you really need. For more information on the beneficial effects of exercise, see Chapter 10.

Relaxation Like exercise, relaxation can help you cope with stressful feelings, preserve adaptation energy stores, dissipate excess hormones associated with GAS, and refocus your energies. Practice relaxation daily until it becomes a habit. You will probably find that you enjoy it.

Once you have learned simple relaxation techniques, you can use them at any time—during a difficult exam or stressful confrontation, for example. If you're facing a tough exam, for example, choose to relax before it or at intervals during it. You can also use relaxation techniques when you face stressful confrontations or assignments. As your body relaxes, your heart rate slows, your blood pressure and metabolic rate decrease, and many other body-calming effects occur, allowing you to channel energy appropriately.

Eating Right Is food really a destressor? Whether foods can calm us and nourish our psyches is a controversial question. Much of what has been published about hyperactivity and its relation to the consumption of candy and other sweets has been shown to be scientifically invalid. High-potency stress-tabs that are supposed to boost resistance against stress-related ailments are nothing more than gimmicks. But it is clear that eating a balanced, healthful diet will help provide the stamina needed to get through problems and stress-proof you in ways that are not fully understood. It is also known that undereating, overeating, and eating the wrong kinds of foods can create distress in the body. For more information about the benefits of sound nutrition, see Chapter 8.

Managing Your Time

Time. Everybody needs more of it, especially students trying to balance the demands of classes, social life, earning money for school, and family obligations. Include the following time management tips in your stress management program:

- *Take on only one thing at a time.* Don't try to pay bills, clean the bathroom, wash clothes, and write your term paper all at once. Stay focused.
- *Clean off your desk.* According to Jeffrey Mayer, author of *Winning the Fight Between You and Your Desk,* most of us spend many stressful minutes each day looking for things that are lost on our desks or in our homes. Go through the things on your desk, toss the unnecessary papers, and put papers for tasks that you must do in folders.
- *Find a clean, comfortable place to work.* Go somewhere where you won't be distracted.
- *Never handle papers more than once.* When bills and other papers come in, take care of them immediately. Write a check and hold it for mailing. Get rid of the envelopes. Read your mail and file it or toss it. If you haven't looked at something in over a year, toss it.
- *Prioritize your tasks.* Make a daily "to do" list and try to stick to it. Categorize the things you must do today, the things that you have to do but not immediately, and the things that it would be nice to do. Prioritize the *Must Do Now* and *Have to Do Later* items, and put deadlines next to each. Only consider the *Nice to Do* items if you finish the others or if the *Nice to Do* list includes something fun for you. Give yourself a reward as you finish each task.
- *Don't be afraid to say no.* All too often we do things out of fear of what someone may think. Set your school and personal priorities. Please yourself as often as you can.
- *Avoid interruptions.* When you've got a project that requires your total concentration, schedule uninterrupted time. Unplug the phone or let your answering machine get it. Close your door and post a *Do Not Disturb* sign. Go to a quiet room in the library or student union where no one will find you.
- *Reward yourself for being efficient.* You've planned to take a certain amount of time to finish a task and you finish early? Take some time for yourself. Have a cup of coffee or hot chocolate. Go for a walk. Start reading something you've wanted to read but haven't had time for. Differentiate between rest breaks and work breaks. Work breaks simply mean switching tasks for awhile. Rest breaks give you time to yourself. Make sure that your rest breaks help you recharge and refresh your energy levels.
- *Become aware of your own time patterns.* Keep a time journal for one week. For many of us, minutes and hours drift by without our even noticing them. Chart your daily schedule, hour by hour, for one week. Note the time that was wasted

and the time spent in productive work or restorative pleasure. Assess how you could be more productive and make more time for yourself.

• *Use time to your advantage.* If you're a morning person, schedule activities to coincide with when you're at your best. Study and write papers in the morning, and take breaks when you start to slow down. Take a short nap when you need it.

• *Break overwhelming tasks into small pieces, and allocate a certain amount of time to each.* If you are floundering in a task, move on and come back to it when you're refreshed.

• *Remember that time is precious.* Many people learn to value their time only when they face a terminal illness. Try to value each day. Time spent not enjoying life is a tremendous waste of potential.

Can St. John's Wort Relieve Stress?

Do an Internet search for information on "herbs and stress," and you'll get 330,000 hits or more. At least 100,000 of them will mention St. John's Wort, one of the most popular herbal remedies; each year Americans buy more than $210 million worth.

St. John's Wort (*Hypericum perforatum*) is a yellow-flowered plant that contains a number of chemical compounds. For centuries the herb has been used as a sedative, malaria treatment, and pain-soothing balm for wounds, burns, and insect bites. Today it is widely prescribed in Europe as a treatment for depression.

In the United States, the FDA has not approved St. John's Wort for any medicinal purpose. However, advertisements and the popular press tout it to relieve stress, counteract depression, and improve mood. It can be readily purchased over the counter (without a prescription) in capsules, teas, or extracts, and many Americans opt to try it. But does it work? The scientific evidence is mixed:

• Several small studies in Europe have indicated that St. John's Wort might be useful in cases of mild to moderate depression.

• A 1996 *British Medical Journal* review of 23 clinical studies concluded that in treating depression, St. John's Wort was more effective than a placebo (a dummy pill) and had fewer side effects than some prescription antidepressants.

• A 2001 U.S. study, published in the *Journal of the American Medical Association,* found that it was not helpful for depression.

A 2002 U.S. clinical trial, one of the largest studies ever conducted on the herb, concluded that St. John's Wort was less effective than either a placebo or the prescription antidepressant Zoloft. First, researchers confirmed patients' diagnosis using standard measures such as the Hamilton Depression Scale, on which scores of 20 or higher indicate major depression. Then they randomly assigned patients to receive treatment with either the placebo, Zoloft (50 to 100 milligrams per day), or the herb (900 to 1,500 milligrams per day.) After eight weeks, the Hamilton scores of people taking St. John's Wort dropped by an average of only 8.7 points, compared to 9.2 points for the placebo and 10.5 points for Zoloft.

Should you take St. John's Wort if you're feeling down? Not without consulting your doctor first. It's tempting to think that herbal remedies are safe, but this is not always the case. While scientists are not sure how St. John's Wort affects the body, it definitely does: Preliminary studies suggest that it might prevent nerve cells in the brain from reabsorbing the chemical serotonin, or that it might reduce the levels of a protein involved in immune function. Possible side effects include dizziness, dry mouth, gastrointestinal problems, fatigue, and increased sensitivity to sunlight.

Furthermore, St. John's Wort can make other drugs less effective by causing the liver to process them more quickly than normal. Drugs that can be affected include oral contraceptives, antibiotics, cardiovascular medications, asthma drugs, medica-

tions to control HIV infection, and drugs that help prevent the body from rejecting transplanted tissue.

Since herbal remedies are not regulated in the United States, it's difficult to know whether that bottle you're buying actually contains St. John's Wort and if so, how strong it is. Levels of hypericin, the plant's active ingredient, vary widely depending on geography and growing conditions. Much of what's sold in stores is picked wild and contains less hypericin than found in commercially farmed plants. Studies have found significant differences in the amount of hypericin, even in batches produced by the same manufacturer, and package labels are frequently inaccurate.

Sources: National Center for Complementary and Alternative Medicine, National Institutes of Health, "Study Shows St. John's Wort Ineffective for Major Depression of Moderate Severity," April 9, 2002 (see http://nccam.nih.gov/news/2002/stjohnswort/pressrelease.htm); National Center for Complementary and Alternative Medicine, National Institutes of Health, "St. John's Wort and the Treatment of Depression," April 9, 2002 (see http://nccam.nih.gov/health/stjohnswort); Cornell University, "Stress Makes St. John's Wort More Effective," *ScienceDaily Magazine,* September 6, 2000 (see http://www.sciencedaily.com/print/2000/09/000904125730.htm); Duke University Medical Center, "Physicians Present Most Comprehensive Clinical Review of St. John's Wort for Treating Depression," *ScienceDaily Magazine,* January 11, 2001 (see http://www.sciencedaily.com/releases/2001/01/010111073255.htm); Duke University, "St. John's Wort Ineffective for Depression, Study Finds," *ScienceDaily Magazine,* April 10, 2002 (see http://www.sciencedaily.com/releases/2002/04/020410075818.htm).

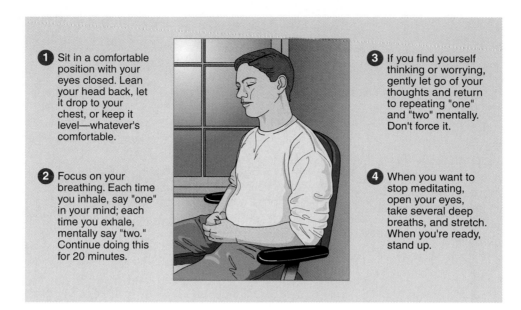

1 Sit in a comfortable position with your eyes closed. Lean your head back, let it drop to your chest, or keep it level—whatever's comfortable.

2 Focus on your breathing. Each time you inhale, say "one" in your mind; each time you exhale, mentally say "two." Continue doing this for 20 minutes.

3 If you find yourself thinking or worrying, gently let go of your thoughts and return to repeating "one" and "two" mentally. Don't force it.

4 When you want to stop meditating, open your eyes, take several deep breaths, and stretch. When you're ready, stand up.

Figure 3.4
A Popular Technique for Meditation

Alternative Stress Management Techniques

Popular "stress fighters" include hypnosis, massage therapy, meditation, and biofeedback. For some people, anti-anxiety medications also serve as a way of controlling stress. See the New Horizon box on St. John's Wort for a discussion of one such medication.

Hypnosis Hypnosis is a process that requires a person to focus on one thought, object, or voice, thereby freeing the right hemisphere of the brain to become more active. The person then becomes unusually responsive to suggestions. Whether self-induced or induced by someone else, hypnosis can reduce certain types of stress.

Massage Therapy If you have ever had someone massage your stiff neck or aching feet, you know that massage is an excellent way to relax. Massage techniques vary from vigorous Swedish massage to the gentler acupressure and Esalen massage. Before selecting a massage therapist, check his or her credentials carefully. The therapist should have training from a reputable program that teaches scientific principles for anatomic manipulation and be certified through the American Massage Therapy Association (AMTA).

Meditation Meditation generally focuses on deep breathing, allowing tension to leave the body with each exhalation. It allows you to get away, to wipe all thoughts out of your mind and turn inward. Practiced by Eastern religions for centuries, meditation is believed to be an important form of personal renewal and introspection. As a stress management tool, it can calm the body and quiet the mind, creating a

sense of peace. There are many different forms of meditation. Most involve sitting quietly for 15 to 20 minutes, focusing on a particular word or symbol, controlling breathing, and getting in touch with the inner self (see Figure 3.4).

Biofeedback Biofeedback involves self-monitoring by machine of physical responses to stress and attempts to control these responses. Perspiration, heart rate, respiration, blood pressure, surface body temperature, muscle tension, and other stress responses are monitored. Then, by trial and error, the person using biofeedback techniques learns to lower his or her stress responses through conscious effort. Eventually, the person develops the ability to lower his or her stress responses at will, without using the machine.

Making the Most of Support Groups

Support groups are an important part of stress management. Friends, family members, and coworkers can provide emotional and physical support. See the Reality Check box for additional information about the beneficial effects of social

Hypnosis A process that allows people to become unusually responsive to suggestion.

Meditation A relaxation technique that involves deep breathing and concentration.

Biofeedback A technique involving machine self-monitoring of physical responses to stress.

Social Connections and Social Support as a Stress Buffer

Although a number of "buffers" may inoculate us from the negative health effects of stress, social support may be more important than all others. Consider the following points, derived from several studies assessing the role of social support and social connections in dealing with stress.

✔ Social environment can have a buffering effect on stress. An example: When a stressor is given to an animal who is alone, its plasma cortisol levels increase by 50 percent; however, when the same stressor is given to an animal surrounded by familiar companions, its plasma cortisol levels do not increase at all.
✔ Being well integrated socially reduces all age-adjusted mortality by a factor of 2, about as much as having low versus high serum cholesterol levels, or being

a smoker versus a nonsmoker. Furthermore, the nature of one's position in the social hierarchy, including relatively higher status within the same social class, has health consequences.
✔ People are statistically more likely to die right after, rather than before, their birthdays and important holidays, as these events include social interactions.
✔ Randomized trials have provided evidence that psychosocial support is associated with longer survival for patients with breast cancer, malignant melanoma, and lymphoma.
✔ Studies looking at the relationship between widowhood (regarded as a high stressor) and depression have found repeatedly that the death of a spouse is more strongly associated with depression among men than women.

How can we explain the final item on the list? Though some argue that men depend more on women for activities of daily living, studies show that widowed men tend to cut off or reduce ties with surviving parents and adult children after

such an event, presumably as they begin to search for a new partner. Women, on the other hand, maintain and in fact increase their social connections during this time, which may serve as a stress buffer.

Sources: From S. Levine, D. M. Lyons, and A. F. Schatzberg, "Psychobiological Consequences of Social Relationships," 1997, *The Annals of the New York Academy of Science* 89 (7), pp. 210–218; M. G. Marmot, R. Fuhrer, S. L. Ettner, N. F. Marks, L. L. Bumpass, and C. D. Ryff, "Contributions of Psychosocial Factors to Socioeconomic Difference in Health," 1998, *Milbank Quarterly* 76, pp. 403–448; D. P. Phillips, T. E. Ruth, and L. M. Wagner, "Psychology and Survival," 1993, *Lancet* 342, pp. 1142–1145; D. Ornish et al., "Intensive Lifestyle Changes for Reversal of Coronary Heart Disease," 1998, *Journal of the American Medical Association* 280, pp. 2001–2007; and D. Spiegel, "Healing Words: Emotional Expression and Disease Outcome," 1999, *Journal of the American Medical Association.*

support. Although the ideal support group differs for each of us, you should have one or two close friends in whom you are able to confide and neighbors with whom you can trade favors. Try to participate in community activities at least once a week. A healthy committed relationship can also provide vital support.

If you do not have a close support group, find out where to turn when the pressures of life seem overwhelming. Family members are often a steady base of support on which you can rely. But if friends or family are unavailable, most colleges and universities have counseling services available at no cost for short-term crises. Clergy, instructors, and dorm supervisors may also be excellent resources. If university services are unavailable or if you are concerned about confidentiality, most communities offer low-cost counseling through mental health clinics.

Developing Your Spiritual Side: Mindfulness

In discussions of spirituality, the concept of mindfulness often emerges. As a meditative technique, mindfulness—the

ability to be fully present in the moment—can aid relaxation, reduce emotional and physical pain, and help us connect more effectively with ourselves, with others, and with nature. The practice of mindfulness includes strategies and activities that contribute to overall health and wellness. In fact, mindfulness and wellness are interconnected and can be developed concurrently, reinforcing each other.

We can think of spirituality as encompassing four dimensions: physical, emotional, social, and intellectual (see Figure 3.5).

The Physical Dimension: Moving in Nature

A delightful way to strengthen the body, build endurance, and bring peace of mind is to interact with the natural environment. Activities such as walking, jogging, biking, and swimming foster this interaction, providing sensory experience (feeling, smelling, touching, listening, and hearing) while strengthening muscles and the cardiovascular system. By focusing on the sounds of birdsong or the crunch of your shoes on freshly fallen snow, you can free yourself of worry or anxious thoughts. Appreciating and absorbing the beauty

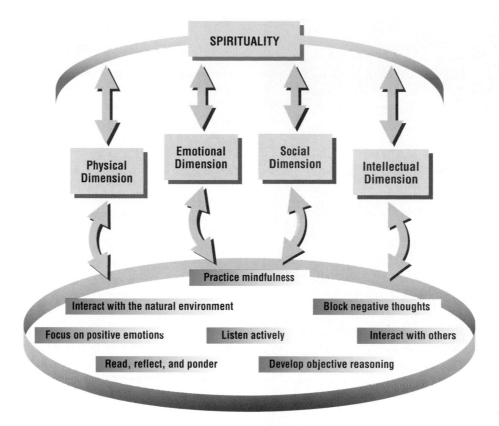

Figure 3.5
Developing Your Spiritual Side

The Emotional Dimension: Dealing with Negative Emotions

Each of us has positive and negative emotions that govern moods and behaviors throughout the day. We often take joy, happiness, and contentment for granted since we tend not to notice the *absence* of stress and distress. However, we typically are aware of negative emotions, such as jealousy, hatred, and anger, because they deplete our energy reserves and cause us problems in interacting with others.

To improve our emotional health and access our spiritual side, we must take notice of the situations that trigger negative emotions, such as anger. (See "Fighting the Anger Urge" earlier in this chapter). Ask yourself these questions:

- What provokes the anger?
- How do you respond to it physiologically? What body parts seem to hold most of the anger?
- Where does your mind focus when angry—on another person or object? On yourself?
- What do you say to yourself when you are angry?

By stopping in the midst of anger and concentrating on physical reactions, we begin to realize the full extent of the dam-age we inflict upon ourselves when we allow negativity to get the best of us. We might ask ourselves, is it worth it? And probably we will conclude: "I don't like allowing this kind of hit on my body. I've got to get a handle on this before I hurt myself or someone else." By practicing thought-stopping, blocking negative thoughts, and focusing on positive emotions via self-talk and other methods of diversion, we can help ourselves through a negative experience.

Just as important as control of negative emotions is the development of spiritual wholeness characterized by faith, hope, and love, the beliefs mentioned in Chapter 2. These beliefs contribute to spiritual growth and lessen the negative effects of stress:

- *Faith* is the belief that helps us realize our purpose in life or the things that are most important to us. It may include faith in a deity, in a particular dogma, or in humanity and the sustaining forces of nature.
- *Hope* is the belief that each of us can look confidently and courageously toward the future. We can easily become trapped in a cynical downhill cycle, focused on the negative and obscuring the positive. By learning to break the negative cycle and cultivate the positive, we will develop our spiritual side more fully.
- *Love* involves accepting, affirming, and respecting ourselves and others, regardless of who they are or how much we might wish them to be different.

The Social Dimension: Interacting, Listening, and Communicating

Developing the spiritual side is not an individual internal process. It is also a social process that enhances relationships with others. The abilities to give and take, speak and listen, forgive and move on are all integral to spiritual development.

Today, life is busier than ever. While constantly juggling responsibilities, it is easy to get so caught up in the stresses of our own lives that we find it difficult to give to others. Here again, we need to stop and think about how being too self-enmeshed can affect relationships and the ability to communicate with others. Communication is a two-way process, in which listening is every bit as important as speaking. The ability to *listen actively* is a potent asset. Active listeners take note of content, intent, and feelings being expressed. They listen to all levels of the communication. Sensitivity and honesty are also essential to the give and take of communication. Ask specific questions, rephrase the speaker's ideas, and focus genuine attention on the speaker. Through such active participation, we gain a greater insight into the other person, who in turn will be encouraged to share more. Sharing becomes more intimate and relationships more connected when people feel that others care for them and are genuinely interested in their well-being. Both parties benefit from such an interchange.

Similar behaviors enhance interactions in a group or work setting, too. How many times in the past week have you sat in class and "totally zoned out" on what was happening? These are lost moments of potential learning and

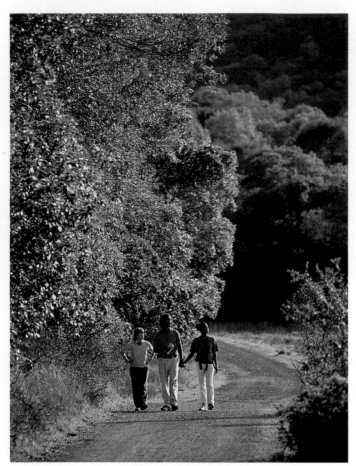

Taking time to relax with friends and enjoy nature can reduce stress and provide perspective on life.

SKILLS FOR BEHAVIOR CHANGE

Beginning Your Own Spiritual Journey

Whether a person's quest for spiritual health takes the form of a love for nature, a weekly visit to a place of religious worship, or some other guise, it is clear that spirituality benefits overall health. While it is possible to achieve spiritual health in many ways, the following ideas have helped a number of people on their spiritual path:

Relaxation and Meditation

"There is no greater source of strength and power for me in my life now than going still, being quiet, and recognizing what real power is," says Oprah Winfrey on the segment of her daily television show called "Remembering Your Spirit." Many people take the time to sit quietly and to meditate; for example, more than 5 million people worldwide practice transcendental meditation, one popular relaxation technique.

Time in Nature

For Henry David Thoreau, who fled civilization to live on Walden Pond, nature was the temple of God and the perennial source of life. A powerfully spiritual moment—and one we have all experienced— is the instant we are confronted with earth's perfection and are filled with awe. The scientist Carl Sagan wrote about his time-in-nature experience: "The wind whips through the canyons of the American Southwest, and there is no one to hear it but us." The crisp, clean smell of the woods after a rainfall, the soothing rhythm of crickets on a summer night, the beauty of freshly fallen snow—these experiences inspire unspeakable awe and humility because of the small but rich part that we, as individuals, play in the larger scheme of the universe.

Intimacy with Others

Loving selflessly is part of spiritual experience. Living life with passion and allowing ourselves to "feel" may be the greatest element of the spiritual journey. Experiencing emotion through a poignant musical passage, feeling the grief of a lost love, and surrendering to love's beauty are all part of human spirituality. By giving, sharing, and loving, we become whole and experience all that we are capable of feeling.

Spiritual Readings

Ranging from inspirational self-help books available at the local bookstore to traditional religious works, the written word has provided insight and guidance throughout human history, during its times of joy and darkest moments. For some, it's the Bible; for others, it may be the Qu'ran; and for still others, it may be a contemporary book such as *Spiritual Healing: Scientific Valida-* *tion of a Healing Revolution* by Daniel J. Benor, M.D. (Vision Publications, 2001). To find books that will foster your personal growth and healing, listen to what others recommend and then search for whatever will move you or speak to you.

Prayer

Prayer may be the oldest spiritual practice and the most popular one in America. Almost all world religions include a form of prayer. Says George Lucas, who plays on religious themes such as good and evil in his blockbuster *Star Wars* series, "Religion is basically a container for faith. And faith is a very important part of what allows us to remain stable, remain balanced." The mental and emotional release, along with a sense of connection to a transcendent dimension, may be at the heart of prayer's effectiveness.

Sources: Elkins and Druckman, "Spirituality: It's What's Missing in Mental Health," *Psychology Today* (September/October 1999), 48; The Transcendental Meditation Program (see http://www.tm.org).

---

experience. What made you withdraw from discussing a particularly hot political topic—fear of rejection? Insecurity? Before you pull away from group activities or connections with others, ask yourself the following questions:

- What prevents me from listening and contributing here? What do I fear? What effect does this situation have on me?
- What thoughts and feelings are getting in the way? Can I put these aside for a moment? What's the worst thing that could happen if I engage in this interaction?
- Are there things that I would feel comfortable sharing with this group? How could I let others know that I have something to say?

The Intellectual Dimension: Sharpening Intuition

Take the time to carefully assess events in life, their causes, and your own involvement in them. This often involves putting aside our emotional dimension for a moment to reflect, read, and ponder. Sometimes this process leads to startling new insights—"Ah-ha! Now I get it; this all makes sense!" Such moments mean so much, but few people include this mental activity in daily rituals. Examining the past, how we've gotten to where we are in the present, and what actions might have changed the course of events is a critical element of spiritual growth. By using our minds for objective reasoning, we develop the intellectual dimension of spiritual health.

Taking Charge

3   3   **3**

Managing Stress

Stress is not something that you can run from or wish into nonexistence. To control stress, meet it head on and use as many resources as you can to fine-tune your coping skills. Following a few simple guidelines will help you become more productive and relaxed.

- *Plan life, not time.* Evaluate all your activities, even the most trivial, to determine whether they contribute to your life. If they don't, eliminate them.
- *Decelerate.* When rushed, ask yourself if you really need to be. What's the worst that could happen if you slow down? Tell yourself at least once a day that failure seldom results from doing a job slowly or too well.
- *Learn to delegate and share.* Don't be afraid to ask others to help or to share the workload and responsibilities.

- *Learn to say no.* Decide what you can do, must do, and want to do, and delegate the rest to someone else either permanently or until you complete your high-priority tasks. Before you take on a new responsibility, finish or drop an old one.
- *Schedule time alone.* Find time each day for quiet thinking, reading, exercising, or other enjoyable activities.

Checklist for Change

Assessing Your Life Stressors

☐ Have you assessed the major stressors in your life? Are they people, events, or specific activities?

☐ Do you often worry about things that never happen? Are you often anxious about nothing?

☐ Have you thought about what you could change to reduce your stress levels?

☐ Do you have a network of friends and family members who can help you reduce your stress levels? Do you know where to get professional advice about reducing them?

☐ Have you thought about what changes you'd like to work on first? Have you developed a plan of action? When do you want to start?

Assessing Community Stressors

☐ Which factors in your environment, campus, and living situation cause stress, both for you and the people around you?

☐ Could these stressors be changed? If so, how? Why would changing them make a difference?

☐ What advice would you give to your school administrators to help them reduce unnecessary stress among students?

Summary

✻ Stress is an inevitable part of our lives. Eustress refers to stress associated with positive events, distress to negative events.

✻ The alarm, resistance, and exhaustion phases of the general adaptation syndrome (GAS) involve physiological responses to both real and imagined stressors and cause a complex cascade of hormones to rush through the body. Prolonged arousal may be detrimental to health.

✻ Undue stress for extended periods of time can compromise the immune system and result in serious health consequences. Psychoneuroimmunology is the science that analyzes the relationship between the mind's reaction to stress and the function of the immune system. While increasing evidence links disease susceptibility to stress, much of this research is controversial. Stress has been linked to numerous health problems including CVD, cancer, and increased susceptibility to infectious diseases.

✻ Multiple factors contribute to stress and to the stress response. Psychosocial factors include change, hassles, pressure, inconsistent goals and behaviors, conflict, overload, and burnout. Other factors are environmental stressors and self-imposed stress. Persons subjected to discrimination or bias due to *isms* may face unusually high levels of stress.

✻ College can be especially stressful. Recognition of the signs of stress is the first step toward better health. Learning to reduce test anxiety and cope with multiple stressors is also important.

✻ Managing stress begins with learning simple coping mechanisms: assessing stressors, changing responses, and learning to cope. Finding out what works best for you—probably some combination of managing emotional responses, taking mental or physical action, downshifting, learning time management, or using alternative stress management techniques—will help you better cope with stress in the long run.

✻ Developing the spiritual side involves practicing mindfulness and its many dimensions. These include the physical dimension—moving in nature; the emotional dimension—identifying and controlling negative emotions and feelings; the social dimension—interacting, listening, and communicating; and the intellectual dimension—sharpening intuition.

Questions for Discussion and Reflection

1. Compare and contrast distress and eustress. Are both types of stress potentially harmful?
2. Describe the alarm, resistance, and exhaustion phases of the general adaptation syndrome and the body's physiological response to stress. Does stress lead to more emotionality, or does emotionality lead to stress? Provide examples.
3. What are some of the health risks that result from chronic stress? How does the study of psychoneuroimmunology link stress and illness?
4. What major factors seem to influence the nature and extent of a person's susceptibility to stress? Explain how social support, self-esteem, and personality can make a person more or less susceptible to stress.

5. Why are some students more susceptible to stress than others? What services are available on your campus to help you deal with excessive stress?
6. What can college students do to inoculate themselves against negative stress effects? What actions can you take to manage your stressors? How can you help others to manage their stressors more effectively?

7. How does anger affect the body? Discuss the steps you can take to fight your own anger urge and help your friends control theirs.
8. What can you do to develop the dimensions of spirituality in your life? How can you apply the social dimension of spirituality to your current relationships?

Application Exercises

Reread the What Do You Think? scenarios at the beginning of the chapter, and answer the following questions:

1. What could the students in the chapter opener have done to inoculate themselves against their negative reactions to stressful events? What services on campus could they have used to help them through their troubles?
2. What factors make stress potentially greater for students whose background or age differs from that of "typical" students on a particular campus?

3. What direct and indirect health effects of stress may these students experience? What symptoms of stress should particularly concern them?
4. What strategies should these students follow to reduce the stress they are experiencing? As a friend, what action could you take to reduce their stress levels?

Accessing Your Health on the Internet

Visit the following Internet sites to explore further topics and issues related to personal health. To visit an organization's website, go to the companion website for *Access to Health, Eighth Edition* at www.aw.com/donatelle, click on the book image, and select "Accessing Your Health on the Internet" from the navigation menu on the left.

1. *Center for Anxiety and Stress Treatment.* Provides resources and services regarding a broad range of stress-related topics.

2. *Hampden-Sydney College.* Links to useful tips for dealing with stressful issues commonly experienced by college students.
3. *Mind Tools.* Focuses on all aspects of stress and stress management.
4. *National Center for Post-Traumatic Stress Disorder.* Research and education on PTSD, offering a variety of links to fact sheets and helpful sites.

Further Reading

Coffey, R. *Unspeakable Truths and Happy Endings.* Sidran Press, 1998 (see *http://www.sover.net/~schwcof/email.html*).

An outstanding resource that focuses on survivors of trauma/stress and recovery from human cruelty. Discussion of effects of war, rape, sexual assault, street crime, terrorism, and domestic violence, all major stressors in contemporary life.

Health and Stress: Newsletter of the American Institute of Stress (see *http://www.stress.org/news.html*).

Excellent monthly resource. Reports on latest developments in all areas of stress research. Each issue contains a listing of meetings of interest and a book review.

Rice, P. L. *Stress and Health.* Monterey, CA: Brooks/Cole, 1998.

An overview of current perspectives on stress and the influence of personal control and behavior on health. Discusses stress management as a factor in controlling pain, anxiety, and depression. An excellent resource for health professionals.

Seaward, B. *Managing Stress.* Philadelphia, PA: Jones & Bartlett, 2002.

Spirituality and stress expert provides complete overview of stress and health effects.

Weil, A. *Ask Dr. Weil.* New York: Random House, 1998.

A new-age author who provides an overview of mind–body health and alternative strategies for coping with life's challenges.

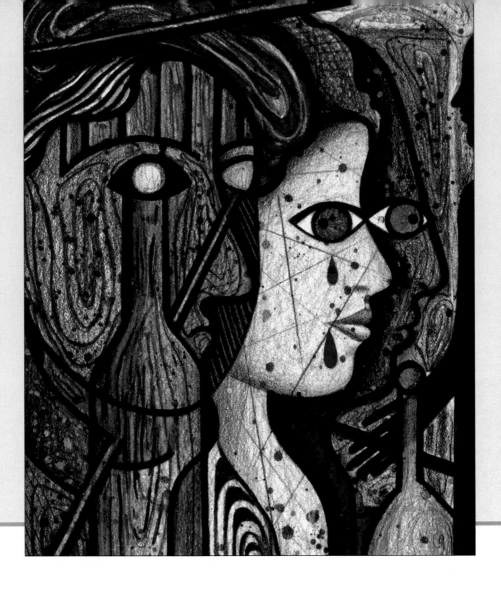

Objectives

* Differentiate between intentional and unintentional injuries, and discuss societal and personal factors that contribute to violence in American society.

* Identify factors that contribute to homicide, domestic violence, sexual victimization, and other intentional acts of violence.

* Explain how terrorism can affect individuals and populations, and summarize practical steps to lower your risk from terrorist attacks.

* Discuss strategies to prevent intentional injuries and reduce their risk of occurrence.

* Identify types of crime that are common on college campuses, and explain how the campus community, law enforcement officials, and individuals can prevent crime.

* Discuss the impact of unintentional injuries on American society, and explain actions that might contribute to personal risk of injuries of all types.

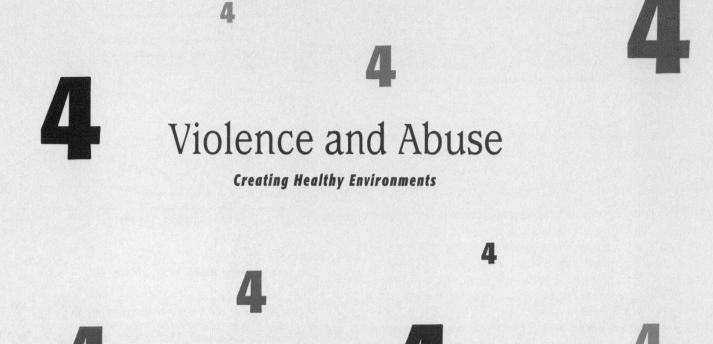

Violence and Abuse

Creating Healthy Environments

What do you think?

The September 11, 2001, terrorist attack on the United States galvanized the country in a burst of patriotic fervor. For many, this horrendous act of violence was incomprehensible, something that had previously seemed possible only on television or in the movies. While reactions of generosity, heroism, goodwill, and other positive behaviors persisted for months after the incident, there was also a darker side to how some Americans reacted. Reports of racist attacks, beatings, and human rights violations became widespread. Some political leaders called for American schools to ban all students from Iran, Afghanistan, Pakistan, and other countries in the Near East. Many compared the treatment of Muslim groups to that of Japanese Americans during World War II.

Can you think of other examples in which religious groups, racial groups, or other segments of society have been the victims of hate crimes and discrimination? ✳ *What types of situations cause such attacks to occur?* ✳ *What role do emotions such as fear and lack of understanding play in these attacks?* ✳ *What underlying beliefs and philosophies ignite such behaviors?* ✳ *What do you think we can do to prevent victimization of entire groups for the actions of a few individuals?*

"Across the land, waves of violence seem to crest and break, terrorizing Americans in cities and suburbs, in prairie towns and mountain hollows."

"To millions of Americans few things are more pervasive, more frightening, more real today than violent crime. . . . The fear of being victimized by criminal attack has touched us all in some way."

"Among urban children ages 10–14, homicides are up 150 percent, robberies are up 192 percent, assaults are up 290 percent."

Y ou might think these are statements from today's newspapers or television news. But they're not. The first quotation comes from President Herbert Hoover's 1929 inauguration speech, the second from the 1860 Senate report on crime, and the third from a 1967 report on children's violence.[1] Clearly, violence and our concern over its rising rates are not new concepts.

The term **violence** is used to indicate a set of behaviors that produce injuries, regardless of whether they are **intentional injuries** (committed with intent to harm) or **unintentional injuries** (committed without intent to harm, often accidentally). Any definition of *violence* implicitly includes the use of force, regardless of the intent, but as you'll see, some forms of violence are also extremely subtle. In this chapter, we focus on the various types of intentional and unintentional violence, the underlying causes of or contributors to these problems, strategies to reduce risk of encountering violence, and possible methods for preventing violence. Although certain indicators of violence, such as murders and deadly assaults, seem to be on the decline, other forms of violence, such as rape and hate crimes, are on the increase. Even more important is that for all we know about violence incidence and prevalence, a great deal remains unknown. Just how many people suffer in silence, failing to report violent acts due to fear of repercussions or accepting violence as "the way it is," remains unknown.

Violence in the United States

Even though violence has long been a major concern in American society, it wasn't until 1985 that the U.S. Public

Violence   A set of behaviors that produce injuries, as well as the outcomes of these behaviors (the injuries themselves).

Intentional injuries   Injuries committed on purpose with intent to harm.

Unintentional injuries   Injuries committed without intent to harm.

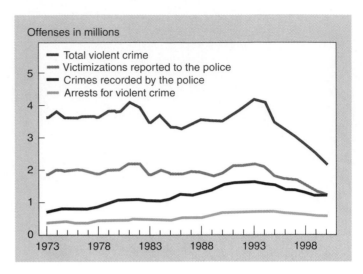

Figure 4.1
Changes in Crime Rates, 1973–2000

*Notes: Total serious violent crime is the number of homicides recorded by police plus the number of rapes, robberies, and aggravated assaults reported in the National Crime Victimization Survey. Victimization is the number of homicides recorded by police plus other serious crimes that respondents to the Victimization Survey said were reported to police. Crimes recorded by police and arrests are based on law enforcement reports to the FBI.

Source: Bureau of Justice Statistics, "Key Crime and Justice Facts at a Glance," 2002 (http://www.ojp.usdoj/bjs/glanc/cv2.htm).

Health Service formally identified violence as a leading public health problem that was contributing to significant death and disability rates. The Centers for Disease Control and Prevention (CDC) created an entire division known as the Division of Violence Prevention and considers violence a form of chronic disease that is pervasive at all levels of American society. Vulnerable populations, such as children, women, black males, and the elderly, were listed as being at high risk.

Recent numbers indicate that we have made dramatic improvements in certain areas. Since 1973, FBI statistics show that overall crime and certain types of violent crime have actually decreased each year (see Figure 4.1). In addition, a recent Department of Justice report on crime and safety on college campuses suggests that colleges and universities are relatively safe.[2] However, many question the accuracy of such reports, since petty theft, date rape, fighting, and other common campus incidents are not always reported to police. Although a person's chances of being murdered or violently assaulted may have declined, the odds of being a victim of crimes such as burglary, theft, and minor assault in general are on the increase.[3]

Unfortunately, violence affects everyone directly or indirectly. While the direct victims of violence and those close to them obviously suffer the most, others suffer in various ways because of the climate of fear that violence generates. Women are afraid to walk the streets at night. The elderly are often afraid to go out even in the daytime. After terrorist attacks such as that in 2001 on the World Trade Center in New

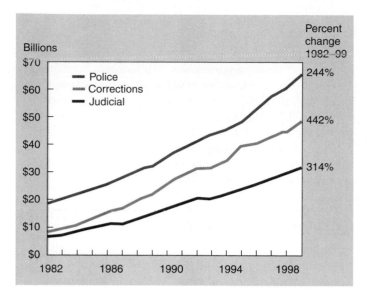

Figure 4.2
Increasing Costs of Crime Control in the United States, 1982–1999

Source: Bureau of Justice Statistics, "Key Crime and Justice Facts at a Glance," 2002 (see http://www.ojp.usdoj/bjs/glanc/exptyp.htm).

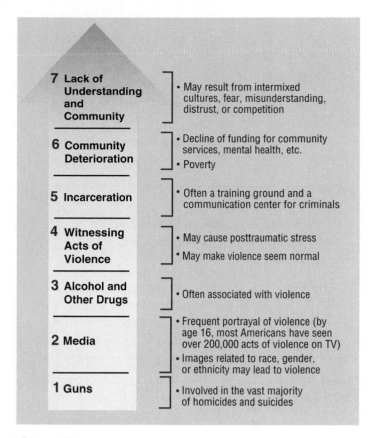

Figure 4.3
Correlates to Violence

York, people are afraid to fly, work in tall buildings, or live in heavily populated areas. The cost of homeland security is staggering. You might be surprised to know that international travelers often fear coming to the United States in much the same way that some Americans fear traveling to other regions of the world where attacks on U.S. citizens have taken place. Tourists are afraid of being brutalized in many of our nation's cities, hearing of children dodging bullets while playing in city neighborhoods or of drivers being "carjacked." Many of these reports are carried in the international news media, depicting the United States as a violent nation.

Even people who live in "safe" areas can become victims of violence within their own homes or at the hands of family members. At the very least, everyone pays higher tax bills for law enforcement and prisons and higher insurance premiums for damage done to others' or their own property. Although the greatest cost of violence lies in human suffering and loss, the direct and indirect financial cost of homicide, suicide, and related injuries on perpetrators and victims is estimated at more than $250 billion. Between 1982 and 1999, the direct costs for police intervention increased 244 percent, corrections costs increased 442 percent, and judicial costs went up 314 percent, a staggering blow to communities that must prioritize services and cope with declining federal and state funding.[4] (see Figure 4.2).

Societal Causes of Violence

Several social, cultural, and individual factors increase the likelihood of violent acts (see Figure 4.3). Commonly listed factors include the following:

- *Poverty.* Low socioeconomic status and poor living conditions can create an environment of hopelessness, leaving one feeling trapped and seeing violence as the only way to obtain what is needed or wanted.
- *Unemployment.* It is a well-documented fact that when the economy goes sour, violent crime, suicide, assault, and other crimes increase.
- *Parental influence.* Violence is cyclical. Children raised in environments in which shouting, slapping, hitting, and other forms of violence are commonplace are more apt to "act out" these behaviors as adults. Horrifying reports in recent years have made this pattern impossible to ignore.
- *Cultural beliefs.* Cultures that objectify women and empower men to be tough and aggressive tend to have increased rates of violence in the home.
- *The media.* A daily dose of murder and mayhem can take a toll on even resistant minds.
- *Discrimination/oppression.* Whenever one group is oppressed by another, seeds of discontent are sown and hate crimes arise.
- *Religious differences.* Religious persecution has been a part of the human experience since earliest times.
- *Breakdowns in the criminal justice system.* Over-crowded prisons, lenient sentences, early releases from prison, and trial errors subtly encourage violence in a number of ways.

- *Stress.* People who suffer from inordinate amounts of stress or are in crisis are more apt to be highly reactive, striking out at others or acting irrationally.
- *Heavy use of alcohol and other substances.* Alcohol and drug abuse are often catalysts for violence, being risk factors for domestic violence, rape, child abuse, homicide, and a multitude of crimes.[5]

In addition to these broad, societally based factors, many personal factors also can lead to violence.

> **What do you think?**
>
> *Why do you think there is so much violent behavior in the United States?* ✻ *Why do you think the rate of violent crime decreased in the six months following the September 11 terrorist attacks?* ✻ *What actions can you take personally to prevent violence from occurring?* ✻ *What could be done to reduce risk on your campus?* ✻ *In your community?*

Personal Precipitators of Violence

If you are like most people, you probably acted out your anger much more readily as a child than you do today. However, even the worst behaved children usually grow up. As we mature, we learn to control outbursts of anger and approach conflict rationally, not aggressively.

Yet others go through life acting out their aggressive tendencies in much the same ways they did as children or their families did. Why do two children from the same neighborhood, or even from the same family, go in different directions when it comes to violence? There are several antecedents or predictors of future aggressive behavior.

Anger Anger is a spontaneous, usually temporary, biological feeling or emotional state of displeasure that occurs most frequently during times of personal frustration. Since life is stressful, anger becomes a part of daily life experiences. Anger can range from slight irritation to rage, a violent and extreme form of anger.[6] When it is acted out at home or on the road, the consequences can be deadly. (See the Skills for Behavior Change box.)

What makes some people flare up at the slightest provocation? Often, people who anger quickly are individuals who have a low tolerance for frustration, believing that they should not have to put up with inconvenience or petty annoyances. The cause may be genetic or physiological; there is evidence that some people are born unstable, touchy, or easily angered.[7] Another cause of anger is sociocultural. Because many people are taught not to express anger in public, many do not know how to handle it when it reaches a level that cannot be hidden. Family background may be the most important factor. Typically, anger-prone people come from families that are disruptive, chaotic, and not skilled in emotional expression.[8] In fact, the single largest predictor of future violence is past violence.[9]

Aggressive behavior is often a key aspect of violent interactions. **Primary aggression** is goal-directed, hostile self-assertion that is destructive in nature. **Reactive aggression** is more often part of an emotional reaction brought about by frustrating life experiences. Whether aggression is reactive or primary in nature, it is most likely to flare up in times of acute stress, during relationship difficulties or loss, or when a person is so frustrated that he or she feels the only recourse is to strike out at others.

> **What do you think?**
>
> *What are some examples of primary aggression?* ✻ *Reactive aggression?* ✻ *Can both of them result in the same degree of harm?* ✻ *Do you think our laws are more lenient when violent acts result from reactive aggression?* ✻ *Why?*

Substance Abuse Although much has been written about a link between substance abuse and violence, we have yet to show that substance abuse actually causes violence. In fact, many violent acts are carefully planned actions that involve no alcohol or drug abuse. In some situations, however, psychoactive substances appear to be a form of "ignition" for violence:

- Consumption of alcohol—by perpetrators of the crime, the victim of the crime, or both—immediately preceded over half of all violent crimes, including murder.[10]
- Chronic drinkers are more likely than others to have histories of violent behavior.[11]
- Criminals using illegal drugs commit robberies and assaults more frequently than nonusing criminals and do so especially during periods of heavy drug use.[12]
- In domestic assault cases, more than 86 percent of the assailants and 42 percent of victims reported using alcohol at the time of the attack. Nearly 15 percent of victims and assailants reported using cocaine at the time of the attack.[13]
- Ninety-two percent of assailants and 42 percent of victims reported using alcohol or other drugs on the day of the assault.[14]
- Mentally ill patients who fail to adhere to prescription drug regimens and abuse alcohol and/or other drugs are significantly more likely to be involved in a serious violent act in the community.[15]
- Substance abuse markedly increases the risk of both homicide and suicide. Problems at work due to drinking, hospitalization for a drinking problem, use of illicit drugs, and arrest for use of illicit drugs all place subjects at risk for violent death by homicide. The combination of depression and use of alcohol or other drugs increases homicide and suicide rates threefold.[16]

Road Rage!

We pulled out into traffic and immediately were serenaded by a blaring horn from a car speeding by in the next lane. Apparently we had pulled out in front of the car, causing the driver to swerve quickly to the left lane to avoid hitting us. We felt bad and were thankful that nothing serious had happened, but the other driver wasn't so quick to forgive. For several miles she maneuvered to make us pull over, or slowed down in the neighboring lane in order to pull alongside our car. I wanted nothing to do with this and slowed down as well to avoid having to face her. Finally, she pulled over as she approached a right-hand turn, and as we went by, she stuck her head out the window and screamed venomous slurs our way. I'll never forget the expression on the woman's face as we went by. It was filled with such hatred and anger, such rage.

—From the author's files

If you drive at all, you have probably encountered road rage. While drunk driving remains a critical problem, the facts about aggressive driving are surely as ominous. According to the National Highway Transportation Safety Association, 41,907 people died on the highways last year. An estimated two-thirds of these fatalities were caused at least in part by aggressive driving behavior.

Why is road rage becoming more common? One reason is sheer overcrowding. In the last decade, the number of cars on the roads has increased by more than 11 percent, and the number of miles driven has increased by 35 percent; however, the number of new road miles has only increased by 1 percent. That means more cars in the same amount of space, and the problem is magnified in urban areas. Also, people have less time and more things to do. When people try to fit more activities into the day, stress levels rise. Stress creates anxiety, which leads to short tempers and road rage.

Are You Immune to Road Rage?

You may think you are the last person who would drive aggressively, but you might be surprised. Have you ever tailgated a slow driver, honked long and hard at another car, or sped up to keep another driver from passing? If you recognize yourself in any of these situations, watch out!

Avoid the "Rage" (Yours and Other Drivers')

Whether you are getting angry at other drivers or another driver is visibly upset with you, there are things you can do to avoid major confrontations. The key is to discharge your emotion in a healthy way. If you are the target of another driver's rage, do everything possible to get away from the other driver safely:

- Avoid eye contact!
- If you need to use your horn, do it sparingly.
- Get out of the way. Even if the other guy is speeding, it's safest to not make a point by staying in your lane.
- If someone is following you after an on-the-road encounter, drive to a public place or the nearest police station.
- Report any aggressive driving incidents to the police department immediately. You may be able to prevent further occurrences by the same driver.
- Above all, always buckle your seat belt! Seat belts save 9,500 lives annually.

Intentional Injuries

Anytime someone sets out to harm other people or their property, the incident may be referred to as one of intentional violence. Such incidents often result in intentional injuries, which come in many forms. Whether the situation entails a simple outburst of anger or a fatal attack with a weapon, the resulting intentional injuries cause pain and suffering at the very least, and disability or death at the worst.

Gratuitous Violence

Violence can manifest itself in many ways. Often the most shocking or gratuitous crimes gain the greatest attention, such as stories of innocent victims of drive-by shootings or young students who turn their internal rage outward on family, classmates, and teachers.

Assault/Homicide Homicide, death that results from intent to injure or kill, accounts for nearly 17,000 premature deaths in the United States.[17] These numbers are down slightly from 1997 but still represent a significant contributor to life lost in certain segments of the population. Although homicide was the fourteenth leading cause of death in the United States among all age groups in 1999, it was the second leading cause of death for persons age 15 to 24. Homicide is the

Primary aggression Goal-directed, hostile self-assertion, destructive in character.

Reactive aggression Emotional reaction brought about by frustrating life experiences.

Homicide Death that results from intent to injure or kill.

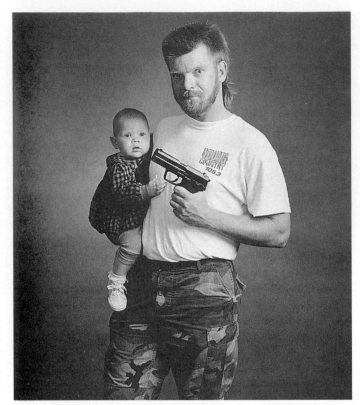

Guns are a common part of life in many households in this country. What effect might this have on the children in these homes?

leading cause of death for black males age 15–24 and the second leading cause of death for young Hispanic males. In 2000 the homicide rate for young black males was 17 times the rate for young non-Hispanic white males. The rate for young Hispanic males was 7 times the rate for young non-Hispanic males.[18] As measured by years of potential life lost, homicide exacted a heavy toll (see Table 4.1).

For every violent death, at least one hundred nonfatal injuries are caused by violence. In 1999, an estimated 28,874 firearm-related deaths occurred, including large numbers of homicides and suicides.[19] For every person shot and killed by a firearm, almost three others were treated annually for non-fatal shootings, many of them children under age 10.[20]

For an American, the average lifetime probability of being murdered is 1 in 153—but the average masks large differences for specific segments of the population. For white women, the risk of murder is 1 in 450; for black men, it is 1 in 28. For a black man in the 20- to 22-year-old age group, the risk is 1 in 3. Combined across races, males represent 77 percent of all murder and nonnegligent manslaughter victims. Black males are 1.14 times more likely than white males to be murder victims; white females are 1.5 times more likely than black females to be victims.[21] Over half of all homicides occur among people who know one another. In two-thirds of these cases, the perpetrator and the victim are friends or acquaintances; in one-third, they belong to the same family.[22]

Living in certain regions of the country also seems to increase one's risk for homicide. Statistics on homicides from other areas of the world provide an interesting comparison of international homicide risk (see Table 4.2).

Bias and Hate Crimes

In spite of national efforts in workplaces, schools, and communities to promote understanding and diversity-related appreciation, intolerance of differences continues to smolder in many parts of U.S. society. The killings of James Byrd and Matthew Shepard, the murder of two gay men in California, and the arson attacks on several U.S. synagogues remind Americans that violence based on race and other "isms" still occurs. International terrorist acts often reflect the hatred of one religious or political group for another that is considered to be "of less value" due to differences in religion, language, or other characteristics. Recent acts of violence against different racial groups by police, beatings in public schools and on the streets that are racially motivated "gang" events, and other hate crimes are common events on the nightly news.

According to the FBI's most recent Hate Crime Statistics Report, nearly 8,000 bias-motivated crimes were reported in 1999, compared to 7,700 in 1998. Of the total reported incidents, 4,300 were motivated by racial bias, 1,400 by religious bias, 1,300 by sexual orientation bias, and over 800 were related to ethnicity/national origin bias.[23]

After the September 11 terrorist attack in the United States, reports of hate-related incidents, beatings, and other physical and verbal assaults escalated, even as other rates of violent crime decreased. In particular, persons of Muslim or Middle-Eastern descent reported civil rights violations at work, in mass transit, and in communities throughout the United States. Many believe that the reported incidents are but the tip of the iceberg and that actual numbers of bias/hate-related crimes are much higher, but people do not report them out of fear of possible retaliation.

Hate crimes vary along two dimensions: (1) the way they are carried out and (2) their effects on victims. Vicious gossip, nasty comments, and devilish pranks may not make campus headlines, but they can hurt nonetheless. Generally, about 30 percent of all hate crimes are against property, with the other 70 percent being against the person. Recent studies have identified three additional characteristics of hate crimes:[24]

- They are excessively brutal.
- They are perpetrated at random on total strangers.
- They are perpetrated by multiple offenders.

In addition, the perpetrators tend to be motivated by thrill, defensive feelings, or a hate-mongering mission.

Academic settings are not immune to hatred and bias. According to a report in the Chronicle of Higher Education, nearly one-third of our nation's campuses have reported incidents of hate crimes. Another study of four campuses found that victimization rates varied widely, from 12 percent of Jewish students to as high as 60 percent of Hispanic

Table 4.1
Years of Potential Life Lost (per 100,000)

Years of Potential Life Lost (YPLL) is a rough measure of the impact of a specific disease or societal event/condition on a given population. It is calculated by subtracting the age at death of a person from the expected life expectancy for this person. In this table, the total years are those lost before age 75 per 100,000 population under the age of 75. It provides a glimpse of the overall impact of a problem on the lives of particular populations.
Some questions to consider: Where are the greatest disparities in YPLL among males? Among females? What factors do you think contribute to the low rates of suicide in some groups? High rates of assault?

	UNINTENTIONAL INJURY	SUICIDE	ASSAULT (HOMICIDE)
MALE			
White	1,475.9	624.7	253.9
Black	1,888.7	388.1	1,753.5
American Indian/Alaska Native	2,771.7	850.8	568.3
Asian/Pacific Islander	637.1	308.8	210.2
Hispanic	1,536.8	346.6	676.8
White, non-Hispanic	1,440.8	657.6	167.1
FEMALE			
White	586.8	154.4	95.0
Black	676.9	67.0	370.2
American Indian/Alaska Native	1,276.8	219.7	205.8
Asian/Pacific Islander	309.6	102.5	80.2
Hispanic	461.8	306.3	121.9
White, non-Hispanic	599.1	164.4	88.2

Note: The groups of white, black, Asian/Pacific Islander, and American Indian/Alaska Native include persons of Hispanic and non-Hispanic origin. Conversely, persons of Hispanic origin may be of any race.
Source: Department of Health and Human Services, National Institutes of Health, Centers for Disease Control, Health U.S. 2001. http://www.cdc.gov

Table 4.2
Homicide Rates and Rankings for Selected Countries (includes gun and nongun rates)

COUNTRY	YEAR	HOMICIDE RATE	RANKING
South Africa	1995	75.30	1
Colombia	1996	64.60	2
Estonia	1994	28.21	3
Brazil	1993	19.04	4
Mexico	1994	17.58	5
Philippines	1996	16.20	6
Taiwan	1996	8.12	7
United States	1997	6.80	8
N. Ireland	1994	6.09	9
Canada	1992	2.19	17
Australia	1994	1.86	20
England/Wales	1992	1.41	25
Sweden	1993	1.30	27
Norway	1993	0.97	35
Japan	1994	0.62	38

Note: These rates are per 100,000 population and are subject to possible errors in reporting and information gathering. For this reason, they are to be used only as indicators of trends, not hard-and-fast data points.
Source: Adapted from "International Homicide Rate Table," by H. Picard, (Online), January 7, 2000; *The Will to Kill,* by J. Fox and J. Levin, 2001, p. 35, Boston: Allyn & Bacon.

Superpredators: A New Generation of Violent Adults?

Criminologists are warning of an impending juvenile crime wave created by a new breed of "superpredators." While homicide rates dropped dramatically during the 1990s, these declines occurred among adult offenders. Between 1985 and the mid-1990s, a very different pattern was emerging among teenagers; in fact, the rate of murder committed by teens tripled. Although many factors are blamed for the sharp rise, experts point to the emergence of crack cocaine as a major culprit. As the market for crack increased, so did the risks for sellers, complete with a form of armed "gun" mentality for protecting precious cargo. Guns in the hands of teenagers who are often impatient, imprudent, impulsive, and willing to act spontaneously without thinking about consequences have greatly increased murder rates.

As guns proliferated to protect the drug traffic, gangs of like-minded, similarly directed teenagers formed to protect individual interests. Instead of killing for serious matters, such as self-defense or protecting a loved one, these teens may kill for trivial matters, such as stealing a letter jacket or an expensive pair of shoes.

The crack market has stabilized since the early 1990s and gangs are beginning to dwindle. Yet a new form of violence is erupting. Fed by pro wrestling role models, a violent media, and a host of other problems, today's youth may be more likely to engage in vicious and seemingly senseless violence than any other generation to date. Dysfunctional families, poor school systems, and a lack of support for positive change often leave communities reeling from youth violence.

Source: James Alan Fox and Jack Levin, *The Will to Kill* © 2001. Published by Allyn & Bacon, Boston, MA. Copyright © 2001 Pearson Education.

---

students. White students were victimized at rates ranging from 5 to 15 percent.[25] The sad truth is, however, that many minor assaults go unreported, so this may be only part of the picture.

The tendency toward violent acts on campus might best be defined as campus **ethnoviolence,** a term that reflects relationships among groups in the larger society and is based on prejudice and discrimination. Although ethnoviolence often is directed randomly at persons affiliated with a particular group, the group itself is specifically targeted apart from other people, and that differentiation is usually ethnic in nature. Typically, the perpetrators agree that "the group is an acceptable target." For example, in a largely Christian community, Jews and Muslims may be considered acceptable targets.[26] Students bring with them attitudes and beliefs from past family and life experiences.

Prejudice and discrimination are always at the base of ethnoviolence. **Prejudice** is a set of negative attitudes toward a group of people. To say that a person is prejudiced against some group is to say that the person holds a set of beliefs about the group, has an emotional reaction to the group, and is motivated to behave in a certain way toward the group. **Discrimination** constitutes actions that deny equal treatment or opportunities to a group of people, often based on prejudice and bias.

Often intolerance stems from a fear of change and a desire to blame others when forces such as the economy and crime seem to be out of control. What can you do to be part of the solution rather than part of the problem?

- Support educational programs that foster understanding and appreciation for differences in people. Many colleges now require diversity classes as part of their academic curriculum.
- Examine your own attitudes and behaviors. Are you intolerant of others? Do you engage in racist, sexist, or similar behaviors meant to demean a group of individuals? If you have problems with a particular group, why?
- Do you discourage hurtful jokes and other forms of social or ethnic bigotry? Do not participate in such behaviors, and express your dissatisfaction with those who do.
- Vote for community leaders who respect the rights of others and who value diversity. Vote against intolerant candidates.
- Educate yourself. Read, interact with, and attempt to understand people who appear to be different from you. Remember that you do not have to like everything about them. Other people may not like everything about you, either. However, respecting people's right to be different is a part of being a healthy, integrated individual.
- Examine your own values in determining the relative worth of your friends and the others in your life. Are you judgmental? Do you judge people on appearances, or do you take time to know them as individuals?
- Encourage your legislators to support antihate and antibias legislation. Vote for those who support antidiscrimination policies and programs.

Ethnoviolence   Violence directed randomly at persons affiliated with a particular group.

Prejudice   A set of negative attitudes and beliefs or an emotional reaction or way of thinking about a group of people.

Discrimination   Actions that deny equal treatment or opportunities to a group, often based on bias and prejudice.

Gang Violence The growing influence of street gangs has had a harmful impact on our country. Drug abuse, gang shootings, beatings, thefts, carjackings, and the possibility of being caught in the middle between gangs at war have led to whole neighborhoods being held hostage by gang members. Once thought to be a phenomenon that occurred only in inner-city areas, gang violence now also occurs in both rural and suburban communities, particularly in the southeastern, southwestern, and western regions of the country.

Why do young people join gangs? Although the reasons are complex, gangs apparently meet many of their needs. Gangs provide a sense of belonging to a "family" that gives them self-worth, companionship, security, and excitement. In other cases, they provide economic security through criminal activity, drug sales, or prostitution. Once young people become involved in the gang subculture, it is difficult for them to leave. Threats of violence or fear of not making it on their own dissuade even those who are most seriously trying to get out.

Who is at risk for gang membership? Membership varies considerably from region to region. The age range of gang members is typically 12 to 22 years. Risk factors include low self-esteem, academic problems, low socioeconomic status, alienation from family and society, a history of family violence, and living in gang-controlled neighborhoods.

The best way to prevent someone from joining a gang is to keep that person connected to positive influences and programs. From a child's early years, the focus should be on establishing bonds among friends, family, and school. Any student who has learning disabilities or other problems that make it hard to keep up should be involved in alternative activities that foster success and prevent a sense of alienation.

Community-based prevention programs that coordinate involvement of families, social service organizations, and law enforcement, school, and city officials have proved effective in keeping students out of gangs. Also, community members must begin to think of gang members not merely as trouble-making delinquents but as people whose circumstances make them susceptible to the gang lifestyle.

In part because the number of gangs and gang-related crimes grows daily, Congress passed a crime bill in the early 1990s that included the hiring of 100,000 additional police officers, a ban on assault weapons, reform of the welfare system, the creation of a national network of neighborhood banks to boost communities' economic development, and the establishment of "boot camps" for young nonviolent offenders. (Similar additions to our national policing and surveillance capabilities have been initiated post–September 11th.) These boot camps were designed to keep offenders out of prison and instill discipline, self-esteem, and respect for the law. Preliminary results indicate that such "tough love" programs are not as effective as many had hoped. Public health professionals have long advocated prevention rather than the current efforts spent on intervention. Examining the

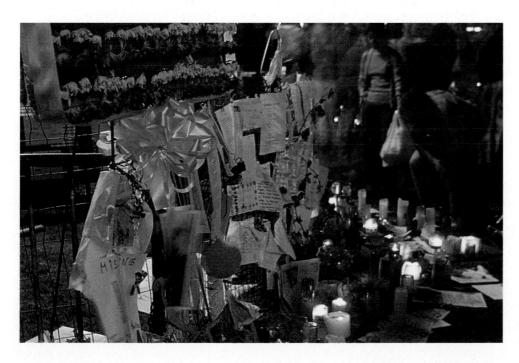

The events of September 11, 2001, were a grim reminder of the power and senselessness of hatred.

Gun Control: Issues and Choices

More than thirty years ago, *Time* magazine ran a feature entitled "The Gun in America," which summarized the feelings of a nation reeling from the murders of John F. Kennedy, Robert Kennedy, and Martin Luther King, Jr. The national disgust that followed led to the Gun Control Act of 1968, a milestone law that banned most interstate gun sales, licensed most gun dealers, and barred felons, minors, and the mentally ill from owning firearms.

Today, gun violence has spread to our nation's playgrounds and schools. Recent statistics suggest that one in two high schoolers is threatened or injured with a weapon each year. While juvenile crime as a whole is down—even more dramatically than the precipitous drop in adult crime—the number of youths murdered by firearms went up 153 percent from 1985 to 1995! In some ways, the recent school killings across the country are aberrations. The percentage of households that own guns is actually declining, from a decades-long average of about 45 percent to approximately 40 percent. Still, there are nearly as many firearms in the United States as people, more than 235 million by some estimates. At a time when crime rates are dropping, gun crime is dropping, too. But gun murders in the United States are still far more common than they were 30 years ago, and much more common than they are in other Western industrialized nations.

Since the 1968 gun control legislation, the only major gun laws to date are the Brady Bill, which requires background checks of purchasers, and the assault-gun ban. Although there is talk about a gun safety-lock law and special "owner-use only" imprinting on guns, Congress is unlikely to pass any major gun control measures in the near future. In fact, the trend is toward more deregulation of guns and laws that permit concealed weapons in many states. The number of states that permit concealed weapons has gone from 8 to 31 since 1985. A recent book, *More Guns, Less Crime: Understanding Crime and Gun Laws,* analyzed crime rates in the 10 states that passed right-to-carry laws between 1977 and 1992. The author contends that after these laws were enacted, murders fell an average of 8 percent, rapes 5 percent, and aggravated assaults by 7 percent at a time when murders, rapes, and assaults were increasing in states without such laws. Criminologists, researchers, and gun control lobbyists say that the book's research has been poorly conducted, its statistics are suspect, and its conclusions, dangerous. Whom are we to believe?

Millions of Americans believe passionately that their right to bear arms, their personal safety against tyranny, and their hunting rights should not be curtailed. Others believe that we have gone too far in "protecting" our rights, that outgunned police forces and the typical citizen on the street face undue risks as others maintain their right to own assault weapons. Some even argue that events such as the school shootings could have been prevented if teachers had the right to carry guns for protection! Many of us have wondered about buying guns for "protection" as violence seems to escalate. Concealed weapons appeal to those who fear for their own safety and want a means to fight back. But what's to say that people won't overreact to perceived threats?

Recent lawsuits against gun manufacturers raise yet another controversial issue. Are gun manufacturers liable for violent homicides, in much the same way that the tobacco industry is being held liable for deaths from cigarette smoking? The attorneys general of several states feel they are and are taking these suits to court as of this writing. They argue that many deaths are preventable through better monitoring of sales and curtailing production of armor-piercing bullets and repeat-style assault weapons. They believe that it is possible to manufacture guns that fire only if the original owner is operating them, but that gun manufacturers refuse to produce them.

In the future, we will all be called upon to make choices that may affect the lives of our families, coworkers, and friends. What can you do?

- Investigate the facts about gun-related violence. Your best data sources are federal or state crime statistics, rather than special interest groups that might have a vested interest in proving their claims.
- Review the points made by the National Rifle Association and compare its data with federal or state crime data and data from groups lobbying for anti-gun protection. Consider the pros and cons of each argument.
- Consider what the antigun movement is really advocating. Would their actions really keep hunters from buying rifles, or homeowners from having handguns in their homes for protection? Would user IDs on guns, which would not allow anyone but the original purchaser to operate the weapon, be acceptable to the NRA? Why or why not?
- Analyze the voting records of your state and national political representatives regarding gun control. Are they voting in ways that support your own beliefs?

Do you feel there should be any additional restrictions on use or ownership of guns? Explain your answer. Do the risks of ownership outweigh the benefits? Do the benefits outweigh the risks?

Source: From R. Lacayo, "Still Under the Gun," *Time,* July 6, 1998, pp. 32–56.

underlying causes of violence should provide evidence for supporting systemwide changes in the social environment. (See the Health Ethics: Conflict and Controversy box.)

Terrorism: Increased Risks from Multiple Sources

Not so long ago, Americans considered acts of terrorism to be limited to isolated events in distant cities, seldom amounting to more than a blip on the evening news. The bombing of the Oklahoma City federal building in 1995 focused national attention on terrorism for a brief moment in time. Most of us, however, went about our daily business after the event, acknowledging that it was the act of a madman and sympathizing with the victims.

On September 11, 2001, Americans got a huge wake-up call. Terrorist attacks on the World Trade Center and Pentagon revealed the vulnerability of our nation to domestic and international threats. The terms terrorist attack, bioterrorism, and biological weapons catapulted us into the new millennium with an emotional reaction unlike any ever seen. America had lost its innocence and its illusion of invulnerability. An undercurrent of fear and anxiety about potential threats from faceless strangers shook many of us in ways that we had never even considered.

What Is Terrorism? According to the FBI, **terrorism** is the use of unlawful force or violence against persons or property to intimidate or coerce a government, the civilian population, or any segment thereof, in furtherance of political or social objectives. Typically, terrorism is of two major types: (1) *domestic terrorism*, which involves groups or individuals whose terrorist activities are directed at elements of our government or population without foreign direction, and (2) *international terrorism*, which involves groups or individuals whose terrorist activities are foreign-based, transcend national boundaries, and are directed by countries or groups outside the United States.

Clearly, terrorist activities may have immediate impact in terms of loss of lives and resources. However, the September 11th attacks resulted in far-reaching effects on the U.S. economy, airlines, and transportation systems. Perhaps most damaging in the aftermath of the attacks was the fear, anxiety, and altered behavior of countless Americans. How many people will fear working in skyscrapers for years to come? How many will fear climbing on a plane, crossing a bridge, or getting on the subway? How many will worry excessively about biological weapons? (See the Health in a Diverse World box). Will worry about future terrorist attacks disrupt our lives and our interactions with others?

As the media spur our anxieties about germ, chemical, and nuclear warfare and the multitude of ways that terrorists can breach our defenses, is it any wonder that an already stressed American public is demonstrating increasing concern? What can we do to reduce our risk of terrorist attack?

Be assured that the U.S. Centers for Disease Control and Prevention (CDC) has a wide range of ongoing programs and services to help Americans respond to terrorist threats and prepare for possible attacks. Information is available on the CDC website and is updated regularly. The FBI and other government agencies have also prepared a sweeping set of procedures and guidelines for ensuring citizen safety. Here are some things you can do to help reduce the risk of terrorist attacks:

- *Be aware of your own reactions to stress, anxiety, and fear.* Try to assess how much of your fear is justifiable in a given situation and how much is a product of media sensationalism. Practice stress reduction techniques, try to determine the source of your stressors, and react as prudently as possible.
- *Be conscious of your surroundings.* If you notice suspicious activities or irregularities, report them to a person in authority. Being a passive observer and not speaking up when warranted may put you and others at risk.
- *Stay informed.* Try to stay on top of the news and understand the underlying roots of violent activity. Persistent poverty, pervasive religious or political fanaticism, and political situations in which there is an imbalance of power can provide ample fodder for violent acts. Consider when a self-righteous contempt for others may lead to persecution and violation of human rights. Be skeptical of acts perpetrated in the name of some cause, and intervene if possible to defuse violence.
- *Seek understanding.* Whenever two opposing groups mentally stop engaging with each other or communication breaks down, hatred, bigotry, and anger may result. Knowing about each other's customs, cultures, and beliefs and keeping the lines of communication open are good steps to avoid separation.
- *Seek information.* When political parties fight for power in election years, know your candidates. What are their underlying beliefs regarding national defense, spending for consumer protection, policies on immigration, human rights violations, diversity issues, hate crimes, gun control, and so forth? Are they more aligned with one ideology than another? What is their stance on government interference and control, punishment of offenders, and other key issues?
- *Know what to do in an emergency.* Whom would you call? How would you access local and regional assistance? Do you have the necessary provisions to keep safe in an emergency—food, water, first aid? What happens when your electricity is off, your phone and communication systems are down, and your access to health care is limited?

Terrorism The use of unlawful force or violence against persons or property to intimidate or coerce a government, the civilian population, or any segment thereof, in furtherance of political or social objectives.

Bioterrorism: Pandora's Box

For many, the threat of any kind of viable attack on the United States was incomprehensible until the World Trade Center and Pentagon attacks on September 11, 2001. As shocking as those events were, they may pale in comparison to the unleashing of a Pandora's box of biological killers, which could threaten the health of the entire global population. Before the terrorist attacks in New York and Washington, D.C., many people had never heard of diseases such as anthrax, but within a few days Americans watched as endless newscasts discussed the potential horrors of biological warfare.

As chilling as these threats might be, the actual potential for bioterrorism is much more far-reaching than any of us might imagine. Included are a wide range of threats from both biological diseases and chemical agents, as indicated below. You can find a complete overview of each of these, plus national initiatives for preventing bioterrorism attacks, on the CDC website (http://www.bt.cdc.gov/).

Biological Agents/Diseases

Category A diseases are pathogens rarely seen in the United States and pose a risk to national security because they (a) can be easily disseminated or transmitted person-to-person; (b) cause high mortality, with potential for major public health impact; (c) might cause widespread panic and social disruption; and (d) require special action for public health preparedness. The Category A threats that are the greatest concern are highlighted in the list that follows; you can find information on others at the CDC website.

• *Bacillus anthracis* (**anthrax**): An acute infectious disease caused by a bacterium, anthrax typically occurs in host animals but can also infect humans.

Three major forms of anthrax may occur: inhalation, cutaneous (skin), and intestinal anthrax, all with symptoms that usually appear within seven days after infection. Early symptoms of inhalation anthrax resemble those of a common cold, followed by respiratory symptoms and shock, which is often fatal. The intestinal form appears initially as nausea, vomiting, loss of appetite, and fever, followed by abdominal pain, bloody vomit, and severe diarrhea. It is believed that direct person-to-person spread of anthrax is very rare; thus, immunization and treatment of contacts are not recommended. If exposed, antibiotics are effective treatments in the early stages. Vaccination is also effective.

• *Clostridium botulinum* toxin (**botulism**): Botulism is an acute muscle-paralyzing disease caused by a toxin that a bacterium produces. There are three major forms of botulism. Foodborne, the most common strain, leads to illness within hours. Infant botulism affects babies who harbor the organism in their intestines. Wound botulism occurs when cuts are infected. Fortunately, botulism is not spread from person to person. Symptoms include double vision, blurred vision, slurred speech, difficulty swallowing, and muscle weakness that descends through the body, eventually paralyzing the ability to breathe and killing the person.

• *Versinia pestis* (**plague**): An infectious disease of animals and humans that is found in many parts of the world, plague is caused by a bacterium carried by rodents and their fleas. The plague organism infects the lungs. Fever, headache, weakness, and a watery, blood-laden cough are frequent symptoms. Pneumonia follows quickly and over two to four days may cause septic shock. Without treatment, plague can be fatal. Person-to-person contact with transfer of respiratory droplets

spreads the disease. A vaccine has not been developed, but several antibiotics are effective if given early.

• *Variola major* (**smallpox**): Although smallpox was eliminated from the world in 1977, stockpiling of the virus that causes this disease has occurred in many regions of the world. Smallpox spreads from person to person by infected saliva droplets and is most contagious during the first week of illness. Initial symptoms include high fever, fatigue, headaches, and backaches. In two to three days a characteristic rash develops, with flat red lesions that evolve into pustules most prominent on the face, arms, and legs. Lesions crust early in the second week. Scabs develop, separate, and fall off after about three or four weeks. Most people who get smallpox recover, but death occurs in up to 30 percent of cases. Although most Americans born prior to 1972 were vaccinated, it is uncertain whether these shots conferred lasting immunity. Although vaccines are effective, the current supply is limited. Treatment for smallpox focuses on relieving symptoms, but new antiviral agents are being tested.

Category B diseases are of concern but are not as easily transmitted and do not have as high a mortality rate as Category A diseases. Examples include *Coxiella burnetii* (Q fever), *Brucella* species (brucellosis), *Burkholderia mallei* (glanders), ricin toxin from *Ricinus communis* (castor beans), epsilon toxin of *Clostridium perfringens,* and staphylococcal enterotoxin B.

Category C diseases are emerging pathogens that could be engineered for bioterrorism in the future because they have the potential for high morbidity and mortality rates and could be easily produced and disseminated. Examples include nipah virus, hantavirus, tick-borne hemorrhagic fever, tick-borne encephalitis viruses, yellow fever, and multi-drug-resistant tuberculosis.

Chemical Agents

These agents are classified by the body system they damage or the effect that they produce in victims. See the CDC website for a complete listing.

Blister/Vesicants
Distilled mustard (HD)
Lewisite
Various forms of nitrogen mustard and lewisite combinations

Blood
Arsine
Cyanogen chloride

Hydrogen chloride
Hydrogen cyanide

Choking/Lung/Pulmonary Damage
Chlorine
Diphosgene
Nitrogen oxide
Zinc oxide

Incapacitating
Agent 15
BZ
Canniboids
Fentanyls
LSD
Phenothiazines

Nervous system
Cyclohexyl sarin
Sarin

Riot control/tearing

Vomiting

Source: Centers for Disease Control and Prevention, Public Health Emergency Preparedness and Response, 2002 (see http://www.bt.cdc.gov).

Domestic Violence

In the 1980s a popular country-western song crooned, "No one knows what goes on behind closed doors." Domestic violence shows us just how true that refrain can be. **Domestic violence** refers to the use of force to control and maintain power over another person in the home environment. It can involve emotional abuse, verbal abuse, threats of physical harm, and actual physical violence ranging from slapping and shoving to beatings, rape, and homicide.

Women as Victims While young men are more apt to become victims of violence from strangers, women are much more likely to become victims of violent acts perpetrated by spouses, lovers, ex-spouses, and ex-lovers. In 2000, more than 6 million women were victims of assault. In fact, 6 of every 10 women in the United States will be assaulted at some time in their lives by someone they know.[27] Every year, approximately 12 percent of married women are the victims of physical aggression perpetrated by their husbands, according to a national survey.[28] This aggression often includes pushing, slapping, and shoving, but it can take more severe forms.

Each year about 4 percent of married women are beaten, threatened, or actually injured by knives or guns.[29] In fact, acts of aggression by a husband or boyfriend are one of the most common causes of death for young women, and roughly 2,200 women in the United States are killed each year by their partners or ex-partners.[30] Over a recent 10-year period, according to the National Crime Survey, on average, more than 2 million assaults on women occurred each year. More than two-thirds of these assaults were committed by someone the woman knew.[31]

The following U.S. statistics indicate the seriousness of this long-hidden problem:[32]

- The most vulnerable women are African American and Hispanic, live in large cities far from their families, and are young and unmarried.
- Every 15 seconds, someone batters a woman.
- Only 1 in every 250 such assaults is reported to the police.
- More than a third of female victims of domestic violence are severely abused on a regular basis.
- About five women are killed every day in domestic violence incidents.
- Three of every four women murdered are killed by their husbands.
- Domestic violence is the single greatest cause of injury to women, surpassing rape, mugging, and auto accidents combined.
- About 25 to 45 percent of all women who are battered sustain such attacks during pregnancy.
- One-quarter of suicide attempts by women occur as a result of domestic violence.

How many times have you heard of a woman who is repeatedly beaten by her partner and wondered, "Why doesn't she just leave him?" There are many reasons why some women find it difficult to break their ties with their abusers.

> **Domestic violence** The use of force to control and maintain power over another person in the home environment, including both actual harm and the threat of harm.

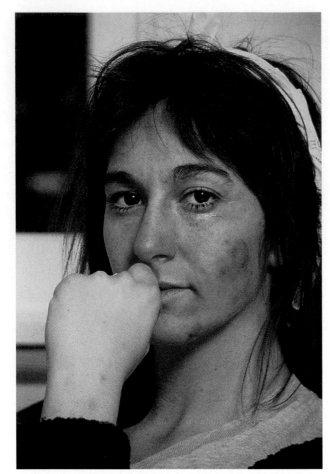

Despite obvious physical and psychological injury, it can be difficult for a woman to leave an abusive partner.

Many women, particularly those with small children, are financially dependent on their partners. Others fear retaliation against themselves or their children. Some women hope that the situation will change with time (it rarely does), and others stay because their cultural or religious beliefs forbid divorce. Finally, some women still love the abusive partner and are concerned about what will happen to him if they leave.[33]

Psychologist Lenore Walker developed a theory known as the "cycle of violence" to explain how women can get caught in a downward spiral without knowing what is happening to them.[34] The cycle has three phases:

1. *Tension building*. In this phase, minor battering occurs, and the woman may become more nurturant, more pleasing, and more intent on anticipating the spouse's needs in order to forestall another violent scene. She assumes guilt for doing something to provoke him and tries hard to avoid doing it again.
2. *Acute battering*. At this stage, pleasing her man doesn't help and she can no longer control or predict the abuse. Usually, the spouse is trying to "teach her a lesson," and when he feels he has inflicted enough pain, he'll stop. When the acute attack is over, he may respond with shock and denial

about his own behavior. Both batterer and victim may soft-pedal the seriousness of the attacks.
3. *Remorse/reconciliation*. During this "honeymoon" period, the batterer may be kind, loving, and apologetic, swearing he will never act violently again. He may "behave" for several weeks or months, and the woman may come to question whether she overreacted to past abuse.

When the tension that precipitated past abuse resurfaces, the man loses control and beats the woman again. Unless some form of intervention breaks this downward cycle of abuse, contrition, further abuse, denial, and contrition, it will repeat itself again and again—perhaps ending only in the woman's—or, rarely, the man's—death.

It is very hard for most women who get caught in this cycle of violence (which may include forced sexual relations and psychological and economic abuse as well as beatings) to summon up the resolution to extricate themselves. Most need effective outside intervention.

Men as Victims   Men are also victims of domestic violence. Some women do abuse and even kill their partners. Approximately 12 percent of men reported that their wives had engaged in physically aggressive behaviors against them in the past year—nearly the same percentage of reported claims as for women. The difference between male and female batterers is twofold. First, although the frequency of physical aggression may be similar, the impact is drastically different: Women are typically injured in domestic incidents two to three times more often than men.[35] These injuries tend to be more severe and have resulted in significantly more deaths. Women do engage in moderate aggression, such as pushing and shoving, at rates almost equal to those of men, but severe aggression that is likely to land the victim in the hospital is almost always male-against-female. Second, a woman who is physically abused by a man is generally intimidated by him: She fears that he will use his power and control over her in some fashion. Men, however, generally report that they do not live in fear of their wives.

Causes of Domestic Violence   There is no single explanation for why people tend to be abusive in relationships. Although alcohol abuse is often associated with such violence, marital dissatisfaction seems to also be a predictor.[36] Numerous studies also point to differences in the communication patterns between abusive and nonabusive relationships.[37] While some argue that the hormone testosterone causes male aggression, studies have failed to show a strong association between physical abuse in relationships and this hormone.[38] Many experts believe that men who engage in severe violence are more likely than other men to suffer from personality disorders.[39]

Regardless of the cause, it is the dynamics that *both* people bring to a relationship that will result in violence and allow it to continue. Community support and counseling services can help determine underlying problems and allow the victim and the batterer to break the cycle. The Assess Yourself box may help you determine if you are a victim of abuse.

Child Abuse   Children raised in families in which domestic violence and/or sexual abuse occur are at great risk for damage to personal health and well-being. The effects of such violent acts are powerful and long-lasting. **Child abuse** refers to the systematic harm of a child by a caregiver, generally a parent.[40] The abuse may be sexual, psychological, physical, or any combination of these. Although exact figures are lacking, many experts believe that over 2 million cases of child abuse occur every year in the United States, involving severe injury, permanent disability, or death.

Child abusers exist in all gender, social, ethnic, religious, and racial groups, but they tend to share certain characteristics: a history of abuse as a child, a poor self-image, feelings of isolation, extreme frustration with life, higher stress or anxiety levels than normal, a tendency to abuse drugs and/or alcohol, and unrealistic expectations of the child. It is estimated that one-half to three-quarters of men who batter their female partners also batter children. In fact, spouse abuse is the single most identifiable risk factor for predicting child abuse. Children with disabilities or other "differences" are more likely to be abused.

Child Sexual Abuse   **Sexual abuse of children** by adults or older children includes sexually suggestive conversations; inappropriate kissing; touching; petting; oral, anal, or vaginal intercourse; and other kinds of sexual interaction. The most frequent abusers are a child's parents or companions or spouses of the child's parents. Next most frequent are grandfathers and siblings. Girls are more commonly abused than boys, although young boys are also frequent victims, usually of male family members. Between 20 and 30 percent of all adult women report having had an unwanted childhood sexual encounter with an adult male, usually a father, uncle, brother, or grandfather. It is a myth that male deviance or mental illness accounts for most of these incidents: "Stories of retrospective incest patients typically involved perpetrators who are 'Everyman'—attorneys, mental health practitioners, businessmen, farmers, teachers, doctors, and clergy."[41]

Most sexual abuse occurs in the child's home. The risk is higher when the following conditions are present:[42]

1. The child lives without one of his or her biological parents.
2. The mother is unavailable either because she is disabled, ill, or working outside the home.
3. The parents' marriage is unhappy.
4. The child has a poor relationship with his or her parents or is subjected to extremely punitive discipline.
5. The child lives with a stepfather.

Two points about the impact of child abuse in later life are worth making: Ninety-nine percent of the inmates in the maximum security prison at San Quentin were either abused or raised in abusive households; and 300,000 children between the ages of 8 and 15 are living on the nation's streets, willing to prostitute themselves to survive rather than return to the abusive households they ran away from.[43]

Although most people who were abused as children do not end up as convicts or prostitutes, many do bear spiritual, psychological, and/or physical scars. Clinical psychologist Marjorie Whittaker has found that "of all forms of violence, incest and childhood sexual abuse are considered among the most 'toxic' because of their violations of trust, the confusion of affection and coercion, the splitting of family alignments, and serious psychological and physical consequences."[44]

Not all child violence is physical. Health can be severely affected by psychological violence—assaults on personality, character, competence, independence, or general dignity as a human being. The negative consequences of this kind of victimization can be harder to discern and therefore harder to combat. They include depression, low self-esteem, and a pervasive fear of doing something that will offend the abuser.

What do you think?

What factors in society lead to child abuse and neglect? ✳ *What are common characteristics of children's abusers?* ✳ *Why are family members often the perpetrators of child abuse and child sexual abuse?* ✳ *What actions can be taken to prevent such behaviors?*

Sexual Victimization

As with all forms of violence, men and women alike are susceptible to sexual victimization. However, sexual violence against women is of epidemic proportions. Therefore much of our focus here is on women as victims. In fact, sexual battering is the single greatest cause of injury to women in the United States, occurring more frequently than car accidents, muggings, and rapes combined.[45] Physical battering and emotional abuse often leave psychological as well as physical scars. One-quarter to one-third of high school and college students report involvement in dating violence, as perpetrators, victims, or both.[46]

Sexual Assault and Rape   **Sexual assault** is any act in which one person is sexually intimate with another person without that other person's consent. This may range from simple touching to forceful penetration and may include such things as ignoring indications that intimacy is not wanted,

---

Child abuse   The systematic harming of a child by a caregiver, typically a parent.

Sexual abuse of children   Sexually suggestive conversations; inappropriate kissing; touching; petting; oral, anal, or vaginal intercourse; and/or other kinds of sexual interaction between a child and an adult or older child.

Sexual assault   Any act in which one person is sexually intimate with another person without that other person's consent.

Are You a Victim of Abuse?

Symptoms of Abuse: Threats, Power Misuse, and Control

Do any of these symptoms describe your life?

Using Emotional Abuse
> Putting the other person down
> Making the other person feel bad about himself or herself
> Calling the other person names
> Making the other person think he or she is crazy
> Playing mind games
> Humiliating the other person
> Making the other person feel guilty

Using Economic Abuse
> Preventing the other person from getting or keeping a job
> Making the other person ask for money
> Giving the other person an allowance
> Taking the other person's money
> Not letting the other person know about or have access to family income

Using Intimidation
> Making the other person afraid by using looks, gestures, or actions
> Smashing things
> Abusing pets
> Displaying weapons

Using Isolation
> Controlling what the other person does, who he or she sees, what's read, and where he or she goes
> Limiting the other person's involvement with others
> Using jealousy to justify actions

Using Privileges
> Treating the other person like a servant
> Making all the big decisions
> Acting like the master of the castle
> Being the one who determines the rules

Using Coercion and Threats
> Making or carrying out threats to do something to hurt the other person
> Threatening to leave the other person or to commit suicide
> Making the other person drop charges
> Making the other person do illegal things

Using Children
> Making the other person feel guilty about the children
> Using the children to relay messages
> Using visitation to harass the other person
> Threatening to take the children away

Minimizing, Denying, and Blaming

Making light of the abuse and not taking the other person's concerns about it seriously

Saying the abuse never happened

Shifting responsibility for abusive behavior

Saying the other person caused it.

Have the Following Ever Happened to You?

Does your partner:

1. Blame everyone else, especially you, for his or her mistakes?

Yes_____   No_____

2. Prevent you from seeing your family or friends?

Yes_____   No_____

3. Curse you, say mean things, mock you, or humiliate you?

Yes_____   No_____

4. Force you to have sex or force you to engage in sex that makes you feel uncomfortable?

Yes_____   No_____

5. Restrain, hit, punch, slap, or kick you?

Yes_____   No_____

6. Intimidate or threaten you?

Yes_____   No_____

7. Prevent you from leaving the house, getting a job, or continuing your education?

Yes_____   No_____

If you answered "yes" to any of these questions, you may be in an abusive relationship. You should seriously examine your relationship and consider counseling.

Source: Metropolitan Nashville Police Department, Domestic Violence, 2002 (see http://www.police.Nashville.org/bureaus/investigative/domestic/symptoms.htm).

threatening force or other negative consequences, and actually using force.

Rape is the most extreme form of sexual assault and is defined as "penetration without the victim's consent."[47] Whether committed by an acquaintance, a date, or a stranger, rape is a criminal activity that usually has serious emotional, psychological, social, and physical consequences for the victim. Typically, victims are young females, with 29 percent under 11 years of age, 32 percent between the ages of 11 and 17, and 22 percent between ages of 18 and 24.[48] Women age 16 to 19 are four times as likely as the general population to be rape victims.[49]

One of the most startling aspects of sex crimes is how many of them go unreported, usually out of a belief that this is a private, personal matter, fear of reprisal by the assailant, or unwarranted guilt or feelings of responsibility. It is thought that one out of every three women is the victim of an attempted or completed rape in her lifetime. Although as many as two-thirds of all rapes are never reported, there were over 261,000 reported cases of rape, attempted rape, or sexual assault in 2001.[50] See Figure 4.4 for more information.

Incidents of rape generally fall into one of two types—aggravated or simple. An **aggravated rape** involves multiple attackers, strangers, weapons, or physical beatings. A **simple rape** is perpetrated by one person, whom the victim knows, and does not involve a physical beating or use of a weapon. Most incidents are classified as simple rapes, with one report suggesting that 82 percent of female rape victims have been victimized by acquaintances (53 percent), current or former boyfriends (16 percent), current or former spouses (10 percent), or other relatives (3 percent). With almost half of all rape charges dismissed before the cases reach trial and a perceived lack of male understanding of how rape affects women, it's easy to understand why experts feel that so-called "simple" rape is seriously underreported and ignored.

Rape   Sexual penetration without the victim's consent.

Aggravated rape   Rape that involves multiple attackers, strangers, weapons, or a physical beating.

Simple rape   Rape by one person known to the victim that does not involve a physical beating or use of a weapon.

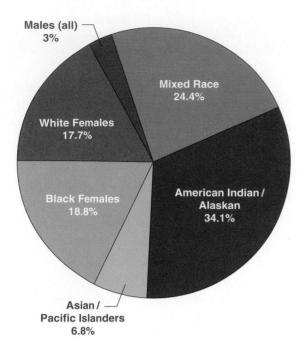

Figure 4.4

Lifetime Rate of Rape or Attempted Rape in the United States

Source: Bureau of Justice Statistics, "2001 Crime Victimization Survey."

Acquaintance or Date Rape Although the terms *date rape*, *friendship rape*, and *acquaintance rape* have become standard terminology, they are typically misused. Not all rapes occur on dates, not all the relationships are friendships, and sometimes the term *acquaintance* is used all too loosely. Many acquaintance rapes occur as the result of incidental contact at a party or when groups of people congregate at one person's house. These are crimes of opportunity, not necessarily a prearranged date. This is an important distinction because the term *date* may suggest some type of reciprocal interaction arranged in advance. While most date or acquaintance rapes happen to women age 15 to 21 years, the 18-year-old new college student is one of the most likely victims.[51]

In a study of 6,000 college students from 32 different universities, researchers found the following:

- More than 50 percent of the college women surveyed had endured some form of sexual abuse.
- More than 25 percent had been the victims of rape or attempted rape.
- Eighty-four percent of the assault victims knew their assailants.
- Fifty-seven percent of the assaults occurred on dates.
- Forty-one percent of the women raped were virgins at the time of the assault.
- Seventy-three percent of the assailants and 55 percent of the victims had used alcohol or drugs prior to the assault.

Sexual harassment Any form of unwanted sexual attention.

- Forty-two percent of the victims indicated that they had sex with the offender again (it is unknown whether the subsequent sex was voluntary).
- Twenty-five percent of the men admitted to some degree of aggressive sexual behavior.
- Men were most likely to commit sexual assaults during their senior year in high school or first year in college.[52]

Date rape is not simply miscommunication; it is an act of violence. Well-known expert on interpersonal relationships Susan Jacoby puts it this way:

> Some women (especially the young) initially resist sex not out of real conviction but as part of the elaborate persuasion and seduction rituals accompanying what was once called courtship. And it is true that many men (again, especially the young) take pride in the ability to coax a woman a step further than she intended to go. But these mating rituals do not justify or even explain date rape. Even the most callow youth is capable of understanding the difference between resistance and genuine fear; between a halfhearted "no, we shouldn't" and tears or screams.[53]

Marital Rape While the legal definition of marital rape varies within the United States, marital rape can be defined as any unwanted intercourse or penetration (vaginal, anal, or oral) obtained by force, threat of force, or when the wife is unable to consent.[54] Some researchers estimate that marital rape may account for 25 percent of all rapes; rape in marriage may be an extremely prevalent form of sexual violence. Although this problem has undoubtedly been common since the earliest origins of marriage as a social institution, it is noteworthy that marital rape did not become a crime in all 50 states until 1993. Even more noteworthy is the fact that in 33 states, there are still exemptions from rape prosecution, effectively meaning that the judicial system may treat it as a lesser form of crime.

Who is most vulnerable to marital rape? In general, women under the age of 25 and those who are from lower socioeconomic groups are at highest risk. Women from homes where other forms of domestic violence are common and where there is a high rate of alcoholism and/or substance abuse also tend to be victimized at greater rates than others. Women who are subjected to marital rape often report multiple offenses over a period of time and that these events are more likely to be forced anal and oral experiences.[55]

Again, abuse of power and an unmitigated need to control and dominate seem to be key factors in the husband-rapist profile. Marital rape can have devastating short- and long-term consequences for women, including injuries to the vaginal and anal areas, lacerations, soreness, bruising, torn muscles, fatigue, panic attacks, sexually transmitted diseases, broken bones, wounds, and other emotional and physical scars.

Sexual Harassment If we think of violence as including verbal abuse and the threat of coercion, then sexual harassment is a form of violence. Under Title VII of the Civil Rights Act, **sexual harassment** is defined as "unwelcomed sexual advances, requests for sexual favors, and other verbal or physical contact of a sexual nature." Despite what might appear to be a clear definition, sexual harassment is often difficult to identify. While many people would say that sexual harassment is anything the offended person *believes* is harassment, others will say that this explanation is too nebulous.

The issue of sexual harassment was brought to the collective consciousness of society in the early 1990s when Anita Hill charged Supreme Court Justice nominee Clarence Thomas with sexual harassment in a previous employment environment. The alleged harassment was partly in the form of sexually offensive humor, not all directed at Hill. What had long been dismissed as harmless behavior became a cause for concern in business, academia, and government. More recently, the Paula Jones and Monica Lewinsky scandals have kept sexual harassment issues in the news and have focused attention on additional aspects such as improper touching, improper suggestions, and inappropriate uses of power. Most colleges and universities now offer courses on identifying and preventing sexual harassment, and most companies have established sexual harassment policies and procedures for dealing with it.

It's always important to watch what you say and how you say it, but nowhere is this more true than at work. Learning what constitutes sexual harassment may save you embarrassment in the future. A simple compliment on a colleague's appearance can be offensive if stated without sensitivity, regardless of the intent. "You look very nice today" can become offensive if stated as, "That dress looks great on your body." Even if the person enjoys your comment, you have to remember that others may overhear. If you become known as someone who makes such comments, you will be considered a risk the next time a promotion comes up.

Most companies now have sexual harassment policies in place, as well as procedures for dealing with it. If you feel you are being harassed, the most important thing you can do is be assertive. Immediately after the incident occurs, follow these guidelines:

- *Tell the harasser to stop.* Be clear and direct about what is bothering you and why you are upset: "I don't like this joke/touch/remark/look. It makes me feel uncomfortable and it makes it hard for me to work/participate/be your friend," and so on. This may be the first indication the person has ever had that such behavior is inappropriate. This will usually stop the harassment.
- *Document the harassment.* Make a record of the incident. If the harassment becomes intolerable, having a record of exactly what occurred (and when and where) will be helpful in making your case.
- *Complain to a higher authority.* Talk to your manager about what happened. If the manager or supervisor doesn't take you seriously, find out what the internal grievance procedures are for your organization.
- *Remember that you have not done anything wrong.* You will likely feel awful after being harassed (especially if you have

to complain to superiors). However, you should feel proud that you are not keeping silent. The person who is harassing you is wrong, not you. If the situation becomes so uncomfortable that you feel you can't work with the harasser, why should you be the one to leave?

What do you think?

Why do you think women are often reluctant to report sexual harassment? ❋ *Why do you think so many men report that they were unaware of their own sexually harassing behaviors?* ❋ *What can be done to increase awareness in this area?*

Social Contributors to Sexual Assault According to many experts, certain common assumptions in our society prevent recognition by both the perpetrator and the wider public of the true nature of sexual assault.[56] These assumptions include the following:[57]

- *Minimization.* It is often assumed that sexual assault of women is rare because official crime statistics, including the Uniform Crime Reports of the FBI, show very few rapes per thousand population. However, rape is the most underreported of all serious crimes. Researchers have found that nearly 25 percent of women in the United States have been raped.
- *Trivialization.* Incredibly enough, sexual assault of women is still often viewed as a jocular matter. During a gubernatorial election in Texas a few years back, one of the candidates reportedly compared a bad patch of weather to rape: "If there's nothing you can do about it, just lie back and enjoy it." (He lost the election—to a woman.)
- *Blaming the victim.* Many discussions of sexual violence against women display a sometimes unconscious assumption that the woman did something to provoke the attack—that she dressed revealingly or flirted outrageously.
- *"Boys will be boys."* According to this assumption, men just can't control themselves once they become aroused.

Over the years, psychologists and others have proposed several theories to explain why many males sexually victimize women. In one of the first major studies to explore this issue, almost two-thirds of the male respondents had engaged in intercourse unwanted by the woman, primarily because of male peer pressure.[58] By all indicators, these trends continue today. Peer pressure is certainly a strong factor, but a growing body of research suggests that sexual assault is encouraged by the socialization processes that males experience daily.[59]

- *Male socialization.* Throughout our lives, we are exposed to social norms that "objectify" women—make them appear as objects that can be used. Media portrayals of half-dressed and undressed women in seductive poses promoting products, for instance, contribute to sex-role stereotyping. These portrayals often show males as aggressors and females as

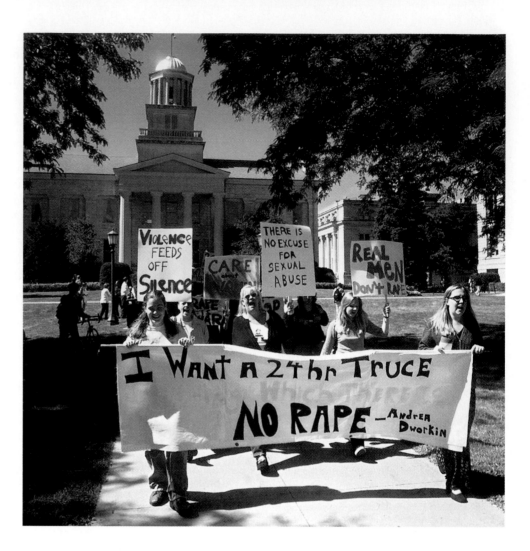

College students can organize vigils, marches, and educational programs to raise awareness about violence against women.

targets. In addition, men are exposed from an early age to antifemale jokes and vulgar and obscene terms for women. These reinforce the idea that females are lesser beings who may be pushed around with impunity.[60] Males are also discouraged from acting in ways that society views as feminine. They are told to act tough and unemotional; strive for power, status, and control; be aggressive and take risks.

• *Male attitudes.* Several studies have confirmed a greater tolerance of rape among men who accept the myth that rape is something women secretly desire, who believe in adversarial relationships between men and women, who condone violence against women, or who hold traditional attitudes toward sex roles. Such men are more apt to blame the victim and more likely to commit rape themselves if they think they can get away with it.[61]

• *Male sexual history and hostility.* Most rapists are not abnormal or psychologically disturbed. Rather, they tend to be people whose childhoods involved early, multiple sexual experiences (both forced and voluntary) and who feel hostility toward women.[62]

• *Male misperceptions.* Men who are convinced that women really want sex even if they say they don't are more likely to perpetrate sexual assaults. They more readily misinterpret women's words and behavior and act on their mispercep-

tions—only to be surprised later when women claim that they have been assaulted.[63]

• *Situational factors.* Several factors increase the likelihood of sexual assault. Dates in which the male makes all the decisions, pays, drives, and in general controls what happens are more likely to end in sexual aggression. Alcohol and drug use increase the risk and severity of sexual assault. Length of relationship is another important situational factor: The more long-standing the relationship, the greater the chance of aggression. Finally, males who belong to a close-knit social group involving intense interaction are more prone to engage in a peer-pleasing assault.

> **What do you think?**
>
> *What factors make men likely to commit sexual assault or rape?* ✳ *What measures might be effective in preventing such behaviors?*

Crime on Campus: A Safe Haven?

Though the majority of crimes on campus still consist of larceny, vandalism, and setting off fire alarms illegally, the rate of violent crime is increasing. Traditionally, most campus crimes were handled internally. This has changed as more states have passed legislation requiring that colleges and universities warn their students about crime and danger both on campus property and in off-campus housing that they recommend.[64] In 1992, Congress passed the Campus Sexual Assault Victim's Bill of Rights, known as the Ramstad Act. The act gives victims the right to call in off-campus authorities to investigate serious campus crimes. In addition, universities must set up educational programs and notify students of available counseling.

Sexual Assault on Campus   Most studies of sexual assault among college students indicate that 25 percent to 60 percent of college men have engaged in some form of sexually coercive behavior.[65] This is consistent with the 27 percent of college women who have reported experiencing rape or attempted rape since they were 14 years old, and the 54 percent who claim to have been sexually victimized (forced to endure unwanted petting, kisses, and other advances).[66] In one survey, only 39 percent of the men sampled denied coercive involvement, 28 percent admitted to having used a coercive method at least once, and 15 percent admitted that they had forced a woman to have intercourse at least once.[67] And according to a large, nationally representative sample of college and university students, 25 percent of the male respondents had been involved in some form of sexual assault since age 14.[68] Since this early national study many smaller studies have reported similar statistics.

As in the general public, the incidence of sexual assault on campuses is believed to be seriously underreported. In a recent report, one major university familiar to the author claimed there were no rapes on campus. But based on national averages, it seems highly unlikely that no forcible sexual encounters would occur in a setting where nearly 16,000 students date, drink, and socialize every week. The fact is that coercive sex or date rape is seldom reported to campus police, and when a rape victim seeks help at the campus health center, the center is not compelled to report the crime. In one study, 20 percent of female respondents at a midwestern university said they had been raped by someone they knew, but only 8 percent of them had reported it to the police. At another midwestern university, 20 percent of 247 women interviewed said they had experienced date rape, but few had reported it.[69] Needless to say, other sexual violations, such as obscene phone calls, stalking, sexual molestation that does not result in penetration, exhibitionism, voyeurism, and attempted rape, go equally unreported.[70]

Sexual Harassment on Campus   How pervasive is sexual harassment at U.S. schools? According to a national study by the American Association of University Women, four out of five students attending public schools have been sexually harassed by other students. Over one-third of these incidents are reported to occur before the seventh grade. Another study indicates that 90 percent of undergraduate women and 52 percent of graduate women report at least one negative experience from male students, and that the students most likely to harass these women are members of fraternities, athletic teams, and all-male groups and cliques; men who are defiant or angry at women; and those who have been abused themselves.[71]

While peers pose a threat of harassment, a study by the Institute of Social and Economic Research at Cornell University found that 61 percent of upperclass and graduate students experienced "unwanted sexual attention from someone of authority within the university."[72] Typically, these attentions come from male professors and may include affairs of male faculty with married and unmarried female students; demands for sex, with threats of lower grades for noncompliance; and sexually offensive and hostile environments in the classroom.[73] Many universities have strict codes of conduct relating to faculty–student consensual as well as nonconsensual relationships. Many of these policies stem from reported difficulties with power and control between faculty and students and the potential for negative consequences.

> **What do you think?**
>
> *What policies does your school have regarding consensual relationships between faculty members and students? ✳ Do you think that consenting adults should have the right to interact, regardless of their positions within a system or workplace? ✳ What are the potential dangers of such interactions?*

Reducing Risks

After a violent act is committed against someone we know, we acknowledge the horror of the event, express sympathy, and go on with our lives. But the person who has been brutalized may take months or years to recover. It is far better to prevent a violent act than to recover from it.

Self-Defense against Rape

Rape can occur no matter what preventive actions you take, but commonsense self-defense tactics can lower the risk. Self-defense is a process that includes learning increased awareness, self-defense techniques, reasonable precautions, and the self-confidence and judgment needed to determine appropriate responses to different situations.[74] Figure 4.5 identifies practical tips for preventing personal assaults.

Taking Control   Most rapes by assailants unknown to the victim are planned in advance. They are frequently preceded by a casual, friendly conversation. Although many women have said that they started to feel uneasy during such a conversation, they denied the possibility of an attack to themselves until it was too late. Listen to your feelings, and trust

In Your Car

- Always keep your doors and windows locked.
- Purchase cars with an alarm system and remote entry.
- Don't stop for vehicles in distress; call for help.
- If your car breaks down, lock the doors and wait for help from the police.
- If you think someone is following you, do not drive to your home; drive to a busy place and attract attention.
- Stick to well-traveled routes.
- Keep your car in good running order and always filled with gas.
- On long trips, don't make it obvious you're traveling alone.
- Do not sleep in your car along interstate highways.
- Carry a cell phone with programmed emergency numbers.

On the Street

- Walk or jog at a steady pace.
- Walk or jog with others.
- At night, avoid dark parking lots, wooded areas, and any place that offers an assailant good cover.
- Listen for footsteps and voices.
- Be aware of cars that keep driving around in your area.
- Vary your running or walking routes.
- Carry pepper spray or other deterrents, or walk or jog with a dog… the bigger, the better!
- Carry change to make a phone call.
- Tell others where you are going, your route, and when you'll return.

Figure 4.5
Preventing Personal Assaults

your intuition. Be assertive and direct to someone who is getting out of line or threatening—this may convince the would-be rapist to back off. Stifle your tendency to be "nice," and don't fear making a scene. Let him know that you mean what you say and are prepared to defend yourself:

- *Speak in a strong voice.* Use statements like "Leave me alone" rather than questions like "Will you please leave me alone?" Avoid apologies and excuses.
- *Maintain eye contact with the would-be attacker.*
- *Sound as if you mean what you say.*
- *Stand up straight, act confident, and remain alert.* Walk as if you own the sidewalk.

Many rapists use certain ploys to initiate their attacks. Among the most common are the following:

- *Request for help.* This allows him to get close—to enter your house to use the phone, for instance.
- *Offer of help.* This can also help him gain entrance to your home: "Let me help you carry that package."
- *Guilt trip.* "Gee, no one is friendly nowadays. I can't believe you won't talk with me for just a little while."
- *Purposeful accident.* He may bump into the back of your car, and then assault you when you get out to see the damage. Don't stop unless you have to in these situations, and if you do stop, stay in your car with the doors locked.
- *Authority.* Many women fall for the old "policeman at the door" ruse. If anyone comes to your door dressed in uniform, ask him to show his ID before you unlock the door. You can also call the police department to confirm his ID.

If you are attacked, act immediately. Don't worry about causing a scene. Draw attention to yourself and your assailant. Scream "Fire" loudly. Research has shown that passersby are much more likely to help if they hear the word *fire* rather than just a scream. Your attacker may also be caught off balance by the action.

To prevent an attack, remember the following points:

- *Always be vigilant.* Even the safest cities and towns have rapes. Don't be fooled by a sleepy-little-town atmosphere.
- *Use campus escort services whenever possible.*
- *Be assertive in demanding a well-lit campus.*
- *Don't use the same routes all the time.* Vary your movement patterns.
- *Don't leave a bar alone with a friendly stranger.* Stay with your friends, and let the friendly stranger come along. Don't give your address to anyone you don't know.
- *Let friends and family know where you are going, what route you'll take, and when to expect your return.*
- *Stay close to others.* Avoid shortcuts through dark or unlit paths. Don't be the last one to leave the lab or library late at night.
- *Keep your windows and doors locked.* Don't open the door to strangers.

What to Do If a Rape Occurs

If you are a rape victim, report the attack. This gives you a sense of control. Follow these steps:

- Call 911 (if available).
- Do not bathe, shower, douche, clean up, or touch anything the attacker may have touched.
- Do not throw away or launder the clothes you were wearing, as they will be needed as evidence.
- Bring a clean change of clothes to the clinic or hospital.
- Contact the rape assistance hotline in your area and ask for advice on therapists or counseling if you need additional help or advice.

If a friend is raped, here's how you can help:

- Believe her and don't ask questions that may appear to implicate her in the assault.

- Recognize that rape is a violent act and the victim was not looking for this to happen.
- Encourage her to see a doctor immediately, as she may have medical needs but feel too embarrassed to seek help on her own. Offer to go with her.
- Encourage her to report the crime.
- Be understanding and let her know you will be there for her.
- Recognize that this is an emotional recovery and it may take six months to a year for her to bounce back.
- Encourage her to seek counseling.

A Campuswide Response to Violence

Increasingly, college campuses have become microcosms of the greater society, complete with the risks, hazards, and dangers people face in the world. Many college administrators have been proactive in establishing violence-prevention policies, programs, and services.[75]

Changing Roles To increase student protection, campus law enforcement has changed over the years in both numbers and authority to prosecute student offenders. Campus police are responsible for emergency responses to situations that threaten safety, human resources, the general campus environment, traffic and bicycle safety, and other dangers. Campus police have the power to enforce laws with students in the same way they are handled in the general community. In fact, many campuses now hire state troopers or local law enforcement officers to deal with campus issues rather than maintain a separate police staff.

Many of these law enforcement groups follow a *community policing* model in which officers have specific responsibilities for certain areas of campus, departments, or events. By narrowing the scope of each officer's territory, officers get to know people in the area and are better able to anticipate and prevent risks. This differs from earlier safety policies, in which campus security typically swooped down only in times of trouble.

Prevention Efforts Many colleges and universities now include crime prevention and safety specialists in their law enforcement agencies. These specialists work to improve university policies and procedures to reduce risk to students and others on campus. They commonly recommend the following activities:

- A rape awareness and education program for members of the campus community.
- A crime prevention orientation program for new faculty and staff as well as students.
- Specialized safety workshops for particular groups, such as commuters, international students, athletes, and students with disabilities.
- Printed and electronic educational messages about personal safety.
- A notification process to distribute information about special hazards.

- Alcohol and drug programs dealing with policy, awareness, education, and enforcement.
- A "grounds safety" program, including measures such as removing shrubs from dark areas and providing good lighting throughout the campus.
- A system of emergency call boxes or telephones across campus.
- Escort services for students who must be out after dark.
- Motorist assistance programs for persons with car trouble.
- Antitheft programs, including regular patrols of parking lots and other areas.
- Victim advocacy programs, such as rape or abuse counseling.

The Role of Student Affairs Although some overlap may exist between law enforcement activities, student affairs offices need to play a vital role in all on-campus programs, both to prevent trouble and to resolve problems that do occur. Student groups should monitor progress, identify potential threats, and advocate for improvements in any areas found to be deficient. A student affairs office can play a key role in making sure that mental health services, student assistance programs, and other services are high quality, easily accessible, and meet student needs. A human services or student affairs office should seek to involve the wider student body and ensure that all are acutely aware of its services. If these programs are not visible or proactive in ensuring campus safety, a careful assessment of their roles and responsibilities should be made. Student leaders can play a major role in shaping such services and advocating for the campus population.

Community Strategies for Preventing Violence

Since the causes of homicide and assaultive violence are complex, community strategies for prevention must be multidimensional. Successful strategies include the following:[76]

- Developing and implementing educational programs to teach people communication, conflict resolution, and coping skills.
- Working with individuals to help them develop self-esteem and respect for others.
- Rewarding youngsters for good behavior, and never spanking a child when angry (Children need to know that anger is sometimes acceptable, but violence never is. Use family meetings to resolve conflicts.)
- Establishing and enforcing policies that forbid discrimination on the basis of gender, religious affiliation, race, sexual orientation, marital status, and age.
- Increasing and enriching educational programs for family planning.
- Increasing efforts by health care and social service programs to identify victims of violence.
- Improving treatment and support for victims.
- Treating the psychological as well as the physical consequences of violence.

Unintentional Injuries

As stated previously, unintentional injuries occur without planning or intention to harm. Examples of unintentional injuries include car accidents, falls, water accidents, accidental gunshots, recreational accidents, and workplace accidents. None of these injuries happen on purpose, yet they may result in pain, suffering, and possibly even death. Most efforts to prevent unintentional injuries focus on changing something about the *person*, the *environment*, or the *circumstances* (policies, procedures) that put people in harm's way.

Residential Safety

Injuries within the home typically take the form of falls, burns, or intrusions by others. Some populations, such as the elderly, are particularly vulnerable to household injuries; however, the elderly are not the only victims. Each year, hundreds of children suffer severe burns or die from accidental fires, falls, and other home-based injuries. To reduce the risk of accidents, consider the following:

Fall-Proof Your Home

- Eliminate clutter, particularly objects you may stumble over in the dark. Leave nothing lying around on the floor.
- Make sure all rugs are securely fastened to the floor and don't slide when stepped on. Inexpensive rubberized mats or strips will hold rugs in place.
- Train your pets to stay out from under your feet. Many an unsuspecting person has ended up on the floor while trying to avoid a pet.
- Make sure handrails are secure and within easy reach. All stairs should have slip-proof treads.
- Install slip-proof mats or decals in showers and tubs. Add handrails and places to grab for stability in tubs and showers.

Avoid Burns

- Extinguish all cigarettes in ashtrays before you go to bed. Don't smoke and drink before bed. In fact, don't smoke in bed at any time! Sparks can smolder in mattresses or upholstered furniture, then flare into flames.
- Don't throw spent matches in the trash with paper and other combustibles. Soak matches in water before discarding.
- Set all lamps away from drapes, linens, and paper, particularly halogen lights or specialty lamps that can get extremely hot.
- Keep all hotpads and kitchen cloths away from stove burners. When not using a cloth, set it on a counter far from the stove.
- Keep candles under control and away from combustibles. While it may seem romantic to go to sleep by candlelight, it is highly risky. Don't do it.

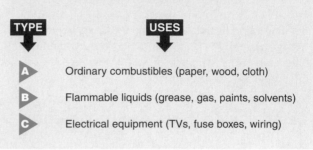

Fire extinguishers are labeled A, B, and C, depending on the kind of fire they are designed to extinguish. They also are numbered according to the size of the fire they can put out. The higher the number, the greater the capacity.

TYPE	USES
A	Ordinary combustibles (paper, wood, cloth)
B	Flammable liquids (grease, gas, paints, solvents)
C	Electrical equipment (TVs, fuse boxes, wiring)

Figure 4.6
Do You Have an Appropriate Fire Extinguisher?

- Whenever possible, purchase stoves and ovens with controls in front so you can avoid reaching over hot pans to change the burner temperature.
- Use caution when lighting barbecue grills and other home-based fires. Never spray combustible fluids such as lighter fluid directly onto the fire.
- Check chimneys and fireplaces regularly for buildup of flammable soot.
- Service furnaces annually, and be sure to change the filters.
- Avoid overloading electrical circuits with appliances and cords. Older buildings are at particular risk for fire from such overloads.
- Program phones with emergency numbers for speed dialing, and keep these numbers in clear sight near phones as well.
- Replace batteries in smoke alarms periodically, and test them regularly to make sure the batteries are working.
- Have the proper fire extinguishers ready in case of fire (see Figure 4.6).

Prevent Unwanted Intruders

- Close blinds and drapes whenever you are away and in the evening when you are home. Remove large bushes and obstructions from around your windows and doors so that anyone lurking outside will be visible.
- Install dead-bolt locks on all doors and locks on windows. Put a peephole in the main entryway to your home, and do not let anyone in without checking.
- If you have a screen door, lock it. If an unfamiliar visitor comes to the door, this door can serve as a barrier.
- If possible, install a home alarm system.
- Rent apartments that require a security code or clearance to gain entry.
- Avoid apartments that are easily accessible, such as first-floor units with large patio doors.
- Don't give information about your home or schedule to telephone solicitors. Try to vary the times of day that you come home for lunch or quick stops to check on things.

- Don't let repairmen in without identification. Preferably, landlords should give information about such visits well in advance. Have someone else with you when repairmen are there working. Just because a person is licensed to fix refrigerators does not mean he can be trusted.
- Avoid dark parking structures, laundry rooms, and the like. Try to use these areas only when others are around.
- Use initials for first names on mailboxes and in phone listings. Keep your address out of phone books.
- Keep a cell phone near your bed and program it to 911. Unlike what you see on TV, many intruders do not cut phone lines. More commonly, they simply pick up the receiver in another room as they walk through, thereby disabling a bedroom phone.
- Get to know your neighbors. Organize a neighborhood watch.
- Be careful of "doggy doors." Some thieves let their smallest associate crawl through and unlock the door.
- Be careful of skylights and other areas that open up from the outside. Keep them locked and bolted.
- When away, put the lights in different rooms on timers set to come on and go off at different times. Stop your mail and newspaper.

Although no amount of security will prevent all threats of intrusion, following these precautions, as well as actively searching for well-maintained housing in low-crime areas, are good steps toward preventing break-ins. Usually intruders are searching for items to sell and enter with theft in mind. If you encounter an intruder, it is far better to give up your money than to fight.

What do you think?

Do a "spot check" of your home. What areas might pose a risk for home accidents or forced entry? ✳ Do you know the numbers of your local fire and police departments? ✳ Do you have a fire extinguisher in your house? ✳ What would you do if the house caught on fire and you needed to escape immediately?

Workplace Safety

American adults spend most of their waking hours on the job. While most job situations are pleasant and productive, others pose physical and emotional hazards. Stress, burnout, hostile or abusive interactions with others, discrimination, power struggles, sexual harassment, and a host of other threats are possible whenever people are cloistered together for prolonged periods of time. The nature of the job itself, the corporate culture, and the policies and procedures that characterize certain professions can add to workplace stress.

Fatal Injuries   Certain industries are inherently more hazardous than others; outdoor occupations show the highest fatality and injury rates. While workplaces have begun serious

programming, policies, and services designed to reduce risks, the following statistics indicate a continuing problem:[77]

- In 1999, job-related fatalities reached their highest levels since record keeping began. Rates have decreased slightly since then but continue to surpass most previous fatality reports. Data released in 2002 is sure to be even higher when the September 11 deaths of police and firefighters are recorded.
- Highway crashes were the leading cause of on-the-job fatalities and accounted for 27 percent of fatal work injury totals in 2000. Most involved truck drivers.
- Sixteen percent of worker fatalities resulted from other types of transportation-related incidents, such as tractors and forklifts overturning in fields or warehouses, workers being struck by vehicles, aircraft and railway crashes, and water vehicles crashing or capsizing.
- Workplace homicides have declined in recent years but continued as a major cause of workplace danger, accounting for over 13 percent of all occupational injuries. Coworker disputes, former coworker disputes, and shootings during the course of robbery led the list. In addition, homicides occur at workplaces as a result of domestic violence carryover, when a violent spouse or former partner comes to work to get revenge on a partner.
- Falls, being struck by objects, and electrocutions are also significant causes of worker fatality.
- On average, about 17 workers were fatally injured each day in 2000. Hundreds more were permanently or temporarily disabled. Overall, there were 2,576,000 workdays lost to injury in 2000.
- Most fatally injured workers under 16 years of age were killed while doing farmwork.
- Men between the ages of 35 and 54 are the most likely victims of fatal occupational injuries.

Nonfatal Work Injuries   Although deaths capture media attention, other workers may be seriously injured or disabled. Chronic, debilitating pain and other injuries can cause great economic strain on organizations due to workers' compensation claims and days lost from work. Injuries that cause the greatest number of lost-work days include carpal tunnel syndrome, hernia, amputation of a limb, fractures, sprains and strains (often of the back), cuts or lacerations, and chemical burns.[78] For example, nearly half of all workers with carpal tunnel syndrome miss 30 days or more of work each year. Because so many work injuries are due to repetitive motion, overexertion, or inappropriate motion, they are largely preventable through training and techniques designed to reduce employees' risks.

What do you think?

What can be done to prevent injuries? ✳ Are students on your campus at risk from any of the problems discussed? ✳ Does your school have programs in place to prevent injuries? ✳ Do you think more can be done, and if so, what?

Managing Campus Safety

Commonsense precautions are themes of this chapter. Follow sensible guidelines on where you go, when, and with whom. What limits do you set when you're out with friends, whether casual or intimate? Most campuses have initiated programs, services, and policies designed to protect students from potential threats against personal health and safety. Answer the following questions to help determine your college administrators' degree of interest in and commitment to a violence-free setting.

Checklist for Change

Making Personal Choices

☐ Do you decide before going on a date to limit your sexual behavior?

☐ Do you travel in groups whenever possible?

☐ Do you avoid being out alone at night?

☐ Do you avoid high-crime areas?

☐ Do you take the precautions necessary to reduce your risk of injury from violence?

Making Community Choices

☐ Does your health center offer workshops on rape prevention and the prevention of other sexual offenses?

☐ Does your campus offer courses focused on understanding human diversity?

☐ Does your campus offer workshops or information for students to help them avoid situations that put them at risk for violent interactions?

☐ Does your campus offer confidential counseling or assistance to victims of sexual assault?

☐ Does your campus offer workshops or educational sessions dealing with suicide?

☐ Does your campus offer information, workshops, or other services dealing with partner and domestic violence?

☐ Does your campus have strict substance abuse policies?

☐ Are services such as rides and escort services available after hours to prevent rapes and assaults? Has your university increased the role of campus security to improve student safety?

☐ Is your campus well-lighted and open in the evenings?

☐ Are campus health educators, counselors, and other professionals trained to spot victimization in clients and recommend appropriate services?

☐ Does your campus have a code of conduct that mandates swift and prudent punishment for alcohol and other drug abuse and acts of campus violence?

Summary

* Intentional injuries result from actions committed with intent to harm. Unintentional injuries are the result of actions involving no intent to harm. Violence is at epidemic levels in the United States. Many factors lead people to be violent. Among them are anger, substance abuse, and root causes of oppression, poor mental health, and economics.

* Acts of terrorism are becoming more common in the United States. In addition to their immediate impact, terrorist activities can exert damaging long-term effects by fostering an atmosphere of fear and anxiety.

* Violence affects everyone in society—from the direct victims, to those who live in fear, to those who pay higher taxes and insurance premiums. Over half of homicides are committed by people who knew their victims. Bias and hate crimes divide people, but teaching tolerance can reduce risks. Gang violence continues to grow but can be combated by programs aimed at reducing the problems that lead to gang membership. Violence on campus may be increasing, but the victims' rights have also increased as a result of major legislation.

* Prevention of violent acts begins with avoiding situations in which harm may occur. There are several avenues available for reducing risks, including community, school, workplace, and individual strategies. Many crimes of general society are now commonplace at universities and colleges, including personal assaults, harassment, hate crimes, and even murder.

* Unintentional injuries frequently occur in homes and work sites and can produce serious consequences, including death. By following commonsense guidelines, you can significantly reduce your risk of falls, burns, and other injuries.

Questions for Discussion and Reflection

1. What major types of crimes are committed in the United States? What is the difference between primary and reactive aggression?
2. What major factors lead to violent acts?
3. Who tends to be susceptible to the appeal of gang membership? What actions can be taken to keep young kids out of gangs?
4. What is terrorism, and why does it occur? What can you do to protect yourself against terrorist attacks?
5. Compare domestic violence against men and against women: What are the differences? What are the similarities? What causes domestic violence?
6. What conditions put a child at risk for abuse? What can be done to prevent or decrease the amount of child abuse?
7. What is sexual harassment, and what factors contribute to it in the workplace?
8. What factors increase risk for sexual assault?
9. What are the most effective violence prevention strategies on your campus?
10. What steps can you take to lower your risk of injury from unintentional violence?

Application Exercises

Reread the What Do You Think? scenarios at the beginning of the chapter and answer the following questions:

1. Why do you think violent incidents occur? What actions could we take as a society to reduce violence?
2. Do you believe that violence is really much worse than it was back in the "good old days"? Or are we just more aware of it due to increased media coverage?
3. How safe is your campus? What policies, procedures, and safeguards are in place to protect you? What other actions could be taken?

Accessing Your Health on the Internet

Visit the following Internet sites to explore further topics and issues related to personal health. To visit an organization's website, go to the Companion Website for *Access to Health, Eighth Edition* at www.aw.com/donatelle, click on the book image, and select "Accessing Your Health on the Internet" from the navigation menu on the left.

1. *Communities Against Violence Network* An extensive, searchable database for information about violence against women, with articles about everything from domestic violence to legal information and statistics.
2. *Crimes on College Campuses* Comprehensive source of information and statistics on colleges and universities across America.
3. *National Center for Injury Prevention and Control* The WISQARS database of this CDC section provides statistics and information on fatal and nonfatal injuries, both intentional and unintentional.
4. *National Center for Victims of Crime* Provides information and resources for victims of crimes ranging from hate crimes to sexual assault.
5. *National Institute for Occupational Safety and Health (NIOSH)* Excellent reference for national statistics on injury and violence, in both the community and the workplace.
6. *Workplace Solutions* Provides information that helps promote well-being by helping people understand the nature of interpersonal conflict, stress, and violence at work.

Further Reading

Hoffman, A., J. Schuh, and R. Fenske. *Violence on Campus.* Gaithersburg, MD: Aspen, 1998.

Overview of violence on campus, unique factors that lead to violence and abuse on college campuses, and current programs and policies designed to reduce risk.

Ottens, A., and K. Hotelling, Eds. *Sexual Violence on Campus: Policies, Programs, and Perspectives.* New York: Springer Publishing, 2001.

Overview of trends, causes, and contributors to violence on campus, as well as policies and programs designed to prevent violence.

U.S. Department of Health and Human Services. "Inventory of Federal Data Systems for Injury, Surveillance, Research and Prevention Activities." Washington, DC: Government Printing Office, 2001.

Excellent reference for data, reporting mechanisms, and instruments used in assessing U.S. violence statistics.

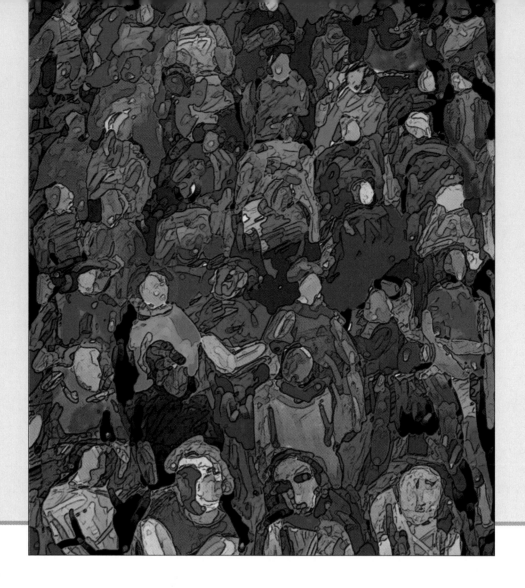

Objectives

* Explain the importance of understanding symbolism and individual perceptions in the communication process.

* Discuss ways to improve communication skills and interpersonal interactions through self-disclosure, effective listening and speaking skills, "I" messages, nonverbal communication, assertive communication, establishing proper climates, and effective conflict management.

* Explain the types and characteristics of intimate relationships, and how they are maintained.

* Discuss similarities and differences between men and women in communication styles and in how they make decisions, choose partners, share feelings, and relate to each other.

* Discuss the barriers to intimate relationships and factors that inhibit successful communication. Explain how these barriers can be overcome.

* Discuss the importance of commitment, honesty, and mutual respect in relationships.

* Examine factors that are important in determining the success of an intimate relationship.

* Discuss factors that affect life decisions such as whether to remain single and whether to have children. Examine child-rearing practices in the United States.

* Describe the warning signs of relationship decline, where to get help, and factors that may lead to relationship problems.

* Discuss actions that can improve interpersonal interactions.

5 Healthy Relationships

Communicating Effectively with Friends, Family, and Significant Others

---

What do you think?

James is a sophomore at Texas Tech. Outgoing and friendly, he likes to talk to anyone who will listen. Mostly, his conversations center on himself—particularly the intimate details of his sexual exploits. Several friends are uncomfortable with his graphic depictions of private information. Sasha, his girlfriend, has no idea that James tells others about these details.

What might you do if James told you about his sexual exploits? ❋ Would you tell Sasha what James said? ❋ Why or why not? ❋ How might you react if you heard such details from a 12-year-old boy or a 70-year-old woman? ❋ Discuss how age, gender, race, and other factors influence your reaction.

Kate, a 26-year-old senior at a large southern university, hopes to become a hospital administrator. She is attractive and accomplished, and several people have asked to date her. But she has clearly indicated that she is *not* interested in a love relationship, wishes to remain single, and also does not want to have children. In spite of her wishes, her family and friends continually try to "fix her up" with someone, which she finds frustrating. Her parents also pressure her about giving them grandchildren.

What difficulties might be faced by someone who wishes to remain single in our society? ❋ How do you react when you hear that someone chooses to remain single or not have children? ❋ Can a healthy person choose to avoid all intimate relationships? ❋ Why or why not? If you were Kate's friend, how might you help her be who she wants to be?

H umans are "social animals"—we have a basic need to belong and to feel loved, appreciated, and wanted.[1] We can't live without relating to others in some way. In fact, a study done by researchers at the Harvard School of Public Health shows that the ability to relate well with people throughout your life can have almost as much impact on your health as exercise and good nutrition.[2] The benefits of healthy relationships are many, although they can also be a source of unhappiness and grief.

All relationships involve a degree of risk. Only by taking these risks, however, can we grow and truly experience all that life has to offer.

In this chapter, we examine healthy relationships and the communication skills necessary to create and maintain them. Why is communication so important? For one thing, the way we communicate influences whether or not we are accepted by others. For another, most of us sincerely want to express ourselves clearly and honestly in our relationships. Clear communication can help us bridge our differences, and it can also affect health. Several studies point to links between the inability to identify and communicate feelings and increased health risks. For example, an ongoing study of 2,500 Finnish men, ages 42–60, has found that the "stoic personality" may in fact promote dramatic increases in mortality. Many other studies have linked suppressed emotions with health problems such as hypertension and inflammatory bowel disease.[3]

Expressing ourselves well and knowing how to understand what others are saying are both vitally important to communication. These abilities lay the groundwork for healthy relationships, and satisfying relationships are significant factors in overall health. In this chapter, we look at communication styles and intimate and nonintimate relationships to gain a better understanding of how we interact with others and express ourselves.

The Communication Process: Getting Started

Many of us find it difficult to tell people what we really think or to express how we feel during a particularly happy or sad moment. Much of this difficulty stems from the complexity of human language itself. How and where we were raised and the perceptions, thoughts, and attitudes we have developed give each of us a unique perspective on language. Even a simple word can cause confusion, send mixed messages, and create misunderstanding. E-mail communication is particularly prone to misinterpretation and resultant problems. Your friend's definition of *happiness* or *love* may differ from yours. Your friend may think of a dog as a barking, smelly animal, while you view dogs as loving companions. The word *dog* has different connotations for each of you. Awareness of the subtleties of language definitely aids the communication process.

Symbolism in Communication

How often have you heard someone say "We just can't communicate" or "You're sending me mixed messages"? These exchanges occur regularly as people struggle to solve a problem, learn a new skill, start a relationship, or work through difficulties in an existing relationship.[4] Whereas people typically use the word **communication** to mean "talking and listening, sending messages with words or your body," communication experts tend to describe this act as "the symbolic process of shared meanings."[5] Symbols transmit messages and represent people, events, places, or objects. Words or verbal expressions, facial expressions, vocal tone, eye contact, gestures, movement, body posture, appearance, context, and spatial distance all reflect various communication symbols. Gifts, food, cards, e-mails, and other objects are also forms of symbolic communication. The multiplicity of symbolic gestures and ways of interpreting them can make communication a challenge. Sometimes we think we are saying something quite clearly, but even an attentive listener may misunderstand the symbols we use and thus our meaning.

Because communication is a process, our every action, word, or other symbol becomes part of our lived history with others—part of the evolving impression we make. If we are nasty and hostile with someone, even for a short period of time, those messages form a permanent part of our shared history. Each time we interact and communicate, this history evolves, for better or for worse. This is complicated by the fact that each person brings "baggage" (both good and bad) from the past into an interaction. For example, a person who has become cynical and distrustful may be critical and guarded during interactions with others. Our interpretations of communication also become part of shared history, and interpretation can be tricky. If someone says, "I love you," it may mean friendship, the love shared by family members, or the passion reserved for a deep and intimate relationship. Knowing how to seek clarification, ask for what you want from others, and interpret words in the context of the situation are critical skills.

How Perception Affects Communication

Perception is the process by which people filter and interpret information from the senses in order to create a meaningful picture of the world.[6] It is the lens through which a person views the world. Gender, culture, educational level, family behaviors, and a host of other factors influence this view.

Communication The transmission of information and meaning from one individual to another.

Perception The process of filtering and interpreting information gathered through the senses.

Self-disclosure The process of revealing one's inner thoughts, feelings, and beliefs to another person.

Important factors that affect your perceptions, and therefore your communication effectiveness, include the way you define yourself (*self-concept*) and the way you evaluate yourself (*self-esteem*). Your self-concept is like a mental mirror that reflects how you view your physical features, emotional states, talents, likes and dislikes, values, and roles.[7] Are you a student, a mother, a Protestant, a young adult, a pianist? How you define yourself is your self-concept. Your assessment of yourself constitutes your self-esteem. You might consider yourself an excellent student, a horrible singer, a great lover, or a "10" in terms of appearance—such judgments indicate your level of self-esteem or self-evaluation.

Self-perceptions influence communication choices. If you feel unattractive, uncomfortable, or inferior to others, you may choose not to interact with them. If you feel self-conscious and ill at ease around people who seem different, you might avoid them. Conversely, if you feel secure in your unique characteristics and talents, that positive self-concept will make it easier to interact with a variety of people in a healthy, balanced way.

What do you think?

Take a few minutes to identify who you are, using characteristics that describe the following:

- *Your moods or feelings.*
- *Your appearance and physical condition.*
- *Your social traits.*
- *The talents you possess or lack.*
- *Your intellectual capacity.*
- *Your strong beliefs or philosophies.*
- *Your social roles.*
- *Your economic status.*

Write your responses, then ask someone you know well and trust to write responses about you. Do your observations match?

Improving Your Communication Skills

All of us can learn to be better communicators. In this life-long process are several challenges and no simple solutions. We can start, however, by learning how to share information through self-disclosure. This form of sharing will allow others to better understand us. Likewise, we can work at becoming better listeners—a critical skill for starting or maintaining any relationship. A third skill involves understanding nonverbal communication—both how we convey nonverbal messages and how others use their bodies and facial expressions to convey information. Through understanding how to deliver and interpret information, we can enhance the relationships in our lives. In order to have healthy interactions with others and keep stress levels under control, it is important to deal

with problems as early as possible. Learning communication skills that quickly resolve fights and misunderstandings can reduce unnecessary stress and lead to happier, more productive relationships.

Learning Appropriate Self-Disclosure

Self-disclosure is the sharing of personal information with others. If you are willing to share personal information with others, they will likely share personal information with you. In other words, if you want to learn more about someone, you have to be willing to share parts of your personal self with that person. Self-disclosure is not storytelling or sharing secrets; rather, it is revealing how you are reacting to the present situation and giving any information about the past that is relevant to the other person's understanding of your current reactions.[8]

Self-disclosure can be a double-edged sword, for there is risk in divulging personal insights and feelings. If you sense that sharing feelings and personal thoughts will result in a closer relationship, you will likely take such a risk. But if you believe that the disclosure may result in rejection or alienation, you may not open up so easily. If the confidentiality of previously shared information has been violated (if a person told others about information you'd asked to be kept private), you may hesitate to disclose yourself in the future.

However, the risk in not disclosing yourself to others is that you will lack close relationships. Psychologist Carl Rogers stressed the importance of understanding yourself and others through self-disclosure. Rogers believed that weak relationships were characterized by inhibited self-disclosure.[9]

If self-disclosure is a key element in creating healthy communication, but fear is a barrier to that process, what can we do? The following suggestions can help:

- *Get to know yourself.* Remember that your self includes your feelings, beliefs, thoughts, and concerns. The more you know about yourself, the more likely it is that you will be able to communicate with others about yourself.
- *Become more accepting of yourself.* No one is perfect or has to be. Even the people you look up to have their flaws. Only by accepting your imperfections can you expect others to accept them, too.
- *Be willing to discuss your sexual history.* In a culture that puts many taboos on discussions of sex in everyday conversation, it's no wonder we find it hard to disclose our sexual feelings to those with whom we are intimate. However, with the soaring numbers of sexually transmitted diseases and the ever-looming threat of AIDS, there has never been a more important time to disclose sexual feelings and history. The long-lasting effects of an unwanted pregnancy or the HIV virus underscore the need to communicate about sex before you become intimate with someone.
- *Choose a safe context for self-disclosure.* Context refers to the setting in which the self-disclosure occurs. Choose a setting in which you feel safe to let yourself be known. When and where you make such disclosures and to whom may greatly influence the response. Select a setting in which you feel safe.

Being a Better Listener

How many times have you been caught not paying attention to what someone close to you is saying? After several moments of nodding and saying "uh-huh" your friend finally asks you a question, and you haven't the faintest idea what has been said. When you are stressed, preoccupied, haven't slept well, or are under the influence of a drug such as alcohol, your listening ability is often impaired. Other sources of difficulty for listeners include:[10]

- Being so interested in what you have to say that you listen mainly to find an opening to get the floor.
- Thinking about or formulating a rebuttal to what is being said rather than listening to what is being said.
- Evaluating or making judgments about the speaker or the message.
- Not asking for clarification when there are things that you are unclear about.
- Nodding or gesturing so wildly that you distract the speaker and he or she gives up the floor.
- External noise, commotion, or distractions that hinder your hearing.
- Lack of familiarity with a language or dialect.
- Not being able to hear the speaker because your own beliefs are so strong and/or you feel so emotional about a given topic.

Listening is a vital part of interpersonal communication; it allows us to share feelings, express concerns, communicate wants and needs, and let our thoughts and opinions be known. We must do the necessary work to improve both our speaking and listeningskills, which will enhance our relationships, improve our grasp of information, and allow us to interpret more effectively what others say. We listen best when (1) we believe that the message is somehow important and relevant to us, (2) the speaker holds our attention through humor, dramatic effect, use of the media, or other techniques, and (3) we are in the mood to listen (free of distractions and worries, happy, etc.). Listening to a technical lecture on the physiology of the brain right after you have just had a fight that ended a relationship would probably be distracting for most people. However, there are things we can do to improve our daily listening. The Skills for Behavior Change box provides some suggestions for improving your listening.

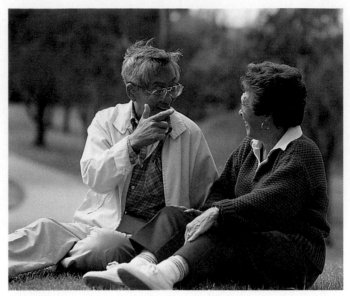

Relationships are strengthened over time as partners develop listening skills and the ability to share their intimate thoughts and feelings.

The Three Basic Listening Modes There are three main ways in which we listen. Knowing when to use each of these will enhance the way in which you listen and improve the outcome.

1. *Competitive* or *combative listening* happens when we are more interested in promoting our own point of view than in understanding or exploring someone else's view. We listen either for openings to take the floor or for flaws and weak points that we can attack. Looking at your watch, sighing, nodding vigorously, staring into space, or other actions are meant to put speakers in their places or cause them to relinquish the floor.

2. *Passive or attentive listening* occurs when we are genuinely interested in hearing and understanding the other person's point of view. By being attentive and passively listening, we provide encouragement for more discussion. We assume that we heard and understand correctly, but we stay passive and don't verify it.

3. *Active or reflective listening* is the single most useful and important listening skill. In active listening, we are also genuinely interested in understanding what the other person is thinking, feeling, and wanting in addition to what the message means, and we are active in checking out our understandings before we respond with our own new message. We restate or paraphrase our understanding of the other person's meaning and reflect it back to the sender for verification. This verification or feedback process is what distinguishes active listening and makes it effective.[11]

Benefits of Active Listening The most obvious benefit of active listening is that it helps remove the chance of a misunderstanding or, if a misunderstanding does occur, makes it immediately apparent. Several other possible benefits include the following:[12]

Learning to Really Listen

Most of us have lamented the fact that someone "never listens" and seems to monopolize the entire conversation. Although we are quick to recognize such listening flaws in others, we are often less likely to spot listening problems of our own. On a daily basis, we all have times when we just "tune out." When the class professor drones on about a subject we don't relate to, we begin doodling or put on a blank facial expression, even though we are thinking about what to wear to the movies that night or planning dinner. When that boring friend tells the same story over and over again, we say "uh-huh," "yes," and worry that we'll be caught when he asks a question and we don't have a clue what he is talking about. We grimace at the thought of certain people calling but dash for the phone when the caller ID indicates that it is someone we love to talk with. What is the difference? Why do we tune out when some people speak and tune in for every word when others talk to us?

We gravitate toward those who seem to understand us and with whom we have a fun and interesting interaction. If the truth be told, most of us are only mediocre listeners at best. We slip in and out of focus in a conversation, hear only the gist of what is being said, and provide only minimal, phony feedback or responses when we are not all that interested. What does it take to be an excellent listener? Practicing the following skills and consciously using them on a daily basis is an important part of improved communication.

- *Be present in the moment.* Contrary to what is often believed, good listeners don't just sit back with their mouths shut and listen. They participate and acknowledge what the other person is saying. (Nodding, smiling, saying "yes" or "uh-huh", and asking questions at appropriate times are all part of this. Take care, however, not to numbly say "uh-huh" to every word, which is distracting and conveys insincerity.)

- *Use positive body language and voice tone.* Show that you are "with" the speaker in the conversation by turning toward him or her and staying focused (wandering eyeballs are a sure sign that your mind is elsewhere). Avoid barrier gestures such as shaking your head "no" or making negative faces; smile at appropriate times and maintain appropriate eye contact (deadpan stares can also be distracting). Voice tone, posture, and an attitude that conveys interest are all key.

- *Show empathy and sympathy.* Watching for verbal and nonverbal clues as to the other person's feelings and trying to relate can be a very useful tool. For example, saying, "That must have been really hard for you. That must have made you feel terrible," can encourage the speaker to talk and feel more comfortable with you as an understanding listener.

- *Ask for clarification.* If you aren't sure where the speaker is going with something or what he or she means, indicate that you aren't sure you've understood or paraphrase and restate what you think you heard. This kind of feedback is invaluable in avoiding misinterpretation and/or lapses in overall communication. As a speaker, you may ask," What did you think I was just saying?" but be sure to say this in a nonthreatening manner.

- *Control that deadly desire to interrupt.* Some people start nodding and gesturing before you ever get a word out of your mouth. If you are like that, squelch it, even if you have to put an inconspicuous hand over your mouth. Try taking a deep breath for two seconds, then hold your breath for another second and really listen to what is being said as you slowly exhale. Don't be so enthusiastically empathetic that you finish the speaker's sentences and/or put words in someone's mouth. Let her finish what she is saying!

- *Avoid snap judgments based on what other people look like or what they are saying.* If you notice some strange quirk in their mannerisms, try to focus on what is being said, not the mannerisms. Avoid stereotyping or labeling and try to hear what is really being said.

- *Resist the temptation to "set the other person straight."* Control your urge to correct errors in conversation or to react defensively. Listen and hear without reacting or trying to rationalize what the speaker is trying to say.

- *Try to focus on the speaker.* Sometimes it is very tough to listen to someone who is trying to talk about a painful situation if we are experiencing or have recently experienced the same thing. Hold back the temptation to "tell all" and fly off into your own rendition of a similar situation. Give the speaker the moment and later, after he or she is done talking, you may want to talk about your own situation as a means of validating the feelings expressed. Don't tell him how he is feeling or how he should feel.

- *Be tenacious.* Stick with the speaker and try to stay on the topic. Offer your thoughts and suggestions, but remember that you should only advise up to a certain point. Clarify statements with "this is my opinion" as a reminder that it is only opinion, rather than fact.

- Sometimes people just need to be heard and acknowledged before they are willing to consider an alternative or soften their position.
- It is often easier for people to listen to and consider the other's position when they know the other is listening and considering their position.
- It helps people to spot the flaws in their reasoning when they hear it played back without criticism.
- Active listening helps identify areas of agreement so that the areas of disagreement are put into perspective and are diminished rather than magnified.

- Reflecting back what we hear each other say helps give each of us a chance to become aware of the different levels of communication that are going on below the surface. This helps to bring things into the open, where they can be resolved more readily.
- If we listen and try to understand other people's points of view, we can more effectively help people see the flaws in their positions or discover the flaws in our own position.

Using Nonverbal Communication

Understanding what someone is saying often involves much more than listening and speaking. Often, what is *not* actually said may speak louder than any words. Rolling the eyes, looking at the floor or ceiling rather than maintaining eye contact, body movements, hand gestures—all these nonverbal clues influence the way we interpret messages.[13] Researchers have found that only 7 percent of the meaning of a message comes from the words spoken. An astounding 93 percent of the meaning comes from nonverbal cues.[14]

Nonverbal communication includes all unwritten and unspoken messages, both intentional and unintentional. Because expressions and actions can mean so many different things and be interpreted in so many different ways, it is easy to be confused by nonverbal messages. This confusion increases when what a person says seems to cotradict what he or she does. How would you interpret the following?

- Ramell assures Becky that she loves her spaghetti sauce, yet only picks at it and leaves most of it on her plate.
- Ramone tells Nicole that he loves her deeply, but whenever they go out, he constantly watches other women and acts detached and uninterested in Nicole.
- Mary tells Joselyn that she has forgiven her for gossiping about her, yet she avoids Joselyn on campus and does not look at her when Joselyn speaks to her.

In most cases, when differences exist between what is being said and what is being done, people tend to agree with the old saying: Actions speak louder than words. Effective communicators learn to observe nonverbal cues and carefully differentiate between what someone is saying and what is really being said.

Expressing Difficult Feelings

How many times have you struggled to find just the right words in an emotionally charged situation? Imagine Sarah has been dating Charles and, while she feels he is a great person, he is not the one she wants to date exclusively. She wants to tell him that she likes him a lot, but she is not in love with him. Like most people, Sarah finds that expressing her feelings in a way that is not hurtful to another person is difficult. Professionals offer the following guidelines for expressing feelings:[15]

- Try to be specific rather than general about how you feel. Consistently using only one or two words to say how you are feeling, such as *unhappy* or *upset*, is too vague and general. Explain what you mean when you say *upset*: irritated, agitated, mad, anxious, uncomfortable, angry, bothered?
- Specify the degree of feelings, and you will reduce the chances of being misunderstood. When you say *angry*, someone may think you are enraged when you are just a bit irritated.
- When expressing anger or irritation, first describe the specific behavior you don't like, then your feelings. The other person may become immediately defensive or intimidated when he or she first hears "I am angry with you" and could miss the message.
- If you have mixed feelings, say so, and express each feeling and explain what each feeling is about. For example: "I really like your sense of humor and your values, but I don't feel comfortable around you 24-7." "I am thankful that I met you and we can be friends, but I don't have the depth of feeling that I think needs to be there for a relationship. We just are too different."

In general, the most tried and true techniques for expressing your feelings involve using **"I" messages** that include feelings like those stated above, rather than "you" statements that imply blame or something that the other person did wrong. "I" messages ("I like being with you"; "I'm sorry that I missed practice") are a direct, clear, and effective way to send information to others. When using "I" messages, the speaker takes responsibility for communicating his or her own feelings, thoughts, and beliefs. People who practice using "I" messages tend to have more positive interactions and generate less defensiveness from listeners.

The opposite of an "I" message is a "you" message. "You" messages are easy to distinguish because they begin with the communicator saying "you" ("You made me so mad"; "You never say you're sorry about anything"). "You" messages leave the receiver of the information on the defensive and ready to attack. The following example illustrates the difference between "I" and "you" messages.

Terry and Jim have been working together on a class project for most of the term. Although they are both supposed to contribute 50 percent to the final product, Jim has done very little work thus far. Terry is very angry, but rather than saying, "Jim, you're really lazy and you are not holding up your part of this assignment," she decides to try another tactic. She says, "Jim, I really am feeling over-burdened by all of the work I've been putting into this project. I don't want to feel 'used' in this process and I want both of us to get as much out of the effort as we can." Because Terry is putting this discussion in terms of how she is feeling (using "I" messages) rather than attacking Jim with "you" statements that make him want to defend himself, they are more likely to communicate constructively. Jim is apt to get the message and start contributing to the project.

To practice using "I" messages, follow these steps:

1. *"When you."* Start by thinking about a problem behavior or situation that you want to discuss. Choose something specific —not a vague, sweeping complaint such as "My roommate is such a slob, and he needs to change." Concentrate on a particular ("When you leave your clothes all over the floor . . .").
2. *"I feel."* Identify how the behavior or incident makes you feel, and state those feelings by starting your sentence with "I." Adding a feeling statement allows you to share your reaction honestly without placing blame or exerting power ("I feel frustrated and angry").
3. *"Because."* Add a statement to explain, from your perspective, why the feeling occurred (". . . because I spend so much time trying to keep the place looking good").

Now let's put these steps together into one simple sentence: "When you leave your clothes on the floor, I feel frustrated and angry because I spend so much time trying to keep the place looking good."

Communicating Assertively

Communicating assertively means using direct, honest communication that maintains and defends your rights in a positive manner. **Assertive communicators** are people who get their points across while at the same time respecting the rights of others. Assertiveness demands both verbal and nonverbal skills. Verbally, assertive communicators speak calmly, directly, and clearly to those around them. Nonverbally, they maintain direct eye contact, sit or stand facing the person they are speaking to, and sit or stand with an erect posture that indicates confidence and control.

Assertiveness is often distinguished from two other styles of communication that produce poor results: *nonassertiveness* and *aggressiveness*. **Nonassertive communicators** tend to be shy and inhibited. Verbally, nonassertive communicators may speak too rapidly, use a tone that is too low to be heard easily, or not say directly what's on their minds. Nonverbally, their body language frequently reveals timidity: Their shoulders slump, they don't face the person they are talking to, or they avoid direct eye contact. Nonassertive people fear that if they really express how they feel, it will upset others. This fear leaves them without positive ways of communicating their needs and concerns. (See the Assess Yourself box.)

Aggressive communicators tend to employ an angry, confrontational, hostile manner in their interactions with others. Their communications are typically loud and verbally abusive, and they often blame others when things don't go their way. Someone who constantly uses "you" messages, causing the receiver of the information to feel on the defensive immediately, is usually an aggressive communicator.

> ### What do you think?
>
> *How would you describe your communication style—nonassertive, assertive, or aggressive? ✳ Do you tend to use more "I" or "you" messages? ✳ Should you alter your communication style in any way? ✳ If so, why?*

Establishing a Proper Climate

An open climate for communication does not simply happen. Although selecting a safe place and a trustworthy confidant are important, carefully consider your own role in establishing a supportive climate for conversation. If you follow these steps when you speak, the other person is more likely to engage in an open, honest conversation with you:[16]

- *Watch judgmental statements.* Words such as *stupid, ridiculous, great, crummy,* or *fantastic* show that an evaluation has already been made. Many of these judgmental statements leave no room for another opinion. Instead, use descriptive statements that reveal your feelings without labeling them as good, bad, right, or wrong. Say, "Your borrowing my car makes me very nervous," rather than, "You stupid thing, you'll wreck my car and hurt yourself!"
- *Keep an open mind.* Since absolute statements tend to close off other opinions, thereby restricting communication, use qualifying statements to give others a chance to state their opinions. Say, "This may not always be true, depending on the circumstances," or, "I could be wrong, but it's what I think."
- *Avoid projecting superiority or lecturing.* If you really want someone's opinion, then respect it as having some value.

Nonverbal communication All unwritten and unspoken messages, both intentional and unintentional.

"I" messages Messages in which a person takes responsibility for communicating his or her own feelings, thoughts, and beliefs by using statements that begin with "I," not "you."

Assertive communicators People who use direct, honest communication that maintains and defends their rights in a positive manner.

Nonassertive communicators Individuals who tend to be shy and inhibited in their communication with others.

Aggressive communicators People who use hostile, loud, and blaming communication styles.

Standing Up for Yourself

You know that sinking feeling. Someone asks you to do something, and your stomach lurches. You don't want to go along, but you can't come up with a good excuse. It's hard to say no. How often are you caught in the "I can't say no" trap? Read the following situations and assess your response according to the following 5-point scale:

1 = never   2 = very seldom   3 = sometimes   4 = frequently   5 = always

1. Friends ask you to ride home with them after they've all been drinking. You know you shouldn't go, but you think one of them is cute, and you don't want to seem like a prude. You take the ride.	1	2	3	4	5
2. Someone says something really nasty about someone you like. You jump to the defense of the person being criticized, even though you are in the minority opinion.	1	2	3	4	5
3. You feel strongly about a political issue, but it is the opposite of the opinion held by your parents. You remain silent rather than getting into an argument.	1	2	3	4	5
4. You start out by saying no to something but get talked into doing it after a short time.	1	2	3	4	5
5. You're stressed out, with too much to do and too little time, but you can't seem to say no when someone asks for a favor.	1	2	3	4	5
6. Someone is critical of something you do. You quickly defend your actions by explaining why you did what you did.	1	2	3	4	5
7. You would describe yourself as assertive and tend to quickly let others know your thoughts about certain issues.	1	2	3	4	5
8. Your decisions can be easily swayed by a strong argument from someone else pushing you in the opposite direction.	1	2	3	4	5

Think about your responses to each statement. Do your responses indicate an assertive communication style in which you stand up for your feelings or beliefs? What factors cause you to hold back when you should probably speak up? How can you work to improve your communication behaviors in this area?

As you learn to show respect for others' opinions, your opinion will become more respected. Monitor your facial expressions, voice pitch and intonation, word choice, and actions to see whether they express true interest and respect.

• *Don't ask for feedback unless you want an honest answer.* How many times have you asked people what they thought only to be hurt or angry when they told you? If you become visibly upset by honest feedback, people won't give it to you.

Look at such feedback as an attempt to help. No one enjoys criticism, but you can't correct a negative action unless you are aware of it.

• *Avoid people who tend to give negative feedback.* Some people have such low self-esteem that they delight in criticizing others. Try to determine the underlying motives of such people and then avoid them if at all possible.

Managing Conflict

A **conflict** is an emotional state that arises when the behavior of one person interferes with the behavior of another. Conflict is inevitable whenever people live or work together. Not all conflict is bad; in fact, airing feelings and coming to some form of resolution over differences can sometimes strengthen strained relationships. **Conflict resolution** and successful conflict management are a systematic approach to resolving differences fairly and constructively, rather than allowing them to fester. The goal of conflict resolution is to solve differences peacefully and creatively.

Conflict An emotional state that arises when the behavior of one person interferes with the behavior of another.

Conflict resolution A concerted effort by all parties to resolve points in contention in a constructive manner.

Intimate relationships Relationships with family members, friends, and romantic partners, characterized by closeness and understanding.

Most conflicts revolve around two message components: content and relationship. *Content* is usually easy to discern, as it is the subject of the sentences used by the participants. It deals with the issues on the surface. *Relationship* is more difficult to discern because it embodies the interactions between the people involved and usually involves issues that are much more deeply rooted. Because of the double-pronged nature of messages, many arguments arise out of seemingly innocuous situations. For instance, a housemate comes home from the library, walks into the kitchen, and asks, "What's for dinner?" The other responds, "Whatever you make! When are you going to take care of yourself for once?" On the surface, the conflict may be about dinner, the content. From a relationship standpoint, however, one roommate feels used and underappreciated.

Prolonged conflict can destroy relationships unless the parties agree to resolve points of contention in a constructive manner. As two people learn to negotiate and compromise on their differences, the number and intensity of conflicts should diminish. Conflict resolution can therefore be a growth process for people as they learn to recognize problems and solutions based on past experiences.

During a heated conflict, try to pause for a moment before responding, consider the possible impact of your comments or actions, and speak slowly and state your point positively and constructively. You can also dismiss yourself from the situation and walk away.

Rude or inconsiderate behavior usually develops in situations in which a person fails to recognize the feelings or rights of another. To avoid this type of behavior, try to see the other person's point of view, listen actively, avoid interrupting, and avoid making gestures, such as head shaking or finger pointing, that indicate disagreement. A key element of managing conflict successfully is to remember to validate others' opinions and to treat others as you would like to be treated. Maintain respect and concern for others' welfare at all times.

Here are some strategies for conflict resolution:[17]

1. *Focus on one topic at a time,* and make other preoccupations clear, such as in, "I may seem angry, but I had a bad day at school today and I'm really worried about my grades." This takes the heat off the other person.
2. *Stop the action and cool down* before things get out of control. One sign of major distress in a couple is escalating hostility, often in the form of nagging that provokes angry responses. The escalation seems unstoppable once it gets started. Never send an e-mail to someone when you are upset. E-mails make it very easy to misinterpret what someone feels or intends. Talk in person: Eye contact, gestures, and body language all speak louder than written words.
3. *Be specific in your criticisms or praises.* Prevent small complaints that you may stew over. You could say, "When I see your clothes on the floor, I feel that you are not doing your share of the work in the house and I feel taken advantage of," instead of, "You're a slob."
4. *Learn to "edit" what you say* before you say it so as to avoid remarks that would be needlessly hurtful. For example,

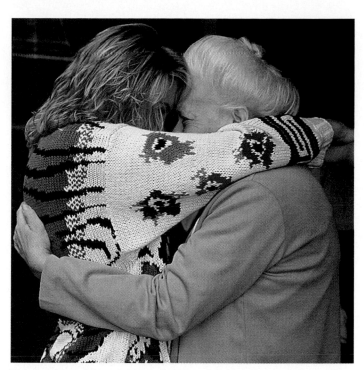

The emotional bonds that characterize intimate relationships know no boundaries.

don't dredge up past events and old grudges during a fight. Don't bring up additional issues before you've resolved the one at hand.
5. *Think about possible solutions* to problems that involve compromises for both parties. Discover options that work for both of you by doing some brainstorming. Consider all the options first, then eliminate those that aren't acceptable to both of you. Be committed to change.
6. *Never think in terms of winning an argument.* Think instead of ways to keep an argument from happening. By doing so, both parties win. Avoid becoming too invested in getting your way. Remember that your reality is not the only reality!

What do you think?

When you have conflicts, does the content of your language accurately represent what you want to convey? ✳ *How could you improve your conflict resolution skills?*

Characterizing and Forming Intimate Relationships

We can define **intimate relationships** in terms of four characteristics: *behavioral interdependence, need fulfillment, emotional attachment,* and *emotional availability.* Each of these characteristics may be related to interactions with family, close friends, and romantic partners.[18]

Behavioral interdependence refers to the mutual impact that people have on each other as their lives and daily activities intertwine. What one person does influences what the other person wants to do and can do. Behavioral interdependence may become stronger over time to the point that each person would find a great void if the other person was gone.

Intimate relationships also fulfill psychological needs and so are a means of *need fulfillment.* Through relationships with others, we fulfill our needs for the following:

- Intimacy—requiring someone with whom we can share our feelings freely.
- Social integration—requiring someone with whom we can share our worries and concerns.
- Nurturance—requiring someone whom we can take care of and who will take care of us.
- Assistance—requiring someone to help us in times of need.
- Reassurance or affirmation of our own worth—requiring someone who will tell us that we matter.

In rewarding, intimate relationships, partners and friends meet each other's needs. They disclose feelings, share confidences, and provide support and reassurance.

In addition to behavioral interdependence and need fulfillment, intimate relationships involve strong bonds of *emotional attachment,* or feelings of love and attachment. Often, when we hear the word *intimacy,* we immediately think of a sexual relationship. Although sex can play an important role in emotional attachment, a relationship can be very intimate and not be sexual. Two people can be emotionally intimate (share feelings) or spiritually intimate (share spiritual beliefs and meanings), or be intimate friends. The intimacy level experienced by any two people cannot easily be judged by those outside the relationship.

Emotional availability, the ability to give to and receive from others emotionally without fear of being hurt or rejected, is the fourth characteristic of intimate relationships. At times, all of us may limit our emotional availability—for example, after a painful breakup we may decide not to jump into another relationship immediately. Holding back can offer time for introspection and healing as well as time to consider the "lessons learned." However, because of intense trauma, some people find it difficult to be fully available. This limits their ability to experience and enjoy intimate relationships.

In the early years of life, families provide the most significant relationships. Gradually, the circle widens to include friends, coworkers, and acquaintances. Ultimately, most of us develop romantic or sexual relationships with significant others. Each of these relationships plays a significant role in psychological, social, spiritual, and physical health.

> **Family of origin** People present in the household during a child's first years of life—usually parents and siblings.
>
> **Nuclear family** Parents (usually married, but not necessarily) and their offspring.

Families: The Ties That Bind

The United Nations defines seven basic types of families, including single-parent families, communal families (unrelated people living together for ideological, economic, or other reasons), extended families, and others. But most Americans think of family in terms of the "family of origin" or the "nuclear family." The **family of origin** includes the people present in the household during a child's first years of life—usually parents and siblings. However, the family of origin may also include stepparents, grandparents, aunts or uncles, partners, and friends. The family of origin has a tremendous impact on the child's psychological and social development. The **nuclear family** consists of parents (usually married, but not necessarily) and their offspring.

The modern American family looks quite different from those of previous generations. The *Leave It to Beaver* type of family encouraged during the 1950s—composed of Mom with her apron, staying at home and content with her role as mother and spouse; Dad with his briefcase, trying to move up the corporate ladder; and two or three happy, well-adjusted children—is not the norm. Over half of today's moms work outside the home, and large numbers of children are cared for by single parents, grandparents, relatives, stepparents, friends, nannies, day care centers, and other "parents."

No particular family structure is inherently good or bad, and neither are particular roles (such as the idealized *Leave It to Beaver* mom) required of certain family members in order for a family to thrive. Families that promote the most positive health outcomes for all members appear to be those that offer a sense of security, safety, and love and the opportunity for members to grow through positive interactions.

If parents are not afraid to share feelings, affection, and love with each other and their offspring, their children are likely to become emotionally connected adults. If the home environment provides stability and seems safe, it is likely that the children will learn to express feelings and develop intimacy skills. Sibling interactions provide a way to learn and practice interpersonal skills. People can practice positive behaviors and learn the rights and wrongs of negative behaviors in a safe and nonjudgmental environment when the family itself is healthy. However, if the family is psychologically or physically unhealthy, it may pose significant barriers to later relationships, as we discuss later in the section on dysfunctional families.

Establishing Friendships

> *A Friend is one who knows you as you are*
> *understands where you've been*
> *accepts who you've become*
> *and still gently invites you to grow.*
> —Author Unknown

Good friends—they can make a boring day fun, a cold day warm, or a gut-wrenching worry disappear. They can make us feel that we matter and we have the strength to get through just about anything. They can also make us angry, disappoint us, or seriously jolt our own comfortable ideas about right and wrong. No friendship is perfect and most need careful attention if they are to remain stable over time. Psychologists believe that people are attracted to and form relationships with people who give them positive reinforcement and that they dislike those who punish them. The basic idea is simple: You like the people who like you. Another factor that affects the development of a friendship is a real or perceived similarity in attitudes, opinions, and background.[19] In addition, true friends have a sense of *equity* in which they share confidences, contribute fairly and equally to maintaining the friendship, and consistently try to give as much as they get back from the interactions.[20]

Though we all know that friends enrich our lives, most people don't realize that real health benefits result from strong social bonds. Social support has been shown to boost the immune system, improve the quality and possibly the length of life, and even reduce the risks of heart disease.[21]

Although most of us have a fairly clear idea of the distinction between a friend and a lover, this difference is not always easy to verbalize. Some people believe that the major difference is that no intimate physical involvement exists between friends. Others have suggested that intimacy levels are much lower between friends than between lovers. But as we have stated, people can be intimate with each other without being sexually involved. Also, many people have sex with others more as friends than as true lovers and partners. Confused? You are probably not alone. Surprisingly, little research has been done to clarify these terms. Psychologists Jeffrey Turner and Laurna Rubinson have described the characteristics that make a good friendship:[22]

- *Enjoyment.* Friends enjoy each other's company most of the time, although temporary states of anger, disappointment, or mutual annoyance may occur.
- *Acceptance.* Friends accept each other as they are, without trying to change or make the other into a different person.
- *Trust.* Friends share mutual trust. Each assumes that the other will act in his or her friend's best interest.
- *Respect.* Friends respect each other in the sense that each assumes that the other exercises good judgment in making life choices.
- *Mutual assistance.* Friends are inclined to assist and support one another. Specifically, they can count on each other in times of need, trouble, or personal distress.
- *Confiding.* Friends share experiences and feelings with each other that they don't share with other people.
- *Understanding.* Friends have a sense of what is important to each and why each behaves as he or she does. Friends are not puzzled or mystified by each other's actions.
- *Spontaneity.* Friends feel free to be themselves in the relationship, without being required to play a role, wear a mask, or inhibit revelation of personal traits.

According to psychologist Dan McAdams, most of us are fortunate to develop one or two lasting friendships in a lifetime.[23]

Significant Others, Partners, Couples

Most people choose at some point to enter into an intimate sexual relationship with another person. Numerous studies have analyzed the ways in which couples form significant partnering relationships. Most couples fit into one of four categories of significant sexual or committed relationships: married heterosexual couples, cohabiting heterosexual couples, lesbian couples, and gay male couples. These groups are discussed in greater detail later in this chapter.

Love relationships in each of these four groups typically include all the characteristics of friendship as well as other characteristics related to passion and caring:[24]

- *Fascination.* Lovers tend to pay attention to the other person even when they should be involved in other activities. They are preoccupied with the other and want to think about, look at, talk to, or merely be with that person.
- *Exclusiveness.* Lovers have a special relationship that usually precludes having the same bond with a third party. The love relationship takes priority over all others.
- *Sexual desire.* Lovers want physical intimacy with the partner, desiring to touch, hold, and engage in sexual activities with each other.
- *Giving the utmost.* Lovers care enough to give the utmost when the other is in need, sometimes to the point of extreme sacrifice.
- *Being a champion or advocate.* Lovers actively champion each other's interests and attempt to ensure that the other succeeds.

For obvious reasons, the best love relationships share friendships, and the best friendships include several love components. Both relationships share common bonds of nurturance, enhancement of personal well-being, and a genuine sense of mutual regard, trust, and security. Healthy friendships and love relationships greatly enhance overall health and lead to sustained personal growth throughout one's life (see Figure 5.1).

This Thing Called Love

What is love? Finding a definition of love may be more difficult than listing characteristics of a loving relationship. The term *love* has more entries in *Bartlett's Familiar Quotations* than any other word except *man*.[25] This four-letter word has been written about and engraved on walls; it has been the theme of countless novels, movies, and plays. There is no one definition of *love,* and the word may mean different things to people depending on cultural values, age, gender, and situation. Yet, we all know what it is when it strikes (see Figure 5.2).

Many social scientists maintain that love may be of two kinds: *companionate* and *passionate*. Companionate love is a secure, trusting attachment, similar to what we may feel for family members or close friends. In companionate love, two people are attracted, have much in common, care about each other's well-being, and express reciprocal liking and

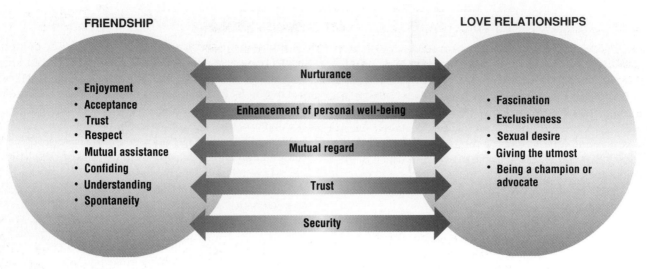

FRIENDSHIP

- Enjoyment
- Acceptance
- Trust
- Respect
- Mutual assistance
- Confiding
- Understanding
- Spontaneity

Nurturance

Enhancement of personal well-being

Mutual regard

Trust

Security

LOVE RELATIONSHIPS

- Fascination
- Exclusiveness
- Sexual desire
- Giving the utmost
- Being a champion or advocate

Figure 5.1
Common Bonds of Friends and Lovers

respect. Passionate love is, in contrast, a state of high arousal, filled with the ecstasy of being loved by the partner and the agony of being rejected.[26] The person experiencing passionate love tends to be preoccupied with his or her partner and to perceive the love object as being perfect.[27] According to Hatfield and Walster, passionate love will not occur unless three conditions are met.[28] First, the person must live in a culture in which the concept of "falling in love" is idealized. Second, a "suitable" love object must be present. If the person has been taught by parents, movies, books, and peers to seek partners having certain levels of attractiveness or belonging to certain racial or social groups or having a certain socioeconomic status and none is available, the person may find it difficult to allow himself or herself to become involved. Finally, for passionate love to occur, there must be some type of physiological arousal that occurs when a person is in the presence of the beloved. Often this arousal takes the form of sexual excitement.

In his article "The Triangular Theory of Love," researcher Robert Sternberg attempts to clarify further what love is by isolating three key ingredients:

- *Intimacy.* The emotional component, which involves feelings of closeness.
- *Passion.* The motivational component, which reflects romantic, sexual attraction.
- *Decision/commitment.* The cognitive component, which includes the decisions you make about being in love and the degree of commitment to your partner.

According to Sternberg's model, the higher the levels of intimacy, passion, and commitment, the more likely a person is to be involved in a healthy, positive love relationship.

According to anthropologist Helen Fisher (and others), attraction and falling in love follow a fairly predictable pattern based on (1) *imprinting,* in which our evolutionary patterns, genetic predispositions, and past experiences trigger a romantic reaction; (2) *attraction,* in which neurochemicals

produce feelings of euphoria and elation; (3) *attachment,* in which endorphins—natural opiates—cause lovers to feel peaceful, secure, and calm; and (4) *production of a cuddle chemical,* in which the brain secretes the chemical *oxytocin,* thereby stimulating sensations during lovemaking and eliciting feelings of satisfaction and attachment.[29]

Lovers who claim that they are swept away by passion may not, therefore, be far from the truth.

> A meeting of the eyes, a touch of the hands or a whiff of scent may set off a flood that starts in the brain and races along the nerves and through the blood. The familiar results—flushed skin, sweaty palms, heavy breathing—are identical to those experienced when under stress. Why? Because the love-smitten person is secreting chemical substances such as dopamine, norepinephrine, and phenylethylamine (PEA) that are chemical cousins of amphetamines.[30]

Although attraction may in fact be a "natural high," with PEA levels soaring, this hit of passion loses effectiveness over time as the body builds up a tolerance. Needing a continual fix of passion, many people may become attraction junkies, seeking the intoxication of love much as the drug user seeks a chemical high.[31]

Fisher speculates that PEA levels drop significantly over a three-to-four-year period, leading to the "four-year itch" that shows up in the peaking fourth-year divorce rates present in over 60 cultures. Romances that last beyond the four-year decline of PEA are influenced by another set of chemicals, known as endorphins, soothing substances that give lovers a sense of security, peace, and calm.[32]

Oxytocin is also being studied for its role in the love formula. Produced by the brain, it sensitizes nerves and stimulates muscle contractions, the production of breast milk, and the desire for physical closeness between mother and infant. Scientists speculate that oxytocin may encourage similar cuddling between men and women. Oxytocin levels have also been shown to increase dramatically during orgasm for both men and women.[33]

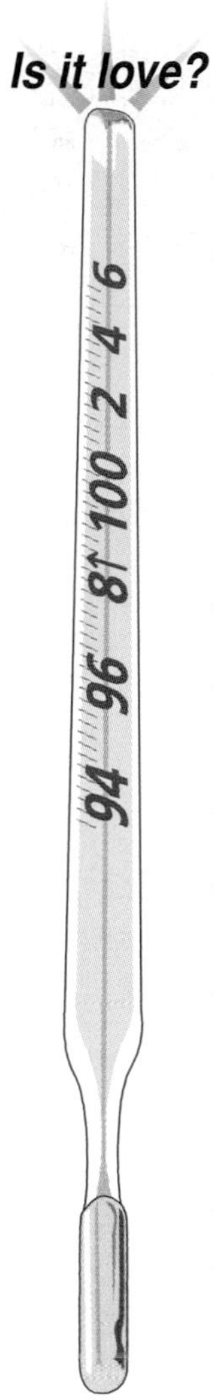

Is it love?

- **Verbally expressing affection,** such as saying "I love you"
- **Offering self-disclosure,** such as revealing intimate facts about oneself
- **Giving nonmaterial evidence,** such as emotional and moral support in times of need, and respecting the other's opinion
- **Expressing nonverbal feelings,** such as feeling happy, more content, more secure when the person is present
- **Giving material evidence,** such as gifts, flowers, small favors, or doing more than one's own share of a task
- **Physically expressing love,** such as hugging, kissing, making love
- **Tolerating the other,** such as accepting his or her idiosyncrasies, peculiar routines, or forgetfulness
- **Wanting to promote** the partner's welfare
- **Feeling happiness** with the partner
- **Holding the partner** in high regard
- **Being able to count on the partner** in time of need
- **Being able to understand** each other
- **Sharing oneself and one's possessions** with the partner
- **Giving emotional support** to the partner
- **Being able to communicate** about intimate things
- **Valuing the partner's presence** in one's own life

Figure 5.2
Common Experiences of Love
Source: From *Human Sexuality* by B. Strong, C. DeVault, and B. Sayad, 1999. Reprinted by permission of The McGraw-Hill Companies.

In addition to such possible chemical influences, past experiences significantly affect our attractions for others. Our parents' modeling of traits we believe are desirable or undesirable may play a role in drawing us to people with similar traits. Many researchers have investigated the possible link between males seeking their own mothers and females seeking their fathers in partners. To date, research on chemical attractions and parent-seeking tendencies is inconclusive and should be viewed only as preliminary. Much more research is needed to confirm these provocative theories.

Gender Issues in Relationships

When it comes to relationships, are men really from Mars and women from Venus? If they are not planets apart, how far apart are they, and what are the implications of the disparities?

In her book *You Just Don't Understand: Women and Men in Conversation,* psychologist Deborah Tannen described sev-

eral basic differences in conversational styles between men and women that can make communication challenging.[34] She coined the term **genderlect** to characterize differences in word choices, interruption patterns, questioning patterns, language interpretations and misinterpretations, and vocal influences based on gender. Tannen is not alone in her research. In fact, communication patterns between women and men have been studied for generations, with similar results.

Recent research validates much of Tannen's work and indicates that women tend to be more expressive, relationship oriented, and concerned with creating and maintaining intimacy; men tend to be more instrumental, task oriented, and concerned with gathering information or with establishing and maintaining social status or power.[35] Unlike women, men tend to believe that they are not supposed to show emotions and are brought up to believe that "being strong" is often more important than having close friendships. As a result, according to research, only 1 male in 10 has a close male friend to whom he divulges his innermost thoughts.[36] Figure 5.3 summarizes some of these characteristics.

> **What do you think?**
>
> *Who are the people with whom you feel most comfortable talking about very personal issues?* ✳ *Do you talk with both males and females about these issues, or do you tend to gravitate toward just one sex?* ✳ *Why do you think you do this?*

Styles in Decision Making

According to Harvard professor Carol Gilligan, men and women may make very different decisions when facing ethical dilemmas.[37] Gilligan believes that women tend to think and speak differently from men because of the two genders' contrasting images of self. Because of these self-image differences, Gilligan believes that there is a feminine ethic of *care* and a masculine ethic of *justice.*[38] Following this line of thinking, she suggests that women view sensitivity to others, loyalty, responsibility, self-sacrifice, and peacemaking as key factors to consider in making ethical decisions. In contrast, men are more interested in individual rights, equality before law, and fair play—factors that are much more impersonal. Because such gender differences would affect both the encoding and decoding of messages, difficulties in communication might result.[39]

Picking Partners

For both males and females, more than just chemical and psychological processes influence the choice of partners. One

Genderlect The "dialect," or individual speech pattern and conversational style, of each gender.

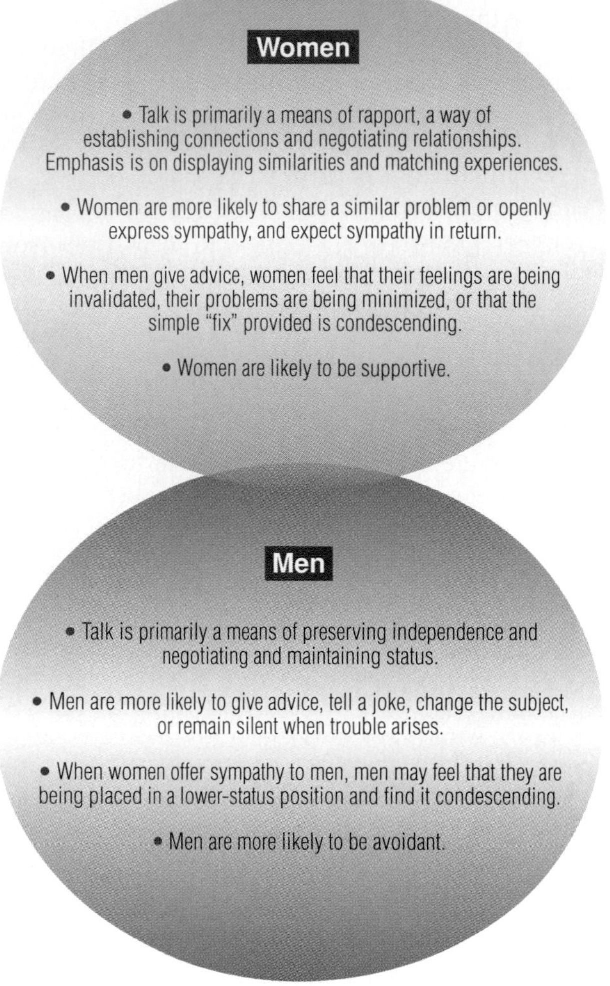

Women

- Talk is primarily a means of rapport, a way of establishing connections and negotiating relationships. Emphasis is on displaying similarities and matching experiences.

- Women are more likely to share a similar problem or openly express sympathy, and expect sympathy in return.

- When men give advice, women feel that their feelings are being invalidated, their problems are being minimized, or that the simple "fix" provided is condescending.

- Women are likely to be supportive.

Men

- Talk is primarily a means of preserving independence and negotiating and maintaining status.

- Men are more likely to give advice, tell a joke, change the subject, or remain silent when trouble arises.

- When women offer sympathy to men, men may feel that they are being placed in a lower-status position and find it condescending.

- Men are more likely to be avoidant.

Figure 5.3

Troubles Talk: How Men and Women Respond
Source: From "Gender Differences in Self-Reported Responses in Troubles Talk," by S. L. Michaud and R. Warner, 1997, *Sex Roles: A Journal of Research* 37 (7–8), p. 527.

important factor is *proximity,* or being in the same place at the same time. The more you see a person in your hometown, at social gatherings, or at work, the more likely that an interaction will occur. Thus, if you live in New York, you'll probably end up with another New Yorker. If you live in northern Wisconsin, you'll probably end up with another Wisconsinite. (With the advent of the Internet, geographic proximity is not always as important. See the Reality Check box.)

You also pick a partner based on *similarities* (in attitudes, values, intellect, and interests); the old adage that "opposites attract" usually isn't true. If your potential partner expresses interest or liking, you may react with mutual regard known as *reciprocity.* The more you express interest, the safer it is for someone else to return the regard, and the cycle spirals onward.

A final factor that apparently plays a significant role in selecting a partner is *physical attraction.* Whether such attraction is caused by a chemical reaction or a socially learned

behavior, males and females appear to have different attraction criteria. Men tend to select their mates primarily on the basis of youth and physical attractiveness. While women also value physical attractiveness, they tend to place higher emphasis on partners who are somewhat older, have good financial prospects, and are dependable and industrious.

> **What do you think?**
>
> *What factors do you consider the most important in a potential partner? ✳ Which are absolute musts? ✳ Are there any differences between what you believe to be important in a relationship and the things your parents feel are important?*

Sharing Feelings

Although men tend to talk about intimate issues with women more frequently than with men, women still complain that men do not communicate enough about what is really on their minds. This may reflect the powerfully different socialization processes experienced by women and men, which influence their communication styles. Throughout their lives, females are offered opportunities to practice sharing their thoughts and feelings with others. In contrast, males receive strong societal messages to withhold their feelings. The classic example of this training in very young males is the familiar saying, "Big boys don't cry." Men learn very early that certain emotions are not to be shared, with the result that they are more information-focused and businesslike in their conversations. Understandably, such differences in communication styles contribute to misunderstandings and conflict between the sexes. (See the Women's Health/Men's Health box.)

Although men are often perceived as being less emotional than women, the question remains whether men really feel less or just have more difficulty expressing their emotions. In one study, when men and women were shown scenes of people in distress, the men exhibited little outward emotion, whereas the women communicated feelings of concern and distress. However, physiological measures of emotional arousal (such as heart rate and blood pressure) indicated that the male subjects were actually as affected emotionally as the female subjects but inhibited the expression of their emotions, whereas the women openly expressed them. In other studies, men and women responded very differently to the same test.[40]

When men are angered, they tend to interpret the cause of their anger as something or someone in their environment and are likely to turn their anger outward in an aggressive manner. Women, on the other hand, tend to see themselves as the source of the problem and turn their anger inward, thereby suppressing direct expression of it.[41] Such differences in expressing anger can easily lead to breakdowns in communication between men and women.

Computer Dating: Issues for the Communication Age

Ten years ago, the thought of sharing intimate life details with a faceless stranger in cyberspace would have been unthinkable. Today, such meetings may lead to excitement, intrigue, or "happily-ever-after" encounters. In increasingly large numbers, however, they may also lead to disappointment as the computer persona turns out to be a rather ordinary, dull person in real life. Occasionally, as recent newspaper headlines point out, chance computer relationships can lead to victimization and death. In one such instance, a woman had been communicating daily with her "computer friend" for several months. When her friend began to use increasingly vivid and kinky sexual references and seemed to know more about

her than she wished, she became uncomfortable and tried to back off. She was relentlessly "stalked" via her home and work computers, and it became evident that her computer stalker knew her address and much about her personal life. Eventually, she was found dead, the result of a vicious attack by the person she knew only via computer.

Though this incident is a dramatic example of computer interactions gone wrong, it is important to remember that there are inherent risks in engaging in communications with people you don't know in any traditional sense. Remembering these key points of computerized communication may save you many hours of worry and frustration.

✔ Never give your real name or vital information (e.g., credit card numbers) to a computer chat partner. Use a screen name only, and avoid giving information that may help chat partners home in on you personally.

✔ If your conversations become suggestive, threatening, or make you uncomfortable in any way, terminate the session. Report such violations to your Internet service provider.

✔ Never arrange to meet strangers at your home or their homes. Pick a safe public meeting place, and bring a friend. Do not give specific identifying information until you know much more about the person. Keep job location and employment information out of the conversation, except in generic terms.

✔ Ask yourself why you are seeking intimacy from strangers on the computer rather than interacting with people you know, particularly if the computer seems to be taking up a disproportionate amount of your time. If your hours online are excessive, you may need to talk to a counselor or friend about your situation.

Communication between Couples

The following techniques can promote good communication between couples:[42]

1. **Leveling** refers to sending your partner a clear, simple, and honest message. The purposes of leveling are to: (1) make communication clear; (2) clarify the expectations partners have of each other; (3) clear up pleasant and unpleasant feelings and thoughts from past incidents; (4) make clear what is relevant and what is irrelevant; and (5) become aware of the things that draw you together or push you apart.

2. **Editing** means censoring remarks that may be hurtful or are irrelevant. Often, when people are upset, they let everything fly, bringing up old issues and incidents that cause pain and put a partner on the defensive. Editing means taking the time and making the effort not to say inflammatory things. Leveling and editing help establish genuine communication characterized by caring and sensitivity.

3. **Documenting** refers to giving specific examples of issues under discussion. Documenting helps you avoid gross generalizations that tend to be accusatory, such as "You always" and "You never." If you provide specific examples of when and how an incident occurred, your partner will gain a concrete understanding of the issue. In documenting, you can also include specific suggestions for changing or improving the situation.

4. **Validating** means letting a partner know that although you may not agree with his or her point of view, you still respect the person's thoughts and feelings ("I don't agree with you, but I can see how you might view things that way"). This does not mean that you are giving in to your partner; you are simply recognizing that your opinions differ.

We All Want to Be Understood

The bottom line is: Both men and women want to be heard and understood in their conversations. Understanding gender differences in communication patterns, rather than casting

---

Leveling   The communication of a clear, simple, and honest message.

Editing   The process of censoring comments that would be intentionally hurtful or irrelevant to the conversation.

Documenting   Giving specific examples of issues being discussed.

Validating   Letting your partner know that although you may not agree with his or her point of view, you still respect the fact that he or she thinks or feels that way.

Men and Women Really Are Different: Recognizing and Acknowledging Uniqueness

Make no mistake about it, men and women learn very different patterns of behavior and communication from their earliest years and carry these tendencies with them throughout their lives. Sometimes this makes understanding each other difficult, such as when we are bothered by mannerisms or habits that we are not even aware of. Recognizing that it is differences that make us unique is a good first step in anticipating potential problems in communication and warding off those problems in advance. Note that these characteristics are not absolute. No doubt you know men who demonstrate traits that are more like those of their female counterparts and vice versa.

Men

Body Language

Occupy more space; gesture away from the body; lean back when listening; less feedback through body language; more forceful gestures (backslapping, stronger handshakes); overt fidgeting

Facial Expression

Often avoid eye contact; show less warmth in facial expression; frown more often

Speech Patterns

More likely to interrupt, mumble, and use fewer speech tones (approximately three); voices are lower and usually louder; sound more abrupt; talk less personally about selves; make more direct statements than feeling statements; use fewer adjectives and descriptive statements; use fewer terms of endearment; tendency to lecture

Behavioral Differences

More inclined to be analytical; give fewer compliments; use more sarcasm and teasing to show affection; cry less often; more argumentative; difficulty in expressing intimate feelings; hold fewer grudges; gossip less; less likely to ask for help; tend to take rejection less personally; apologize less often

Women

Take up less space; movement is light and easy; gesture toward the body; lean forward when listening; provide feedback via body language; less likely to invade another's space; more gentle when touching others

Maintain better eye contact; smile and nod more often

Interrupt less often; articulate more clearly; use more speech tones (five); may sound more emotional; voices are higher pitched and softer; more likely to discuss feelings and disclose more personal information; make more tentative statements ("kind of," "isn't it?")

More emotional approach to issues; give more compliments; show more expression; express feelings more readily; greater tendency to hold grudges; inclined to gossip more; more likely to ask for help; take rejection more personally; apologize more frequently

Sources: "Men and Women are Different!" from Kings Communications website, www.KingsCommunication.com, 10/14/02. Reprinted by permission. Mark L. Knapp and Anita L. Vangelisti, *Interpersonal Communication and Human Relationships* (Boston: Allyn & Bacon/Longman, 2000).

blame at each other, is the first step toward promoting effective communication. Tannen suggests that expec-ting persons of the other sex to change their style of communication is not an effective way to deal with the gender gap. Instead, learn to interpret messages while explaining your own unique way of communicating. Working to understand the different ways in which males and females use language will help us all achieve the goal of clear and honest communication.

What do you think?

Do you believe that men and women really communicate in different styles? ✳ *Are you more comfortable talking with women or men?* ✳ *Why?* ✳ *What can you do to improve your communication with members of the other sex?*

Overcoming Barriers to Intimacy

Obstacles to intimacy include lack of personal identity, emotional immaturity, and a poorly developed sense of responsibility. The fear of being hurt, low self-esteem, mishandled hostility, chronic "busyness" (and its attendant lack of emotional presence), a tendency to "parentify" loved ones, and a conflict of role expectations may be equally detrimental. In addition, individual insecurities and difficulties in recognizing and expressing emotional needs can lead to an intimacy barrier. These barriers to intimacy may have many causes, including miscommunication, a dysfunctional family background, and jealousy.

Barriers to Communication

In today's world of instant messages, cell phones, pagers, and technologically advanced information systems, communication problems have grown exponentially. Our current means of communication differ greatly from those of our ancestors. In addition to physical changes in communication, people around the world must increasingly interact with others of vastly different backgrounds and values. Finding a means of communicating that accommodates everyone can be difficult. Barriers to communication take many forms.

Differences in Background Age, education, social status, gender, culture, political beliefs, and many other variables can lead to differences between communicators. Your closest friends from high school, with whom you grew up, shared many similar experiences with you. Shared experiences contribute to shared meaning and understanding. But at college, you may suddenly find yourself among people having few shared experiences. Remember that the goal of good communication is not necessarily to have everyone agree with you; rather, it is to have others understand you.

Alcohol and Drugs Perhaps nothing stands in the way of effective communication more than alcohol and drugs. With an inhibited ability to encode messages, you may not be understood correctly. With an inhibited ability to decode messages, you may misinterpret someone else's message. Is it any wonder that 90 percent of campus rapes take place under the influence of alcohol? Avoiding date rape depends on a woman's ability to be clear in her own mind about what she wants and then to make herself clearly understood. It also depends on a man's ability to listen and hear what is being said, rather than what he thinks is being said. In most college campus sexual encounters that lead to date rape complaints, alcohol and drugs have interfered with the ability to clearly communicate.

Dysfunctional Families

As noted earlier, the ability to sustain genuine intimacy is largely developed in the family of origin. If you were to examine even the most pristine family under a microscope, you would likely find some problems. No group of people can interact perfectly all the time, but this does not necessarily make them dysfunctional. In a truly **dysfunctional family**, interaction between family members inhibits psychological growth, self-love, emotional expression, and individual development. Negative interactions are the norm rather than the exception.

Children raised in dysfunctional settings tend to face tremendous obstacles to growing up healthy. Coming to terms with past hurts may take years. However, with careful planning and introspection, support from loved ones, and counseling when needed, children from even the worst homes have proved to be remarkably resilient. Many are able to forget the past and to focus on the future, developing into healthy, well-adjusted adults. But some have problems throughout their lives.[43] For example, adults who grew up with alcoholic parents may have serious problems creating and maintaining intimate relationships. The family messages that these children receive are typically contradictory, as the family usually tries to hide the presence of alcohol abuse in the home.

Many adult children of alcoholics (ACOAs) claim that they become involved in unhealthy relationships and have difficulty trusting others, communicating with partners, and defining a healthy relationship.[44] Research supporting this theory is conflicted, and many questions remain concerning how past experiences affect relationships for ACOAs.

Another tragically large group of people struggling with intimacy problems originating in the family of origin are survivors of childhood emotional, physical, and sexual abuse (see Chapter 4). It is important to note that dysfunctional families are found in every social, ethnic, religious, economic, and racial group.

Jealousy in Relationships

"Jealousy is like a San Andreas fault running beneath the smooth surface of an intimate relationship. Most of the time, its eruptive potential lies hidden. But when it begins to rumble, the destruction can be enormous."[45] **Jealousy** has been described as an aversive reaction evoked by a real or imagined relationship involving one's partner and a third person.

Contrary to what many of us may believe, jealousy is not a sign of intense devotion to the person who is its target. Instead, jealousy is often a sign of underlying problems that may prove to be a significant barrier to a healthy intimate relationship. Causes of jealousy typically include the following:

- *Overdependence on the relationship.* People who have few social ties and who rely exclusively on their significant others tend to be fearful of losing them.
- *High value on sexual exclusivity.* People who believe that sexual exclusiveness is a crucial indicator of a love relationship are more likely to become jealous.
- *Severity of the threat.* People may feel uneasy if a person with a fantastic body, stunning good looks, and a great personality appears interested in their partners. But they may brush off the threat if they appraise their rival as "unworthy" in terms of appearance or other characteristics.
- *Low self-esteem.* People who feel good about themselves are less likely to feel unworthy and to fear that someone else is going to snatch their partners away from them. The underlying question that torments people with low self-esteem is "Why would anyone want me?"
- *Fear of losing control.* Some people need to feel in control of the situation. Feeling that they may be losing the attachment of or control over a partner can cause jealousy.

Dysfunctional family A family in which the interaction between family members inhibits rather than enhances psychological growth.

Jealousy An aversive reaction evoked by a real or imagined relationship involving a person's partner and a third person.

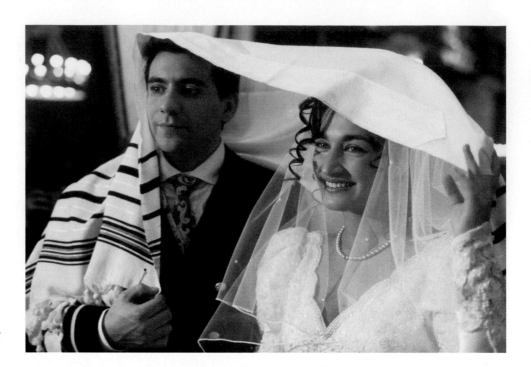

For many people, marriage or commitment ceremonies serve as the ultimate symbol of commitment between two people, validating their love for each other.

In both sexes, jealousy is related to the expectation that it would be difficult to find another relationship if the current one should end. For men, jealousy is positively correlated with self-evaluative dependency, the degree to which the man's self-esteem is affected by his partner's judgments. Though a certain amount of jealousy can be expected in any loving relationship, it doesn't have to threaten a relationship as long as partners communicate openly about it.[46]

What do you think?

"Jealousy is not a barometer by which the depth of love can be read. It merely records the depth of the lover's insecurity" (anthropologist Margaret Mead, 1901–1978). Do you agree or disagree with this statement? ✴ *What other factors may play a role in jealousy?*

Committed Relationships

Commitment in a relationship means that there is an intent to act over time in a way that perpetuates the well-being of the other person, oneself, and the relationship. Polls show that the majority of Americans—as many as 96 percent—strive to develop a committed relationship. These relationships can take several forms, including marriage, cohabitation, and gay and lesbian partnerships.

Marriage

In many societies around the world, traditional committed relationships take the form of marriage. In the United States,

marriage means entering into a legal agreement that includes shared financial plans, property, and responsibility for raising children. Many Americans also view marriage as a religious sacrament that emphasizes certain rights and obligations for each spouse.

Close to 90 percent of all Americans marry at least once. U.S. Census Bureau data shows that we are marrying later than ever before. In 1970 the median age for first marriage was 22.5 years for men and 20.6 years for women; by 1998, this had risen to 26.7 years for men and 25.0 years for women.[47] This trend appears to be continuing.

Many Americans believe that marriage involves **monogamy**, or exclusive sexual involvement with one partner. In fact, the lifetime pattern for many Americans appears to be **serial monogamy**, which means that a person has a monogamous sexual relationship with one partner before moving on to another monogamous relationship. However, some people prefer to have an **open relationship**, or open marriage, in which the partners agree that there may be sexual involvement for each person outside their relationship.

Humans are not naturally monogamous; most of us are capable of being sexually and/or emotionally involved with more than one person at a time. Sexual infidelity is an extremely common factor in divorces and breakups. So why do we continue to get married?

Certainly marriage is socially sanctioned and highly celebrated in our culture, so there are numerous incentives for couples to formalize their relationship with a wedding ceremony. A healthy marriage provides emotional support by combining the benefits of friendship and a loving committed relationship. A happy marriage also provides stability for both the couple and for those involved in the couple's life. Considerable research indicates that married people live longer, feel happier, remain mentally alert longer, and suffer fewer physical and mental health problems.[48] Even people who divorce seem to miss being married: Nearly 80 percent of them remarry.

While a successful marriage can bring much satisfaction, traditional marriage does not work for everyone. Some research suggests that today's women who choose marriage may not be as happy as their mothers were.[49] This may reflect increasing pressure on women to perform multiple roles such as taking care of a family while working outside the home. Other studies suggest that the happiness of never-married men has increased. However, traditional marriage is not the only path to a successful committed relationship.

Cohabitation

Cohabitation is defined as two people with an intimate connection who live together in the same household. For a variety of reasons, increasing numbers of Americans are choosing cohabitation. These relationships can be very stable and happy, with a high level of commitment between the partners. In some states, cohabitation that lasts a designated number of years (usually seven) legally constitutes a **common-law marriage** for purposes of real estate and other financial obligations.

Cohabitation can offer many of the same benefits that marriage does: love, sex, companionship, and the ongoing opportunity to know a partner better over time. In addition to enjoying emotional and physical benefits, some people may cohabit for practical reasons such as the opportunity to share bills and housing costs. While many cohabitors are young, some older adults choose this lifestyle because they would lose income, such as Social Security or a late spouse's pension, if they were to marry.

Successful cohabitations can also offer benefits not found in marriage. Partners may feel greater autonomy and independence than they might find in a traditional arrangement. Furthermore, if they decide to separate, they do not experience the legal problems and expense of a divorce.

Although cohabitation has its advantages, it also has some drawbacks. Perhaps the greatest disadvantage is the lack of societal validation for the relationship. Many cohabitors must deal with pressures from parents and friends, difficulties in obtaining insurance and tax benefits, and legal issues over property. In 1996, Congress reaffirmed tax advantages for married couples, and effectively blocked cohabiting heterosexual and homosexual couples from these benefits through the "Defense of Marriage Bill." Today, controversy continues over whether traditional marriage should remain the only means of eligibility for tax deductions, health insurance, and other benefits. In general, there appears to be a trend toward recognizing the validity of unmarried relationships. The state of Vermont, for example, has passed a law that allows partners to form "civil unions."[50] Some companies now offer insurance benefits to employees' unmarried partners. See the New Horizons in Health box for more on rates of marriage, divorce, and cohabitation.

Gay and Lesbian Partnerships

Whether they are gay or straight, male or female, most adults want intimate, committed relationships. Lesbians and gay men seek the same things in primary relationships that heterosexual partners do: friendship, communication, validation, companionship, and a sense of stability.

The 2000 U.S. Census revealed a significant increase in the number of same-sex partner households across the country—more than three times the total reported in the 1990 Census. The states with the most reported same-sex households are California, New York, Florida, Illinois, and Georgia. According to Lee Badgett, research director of the Institute for Gay and Lesbian Strategic Studies, the actual number of households is probably much higher. Many gay and lesbian partners hesitate to report their relationship due to concerns about discrimination.[51]

Studies of lesbian couples indicate high levels of attachment and satisfaction and a tendency toward monogamous, long-term relationships. Gay men, too, tend to form committed, long-term relationships, especially as they age, much like their heterosexual counterparts.

Challenges to successful lesbian and gay male relationships often stem from discrimination and difficulties dealing with social, legal, and religious doctrines. For lesbian and gay couples, obtaining the same level of "marriage benefits," such as tax deductions, power-of-attorney, and other rights, continues to be a challenge. However, commitment ceremonies and marriage ceremonies are becoming more frequent in some U.S. cities and in several countries. As mentioned above, Vermont now recognizes same-sex civil unions.[52]

Staying Single

Increasing numbers of adults—of all ages—are electing to remain single. In 1970, 18.9 percent of adult men and 13.7 percent of adult women were unmarried. By the late 1990s, the proportion of adult Americans who were single by choice or by chance (sometimes after failed marriages) had increased significantly, to more than 37 percent of men and over 41 percent of women. Other changes are reflected in the following facts:

Monogamy   Exclusive sexual involvement with one partner.

Serial monogamy   A series of monogamous sexual relationships.

Open relationship   A relationship in which partners agree that sexual involvement can occur outside the relationship.

Cohabitation   Living together without being married.

Common-law marriage   Cohabitation lasting a designated period of time (usually seven years) that is considered legally binding in some states.

News from the World of Marriage, Divorce, and Cohabitation Studies

Are you considering marriage? Consider these facts: By age 30, about three-fourths of women in the United States. have been married and about half have cohabited outside of marriage, according to a comprehensive new report on cohabitation, marriage, divorce, and remarriage by the Centers for Disease Control and Prevention. The study was based on interviews with nearly 11,000 women 15–44 years of age and examined individual and community factors that influence whether a person marries, divorces, cohabits, or chooses to remain single. Points of interest from this study include the following:

- Divorce rates are up, but so are the number of second marriages. Divorcees who do remarry usually wait three years before saying "I do" again.
- More women are choosing to remain single. In 1963, 83 percent of women in the age group studied were married; today, just over 66 percent of all women will marry.
- The pre-1950s family pattern of Mom, Dad, and kids living under the same roof is no longer the norm.

- Roughly half of all first marriages for people younger than 45 end in divorce. First marriages that end in divorce typically last about eight years. The "seven-year itch" seems to be validated by statistical data!
- Younger generations of Americans are delaying marriage until later in life. Most people are spending more of their lives unmarried.
- More educated people are more likely to marry and stay married, perhaps because they are more mature and/or financially stable when they tie the knot.
- Overall unmarried cohabitations are less stable than marriages. The probability of a premarital cohabitation breaking up within five years is 49 percent. The probability of a first marriage ending in separation or divorce within five years is 20 percent. After 10 years, the probability of a first marriage ending is 33 percent, compared with 62 percent for cohabitations.
- Cohabitations and marriages tend to last longer under certain conditions such as: a woman's age at the time the cohabitation or marriage began (older is better); whether she was raised throughout childhood in an intact two-parent family that seemed to be happy; whether religion plays an important role in her life; and whether she had a higher family income or lived in a community with high median family income, low male unemployment, and low poverty.

- Marriages that end do not always end in divorce; many end in separation and do not go through divorce. Separated white women are much more likely (91 percent) to divorce after three years, compared with separated Hispanic women (77 percent) and separated black women (67 percent).
- The probability of remarriage among divorced women is 54 percent in five years overall: 58 percent for white women, 44 percent for Hispanic women, and 32 percent for black women. However, there is also a strong probability that second marriages will end in separation or divorce (23 percent after five years and 39 percent after 10 years).
- In the 1950s, if a woman divorced, there was a 65 percent chance that she would remarry. Today, only about 50 percent of divorced women choose to remarry.

Source: National Center for Health Statistics, Centers for Disease Control, "New Report Sheds Light on Trends and Patterns in Marriage, Divorce, and Cohabitation," July 24, 2002, series report 23, number 22 (see http://www.cdc.gov/nchs/releases/02news/div_mar_cohab.htm).

- Over 10 percent of all people say they would never marry.
- People marrying today have more than a 50 percent chance of divorcing.
- As more women enjoy financial independence, they are less likely to remarry after divorce.
- Increasing numbers of widows and widowers are opting not to remarry.

Today, large numbers of people prefer to remain single. Singles clubs, social outings arranged by communities and religious groups, extended family environments, and a large number of social services support the single lifestyle. Many

singles live rich, rewarding lives and maintain a large network of close friends and families. Although sexual intimacy may or may not be present, the intimacy achieved through other interactions with loved ones is a key aspect of the single lifestyle.

Some research indicates that single people live shorter lives, are more unhappy, and are more likely to experience financial and health problems than their married peers. However, other studies refute these conclusions. Few research studies to date have controlled for other confounding variables, such as environmental conditions, past histories, and other factors that may carry more weight than the married or single state.

What do you think?

Although there are advantages and disadvantages in marriage, many people feel that marriage is a desirable option. Are there any advantages in remaining single? ✳ What are potential disadvantages? ✳ Are there any societal or organizational supports for the single lifestyle?

Success in Relationships

Our definition of success in a relationship tends to be based on whether a couple stays together over the years. Learning to communicate, respecting each other, and sharing a genuine fondness are crucial to relationship success. Many social scientists agree that the happiest committed relationships are flexible enough to allow the partners to grow throughout their lives.

Partnering Scripts

Parents often believe that their children will achieve happiness by living much as they have. Accordingly, most children are reared with a very strong script for what is expected of them as adults. Each group in society has its own partnering script that includes similarities of sex, age, social class, race, religion, physical attributes, and personality types. By adolescence, people generally know exactly what type of person they are expected to befriend or date. By which partnering script were you raised? Just picture whom you could or couldn't bring home to meet your family.

Society provides constant reinforcement for traditional couples, but it may withhold this reinforcement from couples of the same sex, mixed race, mixed religion, and mixed age. People who have not chosen an "appropriate" partner are subject to a great deal of external stress. In addition to denying recognition to such couples, friends and family often blame the "inappropriateness" of the couple if the relationship fails. Recognizing that this stress is external to the relationship can help alleviate criticism and distancing between the partners.

Nonetheless, many nontraditional relationships survive and flourish. For example, the number of interracial marriages has quadrupled since the late 1960s, and the number of same-sex partner households has grown from 145,130 to almost half a million over the past ten years.[53]

What do you think?

What characteristics are most important to you in a potential partner? ✳ Which of these would be important to your parents or friends? ✳ If your parents or friends didn't like a potential partner, how important would their opinion be to you? ✳ What would you do in this situation?

Being Self-Nurturant

It is often stated that you must love yourself before you can love someone else. What does this mean? Learning how you function emotionally and how to nurture yourself through all life's situations is a lifelong task. You should certainly not postpone intimate connections with others until you have achieved this state. However, a certain level of individual maturity helps in maintaining a committed relationship. For example, divorce rates are much higher for couples under age 30 than for older couples.

Two concepts that are especially important to a good relationship are accountability and self-nurturance. **Accountability** means that both partners in a relationship see themselves as responsible for their own decisions and actions. They don't hold the other person responsible for positive or negative experiences.

Self-nurturance goes hand in hand with accountability. In order to make good choices in life, a person needs to maintain a balance of sleeping, eating, exercising, working, relaxing, and socializing. When the balance is disrupted, as it will inevitably be, self-nurturing people are patient with themselves and try to put things back on course.

It is a lifelong process to learn to live in a balanced and healthy way. Two people who are on a path of accountability and self-nurturance together have a much better chance of maintaining a satisfying relationship.

Confronting Couple Issues

Couples seeking a long-term relationship have to confront a number of issues that can enhance or ruin their chances of success. Some of these issues involve gender roles and power sharing.

Changing Gender Roles Throughout history, women and men have taken on various roles in their relationships. In agricultural America, gender roles were determined by tradition and each task within a family unit held equal importance.

Our modern society has very few gender-specific roles. Women and men alike drive cars, care for children, operate computers, manage finances, and perform equally well in the tasks of daily living. However, rather than taking on the "traditional" female and male roles, many couples find it makes more sense to divide tasks on the basis of schedule, convenience, and preference. While it may make sense to divide household chores, it rarely works out that the division is

Accountability Accepting responsibility for personal decisions, choices, and actions.

Self-nurturance Developing individual potential through a balanced and realistic appreciation of self-worth and ability.

equal. Today's working woman, living in a dual-career family and coping with the responsibilities of being a partner, a mother, and a professional, is often stressed and frustrated. Men, who may have expected a more traditional role for their partners, may experience difficulties. Even when women work full time, they tend to bear heavy family and household responsibilities. Over time, if couples are unable to communicate about how they feel about performing certain tasks, the relationship may suffer.

Sharing Power Power can be defined as the ability to make and implement decisions. There are many ways to exercise power, but powerful people are those who know what they want and have the ability to attain it. In traditional relationships, men were the wage earners and consequently had decision-making power. Women exerted much influence, but in the final analysis they needed a man's income for survival.

But as women became wage earners in increasing numbers, the power dynamics between women and men changed. As long as men as a group earn substantially more money than women, they will continue to exercise decision-making capacity. Within individual households, however, the dynamics have shifted considerably, with greater numbers of women working and enjoying their own financial resources. Part of the increase in the divorce rate undoubtedly reflects the recognition by working women that they can leave bad relationships in which they previously felt confined. In general, successful couples arrange power relationships that reflect their unique needs rather than popular stereotypes.

Single parents face additional challenges in juggling their work and family responsibilities. Many use community resources such as after school day care centers.

Having Children . . . or Not?

When a couple decides to raise children, their relationship changes. Resources of time, energy, and money are split many ways, and the partners no longer have each other's undivided attention. Babies and young children do not time their requests for food, sleep, and care to the convenience of adults. Therefore, individuals or couples whose own basic needs for security, love, and purpose are already met make better parents. Any stresses that already exist in a relationship will be further accentuated when parenting is added to the list of responsibilities. Having a child does not save a bad relationship—in fact, it only seems to compound the problems that already exist. A child cannot and should not be expected to provide the parents with self-esteem and security.

Changing patterns in family life affect the way children are raised. In modern society, it is not always clear which partner will adjust his or her work schedule to provide the primary care of children. Nearly half a million children each year become part of a blended family when their parents remarry; remarriage creates a new family of stepparents and stepsiblings. In addition, an increasing number of individuals are choosing to have children in a family structure other than a heterosexual marriage. Single women can choose adoption or alternative (formerly called "artificial") insemination as a way to create a family. Single men can choose to adopt or can obtain the services of a surrogate mother. According to the 2000 census, over 9 percent of all U.S. households were headed by a man or woman raising a child alone, reflecting a growing trend in America and in the international community.[54] Regardless of the structure of the family, certain factors remain important to the well-being of the unit: consistency, communication, affection, and mutual respect. See Table 5.1 for emerging trends in childrearing.

Some people become parents without a lot of forethought. Some children are born into a relationship that was supposed to last and didn't. This does not mean it is too late to do a good job of parenting. Children are amazingly resilient and forgiving if parents show respect and communicate about household activities that affect their lives. Even children who grew up in a household of conflict can feel loved and respected if the parents treat them fairly. This means that parents must take responsibility for their own conflicts and make it clear to children that they are not the reason for the conflict.

Today, many families find that two incomes are needed just to make ends meet. That's why more than 80 percent of all mothers with children under the age of 5 work outside the home. Day care, extended family and friends, grandparents, neighbors, and nannies "mind the kids." Some employers offer family leave arrangements that allow parents more latitude in taking time from work.

Table 5.1
The Emerging Twenty-First-Century American Family

PERCENTAGE OF CHILDREN IN VARIOUS TYPES OF FAMILIES

	ONE SINGLE PARENT	TWO PARENT, CONTINUING	TWO PARENT, REMARRIED	TWO ADULTS, EX-MARRIED	ADULT, NEVER MARRIED
1972	4.7	73.0	9.9	3.8	8.6
1978	10.2	65.3	13.6	4.0	6.9
1982	14.3	59.3	13.7	5.2	7.3
1988	18.6	54.7	13.0	5.0	8.7
1990	14.9	56.1	17.9	5.1	6.0
1994	18.4	52.8	14.7	7.1	7.0
1998	18.2	51.7	12.3	8.6	9.2

Note: Single Parent = *only one adult in household;* two parent, continuing = *married couple, never divorced;* two parent, remarried = *married couple, at least one remarried (unknown if children came before or after remarriage);* two adults, ex-married = *two or more adults, previously but not currently* married; adult never married = two or more adults, *never married (this category also includes some other family structures).*
Source: General Social Survey News, Number 13, August 1999. From National Opinion Research Center. Reprinted by permission of NORC.

What do you think?

What characteristics of a healthy family environment are important to you? ✳ *Do you think that day care centers, extended family units, and full-time baby-sitters can provide a positive environment for children?* ✳ *Why or why not?*

When Relationships Falter

Breakdowns in relationships usually begin with a change in communication, however subtle. Either partner may stop listening, ceasing to be emotionally present for the other. In turn, the other feels ignored, unappreciated, or unwanted. Unresolved conflicts increase, and unresolved anger can cause problems in sexual relations. Over time, relationships with such difficulties may end in divorce. Age at first marriage, race, and socioeconomic status also affect the success of relationships (see Figure 5.4).

When a couple who previously enjoyed spending time alone together find themselves continually in the company of others, spending time apart, or preferring to stay home alone, it may be a sign that the relationship is in trouble. Of course, the need for individual privacy and **autonomy** (the ability to care for oneself emotionally, socially, and physically) is not a cause for worry—it's essential to health. If, however, a partner decides to change the amount and quality of time spent together without the input or understanding of the other, it may be a sign of hidden problems.

College students, particularly those who are socially isolated and far from family and hometown friends, may be particularly vulnerable to staying in unhealthy relationships. They may become emotionally dependent on a partner for everything from eating meals to recreational and study time, and

mutual obligations such as shared rental arrangements, transportation, and child care can make it tough to leave.

It's also easy to mistake unwanted sexual advances for physical attraction or love. Without a network of friends and supporters to talk with, to obtain validation for feelings or to share concerns, a student may feel stuck in a relationship that is headed nowhere.

Honesty and verbal affection are usually positive aspects of a relationship. In a troubled relationship, however, they can be used to cover up irresponsible or hurtful behavior. "At least I was honest" is not an acceptable substitute for acting in a trustworthy way. The words "But I really do love you" should not be used as a license to be inconsiderate or rude.

Getting Help

The first place some people look for help for relationship problems is a trusted friend. But although friends can offer support during trying times, few have the training and detachment necessary to resolve serious relationship problems.

Most communities have trained therapists who specialize in relationship difficulties. These practitioners may be psychiatrists, licensed psychologists, social workers, or counselors with advanced degrees. Most student health centers or on-campus counseling centers offer these services at reduced fees for students. If you are unaware of such services, ask your instructor for suggestions.

If a couple's commitment to the relationship is strong, their chances of solving problems increase. The counselor typically interviews the partners separately and together,

---

Autonomy The ability to care for oneself emotionally, socially, and physically.

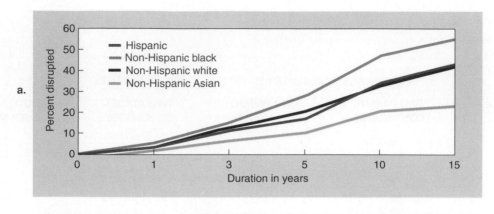

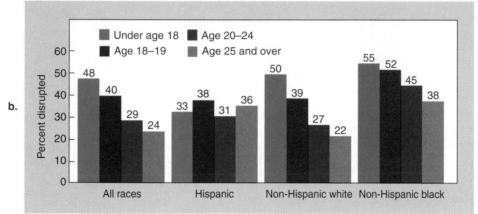

Figure 5.4
Effects of Women's Age and Ethnicity on Marriage Success

(a) Probability that the first marriage breaks up by duration of marriage and women's race/ethnicity: United States, 1995

(b) Probability that the first marriage breaks up within 10 years by women's race/ethnicity and age at beginning of marriage: United States, 1995

Source: "Cohabitation, Divorce, and Remarriage in the United States," Centers for Disease Control and Prevention: Vital and Health Statistics, Series 23, Number 22, July 2002.

gradually helping them recognize and change the behaviors and attitudes that are detrimental to the relationship. Counseling may take a few weeks, several months, or even years as couples examine their values and reestablish their commitment. Beware of the counselor who tells you to drop the relationship on the first visit or who tries to give advice without hearing the full story. Most good counselors will spend a good deal of time letting you tell them what you want to do and helping you work through your feelings rather than adopt theirs.

Trial Separations

Sometimes a relationship becomes so dysfunctional that even counseling cannot bring about significant change. Moving apart for a period of time may allow some preliminary healing and give both parties an opportunity to reassess themselves and their commitment. Trial separations do not guarantee that the situation will improve, nor do they mean the relationship is ending. If both people are involved in

counseling or have other support systems and mutually agree on the need for a trial separation, it may be a way to regroup and save a failing relationship.

When and Why Relationships End

Based on recent statistics, it has been predicted that 20 percent of those who marry today will divorce within 5 years; one-third may divorce within 10 years; and 40 percent will divorce before their fifteenth anniversary. Ultimately, half of all marriages

What do you think?

What factors do you think contribute to a U.S. divorce rate that is higher than any other reported rate? ✳ How would you explain Americans' attitudes about marriage and divorce to a friend from another country?

World Divorce Rates: United States Ranked Number Two

Although many factors contribute to the divorce rates in a given country, the United States has consistently been among the highest. Cultural values, religious values, living patterns, socioeconomic status, customs, social norms, and a host of other factors influence divorce decisions. Some of the countries with the highest rates are highlighted in bold; note that Greece, Italy, Poland, Spain, and Turkey are among the lowest-ranking countries. Divorce is legal in the countries shown in this list; the divorce rates are per 100 marriages.

Austria	43.4
Belarus	**52.9**
Belgium	44.0
Bulgaria	21.1
Canada	37.0
Czech Republic	43.3
Denmark	**44.5**
Finland	**51.2**
France	38.3
Germany	39.4
Greece	15.7
Hungary	37.5
Italy	10.0
Luxembourg	**47.4**

Moldova	28.1
Netherlands	38.3
Norway	40.4
Poland	17.3
Portugal	26.2
Romania	19.1
Russia	**43.3**
Spain	15.2
Sweden	**54.9**
Switzerland	25.5
Turkey	6.0
Ukraine	40.0
United Kingdom	**42.6**
United States	**54.8**

Sources: www.divorcereform.org; "Recent Demographic Developments in Europe, 2001," Council of Europe Publishing, 2001; Jean-Paul Sardon, "Recent Demographic Trends in the Developed Countries," *Population: English Edition* 57 (January-February 2002).

will end in divorce.[55] The Health in a Diverse World box compares the American divorce rate with that of other countries.

While the divorce rate may seem alarming, the actual number of failed relationships is probably much higher. Many people never go through a legal divorce process, and as a result, are not counted in these statistics. Cohabitors and unmarried partners, who raise children, own homes together, and exhibit all the outward appearances of marriage without the license, are also not included.

Why do relationships end? There are many reasons, including illness, financial concerns, and career problems. Other breakups arise from unmet expectations. Many people enter a relationship with certain expectations about how they and their partner will behave. Failure to communicate these expectations to the partner can lead to resentment and disappointment. Differences in sexual needs may also contribute to the demise of a relationship. Table 5.2 shows important factors in relationship failure.

Under stress, communication and cooperation between partners can break down. Conflict and negative interactions as well as a general lack of respect between partners can erode even the most loving relationship.

Coping with Loneliness

When a relationship ends, it is normal to experience painful emotions of anger, guilt, rejection, and unworthiness. No matter how miserable the relationship was, feelings of failure are common. Counselors estimate that it can take at least

a year and often longer to recover from the loss of a major relationship, whether by death or separation.

While it may be painful, reflecting on the past relationship can help prevent similar mistakes in the future. Concentrating on the negative aspects of an ex-partner is a natural tendency, but it is equally important to remember what you loved in the other person and what is lovable about you. When we accept the risk and challenge of close relationships, we accept one of the greatest gifts life has to offer. People who acknowledge the difficulty of what they are going through and share their feelings with others heal faster and more completely than those who are isolated. With time and support from friends, people do recover and establish rewarding new relationships.

Building Better Relationships

Most relationships start with great optimism and true love. So why do so many run into trouble? "We just don't know how to handle the negative feelings that are the unavoidable by-product of the differences between two people, the very differences that attract them to each other in the first place. Think of it as the friction any two bodies would generate rubbing against each other countless times each day," says Howard Markman, Ph.D., professor of psychology at the University of Denver.[56] According to Markman, most unhappy couples don't need therapy; they need education in how relationships work and the special skills that make them work well. Markman and

Table 5.2
Key Factors Predicting Success and Failure in Marriages and Relationships

TRAITS THAT PREDICT SUCCESS

INDIVIDUAL
• High self-esteem
• Flexibility
• Assertiveness
• Sociability

COUPLE
• Similarity
• Long acquaintanceship
• Good communication skills
• Good conflict-resolution skills

CONTEXT
• Older age
• Healthy family-of-origin experiences
• Happy parental marriage
• Parents' and friends' approval
• Significant educational career preparation

COMMON REASONS FOR MARRIAGE AND RELATIONSHIP FAILURE

• Poor communication
• Financial problems
• Lack of commitment to the marriage
• Dramatic change in priorities
• Infidelity
• Failed expectations or unmet needs
• Addictions and substance abuse
• Physical, sexual, or emotional abuse
• Lack of conflict-resolution skills

TRAITS THAT PREDICT FAILURE

INDIVIDUAL
• Neurotic characteristics
• Anxiety
• Depression
• Impulsiveness
• Self-consciousness
• Vulnerability to stress
• Anger/hostility
• Dysfunctional beliefs

COUPLE
• Dissimilarity
• Short acquaintanceship
• Premarital sex with many partners
• Premarital pregnancy
• Cohabitation
• Poor communication and conflict-resolution skills

CONTEXT
• Younger age
• Unhealthy family-of-origin experiences
• Parental divorce or chronic conflict
• Parents' or friends' disapproval
• Pressure to marry
• Little education or career preparation

Source: "Making Marriage Last," American Academy of Matrimonial Lawyers (see http://www.aaml.org/Marriage_Last/MarriageMain.htm).

others promote **psychoeducation**, the teaching of crucial psychological skills—giving people knowledge so they can help themselves. Psychoeducation courses aren't therapy per se, but they typically have a therapeutic effect on couples.

Elements of Healthy Relationships

Relationships that are satisfying and stable share certain characteristics. A key ingredient is **trust**, the degree of

Psychoeducation The teaching of crucial psychological skills, giving people knowledge so they can help themselves.

Trust The degree of confidence felt in a relationship.

confidence felt in a relationship. Without trust, intimacy will not develop and the relationship could fail. Trust includes three fundamental elements:

- *Predictability* means that you can predict your partner's behavior, based on the knowledge that your partner acts in consistently positive ways.
- *Dependability* means that you can rely on your partner to give support in all situations, particularly those in which you feel threatened with hurt or rejection.
- *Faith* means that you feel absolutely certain about your partner's intentions and behavior.

Trust can develop even when it is initially lacking. This requires opening yourself to others, which carries the risk of hurt or rejection.

Other characteristics of happy relationships include the following:

- Partners interpret each other's behavior in the context of their own relationship, without overreacting to behaviors that remind them of past relationships. For example, if a previous partner continually flirted with other people and cheated on you, the sight of your current partner dancing with someone else at a party could trigger unpleasant memories. However, don't assume that your current partner will behave the same way.
- Partners who like each other and find each other interesting are happier than those who don't. Many people describe their partners as their best friends. Although most relationships have their share of ups and downs, members of successful couples are able to talk, listen, and touch each other in an atmosphere of caring. They value a good sense of humor and exhibit clear communication, cooperation, and the ability to resolve conflicts constructively.
- Sexual intimacy is a major component of healthy relationships, but sex is not a major reason for the existence of the relationship. Some couples admit to sexual dissatisfaction but find the relationship itself more important than sexual pleasure. Many couples report that as communication and trust increase, the sexual relationship also improves.
- Another important quality is a shared and cherished history, including private jokes, special places where key events have occurred, nicknames, rituals, emotions, and significant shared time and activities.

After reading this chapter, it should be apparent that relationships—whether with partners, parents, friends, or others—involve complex interactions that don't always work the way you'd like them to. Occasionally, they'll lead to frustrations and disappointments. However, they also will be a source of great joy and fulfillment. Developing skills that will protect you in a relationship and also help your relationship grow and flourish is an important step in achieving relationship health. In addition, learning not to take yourself quite so seriously, to forgive others' slips, and to overcome your own fears and overreactions will help keep relationships on course.

Taking Charge

5 **5** **5**

Creating Healthy Relationships

As you have seen in this chapter, interpersonal interactions and communication skills can have a significant impact on overall health. Think about the relationships in your life. Are you satisfied with the number and types of friendships you have established? Whether you are conversing with intimate partners, friends, family members, or casual acquaintances, the way in which you say things and how you act will affect your message. Are you involved in an intimate relationship, and is it meeting your expectations? Using the information in this chapter, what can you do to enhance the relationships in your life?

Checklist for Change

Making Personal Choices

- ☐ Have you thought about your own communication style? Are you a good listener, or do you like to hold everyone's attention with your own talking?
- ☐ What factors are most important to you in a potential partner? If you have been or are in a relationship, what factors or traits have caused problems?
- ☐ What relationships are most important to you? How have these relationships affected your relationships with others?
- ☐ What positive things do you bring to a relationship?
- ☐ What do you expect in a longterm relationship? What behaviors would you consider acceptable and unacceptable in your partner?
- ☐ What do you think are the three most important attributes of a friend?

Making Community Choices

- ☐ When you communicate information to others, do you

make every attempt to be accurate, unbiased, and unemotional in your delivery?

☐ Is there a place on your campus or in your community where you can work on your communication problems?

☐ Do you make a habit of putting yourself in the other person's shoes when discussing how your actions may have made that person feel or how that person may be feeling in general?

☐ Do you reach out to friends who are having problems in their relationships?

☐ Do you try to work through your problems with others, or do you avoid problems?

Summary

❋ Communication is a complex process that dictates how we interact with others. Understanding each other's words and symbols is an important part of communication. Our perceptions of these words and symbols, or our way of interpreting incoming information, is equally consequential as we forge relationships throughout our lives.

❋ A number of factors need to be addressed in order to improve the ability to communicate with others. These include learning how to use self-disclosure, listen effectively, convey and interpret nonverbal communication, establish a proper climate for communicating, and manage and resolve conflicts.

❋ Intimate relationships have several different characteristics, including behavioral interdependence, need fulfillment, emotional attachment, and emotional availability. These characteristics influence how we interact with others and the types of intimate relationships we form. Family, friends, and partners or lovers provide the most common opportunities for intimacy. Each relationship may include healthy and unhealthy characteristics that may affect daily functioning.

❋ Gender differences in communication can include different conversation styles as well as differences in sharing feelings and disclosing personal facts and fears. These differences explain why men and women may relate differently in intimate relationships. Understanding these differences and learning how to deal with them are important aspects of healthy relationships.

❋ Barriers to intimacy often involve barriers in communication, which could result from a difference in backgrounds

or the effects of alcohol and drugs. Other barriers may include the different emotional needs of both partners, jealousy, and emotional wounds that could result from being raised in a dysfunctional family.

❋ Commitment is an important ingredient in successful relationships for most people. The major types of committed relationships include marriage, cohabitation, and gay and lesbian partnerships.

❋ Success in committed relationships requires understanding the roles of partnering scripts, the importance of self-nurturance, the elements of a good relationship, and the ability to confront couple issues.

❋ Life decisions such as whether to marry or remain single or whether to have children require serious consideration. Remaining single is more common than ever before. Most single people lead healthy, happy, and well-adjusted lives. Those who decide to have or not to have children can also lead rewarding, productive lives as long as they have given this decision the utmost thought, weighing the pros and cons of each in the context of their lifestyle. Today's family structure may look different from that of previous generations, but love, trust, and commitment to a child's welfare continue to be the cornerstones of successful childrearing.

❋ Before relationships fail, often many warning signs appear. By recognizing these signs and taking action to change behaviors, partners may save and enhance their relationships.

❋ There are many strategies for building better relationships. Examining one's own behaviors to determine what to change and how to change it is an important ingredient of success.

Questions for Discussion and Reflection

1. Why are symbolism and individual perception so critical to the communication process?
2. How are self-esteem and stress directly related to physical well-being? How does communication improve self-esteem and reduce stress?
3. Why is self-disclosure so important to mental well-being? At what times is it better not to disclose personal information?
4. What is nonverbal communication, and why is it important to develop skills in this area? Give examples of some things that you do to communicate without words.

5. What are the characteristics of intimate relationships? What are behavioral interdependence, need fulfillment, emotional attachment, and emotional availability, and why is each important in relationship development?
6. Why are relationships with family important? Explain how your family unit was similar to or different from the traditional family unit in early America. Who made up your family of origin? your nuclear family?
7. How can you tell the difference between a love relationship and one that is based primarily on attraction? What characteristics do love relationships share?

8. What problems can form barriers to intimacy? What actions can you take to reduce or remove these barriers?
9. What are common elements of good relationships? Warning signs of trouble? What actions can you take to improve your own interpersonal relationships?
10. Name some common misconceptions about people who choose to remain single and about couples who choose

not to have children. Do you want to have children? Why or why not? What characteristics show that a couple is ready to have children?
11. How have gender roles changed over the past 20 years? Do you view the changes as positive for both men and women?

Application Exercises

Reread the What Do You Think? scenarios at the beginning of the chapter, and answer the following questions.

1. Do most people "grossly exaggerate" the wonders of their newfound loves? Do you know anyone like James, who talks about the intimate sexual details? Do you think this is appropriate? Is it fair to the other person involved in the relationship? How could you communicate a lack of interest in such private details?

2. In spite of society's progress in recognizing that different ways of life can be rewarding, the decision to remain single in America is often difficult. Why do people like Kate face so many challenges in being accepted as a single person? What could be done to improve the status of single people in American society?

Accessing Your Health on the Internet

Visit the following Internet sites to explore further topics and issues related to personal health. To visit an organization's website, go to the Companion Website for *Access to Health, Eighth Edition* at www.aw.com/donatelle, click on the book image, and select "Accessing Your Health on the Internet" from the navigation menu on the left.

1. *ANWeb Resources—Peace and Conflict Resolution.* Provides links to numerous sites dealing with conflict resolution.
2. *Couples National Network.* Link into a network for same-gender couples and singles, with resources about gay and lesbian issues.

3. *Mental Health Notes.* User-friendly information about dysfunctional families from a licensed clinical psychologist. Includes links to related mental health articles.
4. *National Center for Health Statistics.* This division of the Centers for Disease Control and Prevention has up-to-date statistics on trends in marriage, divorce, and cohabitation.
5. *Relationship Growth Online.* Provides information, quizzes, games, advice, and links to more information on how to build better relationships.
6. *University of Missouri Counseling Center Self-Help Area.* Provides a bibliography of books and other resources dealing with intimacy issues.

Further Reading

Busby, D., and V. Loyer-Carlson. *Pathways to Marriage with RELATE Online Relationship Inventory: Premarital and Early Marital Relationships.* Boston: Allyn & Bacon/Longman, 2003.

Step-by-step approach to building better relationships.

Erber, R., and M. Wang-Erber. *Intimate Relationships: Issues, Theories, and Research.* Boston: Allyn & Bacon/Longman, 2001.

Overview of common issues in relationships, theories about why relationships succeed and fail, and discussions of relevant research.

Galvin, K., and P. Cooper. *Making Connections.* Los Angeles: Roxbury Publishing 2000.

Outstanding overview of the importance of interpersonal communication in everyday lives. Provides practical strategies to assist us at all stages of life.

Gray, J. *Men Are from Mars, Women Are from Venus: A Practical Guide for Improving Communication and Getting What You Want in Your Relationships.* San Francisco: HarperCollins, 1998.

Overview of male and female communication styles and practical strategies for improving relationships. Available as both audiocassette and book.

Koman, A. *How to Mend a Broken Heart: Letting Go and Moving On.* Chicago: Contemporary Books, 1997.

A step-by-step program for dealing with the end of a relationship, including working through the emotional stages, strategies for coping, and gaining strength to move on.

Tannen, D. *Gender Discourse.* New York: Oxford University Press, 1996.

A collection of six scholarly essays exploring language and gender.

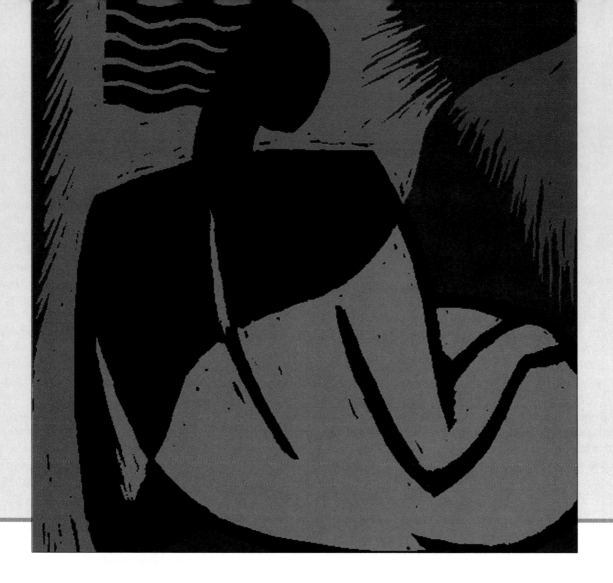

Objectives

* Define sexual identity, and discuss the roles of the major components of sexual identity, including biology, gender identity, gender roles, and sexual orientation.

* Identify the components of male and female reproductive anatomy and physiology and their functions.

* Discuss the options available for the expression of one's sexuality.

* Classify sexual dysfunctions, and describe each disorder.

Sexuality

Choices in Sexual Behavior

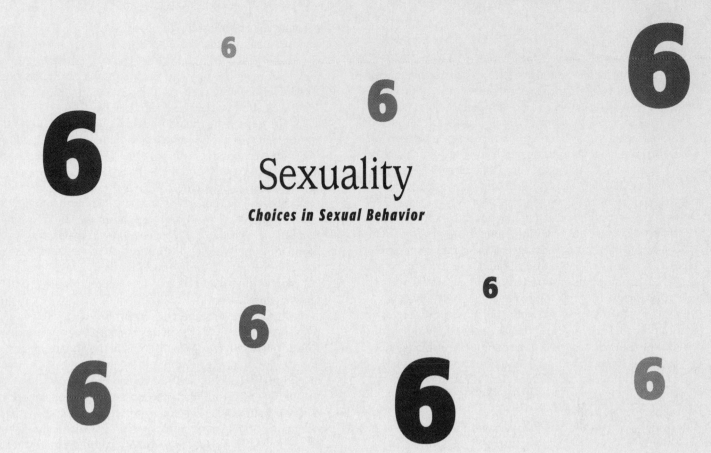

What do you think?

Ben is a bright, articulate athlete who was highly recruited to play college football. By the end of his freshman year he had earned a starting position as a wide receiver. Although on the surface it would appear that he has everything going for him, he has been struggling internally lately. Ben knows he is emotionally, romantically, and sexually attracted to other men, and he is really struggling with the "fag" jokes and other degrading remarks toward gays and lesbians made by his coaches and teammates.

*Should Ben tell his coaches and teammates he is offended by their remarks? * Should Ben tell his coaches and teammates he is gay? * Why might he be afraid to do so? * What are the possible repercussions? * Is homophobia more prevalent in athletic settings than in other settings?*

Todd and Jennifer have been having sexual relations for about six months. Jennifer has found that she is capable of having orgasms when she masturbates or when Todd performs oral sex on her, but she never has an orgasm during intercourse. Jennifer has never told Todd that she is having a problem with orgasms during intercourse. In fact, she fakes an orgasm because she is embarrassed about it and does not want to disappoint him.

*Should Jennifer talk to Todd about her inability to reach orgasm? * How do you think Todd will react if she does? * Is this a fairly typical problem for women? * Should Jennifer seek expert advice from a sex therapist?*

Human sexuality can be fascinating, complex, contradictory, and sometimes frustrating. In reality, sexuality is interwoven into every aspect of being human. No one theory or perspective can explain all its subtleties. It presents challenges in the areas of personal values, interpersonal relationships, cultural traditions, social norms, new technologies, current research findings, and changing political agendas.

Most college students are or have been sexually active. The Spring 2000 National College Health Assessment reports that about 72 percent of respondents said they were sexually active.[1] Other studies found that four out of five college students said that they have had sexual intercourse at some point during their life; one in four reported that they have had six or more sexual partners in their lifetime. About 80 percent of sexually active college students reported using some form of contraception the last time they had intercourse, although only about 38 percent said they used a condom during their last experience of intercourse. Thirty-five percent of college students said they have either been pregnant or gotten someone else pregnant.

In this chapter, we provide information and insights into the major components of sexual identity, including biology, gender identity, gender roles, and sexual orientation. Understanding your sexual identity will prepare you to make healthful, responsible, and satisfying decisions about your sexuality.

Your Sexual Identity

Sexual identity is determined by a complex interaction of genetic, physiological, environmental, and social factors. The beginning of sexual identity occurs at conception with the combining of chromosomes that influence sex. All eggs (ova) carry an X sex chromosome; sperm may carry either an X or a Y chromosome. If a sperm carrying an X chromosome fertilizes an egg, the resulting combination of sex chromosomes (XX) provides the blueprint to produce a female. If a sperm

carrying a Y chromosome fertilizes an egg, the XY combination produces a male. Not all people, however, have XX or XY chromosomes, nor do they all necessarily exhibit exclusively female or male primary and secondary sex characteristics. **Intersexuality** may occur as often as one in 100 live births; see the Health in a Diverse World box.

The genetic instructions included in the sex chromosomes lead to the differential development of male and female gonads at about the eighth week of fetal life. Once the male **gonads** (testes) and the female gonads (ovaries) are developed, they play a key role in all future sexual development because the gonads are responsible for the production of sex hormones. The primary sex hormones produced by females are estrogen and progesterone. In males, the hormone of primary importance is testosterone. The release of testosterone in a maturing fetus signals the development of a penis and other male genitals. If no testosterone is produced, female genitals form.

At the time of **puberty,** sex hormones again play major roles in development. Hormones released by the **pituitary gland,** called gonadotropins, stimulate the gonads (testes and ovaries) to make appropriate sex hormones. The increase of estrogen production in females and testosterone production in males leads to the development of **secondary sex characteristics.** Male secondary sex characteristics include deepening of the voice, development of facial and body hair, and growth of the skeleton and musculature. Female secondary sex characteristics include growth of the breasts, widening of the hips, and the development of pubic and underarm hair.

Thus far, we have described sexual identity only in terms of a person's biology. While biology is an important facet of sexual identity, the relationship of biology and culture is much more complicated than the popular notion of *sex* as biology and *gender* as social. Biological facts are themselves always understood and interpreted within the cultural framework that gives meaning to those facts. See the Health Ethics box on sex testing among athletes for a discussion of

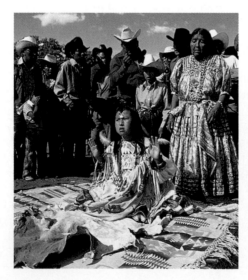
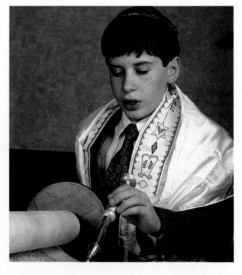

Many cultures mark the onset of puberty in public coming-of-age rituals that celebrate the changes in the young person's life.

situations where "sex" is not always clear cut. The earlier example of intersexuality demonstrates how rigid categories can break down in the face of reality.

Gender is the practice of behaving in masculine or feminine ways as defined by the society in which one lives. In this sense, gender is a performance, something we do rather than something we have, and we learn gender through the process of **socialization.** Through interactions with family, peers, teachers, media, and other social organizations, we learn to act in ways that society deems appropriate.

Each of us expresses our maleness or femaleness to others on a daily basis by the **gender roles** we play. **Gender identity** refers to the personal sense or awareness of being masculine or feminine, a male or a female. It may sometimes be difficult to express one's true sexual identity because of the bounds established by **gender-role stereotypes,** or generalizations about how males and females should express themselves and the characteristics each possesses. Our traditional sex roles are an example of gender-role stereotyping. Men are thought to be independent, aggressive, better in math and science, logical, and always in control of their emotions. Women, on the other hand, are traditionally expected to be passive, nurturing, intuitive, sensitive, and emotional.

Androgyny is the combination of traditional masculine and feminine traits in a single person. Androgynous people do not always follow traditional sex roles but rather choose behaviors based on the given situation. Other people consider themselves to be **transgendered.** These people refuse to follow the sexual and gender scripts prescribed to them based on their biology and resist the division of gender into two distinct categories.[2]

By now you can see that defining sexual identity is not a simple matter. It is a lifelong process of growing and learning. Your sexual identity is made up of the unique combination of your biology, gender identity, chosen gender roles, sexual orientation, and personal experiences. No other person on this earth is exactly like you, and it is up to you to take every opportunity to get to know and like yourself so that you may enjoy your life to the fullest.

What do you think?

How often do you challenge existing gender-role stereotypes? ❋ What is the outcome? ❋ Do you think men and women have the same degree of freedom in gender-role expression?

Sexual Orientation

Sexual orientation is a person's enduring emotional, romantic, sexual, and/or affectional attraction to other persons. You may be primarily attracted to members of the other sex **(heterosexual),** your same sex **(homosexual),** or both sexes **(bisexual). Transsexuals** feel that the bodies they were born with are the wrong sex. Often, they desire to have their bodies surgically altered to fit their internal perception of their sex.

Many homosexual people prefer the terms *gay* and *lesbian* to describe their sexual orientations, as these terms go beyond the exclusively sexual connotation of the term *homosexual.* The term *gay* applies to both men and women, but *lesbian* refers specifically to women.

Sexual identity   Recognition of oneself as a sexual being; a composite of biological sex, characteristics gender identity, gender roles, and sexual orientation.

Intersexuality   Not exhibiting exclusively female or male primary and secondary sex characteristics.

Gonads   The reproductive organs in a male (testes) or female (ovaries).

Puberty   The period of sexual maturation.

Pituitary gland   The endocrine gland controlling the release of hormones from the gonads.

Secondary sex characteristics   Characteristics associated with gender but not directly related to reproduction, such as vocal pitch, degree of body hair, and location of fat deposits.

Gender   The psychological condition of being feminine or masculine as defined by the society in which one lives.

Socialization   Process by which a society communicates behavioral expectations to its individual members.

Gender roles   Expression of maleness or femaleness in everyday life.

Gender identity   Personal sense or awareness of being masculine or feminine, a male or a female.

Gender-role stereotypes   Generalizations concerning how males and females should express themselves and the characteristics each possesses.

Androgyny   Combination of traditional masculine and feminine traits in a single person.

Transgendered   Refusing to follow the sexual and gender scripts prescribed based on biology and resisting the division of gender into two distinct categories.

Sexual orientation   A person's enduring emotional, romantic, sexual, or affectional attraction to other persons.

Heterosexual   Experiencing primary attraction to and preference for sexual activity with people of the other sex.

Homosexual   Experiencing primary attraction to and preference for sexual activity with people of the same sex.

Bisexual   Experiencing attraction to and preference for sexual activity with people of both sexes.

Transsexual   Experiencing the feeling the body one is born into is the wrong sex.

Intersexuality

Intersexual people are born with various levels of male and female biological characteristics, ranging from different chromosomal arrangements to a variety of primary and secondary sex characteristics. While most people are born with either XX or XY chromosomes, some are born with XXY or XO chromosomes. In some people, gonads do not develop fully into ovaries or testicles, and in others external genitalia may be ambiguous. For example, a person may possess a phallus that appears to be a large clitoris or a small penis and a structure that resembles partially fused labia or a split scrotum. Following are some of the more common forms of intersexuality:

- *Androgen Insensitivity Syndrome (AIS):* Two forms of AIS exist: complete and partial. In complete AIS, people with XY chromosomes develop testes, but their bodies cannot respond to androgen, and, therefore, their external genitalia are female. In adolescence, they experience breast development and sparse pubic hair growth but not menses. In partial AIS, external genitalia are ambiguous.
- *Gonadal Dysgenesis:* Like AIS, gonadal dysgenesis has two forms: complete and partial. In complete gonadal dysgenesis, people with XY chromosomes do not develop testes capable of producing androgen, and they have female external genitalia. People with

partial gonadal dysgenesis develop ambiguous external genitalia.
- *Congenital Adrenal Hyperplasia (CAH):* In CAH excess adrenal androgens lead to the development of ambiguous genitalia in people with XX chromosomes. People with CAH have masculine features, such as facial hair, grow quickly but stop growing before they should, have difficulty fighting off infections, and may have difficulty retaining enough salt. People with mild CAH usually have irregular periods and may have trouble becoming pregnant.
- *Turner's Syndrome:* People with Turner's Syndrome have a single X chromosome and a missing or damaged X chromosome. Turner's occurs in about 1 out of 3,000 live births. Symptoms include short stature, webbed neck, absent or retarded development of secondary sex characteristics, absence of menstruation, and drooping eyelids.
- *Klinefelter Syndrome:* People with Klinefelter Syndrome have an extra sex chromosome—XXY instead of XY. This chromosome arrangement occurs in 1 in 500 to 1,000 male births. Not all XXY males will develop Klinefelter Syndrome, and many will never know they have an extra chromosome. Those who do develop Klinefelter Syndrome will have male external genitalia, although the penis may be smaller than in most males. Also, they may develop breasts, lack facial and body

hair, develop rounder bodies, and be overweight. They may also have some degree of language impairment.

Intersexuality has often been treated as a birth defect. Very often parents and physicians make determinations about the sex of a child born with ambiguous genitalia and have surgery performed to make the child's genitalia conform to expectations for the assigned sex. Many members of the intersex community have begun to protest this practice as a form of genital mutilation. They argue that conditions that are not life-threatening should not be surgically altered and that society should become more accepting of the wide range of sexual difference.

Sources: Intersex Society of North America, "Intersexuality Basics" (see www.itpeople.org/frameset.html); S. Shaw, and J. Lee, "Learning Gender in a Diverse Society," *Women's Voices, Feminist Visions: Classic and Contemporary Readings.* (Mountain View, CA: Mayfield Publishing, 2001); The Johns Hopkins Children's Center, "Syndromes of Abnormal Sex Differentiation" (see www.hopkinsmedicine.org/pediatricendocrinology/intersex/index.html); and the National Institute of Child Health and Human Development, "A Guide for SSY Males and Their Families" (see http://156.40.88.3/publications/pubs/klinefelter.htm).

Throughout history, scientists and laypersons alike have debated the mental health status of gays and lesbians. In 1973 the American Psychiatric Association's board of trustees unanimously voted that homosexuality was not a mental illness or psychiatric disorder. This position was affirmed by the American Psychological Association and the Sexuality Information and Education Council of the United States (SIECUS). Recently, the issue of homosexuality as a treatable "disease" has been resurrected. Therapies labeled as conversion or reparative therapies are being promoted in national newspapers and television ads. Mental health professionals have found these ads so troubling that the American Psychological Association passed a resolution reaffirming that homosexuality is *not* a disease in need of a "cure."[3]

Most researchers today agree that sexual orientation is best understood using a multifactorial model, which incorporates biological, psychological, and socioenvironmental factors.[4] Biological explanations focus on research into genetics, hormones (perinatal and postpubertal), and differences in brain anatomy, while psychological and socioenvironmental explanations examine parent–child interactions, sex roles, and early sexual and interpersonal interactions. Collectively, this growing body of research suggests that the origins of homosexuality, like heterosexuality, are complex. To diminish the complexity of sexual orientation to "a choice" is a clear misreprsentation of current research. Homosexuals do not "choose" their sexual orientation any more than heterosexuals do.

Sex Testing among Athletes

Following allegations that some women competitors were really men, sporting federations began the practice of testing the sex of women athletes at the 1966 European Athletics Championships in Budapest. The initial test was a visual examination of the naked athletes. Later, tests screened for chromosomal arrangement.

In 1967, Polish sprinter Ewa Klobukowska became the first woman to fail a sex test and be banned from competi-tion. Later, doctors identified the condition that caused her to fail the test and that would have allowed her to compete.

In 1985, Spanish hurdler Maria Patino traveled to Kobe, Japan, to compete in the World University Games. Although Patino exhibited female sex characteristics and a female body type, her sex test revealed that she did not have two X chromosomes, and the meet officials barred her from the competition. A few months later, she won her event at a meet in Spain. She was then kicked off the Spanish national team, stripped of her titles, and banned from all future competition. Only two and a half years later did she win her fight to be reinstated by the International Amateur Athletics Federation.

Patino has not been alone in her fight against sex testing. Generally, 1 in 400 female athletes will fail the test. After years of activism by women athletes, the International Olympic Committee suspended sex testing for the 2000 Olympic Games, although it retained the right to reinstate the test in the future.

Should women athletes be required to pass a sex test before competing? Do you think Maria Patino is really a woman? Should she have been allowed to compete? Why do you think no equivalent sex test is given to male athletes?

Irrational fear or hatred of homosexuality creates anti-gay prejudice and is expressed as **homophobia**. Homophobic behaviors range from avoiding hugging same-sex friends to name-calling and physical attacks. Herek and colleagues surveyed 2,259 gay and lesbian people and found that one in five women and one in four men had been victimized in the preceding five years because of their sexual orientation.[5]

> **What do you think?**
>
> *Why is sexual orientation so controversial in our society?* ✳ *Do you think homophobic behavior is on the decline in this country?* ✳ *What can you do to help prevent hate crimes?*

Sexual Anatomy and Physiology

An understanding of the functions of the male and female sexual systems will help you derive pleasure and satisfaction from your sexual relationships, be sensitive to your partner's wants and needs, and make responsible choices regarding your own sexual health.

Female Sexual Anatomy and Physiology

The female sexual system includes two major groups of structures, the external genitals (see Figure 6.1) and the internal genitals (see Figure 6.2). The **external female genitals** include all structures that are outwardly visible and are

The process of "coming out" and making one's sexual orientation known takes a great deal of courage for gays and lesbians. Many express a sense of relief after having done so.

Homophobia   Irrational hatred or fear of homosexuals or homosexuality.

External female genitals   The mons pubis, labia majora and minora, clitoris, urethral and vaginal openings, and the vestibule of the vagina and its glands.

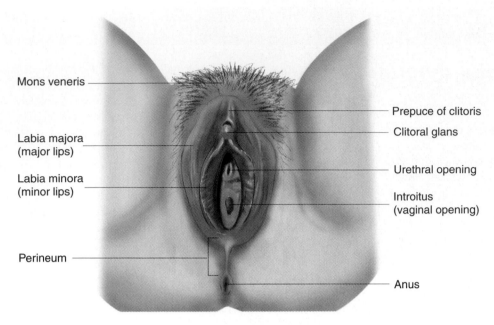

Figure 6.1
External Female Genital Structures
Source: From *Exploring Human Sexuality: Making Healthy Decisions,* by R. D. McAnulty and M. M. Burnette. Published by Allyn & Bacon, Boston, MA. Copyright © 2001 by Pearson Education.

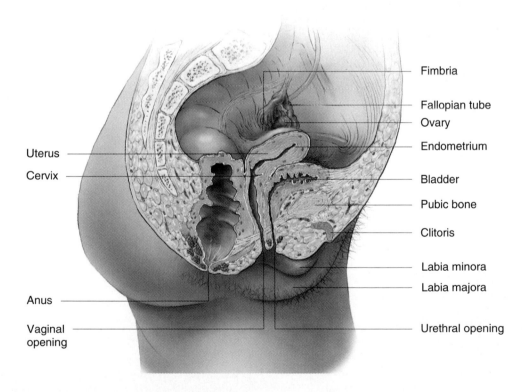

Figure 6.2
Side View of the Female Reproductive Organs

referred to as the vulva. Specifically, the **vulva,** or external genitalia, includes the mons pubis, the labia minora and majora, the clitoris, the urethral and vaginal openings, and the vestibule of the vagina. The **mons pubis** is a pad of fatty tissue covering the pubic bone. The mons serves to protect the pubic bone, and after puberty it becomes covered with coarse hair. The **labia minora** are folds of mucous membrane, and the **labia majora** are folds of skin and erectile tissue that enclose the urethral and vaginal openings. The labia minora are found just inside the labia majora.

The **clitoris** is the female sexual organ whose only known function is sexual pleasure. It is located at the upper end of the labia minora and beneath the mons pubis. Directly below the clitoris is the **urethral opening** through which urine leaves the body. Below the urethral opening is the vaginal opening, or opening to the vagina. In some women, the vaginal opening is covered by a thin membrane called the **hymen.** It is a myth that an intact hymen is proof of virginity. The **perineum** is the area between the vulva and the anus. Although not technically part of the external genitalia, the tissue in this area has many nerve endings and is sensitive to touch; it can play a part in sexual excitement.

The **internal female genitals** of the reproductive system include the vagina, uterus, fallopian tubes, and ovaries. The **vagina** is a tubular organ that serves as a passageway from the uterus to the outside of a female's body. This passageway allows menstrual flow to exit from the uterus during a female's monthly cycle and serves as the birth canal during childbirth. The vagina also receives the penis during intercourse. The **uterus,** also known as the womb, is a hollow, muscular, pear-shaped organ. Hormones acting on the inner lining of the uterus, called the **endometrium,** either prepare the uterus for implantation and development of a fertilized egg or signal that no fertilization has taken place, in which case the endometrium deteriorates and becomes menstrual flow.

The lower end of the uterus, the **cervix,** extends down into the vagina. The **ovaries** are almond-size structures suspended on either side of the uterus. The ovaries produce the hormones estrogen and progesterone and are also the reservoir for immature eggs. All the eggs a female will ever have are present in the ovaries at birth. Eggs mature and are released from the ovaries in response to hormone levels. Extending from the upper end of the uterus are two thin, flexible tubes called the **fallopian tubes.** The fallopian tubes are where sperm and egg meet and fertilization takes place. Following fertilization, the fallopian tubes serve as the passageway to the uterus, where the fertilized egg becomes implanted and development continues.

The Onset of Puberty and the Menstrual Cycle With the onset of **puberty,** the female reproductive system matures, and the development of secondary sex characteristics transforms young girls into young women. The first sign of puberty is the development of breast buds, which occurs around age 11. Under the direction of the endocrine system, the **pituitary gland,** the **hypothalamus,** and the ovaries all secrete hormones that act as chemical messengers among them. Working in a feedback system, hormonal levels in the bloodstream act as the trigger mechanism for release of more or different hormones.

At around the age of 9 ½ to 11 ½ in females, the hypothalamus receives the message to begin secreting **gonadotropin-releasing hormone (GnRH).** The release of

Vulva The female's external genitalia.

Mons pubis Fatty tissue covering the pubic bone in females; in physically mature women, the mons is covered with coarse hair.

Labia minora "Inner lips" or folds of tissue just inside the labia majora.

Labia majora "Outer lips" or folds of tissue covering the female sexual organs.

Clitoris A pea-sized nodule of tissue located at the top of the labia minora.

Urethral opening The opening through which urine is expelled.

Hymen Thin tissue covering the vaginal opening.

Perineum Tissue extending from the vulva to the anus.

Internal female genitals The vagina, uterus, fallopian tubes, and ovaries.

Vagina The passage in females leading from the vulva to the uterus.

Uterus (womb) Hollow, pear-shaped muscular organ whose function is to contain the developing fetus.

Endometrium Soft, spongy matter that makes up the uterine lining.

Cervix Lower end of the uterus that opens into the vagina.

Ovaries Almond-size organs that house developing eggs and produce hormones.

Fallopian tubes Tubes that extend from the ovaries to the uterus.

Puberty The maturation of the female or male reproduction system.

Pituitary gland The endocrine gland located deep within the brain; controls reproductive functions.

Hypothalamus An area of the brain located near the pituitary gland. The hypothalamus works in conjunction with the pituitary gland to control reproductive functions.

Gonadotropin-releasing hormone (GnRH) Hormone that signals the pituitary gland to release gonadotropins.

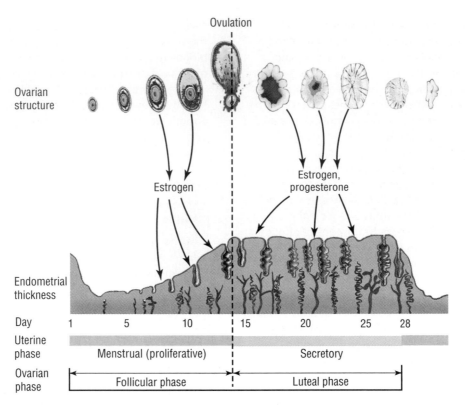

Ovulation

Ovarian
structure

Estrogen

Estrogen,
progesterone

Endometrial
thickness

Day	1	5	10	15	20	25	28

Uterine phase	Menstrual (proliferative)	Secretory

Ovarian phase	Follicular phase	Luteal phase

Figure 6.3
Phases of the Menstrual Cycle
Source: From *Exploring Human Sexuality: Making Healthy Decisions,* by R. D. McAnulty and M. M. Burnette. Published by Allyn & Bacon, Boston, MA. Copyright © 2001 by Pearson Education.

GnRH in turn signals the pituitary gland to release hormones called gonadotropins. Two gonadotropins, **follicle-stimulating hormone (FSH)** and **luteinizing hormone (LH),** signal the ovaries to start producing **estrogens** and **progesterone.** Increased estrogen levels assist in the development of female secondary sex characteristics. In addition, estrogens regulate the reproductive cycle. The normal age range for the onset of the first menstrual period, termed the **menarche,** is 9 to 17 years, with the average age being 11 ½ to 13 ½ years. Body fat heavily influences the onset of puberty, and increasing rates of obesity in children may account for the fact that girls here and in other countries seem to be reaching puberty much earlier than they used to.[6] Very thin girls, such as young athletes, tend to start menstruating later.

The average menstrual cycle is 28 days long and consists of two phases: the *menstrual (proliferative)* (also known as the follicular phase) and the *secretory* or luteal phase (see Figure 6.3). During the proliferative phase, the pituitary gland releases FSH and LH. The FSH acts on the ovaries to stimulate the maturation process of several **ovarian follicles (egg sacs).** These follicles secrete estrogens and, in response to this estrogen stimulation, the lining of the uterus, the endometrium, begins to grow and develop. The inner walls of the uterus become coated with a thick, spongy lining composed of blood and mucous. In the event of fertilization, this endometrial tissue will become a nesting place for the developing embryo. The increased estrogen level also signals the pituitary to slow down FSH production but increase LH secre-

tion. Of the several follicles developing in the ovaries, only one each month normally reaches complete maturity. Under the influence of LH, this one ovarian follicle rapidly matures, and about the fourteenth day of the proliferative phase, it releases an ovum into the fallopian tube—a process referred to as **ovulation.** Just prior to ovulation, the mature egg's follicle begins to increase secretion of progesterone, the first function of which is to spur the addition of further nutrients to the developing endometrium.

After ovulation, the secretory phase begins. The ovarian follicle is converted into the *corpus luteum,* or yellow body, which continues to secrete estrogen and progesterone but in decreasing amounts. In addition, FSH also falls back to preproliferative levels. Essentially, the woman's body is "waiting" to see whether fertilization will occur. During this time, LH declines and progesterone levels begin to rise, causing additional tissue growth in the endometrium.

If fertilization takes place, cells surrounding the developing embryo release a hormone called **human chorionic gonadotropin (HCG).** HCG increases estrogen and progesterone secretion, which maintains the endometrium while signaling the pituitary gland not to start a new menstrual cycle.

When fertilization does not occur, the egg gradually disintegrates within approximately 72 hours. The corpus luteum gradually becomes nonfunctional, causing levels of progesterone and estrogen to decline. As hormonal levels decline, the endometrial lining of the uterus loses its nourishment, dies, and is sloughed off as menstrual flow.

Menstrual Problems Premenstrual syndrome (PMS) comprises the mood changes and physical symptoms that occur in some women during one or two weeks prior to menstruation. Symptoms include breast swelling and tenderness; fatigue; trouble sleeping; upset stomach; bloating; constipation or diarrhea; headache; changes in appetite or food cravings; joint or muscle pain; weight gain; swelling of hands and feet; poor concentration; and feeling blue or irritable.

Treatment for PMS varies, and no one treatment works for everyone. A combination of healthy lifestyle and other treatments may be needed to alleviate symptoms.

As many as 80 percent of women have some negative symptoms associated with the menstrual cycle. Of these, about 3 to 5 percent have symptoms that are similar to but more severe than PMS. Collectively these symptoms are labeled **premenstrual dysphoric disorder,** or **PMDD.** Unlike PMS, PMDD symptoms are severe and difficult to manage. In addition to the physical symptoms described for PMS, PMDD is marked by severe mood disturbances including depressed mood, anxiety, irritability, angry outbursts, and/or periods of sudden tearfulness or sadness. Many PMDD sufferers also experience insomnia and difficulty in concentrating. Women with PMDD experience significantly impaired lives for one to two weeks every month, and the quality of their social relationships is often affected. Only about 25 percent of women who seek medical attention for this disorder are actually diagnosed with this rare condition. Women usually do not develop PMDD until their late 20s or early 30s, and PMDD worsens until menopause.[7]

Many natural approaches to managing PMS can also help PMDD. These strategies include: (1) eating more carbohydrates (grains, fruits, and vegetables); (2) reducing caffeine and salt intake; (3) exercising regularly; and (4) taking measures to reduce stress. Recent investigation into methods of controlling the severe emotional swings has led to the use of antidepressant medications for treating PMDD. A particular type of antidepressant, selective serotonin reuptake inhibitors (SSRIs, e.g., Prozac, Zoloft), has been shown to be very beneficial in reducing the mood disturbances associated with PMDD. Overall, more than 60 percent of women with PMDD respond to SSRIs, even in low doses and when taking them only while premenstrual. Side effects are generally minimal.

Toxic shock syndrome (TSS), although rare today, is still something of which you should be aware. It is caused by a bacterial infection facilitated by tampon or diaphragm use (see Chapters 7 and 17). Since the early 1980s, the Food and Drug Administration (FDA) has mandated that manufacturers of tampons conduct a battery of tests for safety clearance, but regardless of the safeguards, all women who use tampons should be aware of the symptoms of TSS. These symptoms are sometimes hard to recognize because they mimic the flu and include sudden high fever, vomiting, diarrhea, dizziness, fainting, or a rash that looks like sunburn during one's period or a few days after. Proper treatment usually assures recovery in two to three weeks.

Dysmenorrhea is a condition that causes pain or discomfort in the lower abdomen just before or after menstruation. Primary dysmenorrhea usually begins one to two years after a woman's first period, while secondary dysmenorrhea is caused by a specific disease or disorder and may appear years after regular menstruation begins.

Many women find relief for painful menstrual periods through over-the-counter nonsteroidal anti-inflammatory drugs (NSAID) such as ibuprofen and aspirin. Applying a heating pad to the abdomen, taking a hot bath or shower, and massaging the abdomen may also provide relief.

Menopause Just as menarche signals the beginning of a female's potential reproductive years, **menopause**—the permanent cessation of menstruation—signals the end. Generally occurring between the ages of 40 and 60, and at age 51 on average, menopause results in decreased estrogen levels, which may produce troublesome symptoms in some women.

Follicle-stimulating hormone (FSH) Hormone that signals the ovaries to prepare to release eggs and to begin producing estrogens.

Luteinizing hormone (LH) Hormone that signals the ovaries to release an egg and to begin producing progesterone.

Estrogens Hormones that control the menstrual cycle.

Progesterone Hormone secreted by the ovaries; helps keep the endometrium developing in order to nourish a fertilized egg; also helps maintain pregnancy.

Menarche The first menstrual period.

Ovarian follicles (egg sacs) Areas within the ovary in which individual eggs develop.

Ovulation The point of the menstrual cycle at which a mature egg ruptures through the ovarian wall.

Human chorionic gonadotropin (HCG) Hormone that calls for increased levels of estrogen and progesterone secretion if fertilization has taken place.

Premenstrual syndrome (PMS) Comprises the mood changes and physical symptoms that occur in some women during one or two weeks prior to menstruation.

Premenstrual dysphoric disorder (PMDD) Collective name for a group of negative symptoms similar to but more severe than PMS, including severe mood disturbances.

Toxic shock syndrome A potentially life-threatening disease that occurs when specific bacterial toxins are allowed to multiply unchecked in wounds or through improper use of tampons or diaphragms.

Dysmenorrhea Condition that causes pain or discomfort in the lower abdomen just before or after menstruation.

Menopause The permanent cessation of menstruation.

Decreased vaginal lubrication, hot flashes, headaches, dizziness, and joint pain have all been associated with the onset of menopause.

It has long been reported that taking hormones such as estrogen and progesterone through **hormone replacement therapy (HRT)** could relieve women's menopausal symptoms such as bloating and hot flashes, as well as reduce risks of heart disease and osteoporosis. (In 2002 the National Institutes of Health adopted the term **menopausal hormone therapy**, explaining that hormone treatment was never a replacement and did not restore the physiology of youth.) However, several studies in 2000 and 2001 have raised questions about the effect of HRT on cardiovascular disease (CVD). Most recently, results from the Women's Health Initiative (WHI) suggest that there is more potential for harm than good in healthy postmenopausal women taking a combination of estrogen and progesterone to prevent CVD.[8] The early termination of the portion of the WHI that was examining the HRT combination means additional long-term studies are needed. Other questions about increased risks of gall bladder disease, blood clotting disorders, and breast cancer remain unanswered. All women need to discuss the risks and benefits of HRT with their health care provider and come to an informed decision. Finding a doctor who specializes in women's health and carefully studies and keeps up to date with the latest research findings is crucial. Certainly lifestyle changes, such as regular exercise and a diet low in fat and adequate in calcium, can also help protect postmenopausal women from heart disease and osteoporosis.

Male Sexual Anatomy and Physiology

The structures of the male sexual system may be divided into external and internal genitals (see Figure 6.4). The penis and the scrotum make up the **external male genitals.** See the Health Ethics box on circumcision for a discussion of controversy surrounding removal of the foreskin. The **internal male genitals** include the testes, epididymides, vasa deferentia, and urethra and three other structures—the seminal vesicles, the prostate gland, and the Cowper's glands—that secrete components that, with sperm, make up semen. These three structures are sometimes referred to as the **accessory glands.**

The **penis** serves as the organ that deposits sperm in the vagina during intercourse. The urethra, which passes through the center of the penis, acts as the passageway for both semen and urine to exit the body. During sexual arousal, the spongy tissue in the penis becomes filled with blood, making the organ stiff, or erect. Further sexual excitement leads to **ejaculation,** a series of rapid, spasmodic contractions that propel semen out of the penis.

Situated behind the penis and also outside the body is a sac called the **scrotum.** The scrotum serves to protect the testes and also helps control the temperature within the testes, which is vital to proper sperm production. The **testes** (singular: *testis*) are egg-shaped structures in which sperm are manufactured. The testes also contain cells that manufacture **testosterone,** the hormone responsible for the development of male secondary sex characteristics.

The development of sperm is referred to as **spermatogenesis.** Like the maturation of eggs in the female, this process is governed by the pituitary gland. Follicle-stimulating hormone (FSH) is secreted into the bloodstream to stimulate the testes to manufacture sperm. Immature sperm are released into a comma-shaped structure on the back of the testis called the **epididymis** (plural: *epididymides*), where they ripen and reach full maturity.

The epididymis contains coiled tubules that gradually "unwind" and straighten out to become the **vas deferens.** The two vasa deferentia, as they are called in the plural, make up the tubular transportation system whose sole function is to store and move sperm. Along the way, the **seminal vesicles** provide sperm with nutrients and other fluids that compose **semen.**

The vasa deferentia eventually connect each epididymis to the ejaculatory ducts, which pass through the prostate gland and empty into the urethra. The **prostate gland** contributes more fluids to the semen, including

---

Hormone replacement therapy (HRT) or menopausal hormone therapy Use of synthetic or animal estrogens and progesterone to compensate for decreases in estrogens in a woman's body.

External male genitals The penis and scrotum.

Internal male genitals The testes, epididymides, vasa deferentia, ejaculatory ducts, urethra, and accessory glands.

Accessory glands The seminal vesicles, prostate gland, and Cowper's glands.

Penis Male sexual organ that releases sperm into the vagina.

Ejaculation The propulsion of semen from the penis.

Scrotum Sac of tissue that encloses the testes.

Testes Two organs, located in the scrotum, that manufacture sperm and produce hormones.

Testosterone The male sex hormone manufactured in the testes.

Spermatogenesis The development of sperm.

Epididymis A comma-shaped structure atop the testis where sperm mature.

Vas deferens A tube that transports sperm toward the penis.

Seminal vesicles Storage areas for sperm where nutrient fluids are added to them.

Semen Fluid containing sperm and nutrient fluids that increase sperm viability and neutralize vaginal acid.

Prostate gland Gland that secretes nutrients and neutralizing fluids into the semen.

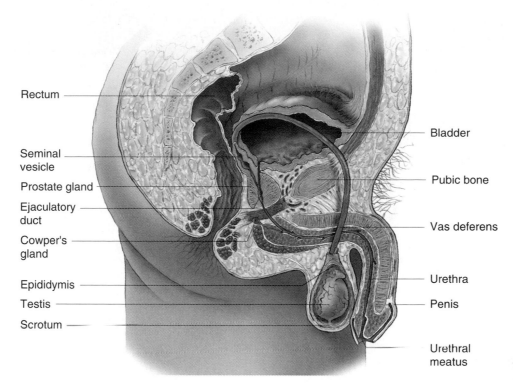

Figure 6.4
Side View of the Male Reproductive Organs

Rectum

Seminal vesicle

Prostate gland

Ejaculatory duct

Cowper's gland

Epididymis

Testis

Scrotum

Bladder

Pubic bone

Vas deferens

Urethra

Penis

Urethral meatus

HEALTH ETHICS: CONFLICT AND CONTROVERSY

Circumcision: Risk versus Benefit

New parents must decide whether their male infant will be circumcised. Circumcision involves the surgical removal of the foreskin, a fold of skin covering the end of the penis. Most circumcisions in the United States have traditionally been performed for religious or cultural reasons or because of concerns of hygiene. The foreskin, which is fully attached to the glans at birth, naturally separates from the glans anywhere from weeks to several years after birth. Once it can be retracted, the glans underneath the foreskin should be cleaned.

Some studies suggest that uncircumcised males may be at slightly greater risk for penile cancer and some sexually transmitted infections, including syphilis, gonorrhea, and HIV. The reason is suspected to be poor hygiene—not cleaning between the foreskin and glans. However, other apparently stronger data suggest that uncircumcised men are no more likely to contract STIs than circumcised men are, and an equal number of deaths occur as a result of circumcision as occur from penile cancer.

According to the American Academy of Pediatrics, overall research does not support the practice of circumcision for health reasons. Thus, circumcision is not a medically necessary procedure. Parents who choose to circumcise do so for religious,

aesthetic, or other personal reasons. What decision do you think you would make for your son? Give your reasons.

Sources: From "Care of the Uncircumcised Penis," by the American Academy of Pediatrics, 2001 (see www.aap.org/family/uncirc.html); "Circumcision Policy Statement," by the American Academy of Pediatrics Task Force on Circumcision, 1999, *Pediatrics* 103, pp. 686–693; "Circumcision in the United States: Prevalence, Prophylactic Effects, and Sexual Practices," by E. O. Laumann, C. M. Masi, and E. W. Zuckerman, 1997, *Journal of the American Medical Association* 277, pp. 1052–1057; "Letter to Dr. Perter Rappo, American Academy of Pediatrics, from the American Cancer Society," by H. Shingleton and C. W. Heath, 1996 (see www.nocirc.org/position/acs.html).

1. Excitement/Arousal Phase

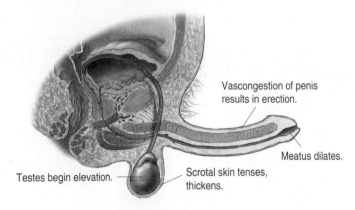

Vascongestion of penis results in erection.

Meatus dilates.

Testes begin elevation.

Scrotal skin tenses, thickens.

2. Plateau Phase

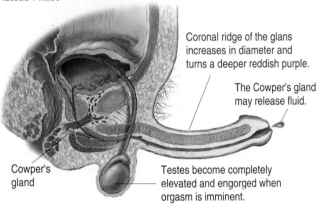

Coronal ridge of the glans increases in diameter and turns a deeper reddish purple.

The Cowper's gland may release fluid.

Cowper's gland

Testes become completely elevated and engorged when orgasm is imminent.

3. Orgasmic Phase

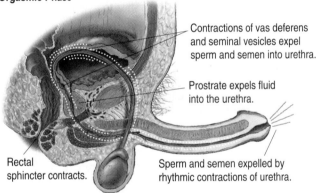

Contractions of vas deferens and seminal vesicles expel sperm and semen into urethra.

Prostrate expels fluid into the urethra.

Rectal sphincter contracts.

Sperm and semen expelled by rhythmic contractions of urethra.

4. Resolution Phase

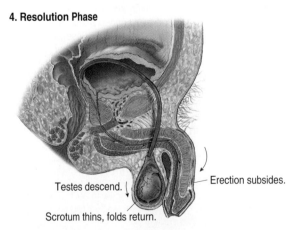

Testes descend.

Erection subsides.

Scrotum thins, folds return.

1. Excitement/Arousal Phase

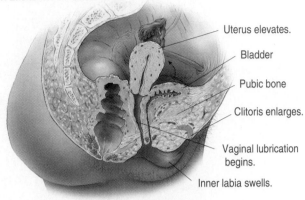

Uterus elevates.

Bladder

Pubic bone

Clitoris enlarges.

Vaginal lubrication begins.

Inner labia swells.

2. Plateau Phase

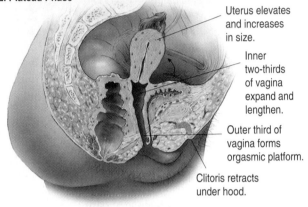

Uterus elevates and increases in size.

Inner two-thirds of vagina expand and lengthen.

Outer third of vagina forms orgasmic platform.

Clitoris retracts under hood.

3. Orgasmic Phase

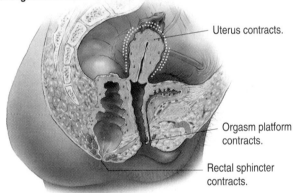

Uterus contracts.

Orgasm platform contracts.

Rectal sphincter contracts.

4. Resolution Phase

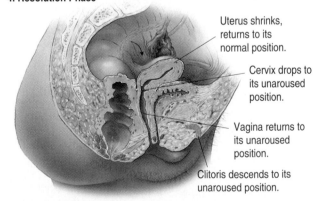

Uterus shrinks, returns to its normal position.

Cervix drops to its unaroused position.

Vagina returns to its unaroused position.

Clitoris descends to its unaroused position.

Figure 6.5

Comparison of Sexual Response between Male and Female

chemicals that aid the sperm in fertilizing an ovum and neutralize the acidic environment of the vagina to make it more conducive to sperm motility (ability to move) and potency (potential for fertilizing an ovum).

Just below the prostate gland are two pea-shaped nodules called the **Cowper's glands.** The Cowper's glands secrete a fluid that lubricates the urethra and neutralizes any acid that may remain in the urethra after urination. Urine and semen do not come into contact with each other. During ejaculation of semen, a small valve closes off the tube to the urinary bladder.

Human Sexual Response

Human psychological traits greatly influence sexual response and sexual desire. Thus, we may find relationships with one partner vastly different from those we might experience with other partners.

Sexual response is a physiological process that generally follows a pattern. Laboratory research has delineated four stages within the response cycle, and researchers agree that each individual has a personal response pattern that may or may not conform to these phases. Both males' and females' sexual responses are somewhat arbitrarily divided into four stages: excitement/arousal, plateau, orgasmic, and resolution (see Figure 6.5). Regardless of the type of sexual activity (stimulation by a partner or self-stimulation), the response stages are the same.

During the first phase, *excitement/arousal,* male and female genital responses are caused by **vasocongestion,** or increased blood flow in the genital region. Increased blood flow to these organs causes them to swell. The vagina begins to lubricate in preparation for penile penetration, and the penis becomes partially erect. Both sexes may exhibit a "sex flush," or light blush all over their bodies. Excitement/arousal can be generated by touching other parts of the body, by kissing, through fantasy, by viewing films or videos, or by reading erotic literature.

During the *plateau phase,* the initial responses intensify. Voluntary and involuntary muscle tensions increase. The female's nipples and the male's penis become erect. A few drops of fluid, which may contain sperm, are secreted from the penis at this time. This fluid is termed *pre-ejaculatory fluid.*

During the *orgasmic phase,* vasocongestion and muscle tensions reach their peak, and rhythmic contractions occur through the genital regions. In females, these contractions are centered in the uterus, outer vagina, and anal sphincter. In males, the contractions occur in two stages. First, contractions within the prostate gland begin propelling semen through the urethra. In the second stage, the muscles of the pelvic floor, urethra, and anal sphincter contract. Semen usually, but not always, is ejaculated from the penis. In both sexes, spasms in other major muscle groups also occur, particularly in the buttocks and abdomen. Feet and hands may also contract, and facial features often contort.

Muscle tension and congested blood subside in the *resolution phase,* as the genital organs return to their pre-arousal states. Both sexes usually experience deep feelings of well-being and profound relaxation. Following orgasm and resolution, many females can become aroused again and experience additional orgasms. However, some men experience a *refractory period,* during which their systems are incapable of subsequent arousal. This refractory period may last from a few minutes to several hours. The length of the refractory period increases with age.

Men and women experience the same stages in the sexual response cycle; however, the length of time spent in any one stage is variable. Thus, one partner may be in the plateau phase while the other is in the excitement or orgasmic phase. Such variations in response rates are entirely normal. Some couples believe that simultaneous orgasm is desirable for sexual satisfaction. Although simultaneous orgasm is pleasant, so are orgasms achieved at different times.

Sexual pleasure and satisfaction are also possible without orgasm or intercourse. Expressing sexual feelings for another person involves many pleasurable activities, of which intercourse and orgasm may only be a part.

> **What do you think?**
>
> *Why do we place so much importance on orgasm?* ✳ *Can sexual pleasure and satisfaction be achieved without orgasm?* ✳ *What is the role of desire in sexual response?*

Sexual Responses among Older Adults

Older adults are commonly stereotyped as being incapable of or uninterested in sexual relations. The truth is, though we do experience some physical changes as we age, these changes generally do not cause us to stop enjoying sex.

In women, the most significant physical changes follow menopause. Skin becomes less elastic; most internal sexual organs, including the uterus and cervix, shrink somewhat; the vaginal walls become thinner; and vaginal lubrication during sexual arousal may decrease. The resulting increased friction during penetration can be painful. The typical physical change during orgasm is that the duration tends to be shorter. In fact, postmenopausal women experience sexual relations much the same as they did prior to menopause, only less intensely and for shorter periods of time.[9] Women who remain sexually active report fewer problems with age-related changes in sexual functioning. The use of artificial lubricants usually resolves the problem of insufficient lubrication. As mentioned earlier,

---

Cowper's glands Glands that secrete a fluid that lubricates the urethra and neutralizes any acid remaining in the urethra after urination.

Vasocongestion The engorgement of the genital organs with blood.

estrogen replacement therapy (ERT) may decrease or prevent these physical changes that follow menopause.

Although men do not experience menopause, their bodies also change as a result of the aging process. They require more direct and prolonged stimulation in order to achieve an erection, and erections become less firm. They are slower to obtain a full erection and to reach orgasm, and their refractory periods are longer. Older men also experience a decrease in the intensity of ejaculation. Semen seeps out during ejaculation rather than being forcefully expelled as is typical in younger men. However, the majority of healthy older men, like healthy older women, maintain a regular and satisfying sex life.

Expressing Your Sexuality

Finding healthy ways to express your sexuality is an important part of developing sexual maturity. Many avenues of sexual expression are available.

Sexual Behavior: What Is "Normal"?

Most of us want to fit in and be identified as normal, but how do we know which sexual behaviors are considered normal? What or whose criteria should we use? These are not easy questions.

Every society sets standards and attempts to regulate sexual behavior. Boundaries arise that distinguish good from bad, acceptable from unacceptable, and result in criteria used to establish what is viewed as normal or abnormal. Common sociocultural standards for sexual behavior in Western culture today include the following:

- *The heterosexual standard.* Sexual attraction should be limited to members of the other sex.
- *The coital standard.* Penile/vaginal intercourse (coitus) is viewed as the ultimate sex act.
- *The orgasmic standard.* All sexual interaction should lead to orgasm.
- *The two-person standard.* Sex is an activity to be experienced by two.

- *The romantic standard.* Sex should be related to love.
- *The safer sex standard.* If we choose to be sexually active, we should act to prevent unintended pregnancy or disease transmission.[10]

These are not laws or rules, but rather social scripts that have been adopted over time. Sexual standards often shift over time, and many people choose not to follow them. We are a pluralistic nation, and that pluralism extends to our sexual practices. Rather than making blanket judgments about normal versus abnormal, try asking the following questions:[11]

- Is a sexual behavior healthy and fulfilling for a particular person?
- Is it safe?
- Does it lead to the exploitation of others?
- Does it take place between responsible, consenting adults?

In this way, we can view behavior along a continuum that takes into account many individual factors. As you read about the options for sexual expression in the pages ahead, use these questions to explore your feelings about what is normal for you. See the Assess Yourself box to examine your own feelings about sexual differences.

Options for Sexual Expression

The range of human sexual expression is virtually infinite. What you find enjoyable may not be an option for someone else. The ways you choose to meet your sexual needs today may be very different from how you meet them two years from now. Accepting yourself as a sexual person with individual desires and preferences is the first step in achieving sexual satisfaction.

Celibacy Celibacy is avoidance of or abstention from sexual activities with others. A completely celibate person also does not engage in masturbation (self-stimulation), whereas a partially celibate person avoids sexual activities with others but may enjoy autoerotic behaviors such as masturbation. Some people choose celibacy for religious or moral reasons. Others may be celibate for a period of time due to illness, the breakup of a long-term relationship, or lack of an acceptable partner. For some, celibacy is a lonely, agonizing state, but others find it an opportunity for introspection, values assessment, and personal growth.

Autoerotic Behaviors Autoerotic behaviors involve sexual self-stimulation. The two most common are sexual fantasy and masturbation.

Sexual fantasies are sexually arousing thoughts and dreams. Fantasies may reflect real-life experiences, forbidden desires, or the opportunity to practice new or anticipated sexual experiences. The fact that you may fantasize about a particular sexual experience does not necessarily mean that you want to, or have to, act that experience out. Sexual fantasies are just that—fantasy.

Celibacy   State of not being involved in a sexual relationship.

Autoerotic behaviors   Sexual self-stimulation.

Sexual fantasies   Sexually arousing thoughts and dreams.

Masturbation   Self-stimulation of genitals.

Erogenous zones   Areas of the body of both males and females that, when touched, lead to sexual arousal.

Cunnilingus   Oral stimulation of a female's genitals.

Fellatio   Oral stimulation of a male's genitals.

Attitudes toward Sexual Differences

How comfortable would you be in the following situations? Why?

	Completely Comfortable			Not at All Comfortable	
1. Your close same-sex friend reveals to you her/his preference for same-sex partners.	1	2	3	4	5
2. Your roommate tells you that she/he likes sexual encounters that involve three or more partners at one time.	1	2	3	4	5
3. Your sister tells you that she would like to have a sex-change operation.	1	2	3	4	5
4. You visit a friend's house, and she/he shows you her/his sexual fantasy room that includes vibrators, sexually explicit magazines, and erotic videos.	1	2	3	4	5
5. Your close friend of another sex reveals to you her/his preference for same-sex partners.	1	2	3	4	5
6. Your 85-year-old grandfather reveals that he is sexually active with his 85-year-old female partner.	1	2	3	4	5
7. A male friend reveals that, although he is heterosexual, he occasionally has sex with other men.	1	2	3	4	5
8. Your lab partner, who looks and acts like a man, reveals that he is really a transgendered woman.	1	2	3	4	5
9. Your blind date tells you that she/he occasionally likes to engage in sadomasochistic sexual play.	1	2	3	4	5
10. Two women from your health class invite you to attend their commitment ceremony at the end of the term.	1	2	3	4	5
11. Your best friend reveals that she/he has made a personal commitment not to engage in sexual activity until marriage.	1	2	3	4	5
12. Your best male friend tells you that he enjoys phone sex.	1	2	3	4	5
13. The person with whom you are romantically involved asks you to tell her/him your sexual fantasies.	1	2	3	4	5
14. You meet someone in an Internet chat room who wants to engage in cybersex.	1	2	3	4	5
15. Your divorced mother reveals that she is dating a man who is your age.	1	2	3	4	5

Masturbation is self-stimulation of the genitals. Although many people feel uncomfortable discussing masturbation, it is a common sexual practice across the life span. Masturbation is a natural, pleasure-seeking behavior in infants and children. It is a valuable and important means for adolescent males and females, as well as adults, to explore sexual feelings and responsiveness.

Kissing and Erotic Touching Kissing and erotic touching are two very common forms of nonverbal sexual communication. Both males and females have **erogenous zones,** areas of the body that when touched lead to sexual arousal. Erogenous zones may include genital as well as nongenital areas, such as the earlobes, mouth, breasts, and inner thighs. Almost any area of the body can be conditioned to respond erotically to touch. Spending time with your partner to explore and learn about his or her erogenous areas is another pleasurable, safe, and satisfying means of sexual expression.

Manual Stimulation Both men and women can be sexually aroused and achieve orgasm through manual stimulation of the genitals by a partner. For many women, orgasm is more likely to be achieved through manual stimulation than through intercourse.

Oral-Genital Stimulation **Cunnilingus** is the term used for oral stimulation of a female's genitals, and **fellatio** refers to oral stimulation of a male's genitals. Many partners find oral-genital stimulation intensely pleasurable. Seventy percent of college-age men and women have had oral sex.[12] For some people, oral sex is not an option because of moral or religious beliefs. It is necessary to remember that HIV and other sexually transmitted infections (STIs) can be transmitted via unprotected oral-genital sex as well as intercourse. Use of an appropriate barrier device is strongly recommended if either partner's health status is in question.

Vaginal Intercourse   The term *intercourse* generally refers to **vaginal intercourse,** or insertion of the penis into the vagina. *Coitus* is another term for vaginal intercourse, which is the most often practiced form of sexual expression. A great variety of positions can be used during coitus. Examples include the missionary position (man on top facing the woman), woman on top, side by side, or man behind (rear entry). Many partners enjoy experimenting with different positions. Knowledge of yourself and your body, along with your ability to communicate effectively, will play a large part in determining the enjoyment or meaning of intercourse for you and your partner. Whatever your circumstance, you should practice safer sex to avoid disease and unwanted pregnancy.

Anal Intercourse   The anal area is highly sensitive to touch, and some couples find pleasure in the stimulation of this area. **Anal intercourse** is insertion of the penis into the anus. Sixteen percent of college-age men and women have had anal sex.[13] Stimulation of the anus by mouth or with the fingers is also practiced. As with all forms of sexual expression, anal stimulation or intercourse is not for everyone. If you do enjoy this form of sexual expression, remember to use condoms to prevent disease transmission. Also, anything inserted into the anus should not be directly inserted into the vagina, as bacteria commonly found in the anus can cause vaginal infections.

Variant Sexual Behavior

Although attitudes toward sexuality have changed radically since the Victorian era, some people still believe that any sexual behavior other than heterosexual intercourse is abnormal or perverted. People who study sexuality prefer to use the neutral term **variant sexual behavior** to describe sexual behaviors that are not engaged in by most people; for example:

- *Group sex.* Sexual activity involving more than two people. Participants in group sex run a higher risk of exposure to AIDS and other sexually transmitted infections.
- *Transvestism.* Wearing the clothing of the opposite sex. Most transvestites are male, heterosexual, and married.
- *Fetishism.* Sexual arousal achieved by looking at or touching inanimate objects, such as underclothing or shoes.

   Some variant sexual behaviors can be harmful to the individual, to others, or to both. Many of the following activities are illegal in at least some states:

- *Exhibitionism.* Exposing one's genitals to strangers in public places. Most exhibitionists are seeking a reaction of shock or fear from their victims. Exhibitionism is a minor felony in most states.

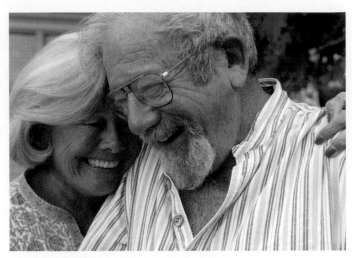

Recent studies indicate that some degree of sexual dysfunction is much more common than once thought. New treatments, such as Viagra, have helped many couples regain satisfying sexual relationships.

- *Voyeurism.* Observing other people for sexual gratification. Most voyeurs are men who attempt to watch women undressing or bathing. Voyeurism is an invasion of privacy and illegal in most states.
- *Sadomasochism.* Sexual activities in which gratification is received by inflicting pain (verbal or physical abuse) on a partner or by being the object of such infliction. A sadist is a person who receives gratification from inflicting pain, and a masochist receives gratification from experiencing it.
- *Pedophilia.* Sexual activity or attraction between an adult and a child. Any sexual activity involving a minor, including possession of child pornography, is illegal.
- *Autoerotic asphyxiation.* The practice of reducing or eliminating oxygen to the brain, usually by tying a cord around one's neck while masturbating to orgasm. Tragically, asphyxiation is usually discovered when people accidentally hang themselves.

> **What do you think?**
>
> *How does our society define "normal" sexual behavior? ✳ What behaviors do you consider normal or abnormal? ✳ Do you consider your own preferred forms of sexual expression to be normal? ✳ Why or why not?*

Difficulties That Can Hinder Sexual Functioning

Research indicates that **sexual dysfunction,** the term used to describe problems that can hinder sexual functioning, is quite common. Don't feel embarrassed if you experience sexual dysfunction at some point in your life. The sexual part of you does not come with a lifetime warranty. You can have breakdowns involving your sexual function just as you can have breakdowns in any of your other body systems. Sexual dysfunction can be divided into five major classes: disorders of sexual desire, sexual performance, sexual arousal, orgasm, and sexual pain. All of them can be treated successfully.

Sexual Desire Disorders

The most frequent reason why people seek out a sex therapist is **ISD,** or **inhibited sexual desire.**[14] ISD is the lack of a sexual appetite or simply a lack of interest and pleasure in sexual activity. In some instances, it can result from stress or boredom with sex. **Sexual aversion disorder** is another type of desire dysfunction, characterized by sexual phobias (unreasonable fears) and anxiety about sexual contact. The psychological stress of a punitive upbringing, a rigid religious background, or a history of physical or sexual abuse may be sources of these desire disorders.

Sexual Performance Anxiety

Sexual performance anxiety arises for a man when he anticipates some sort of problem in the sex act. As a result, he becomes anxious and either is unable to have or maintain an erection or experiences premature ejaculation. When a woman experiences sexual performance anxiety, she may be unable to achieve orgasm or to allow penetration because of the involuntary contraction of muscles in the vagina. People may be able to overcome performance anxiety by learning to focus on immediate sensations and pleasures rather than on orgasm.

Sexual Arousal Disorders

The most common disorder in this category is erectile dysfunction. **Erectile dysfunction,** or **impotence,** is difficulty in achieving or maintaining a penile erection sufficient for intercourse. At some time in his life, every man experiences impotence. Causes are varied and include underlying diseases, such as diabetes or prostate problems; reactions to some medications (for example, medication for high blood pressure); depression; fatigue; stress; alcohol; performance anxiety; and guilt over real or imaginary problems (such as when a man compares himself to his partner's past lovers).

Some 30 million men in this country, half of them under age 65, suffer from impotence. Impotence generally becomes more of a problem as men age, affecting one in four men over the age of 65. Recently the FDA approved the drug Viagra (sildenafil citrate) to treat impotence. Response to the drug's release was record breaking. Taken by mouth one hour before sexual activity, Viagra was reported to successfully manage erectile dysfunction in 60 to 80 percent of cases during clinical trials.[15] The medication is not, however, without risk. The most commonly reported side effects include headache, flushing, stomachache, urinary tract infection, diarrhea, dizziness, rash, and mild and temporary visual changes. In addition, there have been several reported deaths in the United States among Viagra users, prompting more caution in prescribing it to patients with known cardiovascular disease and those taking commonly prescribed short- and long-acting nitrates such as nitroglycerin.[16]

Another drug that can help to prolong erection in men who are able to obtain but not maintain erection is Trazodone, an antidepressant. Several other Viagra-like drugs are being developed that will have different side effects. Another potential treatment is the internal penile pump, a soft-fluid-filled (saline) device that expands and contracts. The saline is transferred by the pump into the penis and causes an erection.[17]

Topical creams and penile injection therapy are also available choices but have not been very popular since the development of Viagra. Topical applications tend to be less effective and more painful than penile injection therapy. Prior to Viagra, injection therapy was the most effective medical treatment available.

Whatever the treatment selected, a supportive partner is the most important factor in regaining a full, healthy sex life.

Orgasm Disorders

Premature ejaculation affects up to 50 percent of the male population at some time in their lives. **Premature ejaculation** is ejaculation that occurs prior to or very soon after the insertion of the penis into the vagina. Treatment for

---

Vaginal intercourse   The insertion of the penis into the vagina.

Anal intercourse   The insertion of the penis into the anus.

Variant sexual behavior   A sexual behavior that is not engaged in by most people.

Sexual dysfunction   Problems associated with achieving sexual satisfaction.

Inhibited sexual desire (ISD)   Lack of sexual appetite or simply a lack of interest and pleasure in sexual activity.

Sexual aversion disorder   Type of desire dysfunction characterized by sexual phobias and anxiety about sexual contact.

Sexual performance anxiety   A condition of sexual difficulties caused by anticipating some sort of problem with the sex act.

Erectile dysfunction (impotence)   Difficulty in achieving or maintaining a penile erection sufficient for intercourse.

Premature ejaculation   Ejaculation that occurs prior to or almost immediately following penile penetration of the vagina.

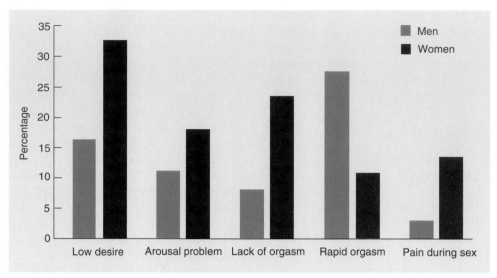

Figure 6.6
Prevalence of Sexual Problems from the National Health and Social Life Survey, 1999
Source: Exploring Human Sexuality: Making Healthy Decisions, by R.D. McAnulty and M.M Burnette. Published by Allyn & Bacon, Boston, MA. Copyright © 2001 by Pearson Education.

premature ejaculation involves a physical examination to rule out organic causes. If the cause of the problem is not physiological, therapy is available to help a man learn how to control the timing of his ejaculation. Fatigue, stress, performance pressure, and alcohol use can all be contributing factors to orgasmic disorders in men.

When a woman is unable to achieve orgasm, termed **female orgasmic disorder,** she often blames herself and learns to fake orgasm to avoid embarrassment or preserve her partner's ego. Contributing to this response are the messages women have historically been given about sex as a duty rather than a pleasurable act for both parties. As with men who experience orgasmic disorders, the first step in treatment is a physical exam to rule out organic causes.

Female orgasmic disorder   The inability to achieve orgasm.

Dyspareunia   Pain experienced by women during intercourse.

Vaginismus   A state in which the vaginal muscles contract so forcefully that penetration cannot be accomplished.

Rohypnol   ("roofies," "rope," "forget pill") A drug that is sometimes used in combination with alcohol to facilitate date rape by making a woman unaware of what is happening to her.

Gamma-hydroxybutrane   (GHB) A "date rape drug" sometimes used in combination with alcohol to facilitate rape by making a woman unaware of what is happening to her.

However, the problem is often solved by simple self-exploration to learn more about what forms of stimulation are arousing enough to produce orgasm.

Masturbation is usually a primary focus in teaching a woman to become orgasmic. Through masturbation, a woman can learn how her body responds sexually to various types of touch. Once a woman has become orgasmic through masturbation, she learns to communicate her needs to her partner.

Sexual Pain Disorders

Two common disorders in this category are dyspareunia and vaginismus. **Dyspareunia** is pain experienced by a female during intercourse. This pain may be caused by diseases such as endometriosis, uterine tumors, chlamydia, gonorrhea, or urinary-tract infections. Damage to tissues during childbirth and insufficient lubrication during intercourse may also cause discomfort. Dyspareunia can also be psychological in origin. As with other problems, dyspareunia can be treated with good results.

Vaginismus is the involuntary contraction of vaginal muscles, making penile insertion painful or impossible. Most cases of vaginismus are related to fear of intercourse or to unresolved sexual conflicts. Treatment involves teaching a woman to achieve orgasm through nonvaginal stimulation. See Figure 6.6 for prevalence data on sexual dysfunction in men and women.

Seeking Help for Sexual Dysfunction

Many theories and treatment models can help people with sexual dysfunction. A first important step is choosing a qualified sex therapist or counselor. A national organization, the

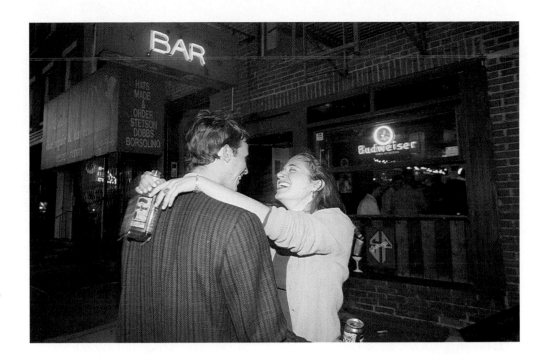

The influence of alcohol can impair judgment and lead to sexual encounters that may not be in a person's best interest.

American Association of Sex Educators, Counselors, and Therapists (AASECT), has been in the forefront of establishing criteria for certifying sex therapists. These criteria include appropriate degree(s) in the helping professions, specialized coursework in human sexuality, and sufficient hours of practical therapy work under the direct supervision of a certified sex therapist. Lists of certified counselors and sex therapists, as well as clinics that treat sexual dysfunctions, can be obtained by contacting AASECT or SIECUS.

Drugs and Sex

Because psychoactive drugs affect the entire physiology, it is only logical that they affect sexual behavior. Promises of increased pleasure make drugs very tempting to those seeking greater sexual satisfaction. Too often, however, drugs become central to sexual activities and damage the relationship.

Alcohol is notorious for reducing inhibitions and promoting feelings of well-being and desirability. At the same time, alcohol inhibits sexual response; thus, the mind may be willing, but not the body.

Perhaps the greatest danger associated with use of drugs during sex is the tendency to blame the drug for negative behavior. "I can't help what I did last night because I was drunk" is a response that demonstrates sexual immaturity. A sexually mature person carefully examines risks and benefits and makes decisions accordingly. If drugs are necessary to increase erotic feelings, it is likely that the partners are being dishonest about their feelings for each other. Good sex should not depend on chemical substances.

Of growing concern in recent years is the increased use of "date rape" drugs. These have become popular among college students and are often used in combination with alcohol.[18] Both **Rohypnol** ("roofies," "rope," "forget pill") and **GHB,** or **gamma-hydroxybutrane** ("Liquid X," "Grievous Bodily Harm," "Easy Lay," "Mickey Finn") have been used to facilitate rape. The dangers of these drugs are discussed in more detail in Chapter 14.

> ### What do you think?
>
> *Why do we find it so difficult to discuss sexual dysfunction in our society?* ✳ *Do you think it is more difficult for men than for women to talk about dysfunction?* ✳ *Have you ever used alcohol or some other drug to enhance your sexual performance?* ✳ *Why are "roofies" of major concern on college campuses?*

Managing Sexual Behavior

Being a sexually healthy adult is a process that requires a commitment to the ongoing assessment of your sexual attitudes and values, your relationships with others, your sexual actions, your communication skills, and all the new information to which you are exposed on a daily basis. Your challenge is to grow as you develop new skills and become more confident with your sexuality. Use the following questions to check your progress.

Checklist for Change

Making Personal Choices

☐ Do you feel comfortable with yourself sexually? Do you know the function and location of the structures that make up the male and female sexual anatomy?

☐ Make a list of the gender roles you have adopted to date. Do you feel limited or bound by any gender-role stereotypes? How might you change them?

☐ Do you know what your options are for expressing your sexuality? Have you reviewed the options and identified those you may be willing to try?

☐ Do you need to work on developing any new skills that will help you reach your goals regarding your sexual self?

Making Community Choices

☐ Have you taken the time to become informed about sexual issues and concerns in your community?

☐ What is your community's stand on sex education in schools?

☐ Do you know what community resources are available to help people with questions about sexuality-related issues?

Summary

* Sexual identity is determined by a complex interaction of genetic, physiological, and environmental factors. Biological sex, gender identity, gender roles, and sexual orientation are all blended into our sexual identity.
* The major components of the female sexual anatomy include the mons pubis, labia minora and majora, clitoris, urethral and vaginal openings, vagina, cervix, fallopian tubes, and ovaries. The major components of the male sexual anatomy are the penis, scrotum, testes, epididymides, vasa deferentia, ejaculatory ducts, and urethra.
* Physiologically, males and females experience four phases of sexual response: excitement/arousal, plateau, orgasmic, and resolution.

* Humans can express their sexual selves in a variety of ways, including celibacy, autoerotic behaviors, kissing and erotic touch, manual stimulation, oral-genital stimulation, vaginal intercourse, and anal intercourse. Sexual orientation refers to a person's enduring emotional, romantic, sexual, or affectionate attraction to other persons. Irrational hatred or fear of homosexuality or gay and lesbian persons is termed *homophobia*.
* Sexual dysfunctions can be classified into sexual desire disorders, sexual performance anxiety, sexual arousal disorders, orgasm disorders, and sexual pain disorders. Drug use can also lead to sexual dysfunction.

Questions for Discussion and Reflection

1. How have gender roles changed over the past 20 years? Do you view the changes as positive for both men and women?
2. Discuss the cycle of changes that occurs in our bodies in response to various hormones (e.g., sexual differentiation while in the womb, secondary sex characteristics at puberty, menopause).
3. What is "normal" sexual behavior? What criteria should we use to determine healthful sexual practice?

4. If scientists finally establish the combination of factors that interact to produce homosexual, heterosexual, or bisexual orientation, will that put an end to antigay prejudice? Why or why not?
5. How can we remove the stigma that surrounds sexual dysfunction so that individuals feel more open to seeking help? Are men and women impacted differently by sexual dysfunction?

Application Exercises

Reread the What Do You Think? scenarios at the beginning of the chapter, and answer the following questions.

1. From what you have learned in this chapter, is Ben justified in being apprehensive about sharing information about his sexual orientation with his coach or teammates? What resources or supports may be available on campus to help Ben deal with this situation?

2. From what you read in this chapter, do you think Jennifer's problem is serious? How might she resolve her problem? How can Todd help her learn to be orgasmic during intercourse?

Accessing Your Health on the Internet

Visit the following Internet sites to explore further topics and issues related to personal health. To visit an organization's website, go to the Companion Website for *Access to Health, Eighth Edition* at www.aw.com/donatelle, click on the book image, and select "Accessing Your Health on the Internet" from the navigation menu on the left.

1. *American Association of Sex Educators, Counselors, and Therapists (AASECT).* Professional organization providing standards of practice for treatment of sexual issues and disorders.
2. *Bacchus and Gamma Peer Education Network.* Student-friendly source of information about sexual and other health issues.

3. *Go Ask Alice.* An interactive question-and-answer resource from the Columbia University Health Services. "Alice" is available to answer questions each week about any health-related issues, including relationships, nutrition and diet, exercise, drugs, sex, alcohol, and stress.
4. *Sexuality Information and Education Council of the United States (SIECUS).* Information, guidelines, and materials for advancement of healthy and proper sex education.
5. *Teen Sexual Health*. Current research and other resources dealing with sexual health for high school and college-age students.

Further Reading

Caron, S. L. *Sex Matters for College Students: Sex FAQ's in Human Sexuality.* Englewood Cliffs, NJ: Prentice Hall, 2002.

   This is a brief, easy-to-read, and affordable paperback designed specifically to answer the basic sexual questions of today's young adults in a friendly and age-appropriate way.

Men's Health Books, ed. *The Complete Book of Men's Health: The Definitive, Illustrated Guide to Healthy Living, Exercise, and Sex.* Emmaus, PA: Rodale Press, 2000.

   A comprehensive and lushly illustrated guide to information on healthy lifestyles for men.

SIECUS (Sexuality Information and Education Council of the United States) Report. 130 West 42nd Street, New York, NY 10036.

   Highly acclaimed and readable bimonthly journal. Includes timely and thought-provoking articles on human sexuality, sexuality education, and AIDS.

Wingood, G. M., and R. DiClemente, eds. *Handbook of Women's Sexual and Reproductive Health.* Boston, Mass. Plenum Publishing, 2002.

   Medical researchers, including those in behavioral sciences and health education, summarize in depth the epidemiology, social and behavioral factors, policies, and effective intervention and prevention strategies related to women's sexual and reproductive health.

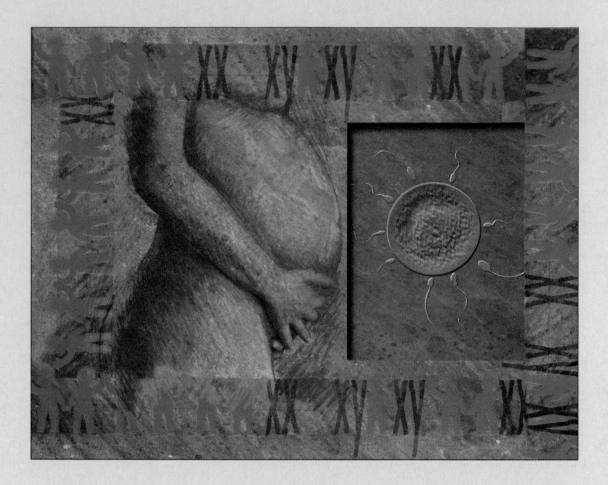

Objectives

* List the different types of contraceptive methods and discuss their effectiveness in preventing pregnancy and sexually transmitted infections.

* Summarize the legal decisions surrounding abortion and the various types of abortion procedures used today.

* Discuss key issues to consider when planning a pregnancy.

* Explain the importance of prenatal care and the physical and emotional aspects of pregnancy.

* Describe the basic stages of childbirth, methods of managing childbirth, and the complications that can arise during labor and delivery.

* Review some of the primary causes of and possible solutions to infertility.

Reproductive Choices

Making Responsible Decisions

What do you think?

Jane and Stephen visited a fertility clinic that recently announced a new service: It allows parents to successfully select the sex of their child from 70 to 90 percent of the time. The process separates male and female sperm so that the preferred type can be used for alternative insemination. The procedure costs $2,500 per trial, and the average couple usually requires three trials to successfully conceive.

Do you think parents should be able to select the sex of their baby? ✳ What are the potential ramifications of this technology? ✳ Should there be any limitations placed on its use? ✳ If so, what would you propose? ✳ How might this and other fertility technologies be abused? ✳ Under what circumstances might you want to select the sex of your child?

Nan is visiting her campus health service for the fourth time this year for emergency contraception. Her health care provider expressed concern that Nan may be using emergency contraception for birth control instead of one of the many contraceptive choices available to her. Nan won't talk about it, nor will she agree to use a contraceptive such as the pill, Norplant, or a diaphragm.

Should limitations be placed on the dispensing of emergency contraception? ✳ If so, what limitations would you propose? ✳ What would be the dangers of using this as one's sole method of contraception? Should a college health service offer access to emergency contraception?

T oday, we not only understand the intimate details of reproduction but also possess technologies that can control or enhance our **fertility.** Along with information and technological advance comes choice, and choice goes hand in hand with responsibility. Choosing if and when to have children is one of our greatest responsibilities. A woman and her partner have much to consider before planning or risking a pregnancy. Children, whether planned or unplanned, change people's lives. They require a lifelong personal commitment of love and nurturing. Are you physically, emotionally, and financially prepared to care for another human being?

One measure of maturity is the ability to discuss reproduction and birth control with one's sexual partner before succumbing to sexual urges. Men often assume that their partners are taking care of birth control. Women often feel that if they bring up the subject, it implies that they are "easy" or "loose." Both may feel that this discussion interferes with romance and spontaneity. You will find embarrassment-free discussion a lot easier if you understand human reproduction and contraception and honestly consider your attitudes toward these matters before you find yourself in a compromising situation.

Methods of Fertility Management

Conception refers to the fertilization of an ovum by a sperm. The following conditions are necessary for conception:

1. A viable egg.
2. A viable sperm.
3. Access to the egg by the sperm.

The term **contraception** (sometimes called *birth control*) refers to methods of preventing conception. These methods offer varying degrees of control over when and whether pregnancies occur. However, since people first associated sexual activity with pregnancy, society has searched for a simple, infallible, and risk-free way to prevent pregnancy. We have not yet found one.

To evaluate the effectiveness of a particular contraceptive method, you must be familiar with two concepts: perfect

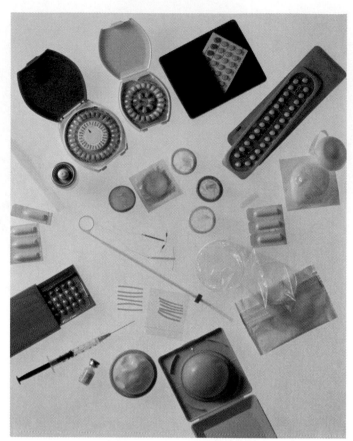

There are many methods of contraception now available. To choose the best one for you and your partner you should consider medical factors, cost, convenience, and other issues important to you.

failure rate and typical use failure rate. *Perfect failure rate* refers to the number of pregnancies that are likely to occur in a year (per 100 uses of the method during sexual intercourse) if the method is used absolutely perfectly, that is, without any error. The *typical use failure rate* refers to the number of pregnancies that are likely to occur with typical use, that is, with the normal number of errors, memory lapses, and incorrect or incomplete use. This information is much more practical for people in helping them make informed decisions about contraceptive methods. See Table 7.1 to find ratings of various contraceptive methods. We'll discuss many of them in this chapter. See the New Horizons in Health box for an overview of some of the new contraceptive options.

Many contraceptive methods can also protect, at least to some degree, against **sexually transmitted infections (STIs).** This is an important factor to consider in choosing a contraceptive. Table 7.1 compares the level of STI protection offered by various contraceptives; see Chapter 17 for more about individual STIs.

Present methods of contraception fall into several categories. **Barrier methods** use a physical or chemical block to prevent the egg and sperm from joining. Hormonal methods introduce synthetic hormones into the woman's system that prevent ovulation, thicken cervical mucous, or prevent a

---

Fertility A person's ability to reproduce.

Conception The fertilization of an ovum by a sperm.

Contraception Methods of preventing conception.

Sexually transmitted infections (STIs) A variety of infections that can be acquired through sexual contact.

Barrier methods Contraceptive methods that block the meeting of egg and sperm by means of a physical barrier (e.g., condom, diaphragm, or cervical cap), a chemical barrier (e.g., spermicide), or both.

News from the World of Contraceptives Research

The introduction of a new contraceptive may take years of research and clinical trials prior to approval by the Food and Drug Administration. However, it appears that within the next few years, our contraceptive options may be expanding. Here's a look at future contraceptives:

New Barrier Methods

- Lea's Shield is a one-size-fits-all silicon rubber device that covers the cervix. The FDA has asked for more clinical studies prior to approval.
- A new vaginal sponge, Protectaid, is made of polyurethane foam and contains a combination of chemicals that serve as spermicide and microbicide to protect against STIs. It is available in Canada.
- FemCap, already available in Europe, covers the cervix and forms a seal against the vaginal wall. It is used with spermicide and contains a groove that traps sperm. FemCap has not yet been approved by the FDA.

Contraceptives for Men

- The oft-discussed "male pill" is probably about five years away.
- An injectable contraceptive that stimulates the production of antibodies to male sex hormones is in the works and will be tested more extensively within the next few years.
- A synthetic testosterone that would be delivered via a skin implant has been developed by the Population Council and is undergoing further testing to determine side effects.

Implant Refinements

- The Population Council, which developed Norplant, is currently working on a single-rod implant delivery system that would inhibit ovulation for two years. The implant contains Nesterone, a synthetic progestin.
- Also being studied are biodegradable implants containing progestin that would be implanted under the skin of the arm or the hip. The hormone is released gradually into the body for 12 to 18 months.

Injections and Vaccines for Women

- Oral or injectable vaccine could stimulate the immune system to create antibodies to a crucial type of protein molecule found on the head of sperm.

Unisex Contraception

- A new group of drugs known as gonadotropin-releasing hormone (GnRH) agonists can be used to prevent the release of FSH and LH from the pituitary gland. Blocking of these hormones will temporarily suppress fertility in men and women.

Sources: Population Council, "Biomedical Research and Products" (see http://www.popcouncil.org/biomed/biomed.html); Johns Hopkins University, "Reproductive Health Online" (see http://www.reproline.jhu.edu).

---

fertilized egg from implanting. Surgical methods can be used to permanently prevent pregnancy. Other methods of contraception may involve temporary or permanent abstinence, or planning intercourse in accordance with fertility patterns. (See the Assess Yourself box to determine what method is right for you and your partner.)

Barrier Methods

The Male Condom The male **condom** is a thin sheath designed to cover the erect penis and catch semen before it enters the vagina. The majority of male condoms are made of latex, although condoms made of polyurethane are now available. "Skin" condoms, made from lamb intestines, are not effective against preventing the spread of STIs. The condom is the only temporary means of birth control available for men and the only barrier that effectively prevents the spread of STIs and HIV. Condoms come in a wide variety of styles: colored, ribbed for "extra sensation," lubricated, nonlubricated, and with or without reservoirs at the tip. All may be purchased with or without spermicide in pharmacies, in some supermarkets and public bathrooms, and in many health clinics. A new condom must be used for each act of intercourse or oral sex.

In addition to helping to prevent some sexually transmitted infections, including genital herpes and HIV, condoms may also slow or reduce the development of cervical abnormalities in women that can lead to cancer. A condom must be rolled onto the penis before the penis touches the vagina, and held in place when removing the penis from the vagina after ejaculation (see Figure 7.1 on page 180). For greatest efficacy, they should be used with a spermicide containing nonoxynol-9, the same agent found in many of the contraceptive foams and creams that women use. If necessary or desired, users can lubricate their own condoms with contraceptive foams, creams, and jellies or other water-based lubricants, such as K-Y jelly, ForPlay Lubricants, Astroglide, or Wet or Aqua Lube, to name just a few. However, never use products such as baby oil, cold cream, petroleum jelly, vaginal

Table 7.1
Contraceptive Effectiveness and STI Prevention

NUMBER OF UNINTENDED PREGNANCIES PER 100 WOMEN DURING FIRST YEAR OF USE

METHOD	TYPICAL USE*	PERFECT USE**	RISK REDUCTION FOR SEXUALLY TRANSMITTED INFECTIONS (STIs)
CONTINUOUS ABSTINENCE	0.00	0.00	Complete
OUTERCOURSE	N/A***	N/A	Some
NORPLANT IMPLANT	0.05	0.05	None
STERILIZATION			
Men	0.15	0.1	None
Women	0.5	0.5	None
DEPO-PROVERA INJECTION	0.3	0.3	None
IUD			
ParaGard (copper T380A)	0.8	0.6	None
Progestasert	2.0	1.5	None
Mirena	0.1	0.1	None
LUNELLE INJECTION	N/A	0.1	None
ORAL CONTRACEPTIVES (THE PILL)			
Combination	5.0	0.1	None
Progestin-only	5.0	0.5	None
MALE CONDOM	14.0	3.0	Good against HIV: reduces risk of others
WITHDRAWAL	19.0	4.0	None
DIAPHRAGM	20.0	6.0	Limited
CERVICAL CAP			
Women who have not given birth	20.0	9.0	Limited
Women who have given birth	40.0	30.0	Limited
FEMALE CONDOM	21.0	5.0	Some
PREDICTING FERTILITY			
Periodic abstinence	20.0		None
Postovulation method		1.0	None
Symptothermal method		2.0	None
Cervical mucous (ovulation) method		3.0	None
Calendar method		9.0	None
FERTILITY AWARENESS METHODS			
With male or female condom	N/A	N/A	None
With diaphragm or cap	N/A	N/A	None
With withdrawal or other methods	N/A	N/A	None
SPERMICIDE	26.0	6.0	Limited
NO METHOD	85.0	85.0	None

EMERGENCY CONTRACEPTON

Emergency contraception pills: Treatment initiated within 72 hours after unprotected intercourse reduces the risk of pregnancy by 75–89 percent (with no protection against STIs). Emergency IUD insertion: Treatment initiated within seven days after unprotected intercourse reduces the risk of pregnancy by more than 99 percent (with no protection against STIs).

Contraceptive effectiveness rates: R. Hatcher et al., Contraceptive Technology—17th Edition, New York: Ardent Media, 1998.

*"Typical Use" refers to failure rates for men and women whose use is not consistent or always correct.

**"Perfect Use" refers to failure rates for those whose use is consistent and always correct.

***N/A means that effectiveness rates are not available.

Contraceptive Comfort and Confidence Scale

These questions are designed to help you assess whether the method of contraception you are using or may consider using in the future is or will be effective for you. Most individuals will have a few yes answers. Yes answers predict potential problems. If you have more than a few yes responses, you may want to talk to a health care provider, counselor, partner, or friend to decide whether to use this method or how to use it so that it will really be effective. In general, the more yes answers you have, the less likely you are to use this method consistently and correctly with every act of intercourse.

Method of contraception you are considering _____

Length of time you used this method in the past _____

Answer Yes or No to the following questions:
___ 1. Have I ever had problems using this method?
___ 2. Have I ever become pregnant while using this method?
___ 3. Am I afraid of using this method?
___ 4. Would I really rather not use this method?
___ 5. Will I have trouble remembering to use this method?
___ 6. Will I have trouble using this method correctly?
___ 7. Do I still have unanswered questions about this method?
___ 8. Does this method make menstrual periods longer or more painful?
___ 9. Does this method cost more than I can afford?
___ 10. Could this method cause serious complications?
___ 11. Am I opposed to this method because of any religious or moral beliefs?
___ 12. Is my partner opposed to this method?
___ 13. Am I using this method without my partner's knowledge?
___ 14. Will using this method embarrass my partner?
___ 15. Will using this method embarrass me?
___ 16. Will I enjoy intercourse less because of this method?
___ 17. If this method interrupts lovemaking, will I avoid using it?
___ 18. Has a nurse or doctor ever told me not to use this method?
___ 19. Is there anything about my personality that could lead me to use this method incorrectly?
___ 20. Am I at risk of being exposed to HIV (the AIDS virus) or other sexually transmitted infections if I use this method?

___ **Total number of Yes answers**

Source: From *Contraceptive Technology*, 17th ed., by R. A. Hatcher et al. (New York: Ardent Media, Inc: 1998), p. 238.

---

yeast infection medications, or hand and body lotion with a condom. These products contain mineral oil and will make the latex begin to disintegrate within 60 seconds.

Condoms are less effective and more likely to break during intercourse if they are old or poorly stored. To maintain effectiveness, store them in a cool place (not in a wallet or hip pocket), and inspect them for small tears before use.

For some people, a condom ruins the spontaneity of sex. Stopping to put it on breaks the mood for them. Others report that the condom decreases sensation. These inconveniences contribute to improper use of the device. Couples who learn to put the condom on together as foreplay are generally more successful with this form of birth control.[1]

Foams, Suppositories, Jellies, and Creams Like condoms, jellies, creams, suppositories, and foam do not require a prescription. Chemically, they are referred to as **spermicides**—substances designed to kill sperm. Foams, suppositories, jellies, and creams usually contain nonoxynol-9, a detergent believed to be effective in also killing viruses, bacteria, and

> **Condom** A single-use sheath of thin latex or other material designed to fit over an erect penis and to catch semen upon ejaculation.
>
> **Spermicides** Substances designed to kill sperm.

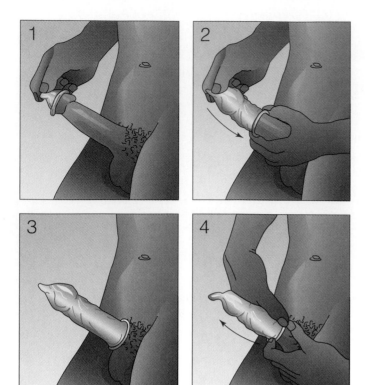

Figure 7.1

How to Use a Condom
The condom should be rolled over the erect penis before any penetration occurs. A small space (about ½") should be left at the end of the condom to collect the semen after ejaculation. Hold the tip of the condom, and unroll it all the way to the base of the penis. Hold the base of the condom before withdrawal to avoid spilling any semen.

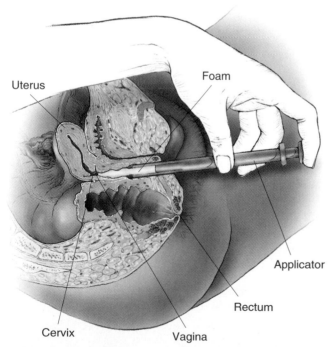

Figure 7.2

The Proper Method of Applying Spermicide within the Vagina

other organisms. Although they are not recommended as the primary form of contraception, spermicides are often recommended for use with other forms of contraception. Though they help prevent the spread of certain STIs, they are most effective when used in conjunction with a condom.

Jellies and creams are packaged in tubes, and foams are available in aerosol cans. All have tubes designed for insertion into the vagina. They must be inserted far enough to cover the cervix, providing both a chemical barrier that kills sperm and a physical barrier that stops sperm from continuing toward an egg (see Figure 7.2).

Suppositories are waxy capsules that are inserted deep in the vagina, where they melt. They must be inserted 10 to 20 minutes before intercourse to have time to melt but no longer than one hour prior to intercourse or they lose their effectiveness. Additional contraceptive chemicals must be applied for each subsequent act of intercourse.

The Female Condom   The **female condom** is a single-use, soft, loose-fitting polyurethane sheath meant for internal use by women. It is designed as one unit with two diaphragm-like rings. One ring, which lies inside the sheath, serves as an insertion mechanism and internal anchor. The other ring, which remains outside the vagina once the device is inserted, protects the labia and the base of the penis from infection. Many women like the female condom because it gives them more control over reproduction than does the male condom. When used correctly, the female condom provides protection against HIV and STIs comparable to that of a latex male condom.

The Diaphragm, with Spermicidal Jelly or Cream   Invented in the mid-nineteenth century, the **diaphragm** was the first widely used birth control method for women.

The diaphragm is a soft, shallow cup made of thin latex rubber. Its flexible, rubber-coated ring is designed to fit snugly behind the pubic bone in front of the cervix and over the back of the cervix on the other side. Diaphragms are manufactured in different sizes and must be fitted to the woman by a trained practitioner. The practitioner should also be certain that the user knows how to insert her diaphragm correctly before she leaves the practitioner's office.

Diaphragms must be used with spermicidal cream or jelly, which is applied to the inside of the diaphragm before insertion. The diaphragm holds the spermicide in place, creating a physical and chemical barrier against sperm. Additional spermicide must be applied before each subsequent act of intercourse, and the diaphragm must be left in place for six to eight hours after intercourse to allow the chemical to kill any sperm remaining in the vagina. When used with spermicidal jelly or cream, it offers significant protection against gonorrhea and possibly chlamydia and human papilloma virus (HPV) (see Figure 7.3).

Using the diaphragm during the menstrual period or leaving it in place beyond the recommended time slightly increases the user's risk of developing **toxic shock syndrome (TSS).** This condition results from the multiplication of bacteria that spread to the bloodstream and cause

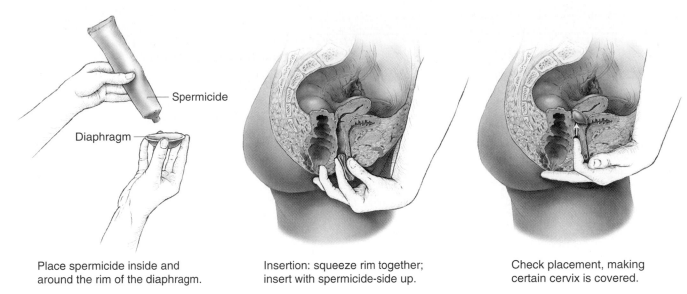

Place spermicide inside and around the rim of the diaphragm.

Insertion: squeeze rim together; insert with spermicide-side up.

Check placement, making certain cervix is covered.

Figure 7.3
The Proper Use and Placement of a Diaphragm

sudden high fever, rash, nausea, vomiting, diarrhea, and a rapid drop in blood pressure. If not treated, TSS can be fatal. The diaphragm (as well as tampons left in place too long) creates conditions conducive to the growth of these bacteria. To reduce the risk of TSS, women should wash their hands carefully with soap and water before inserting or removing the diaphragm.

Another problem with the diaphragm is that it can put undue pressure on the urethra, blocking urinary flow and predisposing the user to bladder infections. A further disadvantage is that inserting the device can be awkward, especially if the woman is rushed. When inserted incorrectly, diaphragms are much less effective.

The Cervical Cap One of the oldest methods used to prevent pregnancy, early cervical caps were made from beeswax, silver, or copper. Today's **cervical cap** is a small cup made of latex that fits snugly over the entire cervix. It must be fitted by a practitioner and is designed for use with contraceptive jelly or cream. It is somewhat more difficult to insert than a diaphragm because of its smaller size.

The cap keeps sperm out of the uterus. It is held in place by suction created during application. Insertion may take place anywhere up to two days prior to intercourse, and the device must be left in place for six to eight hours after intercourse. The maximum length of time the cap can be left on the cervix is 48 hours. If removed and cleaned, it can be reinserted immediately. The cervical cap may offer protection against STIs but not HIV.

Some women report unpleasant vaginal odors after use. Because the device can become dislodged during intercourse, placement must be checked frequently. It cannot be used during the menstrual period or for longer than 48 hours because of the risk of toxic shock syndrome.

Hormonal Methods

Oral Contraceptives Oral contraceptive pills were first marketed in the United States in 1960. Their convenience quickly made them the most widely used reversible method of fertility control.

Most oral contraceptives work through the combined effects of synthetic estrogen and progesterone. Because the levels of estrogen in the pill are higher than those produced by the body, the pituitary gland is never signaled to produce follicle-stimulating hormone (FSH), without which ova will not develop in the ovaries. Progesterone in the pill prevents proper growth of the uterine lining and thickens the cervical mucous, forming a barrier against sperm.

Female condom A single-use polyurethane sheath for internal use by women.

Diaphragm A latex, saucer-shaped device designed to cover the cervix and block access to the uterus; should always be used with spermicide.

Toxic shock syndrome (TSS) A potentially life-threatening disease that occurs when specific bacterial toxins are allowed to multiply unchecked in wounds or through improper use of tampons or diaphragms.

Cervical cap A small cup made of latex that is designed to fit snugly over the entire cervix.

Oral contraceptives Pills taken daily for three weeks of the menstrual cycle that prevent ovulation by regulating hormones.

Table 7.2

Counteracting Reduced Effectiveness of Oral Contraceptives

TYPE OF DRUG	NEED FOR BACKUP CONTRACEPTIVE
Enzyme-inducing drug (i.e., Rifampin, phenobarbital, Dilantin)	Entire duration of treatment plus 7 days, or longer if advised by your clinician.
Nonenzyme-inducing drug (e.g., broad-spectrum antibiotics such as ampicillin, doxycycline, tetracycline)	Entire duration of treatment or 14 days, whichever is shorter, plus 7 days.

Source: From *Contraceptive Technology* (17th ed., p. 457), by R. Hatcher et al., 1998, New York: Ardent Media, Inc.

Pills are meant to be taken in a cycle. At the end of each three-week cycle, the user discontinues the drug or takes a placebo pill for one week. The resultant drop in hormones causes the uterine lining to disintegrate, and the user will have a menstrual period, usually within one to three days. The same cycle is repeated every 28 days. Menstrual flow is generally lighter than it is for women who don't use the pill because the hormones in the pill prevent thick endometrial buildup.

Today's pill is different from the one introduced more than four decades ago. The original pill contained large amounts of estrogen, which caused certain risks for the user, whereas the current pill contains the minimal amount of estrogen necessary to prevent pregnancy.

Because the chemicals in oral contraceptives change the way the body metabolizes certain nutrients, all women using the pill should check with their prescribing practitioners regarding dietary supplements. The nutrients of concern include vitamin C and the B-complex vitamins—B_2, B_6, and B_{12}. A nutritious diet that includes whole grains, fresh fruits and vegetables, lean meats, fish and poultry, and nonfat dairy products is important.

Oral contraceptives can interact negatively with other drugs. For example, some antibiotics diminish the pill's effectiveness and may require an adjustment in dosage (see Table 7.2). Women in doubt should check with their prescribing practitioners or their pharmacists.

Return of fertility may be delayed after discontinuing the pill, but the pill is not known to cause infertility. Women who had irregular menstrual cycles before going on the pill are more likely to have problems conceiving, regardless of pill use.

The pill is convenient and does not interfere with lovemaking. It may lessen menstrual difficulties, such as cramps and premenstrual syndrome (PMS). Oral contraceptives also lower the risk of several health conditions, including endometrial and ovarian cancers, fibrocystic breast disease, ectopic pregnancies, ovarian cysts, pelvic inflammatory disease, and iron deficiency anemia.[2] But possible serious health problems associated with the pill include blood clots, which can lead to strokes or heart attacks, and an increased risk for high blood pressure. The risk is low for most healthy women under 35 who do not smoke; it increases with age and especially with cigarette smoking. See Figure 7.4 for early warning signs of complications associated with oral contraceptive use.

Outside of these risk factors and certain side effects associated with the pill, its greatest disadvantage is that it must be taken every day. If a woman misses taking one pill, she should use an alternative form of contraception for the remainder of that cycle. Another drawback is that the pill does not protect against sexually transmitted infections (STIs). Some teenagers report that the requirement to have a complete gynecological examination in order to get a prescription for the pill is a huge obstacle. Educating young women about what goes on in a gynecological exam would certainly help ease their anxiety. Finally, cost may be a problem for some women. See the Health Ethics box about student health insurance and the pill.

Progestin-Only Pills Progestin-only pills (or minipills) contain small doses of progesterone. Women who feel uncertain about using estrogen pills, who suffer from side effects related to estrogen, or who are nursing may choose these medications rather than combination pills. There is still some

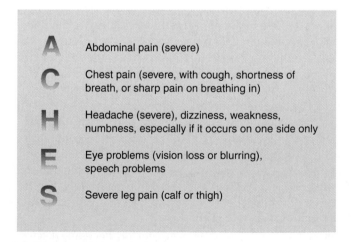

A Abdominal pain (severe)

C Chest pain (severe, with cough, shortness of breath, or sharp pain on breathing in)

H Headache (severe), dizziness, weakness, numbness, especially if it occurs on one side only

E Eye problems (vision loss or blurring), speech problems

S Severe leg pain (calf or thigh)

Figure 7.4
Early Warning Signs for Pill Users
Source: From *Contraceptive Technology* (17th ed., p. 457), by R. Hatcher et al., 1998, New York: Ardent Media, Inc.

Should Prescription Contraceptives Be Covered by Student Health Insurance?

George Washington University (GW) changed its health insurance plan for students in fall 2002 to include coverage of prescription contraceptives after three students said the plan violated a federal law forbidding gender discrimination at institutions receiving federal funds.

The policy change came shortly after advocacy groups representing three female law students at the university sent a letter to school officials urging them to include birth control in the health plan or face a possible lawsuit. The letter was sent jointly by the National Women's Law Center, Trial Lawyers for Public Justice, and Planned Parenthood on behalf of the three students and included a petition signed by more than 100 other students at GW. "The failure to provide coverage for prescription contraceptives is a glaring omission that causes injury to our clients and many other female students at GW, and constitutes sex discrimination," the letter said. "We strongly urge that GW take immediate action to comply with its legal obligation to its students by providing insurance coverage for all FDA-approved prescription drugs and devices, and related medical services, in the health plan it offers to its students."

The letter also cites a lawsuit, *Erickson v. Bartell Drug Co.,* in which a federal court ruled that an otherwise comprehensive health plan cannot exclude prescription contraceptives. The ruling cited Title VII of the Civil Rights Act of 1964, which prohibits employment discrimination based on race, color, religion, sex, or national origin. Although the Erickson case did not involve a college, advocacy groups argue that Title IX of the Education Amendments of 1972, a federal discrimination law, extends the same protection to college students.

After receiving the letter, the university quickly complied, asking its insurance company to add birth-control pills and other prescription contraceptives to its coverage.

Does your student health insurance plan provide coverage for prescription contraceptives? Do you know where to find out information regarding your student health insurance policy? Are you aware of your options for obtaining discounted birth control that may or may not be covered in your student health insurance policy? If your school insurance does not provide coverage for prescription contraceptives, what are some of the steps you and others can take to make a change in the policy? Why do you think some schools might object to adding this coverage?

Source: Jeffrey R. Young, "George Washington Adds Birth Control to Health Plan," *The Chronicle of Higher Education,* September 13, 2002, Student Section, Vol. 49, Issue 3. Copyright © 2002, The Chronicle of Higher Education.

question about the specific ways in which progestin-only pills work. Current thought is that they change the composition of the cervical mucous, thus impeding sperm travel. They may also inhibit ovulation in some women. The effectiveness rate of progestin-only pills is 96 percent, which is slightly lower than that of estrogen-containing pills. Also, their use usually leads to irregular menstrual bleeding. As with all oral contraceptives, the user has no protection against STIs.

Ortho Evra (The Patch)   A hormonal contraceptive patch, **Ortho Evra,** was unveiled in spring 2002. The patch is worn for one week and replaced on the same day of the week for three consecutive weeks, with the fourth week patch-free. The patch is 99 percent effective and works by delivering continuous levels of the hormones estrogen and progestin through the skin and into the bloodstream. This new weekly patch is easy to apply and barely noticeable, with adhesive strong enough even to withstand swimming. The patch can be worn on one of four areas of the body: buttocks, abdomen, upper torso (front or back, excluding the breasts), or upper outer arm.

The contraceptive patch contains hormones similar to those in birth control pills. Some women report experiencing breast symptoms, headache, application site reaction, nausea, upper respiratory infection, menstrual cramps and abdominal pain; most side effects of the contraceptive patch are not serious, and those that are occur infrequently. Serious risks, which can be life threatening, include blood clots, stroke, or heart attacks and are increased by tobacco use. The contraceptive patch does not protect against HIV or other sexually transmitted diseases.

NuvaRing   Introduced in 2002, this effective new contraceptive offers protection for four weeks at a time. **NuvaRing** is a soft, flexible, transparent ring about two inches in diameter that the user inserts into the vagina and leaves in place for three weeks. (The user then removes it for one week for her menstrual period.) Once the ring is inserted, it continuously releases a steady flow of two female hormones, estrogen and progestin.

Ortho Evra   A patch worn for three weeks at a time that releases hormones similar to those in oral contraceptives.

NuvaRing   A soft, flexible ring inserted into the vagina that releases hormones, preventing pregnancy.

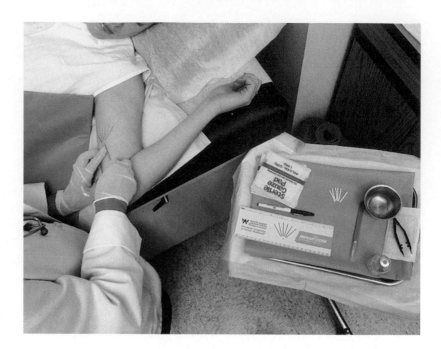

Norplant capsules are surgically implanted into the inside upper arm and provide a safe, long-term contraceptive option for women.

Advantages of NuvaRing include protection against pregnancy for one month; no pill to take daily; no need to be "fitted" by a clinician; no need for spermicide; and that the ability to become pregnant returns quickly when use is stopped. Some of the disadvantages that women might experience include increased vaginal discharge; vaginal irritation or infection; inability to use oil-based vaginal medicine to treat yeast infections when the ring is in place; and inability to use a diaphragm or cervical cap as a backup method for contraception.

Lunelle Lunelle is a low-maintenance monthly shot that requires a visit to a health care practitioner. The monthly injection of the time-released synthetic hormones contains estrogen and progestin. The combination of hormones works in three ways: by keeping the ovaries from releasing an egg (ovulation); thickening the cervical mucous, which prevents sperm from joining with an egg; and preventing a fertilized egg from implanting in the uterus. This form of contraception is 99 percent effective.

Some side effects (which usually clear up after two or three months of use) include bleeding between periods, weight gain or loss, breast tenderness, nausea (rarely), vomiting, and/or changes in mood or sex drive. Lunelle, as with other forms of hormonal contraception, offers no protection from STIs.

Depo-Provera Depo-Provera is a long-acting synthetic progesterone that is injected intramuscularly every three months. Researchers believe that the drug prevents ovulation. Depo-Provera encourages sexual spontaneity because the user does not have to remember to take a pill or insert a device. Those who want to start a family can usually do so without much of a waiting period. There are fewer health problems associated with Depo-Provera than with estrogen-containing pills. The main disadvantage is irregular bleeding, which can be troublesome at first, but within a year, most women are amenorrheic (have no menstrual periods). Weight gain (an average of five pounds in the first year) is common. Other possible side effects include dizziness, nervousness, and headache. Unlike other methods of contraception, this method cannot be stopped immediately if problems arise.

Norplant With **Norplant,** six silicon capsules that contain progestin are surgically inserted under the skin of a woman's upper arm. For five years, they continuously release small amounts of progestin. The progestin in Norplant works the same way as oral contraceptives do; it suppresses ovulation, prevents growth of the uterine lining, and thickens the cervical mucous. Norplant is one of the most effective methods of birth control ever developed.

A trained health care provider can insert Norplant in 10 to 15 minutes. This involves administering a local anesthetic to the upper arm, making a small incision, and with a special needle, placing the six capsules just under the skin in a fan shape. The capsules are similarly removed after five years or, if necessary, at any time after their insertion.

The capsules usually are invisible, and insertion does not leave a scar for most women. At this time, no serious side effects are known. Less serious side effects include irregular bleeding and irregular menstrual periods, acne, weight gain, breast tenderness, headaches, nervousness, depression, and nausea.

Norplant is one of the most effective reversible methods of fertility control and relatively easy for a trained practitioner to implant. A serious disadvantage, however, is its lack of protection against STIs.

Surgical Methods

Sterilization has become the leading method of contraception for women (10.7 million women), closely followed by the oral contraceptive pill (10.4 million women).[3] Although newer surgical techniques make reversal of sterilization theoretically possible, anyone considering sterilization should assume that the operation is *not* reversible. Before becoming sterilized, people should think through possibilities such as divorce and remarriage or a future improvement in their financial status that might make a larger family realistic.

Female Sterilization **Tubal ligation** is one method of sterilization for females. In this surgical procedure, the fallopian tubes are either tied shut or cut and cauterized (burned) at the edges to seal the tubes, blocking sperm's access to released eggs. The operation is usually done in a hospital on an outpatient basis. First, the abdomen is inflated with carbon dioxide gas through a small incision in the navel. The surgeon then inserts a *laparoscope* into another incision just above the pubic bone. This specially designed instrument has a fiberoptic light source that enables the physician to see the fallopian tubes clearly. Once located, the tubes are cut and tied or cauterized.

Ovarian and uterine functions are not affected by a tubal ligation. The woman's menstrual cycle continues, and released eggs simply disintegrate and are absorbed by the lymphatic system. As soon as her incision heals, the woman may resume sexual intercourse with no fear of pregnancy.

As with any surgery, there are risks. Although rare, possible complications of a tubal ligation can include infection, pulmonary embolism, hemorrhage, and ectopic pregnancy. Some patients are given general anesthesia, which itself presents a small risk; others receive local anesthesia. The procedure itself usually takes less than an hour, and the patient is generally allowed to return home within a short time after waking up. Women considering a tubal ligation should thoroughly discuss all the risks with their physician before the operation.

The **hysterectomy,** or removal of the uterus, is a method of sterilization requiring major surgery. It is usually done only when the patient's uterus is diseased or damaged.

Male Sterilization Sterilization in men is less complicated than in women. The procedure, called a **vasectomy,** is usually done on an outpatient basis, using a local anesthetic. The surgeon (generally a urologist) makes an incision on each side of the scrotum, locates the vas deferens on each side, and removes a piece from each. The ends are usually tied or sewn shut.

In a small percentage of cases, serious complications occur: formation of a blood clot in the scrotum (which usually disappears without medical treatment), infection, and inflammatory reactions. Because sperm are stored in other areas of the reproductive system besides the vasa deferentia, couples must use alternative methods of birth control for at least one month after the vasectomy. The man must check with his physician (who will do a semen analysis) to determine when unprotected intercourse can take place. The pregnancy rate in women whose partners have had vasectomies is about 15 in 10,000.

Many men are reluctant to consider sterilization because they fear the operation will affect their sexual performance. However, a vasectomy in no way affects sexual response. Because sperm constitute only a small percentage of the semen, the amount of ejaculate is not changed significantly. The testes continue to produce sperm, but the sperm can no longer enter the ejaculatory duct. After a time, sperm production may diminish. Any sperm that are manufactured disintegrate and are absorbed into the lymphatic system.

Although a vasectomy should be considered permanent, surgical reversal is sometimes successful in restoring fertility. Recent improvements in microsurgery techniques have resulted in annual pregnancy rates of between 40 and 60 percent for women whose partners have had reversals. The two major factors influencing the success rate of reversal are the doctor's expertise and the time elapsed since the vasectomy.

What do you think?

Who do you think is responsible for deciding which method of contraception should be used in a sexual relationship? ✳ *What are some examples of good opportunities for you and your partner to have a discussion about contraceptives?* ✳ *What do you think are the biggest barriers in our society to the use of condoms?*

Lunelle A monthly injection of estrogen and progestin that prevents ovulation and fertilization.

Depo-Provera An injectable method of birth control that lasts for three months.

Norplant A long-lasting contraceptive that consists of six silicon capsules surgically inserted under the skin in a woman's upper arm.

Sterilization Permanent fertility control achieved through surgical procedures.

Tubal ligation Sterilization of the female that involves the cutting and tying off or cauterizing of the fallopian tubes.

Hysterectomy The removal of the uterus.

Vasectomy Sterilization of the male that involves the cutting and tying off of both vasa deferentia.

Other Methods of Contraception

Intrauterine Devices   Women have been using **intrauterine devices (IUDs)** since 1909, but we still are not certain how they work. Although it was once thought that IUDs act by preventing implantation of a fertilized egg, most experts now believe that they interfere with the sperm's fertilization of the egg.

Three IUDs are currently available. The first, Progestasert, is a T-shaped plastic device that contains synthetic progesterone. It slowly releases the progesterone. The practitioner must remove this IUD and insert a new one every year. The second, ParaGard, is also T-shaped, but it has copper wrapped around the shaft and does not contain any hormones. It can be left in place for ten years before replacement. The third, which has just appeared on the market, is Mirena. It is effective for five years and releases small amounts of the progestin levonorgestrel.

A physician must fit and insert the IUD. For insertion, the device is folded and placed into a long, thin plastic applicator. The practitioner measures the depth of the uterus with a special instrument and then uses these measurements to place the IUD accurately so the arms of the T open out across the top of the uterus. One or two strings extend from the IUD into the vagina so the user can check to make sure that her IUD is in place. The device is removed by a practitioner when desired.

Disadvantages of IUDs include discomfort, cost of insertion, and potential complications. The device can cause heavy menstrual flow and severe cramps. Women using IUDs have a higher risk of uterine perforation, ectopic pregnancy, pelvic inflammatory disease, infertility, and tubal infections. If a pregnancy occurs while the IUD is in place, the chance of miscarriage is 25 to 50 percent. The device should be removed as soon as possible. Doctors often offer therapeutic abortion to women who become pregnant while using an IUD because of the serious risks (including premature delivery, infection, and congenital abnormalities) associated with continuing the pregnancy. For a comparison of contraceptive option costs, see Table 7.3.

Withdrawal   This not very effective method of birth control is most commonly used by people who have not taken the time to consider alternatives. The **withdrawal** method involves withdrawing the penis from the vagina just prior to ejaculation. Because there can be up to half a million sperm in the drop of fluid at the tip of the penis before ejaculation, this method is unreliable. Timing withdrawal is also difficult, and males concentrating on accurate timing may not be able to relax and enjoy intercourse.

Emergency Contraceptive Pills   There are more than 2.7 million unintended pregnancies per year in the United States, and nearly half are due to contraceptive failure. According to the Centers for Disease Control and Prevention, more than 11 million American women report using contraceptive methods associated with high failure rates, including condoms, withdrawal, periodic abstinence, and diaphragms.

Emergency contraception can be used when a condom breaks, after a sexual assault, or any time unprotected sexual intercourse occurs. **Emergency contraceptive pills (ECPs)** are ordinary birth control pills containing the hormones estrogen and progestin. Although the therapy is commonly known as the "morning-after pill," the term is misleading; ECPs can be used up to 72 hours after intercourse and can reduce the risk of pregnancy by 75 percent.

Emergency contraceptives require a prescription; the two FDA-approved products are preven and Plan B. After a woman determines she is not already pregnant, by using the pregnancy test included in the kit, the first dose of two light blue emergency pills is taken as soon as possible, within 72 hours after intercourse. The second dose is taken 12 hours later.[4] The most common side effects related to ECPS are nausea, vomiting, menstrual irregularities, breast tenderness, headache, abdominal pain and cramps, and dizziness.

Emergency minipills contain progestin only. Like ECPs, minipills can be used immediately after unprotected intercourse and up to 72 hours beyond. Emergency minipills are equally as effective as ECPs, but nausea and vomiting are far less common. Emergency minipills are an excellent alternative for most women who cannot use ECPs that contain estrogen.

Abstinence and "Outercourse"   Strictly defined, abstinence means deliberately shunning intercourse. This strict definition would allow one to engage in such forms of sexual intimacy as massage, kissing, and solitary masturbation. But many people today have broadened the definition of abstinence to include all forms of sexual contact, even those that do not culminate in sexual intercourse.

Couples who go a step further than massage and kissing and engage in activities such as oral-genital sex and mutual masturbation are sometimes said to be engaging in

---

Intrauterine device (IUD)   A T-shaped device that is implanted in the uterus to prevent pregnancy.

Withdrawal   A method of contraception that involves withdrawing the penis from the vagina before ejaculation. Also called "coitus interruptus."

Emergency contraceptive pills (ECPs)   Drugs taken within three days after intercourse to prevent fertilization or implantation.

Emergency minipills   Contraceptive pills containing only progestin that can be taken up to three days after unprotected intercourse.

Fertility awareness methods (FAMs)   Several types of birth control that require alteration of sexual behavior rather than chemical or physical intervention into the reproductive process.

Table 7.3
Costs of Contraception

METHOD	COST
Continuous abstinence	None
Outercourse (sex play without vaginal intercourse)	None
Withdrawal	None
Sterilization	
Tubal ligation: permanently blocks female's fallopian tubes where sperm join egg	$1,000–$2,500
Vasectomy: permanently blocks male's vas deferens that carry sperm	$240–$520
Norplant	$500–$750/exam, implants, and insertion; $100–$200/removal
Depo-Provera	$20–$40/visits to clinician; $30–$75/injection
IUD (Intrauterine device)	$175–$400/exam, insertion, and follow-up visit
Lunelle	$35–$125/visit and/or examination, if needed; $30–$35/ monthly dose of the injection of Lunelle. The cost usually is less at a clinic and is covered by Medicaid.
Oral contraceptives	$15–$35/monthly pill-pack at drugstores, often less at clinics; $35–$125/exam
NuvaRing	$30–$35/monthly supply of rings; $35–$125/exam
Ortho Evra (patch)	$30–$35/monthly supply of patches; $35–$125/exam
Condoms/female condoms and spermicide	50¢ and up/condom — some family planning centers give them away or charge very little; $2.50/ female condom; $8/applicator kit of spermicide foam and jelly ($4–$8 refills); similar prices for creams, films, and suppositories
Diaphram or cervical cap	$13–$25/diaphragm or cap; $50–$125/examination; $4–$8/ supplies of spermicide jelly or cream
Fertility awareness methods	$5–$8 and up for temperature kits; free classes often available in health and church centers

Note: Some family planning clinics charge for services on a sliding scale according to income.
Source: Reprinted with permission from Planned Parenthood Federation of America, Inc. © 2001 PPFA. All rights reserved.

"outercourse." Like abstinence, outercourse can be 100 percent effective for birth control as long as the male does not ejaculate near the vaginal opening. Unlike abstinence, however, outercourse is not 100 percent effective against sexually transmitted infections (STIs). Oral-genital contact can transmit disease, although the practice can be made safer by using a condom on the penis or a dental dam on the vaginal opening.

Fertility Awareness Methods

Methods of fertility control that rely upon the alteration of sexual behavior are called **fertility awareness methods (FAMs).** These techniques include observing female "fertile periods" and abstaining from sexual intercourse (penis-vagina contact) during these fertile times.

Two decades ago, the "rhythm method" was ridiculed because of its low effectiveness rates. However, it was the only method of birth control available to women belonging to religious denominations that forbade the use of oral contraceptives, barrier methods, and sterilization. Our present reproductive knowledge enables women and their partners to use natural methods of birth control with fewer risks of pregnancy, although these methods remain far less effective than others.

Fertility awareness methods rely upon a knowledge of basic physiology (see Figure 7.5.) A released ovum can survive for up to 48 hours after ovulation. Sperm can live for as

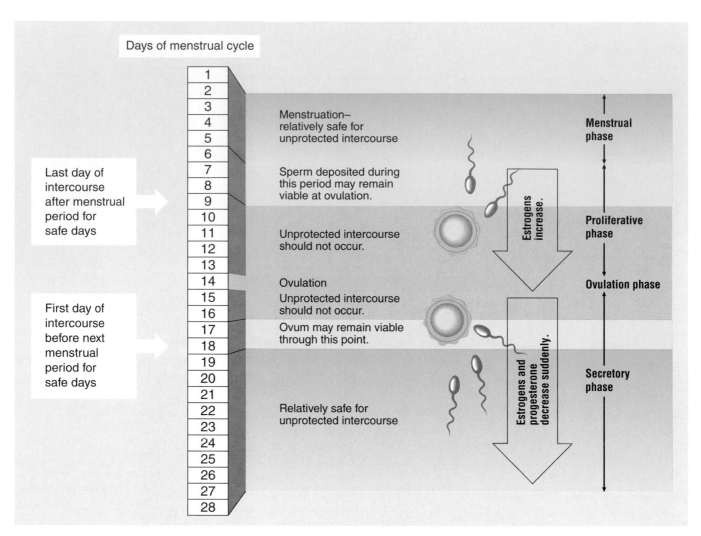

Days of menstrual cycle

1	
2	
3	
4	Menstruation– relatively safe for unprotected intercourse
5	
6	
7	Sperm deposited during this period may remain viable at ovulation.
8	
9	
10	Unprotected intercourse should not occur.
11	
12	
13	
14	Ovulation
15	Unprotected intercourse should not occur.
16	
17	Ovum may remain viable through this point.
18	
19	
20	
21	
22	Relatively safe for unprotected intercourse
23	
24	
25	
26	
27	
28	

Last day of intercourse after menstrual period for safe days

First day of intercourse before next menstrual period for safe days

Estrogens increase.

Estrogens and progesterone decrease suddenly.

Menstrual phase

Proliferative phase

Ovulation phase

Secretory phase

Figure 7.5
The Fertility Cycle
Fertility awareness methods can combine the use of a calendar, the cervical mucous method, and body temperature measurements to identify the fertile period. It is important to remember that most women do not have a consistent 28-day cycle.

Cervical mucous method A birth control method that relies upon observation of changes in cervical mucous to determine when the woman is fertile so the couple can abstain from intercourse during those times.

Body temperature method A birth control method in which a woman monitors her body temperature for the rise that signals ovulation in order to abstain from intercourse around this time.

Calendar method A birth control method in which a woman's menstrual cycle is mapped on a calendar to determine presumed fertile times in order to abstain from penis-vagina contact during those times.

long as five days in the vagina. Natural methods of birth control teach women to recognize their fertile times. Changes in cervical mucous prior to and during ovulation and a rise in basal body temperature are two frequently used indicators. Another method involves charting a woman's menstrual cycle and ovulation times on a calendar. Women may use any combination of these methods to determine their fertile times more accurately.

Cervical Mucous Method The **cervical mucous method** requires women to examine the consistency and color of their normal vaginal secretions. Prior to ovulation, vaginal mucous becomes gelatinous and stretchy, and normal vaginal secretions may increase. Sexual activity involving penis-vagina contact must be avoided while this "fertile mucous" is present and for several days following the mucous changes (see Figure 7.6).

Body Temperature Method The **body temperature method** relies on the fact that the female's basal body temperature

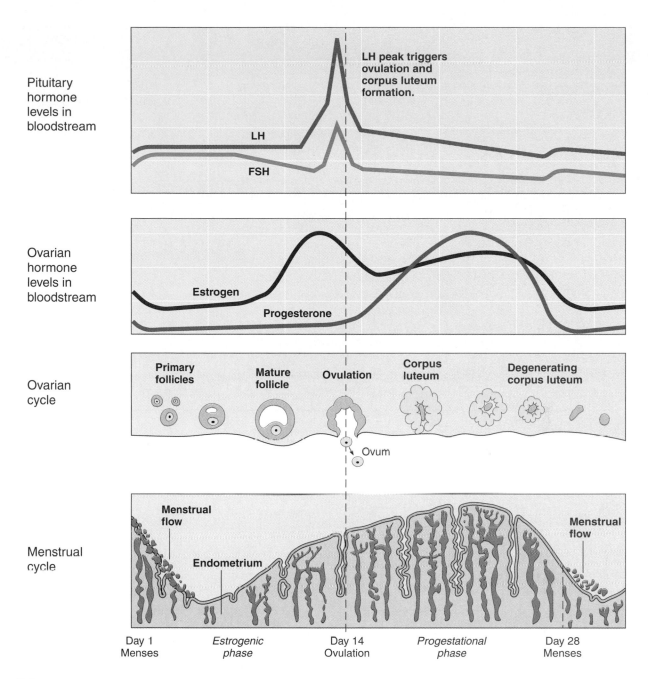

Figure 7.6
Some Bodily Changes That Occur during the Menstrual Cycle

rises between 0.4 and 0.8 degree after ovulation has occurred. For this method to be effective, the woman must chart her temperature for several months to learn to recognize her body's temperature fluctuations. Abstinence from penis-vagina contact must be observed preceding the temperature rise until several days after the temperature rise was first noted.

The Calendar Method The **calendar method** requires the woman to record the exact number of days in her menstrual cycle. Since few women menstruate with complete regularity, this involves keeping a record of the menstrual cycle for 12 months, during which time some other method of birth con-

trol must be used. The first day of a woman's period counts as day 1. To determine the first fertile, unsafe day of the cycle, she subtracts 18 from the number of days in the shortest cycle. To determine the last unsafe day of the cycle, she subtracts 11 from the number of days in the longest cycle. This method assumes that ovulation occurs during the midpoint of the cycle. The couple must abstain from penis-vagina contact during the fertile time.

Women interested in fertility awareness methods of birth control are advised to take supervised classes in their use. Women who are untrained in these techniques run a high risk of unwanted pregnancy.

Facts about Abortion

Because abortion is an issue intensely debated in the media, most of us have heard numerous facts, opinions, and arguments about the subject. How well do the following facts match your understanding of the practice of abortion in the United States and abroad?

✔ Worldwide, more than a quarter of women who become pregnant have either an abortion or an unwanted child.

✔ Each year, an estimated 80,000 women die from complications of unsafe abortion, accounting for 13 percent of the global maternal mortality.

✔ Seventy percent of U.S. abortions are obtained by white women, 20 percent by black women, and 10 percent by other women of color.

✔ Seven percent of abortions are performed in hospitals, 4 percent in private physicians' offices, and 89 percent in clinics.

✔ In the United States, 25 percent of women seeking an abortion must travel more than 50 miles.

✔ In 95 percent of rural U.S. counties, there is no abortion provider.

✔ The National Cancer Institute and the American Cancer Society have concluded that induced abortion *does not* increase the risk of breast cancer.

✔ Ninety percent of all abortions occur by the end of the first 12 weeks of pregnancy.

✔ Of the 46 million abortions that occur worldwide each year, roughly 20 million are performed under unsafe conditions because of poorly trained providers, unsanitary circumstances, and crude and dangerous methods of self-inducement.

Sources: "Facts in Brief: Induced Abortion," Alan Guttmacher Institute, 1999; "Unsafe Abortion around the World," Planned Parenthood Fact Sheet, 2002; Loretta Ross, "Emergency Memorandum to Women of Color" in *From Abortion to Reproductive Freedom* (Boston: South End Press, 1990), p. 149; S. K. Henshaw, "Abortion Incidence and Services in the United States, 1995–1996," *Family Planning Perspectives* 30: (6), 1998; Abortion Access Project, Brochure, 1999; "Induced Abortion Does Not Increase the Risk of Breast Cancer," Fact Sheet No. 240, World Health Organization, June 2000; The Center for Reproductive Law and Policy, "Myths about 'Partial-Birth' Abortion Bans," March 11, 1998.

Abortion

In 1973, the landmark U.S. Supreme Court decision in *Roe v. Wade* stated that the "right to privacy . . . founded on the Fourteenth Amendment's concept of personal liberty . . . is broad enough to encompass a woman's decision whether or not to terminate her pregnancy."[5] The decision maintained that during the first trimester of pregnancy, a woman and her practitioner have the right to terminate the pregnancy through **abortion** without legal restrictions. It allowed individual states to set conditions for second-trimester abortions. Third-trimester abortions were ruled illegal unless the mother's life or health was in danger.

Prior to the legalization of first- and second-trimester abortions, women wishing to terminate a pregnancy had to travel to a country where the procedure was legal, consult an illegal abortionist, or perform their own abortions. Approximately 480,000 illegal abortions were performed in the United States each year, one-third of them on married women. These procedures led to death from hemorrhage or infection in some cases and to infertility from internal scarring in others.

People who oppose abortion believe that the embryo or fetus is a human being with rights that must be protected. The political debate continues as opponents of abortion pressure state and local governments to pass laws prohibiting the use of public funds for abortion and abortion counseling. In recent years, new legislation has given states the right to impose certain restrictions on abortions. Abortions cannot be performed in publicly funded clinics in some states, and other states have laws requiring parental notification before a teenager can obtain an abortion. Although *Roe v. Wade* has not been overturned, it faces many future challenges.

Although many opponents work through the courts and the political process, attacks on abortion clinics and on doctors who perform abortions are increasingly common. Nearly all clinics have faced some form of threats or acts of violence. Recent legal changes, such as the Freedom of Access to Clinic Entrance Act (FACE), offer some relief from the harassment and violence directed at abortion clinics. However, because of such acts, the biggest threat to a woman's access to an abortion now is finding a clinic rather than legal restrictions.[6] See the Reality Check box for more information on abortion access and prevalence.

The best birth control methods can fail. Women may be raped. Pregnancies can occur despite every possible precaution. When an unwanted pregnancy does occur, the decision whether to terminate, carry to term and keep the baby, or carry to term and give the baby away must be made. This is a personal decision that each woman must make, based on her personal beliefs, values, and resources, after carefully considering all alternatives. For a discussion on how abortion is perceived in different countries, see the Health in a Diverse World box.

International Access to Abortion

The United States has had a long struggle over the issue of abortion. A review of laws and guidelines in other countries shows that different cultures have their own customs and beliefs about the practice of abortion. Here's a look at some international differences.

- Over 41 percent of the world's population live in countries that do not require women seeking abortion to meet specific "reason" requirements, meaning that they don't have to explain why they desire an abortion.
- Fourteen countries (including India, Great Britain, and Zimbabwe) have laws that instruct health care providers to consider a woman's economic or social situation in providing abortion services. Women who can show that carrying a baby to term would cause hardship are permitted abortions.
- Thirteen percent of the world's population (53 nations) permit abortion only when the pregnancy poses a threat to the woman's health or safety. Some countries have specific guidelines for determining threat, whereas others allow room for interpretation. For example, in Jamaica, a woman's mental health can be considered, but in Peru there must be a physical threat of permanent injury if the woman carries to term.
- The most stringent laws, those prohibiting abortion completely or allowing abortion only in cases where the mother's life is endangered, are in place in 74 nations (representing 21 percent of the world's population), mainly in Africa and Latin America. In these nations, there can be criminal penalties for both the woman and the abortion provider.
- Fourteen countries require a husband to provide authorization before his wife can receive abortion services. These countries include Japan, Iraq, Syria, and Turkey.

Sources: From "Reproductive Rights 2000: Moving Forward," electronic edition, by The Center for Reproductive Law and Policy (see http://www.crlp.org/ pub_bo_rr2k.html); and "A Global Review of Laws on Induced Abortion, 1985–1997," by A. Rahman, L. Katzive, and S. Fienshaw, 1998, *International Family Planning Perspectives* 24.

Methods of Abortion

The type of abortion procedure is determined by how many weeks the woman has been pregnant. Length of pregnancy is calculated from the first day of her last menstrual period.

If performed during the first trimester of pregnancy, abortion presents a relatively low risk to the mother. The most commonly used method of first-trimester abortion is **vacuum aspiration.** The procedure is usually performed under a local anesthetic. The cervix is dilated with instruments or by placing *laminaria,* a sterile seaweed product, in the cervical canal. The laminaria is left in place for a few hours or overnight and slowly dilates the cervix. After it is removed, a long tube is inserted into the uterus through the cervix, and gentle suction removes fetal tissue from the uterine walls (see Figure 7.7).

Pregnancies that progress into the second trimester can be terminated through **dilation and evacuation (D&E),** a procedure that combines vacuum aspiration with a technique called **dilation and curettage (D&C).** For this procedure, the cervix is dilated with laminaria for one to two days,

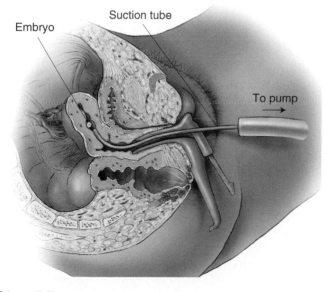

Embryo

Suction tube

To pump

Figure 7.7
Vacuum Aspiration Abortion

Abortion   The medical means of terminating a pregnancy.

Vacuum aspiration   The use of gentle suction to remove fetal tissue from the uterus.

Dilation and evacuation (D&E)   An abortion technique that combines vacuum aspiration with dilation and curettage; fetal tissue is both sucked and scraped out of the uterus.

Dilation and curettage (D&C)   An abortion technique in which the cervix is dilated with laminaria for one to two days, after which the uterine walls are scraped clean.

Emotional Aspects of Abortion

The emotional aftereffects of abortion have been the subject of much interest. Do women who have had abortions suffer symptoms similar to those of post-traumatic stress syndrome? Are they forever haunted by the experience of having had an abortion?

Although a variety of feelings, such as regret, guilt, sadness, relief, and happiness, are normal, no evidence has shown that having an abortion causes long-term psy-

chological trauma for a woman. In a longitudinal study of over 5,000 women who had had abortions, researchers Russo and Dabul found that the best predictor of a woman's emotional well-being following an abortion was her emotional well-being prior to the abortion. Even factors such as marital status or affiliation with a religion that is strongly anti-abortion were found to have no effect on a woman's later sense of self-esteem and well-being.

A small percentage of women who have abortions experience depressive symptoms similar to postpartum blues, but the vast majority express no regrets about

their decision and state they would make the choice again if they found themselves in similar circumstances. Certainly the presence of a support network and the assistance of mental health professionals would be helpful to any woman who is struggling with the emotional aspects of the abortion decision in her own life.

Sources: From "The Relationship of Abortion to Well-Being: Do Race and Religion Make a Difference?" by N. F. Russo and A. J. Dabul, Ph.D., *Professional Psychology: Research and Practice* 28 (1) (2000); Fact Sheet, "The Emotional Effects of Induced Abortion," Planned Parenthood, May 2000.

---

and a combination of instruments and vacuum aspiration is used to empty the uterus. Second-trimester abortions are frequently done under general anesthetic. Both procedures can be performed on an outpatient basis (usually in the physician's office), with or without pain medication. Generally, however, the woman is given a mild tranquilizer to help her relax. Both procedures may cause moderate-to-severe uterine cramping and blood loss.

Two other methods used in second-trimester abortions, though less common than the D&E, are prostaglandin or saline **induction abortions.** Prostaglandin hormones or a saline solution is injected into the uterus, which kills the fetus and initiates labor contractions. After 24 to 48 hours, the fetus and placenta are expelled from the uterus.

The **hysterotomy,** or surgical removal of the fetus from the uterus, may be used during emergencies, when the mother's life may be in danger, or when other types of abortions are deemed too dangerous.

The risks associated with abortions include infection, incomplete abortion (when parts of the placenta remain in the uterus), missed abortion (when the fetus is not actually removed), excessive bleeding, and cervical and uterine trauma. Follow-up and attention to dangerous signs decrease the chances of developing long-term problems. See the Women's Health/Men's Health box for an overview of possible emotional aspects of the decision to abort.

The mortality rate for first-trimester abortions averages 1 death for every 530,000 at eight or fewer weeks. The rate for second-trimester abortions is higher than 1 per 17,000.[7] This higher rate later in the pregnancy is due to the increased risk of uterine perforation, bleeding, infection, and incomplete abortion due to the fact that the uterine wall becomes thinner as the pregnancy progresses.

One surgical method of performing abortion has been the subject of much controversy. **Intact dilation and extraction (D&X),** sometimes referred to by the nonmedical term

"partial-birth abortion," is used only in certain cases, such as when other abortion methods could injure the mother. The procedure generally involves repositioning the fetus to a breech (feet-first) position before extracting most of the body except for the head. The contents of the cranium are then aspirated, resulting in "vaginal delivery of a dead but otherwise intact fetus."[8] Thirty-one states have passed legislation attempting to ban intact dilation and extraction. However, the wording of the legislation in many states has been so general that it could be used to ban all types of abortion. For this reason, such legislation has often been challenged and only 10 states currently fully enforce the laws as written. Professional organizations such as the American College of Obstetrics and Gynecology and the American Medical Association state that physicians, acting in the best interests of their patients, should choose the safest and most appropriate method of abortion in each individual case.

Mifepristone (RU-486)

In September 2000, the U.S. Food and Drug Administration approved **mifepristone,** also known as RU-486, after a 20-year odyssey. Mifepristone is a steroid hormone that induces abortion by blocking the action of progesterone, a hormone produced by the ovaries and placenta that maintains the lining of the uterus. Similar in structure to progesterone, mifepristone binds to cell receptor sites normally occupied by progesterone, causing the uterine lining to break down. As a result, the uterine lining and the embryo are expelled from the uterus, terminating the pregnancy.

Mifepristone's nickname, "the abortion pill," may imply an easy process. However, this treatment actually involves more steps than a clinical abortion, which takes approximately 15 minutes, followed by a physical recovery of about one day. With mifepristone, a first visit to the clinic involves a physical exam and a dose of three tablets, which may cause minor side effects such as nausea, headaches, weakness, and fatigue. The patient returns two days later for a dose of prostaglandins (trade name: misoprostal), which cause uterine contractions that expel the fertilized egg. Women are required to stay under observation at the clinic for four hours.

Ninety-six percent of women who take mifepristone and prostaglandins during the first nine weeks of pregnancy will experience a complete abortion. A return visit is required 12 days later because the pills fail to expel the fetus completely in 4 percent of cases. In such an event, a clinical abortion becomes necessary.[9]

The side effects of this treatment are similar to those reported during heavy menstruation and include cramping, minor pain, and nausea. Approximately 1 in 1,000 women requires a blood transfusion because of severe bleeding. The procedure does not require hospitalization; women may be treated on an outpatient basis.

> **What do you think?**
>
> *If you or your partner unexpectedly became pregnant, would you choose to terminate the pregnancy? ✳ How might an abortion affect your relationship? ✳ What factors would you consider in making your decision? ✳ Why?*

Planning a Pregnancy

The many methods available to control fertility give you choices that did not exist when your parents—and even you—were born. If you are in the process of deciding whether to have children, take the time to evaluate your emotions, finances, and health.

Emotional Health

First and foremost, you need to evaluate why you want to have a child: to fulfill an inner need to carry on the family? To escape loneliness? Are there any other reasons? Can you care for this new human being in a loving and nurturing manner? Are you ready to make all the sacrifices necessary to bear and raise a child?

If you feel, based on your self-evaluation, that you are ready to be a parent, the next step is preparation. You can prepare for this change in your life in several ways: Read about parenthood, take classes, talk to parents of children of all ages, and join a support group. If you choose to adopt, you will find many support groups available to you as well.

Maternal Health

Before becoming pregnant, a woman should have a thorough medical examination. **Preconception care** should include assessment of potential complications. Medical problems such as diabetes and high blood pressure should be discussed,

as should any genetic disorders that run in the family. Additional suggestions for a healthy pregnancy include:

- If you smoke and drink, stop.
- Reduce or eliminate caffeine intake.
- Avoid x-rays and environmental chemicals, such as lawn and garden chemicals.
- Maintain a normal weight; lose weight if necessary.
- Prior to becoming pregnant, get any dental x-rays that will be needed for a checkup.

Paternal Health

It is common wisdom that mothers-to-be should steer clear of toxic chemicals that can cause birth defects. Even women who are trying to conceive are cautioned to avoid toxic environments, eat a nourishing diet, stop smoking and drinking alcohol, and avoid most medications. Now similar precautions are recommended for fathers-to-be. New research suggests that a man's exposure to chemicals influences not only his ability to father a child but also the future health of his child.

Fathers-to-be have been overlooked in past preconception and prenatal studies for several reasons. Researchers assumed that the genetic damage leading to birth defects and other health problems occurred while a child was in the mother's womb. After all, they reasoned, that's where embryonic and fetal development take place. Conventional medical wisdom also held that defective-looking sperm (those with misshapen heads, crooked tails, or retarded swimming ability) were incapable of fertilizing an egg.

Scientists have recently discovered that how sperm look has little to do with how they act. Misshapen sperm can penetrate an egg, and they do not necessarily carry defective genetic goods. Moreover, sperm that look healthy and swim well can be the true genetic culprits. DNA fluorescent

---

Induction abortion   A type of abortion in which chemicals are injected into the uterus through the uterine wall; labor begins and the woman delivers a dead fetus.

Hysterotomy   The surgical removal of the fetus from the uterus.

Intact dilation and extraction (D&X)   A late-term abortion procedure in which the body of the fetus is extracted up to the head and then the contents of the cranium are aspirated.

Mifepristone   A steroid hormone that induces abortion by blocking the action of progesterone.

Preconception care   Medical care received prior to becoming pregnant that helps a woman assess and address potential maternal health.

markers have identified normal-looking, yet genetically flawed, sperm that carry too many or too few chromosomes. Fathers contribute the extra chromosome 21 in about 6 percent of children with Down syndrome, which causes mental retardation; the extra X chromosome in 50 percent of boys with **Klinefelter's syndrome,** which causes abnormal sexual development; and the shortened chromosome 15 in about 85 percent of children with **Prader-Willi syndrome,** a disorder characterized by retardation and obesity.

Although some birth defects are caused by random errors of nature, it now appears that some disorders can be traced to sperm damaged by chemicals. Sperm are naturally vulnerable to toxic assault and genetic damage. Many drugs and ingested chemicals can readily invade the testes from the bloodstream; others ambush sperm after they leave the testes and pass through the epididymides, where they mature and are stored. By one route or another, half of 100 chemicals studied so far (including by-products of cigarette smoke) apparently harm sperm.

Some researchers believe that Vitamin C is nature's way of protecting sex cells from damage. Bad diets, exposure to toxic chemicals, cigarette smoking, and not enough foods rich in vitamin C are probably the biggest culprits in sperm damage.[10]

Financial Evaluation

Another important consideration is finances. First check your medical insurance: Does it provide pregnancy benefits? If not, you can expect to pay between $1,500 and $5,000 for medical care during pregnancy and birth—and substantially more if complications arise. Both partners should find out about their employers' policies concerning parental leave, including length of leave available and conditions for returning to work.

The U.S. Department of Agriculture estimates that it will cost $169,920 to raise a child born in 2001 to the age of 17. Housing costs and food are the two largest expenditures in raising children.[11] Can you afford to give your child the life you would like him or her to enjoy?

The cost of a college education is another consideration. If costs continue to rise by about 5 percent, the four-year cost of a college education at a private college will reach almost $257,000 by the year 2019.[12]

Also consider the cost and availability of quality child care. Prospective parents should realistically assess how much family assistance they can expect with a new baby as well as the availability of nonfamily child care. While you may be aware of the federal tax credit available for child care, you may not realize how little assistance it actually provides: between a maximum of $480 for one child in a family having income of over $28,000 to a maximum of $720 for one child in a family having income of under $10,000. A second child doubles the credit, but no further assistance is provided for a third child or more children. How much does full-time child care cost? It averages between $5,000 and $10,000 a year, depending on your location (urban areas tend to have higher costs).

Contingency Planning

A final consideration is how to provide for the child should something happen to you and your partner. If both of you were to die while the child is young, do you have relatives or close friends who would raise the child? If you have more than one child, would they have to be split up or could they be kept together? Though unpleasant to think about, this sort of contingency planning is very important. Children who lose their parents are heartbroken and confused. A prearranged plan of action will smooth their transition into new families.

What do you think?

What factors will you consider in deciding whether or when to have children? ✳ *Is there a certain age at which you feel you will be ready to be a parent?* ✳ *What goals do you hope to achieve prior to undertaking parenthood?* ✳ *What are your biggest concerns about parenthood?*

Pregnancy

Pregnancy is an important event in a woman's life. The actions taken before a pregnancy begins, as well as behaviors during pregnancy, can have a significant effect on the health of both infant and mother.

Prenatal Care

A successful pregnancy depends on the mother's taking good care of herself and the fetus. It is essential to have regular medical checkups, beginning as soon as possible (certainly within the first three months). Early detection of fetal abnormalities and identification of high-risk mothers and infants are the major purposes of prenatal care. On the first visit, the practitioner should obtain a complete medical history of the mother and her family and note any hereditary conditions that could put a woman or her fetus at risk.

Regular checkups to measure weight gain and blood pressure and to monitor the size and position of the fetus should continue throughout the pregnancy. This early care reduces infant mortality and low birthweight. A study group for the American College of Obstetricians and Gynecologists recommends seven or eight prenatal visits for women with low-risk pregnancies. Unfortunately, prenatal care is not available to everyone. Approximately 30 percent of pregnant teenagers and unmarried women do not receive adequate prenatal attention. Babies of mothers who received no prenatal care are about 10 times more likely to die in the first month of life than babies of mothers who did get prenatal care.

Additional concerns include the mother's physical condition, her level of nutrition, her confidence in her ability to give birth, her use of drugs and medications, and the availability of a skilled practitioner who can oversee the pregnancy

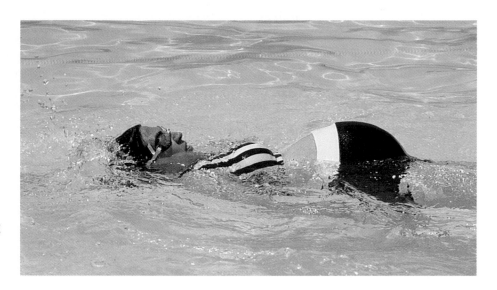

A doctor-approved exercise program during pregnancy can help control weight, make delivery easier, and have a healthy effect on the fetus.

and delivery. A woman planning a pregnancy also needs a support system (spouse or partner, family, friends, community groups) willing to provide love and emotional support during and after her pregnancy.

Choosing a Practitioner   A woman should carefully choose a practitioner to attend her pregnancy and delivery. If possible, this choice should be made before she becomes pregnant. Recommendations from friends are a good starting point. The woman's family physician may also be able to recommend a specialist.

When choosing a practitioner, parents should ask about credentials, professional qualifications, and experience. Besides this information, a pregnant woman must ask questions specific to her condition. Prospective parents should also inquire about the practitioner's experience in handling various complications, commitment to being at the mother's side during delivery, and beliefs and practices concerning the use of anesthesia, fetal monitoring, induced labor, and forceps delivery. What are the practitioner's attitudes toward birth control, abortion, and alternative birthing procedures? The practitioner's approach to nutrition and medication during pregnancy should be similar to the woman's own. Finally, the parents must learn under what circumstances the practitioner would perform a cesarean section.

Two types of physicians can attend pregnancies and deliveries. The *obstetrician-gynecologist* (ob-gyn) is an M.D. who specializes in obstetrics (pregnancy and birth) and gynecology (care of women's reproductive organs). These practitioners are trained to handle all types of pregnancy- and delivery-related emergencies.

A *family practitioner* is a licensed M.D. who provides comprehensive care for people of all ages. The majority of family practitioners have obstetrical experience but will refer a patient to a specialist if necessary. Unlike the ob-gyn, the family practitioner can serve as the baby's physician after attending the birth.

Midwives are also experienced practitioners who can attend both pregnancies and deliveries. *Certified nurse-midwives* are registered nurses having specialized training in pregnancy and delivery. Most midwives work in private practice or in conjunction with physicians. Those who work with physicians have access to traditional medical facilities to which they can turn in an emergency. *Lay midwives* may or may not have extensive training in handling an emergency. They may be self-taught or trained through formal certification procedures.

Alcohol and Drugs   A woman should avoid all types of drugs during pregnancy. Even common over-the-counter medications such as aspirin and beverages such as coffee and tea can damage a developing fetus.

During the first three months of pregnancy, the fetus is especially subject to the **teratogenic** (birth defect–causing) effects of some chemical substances. The fetus can also develop an addiction to or tolerance for drugs that the mother is using. Of particular concern to medical professionals is the use of tobacco and alcohol during pregnancy.

Women who are heavy drinkers may have normal first babies but subsequently deliver children having fetal alcohol syndrome. The symptoms of **fetal alcohol syndrome (FAS)**

Klinefelter's syndrome   A chromosome defect that causes abnormal sexual development.

Prader-Willi syndrome   A disorder characterized by mental retardation and obesity.

Midwives   Experienced practitioners who assist with pregnancy and delivery.

Teratogenic   Causing birth defects; may refer to drugs, environmental chemicals, x-rays, or diseases.

Fetal alcohol syndrome (FAS)   A collection of symptoms, including mental retardation, that can appear in infants of women who drink too much alcohol during pregnancy.

include mental retardation, slowed nerve reflexes, and small head size. The exact amount of alcohol necessary to cause FAS is not known, but researchers doubt that any alcohol is safe. Therefore, they recommend total abstinence from alcohol during pregnancy.

Studies have shown a 25 to 50 percent higher rate of fetal and infant deaths among women who smoke during pregnancy compared with those who do not.[13] Women who smoke more than 10 to 15 cigarettes a day during pregnancy have higher rates of miscarriage, stillbirth, premature births, and low-birthweight babies than do nonsmokers. Smoking restricts the blood supply to the developing fetus and thus limits oxygen and nutrition delivery and waste removal. It appears to be a significant factor in the development of cleft lip and palate, and a significant relationship has been shown between both smoking and "secondhand" smoke and sudden infant death syndrome.[14] Research on the fetal effects of secondhand or sidestream smoke (inhaling smoke produced by others) is inconclusive, but babies whose parents smoke can be twice as susceptible to pneumonia, bronchitis, and related illnesses as other babies. Recent statistics for the United States show that tobacco use among pregnant women has steadily fallen since 1989, when about 20 percent of pregnant women smoked. In 1998, that rate had declined to 12.9 percent.[15]

X-rays   X-rays present a clear danger to the fetus. Although most diagnostic tests produce minimal amounts of radiation, even low levels may cause birth defects or other problems, particularly if several low-dose x-rays are taken over a short time period. Pregnant women are advised to avoid x-rays unless absolutely necessary.

Nutrition and Exercise   Pregnant women need additional protein, calories, vitamins, and minerals, so their diets should be carefully monitored by a qualified practitioner. Special attention should be paid to getting enough folic acid (found in dark, leafy greens), iron (dried fruits, meats, legumes, liver, egg yolks), calcium (nonfat or low-fat dairy products, some canned fish), and fluids.

Vitamin supplements can correct some deficiencies, but there is no substitute for a well-balanced diet. Babies born to poorly nourished mothers run high risks of substandard mental and physical development. Folic acid, when consumed before and during early pregnancy, reduces the risk of spina bifida, a common disabling birth condition resulting from failure of the spinal column to close. Manufacturers of

breads, pastas, rice, and other grain products are now required to add folic acid to their products to reduce neural tube defects in newborns.

Weight gain during pregnancy helps nourish a growing baby. For a woman of normal weight before pregnancy, the recommended weight gain during pregnancy is 25–35 pounds. For obese or overweight women, 15–25 pounds are recommended. Underweight women can gain 28–40 pounds, and women carrying twins should gain about 35–45 pounds. Gaining too much or too little weight can lead to complications. With higher weight gains, women may develop gestational diabetes, hypertension, or increased risk of delivery complications. Gaining too little weight increases the chance of a low-birthweight baby.

Of the total number of pounds gained during pregnancy, about 6–8 are the baby's weight. The baby's birthweight is important, since low weight can mean health problems during labor and the baby's first few months. Pregnancy is not the time to think about losing weight—doing so may endanger the fetus.[16]

As in all other stages of life, exercise is an important factor in weight control during pregnancy and overall maternal health. In one study a balanced 45-minute exercise session three days per week was associated with heavier-birthweight babies, fewer surgical births, and shorter hospital stays after birth. Pregnant women should consult their physicians before starting any exercise program.

Other Factors   A pregnant woman should avoid exposure to toxic chemicals, heavy metals, pesticides, gases, and other hazardous compounds. She should not clean cat-litter boxes because cat feces can contain organisms that cause a disease called **toxoplasmosis**. If a pregnant woman contracts this disease, her baby may be stillborn or suffer mental retardation or other birth defects.

Before becoming pregnant, a woman should be tested to determine if she has had rubella (German measles). If she has not had rubella, she should be immunized for it and wait the recommended length of time before becoming pregnant. A rubella infection can kill the fetus or cause blindness or hearing disorders. If the woman has ever had genital herpes, she should inform her physician. The physician may want to deliver the baby by cesarean section, especially if the woman has active lesions. Contact with an active herpes infection during birth can be fatal to the infant.

Toxoplasmosis   A disease caused by an organism found in cat feces that, when contracted by a pregnant woman, may result in stillbirth or an infant with mental retardation or birth defects.

What do you think?

In looking at your current lifestyle, what behaviors (e.g., nutritional choices, fitness, etc.) would you cease or begin in order to promote a healthy pregnancy? ✳ *What characteristics or skills would you look for in selecting a health care provider for care during your own or your partner's pregnancy?*

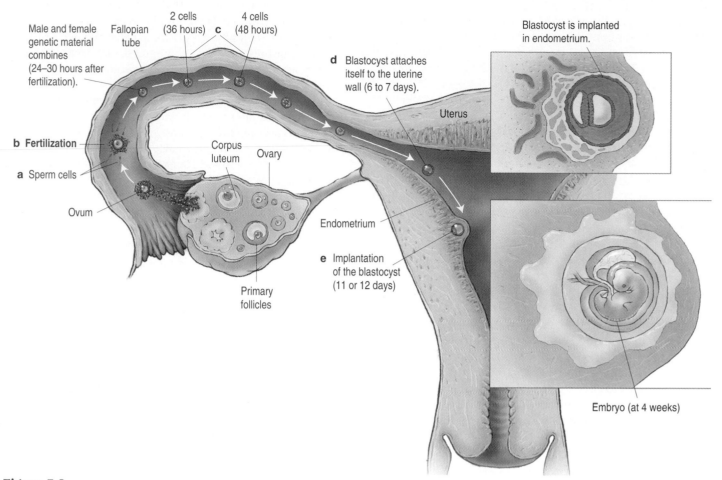

Male and female genetic material combines (24–30 hours after fertilization).

Fallopian tube

2 cells (36 hours) **c** **4 cells (48 hours)**

d Blastocyst attaches itself to the uterine wall (6 to 7 days).

Uterus

Blastocyst is implanted in endometrium.

b Fertilization

Corpus luteum

Ovary

a Sperm cells

Ovum

Endometrium

e Implantation of the blastocyst (11 or 12 days)

Primary follicles

Embryo (at 4 weeks)

Figure 7.8

Fertilization

(a) The efforts of hundreds of sperm may allow one sperm to penetrate the ovum's corona radiata, an outer layer of cells, and then the zona pellucida, a thick inner membrane. (b) The sperm nucleus fuses with the egg nucleus at fertilization, producing a zygote. (c) The zygote divides first into two cells, then four cells, and so on. (d) The blastocyst attaches itself to the uterine wall. (e) The blastocyst implants itself in the endometrium.

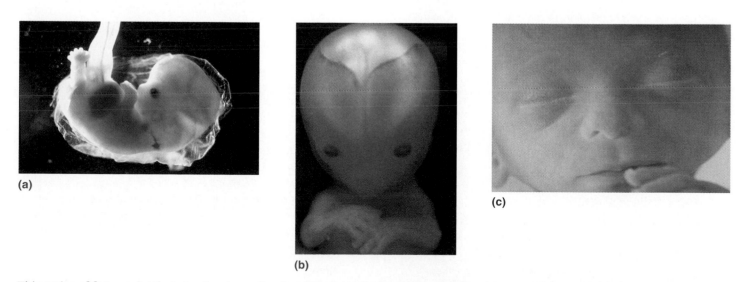

(a)

(b)

(c)

This series of fetoscopic photographs shows the development of a fetus from the first (a), second (b), and third (c) trimesters of pregnancy.

A Woman's Reproductive Years

More than half of the average American woman's expected life span is spent between menarche (first menses) and menopause (last menses), a period of approximately 40 years. Deciding if and when to have children, as well as how to prevent pregnancy when necessary, is a long-term concern.

Today, a woman over 35 who is pregnant has plenty of company. While births to women in their 20s are declining, the rate of first births to women between the ages of 30 and 39 has doubled in the past decade, and births to women over 39 have increased by more than 50 percent. Many women who wait until their 30s to consider having a child find themselves wondering, "Am I too old to have a baby?" Statistically, the chances of having a baby with birth defects do rise after the age of 35. Researchers believe that there is a decline in both the quality and viability of eggs after this age.

Down syndrome, a condition characterized by mild-to-severe mental retardation and a variety of physical abnormalities, is the most commonly occurring genetic condition. One in every 800 to 1,000 live births a year is a child with Down syndrome, representing approximately 5,000 births per year in the United States alone. A common myth is that most children with Down syndrome have older parents. The truth is that 80 percent of children born with Down syndrome are born to women younger than 35. However, the incidence does increase with age. The incidence of Down syndrome in babies born to a mother age 20 is 1 in 10,000

births; it rises to 1 in 400 by age 35, to 1 in 110 by age 40, and to 1 in 35 when she is 45.[17]

Women who delay motherhood until their late 30s also worry about their physical ability to carry and deliver their babies. For these women, a comprehensive exercise program will assist in maintaining good posture and promoting a successful delivery.

Despite these concerns, there are some advantages to having a baby later in life. In fact, many doctors note that older mothers tend to be more conscientious about following medical advice during pregnancy and more psychologically mature and ready to include an infant in their family than some younger women.

Pregnancy Testing

A woman may suspect she is pregnant before she has any pregnancy tests. A typical sign is a missed menstrual period, yet this is not always an accurate indicator. A woman can miss her period for a variety of reasons: stress, exercise, emotional upset. A pregnancy test scheduled in a medical office or birth control clinic will confirm the pregnancy. Women who wish to know immediately can purchase home pregnancy test kits, sold over the counter in drugstores. A positive test is based on the secretion of **human chorionic gonadotropin (HCG),** found in the woman's urine. Home test kits come equipped with a small sample of red blood cells coated with HCG antibodies to which the user adds a small amount of urine. If the concentration of HCG is great enough, it will clump together with the HCG antibodies, indicating that the user is pregnant.

Home pregnancy test kits are about 85 to 95 percent reliable. If done too early in the pregnancy, they may show a false negative. Other causes of false negatives are unclean test tubes, ingestion of certain drugs, and vaginal or urinary tract infections. Accuracy also depends on the quality of the test itself and the user's ability to perform it and interpret the results. Blood tests administered and analyzed by a medical laboratory are more accurate.

The Process of Pregnancy

Pregnancy begins the moment a sperm fertilizes an ovum in the fallopian tubes (see Figure 7.8). From there, the single cell multiplies, becoming a sphere-shaped cluster of cells as it travels toward the uterus, a journey that may last three to four days. Upon arrival, the embryo burrows into the thick, spongy endometrium and is nourished from this carefully prepared lining.

Early Signs of Pregnancy The first sign of pregnancy is usually a missed menstrual period (although some women "spot" in early pregnancy, and such spotting may be mistaken for a period). Other signs of pregnancy include the following:

- Breast tenderness.
- Emotional upset.
- Extreme fatigue.

Down syndrome A condition characterized by mental retardation and a variety of physical abnormalities.

Human chorionic gonadotropin (HCG) Hormone detectable in blood or urine samples of a mother within the first few weeks of pregnancy.

Trimester A three-month segment of pregnancy; used to describe specific developmental changes that occur in the embryo or fetus.

Embryo The fertilized egg from conception until the end of two months' development.

Fetus The name given the developing baby from the third month of pregnancy until birth.

Placenta The network of blood vessels, connected to the umbilical cord, that carries nutrients to the developing infant and carries wastes away.

Fourth trimester The first six weeks of an infant's life outside the womb.

Amniocentesis A medical test in which a small amount of fluid is drawn from the amniotic sac to test for Down syndrome and genetic diseases.

Amniotic sac The protective pouch surrounding the baby.

- Nausea.
- Sleeplessness.
- Vomiting (especially in the morning).

Pregnancy typically lasts 40 weeks. The due date is calculated from the expectant mother's last menstrual period. Pregnancy is typically divided into three phases, or **trimesters,** of approximately three months each.

The First Trimester   During the first trimester, few noticeable changes occur in the mother's body. The expectant mother may urinate more frequently and experience morning sickness, swollen breasts, or undue fatigue. But these symptoms may not be frequent or severe, so she may not even realize she is pregnant unless she has a pregnancy test.

During the first two months after conception, the **embryo** differentiates and develops its various organ systems, beginning with the nervous and circulatory systems. At the start of the third month, the embryo is called a **fetus,** indicating that all organ systems are in place. For the rest of the pregnancy, growth and refinement occur in each major body system so that they can function independently, yet in coordination, at birth. The accompanying photos illustrate physical changes during fetal development.

The Second Trimester   At the beginning of the second trimester, physical changes in the mother become more visible. Her breasts swell and her waistline thickens. During this time, the fetus makes greater demands upon the mother's body. In particular, the **placenta,** the network of blood vessels that carry nutrients and oxygen to the fetus and fetal waste products to the mother, becomes well established.

The Third Trimester   From the end of the sixth month through the ninth is considered the third trimester. This is the period of greatest fetal growth, when the fetus gains most of its weight. During the third trimester, the fetus must get large amounts of calcium, iron, and nitrogen from the food the mother eats. Approximately 85 percent of the calcium and iron the mother digests goes into the fetal bloodstream.

Although the fetus may live if it is born during the seventh month, it needs the layer of fat it acquires during the eighth month and time for the organs (especially the respiratory and digestive organs) to develop to their full potential. Infants born prematurely usually require intensive medical care.

Of course, the process of pregnancy involves much more than the changes in a woman's body. Many important emotional changes occur from the time a woman learns she is pregnant through the "**fourth trimester**" (the first six weeks of an infant's life outside the womb). Table 7.4 on page 200 outlines common emotions and emotional challenges that may arise over the course of pregnancy.

Prenatal Testing and Screening

Modern technology enables medical practitioners to detect health defects in a fetus as early as the fourteenth to eigh-

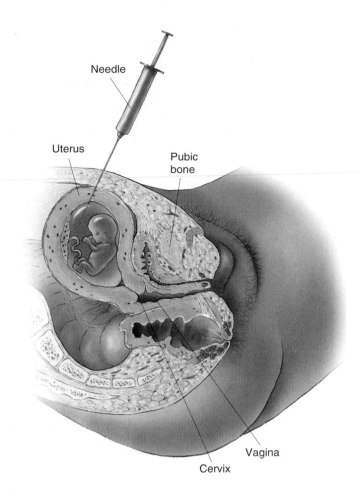

Figure 7.9
Amniocentesis
The process of amniocentesis can detect certain congenital problems as well as the sex of the fetus.

teenth weeks of pregnancy. One common testing procedure, **amniocentesis,** which is strongly recommended for women over age 35, involves inserting a long needle through the mother's abdominal and uterine walls into the **amniotic sac,** the protective pouch surrounding the fetus (see Figure 7.9). The needle draws out 3 to 4 teaspoons of fluid, which is analyzed for genetic information. This test can reveal the presence of 40 genetic abnormalities, including Down syndrome, Tay-Sachs disease (a fatal disorder of the nervous system common among Jewish people of Eastern European descent), and sickle-cell anemia (a debilitating blood disorder found primarily among blacks). Amniocentesis can also reveal gender, a fact many parents choose not to know until the birth. Although widely used, amniocentesis is not without risk. Chances of fetal damage and miscarriage as a result of testing are 1 in 400.

Another procedure, *ultrasound,* or *sonography,* uses high-frequency sound waves to determine the size and position of the fetus. Ultrasound can also detect defects in the central nervous system and digestive system of the fetus. Knowing the position of the fetus assists practitioners in

Table 7.4
Common Emotions Experienced throughout the Pregnancy Process

FIRST TRIMESTER	SECOND TRIMESTER	THIRD TRIMESTER	FOURTH TRIMESTER
Disbelief that one is actually pregnant	Sense that the pregnancy feels "real"	Development of emotional relationship with fetus— beginning to view it as a person as more fetal movement occurs	Sense of being overwhelmed at new responsibility— "What do we do now?"
Fear of miscarriage	Less fear of miscarriage	Fear of labor, labor complications, possible defects	Difficulty in setting limits on friend and family visits; learning to negotiate everyone's roles in baby's life
Feeling of being overwhelmed by changes	Wonder at hearing the heartbeat, beat, feeling movement, bulging tummy	Possible tiredness of pregnancy (Pregnancy seems to take over identity—"Is that all people want to talk about?")	Exhaustion and emotional vacillation due to sleep deprivation, breast-feeding
Tendency to be more emotional —crying more easily, for example	Frustration when symptoms make fulfilling other responsibilities difficult	Impatience for due date to arrive; possible frustration with limited mobility	Surprise at how slow the physical healing process may be; impatient to get back to prepregnancy shape
Apprehension about upcoming decision (screening tests, etc.)	Differing emotions about weight gain (Some enjoy it, others struggle with it.)	Interest in others' birth experiences (especially one's mother's) and parenting styles	Amazement at the birth process
Excitement about telling others about pregnancy if waiting until the end of first trimester	Excitement and anxiety in making plans for future	Excitement in making final preparations for baby, baby showers, which make the event seem more real	Excitement about future; apprehension about post–maternity leave transition, if applicable— "How will I balance everything?"
Anxiety about being a parent	Anxiety about being a parent	Anxiety about being a parent	Anxiety about being a parent

Source: Information for second and fourth trimesters adapted from "Physical and Emotional Changes," by C. M. Peterson and N. L. Stotland, 2000, *Lamaze Parents Magazine,* spring/summer issue.

performing amniocentesis and delivering the infant. New three-dimensional ultrasound techniques clarify images and improve doctors' efforts to detect and treat defects prenatally.

A third procedure, *fetoscopy,* involves making a small incision in the abdominal and uterine walls and inserting an optical viewer into the uterus to view the fetus directly. This device is used with ultrasound to determine fetal age and location of the placenta. This method is still experimental and involves some risk. It causes miscarriage in approximately 5 percent of cases.

A fourth procedure, *chorionic villus sampling (CVS),* involves snipping tissue from the developing fetal sac. CVS can be used at 10 to 12 weeks of pregnancy, and the test results are available in 12 to 48 hours. This test is an attractive option for couples whose offspring would be at high risk for Down syndrome or a debilitating hereditary disease.

If any of these tests reveals a serious birth defect, parents are advised to undergo genetic counseling. In the case of a chromosomal abnormality such as Down syndrome, the parents are usually offered the option of a therapeutic abortion. Some parents choose this option; others research the disability and decide to go ahead with the birth.

> **What do you think?**
>
> *What are your thoughts on prenatal testing?*
> * *Would you want to know if you were carrying a child with a genetic defect or other abnormality?*
> * *Why or why not?*

Childbirth

Making decisions that will affect a newborn baby begins long before the baby is born. Prospective parents need to make a number of key decisions. These include where to have the baby, whether to use drugs during labor and delivery, choice

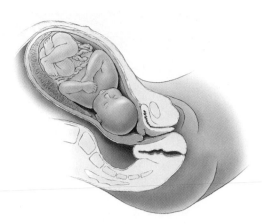

Dilation of the cervix

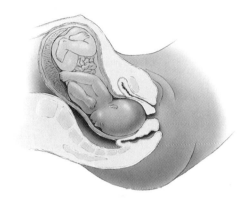

Transition ——————————— **End of Stage I**

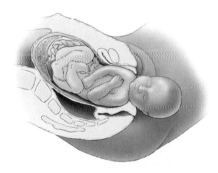

Birth of the baby (Expulsion) ——— **End of Stage II**

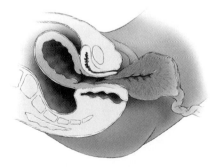

Delivery of the placenta ———— **End of Stage III**

Figure 7.10
The Birth Process

of childbirth method, and whether to breast-feed or bottle-feed. Having answers to these questions will ensure a smoother passage into parenthood.

Choosing Where to Have Your Baby

Today's prospective mothers have many delivery options, ranging from traditional hospital birth to home birth. Parental values are important. Many couples, for instance, feel that the modern medical establishment has dehumanized the birth process; thus they choose to deliver at home or at a *birthing center,* a homelike setting outside a hospital where women can give birth and receive postdelivery care by a team of professional practitioners, including physicians and registered nurses.

However, hospitals have responded to the desire for a more relaxed, less medically oriented birthing process. Many hospitals now offer labor-delivery-postpartum birthing rooms, which allow patients with noncomplicated deliveries to spend the entire process in one room. In addition, "rooming-in," or keeping the baby in the same room with the mother at all times, is encouraged to facilitate bonding and breast-feeding. Partners are generally encouraged to "room-in" with mother and baby as well.

Labor and Delivery

The birth process has three stages (see Figure 7.10). The exact mechanisms that initiate labor are unknown. During the few weeks preceding delivery, the baby normally shifts and turns to a head-down position, and the cervix begins to dilate (widen). The junction of the pubic bones also loosens to permit expansion of the pelvic girdle during birth.

In the first stage of labor, the amniotic sac breaks, causing a rush of fluid from the vagina (commonly referred to as "breaking of the waters"). Contractions in the abdomen and lower back also signal the beginning of labor. Early contractions push the baby downward, putting pressure on the cervix and dilating it further. The first stage of labor may last from a couple of hours to more than a day for a first birth, but it is usually much shorter during subsequent births.

The end of the first stage of labor, called **transition,** is the process during which the cervix becomes fully dilated and the baby's head begins to move into the vagina, or the birth canal. Contractions usually come quickly during transition, which generally lasts 30 minutes or less.

The second stage of labor (the *expulsion stage*) follows transition, when the cervix has become fully dilated. Contractions become rhythmic, stronger, and more painful as the uterus works to push the baby through the birth canal. The

Transition   The process during which the cervix becomes nearly fully dilated and the head of the fetus begins to move into the birth canal.

Tips for Managing Labor

You may not currently be pregnant or the partner of someone who is pregnant, but learning as much as possible about options for managing childbirth provides important skills you can use in the future. The following tips will help make each part of the labor process more manageable:

Early Labor (0–3 centimeters dilation)

- Alternate rest and activity: Take a walk, take a rest.
- Take a warm bath or shower.
- Change positions frequently (upright positions work best).
- Use breathing and relaxation to work through contractions.
- Stay home, where you are most comfortable, for early labor.

Active Labor (4–7 centimeters dilation)

- Change positions frequently.
- Rock in a rocking chair.

- Use gravity: Walking and squatting during contractions will help you continue to progress.
- Dim the lights, use relaxation techniques, and listen to music.

Transition (8–10 centimeters dilation)

- Focus on one contraction at a time.
- Experiment with different positions.
- Focus on breathing, and add vocalization if it helps.
- Deeply relax between contractions.

Birth

- Follow your urge to push as long as your health care provider says it's okay to do so.
- Stay calm, and make sounds if it helps.
- Try to relax the rest of your body (shoulders, neck, jaw, legs).
- Use different positions for pushing (semi-sitting, balancing on all fours, squatting).
- Watch in a mirror if it helps you to feel progress.

Before you decide to take medication during labor, consider the following points:

- If you aren't sure whether you need drugs, you probably don't.
- Don't predict the need for drugs by anticipating future pain.
- Learn the risks and benefits of various medications prior to labor so you can make an informed choice.
- Examine your assumptions and expectations regarding labor pain.

If you experience any of the following situations, medication may help you considerably:

- Your labor is very long and complicated.
- Pain interferes with your ability to concentrate or push.
- Forceps need to be used.
- Labor is progressing too quickly.
- You are too panicked or agitated to participate actively in the process.

Sources: Labor comfort measures adapted from *Prepared Childbirth: The Family Way,* by D. Amis and J. Green, 1999, Plano, TX: Family Way Publications; medication information adapted from *What to Expect When You're Expecting,* by A. Eisenberg, H. Murkoff, and S. Hathaway, 1996, New York: Workman.

---

expulsion stage lasts one to four hours and concludes when the infant is finally pushed out of the mother's body. In some cases, the attending practitioner will do an **episiotomy,** a straight incision in the mother's **perineum,** to prevent the baby's head from tearing vaginal tissues and speed the baby's exit from the vagina. Sometimes women can avoid the need for an episiotomy by exercising and getting good nutrition throughout pregnancy, by trying different birth positions, or by having an attendant massage the perineal tissue. However, the skin's natural elasticity and the baby's size are limiting factors.

After delivery, the attending practitioner cleans the baby's mucous-filled breathing passages, and the baby takes

its first breath, generally accompanied by a loud wail. (The traditional slap on the baby's buttocks, often romanticized in old movies, is no longer a common practice because of the trauma associated with it.) The umbilical cord is then tied and severed. The stump of cord attached to the baby's navel dries up and drops off within a few days.

In the meantime, the mother continues into the third stage of labor, during which the placenta, or **afterbirth,** is expelled from the womb. This stage is usually completed within 30 minutes after delivery.

Most mothers prefer to have their new infants next to them following the birth. Together with their spouse or partner, they feel a need to share this time of bonding with their infant.

Episiotomy   A straight incision in the mother's perineum.

Perineum   The area between the vulva and the anus.

Afterbirth   The expelled placenta.

Managing Labor: Medical and Nonmedical Approaches

Because painkilling drugs given to the mother during labor can cause sluggish responses in the newborn and other complications, many women choose drug-free labor and delivery.

But it is important to keep a flexible attitude about pain relief because each labor is different. Working in partnership with a health care provider to make the best decision for mother and baby is the best plan. Use of painkilling medication during a delivery is not a sign of weakness. One person is not a "success" for delivering without medication while another is a "failure" for using medical measures. Remember, pain is to be expected. In fact, many experts say that the pain of labor is the most difficult in the human experience. However, there is no one right answer in managing that pain. See the Skills for Behavior Change box for more on managing the labor process.

Birth Alternatives

Expectant parents have several options beyond the traditional hospital setting for the process of their infant's birth and their participation in it. Although several of these methods have decreased in popularity, all continue to be used.

The Lamaze Method This birth alternative is the most popular one in the United States. Pre-labor education classes teach the mother to control her pain through special breathing patterns, focusing exercises, and relaxation. Lamaze births usually take place in a hospital or birthing center with a physician or midwife in attendance. The partner (or labor coach) assists by giving emotional support, physical comfort (massage and ice chips), and coaching for proper breath control during contractions. Lamaze proponents discourage the use of drugs.

The Harris Method Parents using this alternative are taught by registered nurses. Gentle touching and controlled breathing are stressed. Partners provide emotional support while a physician-nurse team essentially controls the labor and delivery. Drugs are not prohibited.

Childbirth without Fear Sometimes called the Read Method, this method advocates relaxation and education for understanding the birth process. Mothers are taught to recognize that anticipation of pain creates more pain. The partner provides emotional support, and drugs are not prohibited.

The Leboyer Method Leboyer proponents believe that birth in the standard delivery room is a traumatic experience for the baby. The Leboyer method allows the mother to deliver in a dark and quiet setting. Immediately after delivery, the infant is placed in a warm bath to ease its transition to life outside the womb. Drug use is discouraged.

The Bradley Method The Bradley method emphasizes little to no pain medication and as little medical intervention in the birthing process as possible. Good nutrition and physical activity patterns throughout pregnancy are stressed, and deep relaxation methods are taught. This method also focuses on the partner's role in a satisfying labor experience.

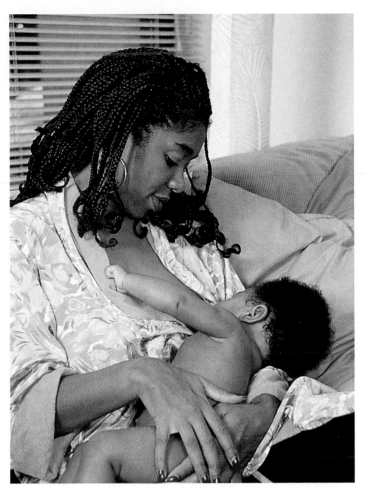

Breast-feeding is one way to enhance the development of intimate bonds between mother and child.

Water Birth Proponents of this method recommend giving birth in a dimly lit, relaxed environment. The mother is placed in a warm tub. The partner may join the woman in the tub to help massage and guide her through contractions. The baby is delivered into the water and then placed at the mother's breast. Many water births take place in the home, generally with no painkillers.

Breast-Feeding and the Postpartum Period

Although the new mother's milk will not begin to flow for two or more days, her breasts secrete a thick yellow substance called *colostrum*. Because this fluid contains vital antibodies to help fight infection, the newborn baby should be allowed to suckle.

The American Academy of Pediatrics strongly recommends that infants should be breast-fed for at least six months, and ideally for 12 months. Scientific findings indicate there are many advantages to breast-feeding. Breast milk is perfectly suited to a baby's nutritional needs. Breast-fed babies have fewer illnesses and a much lower hospitalization rate because breast milk contains maternal antibodies and immunological cells that stimulate the infant's immune system. When breast-fed babies do get sick, they recover more quickly. They are also less likely to be obese than babies fed on formulas, and they have fewer allergies. They may even be more intelligent: A new study finds that the longer a baby was breast-fed, the higher the IQ in adulthood. Researchers theorize that breast milk contains substances that enhance brain development.[18]

This does not mean that breast milk is the only way to nourish a baby. Prepared formulas can provide nourishment that allows a baby to grow and thrive. When deciding whether to breast- or bottle-feed, mothers need to consider their own desires and preferences. Both feeding methods can supply the physical and emotional closeness so essential to the parent-child relationship.

A recent study, by Avery et al., found that women who were able to breast-feed successfully for longer periods of time generally viewed breast-feeding as more positive, had more knowledge about the process, and had higher self-efficacy in their ability to breast-feed.[19]

The *postpartum period* lasts from four to six weeks after delivery. During this time, the mother's reproductive organs revert to a nonpregnant state. Many women experience energy depletion, anxiety, mood swings, and depression during this period. This experience, known as **postpartum depression,** appears to be a normal end product of the birth process. For most women, the symptoms gradually disappear as their bodies return to normal. For others, the symptoms, coupled with the stresses of managing a new family, can cause more severe depression that lasts for several months.

Complications

Complications are a possibility both during pregnancy and at the time of labor and delivery. **Preeclampsia** is a condition that is characterized by high blood pressure, protein in the urine, and edema (fluid retention), which usually causes swelling of the hands and face. This condition complicates approximately 10 percent of pregnancies and is responsible for 18 percent of U.S. maternal deaths each year. Symptoms may include sudden weight gain, headache, nausea or vomiting, changes in vision, racing pulse, mental confusion, and stomach or right shoulder pain. If preeclampsia is not treated, it can cause seizures, a condition called **eclampsia.** Potential problems can include liver and kidney damage, internal bleeding, stroke, poor fetal growth, and fetal and maternal death.

This condition tends to occur in the late second or third trimesters. The cause of preeclampsia is not known; however, the incidence of preeclampsia is higher in first-time mothers, those with a family history of preeclampsia, women over 40 or under 18 years of age, women carrying multiple fetuses, and women with a history of chronic hypertension, diabetes or kidney disorder, or previous history of preeclampsia. Both

men and women who were the product of a pregnancy complicated by preeclampsia are significantly more likely to have a pregnancy affected by preeclampsia. Treatment for women with preeclampsia ranges from bed rest and monitoring for those with mild cases, to hospitalization and close monitoring for more severe cases, which have the potential to be life-threatening for the woman and her fetus.

Problems and complications can also occur during labor and delivery, even following a successful pregnancy. Such possibilities should be discussed with the practitioner prior to labor so the mother understands what medical procedures may be necessary for her safety and that of her child. Although pregnancy still involves a certain amount of risk, the risk is lower than for many other common activities.

Cesarean Section (C-section) If labor lasts too long or if a baby is presenting wrong (about to exit the uterus any way but head first), a **cesarean section (C-section)** may be necessary. This surgical procedure involves making an incision across the mother's abdomen and through the uterus to remove the baby. This operation is also performed in cases in which labor is extremely difficult, maternal blood pressure falls rapidly, the placenta separates from the uterus too soon, the mother has diabetes, or other problems occur.

A cesarean section can be traumatic for the mother if she is not prepared for it. The rate of delivery by cesarean section in the United States increased from 5 percent in the mid-1960s to more than 25 percent by 1988, but it leveled off to approximately 17 percent in 1999.[20] Risks to the mother are the same as for any major abdominal surgery, and recovery from birth takes considerably longer after a C-section. Although a cesarean section may be necessary in certain cases, some physicians and critics, including the federal government's Centers for Disease Control and Prevention (CDC), feel the option has been used too frequently in this country. The CDC had hoped to lower the rate of cesareans in the United States to 15 per 100 births by the year 2000, a level the agency considers to be medically appropriate. Unfortunately, the goal has not been met.

Now, however, surgical techniques allow some women who have had a cesarean section to deliver later children vaginally. Guidelines published by the American College of Obstetricians and Gynecologists give an estimated 50 to 80 percent of women the option of a vaginal birth after cesarean (VBAC). Cesarean sections will still be necessary, however, if the original incision runs from the top to the bottom of the uterus (as opposed to across); if the baby is over 9 pounds; if the birth is multiple; or if the mother has a medical condition that would make vaginal delivery difficult or dangerous, such as a very small pelvis, chronic high blood pressure, or diabetes.

Miscarriage One in 10 pregnancies does not end in delivery. Loss of the fetus before it is viable is called a **miscarriage** (also referred to as *spontaneous abortion*). An estimated 70 to 90 percent of women who miscarry eventually become pregnant again.

Reasons for miscarriage vary. In some cases, the fertilized egg has failed to divide correctly. In others, genetic abnormalities, maternal illness, or infections are responsible. Maternal hormonal imbalance may also cause a miscarriage, as may a weak cervix or toxic chemicals in the environment. In most cases, the cause is not known.

A blood incompatibility between mother and father can cause **Rh factor** problems, sometimes resulting in miscarriage. Rh is a blood protein. Rh problems occur when the mother is Rh-negative and the fetus is Rh-positive. During a first birth, some of the baby's blood passes into the mother's bloodstream. An Rh-negative mother may manufacture antibodies to destroy the Rh-positive blood introduced into her bloodstream at the time of birth. Her first baby will be unaffected, but subsequent babies with positive Rh factor will be at risk for a severe anemia called *hemolytic disease* because the mother's Rh antibodies will attack the fetus's red blood cells.

Medical advances now offer both prevention and treatment for this condition. If testing reveals Rh incompatibility, intrauterine transfusions can be given or an early delivery by cesarean section can be done, depending upon the individual case. Prevention is preferable to treatment. All women with Rh-negative blood should be injected with a medication called RhoGAM within 72 hours of any birth, miscarriage, or abortion. This injection will prevent them from developing the Rh antibodies.

Another cause of miscarriage is **ectopic pregnancy,** or implantation of a fertilized egg outside the uterus. A fertilized egg may implant itself in the fallopian tube or, occasionally, in the pelvic cavity. Because these structures are not capable of expanding and nourishing a developing fetus, the pregnancy cannot continue. Such pregnancies are surgically terminated. Most often, the affected fallopian tube is also removed.

Ectopic pregnancy is generally accompanied by pain in the lower abdomen or aching in the shoulders as the blood flows up toward the diaphragm. If bleeding is significant, blood pressure drops and the woman can go into shock. If an ectopic pregnancy goes undiagnosed and untreated, the fallopian tube will rupture, putting the woman at great risk of hemorrhage, peritonitis (infection in the abdomen), and even death.

Over the past 12 years, the incidence of ectopic pregnancy has tripled, and no one really understands why. We do know that ectopic pregnancy is a potential side effect of pelvic inflammatory disease (PID), which has become increasingly common in recent years. The scarring or blockage of the fallopian tubes characteristic of this disease prevents the fertilized egg from passing to the uterus. About 50 percent of women who have had an ectopic pregnancy conceive again. But women who have had one ectopic pregnancy run a higher risk of having another.

Stillbirth is one of the most traumatic events a couple can face. A stillborn baby is one that is born dead, often for no apparent reason. The grief experienced following a stillbirth is usually devastating. Nine months of happy anticipation have been thwarted. Family, friends, and other children may be in a state of shock, needing comfort and not knowing where to turn. The mother's breasts produce milk, and there is no infant to be fed. A room with a crib and toys is left empty.

The grief can last for years, and both partners may blame themselves or each other. In many cases, no amount of reassurance from the attending physician, relatives, or friends can assuage the grief or guilt. Well-intentioned comments such as "Oh, you'll have another baby someday" may bring no comfort.

Some communities have groups called the Compassionate Friends to help parents and other family members through this grieving process. This nonprofit organization is for parents who have lost a child of any age for any reason.

Sudden Infant Death Syndrome (SIDS)   The sudden death of an infant under one year of age, for no apparent reason, is called **sudden infant death syndrome (SIDS).** Though SIDS is the leading cause of death for children age one month to one year, affecting about 1 in 1,000 infants in the United States each year, it is not a disease. Rather, it is ruled the cause of death after all other possibilities are ruled out.

Postpartum depression The experience of energy depletion, anxiety, mood swings, and depression that women may feel during the postpartum period.

Preeclampsia A complication in pregnancy characterized by high blood pressure, protein in the urine, and edema.

Eclampsia Untreated preeclampsia can develop into this potentially fatal complication that involves maternal strokes and seizures.

Cesarean section (C-section) A surgical procedure in which a baby is removed through an incision made in the mother's abdominal and uterine walls.

Miscarriage Loss of the fetus before it is viable; also called spontaneous abortion.

Rh factor A blood protein related to the production of antibodies. If an Rh-negative mother is pregnant with an Rh-positive fetus, the mother will manufacture antibodies that can kill the fetus, causing miscarriage.

Ectopic pregnancy Implantation of a fertilized egg outside the uterus, usually in a fallopian tube; a medical emergency that can end in death from hemorrhage for the mother.

Stillbirth The birth of a dead baby.

Sudden infant death syndrome (SIDS) The sudden death of an infant under one year of age for no apparent reason.

A SIDS death is sudden and silent; death occurs quickly, often associated with sleep and no signs of suffering.

Because SIDS is a diagnosis of exclusion, doctors do not know what causes it. However, research done in countries including England, New Zealand, Australia, and Norway has shown that placing children on their backs or sides to sleep cuts the rate of SIDS by as much as half. The American Academy of Pediatrics advises parents to lay infants on their backs. Additional precautions against SIDS include having a firm surface for the infant's bed, not allowing the infant to become too warm, maintaining a smoke-free environment, having regular pediatric visits, breast-feeding, and seeking prenatal care.

> ### What do you think?
>
> *What are your thoughts on medical versus natural management of labor and delivery?* ✳ *Do you have strong preferences for how you'd like to manage your own birthing process?* ✳ *If so, what are they?* ✳ *What might be the advantages and disadvantages of breast-feeding?*

Infertility

An estimated one in six American couples experiences **infertility,** or difficulties in conceiving. Reasons include the trend toward delaying childbirth (as a woman gets older, she is less likely to conceive), endometriosis, and the rising incidence of pelvic inflammatory disease.

Causes in Women

Endometriosis is the leading cause of infertility in women in the United States. With this disorder, parts of the endometrial lining of the uterus implant themselves outside the uterus—in the fallopian tubes, lungs, intestines, outer uterine walls or ovarian walls, and/or on the ligaments that support the uterus. The disorder can be treated surgically or with hormonal preparations. Success rates vary.

Another cause of infertility is **pelvic inflammatory disease (PID),** a serious infection that scars the fallopian tubes and blocks sperm migration. PID is a collective name for any extensive bacterial infection of the female pelvic organs, particularly the uterus, cervix, fallopian tubes, and ovaries. PID often results from chlamydia or gonorrheal infections that spread to the fallopian tubes or ovaries. Symptoms of PID include severe pain, fever, and sometimes vaginal discharge.

The past 30 years have brought a tremendous increase in the annual number of PID cases, from 17,800 to about 1 million per year. During the reproductive years, one in seven women reports having been treated for PID,[21] and tens of thousands have been rendered sterile. One episode of PID causes sterility in 10 to 15 percent of women, and 50 to 75 percent become sterile after three or four infections.[22]

Causes in Men

Among men, the single largest fertility problem is **low sperm count.** Although only one viable sperm is needed for fertilization, research has shown that all the other sperm in the ejaculate aid in the fertilization process. There are normally 60 to 80 million sperm per milliliter of semen. When the count drops below 20 million, fertility declines.

Low sperm count may be attributable to environmental factors such as exposure of the scrotum to intense heat or cold, radiation, or altitude, or even to wearing excessively tight underwear or outerwear. However, other factors, such as the mumps virus, can damage the cells that make sperm. Varicose veins above one or both testicles can also render men infertile. Male infertility problems account for around 40 percent of infertility cases.

Treatment

For the couple desperately wishing to conceive, the road to parenthood may be frustrating. Fortunately, medical treatment can identify the cause of infertility in about 90 percent of affected couples. The chances of becoming pregnant range from 30 to 70 percent, depending on the reason for infertility. The countless tests and the invasion of privacy that characterize some couples' efforts to conceive can put stress on an otherwise strong, healthy relationship. Before starting fertility tests, couples should reassess their priorities. Some will choose to undergo counseling to help them clarify their feelings about the fertility process. A good physician or fertility team will take the time to ascertain the couple's level of motivation.

Fertility workups can be very expensive, and the costs are not usually covered by insurance companies. Fertility workups for men include a sperm count, a test for sperm motility, and analysis of any disease processes present. Such procedures should be undertaken only by a qualified urologist. Women are thoroughly examined by an obstetrician/gynecologist for the composition of cervical mucous, extent of tubal scarring, and evidence of endometriosis.

Complete fertility workups may take four to five months and can be unsettling. The couple may be instructed to have sex "by the calendar" to increase their chances of conceiving. In some cases, surgery can correct structural problems such as tubal scarring. In others, administering hormones can improve the health of ova and sperm. Sometimes pregnancy can be achieved by collecting the man's sperm from several ejaculations and inseminating the woman at a later time.

When all surgical and hormonal methods fail, the couple still has some options. These, too, can be very expensive. **Fertility drugs** such as Clomid and Pergonal stimulate ovulation in women who are not ovulating. Ninety percent of women who use these drugs will begin to ovulate, and half will conceive.

Fertility drugs can have many side effects, including headaches, irritability, restlessness, depression, fatigue, edema (fluid retention), abnormal uterine bleeding, breast tenderness, vasomotor flushes (hot flashes), and visual difficulties. Women using fertility drugs are also at increased risk of developing multiple ovarian cysts (fluid-filled growths) and liver damage. The drugs sometimes trigger the release of more than one egg. Thus a woman treated with one of these drugs has a 1 in 10 chance of having multiple births. Most such births are twins, but triplets and even quadruplets are not uncommon.

Alternative insemination of a woman with her partner's sperm is another treatment option. This technique has led to an estimated 250,000 births in the United States, primarily for couples in which the man is infertile. If this procedure fails, the couple may choose insemination by an anonymous donor through a "sperm bank." Many men sell their sperm to such banks. The sperm are classified according to the physical characteristics of the donor (for example, blonde hair, blue eyes) and then frozen for future use. Frozen sperm can survive for up to five years. The woman being inseminated usually chooses sperm from a man whose physical characteristics resemble those of her partner or match her own personal preferences.

In the last few years, concern has been expressed about the possibility of transmitting the AIDS virus through alternative insemination. As a result, donors are routinely screened for the disease.

In vitro fertilization, often referred to as "test tube" fertilization, involves collecting a viable ovum from the prospective mother and transferring it to a nutrient medium in a laboratory, where it is fertilized with sperm from the woman's partner or a donor. After a few days, the embryo is transplanted into the mother's uterus, where, it is hoped, it will develop normally. Until 1984, in vitro fertilization was classified as "experimental." Since then, it has moved into the mainstream of standard infertility treatments. Since 1984, the in vitro process has been responsible for 26,000 births in the United States alone.

In **gamete intrafallopian transfer (GIFT),** the egg is "harvested" from the woman's ovary and placed in the fallopian tube with the man's sperm. Less expensive and time consuming than in vitro fertilization, GIFT mimics nature by allowing the egg to be fertilized in the fallopian tube and migrate to the uterus according to the normal timetable.

Intracytoplasmic sperm injection (ICSI) was first performed successfully in 1992. Basically, a sperm cell is injected into an egg. This complex procedure required researchers to learn how to manipulate both egg and sperm without damaging them. This technique can help men with low sperm counts or motility, and even those who cannot ejaculate or have no live sperm in their semen as a result of vasectomy, chemotherapy, or a medical disorder. Scientists have examined a thousand babies born using this technique and have found no higher rate of birth defects than in the general population. Nonetheless, ICSI is still considered experimental.

In **nonsurgical embryo transfer,** a donor egg is fertilized by the man's sperm and implanted in the woman's uterus. This procedure may also be used in cases involving the transfer of an already fertilized ovum into the uterus of another woman.

In **embryo transfer,** an ovum from a donor's body is artificially inseminated by the husband's sperm, allowed to stay in the donor's body for a time, and then transplanted into the wife's body.

Infertility   Difficulties in conceiving.

Endometriosis   A disorder in which uterine lining tissue establishes itself outside the uterus; the leading cause of infertility in the United States.

Pelvic inflammatory disease (PID)   An infection that scars the fallopian tubes and consequently blocks sperm migration, causing infertility.

Low sperm count   A sperm count below 60 million sperm per milliliter of semen; the leading cause of infertility in men.

Fertility drugs   Hormones that stimulate ovulation in women who are not ovulating; often responsible for multiple births.

Alternative insemination   Fertilization accomplished by depositing a partner's or a donor's semen into a woman's vagina via a thin tube; almost always done in a doctor's office.

In vitro fertilization   Fertilization of an egg in a nutrient medium and subsequent transfer back to the mother's body.

Gamete intrafallopian transfer (GIFT)   Procedure in which an egg harvested from the female partner's ovary is placed with the male partner's sperm in her fallopian tube, where it is fertilized and then migrates to the uterus for implantation.

Intracytoplasmic sperm injection (ICSI)   Fertilization accomplished by injecting a sperm cell directly into an egg.

Nonsurgical embryo transfer   In vitro fertilization of a donor egg by the male partner's (or donor's) sperm and subsequent transfer to the female partner's or another woman's uterus.

Embryo transfer   Artificial insemination of a donor with the male partner's sperm; after a time, the embryo is transferred from the donor to the female partner's body.

Some laboratories are experimenting with **embryo freezing,** in which a fertilized embryo is suspended in a solution of liquid nitrogen. When desired, it is gradually thawed and implanted into the prospective mother. The first U.S. birth of a frozen embryo was reported in 1986. In the future, this technique may make it possible for young couples to produce an embryo and save it for later implantation when they are ready to have a child, thus reducing the risks of fertilizing older eggs.

Infertile couples have another alternative—**embryo adoption programs.** The embryos are originally collected from couples who want children via in vitro fertilization. These couples often donate and freeze extra embryos in case the procedure fails or they want to have more children at a later time. These couples can now donate their unneeded embryos to others. The adopting couple can enjoy the experience of pregnancy and control prenatal care. The cost is approximately $4,000 dollars for the embryos to be thawed and transferred to an infertile woman's uterus or fallopian tubes.

The ethical and moral questions surrounding experimental infertility treatments are staggering. Before moving forward with any of these treatments, individuals need to ask themselves a few important questions. Has infertility been absolutely confirmed? Are reputable infertility counseling services accessible? Have they explored all possible alternatives and considered potential risks? Have all affected parties examined their attitudes, values, and beliefs about conceiving a child in this manner? Finally, they need to consider what and how they will tell the child about their method of conception.

Surrogate Motherhood

Between 60 and 70 percent of infertile couples are able to conceive after treatment. The rest decide to live without children, to adopt, or to attempt surrogate motherhood. In this option, the couple hires a woman to be alternatively inseminated by the male partner. The surrogate then carries the baby to term and surrenders it upon birth to the couple. Surrogate mothers are reportedly paid about $10,000 for their services and are reimbursed for medical expenses. Legal and medical expenses can run as high as $30,000 for the infertile couple.

Couples considering surrogate motherhood are advised to consult a lawyer regarding contracts. Most of these legal

documents stipulate that the surrogate mother must undergo amniocentesis and that if the fetus is defective, she must consent to an abortion. In that case, or if the surrogate miscarries, she is reimbursed for her time and expenses. The prospective parents must also agree to take the baby if it is carried to term, even if it is unhealthy or has physical abnormalities.

Adoption

For couples who have decided that biological childbirth is not an option for them, adoption provides an alternative to bearing a child. Currently, about 50,000 children are available for adoption in the United States every year. This is far fewer than the number of couples seeking adoptions. By some estimates, only 1 in 30 couples receives the children they want. On average, couples spend two years and $100,000 on the adoption process.

In the early 1950s approximately 9 percent of unwed pregnant women gave their child up for adoption. Currently approximately 2 percent of unmarried pregnant women place their children up for adoption. The decline in the number of women placing their children up for adoption results from a number of influences, including the decreased stigma of unwed motherhood, declining number of teens placing their children up for adoption, declining pregnancy rate, and the increased use of contraceptives. There is no research to show that women are choosing to abort their children rather than place them up for adoption.

Women who place their children up for adoption are likely to have greater educational and vocational goals for themselves than those who keep their children. Women who choose adoption come from families who are supportive of the adoption process. If you are pregnant and considering adoption, make sure you think through all the possibilities before you make your decision. Remember: Adoption is permanent. People who can help you think though your options include your partner, friends, family, crisis centers, student health services, family planning clinic, family service agency, or adoption agency.

There are two types of adoption: *confidential* and *open.* In confidential adoption the birth parents and the adoptive parents never know each other. Adoptive parents are given information about the birth parents that they need to take care of the child, such as medical information.

In open adoption, birth parents and adoptive parents know something about each other. There are different levels of openness, ranging from being able to pick from several possible families the one that sounds best for the child to the birth parents and adoptive parents staying in contact over the years. This might include visiting, calling, and writing each other. Both parties must agree to this plan, and it is not available in every state.

Because the number of American children available for adoption is limited, young women who consider placing

---

Embryo adoption programs   A procedure whereby an infertile couple is able to purchase frozen embryos donated by another couple.

Embryo freezing   The freezing of an embryo for later implantation.

their child for adoption have gained new leverage. Increasingly, couples wishing to adopt have turned to independent adoptions arranged by a lawyer, or they may directly negotiate with the birth mother. Independent adoptions now surpass those arranged by social service agencies.

More and more couples are choosing to create families by adopting children from foreign countries. In 2000, U.S. families adopted 18,477 foreign-born children. Intercountry adoption may be a good alternative for many couples, especially those who want to adopt an infant. The cost of intercountry adoption varies greatly, from approximately $7,000 to $25,000 including agency fees, dossier and immigration processing fees, and court costs.

> **What do you think?**
>
> *If you found that you or your partner had infertility problems, how much time and money would you be willing to invest in infertility treatments? ✹ Do you think that single women and lesbians should have equal access to alternative methods of insemination? ✹ Why or why not? ✹ Do you think single women or men and gay males or lesbians should have equal opportunities at adoption? ✹ How do you think society views these types of adoptions? ✹ Why?*

Taking Charge 7 7 7

Reproduction Choices: Making Responsible Decisions

After reading this chapter, you know that pregnancy, childbirth, and reproductive issues are not to be taken lightly. The choices between different types of birth control and the ethical issues surrounding fertility are complex. Take control of your own fertility and share this responsibility in your relationships. Is birth control an option for you? If so, have you considered which birth control options would be most appropriate for you? Be sure to examine all potential side effects and drug interactions. The following questions can help you determine your level of readiness regarding reproduction and sexual health.

Checklist for Change

Making Personal Choices

☐ If you are in a stable relationship and are considering having a child, is it something both you and your partner want?

☐ Do you know and feel comfortable with your philosophical beliefs about children?

☐ Do you feel comfortable discussing birth control with your partner?

☐ Do you feel comfortable choosing a method of birth control that meets the needs of both yourself and your partner?

☐ Are you familiar with the resources available if you have trouble conceiving?

☐ Have you discussed alternatives should you or your partner become pregnant?

Making Community Choices

☐ Have you taken the time to become educated about the issues and concerns related to parenting?

☐ Do you listen with an open mind to issues involving reproduction and sexual health and then make informed decisions?

☐ When you think about having children, do you think in terms of long-range planning?

☐ Do you advocate allowing people to make choices that are in their best interest, regardless of your own personal philosophy or opinions?

☐ Do you believe in providing support for community agencies and social services that assist in meeting the sexual and reproductive health needs of your community?

☐ Do you try to volunteer your time to other people or agencies that may need your assistance?

Summary

* Latex condoms and the female condom, when used correctly for oral sex or intercourse, provide the most effective protection from sexually transmitted infections. Other contraceptive methods include abstinence, "outercourse," oral contraceptives, other hormonal contraceptives, foams, jellies, suppositories, creams, the diaphragm, the cervical cap, intrauterine devices, and withdrawal. Fertility awareness methods rely on altering sexual practices to avoid pregnancy. All of these methods of contraception are reversible. Sterilization is generally permanent, although it can be reversed surgically in some cases.
* Abortion is currently legal in the United States through the second trimester. Abortion methods include vacuum aspiration, dilation and evacuation (D&E), dilation and curettage (D&C), intact dilation and extraction (D&X), hysterotomy, induction abortion, and mifepristone (RU-486).
* Parenting is a demanding job that requires careful planning. Emotional health, maternal health, paternal health, financial evaluation, and contingency planning all need to be taken into account.
* Prenatal care includes a complete physical exam within the first trimester and avoidance of alcohol and drugs, cigarettes, x-rays, and chemicals having teratogenic effects. Full-term pregnancy covers three trimesters.
* Childbirth occurs in three stages. Birth alternatives include the Harris method, Childbirth without Fear, the Leboyer method, the Bradley method, and water birth. Partners should jointly choose a labor method early in the pregnancy to be better prepared for labor when it occurs. Complications of pregnancy and childbirth include miscarriage, ectopic pregnancy, stillbirth, and cesarean section.
* Infertility in women may be caused by pelvic inflammatory disease or endometriosis. In men, it may be caused by low sperm count. Treatment may include alternative insemination, in vitro fertilization, gamete intrafallopian transfer, nonsurgical embryo transfer, and embryo transfer. Surrogate motherhood involves hiring a fertile woman to be alternatively inseminated by the male partner.

Questions for Discussion and Reflection

1. List the most effective contraceptive methods. What are their drawbacks? What medical conditions would keep a person from using them? What are the characteristics of the methods you think would be most effective for you, and why?
2. What are the various methods of abortion? What are the two opposing viewpoints concerning abortion? What is *Roe v. Wade,* and what impact did it have on the abortion debate?
3. What are the most important considerations in deciding whether the time is right to become a parent? What factors will you consider regarding the number of children you will have?
4. Discuss the growth of the fetus through the three trimesters. What medical checkups or tests should be done during each trimester?
5. Discuss the emotional aspects of pregnancy. What types of emotional reactions are common in each trimester and the postpartum period (the "fourth trimester")?
6. Discuss the medical and nonmedical (natural) management of childbirth. What options are available to manage labor? Discuss the various types of alternative birthing practices.

Application Exercises

Reread the What Do You Think? scenarios at the beginning of the chapter and answer the following questions.

1. What are the costs and benefits (both emotional and monetary) of fertility treatment? What factors should couples consider in terms of deciding between fertility treatment options and nonmedical options such as adoption?

Do you think that people like Jane and Stephen should be allowed to select the sex of their child?
2. What contraceptive options might Nan consider other than emergency contraception? What are the positive and negative aspects of these options? What risks is she taking by using only emergency contraception?

Accessing Your Health on the Internet

Visit the following Internet sites to explore further topics and issues related to personal health. To visit an organization's website, go to the Companion Website for *Access to Health, Eighth Edition* at www.aw.com/donatelle, click on the book image, and select "Accessing Your Health on the Internet" from the navigation menu on the left.

1. **Childbirth.Org** Information to encourage parents to be good consumers by knowing their options and how to provide themselves with the best possible care essential to a healthy pregnancy.

2. **The National Parenting Center.** This site invites parents to expand their parenting skills and strengths by sharing information in chat rooms and in an online newsletter.

3. **Safer Sex.** Provides information on safer sex issues. Discusses such issues as what is safer sex, is oral sex safe, women and safer sex, and links to other websites.

Further Reading

Boston Women's Health Collective. *Our Bodies, Ourselves for the New Century: A Book by and for Women.* New York: Simon and Schuster, 1998.

Like its earlier editions, this volume contains information about women's health from a decidedly feminist angle. Every aspect of health is covered, including nutrition, emotional health, fitness, relationships, reproduction, contraception, and pregnancy.

Bullough, V. L., and B. Bullough. *Contraception: A Guide to Birth Control Methods.* 2nd ed. New York: Prometheus Books, 1997.

Historical overview of birth control practices and essential aspects of human reproductive anatomy; contains factual information on all available birth control options and explores the very latest research and testing on contraceptive techniques.

Eisenberg, A., S. Hathaway, and H. Murkoff. *What to Expect When You're Expecting.* 2nd ed. New York: Workman, 1996.

A month-by-month guide to all aspects of pregnancy. Provides information on what the mother can expect regarding physician visits, prenatal testing, physical and emotional changes, and important decisions to be made throughout pregnancy and delivery.

Hatcher, R. A., et al. *Contraceptive Technology.* 17th rev. ed. New York: Ardent Media, Inc., 1998.

Perhaps the best primary reference concerning birth control for physicians, family planning centers, student health services, and educators. Contributors include many staff members of the Centers for Disease Control and Prevention.

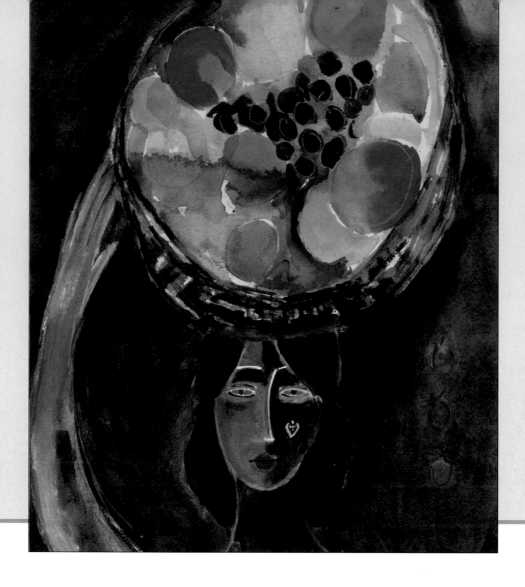

Objectives

* Examine the factors that influence dietary choices.

* Discuss how to change old eating habits, including how to use the Food Guide Pyramids appropriately, eat nutrient-dense foods, prevent dietary deficiencies and excesses, and optimize dietary choices to enhance health.

* Describe the major essential nutrients and their role in maintaining health. Explain any controversies related to these substances and how nutritional guides should influence dietary choices.

* Discuss food as a form of medicine and the facts related to new trends in nutrition, food supplements, and their roles in health and well-being.

* Distinguish among the various forms of vegetarianism, discussing possible health benefits and risks from these dietary alternatives.

* Discuss issues surrounding gender, exercise behaviors, and nutrition. Explain the impact of these issues for your own dietary behaviors now and in the future.

* Discuss how unique situations in your life (pregnancy, stress, illness) can influence dietary needs.

* Discuss the unique problems that college students face when trying to eat healthy foods and the actions they can take to ensure compliance with the Food Guide Pyramids. Explain the role that consumers play in preserving their health through wise nutritional choices.

* Explain some of the food safety concerns facing Americans and people around the world.

Nutrition

Eating for Optimum Health

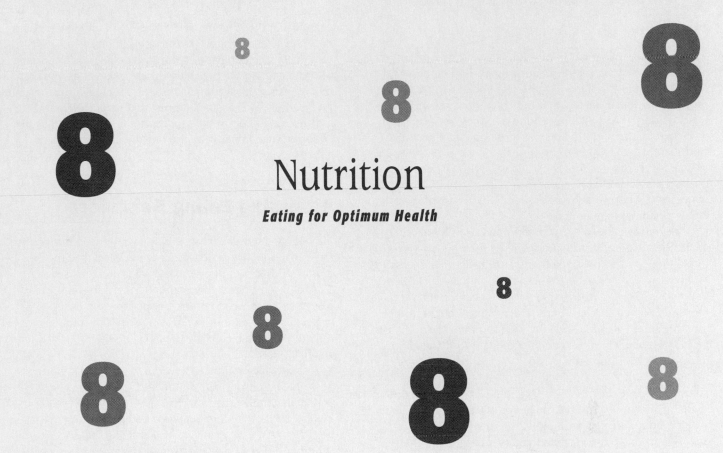

What do you think?

James is chronically thin. Although he eats regular meals and drinks 4–6 cans of a high-calorie supplement daily, he never seems to gain weight. He goes to school full time, has a job for 20 hours per week, and is on the crew team. Lately, James has begun to feel very tired and can't get rid of a persistent cold.

Roberto is a fitness enthusiast who runs 5 to 10 miles daily, lifts weights three to four times per week, and constantly talks about his quest for the perfect body. He criticizes anyone who puts mayonnaise or butter on bread or who eats any kind of fast food.

Jordan is a second grader. When snacks are handed out at school, she strongly objects to eating anything that has fat in it, and she refuses to associate with "piggies" (students who are overweight). Recently, her teacher caught her in the school bathroom, forcing herself to vomit because she had eaten too much and thought she might get fat. Jordan brags that she has never eaten candy and that there are no pesticides or herbicides in the food her family eats.

Martha is a 70-year-old resident of rural northern Wisconsin. She has eaten bacon or sausage with eggs for breakfast nearly every day since she was a child. She is extremely active on the farm and works from morning until sunset. She brags that she has never been sick a day in her life, her cholesterol is normal, and her "ticker" is doing just fine. Her daughter and grandchildren are constantly encouraging her to cut down on saturated fat and dairy products.

How would you assess each individual's dietary behaviors? ✳ *What factors might contribute to them?* ✳ *Which behaviors would you want to change?* ✳ *Why?* ✳ *Which of these individuals has the "healthiest" eating behaviors?* ✳ *If you were to describe someone with healthy eating behaviors, what would that person be like?*

Do you ever get frustrated by conflicting information about diet and nutritional supplements? If so, you are like millions of other Americans. In fact, three out of four Americans say that there is far too much contradictory information about nutrition and they are overwhelmed by the daunting task of trying to distinguish fact from fiction.[1] Just when we think we know the answers, a new research study tells us that what we thought was true probably isn't. We face a steady barrage of new information concerning what we consume as body fuel and what we enjoy as culinary creations.

Today, we face dietary choices and nutritional challenges that our grandparents never dreamed of—exotic foreign foods; dietary supplements; artificial sweeteners; no-fat, low-fat, and artificial-fat alternatives; cholesterol-free, high-protein, high-carbohydrate, and low-calorie products—thousands of alternatives bombard us daily. Caught in the crossfire of advertised claims by the food industry and advice provided by health and nutrition experts, most of us find it difficult to make wise dietary decisions. Knowing where to go for accurate information and how to apply this information takes effort and education. The good news is that, according to the American Dietetic Association, more Americans are seeking out information on food and nutrition and taking action to improve their habits than ever before.[2]

Although most adults want to have healthy diets, this is a formidable task for many college students. Money, time, access to cooking facilities and nutritious foods, and other barriers may make healthy choices more difficult to make. A study of more than 2,000 college students indicated that students often face considerable difficulty planning healthy menus and having the resources to prepare balanced meals.[3] On the other hand, a subsequent study showed that college students and graduates tend to practice more healthful habits and make healthier food choices than nonstudents.[4] Many of the eating behaviors from both of these studies appear to mirror eating patterns that students learned in their homes.

Numerous studies have pointed to the importance of diet and exercise in immune function, risk for chronic disease, and mental functioning and performance. Even simple changes appear to make huge differences. For example, a review in the late 1990s of over 4,500 research studies concluded that widespread consumption of 5–6 servings of fruits and vegetables daily would cause cancer rates to fall by over 20 percent in the global population.[5] Subsequent research has led to increased emphasis on the role of diet and nutrition on cardiovascular disease, diabetes, and a host of other chronic and disabling conditions.[6]

It doesn't take a research study for each of us to know what it feels like to gain weight or be overweight, to feel run down and listless, or to be unhappy with our body, our overall appearance, or our health. Learning fundamental principles designed to help you eat more healthy foods, avoid the problems that so many people face with their weight, and improve general fitness levels is a key focus of the next three chapters. In this chapter, we will help you understand basic nutrition science, as well as the application of sound principles to lifestyle behaviors. Before we begin, it is important that you gain an appreciation for why you eat as you do, the role of your family of origin and basic biology in determining your eating patterns and choices, and resources that you may access to help you be successful in changing negative patterns while building on the healthy choices you are already making.

Assessing Eating Behaviors

Although we have all undoubtedly experienced **hunger** before mealtime, few Americans have experienced the type of hunger that continues for days and threatens survival. Most of us do not eat to sustain physical survival. Instead, we eat because we experience **appetite**—the desire to eat—or because some inner signal tells us that it's time to eat. Appetite may cause people to eat even when they are actually full.

Many factors influence when we eat, what we eat, and how much. Sensory stimulation such as smelling, seeing, and tasting foods can stimulate appetite even if we're not hungry. Finding the right balance between eating to maintain body function (eating to live) and eating to satisfy appetite (living to eat) is a constant struggle for many of us. The following are among the most powerful influences that make us who we are, nutritionally:[7]

- *Personal preferences.* We all choose certain foods because we like the taste. Two widely shared preferences are for the sweetness of sugar and the tang of salt. High-fat foods appear to be another universal preference. Other preferences might be the hot peppers common in Mexican cooking or the curry spices of Indian cuisine. Many of us select foods because they are familiar and provide comfort. How many of you wake up to a certain bowl of cereal, toast, and something else? How many times do you order the same, familiar things when you go out to dinner? Habit is comforting and becomes deeply engrained over time.
- *Cultural heritage or tradition.* People eat the foods they grew up eating. Having been raised on a regimen of an Italian Sunday spaghetti dinner, this author can well understand the influence of tradition and cultural heritage on nutritional choices. Every country and region of the world has its typical foods, from the bratwurst and beer of northern Wisconsin to the Creole seafood of Louisiana. Although some research suggests that genetics may influence such preferences, you need only look to the favorite foods of your family to see what tastes you've become accustomed to.[8]
- *Social interactions.* For many of us, eating and socializing go hand in hand. We go out to eat to take a break from school pressures or just to unwind with people we enjoy.
- *Availability, convenience, and economy.* Economic status may determine the types of foods people purchase. Those with lower incomes find some foods too expensive, whereas

others with higher incomes have more choice. The rampant growth of fast-food establishments across the country makes them easily accessible, and they accommodate most budgets. Most of us eat foods that are readily available, quick and easy to prepare, and friendly to our budgets. The increasing numbers of Americans who opt out of the kitchen and forage for food in fast-food or upscale restaurants show how important convenience and accessibility have become. For students, who may not have access to well-equipped kitchens and lack time for grocery shopping and food preparation, convenience and availability are key factors.

• *Emotional comfort.* Have you ever been stressed out and eaten a whole bag of chips before you realized it? Have you ever felt lonely and found comfort in food because it tasted good and made you feel better? We learn from birth that eating is a pleasant experience associated with warmth, pleasure, and sensory delights. Infants cry and are fed; children are rewarded with food for doing well; weddings, birthdays, and other special occasions center on eating. These rewards carry over into times of disappointment. When we are frustrated, food often becomes our consolation. When we are busy, we reward ourselves with coffee and a snack. "Comfort food" becomes synonymous with enjoyment and pleasure.

• *Values.* Food choices often reflect one's religious or spiritual beliefs, political views, or environmental concerns. For example, many Christians abstain from meat during Lent, the period prior to Easter; some Jewish people abide by kosher dietary laws. Vegetarians often avoid animal products due to animal rights issues; environmentalists buy foods sold in recyclable packages.

• *Body image.* Many people select certain foods because they believe they will enhance appearance, improve health, or act as a preventive agent. Unfortunately, the public is constantly bombarded with misinformation and downright falsehoods, making it hard to discern between false and legitimate claims.

• *Nutrition.* Many people make nutrition choices based purely on health concerns. The new interest in **functional foods,** those products believed to enhance physiological function and improve health, provides substantial evidence of a major interest in this area (see Chapter 23). The old adage "You are what you eat" aptly summarizes the importance of nutritional choices. Scientists have been studying what we eat and why we eat it for centuries.

Nutrition is the science that investigates the relationship between physiological function and the essential elements of the foods we eat. With our country's overabundance of food and vast array of choices, media that "prime" us to want the tasty morsels shown in advertisements, and easy access to almost every type of **nutrient** (proteins, carbohydrates, fats, vitamins, minerals, and water), Americans should have few nutritional problems. However, these "diets of affluence" contribute to several major diseases, including obesity-related problems with heart disease, certain types of cancer, diabetes, hypertension (high blood pressure), cirrhosis of the liver, sleep apnea, varicose veins, gout, gallbladder disease, respiratory problems, abdominal hernias,

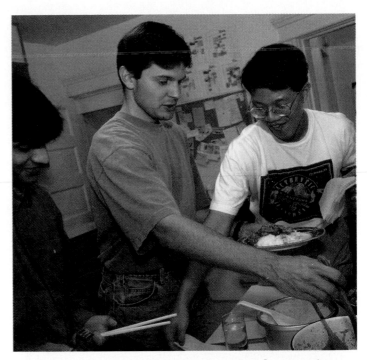

Access to cooking facilities and time to shop for groceries are just two of the many challenges facing college students trying to maintain a healthy diet.

flat feet, complications in pregnancy and surgery, and even higher accident rates, to name but a few.[9] Diabetes, in particular, has reached epidemic proportions in the United States and is largely a product of poor diet, excess weight gain, and lack of exercise. Put in perspective, a weight gain of 11 to 18 pounds increases a person's risk of developing diabetes to twice that of individuals who have not gained weight.[10]

Hunger The feeling associated with the physiological need to eat.

Appetite The desire to eat; normally accompanies hunger, but is more psychological than physiological.

Functional foods Foods believed to be beneficial and/or to prevent disease.

Nutrition The science that investigates the relationship between physiological function and the essential elements of foods eaten.

Nutrients The constituents of food that sustain us physiologically: proteins, carbohydrates, fats, vitamins, minerals, and water.

What's Your EQ (Eating Quotient)?

Keeping up with the latest on what to eat—or not eat—can be a challenge. If you think a few facts might have slipped past you, this quiz should help. There's only one correct answer for each question.

1. Which of these foods is most likely to help prevent the most common form of blindness in older Americans?
   a. carrots
   b. oranges
   c. spinach
   d. tomato juice
   e. zucchini

2. Which is worst for you?
   a. butter
   b. tub margarine
   c. stick margarine
   d. whipped butter
   e. light tub margarine

3. Which claim is backed by the best research?
   a. Hot dogs increase the risk of childhood leukemia.
   b. Carnitine helps you lose weight.
   c. Cranberry juice can help treat urinary tract infections.
   d. Garlic strengthens your immune system.
   e. Coenzyme Q_{10} helps prevent heart disease.

4. Breast cancer kills more women than any other disease.
   a. true
   b. false

5. Which disease has not been linked to diets that are rich in red meat?
   a. colon cancer
   b. heart disease
   c. prostate cancer
   d. stomach cancer

6. A diet rich in fruits and vegetables has not been clearly linked to a lower risk of:
   a. breast cancer
   b. colon cancer
   c. lung cancer
   d. stroke

7. A healthy Mediterranean diet has very little:
   a. bread
   b. olive oil
   c. beans
   d. vegetables
   e. cheese

8. If you're in your 50s or 60s and your blood pressure is normal, it will stay that way.
   a. true
   b. false

9. Four of these strategies have been clearly shown to keep blood pressure from rising. Which hasn't?
   a. cutting salt
   b. losing excess weight
   c. eating potassium-rich foods
   d. getting adequate vitamin C
   e. exercising regularly

10. Which is not a good source of potassium?
    a. cantaloupe
    b. yogurt
    c. brown rice
    d. squash
    e. kidney beans

11. Which has not been linked to a high-salt diet?
    a. stroke
    b. stomach cancer
    c. osteoporosis
    d. diabetes

12. There's evidence that the B vitamin folic acid cuts the risk of all but:
    a. birth defects like spina bifida
    b. stroke
    c. colon cancer
    d. heart disease
    e. prostate cancer

13. Which is not a good source of folic acid?
    a. tuna fish
    b. corn flakes
    c. asparagus
    d. lentils
    e. orange juice

14. The evidence is strongest that vitamin C can:
    a. prevent cancer
    b. lower blood pressure
    c. reduce the duration of colds
    d. prevent colds
    e. prevent cataracts

15. Which isn't dangerous in high doses?
    a. vitamin B_6
    b. vitamin B_{12}

c. niacin
d. vitamin D

16. Most multivitamin supplements contain far less than a day's worth of:
a. zinc
b. vitamin A
c. iron
d. calcium
e. vitamin D

17. Which food poisoning symptoms warrant calling the doctor?
a. bloody diarrhea
b. a stiff neck, severe headache, and fever
c. excessive vomiting
d. any of the above

18. Which is least likely to cause food poisoning?
a. undercooked chicken
b. Caesar salad dressing
c. raw oysters
d. rare hamburger
e. mayonnaise

19. Which is least likely to have contaminants?
a. flounder
b. swordfish
c. raw clams
d. bluefish
e. lake trout

20. What poisons the most children under the age of six?
a. eating moldy food
b. drinking household cleaners
c. taking an overdose of iron pills
d. chewing poisonous houseplant leaves

ANSWERS

1. c. Two carotenoids found in spinach—lutein and zeaxanthin—appear to protect eyes more than beta-carotene and other carotenoids. Other good sources: red bell pepper, okra, and leafy greens like kale, collard greens, and romaine lettuce.

2. a. Butter's saturated fat makes it boost your cholesterol more than margarine will. If you insist on butter, at least get a light whipped brand (some of its fat will be replaced by water and air). As for margarine, a tub always beats a stick, but a light tub or spread has the least cholesterol-raising trans and saturated fat of all.

3. c. In a recent study from Harvard Medical School, women who drank a little over a cup of cranberry juice cocktail a

day were twice as likely to be cured of their urinary tract infections as women who drank a look-alike, taste-alike beverage with no cranberry juice.

4. b. When women of all ages are combined, heart disease kills four times as many women as breast cancer.

5. d. The saturated fat and cholesterol in red meat—especially ground beef—raise the risk of heart disease.

6. a. A few animal studies suggest that something in fruits or vegetables may reduce the risk of breast cancer. But in humans, other cancers are more strongly linked to a lack of fruits and vegetables.

7. e. A true Mediterranean diet is very low in saturated fat. That means very little cheese (and meat, poultry, and butter).

8. b. In the United States, blood pressure rises with age for most people.

9. d. There's convincing evidence for all but the vitamin C. Limiting alcohol to no more than two drinks a day should also keep your blood pressure from rising.

10. c. Most grains aren't rich in potassium. A serving of any of the other four foods will give you at least 500 mg. Most fruits, vegetables, beans, fish, poultry, and milk (but not cheese) are good sources.

11. d. A high-salt diet is most clearly linked to the risk of stroke. But the more salt you eat, the more calcium your body excretes, which can lead to osteoporosis, or brittle bones. While stomach cancer is deadly, the kind that's linked to salty foods is on the decline in the United States.

12. e.

13. a. The best places to get folic acid are fruits, vegetables, beans, fortified cereals, and vitamin supplements.

14. c. Most people think that vitamin C prevents colds, but the research always seems to come up empty. In several studies, though, 1 to 3 grams (1,000 to 3,000 mg) a day reduced the average duration of volunteers' colds from 6 days to 4 ½ days.

15. b. A high dose of B_{12} (500 micrograms a day) can prevent B_{12} deficiency. And it's safe. A high dose of B_6 (possibly as little as 200 mg a day), on the other hand, can cause (reversible) nerve damage. Niacin (about 500 mg a day or more) is considered a drug. While it lowers cholesterol, it can cause side effects like flushing and liver damage. Vitamin D may cause side effects at levels as low as 1,200 IU a day.

(continued on page 218)

16. d. If you want to get close to 100 percent of the U.S. Recommended Daily Allowance from a supplement, you'll need to take calcium separately.

17. d. You should also see a physician if any milder food poisoning symptom lasts for more than three days.

18. e. Despite its reputation for spoiling easily, mayonnaise is not as risky as undercooked poultry, rare hamburger, the raw egg in Caesar salad dressing, and raw shellfish.

19. a. Other low-fat seafood like cod, haddock, Pacific halibut, ocean perch, pollock, sole, and cooked shellfish are also likely to be safe. Ditto for salmon and canned tuna.

20. c. Since 1986, more than 110,000 children have been poisoned by taking an overdose of their parents' (often brightly colored) iron supplements or iron-containing multivitamins, some after swallowing as few as five pills.

Source: Copyright 1995, by Center for Science in the Public Interest. Bonnie Liebman, "What's Your EQ (Eating Quotient)?" *Nutrition Action Healthletter.*

Eating for Health

Americans consume more calories per person than any other population in the world and have the highest rates of obesity. A **calorie** is a unit of measure that indicates the amount of energy we obtain from a particular food. Calories are eaten in the form of *proteins, fats,* and *carbohydrates,* three of the basic nutrients necessary for life. Three other nutrients—*vitamins, minerals,* and *water*—are necessary for bodily function but do not contribute any calories to our diets.

Excess calorie consumption is a major factor in our tendency to be overweight. However, it is not so much the quantity of food we eat that is likely to cause weight problems and resultant diseases as it is the relative proportion of nutrients in our diets and lack of sufficient physical activity to burn the calories we consume. Americans typically get approximately 38 percent of their calories from fat, 15 percent from proteins, 22 percent from complex carbohydrates, and 24 percent from simple sugars.[11] Nutritionists recommend increasing complex carbohydrates to make up 48 percent of our total calories and reducing proteins to 12 percent, simple sugars to 10 percent, and fats to no more than 30 percent of our total diets.

It is the high concentration of fats in the American diet, particularly saturated fats (largely animal fats), that appears to increase our risk for heart disease. Although too much sugar has been implicated in the development of many diseases, much of this information is inaccurate. Contrary to popular opinion, American consumption of sugar has not changed dramatically in recent years. In addition, the only disease associated with long-term excessive sugar intake is dental cavities. Most diet-related diseases result from excess calories and increased consumption of fat. Over the years, several federal agencies have worked to modify the average American's diet through a series of dietary goals and guidelines. How healthy are your eating habits? Find out by completing the quiz in the Assess Yourself box.

The Food Guide Pyramid

The Food Guide Pyramid, promoted by the United States Department of Agriculture (USDA) since 1993, illustrates graphically the importance of grains, cereals, vegetables, and fruits compared to meat, fish, poultry, dairy products, and other foods. Figure 8.1 shows the Food Guide Pyramid with recommended servings and examples of servings from each group.

A Call for a New Pyramid

Researchers have begun a collective movement to significantly "upend" the current pyramid. They favor a pyramid that downplays meat and dairy products and moves whole-grain foods and plant oils to the top of the list of foods that should make up your daily intake. Experts at a recent conference on diet and optimum health have proposed a pyramid that looks much like the guidelines in Figure 8.2 and will be the topic of much debate in the coming years.

Making the Pyramid Work for You

Many people are overwhelmed by their first glance at the pyramid. However, take a look at what the USDA considers a serving: an ounce of ready-to-eat cereal, half a small hamburger bun or bagel, four to five potato chips, or one slice of bread. A normal bowl of cereal has three to four ounces of cereal. When was the last time you ate a quarter of a bowl of cereal? Or only half a hamburger bun? When you consider breakfast, lunch, dinner, and snacks in between, it is really quite easy to get all the servings in this group that you need.

Calorie A unit of measure that indicates the amount of energy obtained from a particular food.

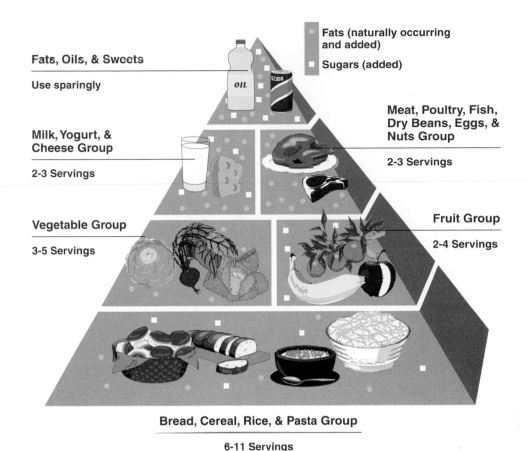

Figure 8.1
Food Guide Pyramid: A Guide to Daily Food Choices
Sources: Food and Nutrition Information Center, "The Interactive Food Guide Pyramid" (2002) (see http:// www.nal.usda.gov:8001/py/pmap.htm); U.S. Department of Agriculture, 1993.

What Counts as a Serving?   The amount of food that counts as one serving is listed below. If you eat a larger portion, count it as more than one serving. For example, 2 cups of milk would count as two servings from the milk, yogurt, and cheese group.

Be sure to eat at least the lowest number of servings from the major food groups; you need them for the nutrients they provide. No specific serving size is given for the fats, oils, and sweets groups because they should be used sparingly.

Bread, Cereal, Rice, and Pasta Group
- 1 slice of bread or medium dinner roll
- ½ cup cooked rice, pasta, or other grains
- 1 ounce ready-to-eat cereal
- 3 cups popped popcorn

Fruit Group
- Whole fruit such as medium apple, banana, or orange
- ½ cup of raw, cooked, or canned fruit
- ¾ cup of fruit juice

Vegetable Group
- 1 cup leafy raw vegetables
- ½ cup chopped fresh, frozen, or canned vegetables

Meat, Poultry, Fish, Dry Beans, Eggs, and Nuts Group
- 2–3 ounces lean, trimmed, and baked or roasted meat, fish, or poultry

The following can substitute for 1 ounce of meat:
- 2 tablespoons peanut butter or other nut or seed butter
- ¼ cup nuts
- ½ cup cooked legumes
- 3 ounces tofu
- 1 egg

Milk, Yogurt, and Cheese Group
- 1 cup milk or yogurt
- 1 ½ ounces natural cheese
- 2 ounces processed cheese
- 1 ½ cups ice cream, ice milk, or frozen yogurt

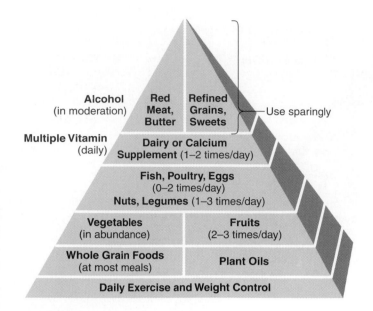

Figure 8.2
Proposed New Food Guide Pyramid
Source: Adapted from *Eat, Drink, and Be Healthy,* by William C. Willet, M.D. (New York: Simon and Schuster, 2001).

Understanding Serving Sizes How much is a "serving"? Is a "serving" different than a "portion"? While these two terms are often used interchangeably, they actually mean different things. A serving is the amount recommended in materials such as the Food Guide Pyramid, while a portion is the amount of food you choose to eat at any one time, which may be more or less than a serving. Most people have trouble judging what a serving looks like and eat two to three servings when they think they are having only one. A national survey found the following:[12]

- Fifty-five percent of those surveyed overestimated the serving size of cooked pasta or rice and took at least two times the amount that they should have.
- Fifty-four percent overestimated the serving size of cooked lean meat, poultry, or fish (2–3 ounces).
- Sixty-eight percent overestimated the serving size of cooked vegetables (½ cup).
- Sixty-eight percent knew that a serving size of bread was just one slice.

To make sure you aren't super-sizing your portions, use these tips to visualize the standard serving size:

- *Cheese:* A 1½ ounce serving is the size of four stacked dice.
- *Fruit, cooked rice or pasta, and cooked vegetables:* Half a cup is the size of a tennis ball cut in half.
- *Raw, leafy vegetables:* One cup is the size of a tennis ball.
- *Cooked lean meat, poultry, or fish:* Two to three ounces is the size of an audiocassette or personal digital assistant.

Making Healthy Choices Although everyone is different, it is generally recommended that you consume foods from the pyramid throughout the day. Try to eat at least two foods

from the bread and cereal group for breakfast. Finding time for a snack of low-fat crackers could take care of another one to two servings during the day. Eating a cup of rice, a muffin, or bread at lunch could take care of two to three more servings, leaving only three to four servings for dinner. A plate of pasta and a slice of reduced-fat, whole-grain bread could just about do it.

With any bread, cereal, or grain product, consider the amount of fat. Many people are duped into thinking that granola is a health food and bran muffins are better than bagels or bread. Sometimes these products are loaded with fat, sugar, and calories. Read the package labels and opt for reduced-fat, whole-grain products (see the Skills for Behavior Change box on whole grains). When eating out, abiding by the guidelines may be challenging. The Reality Check box ("What's Good on the Menu?") offers suggestions.

Today's Dietary Guidelines

With so many changes in the field of nutrition science, the federal government revised its Dietary Guidelines for Americans in 1998 (see Figure 8.3) as follows:

- *Alcohol, in moderation, has health benefits.* Moderation refers to one drink per day for women, two drinks per day for men, preferably with a meal. This dose of alcohol has been consistently linked to higher levels of HDL, or "good" cholesterol, and fewer heart attacks than among people who never drink. However, drinking beyond this magic limit increases the risk for several serious health problems.
- *Vegetarianism is healthful.* The USDA acknowledges for the first time that a vegetarian diet is beneficial. It advocates avoiding organ meat and high-fat processed meats, such as hot dogs and cold cuts.
- *Limit hydrogenated polyunsaturated fats.* The USDA strongly suggests cutting back on foods containing trans-fatty acids, such as margarines and shortenings, which are found in many snack foods.
- *Vitamin and mineral supplements are no substitute for a variety of foods.* In general, it is better to combine foods, especially those that act synergistically with one another, than it is to take supplements. The exceptions include calcium, folate, and vitamin D, which are believed to be okay in supplement form, particularly for those at risk of deficiency.
- *Use sugar and salt sparingly.* Although much of the information about ill-health effects, hyperactivity, and other problems associated with excess sugar is not true, sugar is a major source of excess calories in the average American's diet. While the negative effects of salt may be overexaggerated, some individuals react hypertensively to excess sodium. Because we don't know who will be affected, reduction for all is advised.
- *Weight should* not *increase with age.* Because of increasing levels of information about the relationship between weight gain and premature health risks, maintaining a stable weight throughout life is important.

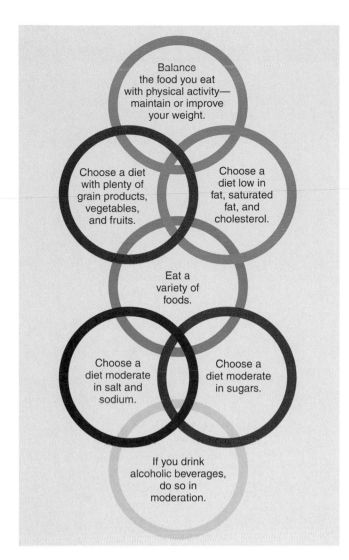

Figure 8.3
Dietary Guidelines for Americans
Source: U.S. Department of Agriculture (1998).

What do you think?

Which food groups from the Food Guide Pyramid are you most likely to eat enough of during a typical day? ✳ Which ones, if any, are you most likely to skimp on? ✳ What are some simple changes that you could make right now in your diet to help meet Pyramid recommendations?

The Digestive Process

Food provides the chemicals we need for energy and body maintenance. Because our bodies cannot synthesize or produce certain essential nutrients, we must obtain them from the foods we eat. Even though we may take in adequate amounts of foods and nutrients, if our body systems are not functioning properly, much of the nutrient value in our food may be lost. Before foods can be utilized properly, the digestive system must break the larger food particles down into smaller, more usable forms. The process by which foods are broken down and either absorbed or excreted by the body is known as the **digestive process.**

Even before you take your first bite of pizza, your body has already begun a series of complex digestive responses. Your mouth prepares for the food by increasing production of **saliva.** Saliva contains mostly water, which aids in chewing and swallowing, but it also contains important enzymes that begin the process of food breakdown, including amylase, which breaks down carbohydrates. *Enzymes* are protein compounds that facilitate chemical reactions but are not altered in the process. From the mouth, the food passes down the **esophagus,** a 9- to 10-inch tube that connects the mouth and stomach. A series of contractions and relaxations by the muscles lining the esophagus gently move food to the next digestive organ, the **stomach.** Here food mixes with enzymes and stomach acids. Hydrochloric acid begins to work in combination with pepsin, an enzyme, to break down proteins. In most people, the stomach secretes enough mucous to protect the stomach lining from these harsh digestive juices.

Eating "Nutrient-Dense" Foods

Although eating the proper number of servings from the food pyramid is important, it is also important to recognize that there are large caloric, fat, and energy differences between food categories within pyramid groups. For example, you might get the same number of calories from a glass of beer as you would from a glass of milk, but you would get many more nutrients from the milk. Likewise, fish and hot dogs provide vastly different fat and energy levels per ounce, with fish providing better energy and calorie value per serving. Nutrient density is even more important for someone who is ill and unable to keep food down. That is why nutrient supplements such as Ensure and others are often provided for cancer patients who need a nutrient "hit" in a small package.

Digestive process   The process by which foods are broken down and either absorbed or excreted by the body.

Saliva   Fluid secreted by the salivary glands; enzymes in the fluid aid in the breakdown of certain foods for digestion.

Esophagus   Tube that transports food from the mouth to the stomach.

Stomach   Large muscular organ that temporarily stores, mixes, and digests foods.

There's More to Whole Grains Than Whole Wheat

It's hard to beat whole grains. They are packed with vitamins, minerals, and fiber that you just don't find in white bread, processed cereals, white rice, or even in many healthful-looking, enriched, "multi-grain" breads, for that matter.

Plus, whole grains have a new health cachet, now that researchers have uncovered disease-fighting properties from the phytonutrients they contain.

Besides their nutritive value, whole grains are loaded with flavor and texture and add interest to meals. Here is *Environmental Nutrition* magazine's guide to some less traditional whole grains and how and why to give them a try.

If you can't find these grains or flours in your local supermarket or health food store, try these mail-order sources:

- Get Healthy Shop—(800) 420-4726; www.gethealthyshop.com
- King Arthur Flour—(800) 827-6836; www.kingarthurflour.com
- True Foods Market—(877) 274-5914; www.truefoodsmarket.com

Grain	What It Is and Nutrients	Flavor Basics and Shopping Tips	Preparation and Serving Suggestions
Amaranth	A high-protein grain that's a good source of fiber and vitamin E. Rich in lysine, an amino acid often missing in grain foods. Tolerated by people sensitive to wheat or gluten-intolerant.	Amaranth seeds have a pleasant, peppery flavor.	• Amaranth flour is higher in fat than wheat, resulting in moister bread; replace no more than ¼ of the flour in bread recipes. • Boil and eat as cereal or use in soups and granolas. The seeds of some varieties can be popped like popcorn. • To prepare: Cook 1 cup amaranth in 3 cups water for ½ hour.
Kasha (buckwheat groats)	Technically, a fruit (the roasted seed of the buckwheat plant), but the food world classifies it as a grain. It's an excellent source of magnesium and a good source of copper and fiber. Like amaranth, it is rich in lysine. Tolerated by people sensitive to wheat or gluten-intolerant, though be careful of mixes that also contain wheat.	Kasha has a hearty, nutty flavor and chewy texture. Kasha comes in whole, coarse, medium, and fine consistencies. Also available as flour. Or make your own by pulverizing whole groats in a food processor or blender until the consistency of flour.	• Great when served as a hot cereal or as a hearty salad with vegetables and paired with a light soup. • Kasha makes an exceptionally flavorful pilaf; prepare with carmelized or browned onions and mushrooms. • Kasha flour makes flavorful, hearty pancakes and pasta. • You can replace up to half the wheat flour in many recipes with kasha flour, but replace only ⅕ the flour in breads. • To prepare: Simmer 1 part groats in 2 parts water for 15 minutes (medium and fine grades cook more quickly).
Quinoa (KEEN-wah)	A staple of ancient Incan culture. It is an excellent source of B vitamins, copper, iron, magnesium, and lysine. It provides a more complete protein than	Quinoa has a mild flavor and a slightly crunchy texture. It comes in different colors, ranging from a pale yellow to red and black. Health food stores sell	• Quinoa flakes are seeds that have been steamed, rolled, then flaked to make an oatmeal-like hot cereal.

Grain	What It Is and Nutrients	Flavor Basics and Shopping Tips	Preparation and Serving Suggestions
	many other grains. A popular alternative for people sensitive to wheat or gluten-intolerant.	pasta and other products made from it.	• Quinoa flour is higher in fat than traditional bread flour, so it tends to make bread moister. Replace up to ¼ of the flour in a bread recipe with it. • Rinse quinoa before cooking to remove its bitter natural coating. • To prepare: Cook 1 cup quinoa in 2 cups water for 20 minutes.
Spelt	Spelt, a distant cousin to wheat, is hearty and grows well without chemical fertilizers, pesticides, and herbicides and therefore is a commonly available organic grain. It is a good source of fiber and B vitamins.	Available as whole berries and whole or refined flour. Also found in bread and pastas in natural food stores.	• Use whole spelt berries as you would rice and barley, in hearty grain salads, pilafs, and fillings. • Use spelt flour to make breads and pastas. Spelt tends to make bread heavier. Experiment by adding a little extra yeast to help bread rise or look for commercial bread mixes. • To prepare: Cook 1 cup berries in 4 cups water for 30–40 minutes.
Teff	This Ethiopian staple is the world's smallest grain and is less refined than many common grains. As a result, it's a nutritional powerhouse, especially rich in protein and calcium. Tolerated by people sensitive to wheat or gluten-intolerant.	Teff has a sweet, nutty flavor and comes in different colors, ranging from creamy white to reddish-brown.	• Serve as a hot breakfast cereal, sprinkled with cinnamon and brown sugar, maple syrup, raisins, or sliced fruit. • To prepare: Cook 1 cup teff in 3 cups water for 15–20 minutes; to add flavor, roast teff with cornmeal for 5 minutes before boiling.
Triticale (Tri-ti-CAY-lee)	This relatively young (only 200 years old) grain is a cross between wheat and rye. It is an excellent source of fiber, B vitamins, and magnesium, plus a good source of iron.	Triticale berries are gray-brown and oval shaped, similar to wheat berries but with a subtle rye flavor. Available as flour, flakes (for cereal), berries, and as part of muesli, granola, or whole-grain cereal combinations.	• Triticale makes wonderful sandwich bread, similar in taste to honey wheat bread. • When making bread, replace no more than half the flour in recipes. Knead gently and let rise only once. • Use triticale flakes like rolled oats to make a hot breakfast cereal. They cook in about 15 minutes. • To prepare: Cook 1 cup berries in 4 cups water for 1 hour.

Source: From "There's More to Whole Grains Than Whole Wheat," by Luanne Hughes, *Environmental Nutrition* (October 2001). Reprinted with permission from Environmental Nutrition, 52 Riverside Drive, New York, NY 10024. For subscription information 800-829-5384.

What's Good on the Menu?

While some restaurants offer hints for health-conscious diners, you're on your own most of the time. To help you order wisely, here are lighter options and high-fat pitfalls. "Best" choices contain fewer than 30 grams of fat, a generous meal's worth for an active, medium-size woman. "Worst" choices have up to 100 grams of fat.

Fast Food

Best Grilled chicken sandwich
Roast beef sandwich
Single hamburger
Salad with light vinaigrette

Worst Bacon burger
Double cheeseburger
French fries
Onion rings

Tips Order sandwiches without mayo or "special sauce." Avoid deep-fried items like fish fillets, chicken nuggets, and French fries.

Italian

Best Pasta with red or white clam sauce
Spaghetti with marinara or tomato-and-meat sauce

Worst Eggplant parmigiana
Fettuccine alfredo
Fried calamari
Lasagna

Tips Stick with plain bread instead of garlic bread made with butter or oil. Ask for the waiter's help in avoiding cream- or egg-based sauces. Try vegetarian pizza, and don't ask for extra cheese.

Mexican

Best Bean burrito (no cheese)
Chicken fajitas

Worst Beef chimichanga
Chile relleno
Quesadilla
Refried beans

Tips Choose soft tortillas (not fried) with fresh salsa, not guacamole. Special-order grilled shrimp, fish, or chicken. Ask for beans made without lard or fat and for cheeses and sour cream provided on the side or left out altogether.

Chinese

Best Hot-and-sour soup
Stir-fried vegetables
Shrimp with garlic sauce
Szechuan shrimp

Wonton soup

Worst Crispy chicken
Kung pao chicken
Moo shu pork
Sweet-and-sour pork

Tips Share a stir-fry; help yourself to steamed rice. Ask for vegetables steamed or stir-fried with less oil. Order moo shu vegetables instead of pork. Avoid fried rice, breaded dishes, egg rolls and spring rolls, and items loaded with nuts. Avoid high-sodium sauces.

Japanese

Best Steamed rice and vegetables
Tofu as a substitute for meat
Broiled or steamed chicken and fish

Worst Fried rice dishes
Miso (very high in sodium)
Tempura

Tips Avoid soy sauces. Use caution in eating sashimi and sushi (raw fish) dishes to avoid possible bacteria or parasites.

Thai

Best Clear broth soups
Stir-fried chicken and vegetables
Grilled meats

Further digestive activity takes place in the **small intestine,** a 20-foot coiled tube containing three sections: the *duodenum, jejunum,* and *ileum.* Each section secretes digestive enzymes that, when combined with enzymes from the liver and the pancreas, further contribute to the breakdown of proteins, fats, and carbohydrates. These nutrients are absorbed into the bloodstream to supply body cells with energy. The liver is the major organ that determines whether nutrients are stored, sent to cells or organs, or excreted. Solid wastes consisting of fiber, water, and salts are dumped into the large intestine, where most of the water and salts are reabsorbed into the system and the fiber is passed out through the anus. The entire digestive process takes approximately 24 hours.

Obtaining Essential Nutrients

Water: A Crucial Nutrient

If you were to go on a survival trip, which would you take with you—food or water? You may be surprised to learn that you could survive for much longer without food than you could without water. Even in severe conditions, the average person can go for weeks without certain vitamins and minerals before experiencing serious deficiency symptoms. **Dehydration,** however, can cause serious problems within a matter of hours; after a few days without water, death is likely.

| **Worst** | Coconut milk
Peanut sauces
Deep-fried dishes |
| **Tips** | Avoid coconut-based curries.
Ask for steamed, not fried,
rice. |

Breakfast

| **Best** | Hot or cold cereal with
2 percent milk
Pancakes or French toast
with syrup
Scrambled eggs with hash
browns and plain toast |
| **Worst** | Belgian waffle with sausage
Sausage and eggs with biscuits
and gravy
Ham and cheese omelette with
hash browns and toast |

| **Tips** | Ask for whole-grain cereal or
shredded wheat with 1 percent
milk or whole-wheat toast with
out butter or margarine. Order
omelettes without cheese,
fried eggs without bacon or
sausage. |

Sandwiches

Best	Ham and Swiss cheese Roast beef Turkey
Worst	Tuna salad Reuben Submarine
Tips	Ask for mustard; hold the mayo and cheese. See if turkey-ham is available.

Seafood

Best	Broiled bass, halibut, or snapper Grilled scallops Steamed crab or lobster
Worst	Fried seafood platter Blackened catfish
Tips	Order fish broiled, baked, grilled, or steamed—not pan-fried or sauteed. Ask for lemon instead of tartar sauce. Avoid creamy and buttery sauces.

Sources: American Dietetic Association (2002) (see http://www.eatright.org); *Health* 10 (November/December 1996): 79.

Just what function does water serve in the body? Between 50 and 60 percent of our total body weight is water. The water in our system bathes cells, aids in fluid and electrolyte balance, maintains pH balance, and transports molecules and cells throughout the body. Water is the major component of our blood, which carries oxygen and nutrients to the tissues and is responsible for maintaining cells in working order.

Individual needs for water vary drastically according to dietary factors, age, size, environmental temperature and humidity levels, exercise, and the effectiveness of the individual's system. Certain diseases, such as diabetes or cystic fibrosis, cause people to lose fluids at a rate necessitating a higher volume of fluid intake. Judging by the large number of people sucking at water bottles today, many Americans seem to fear becoming dehydrated. They also seem to be trying to "flush" their systems with pure water to help organs function more efficiently and enhance their health. Bottled water has become a multimillion-dollar industry that rivals the soda industry. Is all this water consumption really necessary? See the New Horizons in Health box about ongoing research into how much water each of us truly needs.

Is bottled water healthier than city water? In most instances, expensive "spring" and bottled water are no healthier than chlorinated and fluoride-containing city water. In fact, if you look closely at the labels, you'll find that most expensive little bottles don't contain pristine water from natural springs but, rather, purified city water that has been subjected to reverse osmosis. Is it worth the extra cost? Most

experts think not. Have your current water source tested if you doubt its cleanliness. Otherwise, don't spend your money needlessly.

Proteins

Next to water, **proteins** are the most abundant substances in the human body. Proteins are major components of nearly every cell and have been called the "body builders" because of their role in developing and repairing bone, muscle, skin, and blood cells. Proteins are also the key elements of the antibodies that protect us from disease, of enzymes that control chemical activities in the body, and of hormones that regulate bodily functions. Moreover, proteins aid in the transport

Small intestine Muscular, coiled digestive organ; consists of the duodenum, jejunum, and ileum.

Dehydration Abnormal depletion of body fluids; a result of lack of water.

Proteins The essential constituents of nearly all body cells; necessary for the development and repair of bone, muscle, skin, and blood; the key elements of antibodies, enzymes, and hormones.

How Much Water Do We Need?

How much water do we really need? According to a generation of health experts, we should drink eight glasses per day, not including caffeinated beverages. Not until recently had anyone really questioned what scientific evidence there was for that recommendation. That is when Dr. Heinz Valtin, professor emeritus at Dartmouth Medical School and an expert on how the body maintains fluid balance, began to assess the basis for the 64-ounce/day concept. He determined that the advice probably stems from a muddled interpretation of a 1945 Food and Nutrition Board report that said the body needs about 1 milliliter of water for each calorie consumed—almost 8 cups for a typical 2000-calorie diet. That advice is probably sound; however, it does not account for the fact that most of this quantity is contained in prepared foods. (Fruits and vegetables are 80–95 percent water, meats contain over 50 percent water, and even dry bread and cheese are about 35 percent water.) Dr. Valtin was unable to determine how the report came to be interpreted as recommending eight

glasses of pure water per day. Nor did he find any supporting research showing that the average person needs 64 ounces of fluid from any source per day, whether it be from foods or beverages.

Another key finding of Dr. Valtin's group was that, contrary to popular opinion, caffeinated drinks don't dehydrate the person who consumes them; in fact, coffee, tea, and sodas are actually hydrating for people used to caffeine and, thus, should count toward overall fluid intake.

So, should you continue to pay for all those tiny bottles of water? (See the chapter on environmental health for information on the effect of the plastic from all those bottles.) If you're drinking water for the health benefits of those eight additional glasses per day, you may be disappointed. For most of us, adding that much water to what we are already getting just means more trips to the bathroom with little harm done—an expensive habit with few rewards. Furthermore, people with certain medical conditions can put undue stress on the bladder and other systems or can excrete more water soluble-vitamins than they would if they had not been drinking so much. Healthy people who take Ecstasy, which increases thirst dramatically, can drink enough to suffer from *water intoxica-*

tion, which may lead to sodium depletion, cardiac arrhythmias, and other problems.

Concern over Valtin's research has prompted the Food and Nutrition Board to question its own recommendations. Look for official water-intake guidelines in the new future. In the meantime, everyone seems to agree that drinking water is important. The question is whether or not you are already getting close to the right amount with food, juice, milk, soda, coffee, and other fluid sources. Students who aren't eating properly, those who exercise heavily and sweat profusely, and those who aren't getting adequate fluids to compensate for fluid losses may need to pay attention to this. Older people with diminished mental capacity or sensory acuity or those on diuretics for cardiac conditions can also become water depleted and experience serious consequences.

Source: Heinz Valtin, 2002. *American Journal of Physiology,* "Water Consumption Needs: A Look at the Accumulated Evidence," July 12 (5): 88–94.

---

of iron, oxygen, and nutrients to all body cells and supply another source of energy to cells when fats and carbohydrates are not readily available. In short, adequate amounts of protein in the diet are vital to many body functions and ultimately to survival.

Whenever you consume proteins, your body breaks them down into smaller molecules known as **amino acids,** which link together like beads in a necklace to form 20 different combinations. Nine of these combinations are termed **essential amino acids,** meaning that the body must obtain them from the diet; the other 11 are produced by the body.

Dietary protein that supplies all of the essential amino acids is called **complete (high-quality) protein.** Typically, protein from animal products is complete. When we consume foods that are deficient in some of the essential amino acids, the total amount of protein that can be synthesized from the other amino acids is decreased. For proteins to be complete, they must also be present in digestible form and in amounts proportional to body requirements.

What about plant sources of protein? Proteins from plant sources are often **incomplete proteins** in that they are missing one or two of the essential amino acids. Nevertheless, it is relatively easy for the non–meat eater to combine plant foods effectively and eat complementary sources of plant protein (see Figure 8.4). An excellent example of this mutual supplementation process is eating peanut butter on whole-grain bread. Although each of these foods lacks certain essential amino acids, eating them together provides high-quality protein.

Plant sources of protein fall into three general categories: *legumes* (beans, peas, peanuts, and soy products), *grains* (whole grains, corn, and pasta products), and *nuts and seeds.* Certain vegetables, such as leafy green vegetables and broccoli, also contribute valuable plant proteins. Mixing two or more foods from each of these categories during the same meal will provide all of the essential amino acids necessary to ensure adequate protein absorption. People who are not interested in obtaining all of their protein from plants can

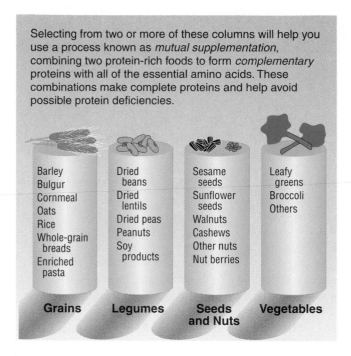

Selecting from two or more of these columns will help you use a process known as *mutual supplementation,* combining two protein-rich foods to form *complementary* proteins with all of the essential amino acids. These combinations make complete proteins and help avoid possible protein deficiencies.

Grains	Legumes	Seeds and Nuts	Vegetables
Barley	Dried beans	Sesame seeds	Leafy greens
Bulgur	Dried lentils	Sunflower seeds	Broccoli
Cornmeal	Dried peas	Walnuts	Others
Oats	Peanuts	Cashews	
Rice	Soy products	Other nuts	
Whole-grain breads		Nut berries	
Enriched pasta			

Figure 8.4

Complementary Proteins

Source: From *Nutrition Concepts and Controversies,* 6th ed., by F.S. Sizer, E.N. Whitney, and E.M. Hamilton, © 1994. Reprinted with permission of Wadsworth, an imprint of the Wadsworth Group, a division of Thomson Learning.

combine incomplete plant proteins with complete low-fat animal proteins such as chicken, fish, turkey, and lean red meat. Low-fat or nonfat cottage cheese, skim milk, egg whites, and nonfat dry milk all provide high quality proteins and have few calories and little dietary fat. Soy provides an excellent option for many people and is growing in popularity as soy products become more flavorful. See the Skills for Behavior Change box for ways to incorporate soy into your diet.

You need to eat enough protein, but make sure you don't consume too much. Eating too much protein, particularly animal protein, can place added stress on the liver and kidneys. It also may increase calcium excretion in urine, which can elevate the risk of osteoporosis and bone fractures.[13]

Recently, several low-calorie diets that practically eliminate carbohydrates and focus on eating large quantities of protein have reemerged in the popular press. Diets that deviate from a balanced nutritional approach are almost certainly flawed. In particular, people who have kidney or liver problems or suffer from fluid imbalances should avoid such diets. See Chapter 9 for more on these and other weight management tactics.

A person might need to eat extra protein if fighting off a serious infection, recovering from surgery or blood loss, or recovering from burns. In these instances, proteins that are lost to cellular repair need to be replaced. There is considerable controversy over whether someone in high-level physical training needs additional protein to build and repair muscle fibers or whether normal daily requirements should suffice.

Although protein deficiency continues to pose a threat to the global population, few Americans suffer from protein deficiencies. In fact, the average American consumes more than 100 grams of protein daily, and about 70 percent of this comes from high-fat animal flesh and dairy products.[14] The recommended protein intake for the average man is only 63 grams, and the average woman needs only 50 grams. (As an example, a 6-ounce broiled sirloin steak contains about 53 grams of protein.) The typical recommendation is that, in a 2,000-calorie diet, about 10 percent of calories should come from protein, 60 percent from carbohydrates, and less than 30 percent from fat. The excess is stored as extra calories, leading to extra fat. See Figure 8.5 to determine your own recommended daily allowance (RDA) for protein.

Carbohydrates

Although the importance of proteins in the body cannot be underestimated, it is **carbohydrates** that supply us with the energy needed to sustain normal daily activity. Long maligned by weight-conscious people, carbohydrates can actually be metabolized more quickly and efficiently than proteins. Carbohydrates are a quick source of energy for the body, being easily converted to glucose, the fuel for the body's cells. These foods also play an important role in the functioning of internal organs, the nervous system, and the muscles. They are the best fuel for endurance athletics because they provide both an immediate and a time-released energy source, as they are digested easily and then consistently metabolized in the bloodstream. For many people, a plate of pasta represents an attractive, healthy alternative to a fatty steak.

There are two major types of carbohydrates: **simple sugars,** which are found primarily in fruits, and **complex carbohydrates,** which are found in grains, cereals, dark green leafy vegetables, yellow fruits and vegetables (carrots, yams), *cruciferous* vegetables (such as broccoli, cabbage, and

---

Amino acids The building blocks of protein.

Essential amino acids Nine of the basic nitrogen-containing building blocks of protein that must be obtained from foods to ensure health.

Complete (high-quality) proteins Proteins that contain all of the nine essential amino acids.

Incomplete proteins Proteins that are lacking in one or more of the essential amino acids.

Carbohydrates Basic nutrients that supply the body with the energy needed to sustain normal activity.

Simple sugars A major type of carbohydrate, which provides short-term energy.

Complex carbohydrates A major type of carbohydrate, which provides sustained energy.

A Consumer's Guide to Soy

Has your interest been piqued by all you've been hearing about soy as a healthy protein alternative? Here's some information that will help you reduce the amount of saturated fat in your diet by increasing your soy intake. Knowing the basic characteristics of these foods is a key to regular use.

The Skinny on Soy

Soy has hit mainstream America in a wave of soy milk, soy burgers, soy dogs, and cheeselike products, totaling nearly $3 billion per year. Interestingly, although touted as a great boon to health-conscious individuals, much of what we believe to be true about soy is still largely in question. Researchers still don't know which of several soybean components provide soy's important health benefits. To date, most (70 to 80 percent) of the health benefits we've seen from soy products appear to be attributable to *isoflavons.* These isoflavons are *phytoestrogens* (plant compounds with estrogen-like activity), which are thought to block human estrogens that may encourage the growth of hormone-sensitive cancers.

However, before you run out and buy soy purely for anti-cancer benefits, it is important to note that phytoestrogens have been found to have both estrogenic and anti-estrogenic effects. Researchers aren't sure why, but it may depend on when in life you get them and in what quantity.

Other benefits of isoflavons in conjunction with soy protein appear to be a reduction in blood cholesterol and overall risk of heart disease, bone building, and protection against some cancers—particularly prostate cancer in men and breast cancer in women. Especially for postmenopausal women, soy seems to be a factor in decreased breast density, which may increase early detection of growing tumors. In general, soy foods naturally contain about two milligrams of isoflavons for every gram of soy protein.

Options for the Soy-Conscious Consumer

Tofu: A soft, cheeselike food made by curdling soy milk that tends to take on the flavor of foods that it is cooked with. Use firm or extra-firm tofu if you want to chunk the tofu for soups, stir fries, or grilling. Choose soft and silky tofu for blending and baking.

Soy nuts: Whole soybeans that have been soaked in water, drained, and baked, usually with salt added. These make great substitutes for peanuts and are loaded with protein and isoflavons.

Tempeh: A tender cake, often a mixture of soybeans and other grains such as rice or millet, that has been fermented to have a smoky or nutty flavor. Can be used in soups, casseroles, or sandwiches.

Edamamé: Green soybeans in their pods or shells; often available frozen. Cook in boiling water and eat like other pea pods with a bit of salt.

Natto: Made of fermented, cooked whole soybeans. Cheeselike texture best used as topping for rice, in soups, and with vegetables.

Soy milk: Soybeans are soaked, ground fine, and strained to produce a milk-like fluid. Often flavored to enhance taste. Unlike milk, doesn't contain calcium (unless fortified).

Soy cheese and yogurt: Made from soy milk and may be substituted as desired.

Source: From *Environmental Nutrition,* May 2002. For subscription information, 800-829-5384.

---

cauliflower), and certain root vegetables, such as potatoes. Most of us do not get enough complex carbohydrates in our daily diets.

A typical American diet contains large amounts of simple sugars. The most common form is *glucose.* Eventually, the human body converts all types of simple sugars to glucose to provide energy to cells. In its natural form, glucose is sweet and is obtained from substances such as corn syrup, honey, molasses, vegetables, and fruits. *Fructose* is another simple sugar found in fruits and berries. Glucose and fructose are **monosaccharides** and contain only one molecule of sugar.

Disaccharides are combinations of two monosaccharides. Perhaps the best-known example is common granulated table sugar (known as sucrose), which consists of a molecule of fructose chemically bonded to a molecule of glucose. Lactose, found in milk and milk products, is another form of disaccharide, formed by the combination of glucose

and galactose (another simple sugar). Disaccharides must be broken down into simple sugars before they can be used by the body.

Controlling the amount of sugar in your diet can be difficult because sugar, like sodium, is often present in food products that you might not expect to contain it. Such diverse items as ketchup, Russian dressing, Coffee-Mate, and Shake 'n' Bake derive between 30 and 65 percent of their calories from sugar. Read food labels carefully before purchasing.

Polysaccharides are complex carbohydrates formed by long chains of saccharides. Like disaccharides, they must be broken down into simple sugars before they can be utilized by the body. There are two major forms of complex carbohydrates: *starches* and *fiber,* or **cellulose.**

Starches make up the majority of the complex carbohydrate group. Starches in our diets come from flours, breads, pasta, potatoes, and related foods. They are stored in

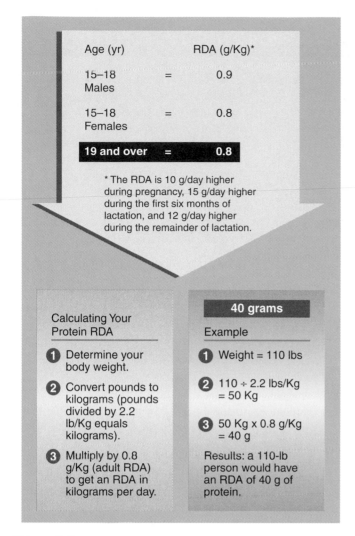

Age (yr)		RDA (g/Kg)*
15–18 Males	=	0.9
15–18 Females	=	0.8
19 and over	**=**	**0.8**

* The RDA is 10 g/day higher during pregnancy, 15 g/day higher during the first six months of lactation, and 12 g/day higher during the remainder of lactation.

Calculating Your Protein RDA

1. Determine your body weight.
2. Convert pounds to kilograms (pounds divided by 2.2 lb/Kg equals kilograms).
3. Multiply by 0.8 g/Kg (adult RDA) to get an RDA in kilograms per day.

40 grams

Example

1. Weight = 110 lbs
2. 110 ÷ 2.2 lbs/Kg = 50 Kg
3. 50 Kg x 0.8 g/Kg = 40 g

Results: a 110-lb person would have an RDA of 40 g of protein.

Figure 8.5
Calculating Your Protein RDA
Source: From *Nutrition Concepts and Controversies,* 6th ed., by F.S. Sizer, E.N. Whitney, and F.M. Hamilton, © 1994. Reprinted with permission of Wadsworth, an imprint of the Wadsworth Group, a division of Thomson Learning.

body muscles and the liver in a polysaccharide form called **glycogen.** When the body requires a sudden burst of energy, it breaks down glycogen into glucose.

Carbohydrates and Athletic Performance Carbohydrates have become the "health foods" of many athletes. Some fitness enthusiasts consume concentrated sugary foods or drinks before or during athletic activity, thinking that the sugars will provide extra energy. This may actually be counterproductive.

One possible problem involves the gastrointestinal tract. If your intestines react to activity (or the nervousness before competition) by moving material through the small intestine more rapidly than usual, undigested disaccharides and/or unabsorbed monosaccharides will reach the colon, which can result in a very inopportune bout of diarrhea.

Consuming large amounts of sugar during exercise can also have a negative effect on hydration. Concentrations ex-

ceeding 24 grams of sugar per 8 ounces of fluid can delay stomach emptying and hence absorption of water. Some fruit juices, fruit drinks, and other sugar-sweetened beverages have more than this amount of sugar. If you use these products, dilute them with ice cubes or water.

Marathon runners and other people who require reserves of energy for demanding tasks often attempt to increase stores of glycogen in the body by *carbohydrate loading.* This process involves modifying the nature of both workouts and diet, usually during the week or so before competition. The athletes train very hard early in the week while eating small amounts of carbohydrates. Right before competition, they dramatically increase their intake of carbohydrates to force the body to store more glycogen, to be used during endurance activities (such as the last miles of a marathon).

The Myth of Sugar and Hyperactivity Contrary to early media reports, extensive research in recent years indicates that sugars *do not* cause hyperactivity.[15] In well-controlled dietary challenge studies, consumption of sugar has not been shown to have negative effects on motor activity, spontaneous behavior, performance in psychological tests, learning, memory, attention span, or problem-solving ability. In addition, sugar intake is not related to violence or criminal activity.

Carbohydrates and Carcinogens The World Health Organization recently labeled *acrylamide,* a compound found in plastics, as a "probable human carcinogen" because it has been shown to cause cancer, as well as genetic, neurological, and reproductive damage, in animals. While some of the concern arises from our use of plastics to cover food in microwaves, the larger issue arose because acrylamide is formed when starchy foods are cooked at high temperatures. University of Stockholm researchers found the highest concentrations of acrylamide in potato chips and crispbreads that were baked or fried, like French fries, crackers, and cereals.[16] Acrylamide was not found in raw foods, meats, or starchy foods that were boiled, such as rice or pasta. Critics of the study say that too few samples were used and that the amounts of acrylamide found were a thousandfold less than levels shown to cause cancer in mice. Follow-up research by

Monosaccharide A simple sugar that contains only one molecule of sugar.

Disaccharide A combination of two monosaccharides.

Polysaccharide A complex carbohydrate formed by the combination of long chains of saccharides.

Cellulose Fiber; a major form of complex carbohydrates.

Glycogen The polysaccharide form in which glucose is stored in the liver.

Flaxseed: The Oat Bran of the Twenty-First Century?

Just as oat bran began to lose its luster as a fiber icon, a new version of good fiber in a small package started arriving in trendy specialty nutrition stores. The blue-flowered flax plant, cultivated since ancient times for its value in clothing (linen fabrics) is part of a growing food enthusiasm. Why all the interest in these little seeds? Largely because the tiny, shiny brown seeds with the mild, nutty flavor are rich in alpha-linolenic acid (ALA), an omega-3 fatty acid that helps reduce blood clotting, primes immune function, and helps prevent abnormal heart rhythms. The seeds are also rich in lignans, phytoestrogens that may hinder hormone-related cancers. The fiber in flax is mostly insoluble, which helps relieve constipation, and partly soluble, which helps lower cholesterol and balance blood sugars.

Although flax is available in pills and liquid form, its highest nutritive value is when it is in its ground, natural form. It is most easily digested and stores best in this medium, particularly when refrigerated, is less likely to become rancid, and, in general, offers consumers the best range of available benefits. Flax can be added to casseroles, meatloafs, and burgers or be mixed in yogurts and breakfast cereals, sprinkled on salads, or added to baked products. Water consumption should be increased to assist in the digestive process. In short, flax is easy to obtain and appears to offer numerous benefits to the health-conscious consumer.

Source: Amy Aubertin, R.D., "Flaxseed Comes of Age: Good Nutrition in a Small Package," *Environmental Nutrition* August 2002. For subscription information, 800-829-5384.

---

the Center for Science in the Public Interest showed that a large order of French fries contained 39–82 micrograms of acrylamide, roughly 300 times what the U.S. Environmental Protection Agency allows in a glass of water.[17] At this writing, the U.S. FDA and other agencies are still deciding on a course of action or whether one is justified.

Fiber

Fiber, often referred to as "bulk" or "roughage," is the indigestible portion of plant foods that helps move foods through the digestive system and softens stools by absorbing water. Fiber also helps to control weight by creating a feeling of fullness without adding extra calories. In spite of all the fiber advocates, the average American consumes only about 12 grams of fiber a day, about half the recommended daily amount of 25 grams.[18]

Insoluble fiber, which is found in bran, whole-grain breads and cereals, and most fruits and vegetables, is associated with these gastrointestinal benefits and has also been found to reduce the risk for several forms of cancer. *Soluble fiber* appears to be a factor in lowering blood cholesterol levels and reducing risk for cardiovascular disease. Major sources of soluble fiber in the diet include oat bran, dried beans (such as kidney, garbanzo, pinto, and navy beans), and some fruits and vegetables. See the New Horizons in Health box for information on the newest fiber source, flaxseed.

The best way to increase intake of dietary fiber is to eat more complex carbohydrates, such as whole grains, fruits, vegetables, dried peas and beans, nuts, and seeds. As with most nutritional advice, however, too much of a good thing can pose problems. Sudden increases in dietary fiber may cause flatulence (intestinal gas), cramping, or a bloated feeling. Consuming plenty of water or other liquids may reduce such side effects.

A few years ago, fiber was thought by some to be the remedy for just about everything. Much of this hope was probably unrealistic, although research does support many benefits of fiber, such as the following:[19]

- *Protection against colon and rectal cancer.* One of the leading causes of cancer deaths in the United States, colorectal cancer is much rarer in countries having diets high in fiber and low in animal fat. Several studies contributed to the theory that fiber-rich diets, particularly those including insoluble fiber, prevent the development of precancerous growths. Whether this was because more fiber helps to move foods through the colon faster, thereby reducing the colon's contact time with cancer-causing substances, or because insoluble fiber reduces bile acids and certain bacterial enzymes that may promote cancer, remained in question. However, although research continues, the latest findings indicate that fiber may not be as protective against colon cancer as once believed.[20] Experts point to the fact that earlier studies failed to adequately control for other factors that may have caused an apparent protective effect. While fiber is still promoted for its possible benefits, more research is necessary.

- *Protection against breast cancer.* Research into the effects of fiber on breast cancer risks is inconclusive. However, some studies indicate that wheat bran (rich in insoluble fiber) reduces blood-estrogen levels, which may affect the risk for breast cancer. Another theory is that people who eat more fiber have proportionally less fat in their diets and this is what reduces overall risk, since fat continues to be implicated in breast cancer risk.

- *Protection against constipation.* Insoluble fiber, consumed with adequate fluids, is the safest, most effective way to prevent or treat constipation. The fiber acts like a sponge, absorbing moisture and producing softer, bulkier stools that are easily passed. Fiber also helps produce gas, which in turn may initiate a bowel movement.

- *Protection against diverticulosis.* About 1 American in 10 over the age of 40 and at least 1 in 3 over age 50 suffers from *diverticulosis,* a condition in which tiny bulges or pouches form on the large intestinal wall. These bulges can become irritated and cause chronic pain if under strain from constipation. Insoluble fiber helps to reduce constipation and discomfort.

- *Protection against heart disease.* Many studies have indicated that soluble fiber (as in oat bran, barley, and fruit pectin) helps reduce blood cholesterol, primarily by lowering LDL ("bad") cholesterol. Whether this reduction is a direct effect or occurs instead through the displacement of fat calories by fiber calories or through intake of other nutrients, such as iron, remains in question.[21]

- *Protection against diabetes.* Some studies suggest that soluble fiber improves control of blood sugar and can reduce the need for insulin or medication in people with diabetes. Exactly why isn't clear, but soluble fiber seems to delay the emptying of the stomach and slow the absorption of glucose by the intestine. The significance of this effect has been downgraded in recent years, however.[22]

- *Protection against obesity.* Because most high-fiber foods are high in carbohydrates and low in fat, they help control caloric intake. Many take longer to chew, which slows you down at the table and makes you feel full sooner.

Most experts believe that Americans should double their current consumption of dietary fiber—to 20 to 30 grams per day for most people and perhaps to 40 to 50 grams for others. (A large bowl of high-fiber cereal with a banana provides close to 20 grams of fiber.) Here are some tips for increasing your fiber intake:

1. Eat a variety of foods. Aim for at least five servings of fruits and vegetables and three to six servings of whole-grain breads, cereals, and legumes per day throughout the day.
2. Consume less processed food.
3. Eat the skins of fruits and vegetables.
4. Get your fiber from foods rather than pills or powders. Pills and powders do not supply enough essential nutrients.
5. Spread out your fiber intake.
6. Drink plenty of liquids—at least 64 ounces of water daily.

Fats

Fats (or *lipids*), another group of basic nutrients, are perhaps the most misunderstood of the body's required energy sources. Fats play a vital role in maintaining healthy skin and hair, insulating body organs against shock, maintaining body temperature, and promoting healthy cell function. Fats make foods taste better and carry the fat-soluble vitamins A, D, E, and K to the cells. They also provide a concentrated form of energy in the absence of sufficient carbohydrates.

If fats perform all these functions, why are we constantly urged to cut back on them?

Although moderate consumption of fats is essential to health, overconsumption can be dangerous. **Triglycerides,** which make up about 95 percent of total body fat, are the most common form of fat circulating in the blood. When we consume too many calories, the liver converts the excess into triglycerides, which are stored throughout our bodies.

The remaining 5 percent of body fat is composed of substances such as **cholesterol,** which can accumulate on the inner walls of arteries, causing a narrowing of the channel through which blood flows. This buildup, called **plaque,** is a major cause of *atherosclerosis* (hardening of the arteries). At one time, the amount of circulating cholesterol in the blood was thought to be crucial. Current thinking is that the actual amount of circulating cholesterol itself is not as important as the ratio of total cholesterol to a group of compounds called **high-density lipoproteins (HDLs).** Lipoproteins are the transport facilitators for cholesterol in the blood. High-density lipoproteins are capable of transporting more cholesterol than are **low-density lipoproteins (LDLs).** Whereas LDLs transport cholesterol to the body's cells, HDLs apparently transport circulating cholesterol to the liver for metabolism and elimination from the body. People with a high percentage of HDLs therefore appear to be at lower risk for developing cholesterol-clogged arteries. Regular vigorous exercise plays a part in reducing cholesterol by increasing high-density lipoproteins.

Fiber The indigestible portion of plant foods that helps move foods through the digestive system and softens stools by absorbing water.

Fats Basic nutrients composed of carbon and hydrogen atoms; needed for the proper functioning of cells, insulation of body organs against shock, maintenance of body temperature, and healthy skin and hair.

Triglycerides The most common form of fat in the body; excess calories consumed are converted into triglycerides and stored as body fat.

Cholesterol A form of fat circulating in the blood that can accumulate on the inner walls of arteries.

Plaque Cholesterol buildup on the inner walls of arteries, causing a narrowing of the channel through which blood flows; a major cause of atherosclerosis.

High-density lipoproteins (HDLs) Compounds that facilitate the transport of cholesterol in the blood to the liver for metabolism and elimination from the body.

Low-density lipoproteins (LDLs) Compounds that facilitate the transport of cholesterol in the blood to the body's cells.

PUFAs and MUFAs: Unsaturated "Good Guys"

Fat cells consist of chains of carbon and hydrogen atoms. Those that are unable to hold any more hydrogen in their chemical structure are labeled **saturated fats.** They generally come from animal sources, such as meats and dairy products, and are solid at room temperature. **Unsaturated fats,** which come from plants and include most vegetable oils, are generally liquid at room temperature and have room for additional hydrogen atoms in their chemical structure. The terms *monounsaturated fat (MUFA)* and *polyunsaturated fat (PUFA)* refer to the relative number of hydrogen atoms that are missing. Peanut and olive oils are high in monounsaturated fats, whereas corn, sunflower, and safflower oils are high in polyunsaturated fats. There is currently a great deal of controversy about which type of unsaturated fat is most beneficial. Although nutritional researchers in the 1980s favored PUFAs, today many believe that they may decrease beneficial HDL levels while reducing LDL levels. PUFAs come in two forms: omega-3 fatty acids and omega 6-fatty acids. MUFAs, such as olive oil, seem to lower LDL levels and increase HDL levels and thus are currently the "preferred," or least harmful, fats. Nevertheless, a tablespoon of olive oil gives you a hefty 10 grams of MUFAs. For a breakdown of the types of fats in common vegetable oils, see Figure 8.6.

Reducing Total Fat in Your Diet Want to cut the fat? These guidelines offer a good place to start:

• *Know what you are putting in your mouth.* Read food labels. Remember that no more than 10 percent of your total calories should come from saturated fat, and no more than 30 percent should come from all forms of fat.
• *Choose fat-free or low-fat versions of cakes, cookies, crackers, or chips.* (Remember, though, that calories still count. Don't eat *more* chips just because they're lower in fat.)
• *Use olive oil for baking and sautéing.* Animal studies have shown that it doesn't raise cholesterol or promote the growth of tumors.
• *If you use margarine, use it in liquid, diet, or whipped forms.* These products have far less trans-fatty acids than solid fat.
• *Choose lean meats, fish, or poultry.* Remove skin. Broil or bake whenever possible. In general, the more well-done the meat, the fewer the calories. Drain off fat after cooking.
• *Choose fewer cold cuts, sausages, hot dogs, and organ meats and less bacon.* Be careful of those products claiming to be "95 percent fat-free" as they may still have high levels of fat.
• *Select nonfat dairy products whenever possible.* Part-skim-milk cheeses such as mozzarella, farmer's, lappi, and ricotta are good choices.
• *When cooking, use substitutes for butter, margarine, oils, sour cream, mayonnaise, and salad dressings.* Chicken broths, wine, vinegar, and low-calorie dressings provide flavor with less fat.
• *Think of your food intake as an average over a day or a couple of days.* If you have a high-fat breakfast or lunch, balance it with a low-fat dinner.

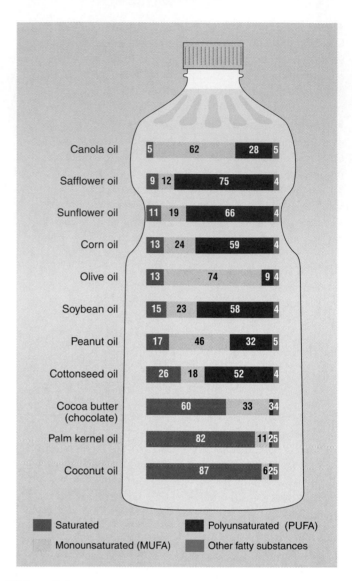

Figure 8.6
Percentages of Saturated, Polyunsaturated, and Monounsaturated Fats in Common Vegetable Oils

Trans-Fatty Acids: Still Bad? Since 1961, Americans have decreased their intake of butter by over 43 percent. Instead, they have substituted margarine, which became known as the "better butter" after reports labeled unsaturated fats the "heart-healthy" alternative. But a widely publicized landmark study in 1990 questioned the benefits of margarine; it indicated that margarine contains fats that raise blood cholesterol at least as much as the saturated fat in butter does.[23] The culprits? **Trans-fatty acids,** fatty acids having unusual shapes, are produced when polyunsaturated oils are *hydrogenated,* a process in which hydrogen is added to unsaturated fats to make them more solid and resistant to chemical change.[24] Besides raising cholesterol levels, trans-fatty acids have been implicated in certain types of cancer.[25]

A more recent study found that the trans-fatty acids found in margarine may in fact pose an even greater risk for heart disease than the saturated fat in butter and lard.[26] But before you dash out and fill your refrigerator with butter, be aware that this research is controversial.

Keep in mind that trans-fatty acids, even monounsaturated acids, alter blood cholesterol the same way as some saturated fats; they raise LDL and lower HDL cholesterol.[27] The American Heart Association has steadfastly stated that because butter is rich in both saturated fat and cholesterol whereas margarine is made from vegetable fat with no dietary cholesterol, margarine is still preferable to butter.[28] Others disagree, claiming that the occasional use of butter is preferable to margarine.[29] Most experts claim that the whole area of trans-fatty acids needs much more research. As a result, they advise that moderation in all fat intake is probably the best rule of thumb.[30] Whenever possible, opt for other condiments on your bread, using jams, fat-free cream cheese, garlic, or other toppings. Some experts advocate using low-fat salad dressings as toppings for bread and pasta, or using olive oil in moderation to add a bit of flavor. If you have high cholesterol, reducing all types of fat and cholesterol in the diet is still sound advice.

New Fat Advice: Is More Fat Ever Better?

Although most of this chapter has promoted the age-old recommendation to reduce saturated fat, avoid trans-fatty acids, and eat more monounsaturated fats, some experts worry that we have gone too far in our anti-fat frenzy (see the New Horizons in Health box on news from the world of nutrition research). In fact, according to some experts, our zeal to eat no-fat or low-fat foods may be one of the greatest causes of obesity in America today. According to the American Heart Association, eating fewer than 15 percent of our calories as fat (less than 34 grams a day on a 2,000-calorie diet) can actually increase blood triglycerides to levels that promote heart disease, while lowering levels of protective HDLs (high-density lipoproteins, or "good" cholesterol). There is also a concern that such very-low-fat diets may lead to shortages of essential fatty acid (EFA) in the diet.[31]

Not all fat is bad. In fact, dietary fat not only transports fat-soluble vitamins such as A, D, E, and K and disease-fighting caratenoids in the blood, it also supplies the two essential fatty acids that we must receive from our diets, *linoleic acid* and *alpha-linolenic acid*. These two fats are needed to make hormonelike compounds that control immune function, pain perception, and inflammation, to name a few key benefits.[32]

Although linoleic acid and alpha-linolenic acid are both polyunsaturated fats, they are actually quite different in what they do. Linoleic acid is a member of the *omega-6* family of fats (found in soybeans, peanuts, corn, and sunflower seeds) and reduces blood levels of total cholesterol and "bad" cholesterol (LDL) when consumed in reasonable amounts. Alpha-linolenic acid is part of the *omega-3* fats, and is found in flax (see the New Horizons in Health box on flax), canola oil, sardines, spinach, kale, green leafy vegetables, walnuts, and wheat germ. Alpha-linolenic acid is converted to two other beneficial omega-3 fats in the body, but you get a much bigger dose of those nutrients by eating cold-water fish such as salmon and tuna that have abundant supplies of omega-3. Today, Americans eat 17 times more omega-6 fats than omega 3s, and most experts agree that we need a more balanced approach.[33]

While both of these essential fats are important, too much linolenic acid may promote blood clots and constrict arteries, leading to inflammation and damaged blood vessels. Consuming more alpha-linolenic acid reduces risks for blood clots and abnormal heart rhythms and may improve immune function. The best rule of thumb is to balance, using the following recommendations:[34]

- Eat fatty fish (bluefish, herring, mackerel, salmon, sardines, or tuna) at least twice weekly.
- Substitute soy and canola oils for corn, safflower, and sunflower. Keep using olive oil, too.
- Add healthy doses of green, leafy vegetables, walnuts, walnut oil, and ground flaxseed to your diet to up intake of alpha-linolenic acid.
- Limit processed and convenience foods, since they often contain harmful saturated and trans fats.
- Pick the MUFA or PUFA with the least amount of calories and most nutrients.

Vitamins

Vitamins are potent, essential, organic compounds that promote growth and help maintain life and health. Every minute of every day, vitamins help maintain nerves and skin, produce blood cells, build bones and teeth, heal wounds, and convert food energy to body energy. And they do all of this without adding any calories to your diet.

Age, heat, and other environmental conditions can destroy vitamins in food. Vitamins can be classified as either *fat soluble,* meaning that they are absorbed through the intestinal tract with the help of fats, or *water soluble,* meaning that they are easily dissolved in water. Vitamins A, D, E, and K

Saturated fats Fats that are unable to hold any more hydrogen in their chemical structure; derived mostly from animal sources; solid at room temperature.

Unsaturated fats Fats that do have room for more hydrogen in their chemical structure; derived mostly from plants; liquid at room temperature.

Trans-fatty acids Fatty acids that are produced when polyunsaturated oils are hydrogenated to make them more solid.

Vitamins Essential organic compounds that promote growth and reproduction and help maintain life and health.

News from the World of Nutrition Research

Recently, nutritional experts from the international community met for a conference titled Diet and Optimum Health. Below, we summarize nutritional research from the last decade and various conclusions from large clinical trials and longitudinal dietary studies.

- Genetics, sedentary lifestyle, and consumption of too much dietary fat are probably not as responsible for our steep increases in obesity in the United States as the recommendation to eat less saturated fat and more carbohydrates. When these recommendations hit the public media, Americans shifted to nonfat or low-fat diets and consumed more refined carbohydrates. One need only look at the ingredients of many nonfat or low-fat foods to see the hefty doses of sugars and refined starches that tempt our palates. Experts believe that in our attempts to reduce saturated fats, we may have actually increased the prevalence of cardiovascular disease (CVD) and obesity.
- There is little support for the theory that increased consumption of dietary fat increases the risk of breast or colon cancer. In fact, the highest rates of these cancers appear to be among those with the lowest overall fat intake. Experts are focusing on the *type* of fat we consume—rather than the total amount consumed—and are recommending greater consumption of monounsaturated, vegetable-based fats, such as olive and canola oil. As a result of these studies, the American Heart Association is likely to move away from recommending nonfat/low-fat products, because they may actually cause people to eat more. Instead, the Association will focus on encouraging more olive oil and plant-based fats in the diet.

- Diets focusing on the glycemic index (a measure of rate of carbohydrate absorption after a meal) seem to be the most effective. Low-glycemic-index foods (which contain more complex carbohydrates, normal levels of monounsaturated fats, and reasonable amounts of proteins) suppress appetite longer, raise HDL cholesterol levels, and seem to protect against disease (hence the call for more olive oil indicated earlier). The new U.S. Dietary Guidelines are likely to be modified to reflect this body of work. Bad news: Potatoes don't fare well on this index. Good news: Pasta remains on the positive side of the index.
- There is dramatic new evidence that eating olive oil and other monounsaturated fats found in certain salad dressings may protect against cardiovascular disease and cancer. If you want super protection, eating olive oil and similar fats with green, leafy vegetables (which contain nutrients that are abundant in chlorophyll) may reduce risk sevenfold.
- Increases in obesity, CVD risks, and certain cancers and diabetes may be attributable in large part to displacing monounsaturated fats (e.g., olive and canola oils) with refined carbohydrates and processed sugars, as well as hydrogenated fat versions found in low-fat and nonfat foods. (Check your labels when purchasing low-fat and nonfat items at the store.)
- White tea is the hottest new food/beverage surfacing as a possible protective mechanism for cancer, particularly colon cancer. Preliminary research is indicating a sevenfold reduction in colon cancer risks and other cancers from two to three servings of white tea per day.
- Lipoic acid and acetyl carnitine (natural, not synthetic forms) have shown amazing results in mice and pig studies. (Natural forms of acetyl carnitine are currently available in health food stores, but natural forms of lipoic acid

are not yet available.) When these substances are combined and given in modest doses to older animals, their brain function reverts to that of younger animals within five to six weeks. The combination of these two seems to have significant effects on the wear-and-tear of aging. Animals fed these substances regenerate brain cells and repair damaged ones. Human trials will begin soon. Doses for effectiveness are not known.
- There seems to be little evidence that supplementing with chromium or selenium is of any benefit.
- Do you take vitamin E supplements? You may want to rethink this practice. According to antioxidant experts at this conference, newer research implicates vitamin E supplementation with reducing HDL levels and a variety of other potential risks, rather than benefits.
- Folic acid has shown promising results in reducing CVD and cancer risks. Deficiencies in folate also lead to chromosome damage.
- Researchers are gaining new information on the importance of iron. Too much or too little iron can impair mitochondria and cause oxidative stress damage to cells.

Source: Linus Pauling Institute, Public Sessions, International Conference on Diet and Optimum Health, May 2001, Portland, Oregon.

are fat soluble; B complex vitamins and vitamin C are water soluble. Fat-soluble vitamins tend to be stored in the body, and toxic accumulations in the liver may cause cirrhosislike symptoms. Water-soluble vitamins are generally excreted and cause few toxicity problems (see Table 8.1).

Despite many media suggestions to the contrary, few Americans suffer from true vitamin deficiencies if they eat a diet containing all of the food groups at least part of the time. Nevertheless, Americans continue to purchase large quantities of vitamin supplements. For the most part, vitamin supplements are unnecessary and, in certain instances, may even be harmful. Overusing them can even lead to a toxic condition known as **hypervitaminosis.**

Minerals

Minerals. (see Table 8.2) are the inorganic, indestructible elements that aid physiological processes within the body. Without minerals, vitamins could not be absorbed. Minerals are readily excreted and are usually not toxic. **Macrominerals** are those minerals that the body needs in fairly large amounts: sodium, calcium, phosphorus, magnesium, potassium, sulfur, and chloride. **Trace minerals** include iron, zinc, manganese, copper, iodine, and cobalt. Only trace amounts of these minerals are needed, and serious problems may result if excesses or deficiencies occur.

Although minerals are necessary for body function, there are limits on the amounts we should consume. Americans tend to overuse or underuse certain minerals.

Sodium   Sodium is necessary for the regulation of blood and body fluids, transmission of nerve impulses, heart activity, and certain metabolic functions. However, we consume much more than we need. It is estimated that the average adult who does not sweat profusely needs only 500 milligrams of sodium (about ¼ teaspoon) per day; yet the average American consumes 6,000 to 12,000 milligrams. The RDA subcommittee recommends restricting sodium to no more than 2,400 milligrams per day; less is better.

The most common form of sodium in the American diet comes from table salt. However, table salt accounts for only 15 percent of sodium intake. The remainder comes from water and from highly processed foods that are infused with sodium to enhance flavor. Pickles, salty snack foods, processed cheeses, many breads and bakery products, and smoked meats and sausages often contain several hundred milligrams of sodium per serving. Many fast-food entrees and convenience entrees pack 500 to 1,000 milligrams of sodium per serving.

Many experts believe that there is a link between excessive sodium intake and hypertension (high blood pressure). Although this theory is controversial, researchers recommend that hypertensive Americans cut back on sodium to reduce their risk for cardiovascular disorders.[35] Osteoporosis researchers are confirming that high sodium intake may increase calcium loss in urine, increasing your risk for debilitating fractures as you age. (See the Women's Health/Men's Health box on page 240.)

Calcium   The issue of calcium consumption has gained national attention with the rising incidence of osteoporosis among elderly women. Although calcium plays a vital role in building strong bones and teeth, muscle contraction, blood clotting, nerve impulse transmission, regulating heartbeat, and fluid balance within cells, most Americans do not consume the 1,200 milligrams of calcium per day established by the RDA.

Because calcium intake is so important throughout life for maintaining strong bones, it is critical to consume the minimum required amount each day. Over half of our calcium intake usually comes from milk, one of the highest sources of dietary calcium. Calcium-fortified orange juice and soy milk provide a good way to get calcium if you do not drink dairy milk. Many green, leafy vegetables are good sources of calcium, but some contain oxalic acid, which makes their calcium harder to absorb. Spinach, chard, and beet greens are not particularly good sources of calcium, whereas broccoli, cauliflower, and many peas and beans offer good supplies (pinto beans and soybeans are among the best). Many nuts, particularly almonds, brazil nuts, and hazelnuts, and seeds such as sunflower and sesame contain good amounts of calcium. Molasses is fairly high in calcium. Some fruits — such as citrus fruits, figs, raisins, and dried apricots—have moderate amounts. Bone meal is not a recommended calcium source due to possible contamination.

Do you consume carbonated soft drinks? Be aware that the added phosphoric acid (phosphate) in these drinks can cause you to excrete extra calcium, which may result in calcium being pulled out of your bones. Calcium/phosphorus imbalance may lead to kidney stones and other calcification problems as well as to increased atherosclerotic plaque.

We also know that sunlight increases the manufacture of vitamin D in the body, and is therefore like having an extra calcium source because vitamin D improves absorption of calcium. Stress, on the other hand, contributes to calcium depletion. It is generally best to take calcium throughout the day, consuming it with foods containing protein, vitamin D, and vitamin C for optimum absorption. Experts vary on which type of supplemental calcium is most readily and efficiently

---

Hypervitaminosis   A toxic condition caused by overuse of vitamin supplements.

Minerals   Inorganic, indestructible elements that aid physiological processes.

Macrominerals   Minerals that the body needs in fairly large amounts.

Trace minerals   Minerals that the body needs in only very small amounts.

Table 8.1
A Guide to Vitamins

VITAMIN	SIGNIFICANT SOURCES	CHIEF FUNCTIONS IN THE BODY
WATER-SOLUBLE VITAMINS		
Thiamin 1.5 mg (RDA+RDI)	Meat, pork, liver, fish, poultry, whole-grain and enriched breads, cereals, pasta, nuts, legumes wheat germs, oats	Helps enzymes realease energy from carbohydrate; supports normal appetite and nervous system function
Riboflavin 1.7 mg (RDA+RDI)	Milk, dark green vegetables, yogurt, cottage cheese, liver, meat, whole-grain or enriched breads and cereals	Helps enzymes release energy from carbohydrate, fat, and protein; promotes healthy skin and normal vision
Niacin 20 mg NE (RDA+RDI)	Meat, eggs, poultry, fish, milk, whole-grain and enriched breads and cereals, nuts, legumes, peanuts, nutritional yeast, all protein foods	Helps enzymes release energy from energy nutrients; promotes health of skin, nerves, and digestive system
Vitamin B_6 2.0 mg (RDA+RDI)	Meat, poultry, fish, shellfish, legumes, whole-grain products, green, leafy vegetables, bananas	Protein and fat metabolism; formation of antibodies and red blood cells; helps convert tryptophan to niacin
Folate 400 μg (DFE+RDA)	Green, leafy vegetables, liver, legumes, seeds	Red blood cell formation; protein metabolism; new cell division; prevents neural tube defects
Vitamin B_{12} 2.4 mg (RDA)	Meat, fish, poultry, shellfish, milk, cheese, eggs, nutritional yeast	Helps maintain nerve cells; red blood cell formation; synthesis of genetic material
Pantothenic acid 5–7 mg (AI)	Widespread in foods	Coenzyme in energy metabolism
Biotin 30 μg (AI)	Widespread in foods	Coenzyme in energy metabolism; fat synthesis glycogen formation
Vitamin C (ascorbic acid) (RDI+RDA) = 60mg	Citrus fruits, cabbage-type vegetables, tomatoes, potatoes, dark green vegetables, peppers, lettuce, cantaloupe, strawberries, mangos, papayas	Synthesis of collagen (helps heal wounds, maintains bone and teeth, strengthens blood vessels); antioxidant; strengthens resistance to infection; helps body's absorption of iron
FAT-SOLUBLE VITAMINS		
Vitamin A 5000 IU	Retinal: Fortified milk and margarine, cream, cheese, butter, eggs, liver Carotene: spinach and other dark leafy greens, broccoli, deep orange fruits (apricots, peaches, cantaloupe) and vegetables (squash, carrots, sweet potatoes, pumpkin)	Vision; growth and repair of body tissues; repro-duction; bone and tooth formation; immunity; cancer protection; hormone synthesis
Vitamin D 400–600 IU (RDA+RD)	Self-synthesis with sunlight, fortified milk, fortified margarine, eggs, liver, fish	Calcium and phosphorus metabolism (bone and tooth formation); aids body's absorption of calcium
Vitamin E 30 IU (RDA+RDI)	Vegetable oils, green, leafy vegetables, wheat germ, whole-grain products, butter, liver, egg yolk, milk fat, nuts, seeds	Protects red blood cells; antioxidant; stabilization of cell membranes
Vitamin K 70–140 μg	Liver, green, leafy, and cabbage-type vegetables, milk	Bacterial synthesis in digestive tract; synthesis of blood-clotting proteins and a blood protein that regulates blood calcium

DEFICIENCY SYMPTOMS	TOXICITY SYMPTOMS
Beriberi, edema, heart irregularity, mental confusion, muscle weakness, low morale, impaired growth	Rapid pulse, weakness, headaches, isomnia, irritability
Eye problems, skin disorders around nose and mouth	None reported, but an excess of any of the B vitamins can cause a deficiency of the others
Pellagra: skin rash on parts exposed to sun, loss of appetite, dizziness, weakness, irritability, fatigue, mental confusion, indigestion	Flushing, nausea, headaches, cramps, ulcer irritation, heartburn, abnormal liver function, low blood pressure
Nervous disorders, skin rash, muscle weakness, anemia, convulsions, kidney stones	Depression, fatigue, irritability, headaches, numbness, damage to nerves, difficulty walking
Anemia, heartburn, diarrhea, smooth tongue depression, poor growth	Diarrhea, insomnia, irritability; may mask a vitamin B_{12} deficiency
Amemia, smooth tongue, fatigue, nerve degeneration progressing to paralysis	None reported
Rare; sleep disturbances, nausea, fatigue	Occasional diarrhea
Loss of appetite, nausea, depression, muscle pain, weakness, fatigue, rash	None reported
Scurvy, anemia, atherosclerotic plaques, depression, frequent infections, bleeding gums, loosened teeth, pinpoint hemorrhages; muscle degeneration, rough skin, bone fragility, poor wound healing, hysteria	Nausea, abdominal cramps, diarrhea, breakdown of red blood cells in persons with certain genetic disorders, deficiency symptoms may appear at first on withdrawal of high doses
Night blindness, rough skin, susceptibility to infection, impaired bone growth, abnormal tooth and jaw alignment, eye problems leading to blindness, impaired growth	Red blood cell breakage, nosebleeds, abdominal cramps, nausea, diarrhea, weight loss, blurred vision, irritability, loss of appetite, bone pain, dry skin, rashes, hair loss, cessation of menstruation, growth retardation
Rickets in children; osteomalacia in adults; abnormal growth, joint pain, soft bones	Raised blood calcium, constipation, weight loss, irritability, weakness, nausea, kidney stones, mental and physical retardation
Muscle wasting, weakness, red blood cell breakage, anemia, hemorrhaging, fibrocystic breast disease	Interference with anticlotting medication, general discomfort
Hemorrhaging	Interference with anticlotting medication; may cause jaundice

Values vary (increase) among women who are pregnant or lactating.
Sources: From *Personal Nutrition, 2d ed.,* by Marie Boyle and Gail Zyla. Reprinted with permission of Wadsworth, an imprint of the Wadsworth Group, a division of Thomson Learning. National Academy Press website under "Reading Room" at http://www Nap.edu (1999).

Table 8.2
A Guide to Minerals

MINERAL	SIGNIFICANT SOURCES	CHIEF FUNCTIONS IN THE BODY
Calcium RDA = 800–1,200 mg+ RDI = 1,000 mg	Milk and milk products, small fish (with bones), tofu, greens, legumes	Principal mineral of bones and teeth; involved in muscle contraction and relaxation, nerve function, blood clotting, blood pressure
Phosphorus RDA = 1,000 mg	All animal tissues	Part of every cell; involved in acid-based balance
Magnesium RDA = 400 mg	Nuts, legumes, whole grains, dark green vegetables, seafood, chocolate, cocoa	Involved in bone mineralization, protein synthesis, enzyme action, normal muscular contraction, nerve transmission
Sodium RDA = 500 mg DRV = 2,400	Salt, soy sauce; processed foods; cured, canned, pickled, and many boxed foods	Helps maintain normal fluid and acid-base balance
Chloride RDA = 750 mg	Salt, soy sauce; processed foods	Part of stomach acid, necessary for proper digestion, fluid balance
Potassium RDA = 2,000 mg DRV = 3,500 mg	All whole foods: meats, milk, fruits, vegetables, grains, legumes	Facilitates many reactions including protein synthesis, fluid balance, nerve transmission, and contraction of muscles
Iodine RDA = 150 µg RDI = 150 µg	Iodized salt, seafood	Part of thyroxine, which regulates metabolism
Iron RDA = 18 mg RDI = 18 mg	Beef, fish, poultry, shellfish, eggs, legumes, dried fruits	Hemoglobin formation; part of myoglobin; energy utilization
Zinc RDA = 15 mg RDI = 15 mg	Protein-containing foods: meats, fish, poultry, grains, vegetables	Part of many enzymes; present in insulin; involved in making genetic material and proteins, immunity, vitamin A transport, taste, wound healing, making sperm, normal fetal development
Copper RDA = 2 mg RDI = 2 mg	Meats, drinking water	Absorption of iron; part of several enzymes
Fluoride 1.5–4.0 mg	Drinking water (if naturally fluoride-containing or fluoridated), tea, seafood	Formation of bones and teeth; helps make teeth resistant to decay and bones resistant to mineral loss
Selenium 50–70 µg	Seafood, meats, grains	Helps protect body compounds from oxidation
Chromium 50–200 µg	Meats, unrefined foods, fats, vegetables oils	Associated with insulin and required for the release of energy from glucose
Molybdenum 75–250 µg	Legumes, cereals, organ meats	Facilitates, with enzymes, many cell processes
Manganese 2.0–5.0 mg	Widely distributed in foods	Facilitates, with enzymes, many cell processes

DEFICIENCY SYMPTOMS

Stunted growth in children; bone loss (osteoporosis) in adults

Unknown

Weakness, confusion, depressed pancreatic hormone secretion, growth failure, behavioral disturbances, muscle spasms

Muscle cramps, mental apathy, loss of appetite

Growth failure in children, muscle cramps, mental apathy, loss of appetite

Muscle weakness, paralysis, confusion; can cause death; accompanies dehydration

Goiter, cretinism

Anemia: weakness, pallor, headaches, reduced resistance to infection, inability to concentrate

Growth failure in children, delayed development of sexual organs, loss of taste, poor wound healing

Anemia, bone changes (rare in human beings)

Susceptibility to tooth decay and bone loss

Anemia (rare)

Diabetes like condition marked by inability to use glucose normally

Unknown

In animals: poor growth, nervous system disorders, abnormal reproduction

TOXICITY SYMPTOMS

Excess calcium is excreted, except in hormonal imbalance states

Can create relative deficiency of calcium

Not known

Hypertension (in salt-sensitive persons)

Normally harmless (the gas chlorine is a poison but evaporates from water); disturbed acid-base balance; vomiting

Causes muscular weakness; triggers vomiting; if given into a vein, can stop the heart

Very high intakes depress thyroid activity

Iron overload: infections, liver injury

Fever, nausea, vomiting, diarrhea

Unknown except as part of a rare hereditary disease (Wilson's disease).

Fluorosis (discoloration of teeth)

Digestive system disorders

Unknown as a nutrition disorder; occupational exposures damage skin and kidneys

Enzyme inhibition

Poisoning, nervous system disorders

Because we have less information about minerals than about vitamins, RDA recommendations are estimates of minimum requirements.
Source: From *Personal Nutrition, 2d ed.,* by Marie Boyle and Gail Zyla and pp. 298–300 of *Nutrition Concepts and Controversies, 6th ed.,* by F.S. Sizer, E.N. Whitney, and E.M. Hamilton, © 1994. Reprinted with permission of Wadsworth, an imprint of the Wadsworth Group, a division of Thomson Learning.

Osteoporosis Prevention: Not for Women Only

Although osteoporosis, a disease characterized by low bone mass and deterioration of bone tissue, is commonly thought of as a woman's disease, men develop it as well. In fact, there has been a surprising increase in the number of cases during the past decade. Whereas four out of every five cases of osteoporosis occur in women, largely due to the depletion of estrogen at menopause, one in three men who are 75 years old or older will develop some degree of the disease.

If estrogen deficiency is a major cause of osteoporosis in women, what causes it in men? Men produce only a little estrogen, yet they resist osteoporosis better than women do. Male hormones must

also play a role because men suffer more fractures after removal of the testes (in cases of disease) or when their testes lose functional ability with aging or disease. Men who have delayed puberty also suffer more fractures, suggesting that time of puberty influences peak bone development in men. Thus, both male and female sex hormones appear to be involved in the development of osteoporosis.

When men do experience osteoporosis, they often have a hard time getting insurance coverage for bone-building medications such as alendronate (Fosamax), and they are often treated with medications developed in response to research done on their female counterparts (an interesting turn of events in the history of male/female treatments). As few as 10 years ago, it was not at all unusual for women to be treated with regimens largely based on research conducted only on men. The Women's

Health Initiative has made significant strides since that time to ensure equality in health research and subsequent treatment based on sex. A recent study conducted at Tufts University indicates that calcium and vitamin D, the nutrients so often recommended to reduce the risk of osteoporotic fractures in women, work just as well in men. This research will pave the way for stronger public health messages indicating that men should consume sufficient calcium, exercise regularly (and, particularly, perform weight-bearing exercises), have bone-density scans at specified intervals, and actively engage in other prevention activities.

Sources: L. Kathleen Mahan and Sylvia Escott-Stump, *Krause's Food, Nutrition, and Diet Therapy* (10th ed.) (Saunders, 2000); E. Whitney and S. Rolfes, *Understanding Nutrition* (8th ed.), (Belmont: Wadsworth, 1999), p. 398.

---

absorbed, although aspartate and citrate salts of calcium are often recommended. The best way to obtain calcium, like all nutrients, is to consume it as part of a balanced diet.

Iron   Worldwide, iron deficiency is the most common nutrient deficiency, affecting more than 1 billion people. In developing countries, more than one-third of the children and women of childbearing age suffer from *iron-deficiency anemia.*[36] In the United States iron deficiency anemia is less prevalent, but still affects 10 percent of toddlers, adolescent girls, and women of childbearing age, making prevention a high priority.[37] In addition to suffering from **anemia,** a problem resulting from the body's inability to produce hemoglobin, the bright red, oxygen-carrying component of the blood, people with iron-deficiency anemia may develop a condition known as **pica,** an appetite for ice, clay, paste, and other nonfood substances that do not actually contain iron and, in fact, may inhibit iron absorption. How much iron do adults need? Females age 19–50 need about 18 milligrams per day, and males age 19–50 need about 10 milligrams.

When iron deficiency occurs, body cells receive less oxygen, and carbon dioxide wastes are removed less efficiently. As a result, the iron-deficient person feels tired and run down. While iron deficiency in the diet is a common cause of anemia, it can also result from blood loss, cancers, ulcers, and other conditions. Generally, women are more

likely to develop iron-deficiency problems because they typically eat less than men and their diets contain less iron. Women having heavy menstrual flow may be at greater risk.

To date, considerable research has linked iron to a host of problems. Iron deficiency may tax the immune system, causing it to function less effectively. Research suggesting a link between cardiovascular disease and elevated iron stores is inconclusive.[38] Likewise, although there appears to be a slight association between iron deficiency and cancer, the mechanism remains inconclusive.[39]

Iron overload (known as **hemochromatosis**), or iron toxicity due to ingesting too many iron-containing supplements, remains the leading cause of accidental poisoning in small children in the United States. Symptoms of toxicity include nausea, vomiting, diarrhea, rapid heartbeat, weak pulse, dizziness, shock, and confusion. As few as five iron tablets containing as little as 200 milligrams of iron have killed dozens of children.

The Medicinal Value of Food

The old adage "you are what you eat" is indeed a motto to live by. Beneficial foods are termed *functional foods* based on the ancient belief that eating the right foods may not only prevent disease, but also actually cure it. This perspective is gaining credibility among the scientific community. (It is also important to be aware of potential interactions between medications you are taking and foods you are eating; see Table 8.3.)

Two major studies, the *Dietary Approaches to Stop Hypertension (DASH) Study* and the *Dietary Intervention Study (DIS)*, provide compelling evidence that diet may be as effective as drugs in bringing borderline hypertension back to the normal range. Diet may also play a role in reducing cholesterol and controlling insulin-dependent diabetes.[40] In these clinically controlled trials, subjects were assigned to two groups: treatment and control. In the treatment group, subjects had to follow recommended diets, which were low in fats and high in fiber and fruits. The control group followed typical American dietary intervention. In each study, subjects in the treatment groups showed significantly improved health indicators (blood pressure, cholesterol, and blood glucose in the DIS study), which reflected the potential benefits of diet in improving health and treating disease.

Antioxidants and Your Health

Antioxidants are substances that are believed to protect active people from *oxidative stress* and resultant tissue damage at the cellular level. This damage is believed to occur in a complex process in which *free radicals* (molecules with unpaired electrons that are produced in excess when the body is overly stressed through exposure to toxic substances or events) either damage or kill healthy cells, cell proteins, or genetic material in the cells. Antioxidants produce enzymes that destroy excess free radicals by scavenging free radicals, slowing their formation, and/or actually repairing oxidative stress damage.

There have been many claims about the benefits of antioxidants in reducing risks of cancer and heart disease, improving vision, and slowing or reversing the aging process. Whether these claims produce scientifically validated evidence that a daily dose of antioxidants is truly beneficial to health remains to be seen. Initial results from numerous research studies appear to support the benefits of at least some of the antioxidant family. For example, the beneficial effects of moderate doses of vitamin C appear to be well substantiated.[41] However, a recent British study of 30 healthy men and women showed that taking a daily 500-milligram supplement of vitamin C had both positive and negative effects on DNA. Similarly, a widely cited Finnish study of 29,000 men reported that for those who smoked a pack of cigarettes a day and took daily beta-carotene supplements, risk of lung cancer actually increased by 18 percent over those who took no supplement.[42]

Other antioxidants that had received initial support in the research have now begun to lose favor in scientific circles. For example, vitamin E, which once had a starring role in the potential prevention of heart disease and cancer, has increasingly received bad reviews from critics who point out that new research doesn't point to any benefits (see the New Horizons in Health box).

In addition to vitamins E and C, other nutrients, including some key minerals, are also important in the destruction of free radicals. Among them are selenium, copper, zinc, iron, and manganese.[43]

Beta-carotene is one of the many compounds classified as **carotenoids.** Carotenoids are part of the red, orange, and yellow pigments found in fruits and vegetables. They are fat soluble, transported in the blood by lipoproteins, and stored in the fatty tissues of the body. Beta-carotene, the most researched carotenoid, is a precursor of vitamin A. This means that vitamin A can be produced in the body from beta-carotene; like vitamin A, beta-carotene has antioxidant properties.[44]

Although there are over 600 carotenoids in nature, two that have received increasing attention recently are *lycopene* (found in tomatoes), and *lutein* (found in green, leafy vegetables such as spinach, broccoli, kale, and brussels sprouts). Both are believed to be more beneficial than beta-carotene in preventing disease.

The National Cancer Institute and the American Cancer Society have endorsed lycopene as a possible means of risk reduction for cancer. A landmark study assessing the effects of tomato-based foods on cancer reported that men who ate 10 or more servings of lycopene-rich foods per week had a 45 percent reduced risk of prostate cancer development.[45]

Lutein is most often touted as a means of protecting aging eyes, particularly from the scourges of age-related macular degeneration (ARMD), a leading cause of blindness for people aged 65 and over. Although researchers don't know for sure what causes ARMD, they do know that older age, light-colored eyes, smoking, and exposure to sunlight increase a person's risk. These same researchers speculate that oxidative damage may be the crux of the problem, and thus, antioxidants have been assessed as a possible means of prevention.[46] Researchers at the National Eye Institute found that those with the highest blood levels of lutein and other antioxidants found in foods were 70 percent less likely to develop ARMD than those with the lowest levels. Researchers in the Nurses Health study found that eating spinach more than five days a week lowered risk by 47 percent and also lowered risk of cataract formation.[47]

Anemia   Iron deficiency disease that results from the body's inability to produce hemoglobin.

Pica   Iron deficiency disease characterized by craving for certain foods and substances.

Hemochromatosis   Iron toxicity due to excess consumption.

Antioxidants   Substances believed to protect active people from oxidative stress and resultant tissue damage at the cellular level.

Carotenoids   Fat-soluble compounds with antioxidant properties.

Table 8.3
Common Food-Medication Interactions

Interactions are listed by drug category, followed by examples of specific medications (with generic and brand names). As always, alert your physician and pharmacists to any over-the-counter medications, herbal remedies, and supplements you are taking.

MEDICATIONS	INTERACTIONS WITH FOODS/NUTRIENTS	WHAT TO DO
ANTIBIOTICS ciprofloxacin (*Cipro*) doxycycline (*Vibramycin*) minocycline (*Minocin*) tetracycline (*Achromycin-V, surrycin*) penicillin (*Ledercillin*)	• Calcium and iron bind with these drugs, inhibiting absorption of the drug plus the calcium and iron. Results in less antibiotic effect, risking the possibility that the bacteria causing the infection will not be killed. • Food slows down absorption of the drug.	• Do not take within three hours of taking calcium-containing antacids, iron supplements, or multivitamins/minerals. • Do not take ciprofloxacin or tetracycline with foods rich in calcium, such as milk and other dairy products. • Take an hour before or two hours after eating.
CARDIOVASCULAR MEDICATIONS **ACE INHIBITORS** captopril (*Capoten*) enalapril (*Vasotec*) lisinopril (*Prinivil, Zestril*) moexipril (*Univasc*)	• Some ACE inhibitors cause hyperkalemia (elevated blood potassium). • Licorice can disrupt potassium balance. • Chili pepper worsens persistent cough side effect. • Food decreases absorption of captopril and moexipril.	• Limit potassium-rich foods (see below) and salt substitutes containing potassium. • Avoid chili pepper. • Take captopril, moexipril an hour before or two hours after eating.
BLOOD THINNERS warfarin (*Coumadin*)	• Vitamin K reduces the effectiveness of anticoagulants. If you maintain a consistent intake of vitamin K, your doctor can adjust your medication level accordingly.	• Keep a consistent intake of vitamin K-rich foods: broccoli, spinach, kale, turnip greens, Swiss chard, cauliflower, Brussels sprouts, asparagus, beets, and chicken liver.
CALCIUM CHANNEL BLOCKERS amlodipine (*Norvasc*) felodipine (*Plendil*) nifedipine (*Adalat, Procardia*)	• Licorice can increase potassium excretion, sodium reabsorption, and raise blood pressure. • Grapefruit can increase blood levels of these drugs up to twofold, causing blood pressure to drop dangerously low.	• Avoid natural licorice • Avoid grapefruit, grapefruit juice, and Seville oranges.
HMG-COA REDUCTASE INHIBITORS ("STATINS") atorvastatin (*Lipitor*) lovastatin (*Mevacor*) simvastatin (*Zocor*)	• Grapefruit significantly increases blood levels of the drug, causing more side effects or toxicity. • Soluble fiber inhibits absorption of lovastatin. • Lovastatin is best absorbed with a big meal containing fat. Works best when asleep.	• Avoid grapefruit, grapefruit juice and Seville oranges. • Don't eat foods rich in fiber, oat bran, or pectin within serveral hours of taking lovastin. • If taken once a day, take lovastatin with the evening meal.

Table 8.3 Continued
Common Food-Medication Interactions

MEDICATIONS	INTERACTIONS WITH FOODS/NUTRIENTS	WHAT TO DO
DIURETICS **POTASSIUM-LOSING DIURETICS** lurosumide (*lasix*) hydrochlorothiazide (*HydroDIURIL*)	• Cause a loss of potassium and magnesium requring extra potassium and magnesium in the diet or supplements. A potassium deficiency can trigger a heart attack. • Licorice can cause a loss of potassium.	• Eat plenty of potassium-rich foods: apricots, bananas, cantaloupe, dairy foods, dried beans, lentils, oranges, tomatoes. • Eat magnesium-rich foods: bananas, dried beans, lentils, nuts. • Avoid natural licorice.
POTASSIUM-SPARING DIURETICS spironolactone (*Aldactone*)	• Prevent kidneys from excreting potassium. Taking in too much potassium can cause irregular heartbeat. • Licorice can disrupt potassium balance.	• Don't overdo foods rich in potassium (see above). • Avoid salt substitutes that contain potassium. • Avoid natural licorice.
PSYCHOTHERAPEUTIC MEDICATIONS buspirone (*Buspar*)—treats anxiety	• Grapefruit significantly increases blood levels of the drug.	• Avoid grapefruit, grapefruit juice, and Seville oranges.
MONOAMINE OXIDASE INHIBITORS (MAOIs) isocarboxazid (*Marplan*) phenelzine (*Nardil*) tranylcypromine (*Parmate*)	• Combining with too much caffeine, beer, or wine (even alcohol-free) or foods rich in tyramine can lead to a dangerous increase in blood pressure.	• Avoid excessive caffeine; use with caution. Avoid foods rich in tyramine: aged cheeses and meats, beer, fava beans, sauerkraut, soy sauce, wine. Use small amounts of beer (one or two 12-oz. bottles a day) and wine (2 to 4 oz. a day) with caution.
OTHER MEDICATIONS cilostazol (*Pletal*)— treats circulatory conditions colchicine –treats gout levodopa (*Dopar, Larodopa, Sinernet*)–treats Parkinson's disease theophylline (*Slo-bid, Theobid, Elixophyllin, Theo-Dur, Uniphyl*)–treats asthma and other pulmonary disorders	• Grapefruit significantly increases blood levels of the drug, causing increased side effects or drug toxicity. • Grapefruit significantly increases blood levels of the drug. • Pyridoxine decreases effectiveness of the drug. Keep pyridoxine (Vitamin B_6) intake to less than 5 mg a day. • Caffeine increases theophylline's side effects: dizziness, nausea, vomiting, convulsions or coma. • Black pepper and chili pepper increase drug blood levels. • Amount of protein and carbohydrate in diet can alter enzyme levels that affect theophylline breakdown.	• Avoid grapefruit, grapefruit juice, and Seville oranges. • Avoid grapefruit, grapefruit juice, and Seville oranges. • Limit foods rich in pyridoxine: chicken, fish, pork, liver, and kidneys. Go easy on legumes, nuts, and whole grains. • Avoid excessive caffeine (e.g., coffee, tea, cola). • Avoid excessive black pepper or chili pepper. • Keep intake of protein and carbohydrate consistent to keep drug levels consistent.

oz = ounces   mg = milligrams

Source: Reprinted by permission of Environmental Nutrition magazine, from K. Neville, "Food, Too, Can Interfere with Medications, If You're Not Careful," *Environmental Nutrition* (November 2001) 52 Riverside Drive, Suite 15A, New York, NY 10024. For subscription information 800-829-5384. Data from *Food Medication Interactions–12th edition* (2002: available at 800-746-2324); *Food & Drug Interactions* (Food and Drug Administration with National Consumers League. 1998, online updated 2000; available at http://~irdilfainter.html): interviews with Zaneta Pronsky, M.S., R.D., F.A.D.A., Sr. Jeanne Crowe, Pharm D., R.Ph. and Dean Elbe, B.Sc.

Vitamin E: Have We Jumped the Gun?

For the past several years, sales of vitamin E have soared. Why? Some studies indicated that it might reduce the risk of heart disease. Even food manufacturers have gotten into the act. Kraft, for example, markets a line of salad dressing, boasting that it is "rich in vitamin E"—"for a healthy body."

Recently, however, a highly regarded study has reported that vitamin E doesn't appear to provide any protection against heart troubles. Researchers from Ontario concluded this after following 9,500 people age 55 and older who were at high risk for cardiovascular "events," such as heart attacks. For nearly five years, half of the group was given 400 international units of vitamin E daily, while the other half took a placebo. In the end, there was no difference in their rates of heart attack, stroke, or death from heart disease. There was no difference, either, in the frequency of other cardiovascular problems such as unstable angina or heart failure.

The Heart Outcomes Prevention Evaluation Study, or HOPE, as it has been dubbed, casts doubt on previous research that pointed to vitamin E as a hedge against heart attack. Those earlier studies indicated that people who eat foods rich in antioxidants such as vitamin E—particularly nuts, oils, and some vegetables—appear to have lower rates of heart disease. Animal studies in which vitamin E appeared to slow the development of atherosclerosis have also been promising. Two large studies from Harvard University particularly boosted hopes when they revealed that people who reported taking 100 units of vitamin E per day had lower rates of heart trouble and less advanced damage to arteries.

One other study, nicknamed CHAOS (The Cambridge Heart Antioxidant Study), used the same rigorous methods as the HOPE trial did and found that people taking 400–800 units of vitamin E significantly reduced their risk of heart attack. However, the average length of the subjects' participation was barely a year and a half, and many of the participants dropped out before conclusive results could be obtained.

The jury is still out on vitamin E. Experts point out that the people in the HOPE study already had severe heart disease, so perhaps vitamin E is most effective as a preventive measure and not as a treatment for advanced atherosclerosis. On the positive side, this study seemed to show that vitamin E, at recommended doses, does not cause any harm to patients. To make a cautious appraisal based on what we know so far, it is wise to note that although safe for consumption, vitamin E can't be counted on to prevent heart attacks.

Source: Reprinted with permission, *Tufts University Health and Nutrition Letter* 18 (1) (2000), 800-274-7581.

Other studies point to additional potential benefits from lutein. A recent study by Tufts University and Korean investigators revealed a dramatic 88 percent drop in breast cancer in women who had the highest blood concentration of lutein. Researchers at the University of Utah Medical School found that the highest consumers of lutein had the lowest risks of colon cancer. In animals, lutein slowed the growth of breast tumors, and in test tubes, it killed cancer cells. Preliminary research has also shown a possible reduction in artery clogging among those consuming highest amounts of lutein.[48]

According to the experts, the answer is moderation. "Antioxidants should always be taken as part of a well-balanced mixture, either as a diet or as a supplement, and not singly," says Dr. John R. Smythies, a researcher at the University of California–San Diego and author of *Every Person's Guide to Antioxidants.*[49] Smythies, like many other experts, advocates for balance in intake and advises that adults take 500 milligrams of daily vitamin C and 400 to 800 I.U. of vitamin E, plus 10 milligrams of beta-carotene. Other antioxidant researchers might go to 1,000 milligrams of vitamin C for the general population and more vitamin E for anyone who exercises intensely for more than an hour each day.[50] Other experts, such as Dr. Balz Frei at the Linus Pauling Institute, indicate that the "200 rule" might be the best option. This recommendation calls for fruits and vegetables in the diet and a supplement of 200 milligrams of vitamin C, 200 I.U. of vitamin E, and 200 micrograms of selenium, along with 400 micrograms of folate and 3 milligrams of vitamin B_6.[51] It is believed that these combinations will reduce the body's overproduction of free radicals, those unstable molecules that can damage healthy cells and turn low-density lipoproteins into artery-clogging compounds.[52] However, even the lowering of free radicals is controversial. Many believe that free radicals are beneficial and work to kill germs in the same way they kill other cells. From this standpoint, killing off free radicals may lower resistance to harmful pathogens.[53]

To find the right balance, keep in mind the following:

- The upper limit for vitamin E, based only on supplements, is 1,000 milligrams. That's roughly equivalent to 1,500 I.U. of "D-alpha-tocopherol," sometimes labeled *natural vitamin E.* More than these amounts could increase risk of stroke and uncontrolled bleeding. Additionally, new research (see the New Horizons in Health box) indicates that the purported benefits of vitamin E may be exaggerated.

- The maximum intake level for selenium from both food and supplements is 400 micrograms per day. More than this amount could cause *selenosis,* a toxic reaction marked by hair loss and brittle nails.

Folate

In 1998, the Food and Drug Administration (FDA) took a major dietary plunge by mandating folate fortification of all bread, cereal, rice, and macaroni products sold in the United States. This practice, which will boost folate intake by an average of about 100 micrograms daily, is expected to decrease the number of infants born with spina bifida and other neural tube defects.

Folate is a form of vitamin B that is believed to be protective for cardiovascular disease and to decrease blood levels of *homocysteine,* an amino acid that has been linked to vascular diseases. Homocysteine results from the breakdown of methionine, an amino acid found in meat and other protein-laden foods. Two B vitamins—folate and B_6—are believed to control homocysteine levels.[54] When intake of folate and B_6 is low, homocysteine levels rise in the blood. Recent studies indicate that when the level of homocysteine rises, arterial walls and blood platelets become sticky, which encourages clotting. (Note: Homocysteine levels tend to rise with age, smoking, and menopause.) When clots develop in areas already narrowed by atherosclerosis, a heart attack or stroke is likely.

Although the amount of folate needed to protect the heart has not been determined, many adults have jumped on the folate bandwagon, taking daily folate supplements of up to 800 micrograms. Recently, a new *dietary folate equivalent (DFE)* was established to distinguish folate in food from its synthetic counterpart, *folic acid.* As a food additive or a supplement, folic acid is absorbed about twice as efficiently as folate. The DFE for folate in women age 19 or over is approximately 400 micrograms, with higher levels for pregnant or lactating women. (See Table 8.2 for daily recommended amounts of other B vitamins.) Potential dangers of taking too much folate include a masking of B_{12} deficiencies and resulting problems, ranging from nerve damage, immunodeficiency problems, anemia, fatigue, and headache, to constipation, diarrhea, weight loss, gastrointestinal disturbances, and a host of neurological symptoms.[55]

Gender and Nutrition

Men and women differ in body size, body composition, and overall metabolic rates. They therefore have differing needs for most nutrients throughout the life cycle (see standard tables on male/female vitamin and mineral requirements) and face unique difficulties in keeping on track with their dietary goals. We have already discussed some of these differences. However, there are some factors that need further consideration. Have you ever wondered why men can eat more than women without gaining weight? Although there are many possible reasons, one factor is that women have a lower ratio of lean body mass to adipose (fatty) tissue at all ages and stages of life. Also, after sexual maturation, rate of metabolism is higher in men, meaning that they burn more calories doing the same things as women.

Different Cycles, Different Needs

In addition to these differences, women have many more "landmark" times in life when their nutritional needs vary significantly from requirements at other times. From menarche to menopause, women undergo cyclical physiological changes that can exert dramatic effects on metabolism and nutritional needs. For example, during pregnancy and lactation, women's nutritional requirements increase substantially. Those who are unable to follow the strict dietary recommendations of their doctors may find themselves gaining more weight during pregnancy and retaining it afterwards. During the menstrual cycle, many women report significant food cravings. Later in life, with the advent of menopause, nutritional needs again change rather dramatically. With depletion of the hormone estrogen, the body's need for calcium to ward off bone deterioration becomes pronounced. Women must pay closer attention to exercise patterns and to getting enough calcium through diet or dietary supplements, or they run the risk of osteoporosis (see this chapter's Women's Health/Men's Health box and Chapter 19 for more information).

Changing the "Meat-and-Potatoes" American

Since our earliest agrarian years, many Americans—especially men—have relied on a "meat-and-potatoes" diet. What's wrong with all those hot dogs, steaks, and hamburgers? Heart disease, stroke, and cancer are probably the greatest threats. Add increased risks for colon and prostate cancers, and the rationale for dietary change becomes even more compelling. Consider the following points:

- Men who eat red meat as a main dish five or more times a week have four times the risk of colon cancer of men who eat red meat less than once a month.
- Heavy red meat eaters are more than twice as likely to get prostate cancer and nearly five times more likely to get colon cancer.
- For every three servings of fruits or vegetables per day, men can expect a 22 percent lower risk of stroke.
- Diets high in fruit and vegetables may lower the risk of lung cancer in smokers from 20 times the risk of nonsmokers

Folate A type of vitamin B that is believed to decrease levels of homocysteine, an amino acid that has been linked to vascular diseases.

to "only" 10 times the risk. They may also protect against oral, throat, pancreatic, and bladder cancers, all of which are more common among smokers.

• The fastest-rising malignancy in the United States is cancer of the lower esophagus, particularly among white men. Though obesity seems to be a factor, fruits and vegetables are the protectors. (The average American male eats less than three servings per day, although five to nine servings are recommended. Women average three to seven servings/day.)

Does something in meat make it inherently bad? Although the fat content of meat and fried potatoes as well as the potential carcinogenic substances produced through cooking have been implicated, probably something more basic is also involved. By eating so much protein, a person fills up sooner and never gets around to the fruits and vegetables. Thus, the potential protective value of consuming these foods is lost. See the Skills for Behavior Change box later in this chapter for tips on incorporating more salads into a meat-and-potatoes diet.

What do you think?

Think about the women that you know who seem to have weight problems. How old are they?
✳ What factors may have influenced them to have problems keeping weight off? ✳ What factors do men have to deal with in controlling their eating and managing their weight?

Determining Your Nutritional Needs

Confused by all of the different recommended nutritional values on food labels? If so, you are not alone. Depending on which sets of guidelines you are following, your age, your sex, and a host of other factors, you could be accurate or totally wrong in your assessment of how much of a given nutrient is right for you. For example, the Dietary Reference Intake of iron for adult women under age 50 is 18 milligrams. For men in the same age range, it is just 8 milligrams. However, if you use the Daily Value for iron, both men and women would need 18 milligrams and, according to the Upper Intake level system, both men and women would be allowed a maximum of 45 milligrams of iron as adults. Why all these differences? Which system should you pay most attention to?

History of Dietary Guidelines and Recommendations

The dietary guidelines that we are most familiar with are the **Recommended Dietary Allowances (RDAs),** which were originally established by the Food and Nutrition board of the National Academy of Sciences' in the early 1940s. These standards have been revised at periodic intervals to reflect changes in nutrition science and were originally designed to prevent nutritional deficiencies in the general population. In recent years, as deficiencies that lead to disease conditions

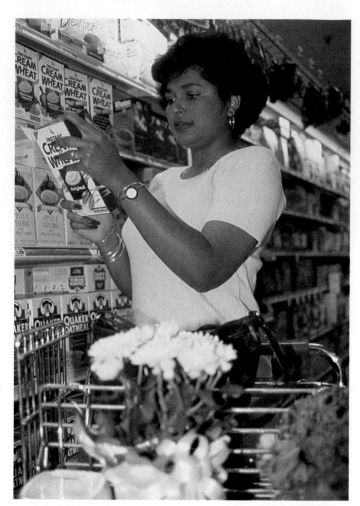

Reading food labels before you purchase food will help you make smart nutritional choices.

have declined, they have been revised to reflect more of a prevention focus. For example, calcium requirements have steadily been increased to reflect concerns about osteoporosis. In the late 1990s, the Food and Nutrition board completed a major overhaul of its guidelines and added these new mechanisms for assessing dietary needs:

> **Adequate Intake (AI)**—a "best guesstimate" of what nutritional needs are likely to be for most people in situations when there hasn't been enough research conducted to fully determine an RDA for a specific nutrient.
>
> **Tolerable Upper Intake Level (UL)**—the highest amount of a nutrient that an individual can safely consume every day without risking adverse health effects.

After a careful analysis of RDAs and the new AI and UL values, a new, combined listing of over 26 essential vitamins and minerals was developed by Canadian and U.S. researchers and is known as the **Dietary Reference Intake (DRI).**[56] Although you seldom see these listings on labels, they are the guidelines recommended for healthy adults and are more comprehensive that RDAs alone because they provide indicators of likely recommendations for nutrients that are currently being studied. Essentially, DRI should be considered the umbrella guidelines under which RDA, AI, and UL will fall.[57]

Reading Labels for Health   To help consumers make choices between similar types of food products that can be incorporated into a healthy diet, the FDA and the U.S. Department of Agriculture developed the **U.S. Recommended Daily Allowances (USRDA)** as a spin-off of RDA recommendations in 1973. The first voluntary food labels with USRDAs were a part of this action. Eventually, in response to consumer demand, the USDA issued mandatory guidelines for food labeling in 1993.[58] These new, mandatory guidelines generally replaced USRDAs with **Reference Daily Intakes (RDIs)** and **Daily Reference Values (DRVs)**. RDIs are the recommended amounts of 19 vitamins and minerals, also known as micronutrients, and DRVs are the recommended amounts for macronutrients, such as total fat, saturated fat, cholesterol, total carbohydrates, dietary fiber, sodium, potassium, and protein.

Together, RDIs and DRVs make up the **Daily Values (DV)** that you will find on food and supplement labels listed as a percentage (% DV); see Figure 8.7 on page 250 for an example. When you look at a label with a % DV listing, you can tell what percentage of a nutrient is found in a serving of food. Although % DV has become widely accepted, it should be noted that it is not as up to date as RDA or DRIs. Although DVs will eventually be updated, they also do not reflect the different needs of older adults, people with conditions such as pregnancy, or gender differences. Advocates of the DV system argue that there isn't enough room for such information on labels, and a basic, easy-to-understand system works best.

Vegetarianism: Eating for Health

For aesthetic, animal rights, economic, personal, health, cultural, or religious reasons, some people choose specialized diets. Between 5 and 15 percent of all Americans today identify themselves as vegetarians. Normally, vegetarianism provides a superb alternative to our high-fat, high-calorie, meat-based cuisine, but without proper information and food choices, vegetarians can also develop dietary problems.

The term **vegetarian** means different things to different people. Strict vegetarians, or *vegans,* avoid all foods of animal origin, including dairy products and eggs. Vegans must be careful to obtain all of the necessary nutrients. Far more common are *lacto-vegetarians,* who eat dairy products but avoid flesh foods. Their diet can be low in fat and cholesterol, but only if they consume skim milk and other low-fat or nonfat products. *Ovo-vegetarians* add eggs to their diet, while *lacto-ovo-vegetarians* eat both dairy products and eggs. *Pesco-vegetarians* eat fish, dairy products, and eggs, while *semivegetarians* eat chicken, fish, dairy products, and eggs. Some people in the semivegetarian category prefer to call themselves "non–red meat eaters."

Generally, people who follow a balanced vegetarian diet have lower weights, better cholesterol levels, fewer problems with irregular bowel movements (constipation and diarrhea), and a lower risk of heart disease than do nonvegetarians. Some preliminary evidence suggests that vegetarians may also have a reduced risk for colon and breast cancer.[59] Whether these lower risks are due to the vegetarian diet per se or to some combination of lifestyle variables remains unclear.

Although in the past vegetarians often suffered from vitamin deficiencies, the vegetarian of the new millennium is usually extremely adept at combining the right types of foods to ensure proper nutrient intake. People who eat dairy products and small amounts of chicken or fish are seldom nutrient-deficient; in fact, while vegans typically get 50 to 60 grams of protein per day, lacto-ovo-vegetarians normally consume between 70 and 90 grams per day, well beyond the RDA. Vegan diets may be deficient in vitamins B$_2$

Recommended Dietary Allowances (RDAs)   The average daily intakes of energy and nutrients considered adequate to meet the needs of most healthy people in the United States under usual conditions.

Adequate intakes (AIs)   Best estimates of nutritional needs.

Tolerable Upper Intake Level (UL)   The highest amount of a nutrient that an individual can safely consume every day without risking adverse health effects.

Dietary Reference Intake (DRI)   A new, combined listing of over 26 essential vitamins and minerals developed by Canadian and U.S. researchers.

U.S Recommended Daily Allowance (USRDA)   Dietary guidelines developed by the Food and Drug Administration (FDA) and the United States Department of Agriculture.

Reference Daily Intake (RDIs)   Recommended amounts of 19 vitamins and minerals, also known as micronutrients.

Daily Reference Values (DRVs)   Recommended amounts for micronutrients such as total fat, saturated fat, and cholesterol.

Daily Values (DVs)   The RDIs and DRVs together make up the Daily Values, seen on food and supplement labels.

Vegetarian   A term with a variety of meanings: vegans avoid all foods of animal origin; lacto-vegetarians avoid flesh foods but eat dairy products; ovo-vegetarians avoid flesh foods but eat eggs; lacto-ovo-vegetarians avoid flesh foods but eat both dairy products and eggs; pesco-vegetarians avoid meat but eat fish, dairy products, and eggs; semivegetarians eat chicken, fish, dairy products, and eggs.

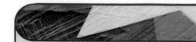

Adding More Salads to Your Diet

Salads and healthful salad toppings add variety to your diet and balance out the average American's meat-and-potatoes diet. Use this information to choose healthful salad greens and toppings for your salad.

Nutritional Comparison of Salad Green Servings

Salad Green	Calories	Vitamin A (IU)	Vitamin C (mg)	Potassium (mg)	Calcium (mg)
Arugula (rocket, roquette)	5	480	3	74	32
Butterhead lettuce (Boston, Bibb)	7	534	4	141	18
Cabbage, red	19	28	40	144	36
Chicory	41	7,200	43	756	180
Endive	8	1,025	3	157	26
Fennel	27	117	10	360	43
Iceberg lettuce	7	182	2	87	10
Leaf lettuce	10	1,064	10	148	38
Romaine lettuce	8	1,456	13	162	20
Spinach	7	2,015	8	167	30*
Watercress	4	1,598	15	112	41

Note: Serving size is one cup; IU = International Units, mg = milligrams
* Much not available to body for use

Nutritional Comparison of Healthful Salad Toppings

Topping	Serving Size	Calories	Bonus Nutrients
Artichoke hearts, in olive oil	1 heart	40	Fiber, folate, potassium, calcium
Avocado, California	¼ of whole fruit	77	Monounsaturated fats, vitamin E, folate, fiber
Beets	½ cup boiled	37	Folate, potassium
Broccoli	½ cup raw	12	Vitamins A and C, calcium, potassium, fiber
Carrots	½ cup raw	31	Vitamin A, beta-carotene, fiber
Cauliflower	½ cup raw	13	Vitamin C
Celery	½ cup raw	6	Vitamin C, potassium
Chicken breast	3 ounces white meat	173	Protein, niacin, vitamin B_6
Chickpeas (garbanzo beans)	½ cup boiled or canned	135	Protein, folate, calcium, potassium, zinc, fiber
Egg	1 whole	78	Vitamins A, E, B_{12}, and D, riboflavin, folate, selenium, zinc. Limit to one egg.
Mushrooms	½ cup	9	Riboflavin, niacin, potassium, selenium
Olives	5 small	20	Monounsaturated fats
Peppers, red, yellow, orange	½ cup raw	14	Vitamins A and C, beta-carotene, fiber
Sardines	3 ounces	160	Protein, omega-3 fatty acids
Sunflower seeds	1 ounce	160	Vitamins E, B_6, niacin, folate, copper, magnesium, zinc, fiber, linoleic acid

Topping	Serving Size	Calories	Bonus Nutrients
Tofu, processed with calcium sulfate	½ cup	94	Protein, calcium, iron, manganese
Tomatoes	½ tomato	13	Vitamins A, C, potassium, lycopene
Tuna, canned in water	3 ounces	99	Protein, niacin, omega-3 fatty acids

Source: "Salads: Going Beyond the Green to Boost Nutrition," Environmental Nutrition, *August 2002.* Reprinted with permission. For subscription information, 800-829-5384.

(riboflavin), B_{12}, and D. Riboflavin is found mainly in meat, eggs, and dairy products; but broccoli, asparagus, almonds, and fortified cereals are also good sources. Vitamins B_{12} and D are found only in dairy products and fortified products such as soy milk. Vegans are also at risk for deficiencies of calcium, iron, zinc, and other minerals, but can obtain these nutrients from supplements. Strict vegans have to pay much more attention to what they eat than the average person does, but by eating complementary combinations of plant products, they can receive adequate amounts of essential amino acids. Examples of complementary combinations are corn and beans, and peanut butter and whole-grain bread. Eating a full variety of grains, legumes, fruits, vegetables, and seeds each day will keep even the strictest vegetarian in excellent health. Pregnant women, the elderly, the sick, and children who are vegans need to take special care to ensure that their diets are adequate. People who take part in heavy aerobic exercise programs (over three hours per week) may need to increase their protein consumption. In all cases, seek advice from a health care professional if you have questions.

The Vegetarian Pyramid

A food guide pyramid has been developed that conveys the essentials of a healthy vegetarian diet (see Figure 8.8). Modeled after the USDA Food Guide Pyramid discussed earlier in this chapter, the vegetarian version clarifies what people who don't eat meat need to do to stay healthy. The vegetarian pyramid defines the following categories. We include examples of single servings in each category:

Grains, Cereal, and Pasta (6–11 servings/day)

- 1 slice bread
- ½ roll or bagel
- 1 tortilla (6")
- 1 ounce cold cereal
- ½ cup cooked cereal, rice, or pasta
- 2 crackers
- 3 cups popcorn

Vegetable Group (2–3 servings/day)

- ½ cup cooked or chopped raw vegetables
- 1 cup raw leafy vegetables
- ¾ cup vegetable juice

Fruit Group (2–3 servings/day)

- 1 medium whole piece of fruit
- ½ cup canned, chopped, or cooked fruit
- ¾ cup fruit juice

Calcium-Rich Foods (4–6 servings/day)

- ½ cup milk or yogurt
- 1 ounce processed cheese

Beans and Alternatives Group (2–3 servings/day)

- ½ cup cooked dry beans, peas, or lentils
- 1 egg
- ⅓ cup bean curd or tofu
- 2–3 tablespoons peanut butter
- 2–3 tablespoons tahini
- 3–4 tablespoons seeds

Other:

- 1 teaspoon flaxseed oil
- vitamins B_{12} and D supplements

> **What do you think?**
>
> *Why are so many people today becoming vegetarians?* ✸ *How easy is it to be a vegetarian on your campus?* ✸ *What concerns about vegetarianism would you be likely to have, if any?*

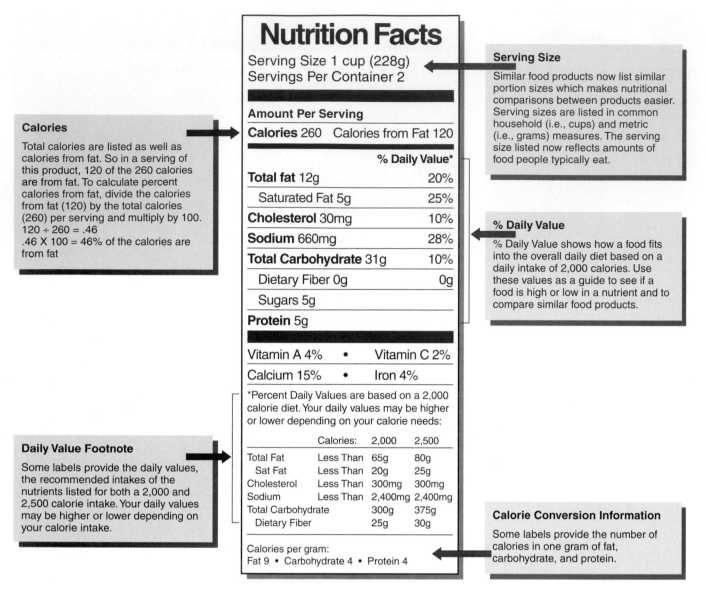

Figure 8.7
Reading a Food Label
Source: Reprinted by permission from Darlene Zimmerman, M.S., R.D., "Hungry for a New Food Label?" *Weight Watchers Thinline* (published by The WW Group Inc.), July–August 1994, 9.

Improved Eating for the College Student

College students often face a challenge when trying to eat healthy foods. Some students live in dorms and do not have their own cooking or refrigeration facilities. Others live in crowded apartments where everyone forages in the refrigerator for everyone else's food. Still others eat at university food services where food choices may be limited. Most students have financial and time constraints that make buying, preparing, and eating healthy food a difficult task. What's a student to do?

Fast Foods: Eating on the Run

If your campus is like many others, you've probably noticed a distinct move toward fast-food restaurants in your student unions so that they now resemble the food courts found in most major shopping malls. These new eating centers fit students' needs for a fast bite of food at a reasonable rate between classes and also bring in money to your school. But many fast foods are high in fat and sodium. Are all fast foods unhealthy?

Not all fast foods are created equal and not all are bad for you. Even at the often-maligned burger chains, menus are healthier than ever before and offer excellent choices for the

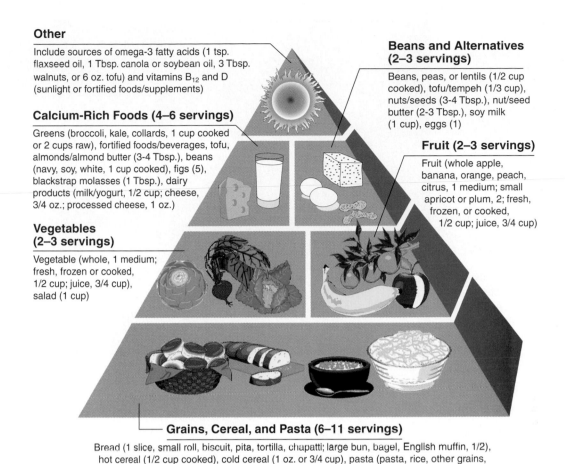

Other

Include sources of omega-3 fatty acids (1 tsp. flaxseed oil, 1 Tbsp. canola or soybean oil, 3 Tbsp. walnuts, or 6 oz. tofu) and vitamins B_{12} and D (sunlight or fortified foods/supplements)

Beans and Alternatives (2–3 servings)

Beans, peas, or lentils (1/2 cup cooked), tofu/tempeh (1/3 cup), nuts/seeds (3-4 Tbsp.), nut/seed butter (2-3 Tbsp.), soy milk (1 cup), eggs (1)

Calcium-Rich Foods (4–6 servings)

Greens (broccoli, kale, collards, 1 cup cooked or 2 cups raw), fortified foods/beverages, tofu, almonds/almond butter (3-4 Tbsp.), beans (navy, soy, white, 1 cup cooked), figs (5), blackstrap molasses (1 Tbsp.), dairy products (milk/yogurt, 1/2 cup; cheese, 3/4 oz.; processed cheese, 1 oz.)

Fruit (2–3 servings)

Fruit (whole apple, banana, orange, peach, citrus, 1 medium; small apricot or plum, 2; fresh, frozen, or cooked, 1/2 cup; juice, 3/4 cup)

Vegetables (2–3 servings)

Vegetable (whole, 1 medium; fresh, frozen or cooked, 1/2 cup; juice, 3/4 cup), salad (1 cup)

Grains, Cereal, and Pasta (6–11 servings)

Bread (1 slice, small roll, biscuit, pita, tortilla, chapatti; large bun, bagel, English muffin, 1/2), hot cereal (1/2 cup cooked), cold cereal (1 oz. or 3/4 cup), pasta (pasta, rice, other grains, 1/2 cup cooked), pancake/waffle (1 small), wheat germ (2 Tbsp.), crackers (2 large)

Figure 8.8

The Vegetarian Food Guide Pyramid

Vegetarians should eat the suggested number of servings from each group daily for a balanced diet. The amount for one serving is listed for selected foods from each group.

Source: Adapted from Melina, V. and J. Forest, *Cooking Vegetarian;* Melina, V. et al., *Becoming Vegetarian.* 2002, www. nutrispeak.com and New York Medical College Vegetarian Pyramid, © 1994 New York Medical College.

discriminating eater. The key word here is *discriminating*. It really is possible to eat healthy fast food if you follow these suggestions:

• Ask for nutritional analyses of items. Most fast-food chains now have them; check their websites or ask at your local outlet.
• Avoid mayonnaise, sauces, and other add-ons. Some places even have fat-free mayonnaise if you ask. Put a hold on extra ketchup.
• Hold the cheese. This extra contributes substantially to total fat while not adding a lot to taste.
• Order single, small burgers rather than large, high-calorie, bacon- or cheese-topped choices. Put on your own ketchup and keep portions small.
• Order salads and be careful how much dressing you put on. Many people think they are being health-smart by eating salad, only to load it with calorie- and fat-rich dressing. Try the vinegar and oil or low-fat alternative dressings. Stay away from eggs and other high-fat add-ons such as bacon bits.
• When ordering a chicken sandwich, order the skinless broiled version rather than the deep-fried version. Many

people think that the deep-fried chicken sandwich is a more healthy choice when it really has more fat than the loaded double burger.

• Check to see what type of oil is used to cook fries if you must have them. Avoid lard-based or other saturated fat products.
• Order wheat buns or bread and ask them to hold the butter.
• Avoid fried foods in general, including hot apple pies and other crust-based fried foods.
• Opt for places where foods tend to be broiled rather than fried.
• Avoid the giant sizes whenever possible and refrain from ordering extra sauces, bacon, and other extras that add additional calories and fat.

When Funds Are Short

Maintaining a nutritious diet within the confines of student life can be challenging. However, if you take the time to plan healthy meals, you will find that you are eating better,

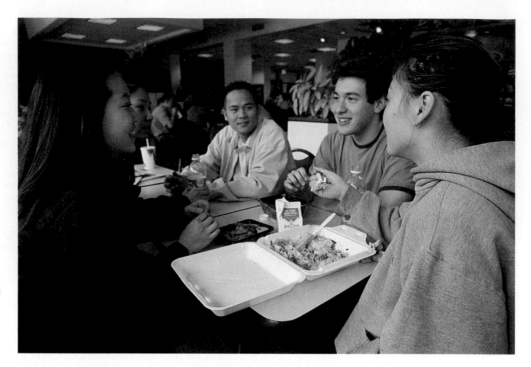

It takes knowledge and planning to make smart menu choices when eating out or in your dining hall. Ask questions to determine which foods offer nutritional value without high fat content.

enjoying it more, and actually saving money. Follow these steps to ensure a healthy but affordable diet:

- Buy fruits and vegetables in season whenever possible for their lower cost, higher nutrient quality, and greater variety.
- Use coupons and specials to get price reductions.
- Shop at discount warehouse food chains; capitalize on volume discounts and no-frills products.
- Plan ahead to get the most for your dollar and avoid extra trips to the store; extra trips usually mean extra purchases. Make a list and stick to it.
- Purchase meats and other products in volume, freezing portions for future needs. Or purchase small amounts of meats and other expensive proteins and combine them with beans and plant proteins for lower cost, calories, and fat.
- Cook large meals, and freeze small portions for later use.
- Drain off extra fat after cooking. Save juices to use in soups and other dishes.
- If you find that you have no money for food, talk to staff at your county or city health department. They may know of ways for you to get assistance.

What do you think?

What problems cause you the most difficulty when you try to eat more healthful foods? ✳ Are these problems typical in your family, or are they unique to your current situation as a student? ✳ What actions can you take to improve your current eating practices?

Supplements: New Research on the Daily Dose

For years, health experts touted the benefits of eating a balanced diet over popping a vitamin and mineral supplement. In fact, we were told that supplements were rarely necessary in the United States and that if we chose to pop those one-a-day pills, most of their water-soluble content would simply be replenishing the nutrient supplies of our underground sewer systems.

So eyebrows were raised in the summer of 2002 when an article in the esteemed *Journal of the American Medical Association (JAMA)* broke with tradition and recommended that "a vitamin/mineral supplement a day just might be important in keeping the doctor away, particularly for some groups of people."[60] Essentially, the article indicated that elderly people, vegans, alcohol-dependent individuals, and patients with malabsorption problems may be at particular risk of deficiency of several vitamins. Although it acknowledged that there may be a risk if you overdose on fat-soluble vitamins, it noted that inadequate amounts of nutrients such as vitamins B_6, B_{12}, D, E, and lycopene are linked to chronic diseases, including coronary heart disease, cancer, and osteoporosis. As a result of this study, *JAMA* indicated that all adults should be taking a basic multivitamin.

So should you rush out and stock up on supplements? Not so fast. According to Dr. David Bender, writing in the *British Medical Journal,*[61] the *JAMA* review article produced little convincing evidence in favor of supplements. According to Dr. Bender, if our dietary intake is adequate, supplements will probably do us little good. Surely there will be much more controversy over supplement utilization in the future. If you are in doubt, make sure you eat from the food groups recommended in the pyramid. If you are facing extreme stressors on the body from physical endurance events, illness, or other nutrient-depleting events, supplements might be beneficial. In all cases, beware of overdosing on ultravitamin supplements and megadoses. Pick the inexpensive varieties and aim to meet minimal levels.

Food Safety: A Growing Concern

As we become increasingly worried that the food we put in our mouths may be contaminated with bacteria, insects, worms, or other substances, the food industry has come under fire. To convince us that their products are safe, some manufacturers have come up with "new and improved" ways of protecting our foods. How well do they work?

Food-Borne Illnesses

Are you concerned that the chicken you are buying doesn't look pleasingly pink, or that your "fresh" fish smells a little *too* fishy or has a grayish tinge? Are you *sure* that your apple juice is free of animal wastes? You may have good reason to be worried. In increasing numbers, Americans are becoming sick from what they eat, and many of these illnesses are life threatening. Scientists estimate, based on several studies conducted over the past 10 years, that food-borne pathogens sicken over 76 million people and cause some 9,000 deaths in the United States annually.[62] Because most of us don't go to the doctor every time we are sick, we may not make a connection between what we eat and later symptoms.

Signs of food-borne illnesses vary tremendously and usually include one or several symptoms: diarrhea, nausea, cramping, and vomiting. Depending on the amount and virulence of the pathogen, symptoms may appear as early as 30 minutes after eating contaminated food or as long as several days or weeks later. Most of the time, symptoms occur five to eight hours after eating and last only a day or two. For certain populations, however, such as the very young, the elderly, or people with severe illnesses such as cancer, diabetes, kidney disease, or AIDS, food-borne diseases can be fatal.

Several factors may be contributing to the increase in food-borne illnesses. According to Michael T. Osterholm, Ph.D., state epidemiologist in Minneapolis,[63] the movement away from a traditional meat-and-potato American diet to "heart-healthy" eating—increasing consumption of fruits, vegetables, and grains—has spurred demand for fresh foods that are not in season most of the year. This means that we must import fresh fruits and vegetables, thus putting ourselves at risk for ingesting exotic pathogens. Depending on the season, up to 70 percent of the fruits and vegetables consumed in the United States come from Mexico alone. The upshot is that a visit to developing countries isn't necessary to be stricken with food-borne "traveler's diarrhea" because the produce does the traveling.[64] Although we are told when we travel to developing countries, "boil it, peel it, or don't eat it," we bring these foods into our kitchens and eat them, often without even washing them.[65] Food can become contaminated by being watered with contaminated water, fertilized with "organic" fertilizers (animal manure), or not subjected to the same rigorous pesticide regulations as American-raised produce. To give you an idea of the implications, studies have shown that *E. coli* (a lethal bacterial pathogen) can survive in cow manure for up to 70 days and can multiply in foods grown with manure unless heat or additives such as salt or preservatives are used to kill the microbes.[66] There are essentially no regulations that say farmers can't use animal manure in growing their crops. Turkey manure, pig manure, and other agribusiness by-products are often sprayed on fields that ultimately grow foods for consumers. *E. coli* 0157:H7 actually increases in summer months in cows awaiting slaughter in crowded, overheated pens. This increases the chances of meat coming to market already contaminated.[67]

Key factors associated with the increasing spread of food-borne diseases include the following:[68]

- Globalization of the food supply. Because food is distributed worldwide, the possibility of exposure to pathogens native to remote regions of the world is greater. For example, a large outbreak of Shigella occurred in Norway, Sweden, and the United Kingdom from lettuce that originated in southern Europe.
- *Inadvertent introduction of pathogens into new geographic regions.* One theory is that cholera was introduced into waters off the coast of the southern United States when a cargo ship discharged contaminated ballast as it came into harbor. Other pathogens may enter into aquatic life in a similar manner.
- *Exposure to unfamiliar food-borne hazards.* Travelers, refugees, and immigrants who move through foreign countries are exposed to food-borne hazards and bring them home with them.
- *Changes in microbial populations.* Changing microbial populations can lead to the evolution of new pathogens. As a result, old pathogens develop new virulence factors or become resistant to antibiotics, making diseases more difficult to treat.
- *Increased susceptibility of varying populations.* People are becoming more vulnerable to disease. The numbers of highly susceptible persons are expanding worldwide because of aging populations, HIV infection, and other underlying medical conditions, such as malnutrition and the compromised health status that results from the use of immunosuppressive drugs. High birth rates and increased longevity have increased the numbers of vulnerable populations at the margins.
- *Insufficient education about food safety.* Increased urbanization, industrialization, and travel, combined with more people eating out, raise the risk of unsafe food handling and illness.

Know what the typical food-borne illnesses are, how you can contract them, and what you can do to prevent infection. Table 8.4 lists common food-borne illnesses and their symptoms.

Table 8.4
Recognizing the Common Food-Borne Illnesses

ILLNESS	SYMPTOMS/RELATED PROBLEMS
Campylobacteriosis	Most common bacterial cause of diarrhea in the United States, affecting over 2 million people a year. Ranges from a mild illness with diarrhea lasting a day, to severe abdominal pain, severe diarrhea (sometimes bloody), sometimes accompanied by fever, occasionally lasting several weeks. Incubation period is 2–5 days, and illness usually lasts 2–10 days. Usually mild, but deaths have been noted among the very young, the very old, or the immunocompromised.
Clostridium perfringens	Typically occurs 6–24 hours after ingestion of food that bears large counts of this bacteria. Usually mild gastrointestinal distress lasting a day or so. Deaths are uncommon.
Escherichia coli O157:H7	Usually a mild gastrointestinal illness that occurs 3–5 days after eating contaminated foods. Severe complications, however, can arise. Hemorrhagic colitis is distinguished by the sudden onset of severe abdominal cramps, little or no fever, and diarrhea that may become grossly bloody. Fewer than 5 percent develop hemolytic uremic syndrome (HUS), a severe, life-threatening illness in which red blood cells are destroyed, kidneys fail, and neurologically based seizures and strokes occur.
Listeria monocytogenes	*Listeria* may be either mild or severe. Milder cases are characterized by sudden onset of fever, severe headache, vomiting, and other flulike symptoms. Listeriosis may appear mild in healthy adults and more sever in fetuses, the elderly, those with kidney disease, users of glucocorticosteroids, and the immunocompromised. Women infected during pregnancy may transmit infection to the fetus, resulting in possible stillbirth or babies born with mental retardation. Over 2,500 people become seriously ill each year, leading to 500 deaths.
Samonella	Usually occurs 6–72 hours after eating contaminated foods and lasts for a day or two. Nausea, diarrhea, stomach pain and vomiting are hallmark symptoms. There are over 40,000 reported cases each year (the actual incidence may be 20 times higher) and about 1,000 deaths.
Staphylococcus aureus	Usually occurs within 1–6 hours following consumption of the toxins produced by the bacteria, but may occur within 30 minutes. Severe nausea and vomiting, cramps, and diarrhea are common. Although the illness generally doesn't last longer than 1–2 days, more serious symptoms may require hospitalization.
Toxoplasmosis	Mild flulike symptoms, or *no* symptoms. Undercooked meat is often the cause. Pregnant women may have stillbirths or babies born with birth defects ranging from heaing or visual impairments to mental retardation.

Source: Centers for Disease Control and Prevention, *"Foodborne Illnesses,"* 2002 (see *http://www.cdc.gov/health/foodill.htm*).

Responsible Use: Avoiding Risks in the Home

Part of the responsibility for preventing food-borne illness lies with consumers—over 30 percent of all such illnesses result from unsafe handling of food at home.

- When shopping, pick up packaged and canned foods first and save frozen foods and perishables such as meat, poultry, and fish till last. Place these foods in separate plastic bags so drippings don't run onto other foods in your cart, contaminating them.
- Check for cleanliness at the salad bar and meat and fish counters. For instance, cooked shrimp lying on the same small bed of ice as raw fish can easily be contaminated.
- When shopping for fish, buy from markets that get their supplies from state-approved sources; stay clear of vendors who sell shellfish from roadside stands or the back of trucks. If you're planning to harvest your own shellfish, check the safety of the water in the area.
- Most cuts of meat, fish, and poultry should be kept in the refrigerator no more than one or two days. They shouldn't be in the grocery store meat counter beyond their dated shelf life, either. If your fish smells particularly "fishy" and your meat has a dark or greenish tinge to it, use caution. Check the shelf life of all products before buying. If expiration dates are close, freeze or eat the product immediately.
- Avoid preparing food if you are sick. Wear latex gloves if you have cuts or burns on your hands. Keep your hands away from your nose, mouth, and eyes. Wash your hands after bathroom trips.
- Eat leftovers within three days.
- Keep hot foods hot and cold foods cold.
- Use a thermometer to ensure that meats are completely cooked. Remember that the rarer the steak, the greater the number of bacteria swarming on the plate. Beef and lamb steaks and roasts should be cooked to at least 145°F; ground meat, pork chops, ribs, and egg dishes to 160°F; ground poultry and hot dogs to 165°F; chicken and turkey breasts to 170°F; and chicken and turkey legs, thighs, and whole birds to 180°F.

- Fish is done when the thickest part becomes opaque and the fish flakes easily when poked with a fork. If you have any concerns, skip seafood such as sushi and raw oysters.
- Never leave cooked food standing on the stove or table for more than two hours. Disease-causing bacteria grow in temperatures between 40°F and 140°F. Cooked foods that have been left standing in this temperature range for more than two hours should be thrown away.
- Never bring your grilled meat into the house on the same plate you took it out on. Raw meat juices are hotbeds for deadly bacteria.
- Never thaw frozen foods at room temperature. Put them in the refrigerator for a day to thaw, or thaw in cold water, changing the water every 30 minutes.
- Wash your hands with soap and water between courses when preparing food, particularly after handling meat, fish, or poultry. Use warm (not hot) water and soap. Don't use antibacterial soap, which only contributes to antibacterial resistance. To wash, rub hands vigorously together for 15–20 seconds. Wash the countertop and all utensils before using them for other foods.

Food Irradiation: How Safe Is It?

Each year, thousands of people get sick from largely preventable diseases such as that caused by *E. coli* as well as other bacteria such as *salmonella* and *listeria*. In response to these concerns, in February 2000 the USDA approved large-scale irradiation of beef, lamb, poultry, pork, and other raw animal foods.

Food irradiation is a process that involves treating foods with gamma radiation from radioactive cobalt, cesium, or other sources of x-rays. When foods are irradiated, they are exposed to low doses of radiation, or ionizing energy, which breaks chemical bonds in the DNA of harmful bacteria, destroying the pathogens and keeping them from replicating. The rays essentially pass through the food without leaving any radioactive residue.[69]

Some companies use cobalt 60, a radioactive substance, for irradiation, but others are beginning to use a new kind of irradiation that dispenses with radioactive compounds and uses electricity as the energy source instead. Thus, as foods pass along a conveyor belt, the energy used to kill bacteria comes from electron beams rather than gamma rays.[70] Irradiation lengthens food products' shelf life and prevents the spread of deadly microorganisms, particularly in high-risk foods such as ground beef and pork. Thus, the minimal costs of irradiation should result in lower overall costs to consumers, in addition to reducing the need for toxic chemicals now used to preserve foods and prevent contamination from external pathogens.

Food irradiation has been approved for potatoes, spices, pork carcasses, and fruits and vegetables since the mid-1980s. Some environmentalists and consumer groups have raised concerns, so irradiated products are not common fare. However, the facts appear to support the use of irradia-

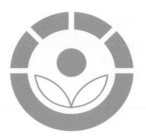

Figure 8.9
Label for Irradiated Foods
The "radura" indicates food that has been irradiated.
Source: USFDA for Food Safety and Applied Nutrition, "Irradiation" (see www.cfsan.fda.gov/~dms/a2z-i.html#irradiation).

tion. Consider the following facts as you decide whether to purchase foods with the "radura" logo (see Figure 8.9):

- Large doses of irradiation can cause an off-taste or color change in meat; however, industry leaders avoid such changes by using low radiation doses.
- Costs may increase by 4–30 cents per pound for irradiated meats in the near future, until the technology improves.
- Not all bacteria are killed using this process, just as all are not killed by pasteurizing milk.
- Consumer groups are concerned about too much cobalt 60 or cesium 137 being released into the environment. Long-term effects are unknown.
- Food that has been irradiated does not differ in nutritional quality from food that has not been irradiated.
- Irradiation creates some by-products, called *radiolytic compounds,* which have been implicated in certain cancers. However, it is not known whether they present increased risk to humans.
- Risks from deadly pathogens in foods increase daily as large meat-producing industries attempt to get product to market quickly. Irradiation appears to be a reasonably safe alternative when weighed against pathogenic risks.
- Some foods, such as apples, pears, and citrus fruits, have actually been shown to spoil faster after irradiation.
- Although the health effects of irradiated food may not be known for many years, the long-term impact of the proliferation of radioactive material on our environment must be considered.

Food irradiation   Treating foods with gamma radiation from radioactive cobalt, cesium, or some other source of x-rays to kill microorganisms.

Food Additives

Additives generally reduce the risk of food-borne illness (i.e., nitrates added to cured meats), prevent spoilage, and enhance the ways foods look and taste. Additives can also enhance nutrient value, especially to benefit the general public. A deficiency can be a terrible public health problem, and a solution is relatively easy to administer. Good examples include the fortification of milk with vitamin D and of grain products with folate. Although the FDA regulates additives according to effectiveness, safety, and ability to detect them in foods, questions have been raised about those additives put into foods intentionally and those that get in unintentionally before or after processing. Whenever such products are added, consumers should take the time to determine what the substances are and if there are alternatives. As a general rule of thumb, the fewer chemicals, colorants, and preservatives, the better. Also, it should be noted that certain foods and additives can interact with medications (see Table 8.3). To be a smart consumer, be aware of these potential dietary interactions. Examples of common additives include the following:

- *Antimicrobial agents.* Substances such as salt, sugar, nitrates, and others that tend to make foods less hospitable for microbes.
- *Antioxidants.* Substances that preserve color and flavor by reducing loss due to exposure to oxygen. Vitamins C and E are among those antioxidants believed to play a role in reduced cancer and cardiovascular disease. BHA and BHT are additives that also are antioxidant in action.
- *Artificial colors.*
- *Nutrient additives.*
- *Flavor enhancers such as MSG.*
- *Sulfites.* Used to preserve vegetable color; some people have severe allergic reactions.
- *Substances that inadvertently get into food products from packaging and/or handling.*
- *Dioxins.* Found in coffee filters, milk containers, and frozen foods.
- *Methylene chloride.* Found in decaffeinated coffee
- *Hormones.* Bovine growth hormone (BGH) found in animal meat.

Food allergies Overreaction by the body to normally harmless proteins, which are perceived as allergens. In response, the body produces antibodies, triggering allergic symptoms.

Food intolerance Adverse effects resulting when people who lack the digestive chemicals needed to break down certain substances eat those substances.

Organically grown Foods that are grown without use of pesticides or chemicals.

Food Allergy or Food Intolerance?

At some point in time, a **food allergy** or **food intolerance** will affect nearly everyone. You eat something, develop gas or have an unpleasant visit to the bathroom, and assume that it is a food allergy. One out of every three people today either say they have a food allergy or avoid something in their diet because they think they have an allergy; in fact, only 3 percent of all children and 1 percent of all adults have real allergic reactions to what they eat.[71] Surprised? Most people are when they hear this.

A food allergy or hypersensitivity is an abnormal response to a food that is triggered by the immune system. Reactions range from minor rashes to severe swelling in the mouth, tongue, and throat, to violent vomiting and diarrhea and occasionally death.

In adults, the most common foods to cause true allergic reactions are shellfish (such as shrimp, crayfish, lobster, and crab); peanuts, which can cause severe anaphylaxis, a sudden drop in blood pressure that can be fatal if not treated promptly; tree nuts such as walnuts; fish; and eggs. In children, food allergens that cause the most problems are eggs, milk, and peanuts.[72]

In contrast to allergies, in cases of food intolerance you may have symptoms of gastric upset, but they are not the result of an immune system response. Probably the best example of a food intolerance is *lactose intolerance,* a problem that affects about 1 in every 10 adults. Lactase is an enzyme in the lining of the gut that degrades lactose, which is in dairy products. If you don't have enough lactase, lactose cannot be digested and remains in the gut to be used by bacteria. Gas is formed and you experience bloating, abdominal pain, and sometimes diarrhea. Food intolerance also occurs in response to some food additives, such as the flavor enhancer MSG, certain dyes, sulfites, gluten, and other substances. In some cases the food intolerance may have psychological triggers.

If you suspect that you have an actual allergic reaction to food, see an allergist to be tested to determine the source of the problem. Because there are several diseases that share symptoms with food allergies (ulcers and cancers of the gastrointestinal tract can cause vomiting, bloating, diarrhea, nausea, and pain), you should have persistent symptoms checked out as soon as possible. If particular foods seem to bother you consistently, look for alternatives or modify your diet. In true allergic instances, you may not be able to consume even the smallest amount safely. For example, people have had severe allergic reactions to peanuts from ingesting as little as a crumb.

Is Organic for You?

Due to mounting concerns about food safety, many people refuse to buy processed foods and mass-produced agricultural products. Instead, they purchase foods that are **organically grown**—foods reported to be pesticide- and chemical-free. Less than a decade ago, buying organic foods meant going to a specialty store and paying premium prices for produce that was wilted, wormy, and smaller in size than its nonorganic

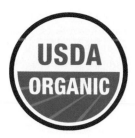

Figure 8.10
Label for Certified Organic Foods
The organic seal indicates that the product is at least 95 percent organic according to USDA guidelines.
Source: USDA Agriculture Marketing Program, The National Organic Program, "Organic Food Standards and Labels: The Facts" (see www.ams.usda.gov/nop/consumerbrochure.htm)

alternative. These products also came with no guarantee that they were really grown in organic environments. People who bought these foods did so out of a desire to eat "healthier" produce and avoid the chemicals that they were increasingly being told caused cancer, immune system problems, and a host of other ailments.

Enter the organics of the twenty-first century—larger, more attractive, and fresher looking but still carrying a hefty price tag. Is buying organic really better for you? Perhaps if

we could put a group of people in a pristine environment and ensure that they never ate, drank, or were exposed to chemicals, we could test this hypothesis; however, it is difficult, if not impossible, to assess the overall impact of organic versus nonorganic food in terms of health outcomes. Nevertheless, the market for organics has been increasing by 15–20 percent per year—five times faster than food sales in general. Nearly 40 percent of U.S. consumers now reach occasionally for something labeled organic, with sales topping $11 billion per year.[73]

More importantly, as of October 2002, any food sold as organic has to meet criteria set by the U.S. Department of Agriculture under the National Organic Rule and can carry a new USDA seal verifying that it is as "certified organic" (Figure 8.10). Under this rule, something that is certified may carry one of the following terms: 100 Percent Organic (100 percent compliance with organic criteria), Organic (must contain at least 95 percent organic materials), Made with Organic Ingredients (must contain at least 70 percent organic ingredients), or Some Organic Ingredients (contains less than 70 percent organic ingredients—usually listed individually). In order to be certified and use any of the above terms, the foods must be produced without hormones, antibiotics, herbicides, insecticides, chemical fertilizers, genetic modification, or germ-killing radiation.

Taking Charge

Managing Eating Behavior

By paying attention, reading, seeking help from reputable trained professionals, and planning ahead, you can improve your own nutritional health.

Checklist for Change

Making Personal Choices

☐ *Eat lower on the food chain.* Substitute fruits, vegetables, nuts, or grains for animal products at least once a day.

☐ *Eat seasonal foods whenever possible.* By eating foods at the peak of harvest, you are most apt to avoid nutrient losses incurred by storage, freezing, canning, and so on.

☐ *Eat lean.* Pay attention to labels, assess your food intake, and balance high-fat meals with low-fat meals. Choose leaner cuts and bake, grill, boil, or broil whenever possible.

☐ *Consume more fruits and vegetables.* Use the real thing instead of juices.

☐ *Combine foods for optimum nutrition.* Identify the best ways to combine grains, beans, fruits, vegetables, nuts, and other foods. You will then be able to optimize dietary returns.

☐ *Practice responsible consumer safety.* Avoid unnecessary chemicals and buy, prepare, and store foods prudently to avoid food-borne illness.

☐ *Eat in moderation.* Learn to separate true hunger feelings from the food cravings that come from boredom. Don't undereat or overeat. Reduce your consumption of sugars and other dietary "extras."

☐ *Keep your systems functioning well.* Even the best diets are doomed to failure if stress, drugs, lack of exercise, sleep deprivation, and other life problems are dragging your body down, particularly your digestive system.

☐ *Keep dietary foods in balance.* Consume appropriate amounts of fats, carbohydrates, proteins, vitamins, minerals, amino acids, fatty acids, and water.

☐ *Pay attention to changing nutrient needs.* Various factors in life may require that you adjust your nutritional intake. Remain informed about new information from reputable sources concerning specific nutrient benefits and hazards.

Making Community Choices

☐ Pay attention to the types of eating establishments available on your campus. If you don't have the options you think you should, take action. Involve your student newspaper and student orga-nizations, talk with food service representatives, involve your student health service, and solicit the support of key people on campus.

☐ Assess your elected officials' priorities regarding nutrition as it pertains to schools, the elderly, pregnant women, and the homeless. Do they support adequate nutrition for high-risk groups? If not, write letters asking for clarification of their positions.

☐ If you patronize certain food establishments, review the food choices. Tell them when they are doing a good job, and request other options.

☐ Be informed about key nutritional concepts. Demand accuracy in reported claims. Speak only from an informed perspective.

Summary

✻ Recognizing that we eat for more reasons than just survival is the first step toward changing our health.
✻ The Food Guide Pyramid provides guidelines for healthy eating.
✻ The major nutrients that are essential for life and health include water, proteins, carbohydrates, fiber, fats, vitamins, and minerals.
✻ Experts are interested in the role of food as medicine and in the benefits of "functional foods." These foods may play an important role in improving certain conditions, such as hypertension.
✻ Men and women have differing needs for most nutrients throughout the life cycle because of different body size and composition.
✻ Vegetarianism can provide a healthy alternative for those wishing to cut fat from their diets or wanting to reduce or eliminate animal consumption. The vegetarian pyramid provides dietary guidelines to help vegetarians obtain needed nutrients.

✻ College students face unique challenges in eating healthfully. Learning to make better choices at fast-food restaurants, eat healthily when funds are short, and eat nutritionally in the dorm are all possible when you use the knowledge contained in this chapter.
✻ Food-borne illnesses, food irradiation, food allergies, organic foods, and other food safety and health concerns are becoming increasingly important to healthwise consumers. Recognizing potential risks and taking steps to prevent problems are part of a sound nutritional plan.

Questions for Discussion and Reflection

1. What are several factors that influence the dietary patterns and behaviors of the typical college student? What factors have been the greatest influences on your eating behaviors? Why is it important to recognize influences on your diet as you think about changing eating behaviors?

2. What are the six major food groups in the USDA Food Guide Pyramid? From which groups do you eat too few servings? What can you do to increase or decrease your intake of selected food groups to improve your health? How can you remember the six groups?

3. What are the major types of nutrients that you need to obtain from the foods you eat? What happens if you fail to get enough of some of them? Are there significant differences between the sexes in particular areas of nutrition?

4. Distinguish between the different types of vegetarianism. Which types are most likely to lead to nutrient deficiencies? What can be done to ensure that even the strictest vegetarian receives enough of the major nutrients?

5. What are functional foods? What are the major functional foods discussed in this chapter? What are their reported benefits, if any?

6. What are the major problems that many college students face when trying to eat the right foods? List five actions that you and your classmates could take immediately to improve your eating.

7. What are the potential benefits and risks of food irradiation? Why is it being used? What are the major risks for food-borne illnesses, and what can you do to protect yourself? How are food illnesses and food allergies different?

Application Exercises

Reread the What Do You Think? scenarios at the beginning of the chapter and answer the following questions.

1. Critique the eating habits of James, Roberto, Jordan, and Martha. What suggestions could you make to help them? How could you make these suggestions in a way that wouldn't offend them?
2. If someone eats a high-fat diet, is 70 years old, and is never sick, why should the person change eating habits?
3. Should children in elementary school be concerned about what they eat? Why or why not?
4. Why is it often difficult to talk with friends or family members about their eating behaviors? How would you approach talking with each of the people listed here?

Accessing Your Health on the Internet

Visit the following Internet sites to explore further topics and issues related to personal health. To visit an organization's website, go to the Companion Website for *Access to Health, Eighth Edition,* at www.aw.com/donatelle, click on the book image, and select "Accessing Your Health on the Internet" from the navigation menu on the left.

1. *American Dietetic Association (ADA).* Provides information on a full range of dietary topics, including sports nutrition, healthful cooking, and nutritional eating; also links to scientific publications and information on scholarships and public meetings.
2. *American Heart Association (AHA).* Includes information about a heart-healthy eating plan and an easy-to-follow guide to healthy eating.
3. *Food and Drug Administration (FDA).* Provides information for consumers and professionals in the areas of food safety, supplements, and medical devices and links to other sources of nutrition and food information.
4. *Food and Nutrition Information Center.* Offers a wide variety of information related to food and nutrition.
5. *National Institutes of Health: Office of Dietary Supplements.* Site of the International Bibliographic Database Information on Dietary Supplements (IBIDS), updated quarterly.
6. *U.S. Department of Agriculture (USDA).* Offers a full discussion of the USDA Dietary Guidelines for Americans.

Further Reading

Nutrition Action Healthletter.

This newsletter, published 10 times a year, contains up-to-date information on diet and nutritional claims and current research issues. The newsletter can be obtained by writing to the Center for Science in the Public Interest, 1501 16th St. NW, Washington, DC 20036.

Nutrition Today.

An excellent magazine for the interested nonspecialist. Covers controversial issues and provides a forum for conflicting opinions. Six issues per year. Order from Williams and Wilkins, 351 West Camden Street, Baltimore, MD 21201-2436.

Schlosser, E. *Fast Food Nation.* Boston: Houghton Mifflin, 2001.

Overview of the influence of the fast food industry and its effect on health and well-being in America.

Tufts University Health and Nutrition Letter.

An excellent source for quick "fixes" on current nutritional topics. Reputable sources and information. E-mail: tufts@tiac.net or phone 1-800-274-7581. The Tufts Nutrition Navigator website (http://navigator.tufts.edu) rates nutrition-related websites for information and accuracy.

U.S. Department of Agriculture.

For information on the proper handling of meat and poultry and other information, call the USDA's Meat and Poultry Hot Line at the toll-free number 1-800-535-4555 between 10:00 A.M. and 4:00 P.M. on weekdays. Write to the Meat and Poultry Hot Line, USDA-FSIS, Room 1165-S, Washington, DC, 20250 for a new booklet, A Quick Consumer's Guide to Safe Food Handling.

Whitney, E., and S. Rolfes. *Understanding Nutrition.* San Francisco: Wadsworth Publishing, 1999.

An introductory college health text that provides an outstanding overview of nutritional information in a highly accessible, easy-to-read format.

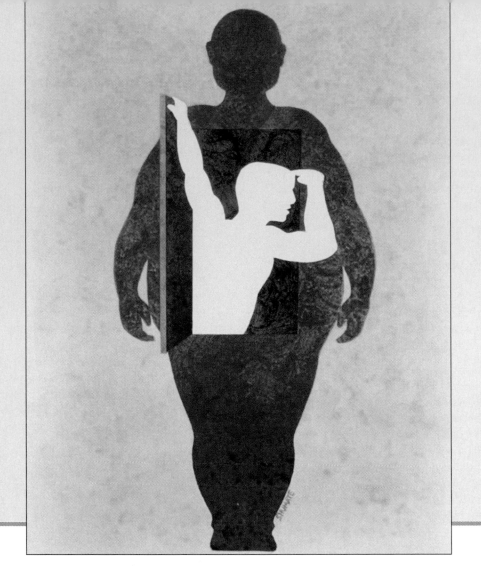

Objectives

* Explain why so many people are obsessed with thinness and body size and how to determine the right weight for you. Define obesity and describe the current epidemic of obesity in the United States.

* Describe the options available for determining percentage body fat content. Indicate which are the most reliable.

* Describe factors that place people at risk for problems with obesity. Indicate which factors a person can control and which cannot be controlled.

* Discuss the roles of exercise, dieting, nutrition, lifestyle modification, fad diets, and other strategies of weight control. Describe the most effective methods of weight management.

* Describe the three major eating disorders, explain the health risks related to these conditions, and indicate the factors that make individuals susceptible to these disorders.

9 Managing Your Weight

In the 1980s and 1990s Americans witnessed unprecedented increases in the rate of obesity. At the same time, they showed little improvement in eating habits or in increasing their physical activity. The Behavioral Risk Factor Surveillance System (BRFSS)[1] showed that the prevalence of obesity among U.S. adults in 2000 was 19.8 percent, which reflects a major increase since 1991. It also found a 49 percent increase between 1990 and 2000 in the number of Americans who have diabetes, a major danger of obesity (see Chapter 18). About 27.3 percent of Americans reported that they did not engage in any physical activity during the 1990s, and only about a quarter of Americans consumed the recommended five or more servings of fruits and vegetables a day.[2] Characteristics of those most prone to obesity indicated a disparate level of risk, based on age, race, and other demographic characteristics (see Table 9.1).

If you think that these statistics are bad, another comprehensive study in 1999, the National Health and Nutrition Examination Survey (NHANES III), reported that an estimated 61 percent of U.S. adults are either overweight or obese, defined as having a body mass index (BMI) of 25 or more, and that the rate of obesity among U.S. adults (defined as BMI greater than or equal to 30) has nearly doubled from approximately 15 percent in 1980 to an estimated 27 percent in 1999.[3]

All indications are that while we were doing better economically, while health professionals promoted lowering fat and cholesterol, while technology swept the nation by storm, and while health education and physical education were downplayed and replaced by other career and academic pursuits in schools, we grew a whole generation of Americans who were more out of shape and fatter than ever before.

Several factors have converged to direct our national attention to health and fitness in a way that supersedes all past efforts. One was the terrorist attack of September 11, 2001. Faced with the threat of fighting unknown adversaries, leaders questioned our collective ability to respond. Second, the national news media publicized the results of these

Table 9.1
Changes in Obesity Rates, 1991 to 2000

	Percent Obese	
Characteristic	**1991**	**2000**
MEN	**11.7**	**20.2**
WOMEN	**12.2**	**19.4**
AGE GROUPS		
18–29	7.1	13.5
30–39	11.3	20.2
40–49	15.8	22.9
50–59	16.1	25.6
60–69	14.7	22.9
>70	11.4	15.5
RACE		
White, non-Hispanic	11.3	18.5
Black, non-Hispanic	19.3	29.3
Hispanic	11.6	23.4
Other	7.3	12.0
EDUCATION		
Less than high school	16.5	26.1
High school degree	13.3	21.7
Some college	10.7	19.5
College or above	8.0	15.2
SMOKING STATUS		
Never smoked	12.0	19.9
Ex-smoker	14.0	22.7
Current smoker	9.9	16.3

Source: CDC Behavioral Risk Factor Surveillance System (BRFSS), "Prevalence of Obesity Among U.S. Adults, by Characteristics," 2001 (see http://www.cdc.gov/nccdphp/dnpa/obesity/trend/prev_char.htm).

national surveys, and third, government officials including the president and the surgeon general publicly proclaimed our need for weight reduction and improved fitness and health. Finally, other studies indicated dramatic increases and bleak forecasts in the rates of several obesity-related diseases, including diabetes, heart disease, and arthritis. For example, some experts have predicted that the numbers of Americans diagnosed with diabetes will increase by a whopping 165 percent, from 11 million in 2000 to 29 million in 2050.[4]

Although we are bombarded with reminders that diet, exercise, and overall lifestyle are important factors in determining quality of life and life expectancy, far too many of us don't seem to get the message. For an indication of just how serious the epidemic of obesity is, see the Health in a Diverse World box in this chapter. Officials estimate that more than 500,000 lives are lost each year to conditions directly related to obesity, and many more deaths may be indirectly related to a history of obesity throughout a person's life.[5] Associated health risks (see Table 9.2) include coronary heart disease, hypertension, diabetes, gallstones, sleep apnea, osteoarthritis, and several cancers. In addition, the relationship between obesity and psychosocial development, including self-esteem, is believed to be significant. The estimated annual health care costs due to obesity in the United States are believed to exceed $100 billion in medical expenses and lost productivity per year.[6] Of course, placing a dollar value on a life lost prematurely due to diabetes, stroke, or heart attack or assessing the cost of social isolation and discrimination against those who are obese or overweight is impossible.

Many of us struggle to know how to eat healthy foods, maintain healthy weight levels, and get adequate amounts of exercise. This chapter is designed to help you better understand why we have such a weight problem in America today and to provide you with simple strategies designed to help you manage your weight. (See the Assess Yourself box to obtain a better understanding of your own dietary habits.) It will also help you understand what underweight, normal weight, overweight, obesity, and eating disorders are, the impact of these conditions on health, and the importance of individual and community actions to reduce overall risk.

Body Image

Most of us think of the obsession with thinness as a recent phenomenon. Beginning with supermodel Twiggy in the 1960s and continuing with supermodel Kate Moss in the late 1990s, the thin look has dominated fashion and the media.

However, an obsession with being thin has been a part of our culture for decades. Anorexia nervosa, an eating disorder, has been defined as a psychiatric illness since 1873. During the Victorian era, women wore corsets to achieve unrealistically tiny waists. By the 1920s, it was common knowledge that obesity was linked to poor health. The American

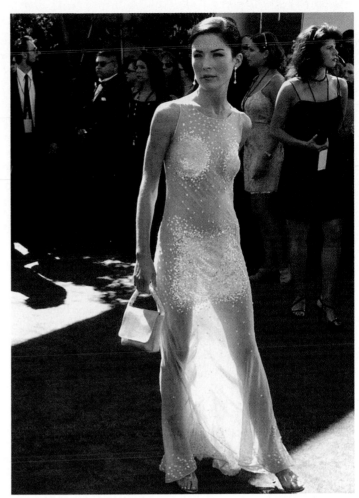

Images in the media, such as this photo of ultra-slim Lara Flynn Boyle, convey the message that a thin body is the ideal body.

Tobacco Company coined the phrase "reach for a Lucky instead of a sweet" to promote the idea that cigarettes dulled appetite.

Today more than ever before, underweight models and TV characters like Ally McBeal exemplify desirability and success, delivering the subtle message that thin is in. In addition, public health warnings that being overweight increases risk for heart disease, certain cancers, and a number of other disorders can send a panic through people when their weight isn't what they think it should be. Some of these distorted views of self-image arise from misinterpreting height-weight charts, making some people strive for the lower readings stipulated for a light-boned person when determining their own normal weight. Sadly, increasing numbers of adolescents, teens, and adults are so preoccupied with trying to be like the size 4 models that they make themselves ill in their quest to be thin. Being overweight has become socially unacceptable in many circles and something to be avoided at all costs, and Americans are looking for fast answers: Should

Are Super-Sized Meals Super-Sizing Americans?

Today, super-sized meals are the norm at many restaurants. Across the country, restaurants and food companies compete with each other to pile it on as customers seek "comfort food" in large portions. Consider the 25-ounce prime rib served at a local steak chain. At nearly 3,000 calories and 150 grams of fat for the meat alone, these dinners serve the dual purpose of slamming shut arteries while adding on pounds. Add a baked potato with sour cream and/or butter, a salad loaded with creamy salad dressing, fresh bread with real butter, and the meal may surpass the 5,000-calorie mark and ring in at close to 300 grams of fat. Keeping in mind that the average daily caloric intake should be closer to 2,000 calories and daily fat consumption should be less than 71 grams, this scale-tipping dinner exceeds what most adults should eat in two days!

And this is just the beginning. Soft drinks, once commonly served in 12-ounce sizes, now come in big gulps and 1-liter bottles. Cinnamon buns at local chains now come in giant, butter-laden, 700-calorie portions. What is the result? Super-sized portions consumed by super-sized Americans. A quick glance at the fattening of Americans provides growing evidence of a significant health problem. According to Donna Skoda, a dietitian and chair of the Ohio State University Extension Service, "People are eating a ton of extra calories. For the first time in history, more people are overweight in America than are underweight. Ironically, although the U.S. fat intake has dropped in the past 20 years from an average of 40 to 33 percent of calories, the daily calorie intake has risen from 1,852 calories per day to over 2,000 per day. In theory, this translates into a weight gain of 15 pounds a year." Skoda and others say that the main reason that Americans are gaining weight is that people no longer know what a normal serving size is. In a recent U.S. Department of Agriculture survey, only 1 percent of the respondents could correctly identify the serving sizes recommended in the Food Guide Pyramid, the visual dietary aid developed by the USDA.

McDonald's super-sized fries weigh 7 ounces and contain 540 calories and 26 grams of fat. Compare that to the 1950s versions your parents and grandparents enjoyed with 220 calories and 12 grams of fat. "Blooming onions" weigh in at over 2,000 calories for a relatively small onion. Grand-sized tacos, huge bagels and muffins, and giant pizzas top off a short list of typical dietary splurging. According to Carrie Wiatt, a Los Angeles dietitian and author of the recently released book *Portion Savvy,* one telling marker of the big-food trend is that restaurant plates have grown from an average of 9 to 13 inches in the past decade. Studies show that people eat 40–50 percent more than they normally would now that large portions are available.

These statistics alone are alarming. However, they are made even worse by a growing trend toward sedentary lifestyles, remote controls, and computer-gazing among far too many Americans. The equation of energy in/energy out is being knocked out of balance on both sides: Americans are taking in more calories and doing less to burn them off. Hence, an epidemic of obesity prevails and is getting worse. Younger and younger kids are eating more and more and picking up lifetime habits that will be hard to change.

To reduce your own risk of super-sizing, follow these simple strategies:

✔ Avoid super-sizing anything. Order the smallest size available when dining out. Focus on taste, not quantity. Get used to eating less and enjoying what you are eating.
✔ Chew your food, and avoid the urge to wash it down with high-calorie drinks. Take time, and let your fullness indicator have a chance to kick in while there is still time to quit.

✔ Serve food on a small or medium plate. Put those big platter-size dinner plates on the top shelf of your cupboard, and leave them there.
✔ Always order dressings, gravies, and sauces on the side. Sprinkle these added calories on carefully, rather than washing your foods down with them. Remember that a tablespoon of gravy could mean an hour on the treadmill to burn off its 200+ calories!
✔ If you order large muffins or bagels, share them with a friend, or bring only half with you and wrap up the rest. Carry a small zip-lock bag, and use it to take home part of those big portions for another day.
✔ Avoid appetizers in restaurants. Often they cost a lot, in terms of money, calories, and fat content.
✔ Share your dinner with a friend, and order a side salad for each of you. Alternatively, put only one-half of your dinner on the "eat now" side of your plate. Save the rest for another day.
✔ Measure portions. Ask for the size of servings before ordering, and always order a size smaller than you really want. When the server tells you it is a "rich dish" or "a lot of food," avoid it.
✔ Avoid buffets and all-you-can-eat establishments. Most of us can eat two to three times what we need—or more.

Source: Some statistics from "Are Super-sized Meals Super-sizing Americans?" by Jane Snow, *Akron Beacon Journal,* May 24, 2000. Reprinted with permission of the Akron Beacon Journal.

Table 9.2
Selected Health Consequences of Overweight and Obesity

Premature Death

- An estimated 300,000 deaths per year may be attributable to obesity.
- The risk of death rises with increasing weight.
- Even moderate weight excess (10 to 20 pounds for a person of average height) increases risk of death.

Cardiovascular Disease

- High blood pressure is twice as common in obese adults as those who are at healthy weights.
- Incidence of all forms of heart disease is increased among overweight and obese people.
- Obesity is associated with elevated triglycerides and decreased "good" cholesterol.

Diabetes

- A weight gain of 11 to 18 pounds increases a person's risk of developing type 2 diabetes to twice that of individuals who have not gained weight.
- Over 80 percent of people with diabetes are overweight or obese.

Cancer

- Overweight and obesity are associated with increased risk of endometrial, colon, gallbladder, prostate, kidney, and postmenopausal breast cancer.
- Women gaining more than 20 pounds between age 18 and midlife double their risk of postmenopausal breast cancer compared to women whose weight remains stable.

Additional Health Consequences

- Sleep apnea and asthma are both associated with obesity.
- For every two-pound increase in weight, the risk of developing arthritis increases by 9 to 13 percent.
- Obesity-related complications during pregnancy include increased risk of fetal and maternal death, labor and delivery complications, and increased risk of birth defects.

Source: U.S. Department of Health and Human Services, "The Surgeon General's Call to Action to Prevent and Decrease Overweight and Obesity" (2001) (see http://www.surgeongeneral.gov/topics/obesity/calltoaction/fact_consequences.htm).

we count calories or carbohydrates? Is dietary fat your biggest enemy? Is Pritikin, Atkins, Weight Watchers, or something else your best weight control strategy? And what is the right weight for you?

Determining the Right Weight for You

Each person's optimal weight depends on a wide range of variables, including body structure, height, weight distribution, and the ratio of fat to lean tissue. In fact, your weight can be a deceptive indicator. Many extremely muscular athletes would be considered overweight based on traditional height-weight charts, while many young women think that they are the right weight based on charts and pride themselves on little weight gain over the years, only to be shocked to discover that 35 to 40 percent of their weight is body fat! In general, weights at the lower end of the range on these charts are recommended for individuals with a low ratio of muscle and bone to fat; those at the upper end are advised

for people with more muscular builds. However, since actual body composition is hard to determine, most charts today simply give a general range for men and women.

Overweight or Obese?

Most of us cringe at the thought of being labeled as one of the "O" words. What is the distinction between the two? **Overweight** refers to increased body weight in relation to height, when compared to a standard such as the height/weight charts in Table 9.3. Historically, nutritionists have defined overweight as being 1–19 percent above one's ideal weight and obese as being over 19 percent above.

> **Overweight** Increased body weight in relation to height.

Readiness for Weight Loss

To see how well your attitudes equip you for a weight loss program, answer the questions that follow. For each question, circle the answer that best describes your attitude. As you complete each of the six sections, tally your score and analyze it according to the scoring guide.

I. GOALS, ATTITUDES, AND READINESS

1. Compared to previous attempts, how motivated are you to lose weight this time?

1	2	3	4	5
Not at all motivated	Slightly motivated	Somewhat motivated	Quite motivated	Extremely motivated

2. How certain are you that you will stay committed to a weight loss program for the time it will take to reach your goal?

1	2	3	4	5
Not at all certain	Slightly certain	Somewhat certain	Quite certain	Extremely certain

3. Considering all outside factors at this time in your life—stress at work, family obligations, and so on—to what extent can you tolerate the effort required to stick to a diet?

1	2	3	4	5
Cannot tolerate	Can tolerate somewhat	Uncertain	Can tolerate well	Can tolerate easily

4. Think honestly about how much weight you hope to lose and how quickly you hope to lose it. Figuring a weight loss of one to two pounds per week, how realistic is your expectation?

1	2	3	4	5
Very unrealistic	Somewhat unrealistic	Moderately unrealistic	Somewhat realistic	Very realistic

5. While dieting, do you fantasize about eating a lot of your favorite foods?

1	2	3	4	5
Always	Frequently	Occasionally	Rarely	Never

6. While dieting, do you feel deprived, angry, and/or upset?

1	2	3	4	5
Always	Frequently	Occasionally	Rarely	Never

IF YOU SCORED:

6 to 16: This may not be a good time for you to start a diet. Inadequate motivation and commitment and unrealistic goals could block your progress. Think about what contributes to your unreadiness and consider changing these factors before undertaking a diet.

17 to 23: You may be close to being ready to begin a program but should think about ways to boost your readiness.

24 to 30: The path is clear: you can decide how to lose weight in a safe, effective way.

II. HUNGER AND EATING CUES

7. When food comes up in conversation or in something you read, do you want to eat, even if you are not hungry?

1	2	3	4	5
Never	Rarely	Occasionally	Frequently	Always

8. How often do you eat because of physical hunger?

1	2	3	4	5
Never	Rarely	Occasionally	Frequently	Always

9. Do you have trouble controlling your eating when your favorite foods are around the house?

1	2	3	4	5
Never	Rarely	Occasionally	Frequently	Always

IF YOU SCORED:

3 to 6: You might occasionally eat more than you should, but it does not appear to be due to high responsiveness to environ-mental cues. Controlling the attitudes that make you eat may be especially helpful.

7 to 9: You may have a moderate tendency to eat just because food is available. Losing weight may be easier for you if you try to resist external cues and eat only when you are physically hungry.

10 to 15: Some or much of your eating may be in response to thinking about food or exposing yourself to temptations to eat. Think of ways to minimize your exposure to temptations so you eat only in response to physical hunger.

III. CONTROL OVER EATING

If the following situations occurred while you were on a diet, would you be likely to eat more or less immediately afterward and for the rest of the day?

10. Although you planned on skipping lunch, a friend talks you into going out for a midday meal.

1	2	3	4	5
Would eat much less	Would eat somewhat less	Would make no difference	Would eat somewhat more	Would eat much more

11. You "break" your plan by eating a fattening, "forbidden" food.

1	2	3	4	5
Would eat much less	Would eat somewhat less	Would make no difference	Would eat somewhat more	Would eat much more

12. You have been following your diet faithfully and decide to test yourself by eating something you consider a treat.

1	2	3	4	5
Would eat much less	Would eat somewhat less	Would make no difference	Would eat somewhat more	Would eat much more

IF YOU SCORED:

3 to 7: You recover rapidly from mistakes. However, if you frequently alternate between eating that is out of control and dieting very strictly, you may have a serious eating problem and should get professional help.

8 to 11: You do not seem to let unplanned eating disrupt your program. This is a flexible, balanced approach.

12 to 15: You may be prone to overeat after an event breaks your control or throws you off the track. Your reaction to these problem-causing events can be improved.

IV. BINGE EATING AND PURGING

13. Aside from holiday feasts, have you ever eaten a large amount of food rapidly and felt afterward that this eating incident was excessive and out of control?

2	0
Yes	No

14. If you answered yes to question 13, how often have you engaged in this behavior during the past year?

1	2	3	4	5	6
Less than once a month	About once a month	A few times a month	About once a week	About three times a week	Daily

15. Have you purged (used laxatives or diuretics, or induced vomiting) to control your weight?

5	0
Yes	No

16. If you answered yes to question 15, how often have you engaged in this behavior during the past year?

1	2	3	4	5	6
Less than once a month	About once a month	A few times a month	About once a week	About three times a week	Daily

(continued on page 268)

IF YOU SCORED:

0: It appears that binge eating and purging are not problems for you.

2 to 11: Pay attention to these eating patterns. Should they arise more frequently, get professional help.

12 to 19: You show signs of having a potentially serious eating problem. See a counselor experienced in evaluating eating disorders right away.

V. EMOTIONAL EATING

17. Do you eat more than you would like to when you have negative feelings such as anxiety, depression, anger, or loneliness?

1	2	3	4	5
Never	Rarely	Occasionally	Frequently	Always

18. Do you have trouble controlling your eating when you have positive feelings—do you celebrate feeling good by eating?

1	2	3	4	5
Never	Rarely	Occasionally	Frequently	Always

19. When you have unpleasant interactions with others in your life, or after a difficult day at work, do you eat more than you'd like?

1	2	3	4	5
Never	Rarely	Occasionally	Frequently	Always

IF YOU SCORED:

3 to 8: You do not appear to let your emotions affect your eating.

9 to 11: You sometimes eat in response to emotional highs and lows. Monitor this behavior to learn when and why it occurs, and be prepared to find alternate activities.

12 to 15: Emotional ups and downs can stimulate your eating. Try to deal with the feelings that trigger the eating and find other ways to express them.

VI. EXERCISE PATTERNS AND ATTITUDES

20. How often do you exercise?

1	2	3	4	5
Never	Rarely	Occasionally	Somewhat frequently	Frequently

21. How confident are you that you can exercise regularly?

1	2	3	4	5
Not at all confident	Slightly confident	Somewhat confident	Highly confident	Completely confident

22. When you think about exercise, do you develop a positive or negative picture in your mind?

1	2	3	4	5
Completely negative	Somewhat negative	Neutral	Somewhat positive	Completely positive

23. How certain are you that you can work regular exercise into your daily schedule?

1	2	3	4	5
Not at all certain	Slightly certain	Somewhat certain	Quite certain	Extremely certain

IF YOU SCORED:

4 to 10: You're probably not exercising as regularly as you should. Determine whether attitude about exercise or your lifestyle is blocking your way, then change what you must and put on those walking shoes!

11 to 16: You need to feel more positive about exercise so you can do it more often. Think of ways to be more active that are fun and fit your lifestyle.

17 to 20: It looks as if the path is clear for you to be active. Now think of ways to get motivated.

After scoring yourself in each section of this questionnaire, you should be able to better judge your dieting strengths and weaknesses. Remember that the first step in changing eating behavior is to understand the conditions that influence your eating habits.

Source: Reprinted from "The Diet Readiness Test," in Kelly D. Brownell, "When and How to Diet," *Psychology Today,* June 1989, 41–46. Reprinted with permission from *Psychology Today* Magazine, copyright © 1989 (Sussex Publishers, Inc.).

Table 9.3
Healthy Weight Ranges for Men and Women

HEIGHT WITHOUT SHOES	WEIGHT* WITHOUT CLOTHES	HEIGHT WITHOUT SHOES	WEIGHT* WITHOUT CLOTHES
4'10"	91–119	5'9"	129–169
4'11"	94–124	5'10"	132–174
5'0"	97–128	5'11"	136–179
5'1"	101–132	6'0"	140–184
5'2"	104–137	6'1"	144–189
5'3"	107–141	6'2"	148–195
5'4"	111–146	6'3"	152–200
5'5"	114–150	6'4"	156–205
5'6"	118–155	6'5"	160–211
5'7"	121–160	6'6"	164–216
5'8"	125–164		

*In pounds
Source: Dietary Guidelines for Americans, 1995, USDA.

Another measurement of overweight and obesity is a mathematical formula known as **body mass index (BMI)**, which represents weight levels associated with the lowest overall risk to health (see the next section to calculate your BMI). Desirable BMI levels may vary with age.[7] Today, you would be classified as being overweight if you have a BMI of 25.0–29.9. About 35 percent of all Americans fit this category.

A person may be classified as overweight using these standards even if the weight gain is due to an increase in lean muscle mass. For example, an athlete may be very lean and muscular, with very little body fat, yet she may weigh a lot more than others of the same height who have little muscle tissue. Conversely, a person may proudly proclaim that he weighs the same amount that he did in high school, but have a much greater proportion of body fat, particularly in the hips, buttocks, or thighs, than he did at a younger age. Body weight alone may not be a good indicator of overall fitness.

Obesity is defined as an excessively high amount of body fat or adipose tissue in relation to lean body mass. It is important to consider both the distribution of fat throughout the body and the size of the adipose tissue deposits. Body fat distribution can be estimated by skinfold measures, waist-to-hip circumference ratios, or techniques such as ultrasound, computed tomography or magnetic resonance imaging, or others. Using traditional standards, people 20–40 percent above their ideal weight are labeled as *mildly obese* (90 percent of the obese fall into this category). Those 41–99 percent above their ideal weight are described as *moderately obese* (about 7–8 percent of the obese fit into this category), and 2–3 percent are identified as fitting the *severely, morbidly, or grossly overweight* category, meaning that they are 100 percent or more above their ideal weight. In the last decade, more and more people fit into the moderate and severe levels of obesity, meaning increased risks at all ages and stages of their lives.[8]

NHANES III defined obesity as having a BMI greater than or equal to 30.0. Nearly 27 percent of Americans are obese; thus the general calculation that over 61 percent of all Americans are overweight or obese.

The difficulty with defining obesity lies in determining what is normal. To date, there are no universally accepted standards for the most "desirable" or "ideal" body weight or *body composition* (the ratio of lean body mass to fat body mass). While sources vary slightly, men's bodies should contain between 11 and 15 percent total body fat and women should be within the range of 18 to 22 percent body fat. At various ages and stages of life, these ranges also vary (see Table 9.4), but generally, when men exceed 20 percent body fat and women exceed 30 percent body fat, they have slipped into obesity.

Why the difference between men and women? Much of it may be attributed to the normal structure of the female body and to sex hormones. Lean body mass consists of the structural and functional elements in cells, body water, muscle, bones, and other body organs such as the heart, liver, and kidneys. Body fat is composed of two types: essential and storage fat. Essential fat is necessary for normal physiological functioning, such as nerve conduction. Essential fat makes up approximately 3 to 7 percent of total body weight

Body mass index (BMI) A technique of weight assessment based on the relationship of weight to height.

Obesity A weight disorder generally defined as an accumulation of fat beyond that considered normal for a person based on age, sex, and body type.

Table 9.4
General Ratings of Body Fat Percentages by Age and Gender

RATING	MALES (AGES 18–30) (PERCENT)	20 OR OVER FEMALES (AGES 18–30) (PERCENT)
Athletic*	6–10	10–15
Good	11–14	16–19
Acceptable	15–17	20–24
Overfat	18–19	25–29
Obese	20 or over	30 or over

*The ratings in the athletic category are general guidelines for those athletes, such as gymnasts and long-distance runners, whose need for a "competitive edge" in selected sports may compel them to try to lose as much weight as possible. However, for the average person, such low body fat levels should be approached with caution.

in men and approximately 15 percent of total body weight in women. Storage fat, the part that many of us try to shed, makes up the remainder of our fat reserves. It accounts for only a small percentage of total body weight for very lean people and between 5 and 25 percent of body weight of most American adults. Female bodybuilders, who are among the leanest of female athletes, may have body fat percentages ranging from 8 to 13 percent, nearly all of which is essential fat.

Too Little Fat?

A certain amount of body fat is necessary for insulating the body, cushioning parts of the body and vital organs, and maintaining body functions. In men, this lower limit is approximately 3 to 4 percent. Women should generally not go below 8 percent. Excessively low body fat in females may lead to amenorrhea, a disruption of the normal menstrual cycle. The critical level of body fat necessary to maintain normal menstrual flow is believed to be between 8 and 13 percent, but there are many additional factors that affect the menstrual cycle. Under extreme circumstances, such as starvation diets and certain diseases, the body utilizes all available fat reserves and begins to break down muscle tissue as a last-ditch effort to obtain nourishment.

The fact is that too much fat and too little fat are both potentially harmful. The key is to find a healthy level at which you are comfortable with your appearance and your ability to be as active as possible. Many options are available for determining your body fat and weight.

Assessing Fat Levels

Today, most weight control authorities believe that getting on the scale to determine your weight and then looking at where you fall on some arbitrary chart may not be helpful. Height-weight charts may lead some to think they are overweight when they are not, or that they are okay when, in fact, they

may be at risk. A number of other measures exist for calculating body content, and some provide a very precise reading or calculation of body fat. They include body mass index, waist-to-hip ratio, and various measures of body fat.

Body Mass Index (BMI)

A useful index of the relationship of height and weight, BMI is the measurement of choice for obesity researchers and health professionals. It is not gender specific, and although it does not directly measure percentage of body fat, it does provide a more accurate measure of overweight and obesity than weight alone.[9]

We find BMI by dividing a person's weight in kilograms by height in meters squared. The mathematical formula is as follows:

$$\text{Weight (kg)} \div \text{height squared (m}^2)$$

To determine BMI using pounds and inches, multiply your weight in pounds by 704.5, then divide the result by your height in inches, and divide that result by your height in inches a second time. (The multiplier 704.5 is used by the National Institutes of Health. Other organizations, such as the American Dietetic Association, suggest multiplying by 700. The variation in outcomes between the two is insignificant, and 700 is easier for most people to remember.) You can also go to the BMI calculator at the National Heart, Lung, and Blood Institute's (NHLBI's) website at http://nhlbisupport.com/bmi/bmicalc.htm.

Healthy weights have been defined as those associated with BMIs of 19 to 25, the range of lowest statistical health risk.[10] The desirable range for females falls between 21 and 23; for males, between 22 and 24.[11] A BMI greater than 25 indicates overweight and potentially significant health risks (see Figure 9.1). A body mass index over 30 is considered obese.[12] Many experts believe that this number is too high, particularly for younger adults.

Calculating BMI is simple, quick, and inexpensive—but it does have limitations. One problem with using BMI as a measurement is that very muscular people may fall into

Normal • Overweight • Obese • Extreme Obesity

Body Weight (pounds)

(BMI 19–24 = Normal; 25–29 = Overweight; 30–39 = Obese; 40–54 = Extreme Obesity)

Height (inches) / BMI	19	20	21	22	23	24	25	26	27	28	29	30	31	32	33	34	35	36	37	38	39	40	41	42	43	44	45	46	47	48	49	50	51	52	53	54
58	91	96	100	105	110	115	119	124	129	134	138	143	148	153	158	162	167	172	177	181	186	191	196	201	205	210	215	220	224	229	234	239	244	248	253	258
59	94	99	104	109	114	119	124	128	133	138	143	148	153	158	163	168	173	178	183	188	193	198	203	208	212	217	222	227	232	237	242	247	252	257	262	267
60	97	102	107	112	118	123	128	133	138	143	148	153	158	163	168	174	179	184	189	194	199	204	209	215	220	225	230	235	240	245	250	255	261	266	271	276
61	100	106	111	116	122	127	132	137	143	148	153	158	164	169	174	180	185	190	195	201	206	211	217	222	227	232	238	243	248	254	259	264	269	275	280	285
62	104	109	115	120	126	131	136	142	147	153	158	164	169	175	180	186	191	196	202	207	213	218	224	229	235	240	246	251	256	262	267	273	278	284	289	295
63	107	113	118	124	130	135	141	146	152	158	163	169	175	180	186	191	197	203	208	214	220	225	231	237	242	248	254	259	265	270	278	282	287	293	299	304
64	110	116	122	128	134	140	145	151	157	163	169	174	180	186	192	197	204	209	215	221	227	232	238	244	250	256	262	267	273	279	285	291	296	302	308	314
65	114	120	126	132	138	144	150	156	162	168	174	180	186	192	198	204	210	216	222	228	234	240	246	252	258	264	270	276	282	288	294	300	306	312	318	324
66	118	124	130	136	142	148	155	161	167	173	179	186	192	198	204	210	216	223	229	235	241	247	253	260	266	272	278	284	291	297	303	309	315	322	328	334
67	121	127	134	140	146	153	159	166	172	178	185	191	198	204	211	217	223	230	236	242	249	255	261	268	274	280	287	293	299	306	312	319	325	331	338	344
68	125	131	138	144	151	158	164	171	177	184	190	197	203	210	216	223	230	236	243	249	256	262	269	276	282	289	295	302	308	315	322	328	335	341	348	354
69	128	135	142	149	155	162	169	176	182	189	196	203	209	216	223	230	236	243	250	257	263	270	277	284	291	297	304	311	318	324	331	338	345	351	358	365
70	132	139	146	153	160	167	174	181	188	195	202	209	216	222	229	236	243	250	257	264	271	278	285	292	299	306	313	320	327	334	341	348	355	362	369	376
71	136	143	150	157	165	172	179	186	193	200	208	215	222	229	236	243	250	257	265	272	279	286	293	301	308	315	322	329	338	343	351	358	365	372	379	386
72	140	147	154	162	169	177	184	191	199	206	213	221	228	235	242	250	258	265	272	279	287	294	302	309	316	324	331	338	346	353	361	368	375	383	390	397
73	144	151	159	166	174	182	189	197	204	212	219	227	235	242	250	257	265	272	280	288	295	302	310	318	325	333	340	348	355	363	371	378	386	393	401	408
74	148	155	163	171	179	186	194	202	210	218	225	233	241	249	256	264	272	280	287	295	303	311	319	326	334	342	350	358	365	373	381	389	396	404	412	420
75	152	160	168	176	184	192	200	208	216	224	232	240	248	256	264	272	279	287	295	303	311	319	327	335	343	351	359	367	375	383	391	399	407	415	423	431
76	156	164	172	180	189	197	205	213	221	230	238	246	254	263	271	279	287	295	304	312	320	328	336	344	353	361	369	377	385	394	402	410	418	426	435	443

Figure 9.1

Body Mass Index Table

Source: Adapted from National Heart, Blood, and Lung Institute. "Clinical Guidelines on the Identification, Evaluation, and Treatment of Overweight and Obesity in Adults: The Evidence Report," 1998 (see http://www.nhlbi.nih.gov/guidelines/obesity/bmi_tbl.htm).

the "overweight" category when they are actually healthy and fit. Another problem is that people who have lost muscle mass, such as the elderly, may be in the "healthy weight" category according to BMI, when they actually have reduced nutritional reserves.[13]

These standards may seem almost impossible for people who consistently exceed the target weights and who have difficulty keeping off any lost weight. Constant failure may lead them to stop trying. The secret lies in establishing a healthful weight at a young age and maintaining it—a task easier said than done. The U.S. Dietary Guidelines for Americans encourage a weight gain of no more than 10 pounds after reaching adult height and endorse small weight losses of one-half to one pound per week, if needed, as well as smaller weight losses of 5 to 10 percent to make a difference toward health.[14]

Waist Circumference

The presence of excess body fat in the abdomen, when out of proportion to total body fat, is considered an independent predictor of risk factors and ailments associated with obesity. Waist circumference measurement is a useful tool for assessing abdominal fat.

What waist size is risky? Men and women have different measures for determining risk. Men who have a waist measurement greater than 40 inches (102 cm) are at risk. Women who have a waist measurement greater than

35 inches (88 cm) are at risk. If a person has a short stature (under 5 feet tall) or has a BMI of 35 or above, waist circumference standards used for the general population might not apply.[15]

Waist circumference is measured by wrapping a tape measure comfortably around the smallest area below the rib cage and above the belly button.

Waist-to-Hip Ratio

Another useful measure is the *waist-to-hip ratio,* a measure of regional fat distribution. Research has shown that excess fat in the abdominal area poses a greater health risk than excess fat in the hips and thighs and is associated with a number of disorders, including high blood pressure, diabetes, heart disease, and certain cancers. A waist-to-hip ratio greater than 1.0 in men and 0.8 in women indicates increased health risks.[16] Therefore, knowing where your fat is carried may be more important than knowing your total fat content.

Men and postmenopausal women tend to store fat in the upper regions of their body, particularly in the abdominal area. Premenopausal women usually store their fat in lower regions of their bodies, particularly the hips, buttocks, and thighs.[17] In fact, waist measurement alone may be a viable way to assess fat distribution. Some research suggests that a waistline greater than 40 inches (102 cm) in men and 35 inches (88 cm) in women may indicate greater health risk.[18]

Measures of Body Fat

Common measures of body fat include hydrostatic weighing, pinch and skinfold measures, girth and circumference measures, soft-tissue roentgenogram, bioelectrical impedance analysis, and total body electrical conductivity.

Hydrostatic Weighing Techniques From a clinical perspective, **hydrostatic weighing techniques** offer the most accurate method of measuring body fat. This method measures the amount of water a person displaces when completely submerged. Because fat tissue is less dense than muscle or bone tissue, a relatively accurate indication of actual body fat can be computed by comparing a person's underwater and out-of-water weights. Although this method may be subject to errors, it is one of the most sophisticated techniques currently available.

Pinch and Skinfold Measures Perhaps the most commonly used method of determining body fat is the **pinch test.** Numerous studies have determined that the triceps area (the back of the upper arm) is one of the most reliable regions of the body for assessing the amount of fat in the subcutaneous (just under the surface) layer of the skin. In making this assessment, a person pinches a fold of skin just behind the triceps with the thumb and index finger and assesses the distance between thumb and finger. It is important to pinch

---

Hydrostatic weighing techniques Methods of determining body fat by measuring the amount of water displaced when a person is completely submerged.

Pinch test A method of determining body fat whereby a fold of skin just behind the triceps is pinched between the thumb and index finger to determine the relative amount of fat.

Skinfold caliper test A method of determining body fat whereby folds of skin and fat at various points on the body are grasped between thumb and forefinger and measured with calipers.

Girth and circumference measures A method of assessing body fat that employs a formula based on girth measurements of various body sites.

Soft-tissue roentgenogram A technique of body fat assessment in which radioactive substances are used to determine relative fat.

Bioelectrical impedance analysis (BIA) A technique of body fat assessment in which electrical currents are passed through fat and lean tissue.

Total body electrical conductivity (TOBEC) Technique using an electromagnetic force field to assess relative body fat.

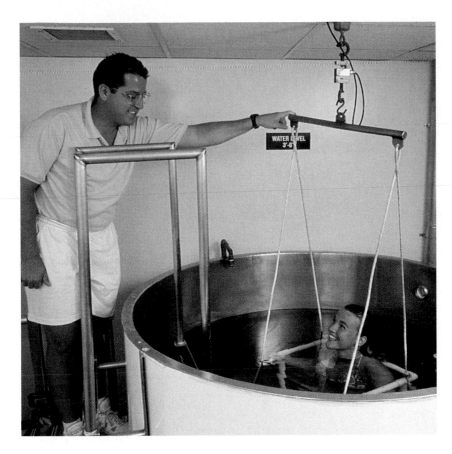

Hydrostatic weighing is the most accurate technique for measuring body fat.

only the fat layer and not the triceps muscle. If the size of the pinch is thicker than 1 inch, the person is generally considered overfat.

Another technique, the **skinfold caliper test,** resembles the pinch test but is much more accurate. This procedure involves pinching folds of skin at various points on the body with the thumb and index finger. A specially calibrated instrument called a *skinfold caliper* is used to measure the fat layer. Besides the triceps, the areas most often measured are the biceps (front of the arm), the subscapular (upper back), and the iliac crest (hip). Special formulas are employed to arrive at a combined prediction of total body fat.

If done by trained technicians, the skinfold caliper test can be fairly accurate. If the person doing the test is inconsistent about the exact locations of the pinch or if it is difficult to distinguish between fat and muscle, the results may be inaccurate. In addition, the heavier a person is, the more prone this technique is to error. For obese people, difficulties in assessment are magnified because of problems in distinguishing between flaccid muscles and fat. Also, most currently available calipers do not expand far enough to obtain accurate measurements on many obese people. Additional errors can result from failure to account for certain age, sex, and ethnic differences in calibrations.

Girth and Circumference Measures

Another common method of body fat assessment is the use of **girth and circumference measures**. Diagnosticians use a measuring tape to take girth, or circumference, measurements at various body sites. These measurements are then converted into constants, and a formula is used to determine relative percentages of body fat. Although this technique is inexpensive, easy to use, and commonly performed, it is not as accurate as many of the others listed here.

Soft-Tissue Roentgenogram

A relatively new technique for determining body fat, the **soft-tissue roentgenogram,** involves injecting a radioactive substance into the body and allowing this substance to penetrate muscle (lean) tissue so that distinctions between fat and lean tissue can be made by means of imaging.

Bioelectrical Impedance Analysis

Another method of determining body fat levels, **bioelectrical impedance analysis (BIA),** involves sending a small electric current through the subject's body. The body's ability to conduct an electrical current reflects the total amount of water in the body. Generally, the more water, the more muscle and lean tissue. The amount of resistance to the current and the person's age, sex, and other physical characteristics are fed into a computer that uses special formulas to determine the total amount of lean and fat tissue. To obtain the most accurate readings, fasting for four hours prior to testing is recommended. BIA may not be as accurate for severely obese individuals.

Total Body Electrical Conductivity

One of the newest (and most expensive) assessment techniques is **total body electrical conductivity (TOBEC),** which uses an electromagnetic

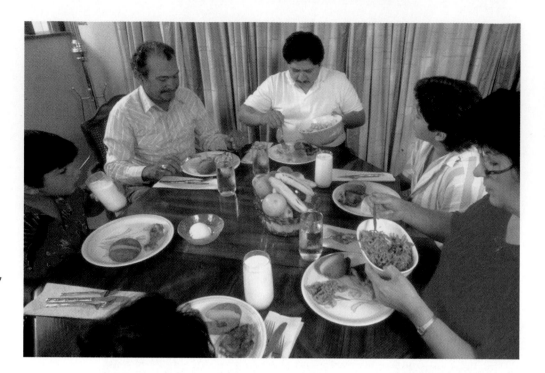

Many factors help determine body type, including heredity and genetic makeup, environmental factors, and learned eating patterns, many of which are connected to habits learned from family.

force field to assess relative body fat. Although based on the same principle as impedance, this assessment requires much more elaborate, expensive equipment, and therefore is not practical for most people.

Although all of these methods can be useful, they can also be inaccurate and even harmful unless the testers are skillful and well trained. Before undergoing any procedure, make sure you understand the expense, potential for accuracy, risks, and training of the tester.

> **What do you think?**
>
> *Calculate your BMI using the formula provided. If possible, try to have your percentage of body fat tested with calipers or one of the other methods listed. Cross-check your results by using the calculator found at the NHLBI website. Which value is most important to you? * Why? * How are they similar?*

Factors Contributing to Obesity

In spite of massive efforts to keep Americans fit and in good health, obesity rates have reached epidemic proportions in America today. Why is this happening in an era where "thin is in" and we are constantly bombarded with the message to "just do it"?

The surgeon general stated it quite simply: "Overweight and obesity result from an energy imbalance. This means eating too many calories and not getting enough exercise."[19] But if it were that simple, Americans would merely reevaluate

their diets, reduce the amount they eat, and exercise more. Unfortunately, it's not that simple. In fact, there are probably many more factors conspiring to make us fat and keep us fat than we have even begun to fathom. Knowing what these factors are, recognizing how they specifically influence our own dietary patterns, and making conscious decisions to change specific lifestyle behaviors is an important first step in beating the "battle of the bulge." For those who don't currently have a weight problem, knowing how to maintain a healthy weight through a lifetime of temptations and metabolic changes is yet another important message to be retained.

What are some of these factors that influence our collective trends toward overweight and obesity? We know that body weight is a result of genes, metabolism, behavior, environment, culture, and socioeconomic status. Of these, behavior and environment are probably easiest to change. See the Health in a Diverse World box for variations in fat levels among different Americans.

Key Environmental Factors

Although there is a long list of potential environmental contributors, the following are currently receiving great attention as influences on our energy intake:

- Bombardment with advertising designed to increase energy intake—ads for high-calorie foods at a low price, marketing larger portion sizes.[20] Prepackaged meals, fast food, and soft drinks are all increasingly widespread. High-calorie drinks such as coffee lattes and energy drinks add to daily calorie intake.
- Changes in the number of working women, leading to greater frequency of restaurant meals and the use of more fast foods and convenience foods.[21]

News about Weight Issues among Americans

During the last year, several national studies have indicated that the epidemic of overweight and obesity is growing rapidly and that certain populations have significant risks. Consider the following and the implications of these findings for you and others:

- Men are considerably more likely than women to be overweight (63 percent of all men, 47 percent of women), but no such difference was found in the prevalence of obesity. *What do you think the reasons for this are?*
- The youngest adults (aged 18–24) and the oldest (65 and over) were about twice as likely as adults in other age groups to be underweight. *Why might this be?*
- Overweight was about twice as prevalent among black non-Hispanic (66 percent) and Hispanic adults (62 percent) than among Asian/Pacific Islanders (32 percent). Slightly more than half of white non-Hispanic adults were overweight. *What factors might contribute to this disparity?*
- Adults in the western region of the United States were less likely to be overweight or obese, while residents of the south-central part of the United States tended to have more weight problems. States with the highest percentages of obese adults were Mississippi (24.3 percent), Alabama (23.5 percent), West Virginia (22.8 percent), Louisiana (22.8 percent), and Texas (22.7 percent). States with the lowest percentages of obese adults were: Hawaii (15.1 percent), Montana (15.2 percent), Delaware (16.2 percent), Massachusetts (16.4 percent), Rhode Island (16.8 percent), and Minnesota (16.8 percent). *What factors might contribute to this pattern?*
- Married men were less likely—but married women more likely—to be in the healthy weight range than those who were single, separated, or divorced. *What are some possible explanations?*
- The "freshman 15" may not be as harmless as once thought. A high BMI in college was linked to cancer deaths, specifically those from breast and prostate cancers. Women who were the most overweight in early adulthood were nearly four times more likely to die from breast cancer than their leanest counterparts. And the most overweight young men faced a 50 percent increased risk of dying from prostate cancer. *What are some possible explanations?*

- Obese individuals tend to eat more meals and eat them later in the day than their nonobese counterparts. Frequent intake episodes tended to be much more common among obese people. *How do you explain these eating patterns?*

Sources: Items 1–5: National Center for Health Statistics, Centers for Disease Control, "Patterns of Body Weight in U.S. Adults" (September 6, 2002) (see http://www.cdc.bov/nchs/realeases/o2facts/adultwght.htm); Item 6: M. Okasha, et al., "College Weight and Later Cancer Risk," *Journal of Epidemiology and Community Health* 56 (2002): 780–784; Item 7: H. B. Forslund, et al., "Meal Patterns and Obesity in Swedish Women," *European Journal of Clinical Nutrition* 56 (8) (2002): 740–747.

- Bottle-feeding of infants, which may increase energy intake relative to breast-feeding.[22]

The following factors contributing to decreased energy expenditure are often cited:

- The increasingly sedentary nature of many jobs.[23]
- Universal use of automated equipment and electronic communications, such as cell phones, remote controls, and other labor-saving devices.[24]
- Spending more time in front of the computer and TV and playing video games.[25]
- Fear of playing or being outside based on the threat of violence.
- Decline in physical education requirements in schools.[26]
- Lack of community resources for exercise.

What do you think?

In addition to those listed, can you think of other environmental factors that contribute to obesity?
✳ *What actions could you take to reduce your risk for each of these factors?*

Heredity

Are some people born to be fat? Several factors appear to influence why one person becomes obese and another remains thin; genes seem to interact with many of these factors.

Body Type and Genes In some animal species, the shape and size of the individual's body are largely determined by its parents' shape and size. Many scientists have explored the role of heredity in determining human body shapes. You need only look at your parents and then glance in the mirror to see where you got your own body type. Children whose parents are obese also tend to be overweight. In fact, a family history of obesity increases one's chances of becoming obese by 25–30 percent.[27] Some researchers argue that obesity has a strong genetic determinant—it tends to run in families. They cite the statistic that 80 percent of children who have two obese parents are also obese.[28] Genes play a significant role in how the body balances calories and energy. Also, by influencing the amount of body fat and fat distribution, genes can make a person more susceptible to gaining weight.

Twin Studies Studies of identical twins who were separated at birth and raised in different environments provide the strongest evidence yet that the genes a person inherits are the major factor determining overweight, leanness, or average weight. Whether raised in family environments with fat or thin family members, twins with obese natural parents tend to be obese in later life.[29] According to another study, sets of identical twins who were separated and raised in different families and who ate widely different diets still grew up to weigh about the same.[30]

Although the exact mechanism remains unknown, it is believed that genes set metabolic rates, influencing how the body handles calories. Some experts believe that this genetic tendency may contribute as much as 25 to 40 percent of the reason for being overweight.[31]

Specific Obesity Genes? In the past decade, more and more research has pointed to the existence of a "fat gene." The most promising candidate is the *Ob* gene (for obesity),

which is believed to disrupt the body's "I've had enough to eat" signaling system and may prompt individuals to keep eating past the point of being comfortably full. Research on Pima Indians, who have an estimated 75 percent obesity rate (nine out of ten are overweight), seems to point to an Ob gene that is a "thrifty gene." It is theorized that because their ancestors struggled through centuries of famine, their basal metabolic rates slowed, allowing them to store precious fat for survival. Survivors may have passed these genes on to their children, which would explain the lower metabolic rates found in Pimas today and their tendency toward obesity.[32] Scientists have found that they can manipulate mice genes and construct an Ob gene that invariably leads to fatness in mice and the development of type 2 diabetes. Many suspect a human counterpart to this gene, but an actual gene formation has yet to be found. In addition, the (beta)-3 adrenergic-receptor gene has been identified and found in human beings and mice. When mutated, it is thought to impede the body's ability to burn fat.[33]

Although the discovery of the Ob gene in mice has provided fertile ground for speculation, researchers have further refined their theories to focus on a protein that the Ob gene may produce, known as leptin, and a new leptin receptor in the brain. According to these studies, leptin is the chemical that signals the brain when you are full and need to stop eating.[34] Although obese people have adequate amounts of leptin and leptin receptors, they do not seem to work properly. Genetic defects have been found to affect levels of leptin. However, it's not clear yet if altering leptin levels would help in treating obesity.[35] Other scientists have isolated a more direct route to appetite suppression, a protein called *GLP-1*, which is known to slow down the passage of food through the intestines to allow the absorption of nutrients. When scientists injected GLP-1 into the brains of hungry rats, the rats stopped eating immediately.[36] Are leptin and GLP-1 key factors in appetite suppression? It is speculated that leptin and GLP-1 might play complementary roles in weight control. Leptin and its receptors may regulate body weight over the long term, calling upon fast-acting appetite suppressants like GLP-1 when necessary.

Yet another chemical influence on weight management may be the hormone ghrelin (see the New Horizons in Health box).

Hunger, Appetite, and Satiety

Theories abound concerning the mechanisms that regulate food intake. Some sources indicate that the hypothalamus (the part of the brain that regulates appetite) closely monitors levels of certain nutrients in the blood. When these levels fall, the brain signals us to eat. In the obese person, it is possible that the monitoring system does not work properly and the cues to eat are more frequent and intense than they are in people of normal weight.

Other sources indicate that thin people may send more effective messages to the hypothalamus. This concept, known as **adaptive thermogenesis**, states that thin people

---

Adaptive thermogenesis Theoretical mechanism by which the brain regulates metabolic activity according to caloric intake.

Brown fat cells Specialized type of fat cell that affects the ability to regulate fat metabolism.

Hunger An inborn physiological response to nutritional needs.

Appetite A learned response that is tied to an emotional or psychological craving for food often unrelated to nutritional need.

Satiety The feeling of fullness or satisfaction at the end of a meal.

Hyperplasia A condition characterized by an excessive number of fat cells.

Hypertrophy The ability of fat cells to swell and shrink.

Ghrelin and the Hungry Hormones: Triggering Your Eat Response?

Recent research suggests that a hormone produced in the stomach known as ghrelin may be among the most important players in our collective difficulties in keeping weight off. Researchers at the University of Washington studied a small group of obese people who had lost weight over a six-month period. They noted that ghrelin levels rose before every meal and fell drastically shortly afterward, suggesting that the hormone plays a role in appetite stimulation. People who lost large amounts of weight via gastric bypass surgery had ghrelin levels that were 72 percent lower than those who lost weight through traditional diets and 77 percent lower than those in a control group. While ghrelin doesn't seem to be a cause of obesity, researchers believe that it may make it more difficult to lose weight once you gain it due to its influence on appetite and eating cues. Subsequent studies will test the impact of ghrelin-blocking drugs in controlling appetite as a form of intervention.

Other hormones that have been implicated in triggering your eat response, but which need much more research before we fully understand their importance, are the following:

- **PYY $_{3-36}$:** A hormone released by cells in the digestive tract in response to food and which seems to signal the brain when you are full. Inadequate amounts of this hormone may lead to eating until you are stuffed and uncomfortable, ultimately leading to obesity.
- **Insulin:** A hormone secreted by the pancreas that serves as the master regulator of glucose in the blood. If sufficient amounts are secreted and if your body is able to utilize it properly, glucose will be burned by the body rather than stored as fat.
- **Cholecystokinin:** As food enters the digestive system, particularly the small intestine, this hormone triggers the release of digestive enzymes to break down foods. It also acts as another signal to stop eating.
- **Leptin:** A hormone secreted by fat cells in the body that serves to keep fat levels constant. If there are excess levels of leptin in the blood, appetite levels drop and calories are burned more rapidly. Although most adults have adequate levels of leptin in the blood, researchers are investigating how enhanced leptin levels will aid in controlling appetite and how leptin works in combination with other hunger hormones.

Sources: D. E. Cummings et al., "Plasma Ghrelin Levels after Diet-Induced Weight Loss or Gastric Bypass Surgery," *New England Journal of Medicine* 346 (21) May 23, 2002; Mohammed Saad, et al., "Genes for Hunger Hormones Play Role in Obesity," *Journal of Clinical Endocrinology and Metabolism* 87 (2002): 3997–4000, 4005–4008.

---

can consume large amounts of food without gaining weight because the appetite center of their brains speeds up metabolic activity to compensate for the increased consumption. Older studies have indicated that specialized types of fat cells, called **brown fat cells,** may send signals to the brain, which controls the thermogenesis response.

The hypothesis that food tastes better to obese people, thus causing them to eat more, has largely been refuted. Scientists do distinguish, however, between **hunger,** an inborn physiological response to nutritional needs, and **appetite,** a learned response to food that is tied to an emotional or psychological craving often unrelated to nutritional need. Obese people may be more likely than thin people to satisfy their appetite and eat for reasons other than nutrition.

In some instances, the problem with overconsumption may be more related to **satiety** than to appetite or hunger. People generally feel satiated, or full, when they have satisfied their nutritional needs and their stomach signals "no more." For undetermined reasons, obese people may not feel full until much later than thin people. The leptin and GLP-1 studies seem to support this theory.

Developmental Factors

Some obese people may have excessive numbers of fat cells. This type of obesity, **hyperplasia,** usually appears in early childhood and perhaps, due to the mother's dietary habits, even prior to birth. The most critical periods for the development of hyperplasia seem to be the last two to three months of fetal development, the first year of life, and between the ages of 9 and 13. Parents who allow their children to eat without restrictions and become overweight may be setting them up for a lifelong excess of fat cells. Central to this theory is the belief that the number of fat cells in a person's body does not increase appreciably during adulthood. However, the ability of each of these cells to swell and shrink, known as **hypertrophy,** does carry over into adulthood. Weight gain may be tied to both the number of fat cells in the body and the capacity of individual cells to enlarge.

An average-weight adult has approximately 25 billion to 30 billion fat cells, a moderately obese adult about 60 billion to 100 billion, and an extremely obese adult as many as 200 billion.[37] People who add large numbers of fat cells to

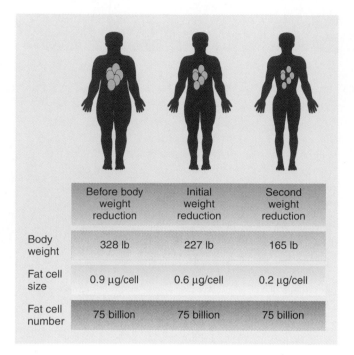

	Before body weight reduction	Initial weight reduction	Second weight reduction
Body weight	328 lb	227 lb	165 lb
Fat cell size	0.9 µg/cell	0.6 µg/cell	0.2 µg/cell
Fat cell number	75 billion	75 billion	75 billion

Figure 9.2
One Person at Various Stages of Weight Loss
Note that, according to theories of hyperplasia, the number of fat cells remains constant but their size decreases when weight is gained.

their bodies in childhood may be able to lose weight by decreasing the size of each cell in adulthood, but the total number of cells will remain the same. With the next calorie binge, the cells swell and sabotage weight loss efforts (see Figure 9.2). Additional research is needed to test these theories.

Setpoint Theory

In 1982, nutritional researchers William Bennett and Joel Gurin presented the **setpoint theory,** which stated that a person's body has a setpoint of weight at which it is programmed to be comfortable. If your setpoint is around 160 pounds, you will gain and lose weight fairly easily within a given range of that point. For example, if you gain 5 to 10 pounds on vacation, it will be fairly easy to lose that weight and remain around the 160-pound mark for a long period of time. Through a process of *adaptive thermogenesis,* the body actually tries to maintain this weight. Some people have equated this point with the **plateau** that dieters sometimes reach after losing a certain amount of weight. The setpoint theory proposes that after losing a predetermined amount of weight, the body will actually sabotage additional weight loss by slowing down metabolism. In extreme cases, the metabolic rate will decrease to a point at which the body will maintain its weight on as little as 1,000 calories per day.

Can a person change this predetermined setpoint? Proponents of this theory argue that it is possible to raise one's setpoint over time by continually gaining weight and failing to exercise. Conversely, reducing caloric intake and exercising regularly can slowly decrease one's setpoint. Exercise seems to be the most critical factor in readjusting setpoint, although diet may also be important.

The setpoint theory remains controversial. Perhaps its greatest impact was the sense of relief it provided for people who have lost weight, plateaued, and regained weight time and time again. It told them that their failure was not due to lack of willpower alone. The setpoint theory also prompted nutritional experts to look more carefully at popular methods of weight loss. If it is correct, an extremely low-calorie diet isn't just dangerous; it may also cause the body to protect the dieter from "starvation" by slowing down metabolism, making weight loss even more difficult.

Endocrine Influence

Over the years, many people have attributed obesity to problems with their **thyroid gland.** They believed that an underactive thyroid impeded their ability to burn calories. However, most authorities agree that less than 2 percent of the obese population have a thyroid problem and can trace their weight problems to a metabolic or hormone imbalance.[38]

Psychosocial Factors

The relationship of weight problems to deeply rooted emotional insecurities, needs, and wants remains uncertain. Food is often used as a reward for good behavior in childhood. As adults face unemployment, broken relationships, financial uncertainty, fears about health and other problems, the bright spot in the day is often "what's on the table for dinner" or "we're going to that restaurant tonight." Again, the research underlying this theory is controversial. What is certain is that eating tends to be a focal point of people's lives, and the comfort foods of childhood may provide a salve for painful social pressures. Eating is essentially a social ritual associated with companionship, celebration, and enjoyment. For many people, the social emphasis on the eating experience is a major obstacle to successful dieting. Although some restaurants offer menu items designed to aid dieters, many people have difficulty choosing responsibly when confronted with an entire menu of delicious, fattening foods.

Some theorists contend that obese people ignore internal cues of hunger and are more likely to use the clock as a guide for "time to eat" than real hunger cues. Other studies refute this hypothesis.

Early Sabotage: Obesity in Youth

One major factor in our preoccupation with food is the pressure placed on us by the food industry's sophisticated marketing campaigns. There may be salad bars at the local fast-food joints, but customers have to run the gauntlet of starchy, beefy delights and high-fat fries to find them. According to the USDA, the food and restaurant industries spend in excess of $40 billion a year on ads to entice hungry people to forgo fresh fruit and sliced vegetables for Ring Dings and Happy Meals.[39] Children are among the most vulnerable to these ads.

Children's impulses to eat junk food haven't changed much in recent decades. However, as noted earlier, they are eating larger portions. Social forces mentioned earlier, including the decline of home cooking, increased production of calorie- and fat-laden fast foods, and video technology that encourages kids to surf the Internet rather than ride their bicycles, have converged to increase the number of overweight young Americans. As a direct consequence, over 6 million American children are now fat enough to endanger their health. An additional 5 million are on the threshold, and the problem is growing more extreme daily. Obese children suffer both physically and emotionally throughout childhood, and those who stay heavy in adolescence tend to stay fat as adults.[40]

Dietary Myth and Misperception

A recent study compared the self-reported and actual caloric intakes and amounts of exercise among a group of overweight adults. The researchers carefully followed obese people who had been unsuccessful on as many as 20 diets, though they claimed that they consumed fewer than 1,200 calories per day. They blamed their failure to lose weight on "metabolism." It turned out that their metabolism levels were normal, but they were actually eating nearly twice as much as they thought they were and exercising only three-quarters as much as they reported.[41]

Does this mean that obesity is simply the result of gluttony and sloth? No. In fact, many studies have shown that obese individuals do not eat much more than their normal-weight counterparts. However, it should be noted that they do exercise less. The majority of overweight individuals are less active than nonobese people. Of course, it could be argued that it is their obesity that leads to their sedentary lifestyle. Much more research is necessary before scientists have a clear profile of both the obese and nonobese.

Metabolic Changes

Even when completely at rest, the body consumes a certain amount of energy. The amount of energy your body uses at complete rest is your **basal metabolic rate (BMR).** About 60 to 70 percent of all the calories you consume on a given day go to support your basal metabolism: heartbeat, breathing, maintaining body temperature, and so on. So if you consume 2,000 calories per day, between 1,200 and 1,400 of those calories are burned without your doing any significant physical activity. But unless you exert yourself enough to burn the remaining 600 to 800 calories, you will gain weight.

Your BMR can fluctuate considerably, with several factors influencing whether it slows down or speeds up. In general, the younger you are, the higher your BMR, partly because in young people cells undergo rapid subdivision,

which consumes a good deal of energy. BMR is highest during infancy, puberty, and pregnancy, when bodily changes are most rapid. BMR is also influenced by body composition. Muscle tissue is highly active—even at rest—compared to fat tissue. In essence, the more lean tissue you have, the greater your BMR, and the more fat tissue you have, the lower your BMR. Men have a higher BMR than women do, at least partly because of their greater proportion of lean tissue.

Age is another factor. After age 30, BMR slows down by about 1 to 2 percent a year. Therefore, people over 30 commonly find that they must work harder to burn off an extra helping of ice cream than they did when in their teens. "Middle-aged spread," a reference to the tendency to put on weight later in life, is partly related to this change. A slower BMR, coupled with less activity and shifting priorities (family and career become more important than fitness), puts the weight of many middle-aged people in jeopardy.

In addition, the body has a number of self-protective mechanisms that signal BMR to speed up or slow down. For example, when you have a fever, the energy needs of your cells increase, which generates heat and speeds up your BMR. In starvation situations, the body protects itself by slowing down BMR to conserve precious energy. Thus, when people repeatedly resort to extreme diets, it is believed that their bodies "reset" their BMRs at lower rates. **Yo-yo diets,** in which people repeatedly gain weight and then starve themselves to lose it, are doomed to failure. When dieters resume eating after their weight loss, their BMR is set lower, making it almost certain that they will regain the pounds they just lost. After repeated cycles of dieting and regaining weight, these people find it increasingly hard to lose weight and increasingly easy to regain it, so they become heavier and heavier.

According to a recent study by Kelly Brownell of Yale University, middle-aged men who maintained a steady weight (even if they were overweight) had a lower risk of

---

Setpoint theory   A theory of obesity causation that suggests that fat storage is determined by a thermostatic mechanism in the body that acts to maintain a specific amount of body fat.

Plateau   That point in a weight loss program at which the dieter finds it difficult to lose more weight.

Thyroid gland   A two-lobed endocrine gland located in the throat region that produces a hormone that regulates metabolism.

Basal metabolic rate (BMR)   The energy expenditure of the body under resting conditions at normal room temperature.

Yo-yo diets   Cycles in which people repeatedly gain weight, then starve themselves to lose weight. This lowers their BMR, which makes regaining weight even more likely.

heart attack than men whose weight cycled up and down in a yo-yo pattern. Brownell found that smaller, well-maintained weight losses are more beneficial for reducing cardiovascular risk than larger, poorly maintained weight losses.[42]

In addition, new research supports the theory that by increasing your muscle mass, you will increase your metabolism and burn more calories each time you exercise (see Chapter 10).

Lifestyle

Of all the factors affecting obesity, perhaps the most critical is the relationship between activity levels and calorie intake. Obesity rates are rising. But how can this be happening? Aren't more people exercising than ever before? Though the many advertisements for sports equipment and the popularity of athletes may give the impression that Americans love a good workout, the facts are not so positive. Data from a newly released National Health Interview Survey show that 4 in 10 adults in the United States never engage in any exercise, sports, or physically active hobbies in their leisure time.[43] Women (43.2 percent) were somewhat more likely than men (36.5 percent) to be sedentary, a finding that was consistent across all age groups. Among both men and women, black and Hispanic adults were more sedentary than white adults.[44] Leisure-time physical activity was also strongly associated with level of education. About 72 percent of adults who never attended high school were sedentary, declining steadily to 45 percent among high school graduates and about 24 percent among adults with graduate-level college degrees.[45]

Do you know people who seemingly can eat whatever they want without gaining weight? With few exceptions, if you were to follow them around for a typical day and monitor the level and intensity of their activity, you would discover the reason. Even if their schedule does not include jogging or intense exercise, it probably includes a high level of activity. Walking up a flight of stairs rather than taking the elevator, speeding up the pace while mowing the lawn, getting up to change the TV channel rather than using the remote, and doing housework all vigorously burn extra calories.

Actually, it may even go beyond that. In studies of calorie burning by individuals placed in a controlled respiratory chamber environment where calories consumed, motion, and overall activity were measured, it was found that some people are better fat burners than others. It is possible that low fat burners may not produce as many of the enzymes needed to convert fat to energy. Or they may not have as many blood vessels supplying fatty tissue, making it tougher for them to deliver fat-burning oxygen. Or perhaps in subtle ways, these people burn more calories through extra motions. Clearly, any form of activity that burns additional calories helps maintain weight.

Smoking   Women who smoke tend to weigh 6–10 pounds less than nonsmokers. After quitting, weight generally increases to the level found among nonsmokers. Weight gain after smoking cessation may be partly due to nicotine's ability to raise metabolic rate. When smokers stop, they burn fewer calories. Another reason former smokers often gain weight is that they generally eat more after they quit, to satisfy free-floating cravings.[46]

What do you think?

Why do you think men and women differ so much in their physical activity patterns? ✳ *Why are certain minority groups less likely to exercise than other groups?* ✳ *What might be done in terms of policies, programs, and services to change these statistics?*

Gender and Obesity

Throughout a woman's life, issues of appearance and beauty are constantly in the foreground. Only recently have researchers begun to understand just how significant the quest for beauty and the perfect body really is.

Of increasing interest is another emerging problem seen in both young men and women, known as **social physique anxiety (SPA),** in which the desire to "look good" has a destructive and sometimes disabling effect on one's ability to function effectively in relationships and interactions with others. People suffering from SPA may spend a disproportionate amount of time "fixating" on their bodies, working out, and performing tasks that are ego-centered and self-directed, rather than focusing on interpersonal relationships and general tasks.[47] Incessant worry about their bodies and their appearance permeates their lives. Overweight and obesity are clear risks for these people, and experts speculate that this anxiety may contribute to eating-disordered behaviors.

Researchers have determined that being severely overweight in adolescence may influence one's social and economic future—particularly for females. Researchers found that obese women complete about half a year less schooling, are 20 percent less likely to get married, and earn $6,710 on average less per year than their slimmer counterparts. Obese women also have rates of household poverty 10 percent higher than those of women who are not overweight. In contrast, the study found that overweight men are 11 percent less likely to be married than thinner men but suffer few adverse economic consequences.

It may be that women suffer such negative consequences of obesity because the social stigma of being overweight is more severe for women than for men. Women are also disadvantaged biologically when it comes to losing weight. Compared to men, women have a lower ratio of lean body mass to fatty mass, in part due to differences in bone size and mass, muscle size, and other variables. Muscle uses more energy than fat does. Because men have more muscle, they burn 10–20 percent more calories than women do during rest.[48] See Chapter 10 for an overview of the role that increased muscle mass has on weight reduction. For all ages, after sexual maturity, men have higher metabolic rates, making it easier for them to burn off excess calories. Women also face greater potential for weight fluctuation due to hormonal changes, pregnancy, and other conditions that increase the likelihood of weight gain. Also, as a group, men are more socialized into physical activity from birth. Strenuous activity in both work and play are encouraged for men, whereas women's roles have typically been more sedentary and required a lower level of caloric expenditure.

Not only are women more vulnerable to weight gain, but also pressures to maintain and/or lose weight make them more likely to take dramatic measures to lose weight. Examples include the predominance of eating disorders among women and the greater numbers of women taking diet pills. However, males experience these pressures, too. The male image is becoming more associated with the bodybuilder shape and size, and men are becoming more preoccupied with their own physical form. Thus eating disorders, exercise addictions, and other maladaptive responses among men are on the increase.

Individuality

Although researchers have learned a great deal in recent years about the factors that predispose people to gain or lose weight, controversy remains. Perhaps the most overlooked element is the individual. Just as no two people are exactly alike physiologically, we are not psychologically identical. Each person is a unique result of genetic background, environment, lifestyle, and emotional responses to a lifetime of experiences.

It is highly possible that the causes of obesity are as varied as the people who are obese. If this is so, there can be no universal cure for weight problems. Instead, we must look for a mechanism of prevention or intervention for each individual that is based upon appropriate cultural, social, environmental, and other factors.

What do you think?

Can you think of other reasons why men and women may differ in how much weight they gain and how easily they are able to lose it? ✷ What historical patterns may have contributed to this trend?

Managing Your Weight

At some point in our lives, almost all of us will decide to go on a diet, and many will meet with mixed success. The problem is probably related to the fact that we think about losing weight in terms of "dieting" rather than adjusting lifestyle and eating behaviors. It is well documented that hypocaloric

(low-calorie) diets produce only temporary losses and may actually lead to disordered binge eating or related problems.[49] While repeated bouts of restrictive dieting may be physiologically harmful, the sense of failure that we get each time we try and fail can exact far-reaching psychological costs.[50] Drugs and intensive counseling can contribute to positive weight loss, but even then, many people regain weight after treatment.

Keeping Weight Control in Perspective

Although experts say that losing weight simply requires burning more calories than are consumed, putting this principle into practice is far from simple. According to William W. Hardy, M.D., president of the Michigan-based Rochester Center for Obesity,

> to say weight control is simply a matter of pushing away from the table is ludicrous. Nature is a cheat. Sure, calories in minus calories out equals weight, but people of the same age, sex, height, and weight can have differences of as much as 1,000 calories a day in "resting metabolic rate"—this may explain why one person's gluttony is another's starvation, even if it results in the same readout on the scale. And while people of normal weight average 25–35 billion fat cells, obese people can inherit a billowing 135 billion. A roll of the genetic dice adds more variety: at least 240 genes affect weight.[51]

Weight loss is more difficult for some people, and may require more supportive friends and relatives more community resources designed to assist, plus extraordinary efforts to prime the body for burning extra calories. Being overweight does not mean people are weak-willed or lazy. As scientists unlock the many secrets of genetic messengers that influence body weight and learn more about the role of certain foods in the weight loss equation, dieting may not be the same villain in the future that it is today.

To reach and maintain the weight at which you will be healthy and feel best, you need to develop a program of exercise and healthy eating behaviors that will work for you now and in the long term. See the Skills for Behavior Change box for strategies to make your weight management program successful. As well, to become a wise food consumer, you need to become familiar with important concepts in weight control.

What Is a Calorie?

A *calorie* is a unit of measure that indicates the amount of energy we obtain from a particular food. One pound of body fat contains approximately 3,500 calories. So each time you consume 3,500 calories more than your body needs to

Social physique anxiety (SPA) A desire to look good that has a destructive effect on a person's ability to function effectively socially.

Tips for Sensible Weight Management

If you've never met a cookie you didn't like, or if "biggie" and "super-size" have become your favorite words, now might be the time for you to get a handle on what is going into your mouth. Rather than thinking about the best diet for you, the key is to find a livable, sustainable way to control food that will work for you. Use the following strategies for developing a weight management plan and making changes in your diet and your activity level to create a plan that is right for you. The Behavior Change Contract will help you make a commitment to your plan.

Making a Plan

- **Think of it as a way of life.** This is a way of improving your body and your health rather than a punishment or a diet. Remember that you are worth it.
- **Assess where you are.** Monitor your eating habits for two or three days, taking careful note of the good things you are doing and the things that need improvement.
- **Set realistic goals.** No matter what you do, you may not have a perfect body. What do you realistically want your body to look like? How do you want to feel when you move? How do you want your clothes to feel on you? Set either a weight or a BMI level that you want to achieve. Establish short-term goals on the way to the final goal.
- **Establish a plan.** What are three dietary changes you can make today? What exercise will you do tomorrow, the next day, and sustain for one week? Once you do one week, plot a course for two weeks. Jot down how you feel after each week's activity.
- **Be consistent.** Make a number of small changes in what you regularly eat and drink and in your daily activity lev-

els. Make changes that you can stick with and that are comfortable for you (parking farther from a destination and walking, eating cereal and juice for breakfast, walking three days per week, swimming once per week, and so on). Set a schedule and try to stick to it, with an alternative time each day in case your plans change. Always have a fallback option for your scheduled exercise.

- **Look for balance in what you do.** Remember that it's more about a balance than about giving things up. If you must have that piece of pizza or chocolate cake, have it, but then be responsible for doing the extra exercise it takes to burn off the calories or for limiting caloric intake the next day. Remember that it's calories taken in and burned over time that makes the difference.
- **Stay positive.** A healthy lifestyle isn't about being "bad" or "good"; none of us is perfect. Focus on the positive steps you are taking and the healthy things you do each week rather than the less healthy things.
- **Be patient and persistent.** You didn't develop a weight problem overnight. Don't expect instant results. Assess other gains that you make each week: gains in energy level, the fit of your clothes, and how you feel in your body.
- **Reward successes.** Set short-term goals and reward yourself when you've reached them. If your first goal is to lose 10 pounds, reward yourself with something fun, new shoes, a new CD—whatever it takes to keep you motivated.

Changing Your Diet

- **Be adventurous with your food choices.** Expand your usual meals and snacks to enjoy a wide variety of different options (consider the whole grains and salad options described in Chapter 8). Explore different smells, textures,

spices, and colors in foods. Focus on the quality of the food rather than the amount you get. Avoid buffets that allow you to replenish your plate several times.

- **Do not constantly deprive yourself of favorite foods or set unrealistic dietary rules or guidelines.** If you slip and eat something you know you shouldn't, be more careful in what you eat the next day. Balance over a week's time is important. Allow slips and reward successes.
- **Be sensible with your knife and fork.** Enjoy all foods, just don't overdo. When you eat out, eat slowly, cut food into smaller pieces, and think about taking some home for tomorrow's lunch or dinner. Resist the urge to clean your plate. Share entrées with a friend and order salads with dressings on the side.
- **Eat on a regular schedule.** Do not skip meals or let yourself get too hungry.
- **Eat breakfast.** This will prevent you from being too hungry and overeating at lunch.
- **Plan ahead and be prepared for when you might get hungry.** Always have good food available when and where you get hungry.

Changing Your Level of Activity

- **Be active and slowly increase activity.** If you stick to something, it will gradually take less and less effort to walk that mile, for example. Gradually increase the speed of your walk and/or the distance (see Chapter 10). Move more, sit less. If you find that you are always gravitating toward the chair or couch or looking for a place to sit, consciously work toward standing or moving. Remember, every step counts. Purchasing an inexpensive pedometer and recording your daily steps is an excellent way to monitor and improve your level of activity.

- **Be creative with your physical activity.** Find activities that you really love and stick to them. If you hate to walk in the rain and love to shop, walk in a covered mall and then shop! Try things you haven't tried before. Today, options such as yoga, Pilates, dancing, swimming, skiing, and gardening are available.

- **Pick an activity that is inexpensive and does not require fancy equipment.** This means you will maintain your fitness program even when you are traveling away from home.

- **Find an exercise partner to help you get started and motivate you.** Don't pick your fittest friend. Find someone who is patient, understanding, and can take the time necessary to be a supporter. One of the worst mistakes you can make is to take your first bike ride with an avid bicyclist. You'll always feel like you can't keep up. Be patient with yourself. Pick other people who need help and commit to helping them. It will also help you get through the difficult days until exercise is a part of your lifestyle.

Source: Adapted in part from Melinda Manore and Janice Thompson, "Table 15.3: Techniques to Help an Active Individual Identify and Maintain a Healthy Body Weight Throughout the Life Cycle" in *Sport Nutrition for Health and Performance* (Champaign, IL: Human Kinetics Publishing, 2000), 417.

---

maintain weight, you gain a pound. Conversely, each time your body expends an extra 3,500 calories, you lose a pound. So if you add a can of Coca-Cola (140 calories) to your daily diet and make no other changes in diet or activity, you would gain a pound in 25 days (3,500 calories ÷ 140 calories/day = 25 days). Conversely, if you walked for half an hour each day at a pace of 15 minutes per mile (172 calories burned), you would lose a pound in 20 days (3,500 calories ÷ 172 calories/day = 20.3 days).

The two ways to lose weight, then, are to lower caloric intake (through improved eating habits) and to increase exercise (expending more calories).

Don't forget, it took time to gain weight; it will take time to lose it. The best strategy is to go slow, set short-term goals, and stick to them.

Exercise

Approximately 90 percent of the daily calorie expenditures of most people occurs as a result of the **resting metabolic rate (RMR).** The RMR is slightly higher than the BMR; it includes the BMR plus any additional energy expended through daily sedentary activities, such as food digestion, sitting, studying, or standing. The **exercise metabolic rate (EMR)** accounts for the remaining 10 percent of all daily calorie expenditures; it refers to the energy expenditure that occurs during physical exercise. For most of us, these calories come from light daily activities, such as walking, climbing stairs, and mowing the lawn. If we increase the level of physical activity to moderate or heavy, however, our EMR may be 10 to 20 times greater than typical resting metabolic rates and can contribute substantially to weight loss.

Increasing BMR, RMR, or EMR levels will help burn calories. An increase in the intensity, frequency, and duration of daily exercise levels can have a significant impact on total calorie expenditure.

Physical activity makes a greater contribution to BMR when large muscle groups are used. The energy spent on physical activity is the energy used to move the body's muscles—the muscles of the arms, back, abdomen, legs, and so on—and the extra energy used to speed up heartbeat and respiration rate. The number of calories spent depends on three factors:

1. The amount of muscle mass moved.
2. The amount of weight moved.
3. The amount of time the activity takes.

An activity involving both the arms and legs burns more calories than one involving only the legs, an activity performed by a heavy person burns more calories than one performed by a lighter person, and an activity performed for 40 minutes requires twice as much energy than if performed for only 20 minutes. Thus, obese persons walking for one mile burn more calories than slim people walking the same distance. It may also take overweight people longer to walk the mile, which means that they are burning energy for a longer time and therefore expending more overall calories than the thin walkers.

Changing Your Eating Habits

At any given time, many Americans are trying to lose weight. Given the hundreds of different diets and endless expert advice available, why do we find it so difficult?

Resting metabolic rate (RMR) The energy expenditure of the body under BMR conditions plus other daily sedentary activities.

Exercise metabolic rate (EMR) The energy expenditure that occurs during exercise.

What Triggers Your "Eat" Response?		What Stops Your "Eat" Response?	

• Time of day
• Mood
• Boredom
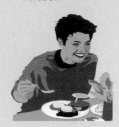
	• Nervousness/
	  anxiety/stress
	• Hormonal fluctuations
	• Peer/family pressure
	• Inattentiveness
	• Habit
	• Hunger/appetite
	• Low self-esteem
	• Environment
	• Sight and smell
	  of favorite foods
		• Acting responsibly in
		  assessing foods
		• Practicing stress
		  management
		• Breaking the habit
		• Remaining active
		• Analyzing emotional
		  problems
		• Making a conscious effort
		• Recognizing true hunger
		• Avoiding environment that
		  causes "eat" response
			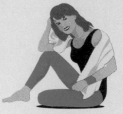
			• Selecting alternatives
			• Recognizing triggers
			• Planning

Figure 9.3
The "Eat" Response
Learn to understand what triggers and stops your "eat" response. Keep a daily log of your responses.

Determining What Triggers an Eating Behavior Before you can change a behavior, you must first determine what causes it.

Many people have found it helpful to keep a chart of their eating patterns: when they feel like eating, where they are when they decide to eat, the amount of time they spend eating, other activities they engage in during the meal (watching television or reading), whether they eat alone or with others, what and how much they consume, and how they felt before they took their first bite. If you keep a detailed daily log of the triggers listed in Figure 9.3 for at least a week, you will discover useful clues about what in your environment or your emotional makeup causes you to want food. Typically, these dietary "triggers" center on problems in everyday living rather than on real hunger pangs. As you record this information, your reasons for eating will often become apparent. Many people find that they eat compulsively when stressed or when they have problems in their relationships. For other people, the same circumstances diminish their appetite, causing them to lose weight.

Changing Your Triggers Once you recognize the factors that cause you to eat, removing the triggers or substituting other activities for them will help you develop more sensible eating patterns. Here are some examples of substitute behaviors:

• When eating dinner, turn off all distractions, including the television and radio.
• Replace snack breaks or coffee breaks with exercise breaks.
• Instead of gulping your food, force yourself to chew each bite slowly.
• Vary the time of day when you eat. Instead of eating by the clock, do not eat until you are truly hungry. Allow yourself only a designated amount of time for eating—but do not rush. Try to become more aware of true feelings of hunger.

• If you find that you generally eat all that you can cram on a plate, use smaller plates. Put your dinner plates away, and use the salad plates instead.
• Stop buying high-calorie foods that tempt you to snack, or store them in an inconvenient place. (Having to run upstairs for the potato chips will force you to think twice before munching them.)

These are just suggestions. After recording your daily intake for a week, you will be able to devise a list of substitutes that are geared toward your particular eating behaviors. You will find more weight management tips in the Skills for Behavior Change box on pages 282–283.

What do you think?

If you were going to try to lose weight, what strategies would you most likely choose? ❋ *Which strategies offer the lowest health risk and the greatest chance for success?* ❋ *What factors might serve to support or sabotage your weight loss efforts?*

Selecting a Nutritional Plan

Once you have discovered what factors tend to sabotage your weight loss efforts, you will be well on your way to healthy weight control. To succeed, however, you must plan for success. By setting goals that are unrealistic or too far in the future, you will doom yourself to failure. Do not try to lose 40 pounds in two months. Try, instead, to lose a healthy 1 to 2 pounds during the first week, and stay with this slow and easy regimen. Reward yourself when you lose pounds, and if you binge and go off your nutrition plan, get right back on it the next day. Remember that you did not gain 40 pounds in eight weeks, so it is unrealistic to punish your body by trying to lose that amount of weight in such a short time.

Seek assistance from reputable sources in selecting a dietary plan that is nutritious and easy to follow. Registered dietitians, some physicians (not all physicians have a strong background in nutrition), health educators and exercise physiologists with nutritional training, and other health professionals can provide reliable information. Beware of people who call themselves "nutritionists." There is no such official designation, leaving the door open for just about anyone to call himself or herself a nutritional expert. Avoid weight loss programs that promise quick, miracle results. They are expensive, and most people regain the weight soon after completing the program.

For any weight loss program, ask about the credentials of the adviser, assess the nutrient value of the prescribed diet, verify that dietary guidelines are consistent with reliable nutrition research, and analyze the suitability of the diet to your tastes, budget, and lifestyle. Any diet that requires radical behavior changes is doomed to failure. The most successful plans allow you to make food choices and do not ask you to sacrifice everything you enjoy (see the "Analyzing Popular Diets" Reality Check box).

Ultimately, the decision to practice responsible weight management is yours. To be successful, choose a combination of exercise and eating that fits your needs and lifestyle. Find a workable plan, stick to it, and you will succeed.

Drastic Weight Loss Measures

When faced with weight gain and loss, when nothing seems to work, people often become willing to take significant risks in order to achieve weight loss. Dramatic weight loss may be recommended in cases of high-risk hypertension, cardiac strain, imperiled lung capacity, gastrointestinal difficulties, crippling strain on bones and joints, surgical risk, and other problems. Even in such situations, opting for drastic dietary, pharmacological, or surgical measures should be considered carefully and discussed with several knowledgeable health professionals and with full awareness of potential adverse effects.

"Miracle" Diets   Fasting, starvation diets, and other forms of **very low calorie diets (VLCDs)** have been shown to cause significant health risks. Typically, depriving the body of food for prolonged periods forces it to make adjustments to prevent the shutdown of organs. The body depletes its energy reserves to obtain necessary fuels. One of the first reserves the body turns to in order to maintain its supply of glucose is lean, protein tissue. As this occurs, weight is lost rapidly because protein contains only half as many calories per pound as fat. At the same time, significant water stores are lost. Over time, the body begins to run out of liver tissue, heart muscle, blood, and so on, as these readily available substances are burned to supply energy. Only after depleting the readily available proteins from these sources does the body begin to burn fat reserves. In this process, known as **ketosis,** the body adapts to prolonged fasting or carbohydrate deprivation by converting body fat to ketones, which can be used as fuel for some brain cells. Within about 10 days after the typical adult begins a complete fast, the body will have used many of its energy stores, and death may occur.

In very low calorie diets, powdered formulas are usually given to patients under medical supervision. These formulas have daily values of 400 to 700 calories plus vitamin and mineral supplements. Although these diets may be beneficial for people who have failed at all conventional weight loss methods and who face severe health risks due to obesity, they should never be undertaken without strict medical supervision. Problems associated with fasting, VLCDs, and other forms of severe calorie deprivation include blood sugar imbalances, cold intolerance, constipation, decreased BMR, dehydration, diarrhea, emotional problems, fatigue, headaches, heart irregularity, ketosis, kidney infections and failure, loss of lean body tissue, weakness, and eventual weight gain due to the yo-yo effect and other variables.

Drug Treatment   Experts reason that if obesity is a chronic disease, it should be treated as such, and the treatment for most chronic diseases includes drugs.[52] The challenge is to develop an effective drug that can be used over time without adverse effects or abuse, and no such drug currently exists.

A classic example of a supposedly safe set of drugs that later were found to have dangerous side effects were Pondimen and Redux, known as *Fen Phen,* two of the most widely prescribed diet drugs in U.S. history.[53] When the drugs were found to damage heart valves and contribute to pulmonary hypertension, a massive recall and lawsuit occurred.

Other diet drugs that you should view with caution include the following:

• *Sibutramine:* Suppresses appetite by inhibiting the uptake of serotonin. It works best with a reduced calorie diet and exercise, but side effects are not to be taken lightly. They include dry mouth, headache, constipation, insomnia, and high blood pressure. As many obese individuals have high blood pressure, this is an obvious concern.
• *Orlistat (Xenical):* Works by inhibiting the action of lipase, an enzyme that helps digest fats. About 30 percent of fats consumed pass through the system undigested, leading to reduced overall caloric intake. Known side effects include

---

Very low calorie diets (VLCDs)   Diets with a caloric value of 400 to 700 calories.

Ketosis   A condition in which the body adapts to prolonged fasting or carbohydrate deprivation by converting body fat to ketones, which can be used as fuel for some brain activity.

Analyzing Popular Diets

In our ongoing quest to find an effective way to lose weight, Americans consider many seemingly reputable options. Are any of these diet plans really the "miracles" that they often claim to be? Don't count on it. Some are quite good, but others produce no long-term effects and may even be dangerous. Each year, "new and improved" versions of the same old dietary ploys surface in bookstores, where they sell millions of copies. Then there are reports of successes and dangers, and finally professional groups jump into the fray to label these diets as ineffective or dangerous. Just when we think we've seen the last of a fad, its authors reinvent themselves and capture our interest yet again. Dr. Kelly Brownell, noted obesity researcher at Yale University, describes this pattern: "When I get calls about the latest diet fad, I imagine a trick birthday cake candle that keeps lighting up and we have to keep blowing it out over and over again."

Virtually anyone can write a book making diet claims. Just because the authors may have Ph.D.s or other credentials, they may not have expertise in the area that they write about. If they do have the expertise, they may base their arguments on unproven science or faulty scientific reasoning. Although health claims should be published only after solid research has proven the results repeatedly with different populations, this happens all too infrequently.

The following is a summary of some of the popular diets and the consensus opinions of the U.S. Department of Agriculture, the American Heart Association, the Center for Science in the Public Interest, and several other professional groups and individuals on the diets' effectiveness and safety.

Book/Program and Author	Premise of the Diet	How It Claims to Work	Experts' Opinions	Comments
The Atkins Diet Robert Atkins, M.D.	Says overweight people eat too many carbohydrates. High-protein diet allows you to eat all the protein you want (meat, eggs, cheese, and more) and restricts refined sugar, milk, white rice, and white flour.	Restrict carbohydrates, and the body goes into ketosis. In ketosis, the body gets energy from ketones, little carbon fragments that are the fuel created by breakdown of fat stores. You feel less hungry.	Highly controversial in spite of claims. Too much fat, no attention to Pyramid guidelines. Few published results and no long-term studies of effects on cardiovascular system or cholesterol. American Dietetic Association and other groups dispute claims. Low intake of fruits and vegetables a problem.	Possible side effects: nausea, fatigue, low blood pressure, elevated uric acid/kidney problems, bad breath, constipation, fetal harm if pregnant.
Carbohydrate Addict's Diet, Richard Heller, M.D. and Rachel Heller, M.D.	Overweight people are "carbohydrate addicts." Their biological processes don't work right when converting food to energy; insulin levels stay high and people crave food. Diet cuts back on carbohydrates and prescribes two-week eating regimens. High in protein and fat.	By restricting carbohydrate intake drastically most of the day, the body releases far less insulin than if you ate carbohydrates at each meal. Lower insulin levels result in smaller appetite.	Science is unsupported. May trick people into eating certain foods for a short time, but saying we are carbohydrate addicts makes as much sense as saying we are oxygen or water addicts. The reward structure of the diet promotes unhealthy eating.	Most health experts dispute the value of this diet. Not realistic for long-term weight maintenance.
Dean Ornish Diet, Dean Ornish, M.D.	Diet and exercise are important. Watch *what* you eat; there are foods you should eat all of the time, some of the time, and none of the time. Less than 10 percent of your calories should come from fat. Eat lots of little meals.	Metabolism is a result of our ancestors. We need to change old metabolic patterns. Meditation is a part of this: When your soul is fed, you have less need to overeat.	Mostly positive for highly restrictive diet and healthy lifestyle regimen. Documented studies show heart blockage reversal. Drawbacks are that it is tough to stick to this diet and new eating patterns must be learned. Only the most committed will stick to this rigid diet.	May be tough for all but strict vegans to adhere to this plan. Eating smaller, more frequent meals may be difficult. Otherwise, a good model.

Book/Program and Author	Premise of the Diet	How It Claims to Work	Experts' Opinions	Comments
Eating Well for Optimum Health, Andrew Weil, M.D.	Eat less, exercise more. Take a more Eastern than Western approach. Avoid quick fixes and set a realistic goal of one to two pounds of weight loss per week. Balance the amount and type of food. Describes meats as "flesh foods." Minimize dairy and take a Mediterranean dietary approach.	Keeps it simple. Criticizes high protein diets because of rise in cholesterol and calcium depletion. Moderation is a key.	A more holistic approach to dieting than most. Considers exercise and stress as factors.	May not be sustainable for those who are used to diets high in dairy or meat. Nutrition experts support this common-sense approach. Vegetarian emphasis substantiated as healthy by numerous studies.
The Zone, Barry Sears, Ph.D.	Offers a wellness philosophy to develop a metabolic state in which the body works efficiently. Recommends eating different calories than you do now and a small amount of protein. Identifies favorable versus unfavorable carbohydrates.	Claims that his percentages of fat, protein, and carbohydrates are the best ratios for health.	Superiority of given ratios is unsubstantiated by research. Mixed reviews from experts: easy to follow, but don't count on results. Some recommendations (eating high-fat ice cream) are questionable.	Not a lot of do's and don'ts. Dieters may find it easy to follow.
The Pritikin Principle, Robert Pritikin	Concern not for calories, but for density of calories. Fat more foods that are not calorie dense, such as apples and oatmeal.	Fill up on foods that have fewer calories. Large volume of fiber and water will keep you full. Emphasis on vegetables, fruits, beans, unprocessed grains; exercise strongly recommended.	Weight loss will occur, but so will frequent feelings of hunger. Weight will usually creep back. Low in fat so healthy in general, except when taken to extreme or for certain groups of people.	Strict limitations of animal products a plus. Incorporates exercise and stress management. Not an easy plan to stick to.
Protein Power, Mary and Michael Eades, M.D.s	Argues that carbohydrate-based diets—fruits, vegetables, and starches—are responsible for rampant obesity. Plan calls for lots of protein, some fiber, not many carbohydrates.	Controlling insulin helps regulate blood pressure and blood fats.	Same problems as other high-protein, low-carb diets. May work in short term, but body can't keep it up and there are health risks.	Can be deficient in important nutrients. Requires a reduction in types of foods one can eat, which is difficult to maintain.
Sugar Busters, H. Leighton Steward, Morrison Bethea, M.D., Samuel Andrews, M.D., and Luis Balart, M.D.	Cut sugar to trim fat. Pay attention to portion size. Eliminate potatoes, corn, rice, bread, carrots, refined sugar, honey, colas, and beer.	Glucose, insulin production theory: The more insulin produced, the more fat.	Most don't like this diet. When you gain weight, it doesn't matter where calories come from; it is total calorie intake that is most important.	You'll lose weight due to decreased calorie intake, but this is not a good long-term strategy.
Weight Watchers	Eat from food groups, tally points to monitor intake. Based on weight and dietary goals. Eat what you want, but use discretion in amount.	Based on calories in, calories out. Includes exercise and social support.	Life focus rather than diet focus. Has support of most national organizations. One of the most highly recommended diets.	Works well for many people, particularly those for whom social support is important.

Sources: United States Department of Agriculture, "The Great Nutrition Debate" (2000) (see http://www.usda.gov/cnpp).

oily spotting; gas with watery fecal discharge; fecal urgency; oily stools; frequent, often unexpected, bowel movements; and possible deficiencies of fat-soluble vitamins.[54]

• *Over-the-counter (OTC) drugs:* Only one OTC medication to help with weight loss has FDA approval. It contains *benzocaine* (in candy or gum form), which anesthetizes the tongue, reducing taste sensation. In 2000, the FDA recommended banning OTCs containing *phenylpropanolamine,* an appetite suppressant, due to problems with rapid pulse, insomnia, hypertension, irregular heartbeats, and kidney failure.[55]

• *Herbal weight loss aids:* St. John's wort (SJW) and other substances that enhance serotonin and suppress appetite have been widely marketed for weight loss. Be aware that SJW is often combined with ephedrine, a stimulant found in certain cold and allergy pills and believed to cause heart attacks, seizures, and strokes.[56] Before you take any herbal medication, make sure you know its possible ingredients and their risks (see Chapter 23).

Surgery   When all else fails, a relatively permanent, yet risky, solution may lie in surgical stapling or tying off of the stomach. In this procedure, the stomach is effectively reduced in size to about the size of an egg and holds only a few tablespoons of food. Patients can't eat enough calories, so they lose weight. Make no mistake about it, this is not a procedure for the typical obese person and should be reserved only for the morbidly obese who face imminent

risks from other health problems. Complications are many, and include infections, nausea, vomiting, and dehydration. (Imagine being really thirsty and only being able to drink a few tablespoons of water at a time.) Patients also face a lifetime of taking only a couple of bites of food at each meal. Vitamin and mineral deficiencies and difficulty eating enough small meals to maintain a normal body weight once excess weight is gone are also complications.

Lifelong medical and sometimes psychological monitoring is needed for those who have this procedure. Because it is costly to undergo and difficult to undo, it should be considered only in the most extreme circumstances.

Liposuction is another surgical procedure for spot reducing. Although this technique has garnered much attention, it, too, is not without risk. Infections, severe scarring, and even death have resulted when the qualifications of the plastic surgeon or medical facilities have not been up to par. In many cases, people who have liposuction regain fat in the areas that it was removed from or need to have multiple surgeries to repair lumpy, irregular surfaces from which the fat was removed.

Trying to Gain Weight

Although trying to lose weight poses a major challenge for many, a smaller group of Americans, for a variety of metabolic, hereditary, psychological, and other reasons, inexplica-

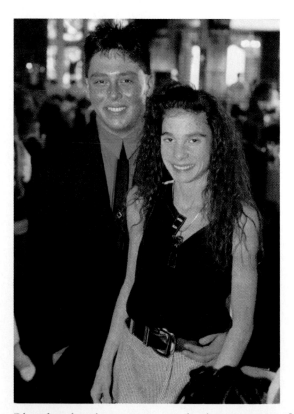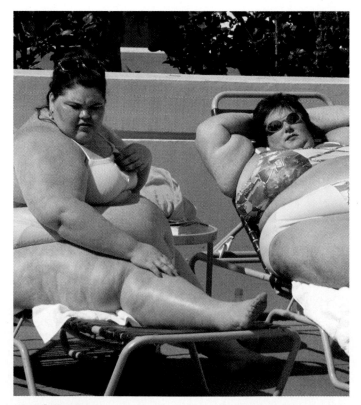

Disordered eating patterns can lead to extremes of anorexia nervosa or of obesity.

bly start to lose weight or can't seem to gain weight no matter how hard they try. If you are one of these individuals, determining the reasons for your difficulty in gaining weight is a must. For example, among older adults, senses of taste and smell may decline, which makes food taste differently and be less pleasurable. Visual problems and other disabilities may make food more difficult to prepare, and dental problems may make eating certain foods more difficult. People who engage in extreme sports that require extreme nutritional supplementation may be at risk for nutritional deficiencies, which can affect immune system and organ functioning, cause weakness that leads to falls and fractures, slow recovery from diseases, and cause a host of other problems.

Once you know what is causing a daily caloric deficit, there are steps you can take to gain extra weight:

- Eat at regularly scheduled times, whether hungry or not.
- Eat more. Obviously, you are not taking in enough calories to support whatever is happening in your body. Eat more frequently, spend more time eating, eat the high-calorie foods first if you fill up fast, and always start with the main course. Take time to shop, to cook, to eat slowly. Put extra spreads such as peanut butter, cream cheese, or cheese on your foods. Make your sandwiches with extra-thick slices of bread, and add more filling. Take seconds whenever possible, and eat high-calorie snacks during the day.
- Supplement your diet. Add high-calorie drinks that have a healthy balance of nutrients.
- Try to eat with people you are comfortable with. Avoid people who you feel are analyzing what you eat or make you feel like you should eat less.
- If you aren't exercising, exercise can increase appetite. If you are exercising or exercising to extreme, moderate your activities until weight gain is evident.
- Avoid diuretics, laxatives, and other medications that cause you to lose body fluids and nutrients.
- Relax. Many people who are underweight operate at high gear most of the time. Slow down, get more rest, and control stress.

Eating Disorders

On occasion, over one-third of all Americans fit the descriptions of obesity and diet obsessiveness. For an increasing number of people, particularly young women, this obsessive relationship with food develops into **anorexia nervosa,** a persistent, chronic eating disorder characterized by deliberate food restriction and severe, life-threatening weight loss. **Bulimia nervosa,** or a variation known as **binge eating disorder (BED),** involves frequent bouts of binge eating followed by purging (self-induced vomiting), laxative abuse, or excessive exercise. In the United States more than 10 million people, 90 percent of whom are women, meet the established criteria for one of these disorders, and their numbers appear to be increasing.[57] Many more suffer from minor forms of

these conditions—not serious enough for a true diagnosis, but dangerously close to the precipice that will ultimately lead to life-threatening results (see Table 9.5).

Anorexia Nervosa

Anorexia involves self-starvation motivated by an intense fear of gaining weight along with an extremely distorted body image. When anorexia occurs in childhood, failure to gain weight in a normal growth pattern may be the key indicator; later, this typically results in actual weight loss. Nearly 1 percent of girls in late adolescence meet the full criteria for anorexia; many others suffer from significant symptoms.

Usually people with anorexia achieve their weight loss through initial reduction in total food intake, particularly of high-calorie foods, eventually leading to restricted intake of almost all foods. What they do eat, they often purge through vomiting or using laxatives. Although they lose weight, people with anorexia never seem to feel "thin enough" and constantly identify body parts that are "too fat."

Bulimia Nervosa

People with bulimia often binge and then take inappropriate measures, such as secret vomiting, to lose the calories they have just acquired. Up to 3 percent of adolescents and young female adults are bulimic, with male rates being about 10 percent of the female rate. People with bulimia are also obsessed with their bodies, weight gain, and how they appear to others. Unlike those with anorexia, people with bulimia are often "hidden" from the public eye because their weight may vary only slightly or fall within a normal range. Also, treatment appears to be more effective for bulimia than for anorexia.

Binge Eating Disorder (BED)

Individuals with binge eating disorder also binge like their bulimic counterparts, but do not take excessive measures to lose the weight that they gain. Often they are clinically obese, and they tend to binge much more often than the

Anorexia nervosa   Eating disorder characterized by excessive preoccupation with food, self-starvation, and/or extreme exercising to achieve weight losses.

Bulimia nervosa   Eating disorder characterized by binge eating followed by inappropriate measures to prevent weight gain.

Binge eating disorder (BED)   Eating disorder characterized by recurrent binge eating, without excessive measures to prevent weight gain.

Table 9.5
DSM-IV Eating Disorder Criteria

ANOREXIA

According to the *DSM-IV*, people who meet the criteria for anorexia nervosa experience all of the following symptoms:

- Refusal to maintain the minimum body weight for one's height and age
- Intense fear of gaining weight even though underweight
- Disturbed perception of one's body weight or size
- In postpubescent women, the absence of at least three consecutive menstrual cycles (In some women, the loss of periods precedes any significant weight loss.)

BULIMIA

People with bulimia experience all of the following:

- Recurrent episodes of consuming a much larger amount of food than most people would during a similar time period (this is usually about two hours) and a sense of loss of control over eating during each episode
- Accompanying attempts to compensate for eating binges by vomiting, abusing laxatives or other drugs, or by fasting or excessive exercise
- Both the binge eating and purging occur at least twice a week for three months
- A negative perception of one's shape and weight

Source: From *DSM-IV,* reported in "Treating Eating Disorders," *Harvard Women's Health Watch,* May 1996, 4–5. Reprinted with permission from Diagnostic and Statistical Manual of Mental Disorders, Fourth Edition. Copyright 1994 American Psychiatric Association.

typical obese person, who may consume too many calories but spaces his or her eating over a more normal daily eating pattern. To date, binge eating disorder is still under consideration as a psychiatric disorder.

Who's at Risk?

There's no simple explanation for why intelligent, often highly accomplished people spiral downward into the destructive behaviors associated with eating disorders. Obsessive-compulsive disorder, depression, and anxiety can all play a role, as can a desperate need to win social approval or gain control of their lives through food.

Sufferers tend to be women from white middle-class or upper-class families in which there is undue emphasis on achievement, body weight, and appearance. Contrary to popular thinking, however, eating disorders span social class, gender, race, and ethnic backgrounds and are present in countries throughout the world. In addition, increasing numbers of males suffer from various forms of eating disorders.

Some studies have shown possible associations between identical twins, and others have pointed to the large numbers of eating disordered persons who have a mother or sister with the disease. Many persons with disordered eating patterns also suffer from other problems: Fifty percent are clinically depressed, 25 percent are alcoholics, and large numbers have other problems, such as compulsive stealing, gambling, or other addictions.[58]

Treatment for Eating Disorders

Because eating disorders result from many factors, spanning many years of development, there are no quick or simple solutions. Treatment often focuses on reducing the threat to life; once the patient is stabilized, long-term therapy involves family, friends, and other significant people in the individual's life. Therapy focuses on the psychological, social, environmental, and physiological factors that have led to the problem. Finding a therapist who really understands the multidimensional aspects of the problem is a must. Therapy allows the patient to focus on building new eating behaviors, recognizing threats, building self-confidence, and finding other ways of dealing with life's problems. Support groups often help the family and the individual gain understanding and emotional support and learn self-development techniques designed to foster positive reactions and actions. Treatment of underlying depression may also be a focus.

What do you think?

Which groups or individuals on your campus appear to be at greatest risk for eating disorders? What social factors might encourage this? ✴ *Why do you think society tends to overlook eating disorders in males?* ✴ *What programs or services on your campus are available for someone with an eating disorder?*

Taking Control of Your Weight

Controlling your weight involves gaining control over food, modifying behaviors, increasing muscle mass, and making exercise a priority. To ensure success, look at weight control as a lifelong commitment rather than a temporary diet. The first step is an honest self-assessment of where you are. What did you find out about yourself as you read this chapter? Are you satisfied with your weight? If not, what can you do to make a change? Next, set a realistic goal. Ask yourself, why do I want to meet this goal? What will I do when I reach it? Then develop a plan to reach your goal. Each person must find his or her own best strategy, recognize potential difficulties, and work to modify behaviors to help bring weight under control. Your school and community have resources to help. If in doubt, ask your instructor or your student health center. Here are some suggestions to help you get started.

Checklist for Change

Making Personal Choices

☐ Design your plan based on your needs. It must fit your personality, your priorities, and your work and recreation schedules. Allow for sufficient rest and relaxation.

☐ Include nutrient-dense foods. Get the most from the foods you eat by selecting foods with high nutritional value.

☐ Balance food intake throughout the day. Rather than gorging yourself at one main meal, you are probably better off eating several smaller meals throughout the day.

☐ Plan for plateaus. If you prepare yourself psychologically for plateaus, you will be less likely to become discouraged. Exercise is probably the critical factor in getting past a plateau.

☐ Chart your progress. Weigh yourself weekly, not daily, to avoid frustration. After all, it is long-range success you are after.

☐ Chart your setbacks. Rather than thinking in terms of failure and punishment, think in terms of temporary setbacks and how to accommodate them. By carefully recording your emotional states when eating, eating habits, environmental cues, and feelings, you may determine why you needed that ice cream cone or why you chose a pizza instead of a salad. Women may need to take into account weight fluctuations due to hormonal changes over the course of the monthly cycle.

☐ Become aware of your feelings of hunger and fullness. For many of us, eating is time-dependent, and we stop eating only when the food is gone (the "clean your plate" syndrome). Long years of "eating when it is time" instead of eating when it is necessary cost us the ability to tell when we are really hungry and when we are really full. By training yourself to become more aware of the eating process, by learning to recognize true hunger pangs and the first signals that you have eaten enough, you will be able to change your eating patterns.

☐ Accept yourself. For many people, this is the most important aspect of successful weight management. It is important to keep weight in perspective. Unless you feel good about who you are inside, exterior changes will not help you very much.

☐ Exercise, exercise, exercise. Although we would all like to wish away our extra pounds, losing weight requires effort and concentration. Different people benefit from different types of activities. Select an exercise program that you consider fun, not a daily form of punishment for overeating. Remember, every little effort contributes toward long-term results.

Summary

* Overweight, obesity, and weight-related problems appear to be on the rise in the United States. Obesity is now defined in terms of fat content rather than in terms of weight alone.
* There are many different methods of assessing body fat. BMI is one of the most commonly accepted measures of weight based on height. Body fat percentages more accurately indicate how fat or lean a person is.
* Many factors contribute to one's risk for obesity, including genetics, developmental factors, setpoint, endocrine influences, psychosocial factors, eating cues, lack of awareness, metabolic changes, lifestyle, and gender. Women often have considerably more difficulty in achieving weight loss.
* Exercise, dieting, diet pills, and other strategies are used to maintain or lose weight. However, sensible eating behavior and adequate exercise probably offer the best options.
* Eating disorders consist of severe disturbances in eating behaviors, unhealthy efforts to control body weight, and abnormal attitudes about body and shape. Anorexia nervosa, bulimia nervosa, and binge eating disorder are the three main eating disorders. Though prevalent among white women of upper- and middle-class families, eating disorders affect women of all backgrounds as well as a number of men.

Questions for Discussion and Reflection

1. Discuss the pressures, if any, you feel to improve your personal body image. Do these pressures come from media, family, friends, and other external sources, or from concern for your personal health?
2. What type of measurement would you choose in order to assess your fat levels? Why?
3. List the risk factors for obesity. Evaluate which seem to be most important in determining whether you will be obese in middle age.
4. Create a plan to help someone lose the "freshman 15" over the summer vacation. Assume that the person is male, 180 pounds, and has 15 weeks to lose the excess weight.
5. Differentiate among the three eating disorders. Then give reasons why females might be more prone to anorexia and bulimia than males are.

Application Exercises

Reread the What Do You Think? scenarios at the beginning of the chapter and answer the following questions:

1. In cases like those of Beth, John, and Bill, what issues might contribute to their eating problems? Do you know of others who have similar problems? Describe those problems and possible solutions.
2. What factors contribute to obesity? In the Bertrands' situation, what factors might they be responsible for, if any? Which would be totally out of their control?
3. What concerns would you have about separating morbidly obese children from their parents? Can you think of a less drastic alternative?

Accessing Your Health on the Internet

Visit the following Internet sites to explore further topics and issues related to personal health. To visit an organization's website, go to the Companion Website for *Access to Health, Eighth Edition* at www.aw.com/donatelle, click on the book image, and select "Accessing Your Health on the Internet" from the navigation menu on the left.

1. ***American Dietetic Association.*** Recommended dietary guidelines and other current information about weight control.
2. ***Duke University Diet and Fitness Center.*** Information about one of the best programs in the country focused on helping people live healthier, fuller lives through weight control and lifestyle change.

3. **Helping to End Eating Disorders (HEED).** The website of an organization dedicated to fighting eating disorders and helping individuals through the ordeal. Includes a chatroom for people to exchange thoughts and share support.

4. **Mayo Health O@sis.** Summary of many weight control issues and concerns.
5. **Shape Up America.** Strategies and ideas for getting in shape and staying at your optimal weight.

Further Reading

Gaesser, G. *Big Fat Lies.* New York: Fawcett Columbine Press, 1997.

Excellent overview of leading theories on fat, obesity, and a host of related problems and issues. Also gives an excellent overview of potential weight loss strategies that are "keepers" for life.

Piscatella, J. *The Fat-Gram Guide to Restaurant Food, 3rd ed.* New York: Workman Press, 2000.

Useful guide to fast foods and restaurant fat content.

United States Department of Agriculture. "The Great Nutrition Debate." 2000 (see http://www.usda.gov/cnpp).

An online transcript of a day of presentations and panel discussions by leading obesity experts and authors of fad diet books.

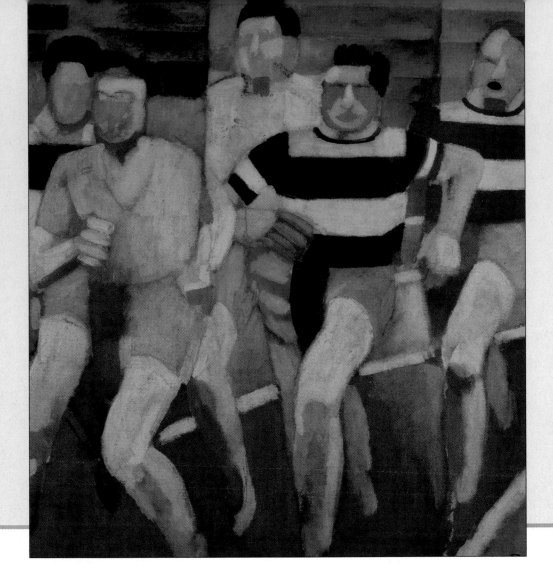

Objectives

* Describe physical fitness and the benefits of regular physical activity, including improved cardiorespiratory fitness, muscular fitness, bone mass, weight control, stress management, mental health, and life span.

* Describe the components of an aerobic exercise program and how to determine the best frequency, intensity, and duration of exercise for people who are fit and those trying to get fit.

* Describe different stretching and strength exercises designed to improve strength and flexibility.

* Compare the various types and benefits of resistance exercise programs.

* Describe common fitness injuries, suggest ways to prevent injuries, and list the treatment process.

* Discuss the factors that contribute to obsessive exercise patterns and suggest strategies for preventing them.

* Summarize the key components of a personal fitness program.

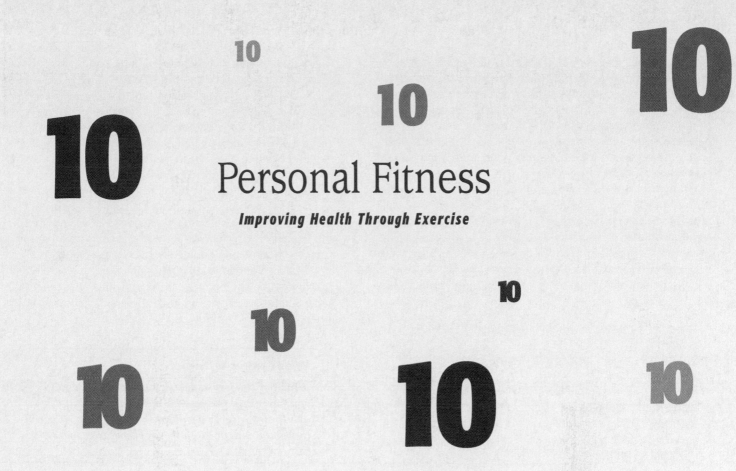

Personal Fitness

Improving Health Through Exercise

What do you think?

Shawn hasn't ever been physically active. In high school he didn't enjoy physical education classes because he didn't have the fitness level or skills needed for competitive activities like basketball and soccer. Now 20 years old and a sophomore in college, Shawn typically drives his car to campus rather than walking the six blocks from his apartment. His idea of a complete meal is a large pepperoni pizza delivered to his door and washed down with a large soda. To relax, he'll play a computer game. Recently Shawn heard about the adverse health effects of a sedentary lifestyle, and he now no longer wants to be a couch potato.

Now that Shawn is ready for a more active lifestyle, how should he begin? ✳ *After years of inactivity, what types of exercises should he choose?* ✳ *Should Shawn see a physician before he starts his exercise program? How soon will he notice positive results?*

Lindsay is an avid runner. She would run five miles daily under any conditions: rain, snow, heat, or cold. When she started developing pain in the heel of her foot during her freshman year at college, she decided to ignore it and work right through it, but the pain got worse. It got so bad, in fact, that she had trouble walking first thing in the morning. Finally, she visited the doctor, who said Lindsay had plantar fasciitis. She gave Lindsay some exercises to do and recommended that she avoid running on hills and buy running shoes that offered more support.

What could Lindsay have done to prevent plantar fasciitis? ✳ *Was it wise for her to try to work through the pain?* ✳ *What risk was she taking?* ✳ *What do you think she should do now?*

A century ago in the United States, simple survival required performing heavy physical labor for several hours each day. A trip to the store meant hitching up the horses or walking, without the benefit of cross-trainer shoes or special walking shoes; in fact, long walks were often taken barefoot or in hand-me-down shoes. Today, "taking a walk" is something we do for recreation, rather than a part of our everyday existence or for necessity. Transportation is provided by motorized vehicles, and even bicycles are designed to minimize effort by the person riding them. Science and technology have transformed our lives in ways that our ancestors could not have imagined. They have also contributed to our growing epidemic of obesity (see Chapter 9), diabetes, and other diseases related to low fitness levels.[1] Consider the following facts about the U.S. population in the early twenty-first century:[2]

- Roughly 13.5 million people have coronary heart disease.
- About 1.5 million people suffer from a heart attack in any given year.
- Some 8 million people have adult-onset (non-insulin-dependent) diabetes.
- About 95,000 people are newly diagnosed with colon cancer each year.
- About 250,000 people suffer from hip fractures each year.
- Fifty million people have high blood pressure.
- Over 60 million people are overweight.
- Large numbers of people suffer from depression and other problems with self-esteem and interpersonal relationships. Although many factors contribute to these problems, being unfit, overweight, or obese may cause increased difficulties for these individuals.

What Is Physical Fitness?

Physical fitness is the ability to perform moderate-to-vigorous levels of physical activity on a regular basis without excessive fatigue. **Exercise training** is the systematic performance of exercise at a specified frequency, intensity, and duration to achieve a desired level of physical fitness.[3] Major health-related components of physical fitness include cardiorespiratory fitness, muscular strength and endurance, flexibility, and better body composition. These components play a vital role in overall health (see Table 10.1). To be considered physically fit, you generally need to attain (and then maintain) certain minimum standards for each component that have been established by exercise physiologists and other fitness experts. Some people have physical limitations that make achieving one or more of these standards difficult. That doesn't mean they can't become physically fit. For example, a woman with limited flexibility due to

arthritis in the knee and hip joints may be unable to jog without extreme pain. Yet by exercising in a swimming pool, where the buoyancy of the water will relieve much of the stress on her joints, she can improve her range of motion. She can also develop muscular strength and cardiovascular fitness by "jogging" at the deep end of a swimming pool while wearing a flotation device. Similarly, a man who needs to use a wheelchair may be unable to run or walk a mile, as required in some fitness tests, but he can stay physically fit by playing wheelchair basketball.

Athletic skill is not a requirement for physical fitness—you do not have to possess the talents of an Olympic athlete to achieve health benefits from regular physical activity and exercise. Many healthy activities, such as walking, running, swimming, and cycling, require no special skill to be performed and enjoyed. Our definition of physical fitness should be adapted to address individual differences in capabilities. There are several different types of physical fitness.

> **What do you think?**
>
> *Which of the key aspects of physical fitness do you currently possess? ✳ Which ones would you like to improve or develop? ✳ What types of activities could you do to improve your fitness level?*

Benefits of Regular Physical Activity

Physical activity is any force exerted by skeletal muscles that results in energy usage above the level used when the body's systems are at rest.[4] Higher levels of physical activity reduce the following:

- The risk of dying prematurely.
- The risk of dying prematurely from heart disease.
- The risk of developing diabetes.
- The risk of developing high blood pressure.
- Blood pressure in people who already have high blood pressure.
- The risk of developing colon cancer.
- Feelings of depression and anxiety.

Other ways in which physical activity is beneficial include the following:

- It helps control weight.
- It helps build and maintain healthy bones, muscles, and joints.
- It helps older adults become stronger and better able to move about without falling.
- It promotes psychological well-being.
- It reduces surgical risks.

Table 10.1
Major Components of Physical Fitness

Cardiorespiratory fitness	Ability to sustain moderate-intensity whole-body activity for extended time periods
Muscular strength and endurance	Maximum force applied with a single muscle contraction. Ability to perform repeated high-intensity muscle contractions
Flexibility	Range of motion at a joint or series of joints
Body composition	A composite of total body mass, fat mass, fat-free mass, and fat distribution

Source: From "ACSM Position Stand on the Recommended Quantity and Quality of Exercise for Developing and Maintaining Cardiorespiratory and Muscular Fitness and Flexibility in Adults," by the American College of Sports Medicine, 1998, *Medicine and Science in Sports and Exercise* 30, pp. 975–991.

- It reduces complications from bone and joint disorders, respiratory disorders, etc.
- It helps immune functioning.

A recent study indicated that regular physical exercise (four hours a week or more) beginning in adolescence and continuing into adulthood can significantly reduce the risk of breast cancer in women age 40 and younger.[5] The recent Surgeon General's report on physical activity and health[6] indicates that physical activity need not be strenuous in order to achieve health benefits and that women and men of all ages benefit from a moderate amount of *daily* activity.

The benefits of moderate physical activity as listed above, are well known and often cited. In fact, regular physical activity improves more than 50 different physiological, metabolic, and psychological aspects of human life. There is no better time than now to begin an exercise plan that will help you reap many of these benefits.[7]

In addition to the physical and psychological benefits of fitness, researchers at the Centers for Disease Control and Prevention (CDC) have documented another major advantage: lower national health care expenditures.[8] Specifically, researchers found that physically active individuals had lower annual direct medical costs than did inactive people. The cost difference was $330 per person, and the potential savings if all inactive American adults became physically active could be in excess of $77 billion.

Improved Cardiorespiratory Fitness

Cardiorespiratory fitness refers to the ability of the circulatory and respiratory systems to supply oxygen to the body during sustained physical activity.[9] Regular exercise will make these systems more efficient by enlarging the heart muscle, enabling more blood to be pumped with each stroke, and increasing the number of *capillaries* (small arteries) in trained skeletal muscles, which supply more blood to working muscles. Exercise improves the respiratory system by increasing the amount of oxygen that is inhaled and distributed to body tissues.[10]

Reduced Risk of Heart Disease Your heart is a muscle made up of highly specialized tissue. Because muscles become stronger and more efficient with use, regular exercise strengthens the heart, enabling it to pump more blood with each beat. This increased efficiency means that the heart requires fewer beats per minute to circulate blood throughout the body. A stronger, more efficient heart is better able to meet the ordinary demands of life.

Prevention of Hypertension *Blood pressure* refers to the force exerted by blood against blood vessel walls, generated by the pumping action of the heart. Hypertension, the medical term for abnormally high blood pressure, is a significant risk factor for cardiovascular disease and stroke.

Hypertension is particularly prevalent among adult African Americans, who develop it about 1.5 times more frequently than white adults.[11] If your working **systolic blood pressure** is consistently 160 millimeters of mercury (mm Hg) or higher, your risk of coronary heart disease is four times greater than normal. If your resting **diastolic blood pressure** regularly exceeds 95 mm Hg, your risk of heart disease is six

Physical fitness The ability to perform regular moderate-to-rigorous physical activity without great fatigue.

Exercise training The systematic performance of exercise at a specified frequency, intensity, and duration to achieve a desired level of physical fitness.

Cardiorespiratory fitness The ability of the heart, lungs, and blood vessels to supply oxygen to skeletal muscles during sustained physical activity.

Systolic blood pressure The pressure in the arteries during a heartbeat; abnormal if consistently 160 mm Hg or above.

Diastolic blood pressure The pressure in the arteries during the period between heartbeats; abnormal if consistently 95 mm Hg or above.

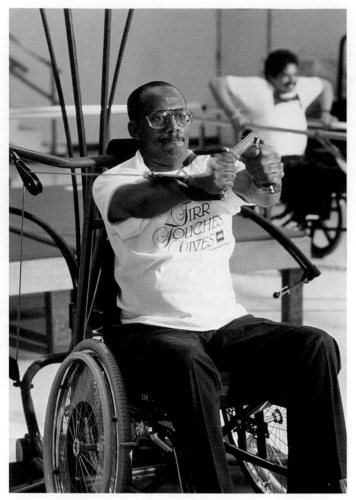

Everyone can attain cardiovascular fitness and muscular strength.

times greater than normal.[12] Low-to-moderate intensity exercise training lowers both systolic and diastolic blood pressure by about 10 mm Hg in people with mild-to-moderate hypertension.[13] (See Chapter 15 for the newest blood pressure guidelines.)

Improved Blood Lipid and Lipoprotein Profile Lipids are fats that circulate in the bloodstream and are stored in various places in the body. Regular exercise is known to reduce the levels of low-density lipoproteins (LDLs—"bad" cholesterol) while increasing the number of high-density lipoproteins (HDLs—"good" cholesterol) in the blood. Higher HDL levels are associated with lower risk for artery disease because they remove some of the "bad cholesterol" from artery walls and hence prevent clogging. The bottom

line: Regular exercise lowers the risk of cardiovascular disease. (For more on cholesterol and blood pressure, see Chapter 15.)

Improved Bone Mass

A common affliction among older adults is **osteoporosis**, a disease characterized by low bone mass and deterioration of bone tissue, which increase fracture risk. Osteoporosis currently affects 20–25 million Americans, 90 percent of them women. About 50 percent of all women eventually develop osteoporosis. Men are not immune; nearly 2 million men have the disease.

Osteoporosis is more common among women than among men for at least three reasons: Women live longer, they have lower peak bone mass than men, and women lose bone mass at a faster rate after menopause as their estrogen levels decrease. Thus, the incidence of osteoporosis and fractures increases substantially with age in both women and men. In the United States alone, nearly 1.5 million osteoporosis-related fractures occur every year![14] The annual cost of medical care related to hip fractures in the United States may exceed $240 billion by the mid-twenty-first century.[15]

Bone, like other human tissues, responds to the demands placed upon it. Women (and men) have much to gain by remaining physically active as they age—bone mass levels are significantly higher among active than among sedentary women.[16] New research indicates that by "surprising" bone (by jumping and other sudden activities), young children may improve their bone density.[17] Regular weight-bearing exercise, when combined with a balanced diet containing adequate calcium, will help keep bones healthy.[18]

Improved Weight Control

Many people start exercising because they want to lose weight. Level of physical activity does have a direct effect upon metabolic rate, even raising it for several hours following a vigorous workout. According to the American College of Sports Medicine, if you want to lose weight through exercise alone without decreasing the amount of food you eat, you should exercise frequently (at least four days a week) for extended time periods (at least 50 minutes per workout).[19] An even more effective method for losing weight combines regular endurance-type exercises with a moderate decrease in food intake. Cutting daily caloric intake beyond this range ("severe dieting") actually decreases metabolic rate by up to 20 percent and makes weight loss more difficult.

A recent meta-analysis challenges the commonly held view that exercise alone is not a useful strategy for obesity reduction. Moderately obese white men who participated in daily exercise of moderate intensity (brisk walking) for 45 to 60 minutes per day, without decreasing their caloric intake, made rapid improvements in cardiovascular fitness and lost weight.[20] Regular exercise also reduced the incidence of heart disease and type 2 diabetes in these participants and reduced the overall death rate.[21]

Osteoporosis A disease characterized by low bone mass and deterioration of bone tissue, which increase risk of fracture.

Table 10.2
The Effect of Physical Activity (PA) on Mental Health

TRAIT OR DISORDER	EFFECT	COMMENTS
Depression	Moderate decrease	Decreases symptoms; efficacy similar to psychotherapy in patients with mild-to-moderate depression; unclear whether PA prevents onset of depression, but it may reduce symptom severity
Anxiety	Small-to-moderate decrease	Reduces state anxiety but unclear whether it improves trait anxiety
Panic disorder	Small decrease	Often produces transient increase in anxiety, but anxiety dissipates with time if patient adheres to regimen of activity
Energy/vigor	Large increase	Intensive PA increases perceived energy level; unclear whether regular PA influences habitual energy levels
Self-esteem	Small-to-moderate increase	Greatest improvement found in those with low self-esteem before PA
Positive affect	Small-to-moderate increase	Effect most pronounced if PA involves social interaction
Eating disorders	Unclear	Intensive PA or exercise may be symptom of an eating disorder

Source: From "Physical Activity Improves Mental Health," by K. R. Fontaine, 2000, *The Physician and Sports Medicine* 28, pp. 83–84.

Improved Health and Life Span

Prevention of Diabetes Non-insulin-dependent diabetes (type 2 diabetes) is a complex disorder that affects millions of Americans, many of whom have no idea that they have the disease. (See Chapter 18.) Risk factors for diabetes include obesity, high blood pressure, and high cholesterol, as well as a family history of the disease.[22] Physicians suggest exercise combined with weight loss and proper diet to manage diabetes. A recent large study found that for every 2,000 calories of energy expended during leisure time activities, the incidence of diabetes was reduced by 24 percent. Perhaps the most encouraging finding was that the protective effect of exercise was greatest among those individuals who were at the highest risk.[23]

Longer Life Span A landmark study conducted at the Institute for Aerobics Research in Texas found that exercise does increase longevity. More than 13,000 white men and women of ages 20 to 80 were followed for eight years. Participants were assigned fitness levels based upon their age, sex, and results of exercise tests. The death rate in the least physically fit group was more than three times higher than that of the most fit group. How much physical activity was required to produce a difference? Sedentary participants who started taking a brisk 30- to 60-minute walk each day experienced significant increases in life expectancy.[24]

Improved Immunity to Disease Recent research suggests that regular moderate exercise makes people less susceptible to disease, although this benefit may depend upon whether they perceive exercise as pleasurable or stressful.[25] However, extreme exercise may actually be detrimental. For example, athletes engaging in marathon-type events or very intense physical training have an increased risk of colds and flu.[26] In a recent study of 2,300 marathon runners, those who ran more than 60 miles per week suffered twice as many upper respiratory tract infections as those who ran fewer than 20 miles per week.[27]

Just how exercise alters immunity is not well understood. We do know that brisk exercise temporarily increases the number of white blood cells (WBCs), the blood cells responsible for fighting infection. Generally speaking, the less fit the person and the more intense the exercise, the greater the increase in WBCs.[28] After brief periods of exercise (without injury), the number of WBCs typically returns to normal levels within one to two hours. After exercise bouts lasting longer than 30 minutes, WBCs may be elevated for 24 hours or more before returning to normal levels.[29] An increased number of WBCs suggests greater immunity to disease and infection.

Improved Mental Health and Stress Management

People who engage in regular physical activity also notice psychological benefits (see Table 10.2). Regular vigorous exercise has been shown to "burn off" the chemical by-products released by the nervous system during normal response to stress. This reduces stress levels by accelerating the body's return to a balanced state. Regular exercise improves physical appearance by toning and developing muscles and reducing body fat. Feeling good about personal appearance boosts self-esteem. At the same time, as people come to appreciate the

The Female Athlete Triad: When Exercise Becomes Obsession

In a quest to be thin and achieve the ideal body, many women, particularly those who are physically active, are at risk for a group of symptoms called the Female Athlete Triad. This often unrecognized disorder is a combination of conditions: disordered eating, amenorrhea (lack of menstrual periods), and osteoporosis.

Combining disordered eating behaviors (anorexia, bulimia, or other forms of binging, purging, or restricted eating) with excessive exercise can lead to changes in normal body functions. If the disordered eating is prolonged or without effective intervention, serious calcium depletion, changes in body hormones, and other negative effects may cause weakening of bone and other problems. Severe cases can lead to disability or even death.

Although men can suffer from many of these symptoms, the problem tends to be much more common in females, particularly those in highly competitive sports where self-discipline and perfection are valued. Athletes in gymnastics, ice skating, cross-country running, and swimming programs and ballet dancers are at the highest risk for the Female Athlete Triad.

Physical Warning Signs

Fatigue
Anemia
Tendency toward stress fractures and injury
Cold intolerance
Sore throat
Erosion of dental enamel from frequent vomiting
Abdominal pain and bloating
Constipation
Dry skin
Lightheadedness/fainting
Chest pain
Irregular or absent menstrual periods
Lanugo (fine, downy hair covering the body)
Changes in endurance, strength, or speed

Behavioral Warning Signs

Use of weight loss products and/or laxatives
Depression
Decreased ability to concentrate
Excessive and compulsive exercise
Preoccupation with food and weight
Trips to bathroom during or after eating
Increasing self-criticism and hostility to self

The American College of Sports Medicine and other groups are noticing a growing incidence of the Female Athlete Triad in physically active girls and women who don't compete athletically but want to look and feel their best. Vigilance by parents, friends, and others is important. If you wonder whether a friend or family member may be experiencing the symptoms of the Female Athlete Triad, ask her about her behavior. A key is to pay attention and notice what is happening. If symptoms are present, a multidisciplinary approach involving parents, coaches, friends, physicians, dietitians, and mental health professionals is warranted.

Sources: Brown University Health Education Office, "Nutrition: Eating Concerns: The Female Athlete Triad" (2002) (see www.brown.edu/Student_Services/Health_Services); Nebraska Cooperative Extension, "NEB Facts: The Female Athlete Triad" (1998) (see http://www.ianr.unl.edu/pubs/foods/nf361.htm).

---

improved strength, conditioning, and flexibility that accompany fitness, they often become less obsessed with physical appearance.[30] They learn new skills and develop increased abilities in favorite recreational activities, which also raise self-esteem. For some, however, the quest for fitness can lead to obsessive exercise patterns, such as the Female Athlete Triad (see the Women's Health/Men's Health box).

What do you think?

Among the many benefits to be derived from physical activity, which two are most important to you? * *Why?* * *After exercising regularly for several days, what benefits do you notice?*

Improving Cardiorespiratory Fitness

The number of walkers, joggers, bicyclists, step aerobics performers, and swimmers is tangible evidence of Americans' increased interest in cardiorespiratory fitness. The primary category of physical activity known to improve cardiorespiratory endurance is **aerobic exercise.** The term *aerobic* means "with oxygen" and describes any type of exercise, typically performed at moderate levels of intensity for extended periods of time, that increases your heart rate. A person said to be in "good shape" has an above-average **aerobic capacity**— a term used to describe the functional status of the cardiorespiratory system (i.e., heart, lungs, blood vessels). Aerobic capacity (commonly written as $VO_{2\ max}$) is defined as the maximum volume of oxygen consumed by the muscles during exercise.

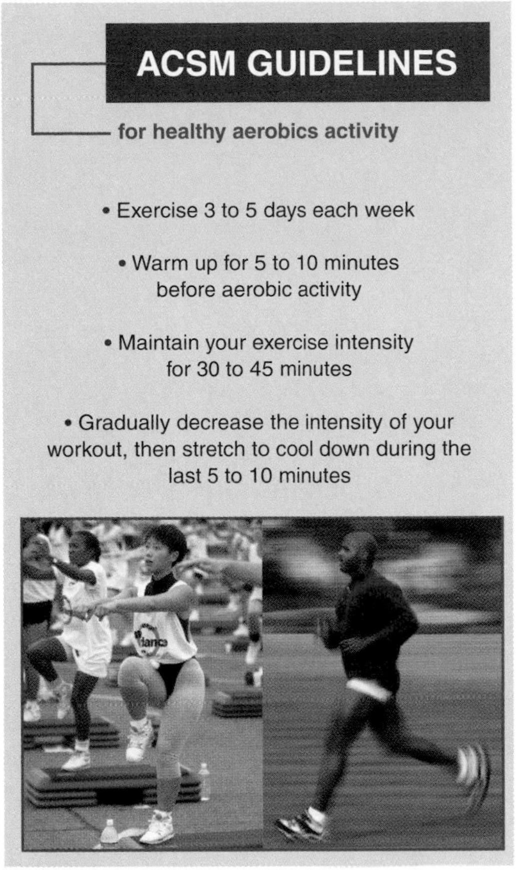

Figure 10.1
ACSM Guidelines for Aerobic Activity
Source: Reprinted with permission of the American College of Sports
Medicine © American College of Sports Medicine 2003.

To measure your maximal aerobic capacity, an exercise physiologist or physician will typically have you exercise on a treadmill. He or she will initially ask you to walk at an easy pace, and then, at set time intervals during this **graded exercise test,** will gradually increase the workload (i.e., a combination of running speed and the angle of incline of the treadmill). Generally, the higher your cardiorespiratory endurance level, the more oxygen you can transport to exercising muscles and the longer you can exercise without becoming exhausted. In other words, the higher the $VO_{2\ max}$ value, the higher your level of aerobic fitness.

You can test your own aerobic capacity by using either the 1.5-mile run or the 12-minute run endurance test described in the Assess Yourself box. However, you should not use these endurance-run tests if you are just starting to exercise.[31] Progress slowly through a walking/jogging program at low intensities before measuring your aerobic capacity with one of these tests. If you're new to exercise, or you have any medical conditions such as asthma, diabetes, heart disease, or obesity, consult your physician before beginning an exercise program.

Aerobic Fitness Programs

What level of activity is required to improve aerobic fitness? There are numerous variables in any particular aerobic activity, but for healthy young adults, aerobic activity that works your heart at a moderate intensity (approximately 70 percent of your maximum heart rate, or about 140 to 160 beats per minute) for prolonged periods of time (20 to 60 minutes of continuous activity) will improve your fitness level.

The most beneficial aerobic exercises are total body activities involving all the large muscle groups of your body; for example, swimming, cross-country skiing, and rowing. If you have been sedentary for quite a while, simply initiating a physical activity program may be the hardest task you'll face. Don't be put off by the next-day soreness you are likely to feel. The key is to begin at a very low intensity, progress slowly, and stay with it!

Determining Exercise Frequency If you are a newcomer to regular physical activity, try to exercise at least three times per week. If you exercise less frequently, you will achieve fewer health benefits. The surgeon general recommends moderate amounts of daily physical activity.[32] As your fitness level improves, your goal should be to exercise 20 to 30 minutes per day, five days a week. Figure 10.1 provides the American College of Sports Medicine guidelines for healthy aerobic activity.

Determining Exercise Intensity Your aerobic exercise program should employ activities of moderate intensity that use large muscle groups and can be maintained for prolonged periods of time. The measure of such a workout is your **target heart rate,** which is a percentage of your maximum heart rate. To calculate target heart rate, subtract your age from 220 for females or from 226 for males. The result is your maximum heart rate. You determine your target heart rate by calculating a desired percentage of

Aerobic exercise Any type of exercise, typically performed at moderate levels of intensity for extended periods of time (typically 20 to 30 minutes or longer), that increases heart rate.

Aerobic capacity The current functional status of a person's cardiovascular system; measured as $VO_{2\ max}$.

Graded exercise test A test of aerobic capacity administered by a physician, exercise physiologist, or other trained person; two common forms are the treadmill running test and the stationary bike test.

Target heart rate Calculated as a percentage of maximum heart rate (226 or 220 minus age); heart rate (pulse) is taken during aerobic exercise to check if exercise intensity is at the desired level (e.g., 70 percent of maximum heart rate).

Self-Assessment of Cardiorespiratory Endurance

After you have exercised regularly for several months, you might want to assess your cardiorespiratory endurance level. Find a local track, typically one-quarter mile per lap, to perform your test. You may either run or walk for 1.5 miles and measure how long it takes to reach that distance, or run or walk for 12 min-utes and determine the distance you covered in that time. Use the chart below to estimate your cardiorespiratory fitness level based upon your age and sex. Note that women have lower standards for each fitness category because they have higher levels of essential fat than men do.

Age*	1.5-Mile Run (min:sec)		12-Minute Run (miles)	
	Women (min:sec)	Men (min:sec)	Women (miles)	Men (miles)
Good				
15–30	<12:00	<10:00	>1.5	>1.7
35–50	<13:30	<11:30	>1.4	>1.5
55–70	<16:00	<14:00	>1.2	>1.3
Adequate for most activities				
15–30	<13:30	<11:50	>1.4	>1.5
35–50	<15:00	<13:00	>1.3	>1.4
55–70	<17:30	<15:30	>1.1	>1.3
Borderline				
15–30	<15:00	<13:00	>1.3	>1.4
35–50	<16:30	<14:30	>1.2	>1.3
55–70	<19:00	<17:00	>1.0	>1.2
Need extra work on cardiovascular fitness				
15–30	>17:00	>15:00	<1.2	<1.3
35–50	>18:30	>16:30	<1.1	<1.2
55–70	>21:00	>19:00	<0.9	<1.0

*Cardiorespiratory fitness declines with age.

If you are now at the Good level, congratulations! Your emphasis should be on maintaining this level for the rest of your life. If you are now at lower levels, set realistic goals for improvement.

Source: Reprinted by permission from Edward T. Howley and B. Don Franks, *Health Fitness Instructor's Handbook,* 3rd ed. (Champaign, IL: Human Kinetics Publishers, 1997), 85.

maximum heart rate, often 60 percent. Thus, if you are a 20-year-old female, your 60 percent target heart rate would be 120 [(220 − 20) x 0.60].

People in poor physical condition should set a target heart rate between 40 and 50 percent of maximum. As your condition improves, you can gradually increase your target heart rate. Increases should be made in small increments, from 40 to 45 percent, then from 45 to 50 percent.

Heart rate reserve is another way to determine target heart rate. First, subtract your resting heart rate (bpm taken after 10 minutes of complete rest) from your maximum heart rate. This is your heart rate reserve. Then take a percentage of this figure (often 60 percent) and add it to your resting heart rate. The result is your target heart rate.

Once you know your target heart rate, you can take your pulse to determine how close you are to this value during your workout. As you exercise, lightly place your index and middle fingers (don't use your thumb) on your radial artery (inside your wrist, on the thumb side). Using a watch or clock, take your pulse for six seconds and multiply this number by 10 (just add a zero to your count) to get the number of beats per minute (bpm). Your pulse should be within a range of 5 bpm above or below your target heart rate. If necessary, adjust the pace or intensity of your workout to achieve your target heart rate.

A target heart rate of 70 percent of maximum is sometimes called the "conversational level of exercise" because you are able to talk with a partner while exercising.[33] If you are breathing so hard that talking is difficult, your intensity of exercise is too high. If you can sustain a conversational level of aerobic exercise for 20 to 30 minutes, you will improve your cardiorespiratory fitness.

Determining Exercise Duration Duration refers to the number of minutes of activity performed during any one session. The Centers for Disease Control and Prevention (CDC) and the American College of Sports Medicine (ACSM) suggest that every adult engage in 20 to 60 minutes of continuous or intermittent (if intermittent, bouts of at least 10-minutes duration) moderate-intensity physical activity most days of the week.[34] Activities that can contribute to this total include dancing, walking up stairs (instead of taking the elevator), gardening, and raking leaves, as well as planned physical activities such as jogging, swimming, and cycling. One way to meet the CDC/ACSM recommendation is to walk two miles briskly.

The lower the intensity of your activity, the longer the duration you'll need to get the same caloric expenditure. For example, a 120-pound woman will burn 180 calories walking for one hour at 2.0 miles per hour but will burn 330 calories if she walks for an hour at a pace of 4.5 miles per hour. A 180-pound man will expend 288 calories per hour playing golf if he carries his clubs but will burn 805 calories per hour cross-country skiing.[35] Your goal should be to expend 300 to 500 calories per exercise session, with an eventual weekly goal of 1,500 to 2,000 calories. As you progress, add to your exercise load by increasing duration or intensity, but not both at the same time. From week to week, don't increase duration or intensity by more than 10 percent.

A program of repeated sessions of exercise over several months or years—exercise training—changes the way your cardiovascular system meets your body's oxygen requirements at rest and during exercise. Since many of the health benefits associated with cardiorespiratory fitness activities take about one year of regular exercise to achieve, don't expect improvements overnight.[36] However, any physical activity of low-to-moderate intensity will benefit your overall health almost from the start (see Figure 10.2). If you are reluctant to start an exercise program, see the two Skills for Behavior Change boxes in this chapter for strategies.

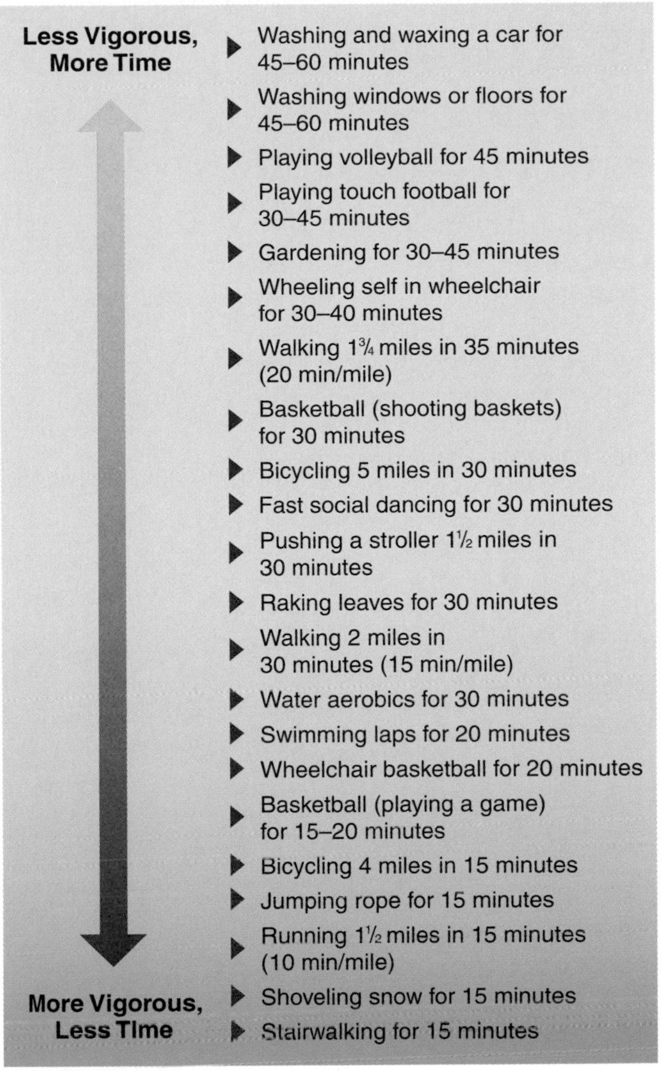

Less Vigorous, More Time

- Washing and waxing a car for 45–60 minutes
- Washing windows or floors for 45–60 minutes
- Playing volleyball for 45 minutes
- Playing touch football for 30–45 minutes
- Gardening for 30–45 minutes
- Wheeling self in wheelchair for 30–40 minutes
- Walking 1¾ miles in 35 minutes (20 min/mile)
- Basketball (shooting baskets) for 30 minutes
- Bicycling 5 miles in 30 minutes
- Fast social dancing for 30 minutes
- Pushing a stroller 1½ miles in 30 minutes
- Raking leaves for 30 minutes
- Walking 2 miles in 30 minutes (15 min/mile)
- Water aerobics for 30 minutes
- Swimming laps for 20 minutes
- Wheelchair basketball for 20 minutes
- Basketball (playing a game) for 15–20 minutes
- Bicycling 4 miles in 15 minutes
- Jumping rope for 15 minutes
- Running 1½ miles in 15 minutes (10 min/mile)
- Shoveling snow for 15 minutes
- Stairwalking for 15 minutes

More Vigorous, Less Time

Figure 10.2
Levels of Physical Activity
A moderate amount of physical activity is roughly equivalent to physical activity that uses approximately 150 calories (kcal) of energy per day, or 1,000 calories per week. Some activities can be performed at various intensities: The suggested durations correspond to expected intensity of effort.
Source: From "A Report of the Surgeon General: Physical Activity and Health," by the Surgeon General's Office, 1996, U.S. Department of Health and Human Services.

What do you think?
Calculate your maximum heart rate. Pick an intensity of exercise that suits your fitness level, for example, 60, 70, or 80 percent of your maximum heart rate. Using a familiar physical activity and monitoring your pulse, experiment by exercising at three different intensities. ✳ *Did you notice any difference in the way you felt while exercising?* ✳ *Afterward?*

Starting an Exercise Routine

Beginners often start their exercise programs too rigorously. The most successful exercise program is one that is realistic and appropriate for your skill level and needs. Be realistic about the amount of time you will need to get into good physical condition. Perhaps the most significant factor early on in an exercise program is personal comfort. Experiment and find an activity that you truly enjoy. Be open to exploring new activities and new exercise equipment.

- *Start slow.* For the sedentary, first-time exerciser, any type and amount of physical activity will be a step in the right direction. If you are extremely overweight or out of condition, you might only be able to walk for five min-

utes at a time. Don't be discouraged; you're on your way!

- *Make only one life change at a time.* Success at one major behavioral change will encourage you to make other positive changes.
- *Set reasonable expectations for yourself and your fitness program.* Many people become exercise dropouts because their expectations were too high to begin with. Allow sufficient time to reach your fitness goals.
- *Choose a specific time to exercise and stick with it.* Learning to establish priorities and keeping to a schedule are vital steps toward improved fitness. Experiment by exercising at different times of the day to learn what schedule works best for you.
- *Exercise with a friend.* It's easier to keep your exercise commitment if you exercise with someone else. Partners

can motivate and encourage each other, provided they remember that the rate of progress will not be the same for them both.

- *Make exercise a positive habit.* Usually, if you are able to practice a desired activity for three weeks, you will be able to incorporate it into your lifestyle.
- *Keep a record of your progress.* Include various facts about your physical activities (duration, intensity) and chronicle your emotions and personal achievements as you progress.
- *Take lapses in stride.* Physical deconditioning—a decline in fitness level—occurs at about the same rate as physical conditioning. Renew your commitment to fitness, and then restart your exercise program.

Why Are Flexibility and Strength Exercises Important?

Stretching Exercises and Well-Being

Who would guess that improved flexibility can give you a sense of well-being, help you deal with stress better, or stop your joints from hurting as much as they used to? But that's just what people who have improved their flexibility are saying. Stretching exercises have become the main highway to improved flexibility. Today, they are extremely popular, both because they work and because people can begin them at virtually any age and enjoy them for a lifetime. We'll look at three especially popular forms of exercise that focus on stretching and developing core muscle strength: yoga, tai chi, and Pilates.

A major objective of stretching exercises is to improve **flexibility,** a measure of the range of motion, or the amount of movement possible, at a particular joint. Improving the range of motion enhances efficiency, extent of movement, and posture. In addition, flexibility exercises have been shown to be effective in reducing the incidence and severity of lower back problems and muscle or tendon injuries that can occur during sports or everyday physical activities.[37] Improved flexibility can also mean less tension and pressure on joints, resulting in less joint pain and joint deterioration.

Flexibility is enhanced by the controlled stretching of muscles and muscle attachments that act on a particular joint. Each muscle involved in a stretching exercise is attached to our skeleton by tendons. Figure 10.3 illustrates an example of the connection between muscle, bone, and tendons. The goal of stretching is to decrease the resistance of a muscle and its tendons to tension, that is, to reduce resistance to being stretched. Stretching exercises gradually result in greater flexibility. In stretching exercises a muscle or group of muscles is stretched to a point of slight discomfort and that position is held for 20 to 30 seconds or more. For many people a regular program of stretching exercises enhances psychological as well as physical well-being.

Types of Stretching Exercises

In the language of exercise science, all of the commonly practiced stretching exercises fall into two major categories: static and proprioceptive neuromuscular facilitation (PNF).[38] **Static stretching** techniques involve the slow, gradual stretching of muscles and their tendons, then holding them at a point. During this holding period—the stretch—participants may feel mild discomfort and a warm sensation in the stretched muscles. Static stretching exercises involve specialized tension receptors in our muscles. When done properly, static stretching slightly lessens the sensitivity of tension receptors, which allows the muscle to relax and be stretched to

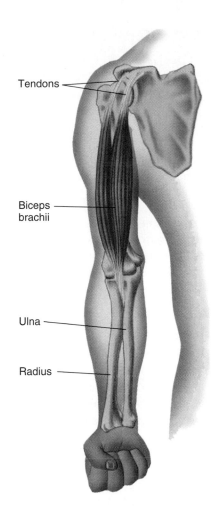

Figure 10.3
Muscles, Bones, and Tendons
Source: From Sharon A. Plowman and Denise L. Smith *Exercise Physiology for Health, Fitness, and Performance, Second Edition* (San Francisco, CA: Benjamin Cummings, 2003).

greater length.[39] The stretch is followed by a slow return to the starting position. The physical aspect of yoga and tai chi is largely composed of static techniques, as are some of the exercises in Pilates programs. (See next section.)

The second major type of stretching exercise, **proprioceptive neuromuscular facilitation (PNF),** is relatively new. While PNF techniques have been shown to be superior to other stretching techniques for improving flexibility, they are, unfortunately, quite complex in their original form. A certified athletic trainer or physical therapist may be required to help in performing PNF exercises correctly; however, several have been simplified to the point that they can be performed with an exercise partner or even alone. PNF techniques involve contraction of a muscle followed by a stretch.

Ballistic stretching involves repeated bouncing motions, during which the muscle and tendon are rapidly stretched and returned to resting length. This process can be likened to taking a rubber band between two fingers, rapidly pulling it apart, and then releasing the tension, again and again. And just as a rubber band can snap in your fingers if you apply too much tension, the muscle fibers being stretched in this way can be torn during these rapid movements. The risk of injury with ballistic stretching is so high that this type of stretching is no longer recommended.

Yoga, Tai Chi, and Pilates

Three major styles of exercise that include stretching have become widely practiced in the United States and other Western countries. **Yoga** originated in India about 5,000 years ago. **Tai chi** is an ancient Chinese form of exercise that, like yoga, combines stretching, balance, coordination, and meditation. Yoga and tai chi are excellent for improving flexibility and muscular coordination. **Pilates** combines stretching with movement against resistance, which is aided by devices such as tension springs or heavy rubber bands. All three of these popular exercise programs include a joining of mind and body as a result of intense concentration on breathing and body position.

Yoga has become one of the most popular fitness and static stretching activities. Yoga blends the mental and physical aspects of exercise, a union of mind and body that participants find rewarding and satisfying. Done regularly, its combination of mental focus and physical effort improves vitality, posture, agility, and coordination.

The practice of yoga focuses attention on controlled breathing as well as purely physical exercise. In addition to its mental dimensions, yoga incorporates a complex array of static stretching exercises expressed as postures (*asanas*). Over 200 postures exist, but only about 50 are commonly

Flexibility   The measure of the range of motion, or the amount of movement possible, at a particular joint.

Static stretching   Techniques that gradually lengthen a muscle to an elongated position (to the point of discomfort) and hold that position for 10 to 30 seconds.

Proprioceptive neuromuscular facilitation (PNF) stretching   Techniques that involve the skillful use of alternating muscle contractions and static stretching in the same muscle.

Yoga   A variety of Indian traditions geared toward self-discipline and the realization of unity; includes forms of exercise widely practiced in the West today that promote balance, coordination, flexibility, and meditation.

Tai chi   An ancient Chinese form of exercise widely practiced in the West today that promotes balance, coordination, stretching, and meditation.

Pilates   Exercise programs that combine stretching with movement against resistance, aided by devices such as tension springs and heavy bands.

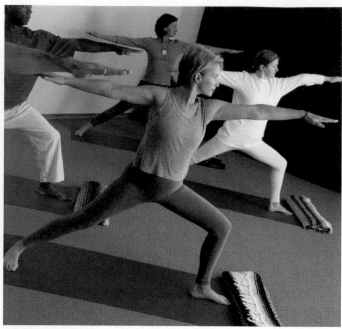

Styles of exercise that involve stretching and strengthening of core body muscles help enhance flexibility and lower stress levels.

practiced. During a session participants move to different asanas and hold them for 30 seconds or more. Yoga not only enhances flexibility, it has the great advantage of being flexible itself. Asanas and combinations of asanas can be changed and adjusted for young and old and to accommodate people with physical limitations or disabilities. Asanas can also be combined to provide even conditioned athletes with challenging sessions.

A typical yoga session will move the spine and joints through their full range of motion. Yoga postures lengthen, strengthen, and balance musculature, leading to increased flexibility, stamina, and strength—and many people report a psychological sense of general well-being.

There are many styles of yoga. Here are three of the most popular:

• *Iyengar yoga* focuses on precision and alignment in the poses. Standing poses are basic to this style, and poses are often held longer than in other styles.
• *Ashtanga yoga* in its pure form is based on a specific flow of poses that creates internal heat. The copious sweating that results is said to have a cleansing effect. Power yoga, a style growing in popularity, is a derivative of Ashtanga yoga.
• *Bikram's yoga* is similar to power yoga but does not incorporate a specific flow of poses. Literally the hottest yoga going, it is performed in temperatures of 100° Fahrenheit, or even a bit higher.

Tai chi is an exercise regimen that is designed to increase range of motion and flexibility while reducing muscular tension. Based on Chi Kung, a Taoist philosophy dedicated to spiritual growth and good health, tai chi was developed about

1000 A.D. by monks to defend themselves against bandits and warlords. It involves a series of positions called *forms* that are performed continuously.

Compared to yoga and tai chi, Pilates is the new kid on the exercise block. It was developed by Joseph Pilates, who came from Germany to New York City in 1926. Shortly after his arrival, he introduced his exercise methodology, which emphasizes flexibility, coordination, strength, and tone. Pilates differs in part from yoga and tai chi in that it includes a component designed to increase strength. The method consists of a sequence of carefully performed movements. Some are carried out on specially designed equipment, while others are performed on mats. Each exercise stretches and strengthens the muscles involved and has a specific breathing pattern associated with it. A class will focus on strengthening specific muscle groups, using equipment that provides resistance.

> **What do you think?**
>
> *Why is it so important to have good flexibility throughout life?* ❋ *Describe some situations in which improved flexibility would help you perform daily activities with less effort.* ❋ *What actions can you take to become more flexible?*

Designing Your Own Stretching Exercise Program: General Guidelines

If participation in formal classes isn't for you, you can easily design your own stretching exercise program. Figure 10.4 shows a selection of exercises that will stretch the major muscle groups of your body, and can be used as a warm-up for other physical activities and exercise programs such as jogging and tennis.

A program of regular stretching exercise doesn't need to take a great deal of time and doesn't require expensive equipment. You can reap the benefits of stretching with just two or three 10-minute sessions per week. Start off slowly with a five-minute session for the first week, then add a five-minute session each week, until you reach a schedule and comfort level that suit you. A hefty program would consist of five 30-minute sessions each week. Sessions get longer as you slowly increase the time you hold a particular stretch and how many times you repeat each type of stretch.

Improving Muscular Strength and Endurance

To get a sense of what resistance training is about, do a resistance exercise. Start by holding your right arm straight down by your side, then turn your hand palm up and bring it up toward your shoulder. That's a resistance exercise, using a

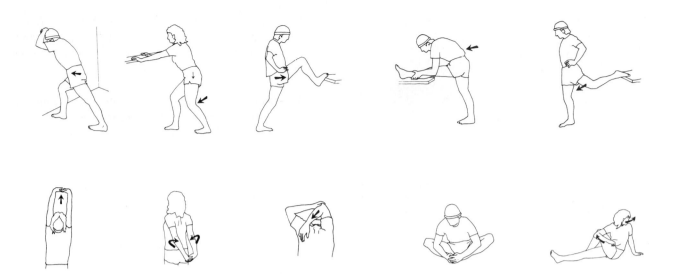

Figure 10.4
Stretching Exercises to Improve Flexibility
Source: Drawings from *Stretching, 20th Anniversary* revised Edition © 2000 Shelter Publications, Box 279, Bolinas, CA 94924.
Reprinted by permission.

muscle (your biceps) to move a resistance (in this case, just the weight of your hand)—not very much resistance. (Refer again to Figure 10.3.) Resistance training usually involves more weight or tension than this, but unlike flexibility training, resistance training is usually equipment intense. You don't get to look like Arnold Schwarzenegger doing these exercises empty handed. Free weights such as dumbbells and barbells and all sorts of tension-producing machines are usually part of resistance training. It's not just bodybuilding that uses this type of exercise, either. Fitness programs and many sports employ resistance training to improve strength and endurance, and many rehabilitation programs for recovery from injuries to muscles and joints are designed around resistance exercises.

Strength and Endurance

In the field of resistance training, **muscular strength** refers to the amount of force a muscle or group of muscles is capable of exerting. The most common way to assess strength in a resistance exercise program is to measure the **one repetition maximum (1 RM),** which is the maximum amount of weight a person can move one time in a particular exercise. For example, 1 RM for the simple exercise done at the beginning of this section is the maximum weight you lift to your shoulder one time. **Muscular endurance** is the ability of muscle to exert force repeatedly without fatiguing. If you can perform the exercise described earlier holding a five-pound weight in your hand and lifting 10 times, you will have greater endurance than someone who attempts that same exercise but is only able to lift the weight seven times.

Some resistance programs are designed primarily for increasing strength; others are aimed more at increasing endurance. Winning an Olympic weight-lifting event depends on the amount of weight that is lifted in just a few seconds. Endurance doesn't play a large role. Conversely, a soccer event lasts much longer and requires enormous endurance but not as much instantaneous brute strength as weight lifting. In football, strength and endurance are both important. Training for endurance uses smaller weights, but repeats an exercise more times than training for strength. If you were endurance training for performing our hand-to-shoulder exercise (called a curl in weight-training circles), you might hold a five-pound weight in each hand and curl 15 times per exercise segment. In training for strength, 40-pound weights might be used for a five-time curl.

Principles of Strength Development

An effective **resistance exercise program** involves three key principles: tension, overload, and specificity of training.[40]

The Tension Principle The key to developing strength is to create tension within a muscle or group of muscles. Tension is created by resistance provided by weights such as barbells or dumbbells, specially designed machines, or the weight of the body.

> **Muscular strength** The amount of force that a muscle is capable of exerting.
>
> **One repetition maximum (1 RM)** The amount of weight/resistance that can be lifted or moved once, but not twice; a common measure of strength.
>
> **Muscular endurance** A muscle's ability to exert force repeatedly without fatiguing.
>
> **Resistance exercise program** A regular program of exercises designed to improve muscular strength and endurance in the major muscle groups.

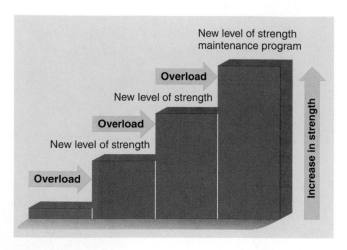

Figure 10.5
The Overload Principle
The overload principle contributes to an increase in strength. Notice that once the muscle has adapted to the original overload, a new overload must be placed on the muscle for subsequent strength gains to occur.
Source: From Philip A. Sienna, *One Rep Max: A Guide to Beginning Weight Training,* Fig. 2.1, 8. Copyright © 1989. William C. Brown Communications, Inc., Dubuque, Iowa. Reprinted by permission of Times Mirror Higher Education Group, Inc., Dubuque, Iowa. All rights reserved.

The Overload Principle   The overload principle is the most important of our three key principles. Overload doesn't mean forcing a muscle or group of muscles to do too much, which could result in injuries. Rather, overload in resistance training requires muscles to do more than they are used to. Everyone begins a resistance training program with an initial level of strength. To become stronger, you must regularly create a degree of tension in your muscles that is greater than you are accustomed to. This overload will cause your muscles to adapt to a new level. As your muscles respond to a regular program of overloading by getting larger, they become stronger. Figure 10.5 illustrates how a continual process of overload and adaptation to the overload improves strength.

Remember that resistance training exercises cause microscopic damage (tears) to muscle fibers, and the rebuilding process that increases the size and capacity of the muscle

---

Hypertrophy   Increased size (girth) of a muscle.

Isometric muscle action   Force produced without any resulting joint movement.

Concentric muscle action   Force produced while the muscle is shortening.

Eccentric muscle action   Force produced while the muscle is lengthening.

---

takes about 24 to 48 hours. Thus resistance training exercise programs should include at least one day of rest and recovery between workouts before overloading the same muscles again.

The Specificity-of-Training Principle   According to the specificity principle, the effects of resistance exercise training are specific to the muscles being exercised. Only the muscle or muscle group that you exercise responds to the demands placed upon it. For example, if you regularly do curls, the muscles involved—your biceps—will become larger and stronger, but the other muscles in your body won't change.

Gender Differences in Weight Training   The results of resistance training in men and women are quite different. Women don't normally develop muscle to the same extent that men do. The main reason for this difference is that men and women have different levels of the hormone testosterone in their blood. Before puberty, testosterone levels in blood are similar for both boys and girls. During adolescence, testosterone levels in boys increase dramatically, about tenfold, while testosterone levels in girls remain unchanged. Muscles will become larger **(hypertrophy)** as a result of resistance training exercise; typically this change is not as dramatic in women as it is in men. To enhance muscle bulk, some bodybuilders (both men and women) take synthetic hormones (anabolic steroids) that mimic the effects of testosterone. However, using anabolic steroids is a dangerous and illegal practice. (See Chapter 14.)

Types of Muscle Activity

Your skeletal muscles act in three different ways: isometric, concentric, and eccentric.[41] In **isometric muscle action,** force is produced through tension and muscle contraction, not movement. Figure 10.6(a) shows an isometric contraction. A **concentric muscle action,** shown in Figure 10.6(b), causes joint movement and a production of force while the muscle shortens. The empty-hand curl we did at the beginning of this section is a concentric exercise, with joint movement occurring at the elbow. In general, concentric muscle actions produce movement in a direction opposite to the downward pull of gravity. **Eccentric muscle action** describes the ability of a muscle to produce force while lengthening. Typically, eccentric muscle actions occur when movement is in the same direction as the pull of gravity; see Figure 10.6(c). Once you've brought a weight up during a curl, an eccentric muscle action would be to lower your hand and the weight back to their original position.

Methods of Providing Resistance

There are four commonly used resistance exercise methods: body weight resistance, fixed resistance, variable resistance, and the use of accommodating resistance devices.

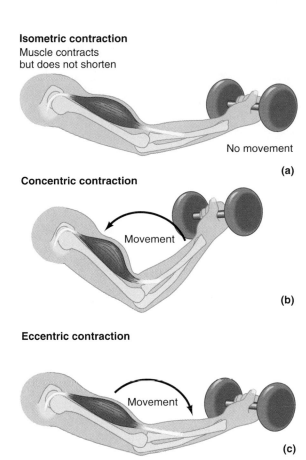

Isometric contraction
Muscle contracts
but does not shorten

No movement

(a)

Concentric contraction

Movement

(b)

Eccentric contraction

Movement

(c)

Figure 10.6
Isometric, Concentric, and Eccentric Muscle Actions
Source: S. Powers, and E. Howley, *Exercise Physiology: Theory and Application to Fitness and Performance* (Madison, WI: Brown and Benchmark, 1997).

Body Weight Resistance (Calisthenics)   Strength and endurance training doesn't always have to rely on equipment. You can use your own body weight to develop skeletal muscle fitness. Calisthenics use part or all of your body weight to offer resistance during exercise. While less effective than other resistance methods in developing large muscle mass and strength, calisthenics are quite adequate for improving general muscular fitness and generally sufficient to improve muscle tone and maintain a level of muscular strength.

Fixed Resistance   Fixed resistance exercises provide a constant amount of resistance throughout the full range of movement. Barbells, dumbbells, and some machines provide fixed resistance because their weight, or the amount of resistance, does not change during an exercise. Fixed resistance equipment has the potential to strengthen all the major muscle groups in the body.

One advantage of dumbbells and barbells is that they are relatively inexpensive. Fixed resistance exercise machines are commonly available at college recreation/fitness facilities, health clubs, and many resorts and hotels.

Variable Resistance   Variable resistance equipment alters the resistance encountered by a muscle during a movement, so that the effort by the muscle is more consistent throughout the full range of motion. Variable resistance machines, such as Nautilus™ and Hammer Strength™, are typically single-station devices; a person stays on the same machine throughout the whole series of exercises. Other types of machines, such as Soloflex™, have multiple stations and the person using them moves from one machine to another. While some of these machines are expensive and too big to move easily, others are affordable and more portable. Many forms of variable resistance devices are sold for home use.

Accommodating Resistance Devices   These machines adjust the resistance according to the amount of force generated by the person using the equipment. The exerciser performs at maximal level of effort, while the device controls the speed of the exercise. The machine is set to a particular speed, and muscles being exercised must move at a rate faster than or equal to that speed in order to encounter resistance.[42]

The Benefits of Strength Training

You may wonder about the benefits associated with strength training beyond that of simply getting stronger. It turns out that regular strength training has many other benefits as well. It can reduce the occurrence of lower back pain and joint and muscle injuries. It can also postpone loss of muscle tissue due to aging and a sedentary lifestyle and help prevent osteoporosis.

Strength training enhances muscle definition and tone and improves personal appearance. This, in turn, enhances self-esteem. Strength training even has a hidden benefit: Muscle tissue burns calories faster than most other tissues, even when it is resting. So, increasing your muscle mass can help you lose pounds and maintain a healthy weight.

Getting Started

When beginning a resistance exercise program, always consider your age, fitness level, and personal goals. Strength training exercises are done in a *set,* or a single series of multiple repetitions using the same resistance. The American College of Sports Medicine[43] recommends single-set resistance programs of up to 15 repetitions per exercise, performed at least two days per week. For instance, one set of curls could be 15 repetitions using 10-pound dumbbells. Each workout session should include 8 to 10 different resistance exercises that involve the major muscle groups of the upper and lower extremities and the trunk. Table 10.3 contains the essential information for a program to build muscular strength and muscular endurance. Remember, experts suggest allowing at least one day of rest and recovery between workouts. See the New Horizons in Health box for information on new research about beginning an exercise program.

Table 10.3
Resistance Training Program Guidelines

- Resistance training should be an integral part of an adult fitness program and of sufficient intensity to enhance strength, muscular endurance, and maintain fat-free mass.
- Resistance training should be progressive in nature, individualized, and provide a stimulus (overload) to all major muscle groups in the body.
- One set of 8 to 10 different resistance exercises that condition the major muscle groups two to three days per week is recommended.
- The goal of this type of resistance training program is to develop and maintain a significant amount of muscle mass, endurance, and strength to contribute to overall fitness and health throughout the life span.
- If sufficient time is available, multiple-set resistance exercise regimens using heavier weights and fewer repetitions will result in greater strength gains and fitness benefits.

Source: From "ACSM Position Stand of the Recommended Quantity and Quality of Exercise for Developing and Maintaining Cardiorespiratory and Muscular Fitness and Flexibility in Adults," by the American College of Sports Medicine, 1998, *Medicine and Science in Sports and Exercise* 30, pp. 975–991.

What do you think?

What types of resistance equipment can you currently access? ✳ Based on what you've read, what actions can you take to increase your muscular strength? ✳ Muscular endurance? ✳ How would you measure your improvement?

Body Composition

Body composition is the fifth and final component of a comprehensive fitness program. Body composition parameters that can be influenced by regular physical activity include total body mass, fat mass, fat-free mass, and regional fat distribution.[44] Body composition is significantly different between women and men, since women have a higher percentage of body fat and a significantly lower percentage of fat-free mass (such as muscle and bone) and bone mineral density.[45]

The most successful weight loss programs combine diet and exercise effectively (see Chapter 9). When participating in endurance training programs for the purpose of losing weight, total body mass and fat mass generally decrease while fat-free mass remains constant. If your main reason for exercising is to lose weight, then you'll need to combine diet with at least three workouts per week that expend 250 to 300 kcal per session (at least 30 to 45 minutes of continuous low-to-moderate–intensity activity, depending on your body weight) in order to see significant reductions in your total body mass and fat mass.[46]

Fitness Injuries

Overtraining is the most frequent cause of injuries associated with fitness activities. Enthusiastic but out-of-shape beginners often injure themselves by doing too much too soon. Pay attention to your body's warning signs. To avoid injuring a particular muscle group or body part, vary your fitness activities throughout the week to give muscles and joints a rest. Set appropriate short-term and long-term training goals. Establishing realistic but challenging fitness goals can help you stay motivated without overdoing it. Overtraining injuries occur most often in repetitive activities like swimming, running, bicycling, and step aerobics. However, use common sense and you're likely to remain injury-free.

Causes of Fitness-Related Injuries

There are two basic types of injuries stemming from participation in fitness-related activities: overuse and traumatic injuries. **Overuse injuries** occur because of cumulative, day-after-day stresses placed on tendons, bones, and ligaments during exercise. The forces that occur normally during physical activity are not enough to cause a ligament sprain or muscle strain, but when these forces are applied on a daily basis for weeks or months, they can result in an injury. Common sites of overuse injuries are the leg, knee, shoulder, and elbow joints.

Overuse injuries Injuries that result from the cumulative effects of day-after-day stresses placed on tendons, muscles, and joints.

Traumatic injuries Injuries that are accidental in nature, which occur suddenly and violently (e.g., fractured bones, ruptured tendons, and sprained ligaments).

What's New in the World of Exercise?

Two recent studies cast an interesting light on the benefits of exercise.

The first, a study of 2,428 adults over a six-year period, examined the risks that those of us who are out of shape face when we suddenly decide to don exercise clothes, lace up the shoes, and hit the exercise trail. The research team studied heart-rate changes in the first minute after exercise among patients who had previous symptoms of heart disease. They found that people whose hearts took longer to slow down, or recover, after exercise were nearly four times more likely to die during the six-year study period than participants with normal recovery times. While just 26 percent of all people in the study had abnormal recovery times, these people constituted 56 percent of all deaths during the course of the study. In addition, the study indicated that people who demonstrated good heart-rate recovery are more likely to benefit from heart surgery and other corrective procedures in the event of cardiovascular problems.

Results of the study indicate that people who have high blood pressure, are obese, take heart medications, and are out of condition physically face significant risks of heart failure when they begin unsupervised, strenuous physical activity. For someone out of shape, getting back into shape should be viewed as a serious behavioral change. Efforts to lose weight, reduce blood pressure, and work up to

high-energy expenditures should be done gradually and under a doctor's supervision. Although this has long been the recommended plan of action, this study confirmed the importance of following that plan. Most important, however, the study identified heart-rate recovery as a significant indicator of benefits and risks.

The second landmark study followed the exercise behavior patterns of over 14,000 female participants in the Nurses' Health Study. Although physical activity has long been associated with a lower risk of coronary heart disease, little has been known about the benefits of certain types of exercise, particularly for women. Walking, in particular, has long been believed to be highly beneficial and often has been recommended as part of a rehabilitation program for people recovering from heart problems and other serious illnesses, but questions still arose about its specific benefits. Until the Nurses' Health Study, the role of walking in the battle against heart disease had not been carefully analyzed, despite being the most common form of exercise among women.

In the Nurses' Health Study, women's risk factors and exercise behaviors were assessed every two years for a period of 14 years. Results of the study provide compelling evidence of the benefits of walking. Brisk walking may, in fact, be just as beneficial for reducing cardiovascular disease as vigorous exercise. Results suggested that a regimen of brisk walking for a total of three or more hours per week (an average of 30 minutes per day) could reduce the risk of coronary events by 30 percent to 40 percent. Increasing this time

provided even greater benefits. This is in line with the most recent recommendations from the Centers for Disease Control and Prevention, the American College of Sports Medicine, and the Surgeon General's Report on Physical Activity and Health.

What we have long suspected is true: Walking makes good sense! It is relatively available to everyone, requires no special equipment, can be done alone or in groups, and may be less damaging to joints over time than repetitive jogging or other strenuous activities. So put on those walking shoes, and let's get going!

Sources: From "Heart-Rate Recovery Immediately After Exercise as a Predictor of Mortality," by M. S. Lauer, E. Blackstone, F. J. Pashkow, C. Snader, and C. Cole, *The New England Journal of Medicine* 341 (1999): 1351–1357; and "A Prospective Study of Walking as Compared with Vigorous Exercise in the Prevention of Coronary Heart Disease in Women," by J. E. Manson et al., *The New England Journal of Medicine* 341 (1999): 650–659.

Traumatic injuries occur suddenly and violently, typically by accident. Typical traumatic injuries are broken bones, torn ligaments and muscles, contusions, and lacerations. Some traumatic injuries occur quickly and are difficult to avoid—for example, spraining your ankle by landing on another person's foot after jumping up for a rebound in basketball. If your traumatic injury causes a noticeable loss of function and immediate pain or pain that does not go away after 30 minutes, you should have a physician examine it.

Prevention

Your exercise clothing is more than a fashion statement—smart choices can help you prevent injuries. For some types of physical activity, you need clothing that allows body heat to dissipate—for example, light-colored nylon shorts and mesh tank top while running in hot weather. For other types, you need clothing that retains body heat without getting you sweat-soaked—for example, layers of polypropylene and/or wool clothing while cross-country skiing.

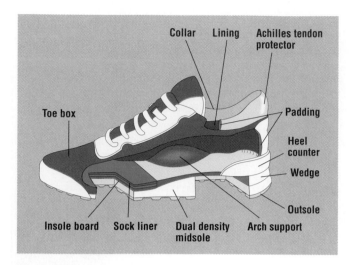

Figure 10.7
Anatomy of a Running Shoe
Source: Reprinted with permission of the American Council on Exercise (www.ACEfitness.org).

Appropriate Footwear When you purchase running shoes, look for several key components. Biomechanics research has revealed that running is a "collision" sport—that is, the runner's foot collides with the ground with a force three to five times the runner's body weight with each stride.[47] The 150-pound runner who takes 1,000 strides per mile applies a cumulative force to his or her body of 450,000 pounds per mile. The force not absorbed by the running shoe is transmitted upward into the foot, leg, thigh, and back. Our bodies are able to absorb forces such as these, but may be injured by the cumulative effects of repetitive impacts (e.g., running 40 miles per week). Therefore, the ability of running shoes to absorb shock is critical.

The midsole of a running shoe must absorb impact forces but must also be flexible (see Figure 10.7). To evaluate the flexibility of the midsole, hold the shoe between the index fingers of your right and left hand. When you push on both ends of the shoe with your fingers, the shoe should bend easily at the midsole. If the force exerted by your index fingers cannot bend the shoe, its midsole is probably too rigid and may irritate your Achilles tendon, among other problems.[48] Other basic characteristics of running shoes include a rigid plastic insert within the heel of the shoe (known as a heel counter) to control the movement of your heel; a cushioned foam pad surrounding the heel of the shoe to prevent Achilles tendon irritation; and a removable thermoplastic innersole that customizes the fit of the shoe by using your body heat to mold it to the shape of your foot. Shoes are the runner's most essential piece of equipment, so carefully select appropriate footwear before you start a running program.

Shoe companies also sell cross-training shoes to help combat the high cost of having to buy separate pairs of running shoes, tennis shoes, weight-training shoes, and so on.

Although the cross-training shoe can be used for participation in several different fitness activities by the novice or recreational athlete, a distance runner who runs 25 or more miles per week needs a pair of specialty running shoes to prevent injury.

Appropriate Exercise Equipment Some activities require special protective equipment to reduce chances of injury. Eye injuries can occur in virtually all fitness-related activities, although some are more risky than others. As many as 90 percent of the eye injuries resulting from racquetball and squash could be prevented by wearing appropriate eye protection—for example, goggles with polycarbonate lenses.[49] Nearly 100 million people in the United States ride bikes for pleasure, fitness, or competition. Head injuries used to account for 85 percent of all deaths attributable to bicycle accidents; however, bike helmets have significantly reduced the number of skull fractures and facial injuries.[50] Look for helmets that meet the standards established by the American National Standards Institute (ANSI) and the Snell Memorial Foundation (SNELL).

> **What do you think?**
>
> *Given your activity level, what injury risks are you exposed to on a regular basis?* ✷ *What changes can you make in your equipment and clothing to reduce these risks?*

Common Overuse Injuries

Body movements in physical activities such as running, swimming, and bicycling are highly repetitive, so participants are susceptible to overuse injuries. In fitness activities, the joints of the lower extremities (foot, ankle, knee, and hip) tend to be injured more frequently than the upper-extremity joints (shoulder, elbow, wrist, and hand). Three of the most common overuse injuries are plantar fasciitis, "shin splints," and "runner's knee."

Plantar Fasciitis Plantar fasciitis is an inflammation of the plantar fascia, a broad band of dense, inelastic tissue (fascia) that runs from the heel to the toe on the bottom of the foot. The main function of the plantar fascia is to protect the nerves, blood vessels, and muscles of the foot from injury. Repetitive weight-bearing fitness activities such as walking and running can inflame the plantar fascia. Common symptoms are pain and tenderness under the ball of the foot, at the heel, or at both locations.[51] The pain of plantar fasciitis is particularly noticeable during the first steps out of bed in the morning. If not treated properly, this injury may progress to the point that weight-bearing exercise is too painful to endure. Uphill running is not advised, since each uphill stride severely stretches (and thus irritates) the already inflamed plantar fascia. This injury can often be prevented by regularly stretching the plantar fascia prior to exercise and by wearing athletic shoes with good arch support and shock absorbency. Stretch the plantar fascia by slowly pulling all five toes upward toward your head, holding for 10 to 15 seconds. Repeat this three to five times on each foot prior to exercise.

Shin Splints A general term for any pain that occurs below the knee and above the ankle is "shin splints." This broad description includes more than 20 different medical conditions. Problems range from stress fractures of the tibia (shinbone) to severe inflammation in the muscles of the lower leg, which can interrupt the flow of blood and nerve supply to the foot. The most common type of shin splints occurs along the inner side of the tibia and is usually a combination of muscle irritation and irritation of the tissues that attach the muscles to the bone in this region. Typically, there is pain and swelling along the middle third of the posteromedial tibia in the soft tissues, not the bone.

Sedentary people who start a new weight-bearing exercise program are at the greatest risk for shin splints, though well-conditioned aerobic exercisers who rapidly increase their distance or pace may also develop them.[52] Running is the most frequent cause of shin splints, but those who do a great deal of walking (e.g., mail carriers, waitresses) may also develop this injury.

To help prevent shin splints, wear athletic shoes with good arch support and shock absorbency. If the pain continues, see your physician. You may be advised to substitute a non-weight-bearing activity such as swimming during your recovery period.

Runner's Knee *Runner's knee* describes a series of problems involving the muscles, tendons, and ligaments about the knee. The most common problem identified as runner's knee is abnormal movement of the kneecap, which irritates the cartilage on the back side of the kneecap as well as nearby tendons and ligaments.[53] Women experience this more often than men (see the Women's Health box).

The main symptom of this kind of runner's knee is the pain experienced when downward pressure is applied to the kneecap after the knee is straightened fully. Additional symptoms may include swelling, redness, tenderness around the kneecap, and a dull, aching pain in the center of the knee.[54] If you have these symptoms, your physician will probably recommend that you stop running for a few weeks and reduce daily activities that compress the kneecap (e.g., exercise on a stair-climbing machine or doing squats with heavy resistance) until you no longer feel any pain.

Treatment

First-aid treatment for virtually all personal fitness injuries involves **RICE**: **r**est, **i**ce, **c**ompression, and **e**levation. *Rest,* the first component of this treatment, is required to avoid further irritation of the injured body part. *Ice* is applied to relieve pain and constrict the blood vessels in order to stop any internal or external bleeding. Never apply ice cubes,

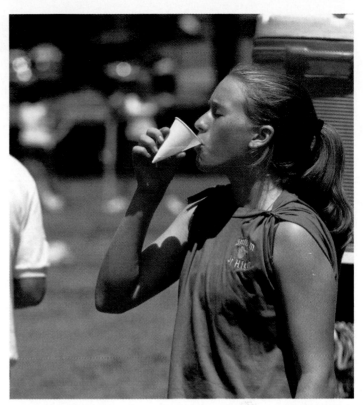

Any form of exercise done during hot weather carries the risk of heat exhaustion or heat stroke.

reusable gel ice packs, chemical cold packs, or other forms of cold directly to your skin. Instead, place a layer of wet toweling or elastic bandage between the ice and your skin. Ice should be applied to a new injury for approximately 20 minutes every hour for the first 24 to 72 hours. *Compression* of the injured body part can be accomplished with a 4- or 6-inch-wide elastic bandage; this applies indirect pressure to damaged blood vessels to help stop bleeding. Be careful, though, that the compression wrap does not interfere with normal blood flow. A throbbing, painful hand or foot is an indication that the compression wrap should be loosened. *Elevation* of the injured extremity above the level of your heart also helps to control internal or external bleeding by making the blood flow uphill to reach the injured area.

Exercising in the Heat

Heat stress, which includes several potentially fatal illnesses resulting from excessive core body temperatures, should be a concern when you are exercising in warm, humid weather. In these conditions, your body's rate of heat production can exceed its ability to cool itself.

RICE Acronym for the standard first-aid treatment for virtually all traumatic and overuse injuries: rest, ice, compression, and elevation.

Female Athletes and Knee Injuries

As women continue to raise the bar in the world of sports, we learn more and more about their potential. At the same time, however, we also learn more about their tendencies toward injury. Although medical experts are unsure of the reasons, female athletes appear to be more susceptible to knee injuries, particularly injuries to the anterior cruciate ligaments (ACLs). Recent studies indicate that women are five to eight times more likely than men to suffer painful, disabling ACL injuries at some point in their lives.

The ACL is a strand of soft tissue that, along with other ligaments, muscles, and tendons, helps stabilize the knee joint. Its role in pivoting, jumping, and sudden changes of direction is critical. Once it is damaged, mobility is often reduced. This ligament is most severely compromised when women partake in contact sports, such as soccer, basketball, and volleyball, although injuries have occurred in non-contact activities as well.

Once injured, the ACL must be repaired surgically and requires months of painful rehabilitation for any chance of a return to normal athletic levels. Even with therapy, ACL injuries can predispose people to later bouts of immobility, injuries due to lingering instability, and various forms of arthritis.

Why are we seeing this trend? Is it because female participation in sports has increased, or are female athletes truly more susceptible to these injuries? According to the American Academy of Orthopedic

Surgeons, the answer lies in physiological differences between males and females. Female athletes are thought to be at a disadvantage because of an imbalance in strength between the hamstring muscles behind the thigh and the quadriceps muscles in front of the thigh. When these two muscle groups work together, they act antagonistically to protect each other and supporting ligature, including that around the knee, from damage. Some researchers suggest that women tend to have underdeveloped or weak hamstrings, which increases the stress placed on the ACL, particularly during unusual movements. In addition, during actions such as jumping and landing, it is felt that women tend to land more straight-legged and flat-footed, a tendency related to weaker thigh muscles. In contrast, men often have much stronger quadriceps and hamstrings and tend to bend their knees and cushion the shock when jumping, causing less stress on supporting structures. Thus, in women who are underexercised or have a severe imbalance between their quadriceps and hamstrings, the risk of ACL injury increases. In addition to weaker muscles, sports medicine officials speculate that structural characteristics, such as wider hips, put greater pressure on the inside of the knee and less on the leg muscle.

Another hypothesis is that women are more prone to ACL injuries during ovulation, when increased estrogen reduces the production of collagen, the body's connective tissue. Orthopedic surgeon Dr. Edward M. Wojtys put this theory to the test by evaluating 40 young women with acute ACL injuries. He discovered that a majority of them did in fact sustain their injuries during ovulation, pointing to the need for further investigation.

So what can women do to protect themselves from ACL injuries? At this point, Dr. Wojtys says that there is no evidence that hormone supplements will protect women against ACL injuries. Doctors advise women to get involved in sports at an early age and partake in weight training and other types of conditioning that will build the hamstring muscles. When knee injuries do occur, they must be taken seriously and treated with rest, ice, compression, and elevation (RICE). If pain doesn't subside, a visit to an orthopedic surgeon may be necessary.

Sources: Johns Hopkins Health website, Health News Zone, http://www.intelihealth.com, "Keeping in the Game: Young Women and Their Knees"; The Doctor's Guide to Medical and Other News, "Link Found Between Menstrual Cycle and Knee Injuries," June 25, 1997.

You can help prevent heat stress by following certain precautions. First, proper acclimatization to hot and/or humid climates is essential. The process of heat acclimatization, which increases your body's cooling efficiency, requires about 10 to 14 days of gradually increased activity in the hot environment. Second, avoid dehydration by replacing the fluids you lose during and after exercise. Third, wear clothing appropriate for your activity and the environment. And finally, use common sense—for example, on an 85-degree, 80 percent humidity day, postpone your usual lunchtime run until the cool of evening.

The three different heat stress illnesses are progressive in severity: heat cramps, heat exhaustion, and heat stroke. **Heat cramps** (heat-related muscle cramps), the least serious problem, can usually be prevented by warm-ups, adequate fluid replacement, and a diet that includes the electrolytes lost during sweating (sodium and potassium). (For general information on cramps, see the next section.) **Heat exhaustion** is caused by excessive water loss resulting from prolonged exercise or work. Symptoms of heat exhaustion include nausea, headache, fatigue, dizziness and faintness, and, paradoxically, "goosebumps" and chills. If you are suffering from heat exhaustion, your skin will be cool and moist. Heat exhaustion is actually a mild form of shock, in which the blood pools in the arms and legs away from the brain and major organs of the body, causing nausea and fainting. **Heat stroke**, often called sunstroke, is a life-threatening emergency condition having a 20 to 70 percent death rate.[55] Heat stroke occurs during vigorous exercise when the body's heat production significantly exceeds its cooling capacities. Body core temperature can rise from normal (99.6°F) to 105°F to 110°F within minutes after the body's cooling mechanism shuts down. With no cooling taking place, rapidly increasing core temperatures can cause brain damage, permanent disability, and death. Common signs of heat stroke are dry, hot, and usually red skin; very high body temperature; and a very rapid heart rate.

If you experience any of the symptoms mentioned here, stop exercising immediately, move to the shade or a cool spot to rest, and drink large amounts of cool fluids. Be aware that heat stress can strike in situations in which the danger is not obvious. Serious or fatal heat strokes may result from prolonged sauna or steam baths, prolonged total immersion in a hot tub or spa, or exercising in a plastic or rubber head-to-toe "sauna suit."[56]

What are the best fluids to drink? The American College of Sports Medicine (ACSM) found little difference in human performance during exercise sessions lasting less than one hour when drinking plain water or "sports drinks" (carbohydrate-electrolyte drinks).[57] However, a recent study suggests otherwise. In a laboratory study requiring intense stationary bicycling (50 minutes of high-level activity followed by a 9- to 12-minute "sprint to the finish"), subjects' cycling performance improved by 6 percent when they drank enough water to replace 80 percent of the fluid they lost as sweat—and by 12 percent when they consumed a similar amount of a sports drink.[58]

Remember that dehydration of 1 to 2 percent of body weight quickly affects physiological function and performance. Dehydration of greater than 3 percent of body weight increases the risk of heat cramps, heat exhaustion, and heat stroke.[59] During intense exercise lasting longer than one hour, the ACSM recommends drinking fluids that contain 4 percent to 8 percent carbohydrates (to delay muscular fatigue) and a small amount of sodium (to improve taste and promote fluid retention). Fluid intake *following* physical activity is also important to prevent dehydration—be sure to drink at least a pint of fluid for every pound of body weight lost during your exercise session.

Exercising in the Cold

When you exercise in cool weather, especially in windy conditions, your body's rate of heat loss is frequently greater than its rate of heat production. Under these conditions, **hypothermia**—a potentially fatal condition resulting from abnormally low body core temperature, which occurs when body heat is lost faster than it is produced—may result. Hypothermia can occur as a result of prolonged, vigorous exercise (e.g., snowboarding or rugby) in 40°F to 50°F temperatures, particularly if there is rain, snow, or a strong wind.

In mild cases of hypothermia, as body core temperature drops from the normal 99.6°F to about 93.2°F, you will begin to shiver. Shivering—the involuntary contraction of nearly every muscle in the body—increases body temperature by using the heat given off by muscle activity. During this first stage of hypothermia, you may also experience cold hands and feet, poor judgment, apathy, and amnesia.[60] Shivering ceases in most hypothermia victims as body core temperatures drop to between 87°F and 90°F, a sign that the body has lost its ability to generate heat. Death usually occurs at body core temperatures between 75°F and 80°F.

To prevent hypothermia, follow these commonsense guidelines:

- Analyze weather conditions and your risk of hypothermia before you undertake an outdoor physical activity. Remember that wind and humidity are as significant as temperature.
- Use the "buddy system"—have a friend join you for cold weather outdoor activities.
- Wear layers of appropriate clothing to prevent excessive heat loss (e.g., polypropylene or woolen undergarments, a windproof outer garment, and wool hat and gloves).
- Finally, don't allow yourself to become dehydrated.[61]

Cramps: Taking Action to Prevent Problems

Although most of us have experienced the quick, intense pain of having a cramp in our foot, calf, or other body part,

---

Heat cramps Muscle cramps that occur during or following exercise in warm or hot weather.

Heat exhaustion A heat stress illness caused by significant dehydration resulting from exercise in warm or hot conditions; frequent precursor to heat stroke.

Heat stroke A deadly heat stress illness resulting from dehydration and overexertion in warm or hot conditions; can cause body core temperature to rise from normal to 105°F to 110°F in just a few minutes.

Hypothermia Potentially fatal condition caused by abnormally low body core temperature.

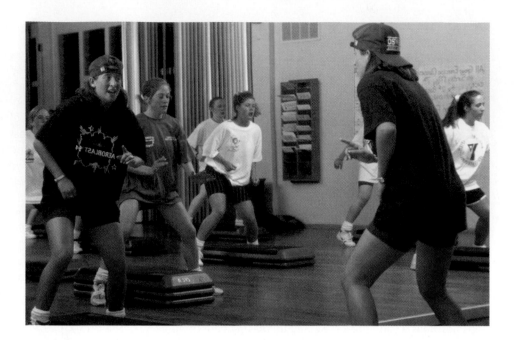

Most college campuses provide a recreation facility so that students and staff can stay fit.

knowing what causes them and what to do about them isn't always so obvious. Muscle cramps are poorly understood. We know that muscle cramps commonly occur among athletes who work their muscles to the point of exhaustion. The overexertion theory of muscle cramps says that when a muscle gets tired, the numerous muscle fibers that comprise the muscle fail to contract in a synchronized rhythm, probably due to overstimulation from the nerves that trigger the muscles to contract.[62]

Previous theories suggested that cramping is related to fluid loss and electrolyte imbalance, but these theories have not held up. For example, musicians, who do not often get sweaty, complain of muscle cramps.[63] Even if dehydration is not the only cause, it is clearly a problem for those who exercise heavily and tend to sweat a lot over prolonged periods of time. Drinking enough fluids before, during, and after such activity is important. On a daily basis, drink enough fluids so you have to urinate every two to four hours. Your urine should be pale and there should be lots of it. During extended exercise, it is recommended that you drink as much as you can tolerate, ideally eight ounces every 15–20 minutes.[64]

Although calcium plays a role in muscle contraction and people with a tendency to have cramps are often calcium deficient, exercise physiologists question the validity of the low-calcium theory. However, because calcium has many health benefits, experts continue to recommend it for anyone who has a tendency toward cramping.

Lack of sodium is yet another possible reason for cramps. If you exercise a lot and sweat a lot, you will lose sodium through sweat and may develop a sodium imbalance and experience cramps. This is most likely to occur in extreme sports such as Ironman triathlons or 100-mile trail runs, particularly in athletes who have consumed only plain water (not sodium-containing food or beverages)

during the event.[65] Many health-conscious athletes restrict their salt intake on a regular basis in an attempt to keep blood pressure under control, but clearly there is a risk in doing so.

Although paying attention to the above nutrients is important to avoid cramping, it is probably more important to make sure that muscles are warmed up and not strained beyond their limit.

If you get cramps, what should you do? Although different things work for different body parts, generally, massage, stretching, putting pressure on the muscle that is cramping, and deep breathing are useful remedies.

What do you think?

Given what you've read about the symptoms of common fitness injuries, are you currently developing any overuse injuries? ✳ If so, what can you do to prevent these problems from getting more serious?

Planning a Fitness Program

Identify Your Fitness Goals

Before you start a fitness program, analyze your personal needs, limitations, physical activity likes and dislikes, and daily schedule. Do you want to improve your quality of life? Lose weight? Lower your risk of health problems? Your specific goal may be to achieve (or maintain) healthy levels of body fat, cardiovascular fitness, muscular strength and endurance, or flexibility and mobility.

Starting an Exercise Program When You Are Overweight or Out of Shape

It isn't surprising that people who are overweight or obese may find it more difficult than their fit friends to start an exercise program. For an overweight person, exercise is like what an average-weight person would experience if she had to jog a mile, get on an elliptical trainer and go for miles, or even walk at a fast pace with 30, 50, or 100 extra pounds strapped on her body. If you are struggling with weight, you face this challenge every day. Carrying around extra pounds creates exercise pain, difficulty in breathing, easy fatigue, blood pressure problems, a greater tendency to get injured, and a host of other things that may serve to keep you away from exercise. Some people get physically sick and feel like throwing up or feel dizzy doing things that fit individuals may do without even increasing their heart rate. Additionally, problems with low self-esteem, poor self-concept, self-consciousness about appearance, and other factors may keep overweight individuals from getting out and getting moving.

Before starting an exercise routine, it's important to recognize the likely barriers and work on possible solutions.

Barriers	Possible Solutions
Concerns over health problems or injuries	Consult with your health care provider before starting a vigorous exercise program, particularly if you have had heart problems, blood pressure issues, chest pain, dizziness or fainting, arthritislike pain in weight-bearing joints, respiratory problems from asthma, or if you are over the age of 40 (men) or 50 (women). Bottom line: If you are worried that exercise will result in a health problem, get yourself checked. Invest in good, supportive shoes; they are worth the investment.
Lack of motivation or confidence	Exercise with a friend or group for positive feedback. Finding a friend at or near your own level of fitness is best. Keep a log of minutes per day of exercise; celebrate progress, even the little improvements. Document health-related changes, such as feeling like you have more energy after exercise. Join a group-exercise program to make you feel accountable (paying for it may make you more likely to go). Reward yourself for improvements. What things (besides food!) can be rewards? Phase in your activity, beginning with several short intervals of activity. Try to do something every day, working up to an hour a day of exercise.
Lack of time	Fill in your Behavior Change Contract with specific daily and weekly goals. Seek support from significant others. Think of exercise time as time for you. This time is yours to energize you, help you cope with stress, and get out in nature. Make exercise a priority.
Lack of access to facilities or equipment	Get a pedometer and work on increasing your steps in everyday activities. Walking requires no special equipment or facilities. If weather is a problem, go to a local mall and shop and walk.
Previous negative experiences	Start slow and make small gains in intensity and duration of exercises. Determine the source of your negativity in order to work through it. Make note of positive experiences, so that you can build more.
Weight	Know that activity becomes easier over time. Choose activities more suited to larger bodies, such as biking, swimming, and walking.
Poor balance	Switch to an exercise that feels more natural and comfortable. Work on strengthening body core muscles through Pilates or yoga.
Anxiety	Progress slowly at a pace that is comfortable. Make exercise fun by varying the activities that you do. Make exercise social. Talk to your friends either by getting them to exercise with you or by bringing your cell phone along and talking to someone while walking. Listen to relaxing music while exercising.
Discomfort, pain, or injury	Switch to an exercise that is less weight bearing, such as biking or swimming. Slow it down a bit.

Source: Richard Parr, "Exercising When You're Overweight: Getting in Shape and Shedding Pounds," *The Physician and Sportsmedicine* October 1996. Exercise Advisor 24 (10): 81–82. © The McGraw-Hill Companies.

Avoiding the Muscle Hustle: Tips for Buying Exercise Products and Services

Exercise Equipment

If you have a treadmill that you use as a clothes hanger or a room full of dusty exercise equipment representing the unfulfilled promises of the latest infomercial, you are not alone. Many people buy great equipment and don't get motivated to get moving, but others buy products and equipment that don't have a ghost's chance of being useful.

If you are considering buying exercise equipment, the Federal Trade Commission (FTC) urges you to evaluate advertising claims for fitness products carefully. The FTC has sued marketers of electronic abdominal exercise belts for claiming that users could get "six-pack abs" and lose inches in a short time. The FDA has never approved any kind of electronic muscle stimulator for weight loss, for losing your double chin, or similar results. While some electronic muscle stimulators may temporarily strengthen, tone, or firm muscles, they will not lead to major muscle toning or a significant change in appearance.

The FTC advises consumers to do the following:

✔ Ignore claims that an exercise machine or device can provide lasting, "no sweat" results in a short time. These claims are false. To get results, you must exercise.
✔ Disbelieve claims that a product can burn fat off a particular part of the body. Achieving a major change in body contour or appearance requires sensible eating and regular exercise that works the whole body and causes caloric deficiencies that affect the entire body.
✔ Read the ad's fine print. Advertised results may be based on more than

just using a machine; they may also be based on caloric restriction.
✔ Be skeptical of testimonials and before and after pictures from "satisfied" customers.
✔ Get details on warranties, guarantees, and return policies.
✔ Check out the company's customer support and service sections. Call the number to see how helpful the person on the other end really is.

Health Clubs

While there are some excellent facilities and many well-trained and professionally certified fitness trainers out there, carefully checking out the staff's credentials may help ensure that your trainer is offering scientifically solid, safe advice. Taking a tour of the facilities before signing up will answer many of your questions.

✔ Ask about the training that a person must have to advise you about use of machines and fitness programs in a particular club. Sometimes staff members take only a one- or two-week training program from club managers or outside trainers.
✔ Look for trainers who have graduated with majors in exercise physiology, nutrition, athletic training, physical education, health promotion and education, health education, or other health-related disciplines. The higher the degree, the better.
✔ Look for trainers with American College of Sports Medicine (ACSM) certification. These individuals must pass a national exam to verify their knowledge about basic physiology and performance.
✔ Ask the trainer about his or her basic first aid and CPR certifications. Are they current? What emergency plans are in place in case someone is injured in the club?
✔ What are the fees to join and monthly fees? What do they entitle you to? Will you get individual attention and specialized training?

✔ When are the machines the busiest? Can you pay a reduced fee to come at nonpeak times?
✔ What are their provisions for family members? Guests?
✔ Ask how regularly the machines and mats are cleaned with antibiotic washes and cleansers.
✔ Avoid the hot tubs and whirlpools unless users are required to shower to get rid of sweat, makeup, and other body debris before hopping in. One of the most germ-laden spots you'll ever encounter is a whirlpool where a bunch of sweaty exercisers have jumped in to refresh themselves after a heavy workout.
✔ If you do use the whirlpools or tubs, find out how often the water is completely changed, who monitors the chemicals in the water, and so on.
✔ If there is a pool on site, ask who monitors the number of people who can use the pool per hour, who regulates the chemicals, how often the water is changed, what the policies are about showering before entry, and other issues.
✔ Check on the frequency of machine repairs and maintenance policies.
✔ What are the locker rooms like? Are they clean and odor-free? What are the club's policies about footwear and swimwear?

Source: Federal Trade Commission, Bureau of Consumer Protection, "FTC Consumer Alert" (May 2002) (see http://www.ftc.gov).

Once you become committed to regular physical activity and exercise, you will observe gradual improvements in your functional abilities and note progress toward your goals. Perhaps your most vital goal will be to become committed to fitness for the long haul—to establish a realistic schedule of diverse exercise activities that you can maintain and enjoy throughout your life.

Design Your Program

Once you commit yourself to becoming physically active, decide what type of fitness program is best suited to your needs. The amounts and types of exercises required to yield beneficial results vary with the age and physical condition of the exerciser. Men over age 40 and women over age 50 should consult their physicians before beginning any fitness program. See the Skills for Behavior Change box for strategies to help out-of-shape and overweight people create an exercise plan.

Good fitness programs are designed to improve or maintain cardiorespiratory fitness, flexibility, muscular strength and endurance, and body composition. A comprehensive program could include a warm-up period of easy walking followed by stretching activities to improve flexibility, then selected strength development exercises, followed by an aerobic activity for 20 minutes or more, and concluding with a cool-down period of gentle flexibility exercises.

The greatest proportion of exercise time should be spent developing cardiovascular fitness, but you should not exclude the other components. Choose an aerobic activity you think you will like. Many people find cross training—alternate-day participation in two or more aerobic activities (i.e., jogging and swimming)—less monotonous and more enjoyable than long-term participation in only one aerobic activity. Cross training is also beneficial because it strengthens a variety of muscles, thus helping you avoid overuse injuries to muscles and joints.

Jogging, walking, cycling, rowing, step aerobics, and cross-country skiing are all excellent activities for developing cardiovascular fitness. Most colleges and universities have recreation centers where students can use stair-climbing machines, stationary bicycles, treadmills, rowing machines, and ski-simulators. See the Reality Check box for tips on selecting exercise equipment and health club memberships.

Taking Charge

10 **10** **10**

Managing Your Fitness Behaviors

Do you want to improve your fitness level? Begin by making a list of your favorite physical activities that can increase strength, flexibility, and cardiorespiratory fitness. Choose which you would like to make part of a regular routine. Then identify specific times to exercise. Consider how exercise could become part of your daily activities. Fill out your Behavior Change Contract, then do it!

Checklist for Change

Making Personal Choices

☐ Try walking as a great way to be active. You don't need special skills or training to be physically active.

☐ Initiate physical activity slowly, and increase the intensity gradually (e.g., start with a 10-minute walk three times a week and work your way up to 30 minutes of brisk walking or other form of moderate activity five times a week).

☐ Split activities can be split into several short periods (e.g., 10 minutes, three times a day, instead of one longer period (e.g., 30 minutes a day).

☐ Select activities that you enjoy and can fit into your daily life. Find a time that fits your schedule and your internal clock.

☐ It may take time to incorporate more activity into your daily life. Don't get discouraged if at first, you miss a day or two; just keep trying and do your best to make it a regular part of your life. You will soon realize how good it feels to be physically active and more fit.

☐ Ask for support from friends and family; likewise, support the people in your life who are trying to be physically active. Sometimes, finding someone who is more out of shape than you and committing to helping him or her will increase your motivation.

☐ Make fitness a priority. Keep a journal of how you feel and what you do.

☐ Try to change your attitude. Think of exercising rather than going to dinner or sitting in front of the TV, as your fun time.

☐ Give yourself two hours of day just for you. At least 30 minutes of that time should be devoted to exercise; the other time can be spent watching TV, reading, talking on the phone, or visiting with friends.

Making Community Choices

☐ Does your college have facilities for exercise? Are there special student rates? What hours are those facilities available?

☐ What community facilities does your hometown have available for exercise? Have you ever considered using these facilities?

☐ Are opportunities available for you to volunteer at a local exercise facility? Have you considered volunteering to help low-income individuals? Children? Why or why not?

Summary

✳ The physiological benefits of regular physical activity include reduced risk of heart attack, hypertension, and diabetes; and improved blood profile, skeletal mass, weight control, immunity to disease, mental health and stress management, and physical fitness. Regular activity can also increase life span.

✳ An aerobic exercise program improves cardiorespiratory fitness. Exercise frequency begins with three days per week and eventually moves up to five. Exercise intensity involves working out at target heart rate. Exercise duration should increase to 30 to 45 minutes; the longer the exercise period, the more calories burned and the bigger improvement in cardiovascular fitness.

✳ Flexibility exercises should involve static stretching exercises performed in sets of four or more repetitions held for 10 to 30 seconds, at least two to three days a week. Popular forms of stretching exercise include yoga, tai chi, and Pilates.

✳ The key principles for developing muscular strength and endurance are the tension principle, the overload principle, and the specificity of training principle. The different types of muscle actions include isometric, concentric, and eccentric. Resistance training programs include body weight resistance (calisthenics), fixed resistance, variable resistance, and use of accommodating resistance devices.

✳ Fitness injuries are generally caused by overuse or trauma; the most common ones are plantar fasciitis, shin splints, and runner's knee. Proper footwear and equipment can help prevent injuries. Exercise in the heat or cold requires special precautions.

✳ Planning a fitness program involves setting goals and designing a program to achieve these goals.

Questions for Discussion and Reflection

1. How do you define physical fitness? What are the key components of a physical fitness program? What might you need to consider when beginning a fitness program?

2. How would you determine the proper intensity and duration of an exercise program? How often should exercise sessions be scheduled?

3. Why is stretching vital to improving physical flexibility?

4. Identify at least four physiological and psychological benefits of physical fitness. What is the significance of the latest fitness report from the Surgeon General's office? How might it help more people realize the benefits of physical fitness?

5. Describe the different types of resistance employed in an exercise program. What are the benefits of each type of resistance?

6. Your roommate has decided to start running first thing in the morning in an effort to lose weight, tone muscles, and improve cardiorespiratory fitness. What advice would you give to make sure your roommate begins properly and doesn't get injured?

7. What key components would you include in a fitness program for yourself?

Application Exercises

Reread the What Do You Think? scenarios at the beginning of the chapter and answer the following questions.

1. Assume for a moment that you are Shawn, thinking about starting an exercise program after a period of inactivity. Create an outline for a three-month program that starts slowly and gradually progresses.

2. One of the hardest obstacles for Shawn will be breaking his old habits: driving instead of walking, watching TV,

playing computer games, and eating unhealthy foods. What advice would you give to Shawn to help him break his habits?

3. How should Lindsay have dealt with her injury? Did she do anything wrong?

4. What risks did Lindsay take by continuing to run on her sore foot? What would you have recommended that she do in light of her discomfort?

Accessing Your Health on the Internet

Visit the following Internet sites to explore further topics and issues related to personal health. To visit an organization's website, go to the Companion Website for *Access to Health, Eighth Edition* at www.aw.com/donatelle, click on the book image, and select "Accessing Your Health on the Internet" from the navigation menu on the left.

1. ***ACSM Online.*** A link with the American College of Sports Medicine and all its resources.

2. ***American Council on Exercise.*** Information on exercise and disease prevention.

3. ***Just Move.*** The American Heart Association's fitness website has the latest information on heart disease and exercise, plus a guide to local, regional, and national fitness events.

Further Reading

Fahey, T. D. *Super Fitness for Sports, Conditioning, and Health.* Boston: Allyn & Bacon, 2000.

A brief guide to developing fitness that emphasizes training techniques for improving sports performance.

Getchell, B., et al. *Physical Fitness: A Way of Life.* 5th ed. Boston: Allyn & Bacon, 1998.

A practical guide for improving all areas of fitness, complying with the latest standards of the ACSM.

Schlosberg, S. *The Ultimate Workout Log: An Exercise Diary and Fitness Guide.* Boston: Houghton Mifflin, 1999.

A six-month log that also provides fitness definitions, training tips, and motivational quotes.

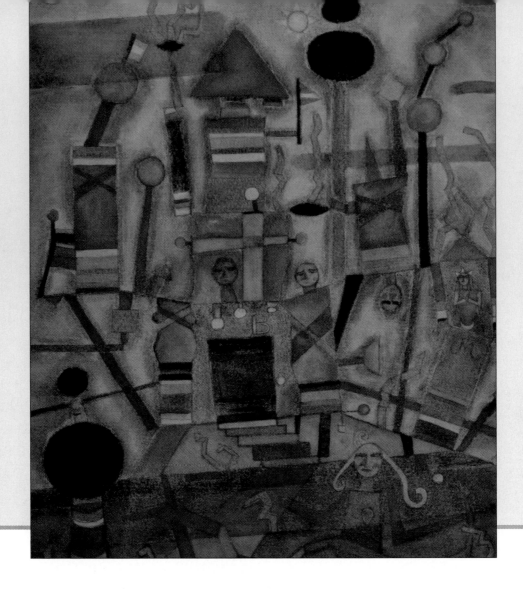

Objectives

* Define *addiction*.

* Distinguish addictions from habits, and identify the signs of addiction.

* Discuss the addictive process, the physiology of addiction, and the biopsychosocial model of addiction.

* Describe the types of addictions, including money, work, exercise, sexual, and Internet addictions, as well as codependence.

* Evaluate treatment and recovery options for addicts, including individual therapy, group therapy, family therapy, and 12-step programs.

11

Addictions and Addictive Behavior

Threats to Wellness

What do you think?

Evan is a college sophomore who likes to bet on football with his friends. Most of the time his bets have been small—$5 here, $10 there. Lately, he's been spending more time and money on betting. He and his roommate have running bets on all aspects of the weekly football contests, leading to increased gambling expenditures that reached $100 over the past weekend. For the first time, Evan dipped into his savings to cover his bets. He's also been skipping his evening class since it's on a Monday night and pro football is on TV. He received D's on two recent tests. His roommate has been less willing to bet with him because of Evan's increasing irritability when he loses.

Is Evan addicted to gambling? ✷ *What signs of possible addiction is he exhibiting?* ✷ *Should his roommate confront him more directly about his gambling?* ✷ *If so, how would you suggest approaching the issue?*

Kelly is at home for the summer after her first year of college. She notices that alcohol is a constant presence in her family. Kelly's father has used alcohol for as long as she can remember. He has never been arrested or been violent, but he spends most evenings at the local bar. When Kelly came home this year during school vacations, she felt hurt that her father spent time at the bar rather than with her, but she never said anything. Kelly's mother doesn't directly discuss his drinking, but she gives him the "cold shoulder" the day after a particularly long visit to the bar.

Is Kelly's father dependent on alcohol? ✷ *How has his drinking affected Kelly?* ✷ *What communication patterns are present in the family that either help or hinder dealing with the issue?* ✷ *How might Kelly's family history affect her own decisions about alcohol?*

I t isn't difficult these days to find numerous high-profile cases of compulsive and destructive behavior. Stories of celebrities and politicians struggling with addictions to alcohol, drugs, and sex are splashed in the headlines and profiled on television news programs. But millions of "everyday" people throughout the world are staging their own battles with addiction as well. (See the Health in a Diverse World box.) Addictions can be perplexing, since many potentially addictive activities may actually enhance the lives of the people who engage in them moderately. The most commonly recognized objects of addiction besides alcohol and drugs are food, sex, relationships, spending money, work, exercise, gambling, and using the Internet.

Defining Addiction

Addiction is continued involvement with a substance or activity despite ongoing negative consequences. Addictive behaviors initially provide a sense of pleasure or stability that is beyond the addict's power to achieve in other ways. Eventually, the addicted person needs to be involved in the behavior in order to feel normal.

Physiological dependence is only one indicator of addiction. Psychological dynamics play an important role, which explains why behaviors not related to the use of chemicals—gambling, for example—may also be addictive. In fact, psychological and physiological dependence are so intertwined that it is not really possible to separate the two. For every psychological state, there is a corresponding physiological state. In other words, everything you feel is tied to a chemical process occurring in your body.[1] Thus, addictions once thought to be entirely psychological in nature are now understood to have physiological components.

To be addictive, a behavior must have the potential to produce a positive mood change. Chemicals are responsible for the most profound addictions, not only because they produce dramatic mood changes, but also because they cause cellular changes to which the body adapts so well that it eventually requires the chemical in order to function normally. Yet other behaviors, such as gambling, spending money, working, and sex, also create changes at the cellular level along with positive mood changes. Although the mechanism is not well understood, all forms of addiction probably reflect dysfunction of certain biochemical systems in the brain.[2]

Traditionally, diagnosis of an addiction was limited to drug addiction and was based on three criteria: (1) the presence of an abstinence syndrome, or **withdrawal**—a series of temporary physical and psychological symptoms that occurs when the addicted person abruptly stops using the drug; (2) an associated pattern of pathological behavior (deterioration in work performance, relationships, and social interaction); and (3) **relapse,** the tendency to return to the addictive behavior after a period of abstinence.

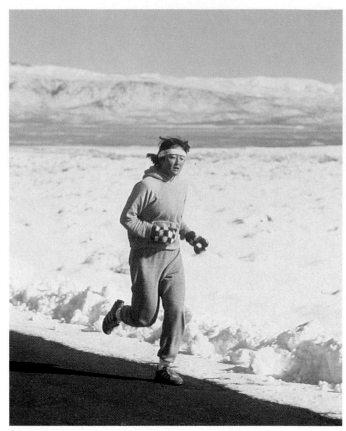

Obsession with a substance or a behavior, even a generally positive activity such as exercise, can eventually develop into an addiction.

Furthermore, until recently, health professionals were unwilling to diagnose an addiction until medical symptoms appeared in the patient. Now we know that although withdrawal, pathological behavior, relapse, and medical symptoms are valid indicators of addiction, they do not characterize all addictive behavior.

Habit versus Addiction

How do we distinguish between a harmless habit and an addiction? The stereotypical image of the addict is of someone desperately seeking a fix 24 hours a day. People have the notion that if you aren't doing the behavior every day, then you're not addicted. The reality is somewhere between these two extremes.

Addiction certainly involves elements of **habit,** a repeated behavior in which the repetition may be unconscious. A habit can be annoying, but it can be broken without too much discomfort by simply becoming aware of its presence and choosing not to do it. Addiction also involves repetition of a behavior, but the repetition occurs by **compulsion,** and considerable discomfort is experienced if the behavior is not performed. An addiction is a habit that has gotten out of control and has negative health effects.

To understand addiction, we need to look beyond the amount and frequency of the behavior, for what happens

Addiction across Cultures

Although alcohol is considered the typical drug of addiction in the United States, many countries are struggling with epidemic rates of dependence on other drugs. In fact, demand for addiction treatment services is increasing in many nations. Here's a look at some current drug addiction treatment data from around the world:

- In India, more people are seeking treatment for heroin addiction, based on estimates that up to 1 million Indians became addicted to the substance during the 1980s.

- Political upheaval and the resulting disintegration of the family appear to be strongly related to rising drug abuse. A study in Ireland found that as many as 10 percent of young people (ages 15–20) in Dublin were addicted to heroin.
- In the Americas as a whole, cocaine and cocaine derivatives account for almost 60 percent of the demand for drug treatment.
- In contrast, in European nations, opiates, primarily heroin, are the drug of choice for nearly three-quarters of individuals seeking treatment.
- Opiates are also the drug of choice for about two-thirds of addicted individuals in Asian nations.

- Amphetamine use is higher in Nordic nations such as Sweden and Finland, where it accounts for 20 percent and 40 percent of treatment needs, respectively.
- Treatment for cannabis (marijuana, hashish) dependence is much higher in the Caribbean, including Jamaica, where it accounts for over 50 percent of treatment demand.

Sources: From "The Social Impact of Drug Abuse," 1995, United Nations Office for Drug Control and Crime Prevention, New York; and "Global Illicit Drug Trends," 1999, United Nations Office for Drug Control and Crime Prevention, New York.

---

when a person is involved in the behavior is far more meaningful. For example, someone who drinks only rarely, and then in moderation, may experience personality changes, blackouts (drug-induced amnesia), and other negative consequences (e.g., failing a test, missing an important appointment, getting into a fight) that would never have occurred had the person not taken a few drinks. On the other hand, someone who has a few martinis every evening may never do anything out of character while under the influence of alcohol but may become irritable, manipulative, and aggressive without those regular drinks. For both of these people, alcohol appears to perform a function (mood control) that people should be able to perform without the aid of chemicals, which is a possible sign of addiction. Habits are behaviors that occur through choice and typically do not cause negative health consequences. In contrast, no one decides to become addicted, even though people make choices that contribute to the development of an addiction.

Signs of Addiction

If you asked 10 people to define addiction, you would quite possibly get 10 different responses. Studies show that all animals share the same basic pleasure and reward circuits in the brain that turn on when they come into contact with addictive substances or engage in something pleasurable, such as eating or orgasm. We all engage in potentially addictive behaviors to some extent because some are essential to our survival and are highly reinforcing, such as eating, drinking, and sex. At some point along the continuum, however, some individuals are not able to engage in these or other behaviors moderately and become addicted.

Although different opinions exist as to the cause of addiction, most experts agree on some universal signs of addiction. All addictions are characterized by four common symptoms: (1) compulsion, which is characterized by **obsession,** or excessive preoccupation with the behavior and an overwhelming need to perform it; (2) **loss of control,** or the inability to predict reliably whether any isolated occurrence

---

Addiction   Continued involvement with a substance or activity despite ongoing negative consequences.

Withdrawal   A series of temporary physical and biopsychosocial symptoms that occur when the addict abruptly abstains from an addictive chemical or behavior.

Relapse   The tendency to return to the addictive behavior after a period of abstinence.

Habit   A repeated behavior in which the repetition may be unconscious.

Compulsion   Obsessive preoccupation with a behavior and an overwhelming need to perform it.

Obsession   Excessive preoccupation with an addictive object or behavior.

Loss of control   Inability to predict reliably whether a particular instance of involvement with the addictive object or behavior will be healthy or damaging.

of the behavior will be healthy or damaging; (3) **negative consequences,** such as physical damage, legal trouble, financial problems, academic failure, and family dissolution, which do not occur with healthy involvement in any behavior; and (4) **denial,** or the inability to perceive that the behavior is self-destructive.

These four components are present in all addictions, whether chemical or behavioral.

> ## What do you think?
>
> *Have you ever seen signs of addiction in a friend or family member? ✳ What types of negative consequences have you witnessed? ✳ Can you think of any habits you have that could potentially become addictive?*

The Addictive Process

Addiction is a process that evolves over time. It begins when a person repeatedly seeks the illusion of relief to avoid unpleasant feelings or situations. This pattern is known as **nurturing through avoidance** and is a maladaptive way of taking care of emotional needs. As a person becomes increasingly dependent on the addictive behavior, there is a corresponding deterioration in relationships with family, friends, and coworkers; in performance at work or school; and in personal life. Eventually, addicts do not find the addictive behavior pleasurable but consider it preferable to the unhappy realities they are seeking to escape. Figure 11.1 illustrates the cycle of psychological addiction.

The Physiology of Addiction

Virtually all intellectual, emotional, and behavioral functions occur as a result of biochemical interactions between nerve cells in the body. Biochemical messengers, called **neurotransmitters,** exert their influence at specific receptor sites on nerve cells. Drug use and chronic stress can alter these receptor sites and cause the production and breakdown of neurotransmitters.

Mood-altering chemicals, for example, fill up the receptor sites for the body's natural "feel-good" neurotransmitters (endorphins) so that nerve cells are fooled into believing they have enough neurotransmitters and shut down production of these substances temporarily. When the drug use stops, those receptor sites become emptied, resulting in uncomfortable feelings that remain until the body resumes neurotransmitter production or the person consumes more of the drug. Some people's bodies always produce insufficient quantities of these neurotransmitters, so they naturally seek out chemicals such as alcohol as substitutes, or they pursue behaviors such as exercise that increase natural production. Thus, we may be "wired" to seek out substances or experiences that increase pleasure or reduce discomfort.

Mood-altering substances and experiences produce **tolerance,** a phenomenon in which progressively larger doses of a drug or more intense involvement in an experience are needed to obtain the desired effects. All of us develop some degree of tolerance to any mood-altering experience. But because addicts tend to seek intense mood-altering experiences, they eventually increase the amount and intensity to the point of causing negative side effects.

Withdrawal is another phenomenon associated with mood-altering experiences. The drug or activity replaces or causes an effect that the body should normally provide on its own. If the experience is repeated often enough, the body adjusts: It starts to require the drug or experience to obtain the effect it used to be able to produce itself, but no longer can. Stopping the behavior will therefore cause a withdrawal syndrome.

Withdrawal symptoms of chemical dependencies are generally the opposite of the effects of the drug being withdrawn. For example, a cocaine addict experiences a characteristic "crash" (depression and lethargy), while a barbiturate addict experiences trembling, irritability, and convulsions upon withdrawal. Withdrawal symptoms for addictive behaviors are usually less dramatic. They usually involve psychological discomforts such as anxiety, depression, irritability, guilt, anger, and frustration, with an underlying preoccupation with or craving for another exposure to the behavior.

Withdrawal syndromes range from mild to severe. The most severe form of withdrawal syndrome is delirium tremens (DTs), which occurs in approximately 5 percent of dependent individuals withdrawing from alcohol.

A Model of Addiction

Theories abound concerning the cause of addictions, and most of them focus on a single causative factor. Biological or disease models have been proposed since ancient times. However, it has become clear through time that psychological and environmental factors may also be involved in the development of addiction. The most effective treatment today is being provided by those who rely on the **biopsychosocial model of addiction,** which proposes that addiction is caused by a variety of factors operating together, thereby lending credibility to all the other theories. The biopsychosocial model is not a compromise solution to a theoretical controversy. Rather, it represents a reasonable comprehension of all that we have learned about addiction.

Biological or Disease Influences Studies show that people addicted to mood-altering substances metabolize these substances differently than nonaddicted people do. For example, studies of adult children of alcoholics have found that these people have abnormal concentrations or activity of various neurotransmitters related to mood—specifically norepinephrine, serotonin, endorphin, and enkephalin.[3] Abnormal levels of any of these neurotransmitters may create a biochemically based mood disorder. To obtain relief from the disorder, people may turn to mood-altering chemicals or behaviors.

significant others. The effects of modeling, imitation, and identification with behavior from early childhood on are well documented. Modeling is especially influential when it involves behavior that is mood-altering. Many studies show that modeling by parents and by idolized celebrities exerts a profound influence on young people.[7]

On an individual level, major stressful life events, such as marriage, divorce, change in work status, and death of a loved one, may trigger addictive behaviors. The death of a spouse is the most common trigger event for excessive drinking among the elderly. Traumatic events in general often instigate addictive behaviors, as traumatized people seek to medicate their pain—pain they may not even be aware of because they've repressed it. One thing that makes addictive behaviors so powerfully attractive is that they reliably alleviate personal pain. However, the relief of pain from addictive behaviors is only temporary; addictive behaviors cause more pain than they relieve. Family members whose needs for love, security, and affirmation are not consistently met; who are refused permission to express their feelings, desires, or needs; and who frequently submerge their personalities to "keep the peace" are prone to addiction. Children whose parents are not consistently available to them (physically or emotionally); who are subjected to sexual abuse, physical abuse, neglect, or abandonment; or who receive inconsistent or disparaging messages about their self-worth may experience psychosocial or physical illness and addiction in adulthood.

Psychological Factors

A person's individual psychological makeup also factors into the potential for addiction. People with low self-esteem, a tendency toward risk-taking behavior, or poor coping skills are more likely to develop addictive patterns of behavior. Individuals who consistently look outside themselves (who have an external locus of control) for solutions and explanations for life events are more likely to experience addiction.[8]

The complexity of addiction and consistent evidence of multiple contributing factors lead us to conclude that addiction is not the result of a single influence but rather of a variety of influences working together. Biological, psychological, and environmental factors all contribute to its development. Although one factor may play a larger role than another in a specific individual, a single factor is rarely sufficient to explain an addiction. Figure 11.2 lists risk factors for addiction.

> **What do you think?**
>
> *Which factors discussed in this section do you think play the biggest role in addiction? ✳ Do you think some addictions have a biological basis? ✳ Why?*

Types of Addiction

It is difficult to document the incidence of addictions of any kind because involvement with a chemical or a behavior does not, by itself, indicate addiction. Nevertheless, many studies on morbidity and mortality associated with a substance or behavior provide reasonable estimates. Another indication of the possible prevalence of addictions is that an estimated 10 million people are actively involved in self-help groups in the United States,[9] although, of course, not all of these groups address addiction.

Clearly, tobacco, alcohol, and other drugs are addictive, and addictions to these drugs create multiple problems for addicted individuals as well as their families and society. In this chapter we examine the fundamental concepts and process of addiction, as well as its associated problems. Later chapters in this book will discuss specific addictions. Our discussion of specific forms of addiction focuses on what are commonly called **process addictions**—behaviors known to

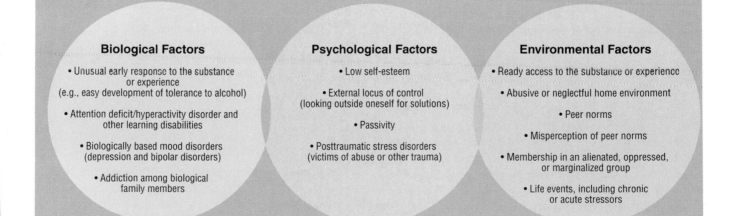

Biological Factors

- Unusual early response to the substance or experience (e.g., easy development of tolerance to alcohol)
- Attention deficit/hyperactivity disorder and other learning disabilities
- Biologically based mood disorders (depression and bipolar disorders)
- Addiction among biological family members

Psychological Factors

- Low self-esteem
- External locus of control (looking outside oneself for solutions)
- Passivity
- Posttraumatic stress disorders (victims of abuse or other trauma)

Environmental Factors

- Ready access to the substance or experience
- Abusive or neglectful home environment
- Peer norms
- Misperception of peer norms
- Membership in an alienated, oppressed, or marginalized group
- Life events, including chronic or acute stressors

Figure 11.2
Risk Factors for Addiction

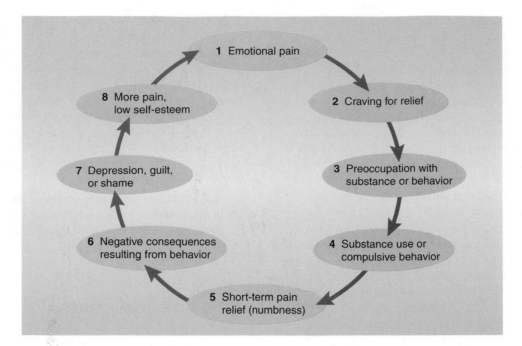

Figure 11.1

Cycle of Psychological Addiction

Source: Adapted from R. Goldberg, *Drugs Across the Spectrum*, 3rd ed., 2000. Reprinted with permission of Wadsworth, a division of Thomson Learning.

Genetic studies support a genetic influence for addiction. It has been known for centuries that alcoholism runs in families. Research on family members and twins has repeatedly confirmed the existence of a genetic factor in alcoholism. In the past decade, other studies have shown that the children of drug-addicted parents are more likely to engage in addictive behaviors than are the children of non-addicted parents. These findings hold true whether or not the children lived with their addicted parents.[4]

Environmental Influences   Cultural expectations and mores help determine whether people engage in certain behaviors. For example, although many native Italians use alcohol abundantly, there is a low incidence of alcoholism in this culture. Low rates of alcoholism typically exist in cultures such as the Italian one, where children are gradually introduced to alcohol in diluted amounts, on special occasions, and within a strong family group. There is deep disapproval of intoxication, which is not viewed as socially acceptable, stylish, or funny.[5] Such cultural traditions and values are not widespread in the United States, where the incidence of alcohol addiction and alcohol-related problems is very high.

Societal attitudes and messages also influence addictive behavior. The media's emphasis on appearance and the "ideal body" plays a significant role in exercise addiction. Media messages associating alcohol use with holidays, celebrations, romance, sports, and special achievements make it difficult for some people to believe it is possible to have fun without using substances. Societal glorification of money and materialism can lead to work addiction, which is often admired. Societal changes, in turn, influence individual norms.

People living in cities characterized by rapid social change or social disorganization often feel less connected to social, religious, and civic institutions. The resulting disenfranchisement leads to increased destructive behaviors, including addiction.[6]

Social learning theory proposes that people learn behaviors by watching role models—parents, caregivers, and

Negative consequences   Physical damage, legal trouble, financial ruin, academic failure, family dissolution, and other severe problems associated with addiction.

Denial   Inability to perceive or accurately interpret the effects of the addictive behavior.

Nurturing through avoidance   Repeatedly seeking the illusion of relief to avoid unpleasant feelings or situations, a maladaptive way of taking care of emotional needs.

Neurotransmitters   Biochemical messengers that exert influence at specific receptor sites on nerve cells.

Tolerance   Phenomenon in which progressively larger doses of a drug or more intense involvement in a behavior is needed to produce the desired effects.

Biopsychosocial model of addiction   Theory of the relationship between an addict's biological (genetic) nature and psychological and environmental influences.

Social learning theory   Theory that people learn behaviors by watching role models—parents, caregivers, and significant others.

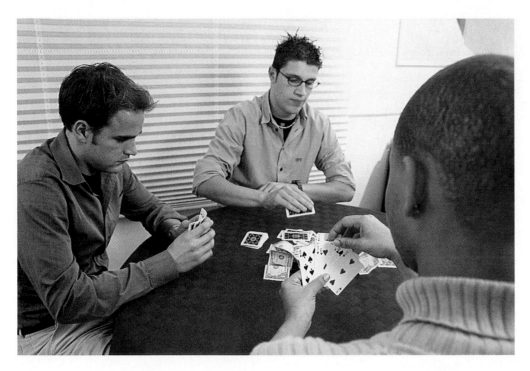

Though many people gamble occasionally as a form of recreation, others become addicted and may face grave financial and personal consequences.

be addictive because they are mood-altering, such as money, work, exercise, Internet, and sexual addictions.

Money Addictions

Money addictions include compulsive gambling, spending, and borrowing. Research has shown that, among susceptible individuals, the various money addictions produce profound mood elevations resulting from synthesis of the neurotransmitters that regulate stimulation, excitement, and pleasure.[10] Money addicts develop tolerance and also experience the phenomenon of withdrawal. Withdrawal symptoms include extreme restlessness, agitation, insomnia, depression, anxiety, and anger.[11] Money addictions are common to both genders and across all ages, races, religions, and socioeconomic groups.

Compulsive Gambling Gambling is a healthy form of recreation and entertainment for millions of Americans. Most people who gamble do so casually and moderately to experience the excitement of anticipating a win.

But over 5 million Americans are **compulsive gamblers** (addicted to gambling), and 15 million more are considered to be at risk for developing a gambling addiction.[12]

Men are more likely to have gambling problems than women are. Gambling prevalence is also higher among lower-income individuals, those who are divorced, African Americans, and individuals residing within 50 miles of a casino. Residents of southern states, where opportunities to gamble have increased significantly in the past 20 years, also have higher problem gambling rates.[13] For these people, gambling is a compulsion that rules, and often ruins, their lives (see the Reality Check box). While casual gamblers can stop anytime they wish and are capable of seeing the necessity to do so, compulsive gamblers are unable to control the

urge to gamble even in the face of devastating consequences: high debt, legal problems, and the loss of everything meaningful, including homes, families, jobs, health—and even their lives. Cardiovascular problems affect 38 percent of compulsive gamblers, and their suicide rate is 20 times higher than that of the general population.[14]

Compulsive Shopping and Borrowing Although compulsive spending has been a pervasive problem in the United States for some time, a more insidious form of the addiction lurks in the new "plastic generation." Credit card companies entice you with fantasies of having it all, right now—whether or not you can afford it.

The credit card companies seem to be succeeding. There are 400 million MasterCards and Visas out there. Add to that cable shopping stations, catalog shopping, and now e-commerce, or shopping over the Internet, and the opportunity to overspend is greater than ever before. The resulting debt from all this spending is phenomenal. Bankruptcies, formerly a last resort, have become almost run of the mill—almost 1.3 million were recorded for 2000. On average, compulsive spenders are $23,000 in debt, usually in the form of credit card debt or mortgages against their homes.[15]

Although most people can manage debt with careful planning, some use spending to meet emotional needs they

---

Process addictions Behaviors such as money addictions, work addiction, exercise addiction, and sex addictions that are known to be addictive because they are mood-altering.

Compulsive gambler A person addicted to gambling.

Gambling and College Students

The Final Four, the Super Bowl, Saturday college football games—there are numerous opportunities for gambling, and recent trends tell us that many college students are taking part. The National Collegiate Athletic Association (NCAA) estimated that during March Madness (the men's college basketball tournament) each year, there are over 1.2 million active gambling pools, with over $2.5 billion gambled. More and more of these dollars are coming from the pockets of college students. There is growing evidence, in fact, that betting on college campuses is interfering with some students' financial and academic futures. Consider the following:

- ✔ Almost 80 percent of college students have participated in most forms of gambling, including casino gambling, lottery tickets, racing, and sports betting.
- ✔ At least 78 percent of youths have placed a bet by the age of 18.
- ✔ Roughly 8 to 20 percent of college students have experienced a gambling problem and about 4.8 percent have gambled compulsively.
- ✔ Student athletes have come under increased scrutiny for their association with gambling. Student athletes who report having gambled also report risk-taking behaviors.
- ✔ The three most common reasons college students give for gambling are risk, the chance to make money, and the excitement.

Although most college students who gamble are able to do so without developing a problem, warning signs of problem gambling include:

- ✔ Missing class or work to participate in gambling.
- ✔ Spending more money than intended on bets.
- ✔ Lying to roommates, friends, and family about betting, amounts spent, and losses.
- ✔ Using tuition money, savings, or money set aside for living expenses to bet.
- ✔ Taking cash advances on credit cards or dipping into savings for betting money.

Source: "Sports Betting by College Students: Who Bets and How Often?" by T. J. Knapp, 1998, *College Student Journal* 32 (2); "Survey on College Gambling," by Penn State University, November 1999; "I Can Make That Shot!" *The Wager,* March 6, 2002 7 (2) (see http://www.thewager.org).

---

can't fulfill elsewhere. Anxiety, self-doubt, and anger all lead to spending as a way of coping with daily stressors. College students may be particularly vulnerable to spending problems because advertisers and credit card companies heavily target them.

Compulsive gambling and shopping can frequently lead to compulsive borrowing to help support the addiction. Irresponsible investments and purchases lead to debts that the addict tries to repay by borrowing more. Compulsive debtors borrow money repeatedly from family, friends, or institutions in spite of the problems this causes. While most people incur overwhelming debt through a combination of hardship and ignorance about financial management, compulsive debtors incur debt primarily as a result of buying or gambling behaviors in which they have engaged to relieve painful feelings.

Work Addiction

In order to understand work addiction, we need to understand the concept of healthy work. Healthy work provides a sense of identity, helps develop our strengths, and is a means of satisfaction, accomplishment, and mastery of problems. Healthy workers may work passionately for long hours. Although they have occasional projects that keep them away from family, friends, and personal interests for short periods of time, they generally maintain balance in their lives and full control of their schedules. Healthy work does not "consume" the worker.

Conversely, **work addiction** is the compulsive use of work and the work persona to fulfill needs of intimacy, power, and success. It is characterized by obsession, perfectionism, rigidity, fear, anxiety, feelings of inadequacy, low self-esteem, and alienation. Work addiction is more than being unable to relax when not doing something considered "productive." It is the pursuit of the "work persona"—the image that work addicts wish to project onto others.

Work addiction is found among all age, racial, and socioeconomic groups, but it typically develops in people in their 40s and 50s. Male work addicts outnumber female work addicts, but women are catching up fast as they gain more equality in the workforce.

Although work addicts tend to be admired in our society, the effects on individuals and those around them are far reaching. Work addiction is a major source of marital discord and family breakup. In fact, most work addicts come from homes that were alcoholic, rigid, violent, or otherwise dysfunctional. A survey of grandchildren of alcoholics revealed that 64 percent identified work addiction as the most common compulsion in one or both of their parents.[16]

Whether or not they lose their families, work addicts do compromise their emotional and physical health. They may become emotionally crippled, losing the communication and human interaction skills critical to living and working with other people. They are often riddled with guilt and chronic fear—of failure, boredom, laziness, persecution, or being found out. Because they are unable to relax and play, they commonly suffer from chronic fatigue. The excessive

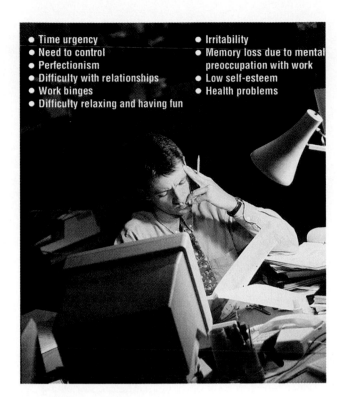

- Time urgency
- Need to control
- Perfectionism
- Difficulty with relationships
- Work binges
- Difficulty relaxing and having fun
- Irritability
- Memory loss due to mental preoccupation with work
- Low self-esteem
- Health problems

Figure 11.3
Signs of Work Addiction

pumping of adrenaline that is part of the addiction causes fatigue, hypertension and other cardiovascular diseases, nervousness, trembling, and increased sweating. Work addicts commonly suffer from disorders of the gastrointestinal tract, and they often report a feeling of pressure in the chest, constricted breathing, dizziness, and lightheadedness. Figure 11.3 identifies other typical signs of work addiction.

Exercise Addiction

It may seem odd that a personal health text that advocates exercise would also identify it as a potential addiction. Yet, as a powerful mood enhancer, exercise can be addictive. Statistics on the incidence of this addiction are not available, but it is clear that a large portion of America's 2 million people with anorexia and/or bulimia use exercise as a purge instead of or in addition to self-induced vomiting.

Addictive exercisers abuse exercise in the same way that alcoholics abuse alcohol or addictive spenders abuse money. They use it compulsively to try to meet needs that cannot truly be met by an object or activity: nurturance, intimacy, self-esteem, and self-competency. As a result, addictive exercise results in negative consequences similar to those found in other addictions: alienation of family and friends, injuries from overdoing it, and a craving for more.

Traditionally, women have been perceived as more at risk for exercise addiction. However, evidence is growing that more men are developing unhealthy exercise patterns. Media images promoting "six-pack abs" and lean, muscular male bodies have influenced society's view of the masculine ideal.

However, that body type is as unrealistic for most men as the stick-thin fashion model figure is for most women. Meanwhile, more men are abusing steroids and overexercising to attain the desired frame. **Muscle dysmorphia,** sometimes referred to as "bigarexia," is a pathological preoccupation with being larger and more muscular.[17] Sufferers view themselves as small and weak even though they may be quite the opposite.[18] Consequences of muscle dysmorphia include excessive weight lifting and exercising as well as steroid or supplement abuse.

Internet Addiction

There are enormous numbers of Internet users in the United States, with virtually unlimited access to all types of information.[19] It is no wonder that Internet use is becoming a serious problem for some people. **Internet addiction** is a blanket term that encompasses various compulsive behaviors related to computer use. They include viewing sexually explicit materials, playing fantasy games or other computer games, online stock trading, and spending hours in chatrooms or on discussion boards.

Current research indicates that the Internet can be addictive for several reasons:

- *It is accessible.* A person doesn't have to travel or leave the house to chat with people, shop, trade, or play games.
- *It provides control.* A person can trade stocks without a broker, and online auction sites allow users to bid on items without an auctioneer. The Internet also provides the illusion of privacy, meaning that people feel more comfortable having open or explicit conversations that they might not have face to face.
- *It is exciting.* Placing the winning bet, watching stocks rise, winning a fantasy game, and making the highest bid all provide a rush of excitement that reinforces the behavior.[20]

Psychologists and other treatment professionals report an increase in the number of clients who exhibit symptoms of Internet addiction and experience subsequent problems in their relationships, work, and other areas of their lives.[21] See the Assess Yourself box to analyze your Internet use.

Work addiction   The compulsive use of work and the work persona to fulfill needs for intimacy, power, and success.

Addictive exercisers   People who exercise compulsively to try to meet needs of nurturance, intimacy, self-esteem, and self-competency.

Muscle dysmorphia   Sometimes referred to as "bigarexia," a pathological preoccupation with being larger and more muscular, which can lead to exercise addiction.

Internet addiction   Compulsive use of computer activities such as fantasy games, online shopping, and chatrooms.

Are You Addicted to the Internet?

How do you know if you're already addicted or rapidly tumbling toward trouble? Everyone's situation is different, and it's not simply a matter of time spent online. Some people indicate they are addicted with only 20 hours of Internet use, while others who spend much more time online insist it is not a problem for them. It's more important to measure the damage your Internet use causes in your life. What conflicts have emerged in family, relationships, work, or school?

Let's find out. This simple exercise will help you in two ways: (1) If you already know or strongly believe you are addicted to the Internet, this guide will assist you in identifying the areas in your life most impacted by your excessive Net use; and (2) If you're not sure whether you are addicted or not, this will help determine the answer and begin to assess the damage done. Remember, when answering, consider only the time you spend online for nonacademic or non-job-related purposes.

Circle the answer that most closely describes your behavior:

1. How often do you find that you stay online longer than you intended?
   1 = Rarely
   2 = Occasionally
   3 = Frequently
   4 = Often
   5 = Always

2. How often do you neglect household chores to spend more time online?
   1 = Rarely
   2 = Occasionally
   3 = Frequently
   4 = Often
   5 = Always

3. How often do you prefer the excitement of the Internet to intimacy with your partner?
   1 = Rarely
   2 = Occasionally
   3 = Frequently
   4 = Often
   5 = Always

4. How often do you form new relationships with fellow online users?
   1 = Rarely
   2 = Occasionally
   3 = Frequently
   4 = Often
   5 = Always

5. How often do others in your life complain to you about the amount of time you spend online?
   1 = Rarely
   2 = Occasionally
   3 = Frequently
   4 = Often
   5 = Always

6. How often do your grades or school work suffer because of the amount of time you spend online?
   1 = Rarely
   2 = Occasionally
   3 = Frequently
   4 = Often
   5 = Always

7. How often do you check your e-mail before something else that you need to do?
   1 = Rarely
   2 = Occasionally
   3 = Frequently
   4 = Often
   5 = Always

8. How often does your job performance or productivity suffer because of the Internet?
   1 = Rarely
   2 = Occasionally
   3 = Frequently
   4 = Often
   5 = Always

9. How often do you become defensive or secretive when anyone else asks you what you do online?
   1 = Rarely
   2 = Occasionally
   3 = Frequently
   4 = Often
   5 = Always

10. How often do you block out disturbing thoughts about your life with soothing thoughts about the Internet?
    1 = Rarely
    2 = Occasionally
    3 = Frequently
    4 = Often
    5 = Always

11. How often do you find yourself anticipating when you will go online again?
    1 = Rarely
    2 = Occasionally
    3 = Frequently
    4 = Often
    5 = Always

12. How often do you fear that life without the Internet would be boring, empty, and joyless?
    1 = Rarely
    2 = Occasionally
    3 = Frequently
    4 = Often
    5 = Always

13. How often do you snap, yell, or act annoyed if someone bothers you while you are online?
    1 = Rarely
    2 = Occasionally
    3 = Frequently
    4 = Often
    5 = Always

14. How often do you lose sleep to late-night log-ons?
    1 = Rarely
    2 = Occasionally
    3 = Frequently
    4 = Often
    5 = Always

15. How often do you feel preoccupied with the Internet when off-line, or fantasize about being online?
    1 = Rarely
    2 = Occasionally
    3 = Frequently
    4 = Often
    5 = Always

16. How often do you find yourself saying "just a few more minutes" when online?
    1 = Rarely
    2 = Occasionally
    3 = Frequently
    4 = Often
    5 = Always

17. How often do you try to cut down the amount of time you spend online and fail?
    1 = Rarely
    2 = Occasionally
    3 = Frequently
    4 = Often
    5 = Always

18. How often do you try to hide how long you've been online?
    1 = Rarely
    2 = Occasionally
    3 = Frequently
    4 = Often
    5 = Always

19. How often do you choose to spend more time online over going out with others?
    1 = Rarely
    2 = Occasionally
    3 = Frequently
    4 = Often
    5 = Always

20. How often do you feel depressed, moody, or nervous when you are off-line, which goes away once you are back online? Do these feelings go away once you are back online?
    1 = Rarely
    2 = Occasionally
    3 = Frequently
    4 = Often
    5 = Always

After you have answered all the questions, add the numbers you selected for each response to obtain a final score. The higher your score, the greater your level of addiction and the problems your Internet usage causes.

20–49 points: You are an average Internet user. You may surf the Web a bit too long at times, but you have control over your usage.

50–79 points: You are experiencing occasional or frequent problems because of the Internet. You should consider the Internet's full impact on your life.

80–100 points: Your Internet usage is causing significant problems in your life. You should evaluate the impact of the Internet on your life and address the problems directly caused by your Internet usage.

Source: Reprinted by permission of Dr. Kimberly S. Young, director of Center for Online Addiction, 2002 (see http://www.netaddiction.com).

Sexual Addiction

Everyone needs love and intimacy, but the sexual practices of people addicted to sex involve neither. In **sexual addiction,** people confuse the intensity of physical arousal with intimacy.[22] They do not feel nurtured by the person with whom they have sex but by the activity itself. Likewise, they are incapable of nurturing another because sex, not the person, is the object of their affection. In fact, people with sexual addictions do not necessarily seek partners to obtain sexual arousal; they may be satisfied by masturbation, whether alone or during phone sex or while reading or watching erotica. They may participate in a wide range of sexual activities, including affairs, sex with strangers, prostitution, voyeurism, exhibitionism, cross-dressing, rape, incest, and pedophilia.

People addicted to sex frequently experience crushing episodes of depression and anxiety, fueled by the fear of discovery. Suicide is high among people who have problems with sexual control. The toll that these addictions exacts is most clearly seen in loss of intimacy with loved ones, which frequently leads to family disintegration.

No group of people is more or less likely than another to become involved in sexual addictions. They affect men and women of all ages, including married and single people, and people of any sexual preference. Most people with sexual addictions share a similar background: a dysfunctional childhood family, often characterized by chemical dependency or other addictions. Many were physically and emotionally abused. People addicted to sex tend to have a history of sexual abuse.

Multiple Addictions

Treatment centers for addiction often find that addicts depend on more than one chemical and/or behavior. Though they tend to have a "drug of choice" or a "behavior of choice," one that they prefer because it is more effective at meeting their needs, as many as 60 percent of people in treatment have problems with more than one addiction. The figure may be as high as 75 percent for people addicted to chemicals. For example, alcohol addiction and eating disorders are commonly paired in women. Both chemically dependent women and men frequently resort to compulsive eating to keep themselves abstinent from drugs. One study showed that 49 percent of compulsive gamblers are also alcoholics.[23] While multiple addictions certainly complicate recovery, they do not make it impossible. As with single addictions, recovery begins with the recognition that there is a problem.

> **What do you think?**
>
> *We have used a broad definition of the concept of addiction in this text. Do you think any behavior can be addictive? ✳ Can one be a chocolate addict or a study addict? ✳ What potential dangers lie in using the term addiction too loosely?*

How Addiction Affects Family and Friends

The family and friends of an addicted person also suffer many negative consequences. Often they struggle with **codependence,** a self-defeating relationship pattern in which a person is "addicted to the addict." It is the primary outcome of dysfunctional relationships or families. Codependence is not accurately defined by isolated incidents but rather by a pattern of behavior. Codependents find it hard to set healthy boundaries and often live in the chaotic, crisis-oriented mode that naturally occurs around addicts. They assume responsibility for meeting others' needs to the point that they subordinate or even cease being aware of their own needs. They may be unable to perceive their needs because they have repeatedly been taught that their needs are inappropriate or less important than someone else's. Their behavior goes far beyond performing kind services for another person. Codependents feel less than human if they fail to respond to the needs of someone else, even when their help was not requested. Although the term *codependent* is used less frequently today, treatment professionals still recognize the importance of helping addicts recognize how their behavior affects those around them and working with family and friends to establish healthier relationships and boundaries.

Family and friends can play an important role in getting an addict to seek treatment. They are most helpful when they refuse to be enablers. **Enablers** are people who knowingly or unknowingly protect addicts from the natural consequences of their behavior. If they don't have to deal with the consequences, addicts cannot see the self-destructive nature of their behavior and will therefore continue it. Codependents are the primary enablers of their addicted loved ones, although anyone who has contact with an addict can be an enabler and thus contribute (perhaps powerfully) to continuation of the addictive behavior. Enablers are generally unaware that their behavior has this effect. In fact, enabling is rarely conscious and certainly not intentional.

> **What do you think?**
>
> *Why do we tend to protect others from the natural consequences of their destructive behaviors? ✳ Have you ever confronted someone you were concerned about? ✳ If so, was the confrontation successful? ✳ What tips would you give someone who wants to confront a loved one about an addiction?*

Treatment For and Recovery From Addiction

A key step in the recovery process is to recognize the addiction. This can be difficult because of the power of denial. Denial—the inability to see the truth—is the hallmark of

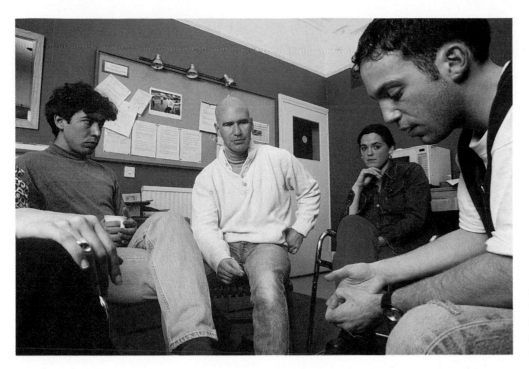

Group therapy provides a safe environment for people to learn how to be honest with themselves and others about the reality and consequences of their addictions.

addiction. It can be so powerful that intervention is sometimes necessary to break down the addict's denial system.

Intervention

Intervention is a planned process of confrontation by people who are important to the addict, including spouse, parents, children, boss, and friends. Its purpose is to break down the denial compassionately so that the addict can see the destructive nature of the addiction. It is not enough to get the person to admit that he or she is addicted. The addict must come to perceive that the addiction is destructive and requires treatment.

Individual confrontation is difficult and often futile. However, an addict's defenses generally crumble when significant others collectively share their observations and concerns about the addict's behavior. It is critical that those involved in the intervention clarify how they plan to end their enabling. For example, a wife may state that she will no longer cover bounced checks or make excuses for her money-addicted husband's antisocial behavior. She may even close their joint account and open a personal account so she will not be legally responsible for his irresponsible acts. All parties involved in the intervention must choose consequences they are ready to follow through with, in the event that the addict refuses treatment. Significant others must also be ready to give support if the addict is willing to begin a recovery program. Components of effective intervention include the following:

- Emphasizing care and concern for the addicted person.
- Describing the behavior that is the cause for concern.
- Expressing how the behavior affects the addict, each person taking part in the intervention, and others.
- Outlining specifically what you would like to see happen.

Intervention is a serious step toward helping someone who probably does not want help. It should therefore be well planned and rehearsed. Most addiction treatment centers have specialists on staff who can help plan an intervention. In addition, books on the subject are available for families and friends who are concerned about someone who may be addicted. Once the problem has been recognized, recovery can begin.

Treatment

Treatment and recovery for any addiction generally begin with **abstinence**—refraining from the addictive behavior. While literal abstinence is possible for people addicted to chemicals, it obviously is not for people addicted to behaviors like work and sex. For these addicts, abstinence means restoring balance to their lives through noncompulsive engagement in the behaviors, such as avoiding certain activities.

Over the years, a movement toward moderation-based treatments has emerged. This approach proposes that many

---

Sexual addiction   Compulsive involvement in sexual activity.

Codependence   A self-defeating relationship pattern in which a person is "addicted to the addict."

Enablers   People who knowingly or unknowingly protect addicts from the natural consequences of their behavior.

Intervention   A planned process of confronting an addict, carried out by significant others.

Abstinence   Refraining from an addictive behavior.

Abstinence or Moderation?

When Bill Wilson founded Alcoholics Anonymous in 1935, complete abstinence from alcohol was the foundation of his program. Most modern, mainstream addiction treatments are still based on abstinence as the key to success. However, over the past 10 years, offshoot treatment programs focusing on moderate use of alcohol have gained a foothold among the general public. Although the moderation philosophy has never been accepted by most treatment centers, a group called Moderation Management, founded by Audrey Kishline, has been gaining popularity, primarily through an extensive Internet presence.

Proponents of the moderation movement say that alcohol addiction should be seen as a continuum, similar to the way other health conditions, such as high blood pressure, are viewed. They claim that just as not everyone with high blood pressure needs the most extreme form of treatment, not all problem drinkers need to stop drinking completely to avoid further problems. They believe that a strict abstinence approach may just turn off people who could benefit from treatment.

Recently, however, the moderation movement took a huge blow when Kishline was sentenced to four and a half years in prison for killing two people while driving under the influence of alcohol. Kishline, whose blood alcohol concentration was .26, crossed the centerline, killing a 38-year-old man and his 12-year-old daughter. A few weeks before, Kishline had posted a message on the Moderation Management website, saying she could no longer moderate her own alcohol use and, although she still believed in the movement, would be seeking 12-step, abstinence-based treatment for herself. Just after Kishline's accident, the director of a leading treatment center in New York resigned after failing to gain his staff's support for offering moderation-based treatment to some clients.

Critics of the moderation movement cite these incidents as poignant evidence that the approach is flawed and simply another way for alcoholics to deny their problem and delay recovery. According to those in the traditional treatment industry, telling alcoholics they can get better while drinking is simply setting them up for failure.

With over 700,000 people in the United States seeking some form of treatment for alcohol problems daily, it is certain that the moderation/abstinence debate will continue for years to come.

Sources: From "License to Drink," by E. Rivera, *Time,* July 31, 2000; and "10th Special Report to the U.S. Congress on Alcohol and Health," by the National Institute on Alcohol Abuse and Alcoholism, July 2000.

---

addicts can learn to moderate their use of substances and activities without stopping entirely. However, this movement has not been without detractors. See the Health Ethics box for more information.

Detoxification refers to the early abstinence period during which an addict adjusts physically and cognitively to being free from the influence of the addiction. It occurs in virtually every recovering addict, and whereas it is uncomfortable for them all, it can be dangerous for some. This is primarily true for those addicted to chemicals, especially alcohol, heroin, and tranquilizers such as Valium. For these people, early abstinence may involve profound withdrawal symptoms that require medical supervision. Therefore, most inpatient treatment programs provide a pretreatment component of supervised detoxification to achieve abstinence safely before treatment begins.

Abstinence alone does little to change the psychological, biological, and environmental dynamics that underlie the addictive behavior. Without recovery, an addict is apt to relapse time and again or simply to change addictions. Recovery involves learning new ways of looking at oneself, others, and the world. It may require exploring a traumatic past so that psychological wounds can be healed. It also involves learning *interdependence* with significant others and new ways of taking care of oneself, physically and emotionally. And involves developing communication skills and new ways of having fun.

Recovery programs are the fuel that gives addicts the energy to resist relapsing. For a large number of addicts, recovery begins with a period of formal treatment. A good treatment program includes the following characteristics:

- Professional staff familiar with the specific addictive disorder for which help is being sought.
- A flexible schedule of both inpatient and outpatient services.
- Access to medical personnel who can assess the addict's health and treat all medical concerns as needed.
- Medical supervision of addicts who are at high risk for a complicated detoxification.
- Involvement of family members in the treatment process.
- A team approach to treating addictive disorders (e.g., medical personnel, counselors, psychotherapists, social workers, clergy, educators, dietitians, and fitness counselors).
- Both group and individual therapy options.
- Peer-led support groups that encourage the addict to continue involvement after treatment ends.
- Structured after-care and relapse-prevention programs.
- Accreditation by the Joint Commission for the Accreditation of Healthcare Organizations (JCAHO) and a license from the state in which it operates.

Detoxification The early abstinence period during which an addict adjusts physically and cognitively to being free from the influences of the addiction.

Addiction Treatment for Women: Still Confronting Barriers

The addiction treatment industry as a whole was built using a "male model" and has only recently begun to address the unique needs of women. Unfortunately, significant barriers remain for women seeking addiction treatment.

Although women entering treatment generally have fewer addiction-related legal problems (arrests for public intoxication or drug dealing, for example) than men do, they face more psychological issues and family, financial, and medical problems. Studies consistently indicate that the two primary barriers women face in successfully completing treatment are child care and transportation. One study found that women who were able to bring their children to inpatient treatment were more likely to remain healthy at six months after treatment. Additional barriers for women seeking addiction treatment include the following:

Individual

- Lack of insurance or inadequate coverage.
- Fear of losing child custody.
- Low self-esteem.
- Low feelings of self-efficacy.

Family

- Too many responsibilities.
- Lack of family support for treatment.
- Abuse in the family environment.

Community

- Lack of support from employer.
- Lack of gender-sensitive treatment options.

A "women-friendly" treatment center should offer the following:

- Educational programs on self-worth, assertiveness, family issues, parenting, and anger management.
- Women-only groups, especially for addressing issues of rape, incest, and abuse.
- Networking with and support from other women in recovery.
- Housing and day care.

Women clearly have different treatment needs than men do. Finding a program that addresses these needs improves the likelihood of long-term success and recovery.

Sources: From "How Are Women Who Enter Substance Abuse Treatment Different Than Men? A Gender Comparison from the Drug Abuse Treatment Outcome Study," by W. Weschberg, S. Craddock, and R. Hubbard. In *Women and Substance Abuse: Gender Transparency,* edited by S. Stevens and H. Wexler (New York: Haworth, 1998).

Most programs apply a combination of family, individual, and group counseling, supplemented with attendance at a 12-step support group. Individuals may also wish to explore alternatives to 12-step groups. Organizations such as Rational Recovery and the Secular Organization for Sobriety provide support without the spiritual emphasis of 12-step groups such as Alcoholics Anonymous.

Choosing a Treatment   The National Institute on Alcohol Abuse and Alcoholism (NIAAA) recently completed Project MATCH (Matching Alcoholism Treatment to Client Heterogeneity), a large-scale study designed to determine if certain types of patients respond better to particular treatments.

The investigators studied three strategies: cognitive-behavioral therapy, motivational psychology, and a facilitated 12-step program with sessions run by a therapist. Results showed that patients did equally well in each of the treatment approaches. This outcome was somewhat surprising, given that it has been common practice for treatment professionals to match patients to certain approaches. Researchers concluded that the focus, therefore, should simply be on selecting a competently run treatment program. Large-scale studies on other addictions have yet to occur.[24]

The Women's Health/Men's Health box describes factors that are important to address when treating female addicts.

Relapse

Relapse is an isolated occurrence of or full return to addictive behavior. It is one of the defining characteristics of addiction. A person who does not relapse or have powerful urges to do so was probably not addicted in the first place. Relapse is proof that a person is addicted and has abandoned the practice of an ongoing recovery program. Addicts are set up to relapse long before they actually do so because of their tendency to meet change and other forms of stress in their lives with the same kind of denial they once used to justify their addictive behavior (e.g., "I don't have a problem, I can handle this"). This sets off a series of events involving immediate or gradual abandonment of structured recovery plans. For example, the addict may quit attending support group meetings and slip into situations that previously triggered the addictive behavior.

Because treatment programs recognize this strong tendency to relapse, they routinely teach clients and significant others concepts of relapse prevention. Relapse prevention teaches people to recognize the signs of imminent relapse and to develop a plan for responding to these signs. Without such a plan, recovering addicts are likely to relapse more frequently, more completely, and perhaps more permanently.

Relapse should not be interpreted as failure to change or lack of desire to stay well. The appropriate response to relapse is to remind addicts that they are addicted and to redirect them to the recovery strategies that have previously worked for them.

In addition to teaching skills, relapse prevention may involve after-care planning such as connecting the recovering person with support groups, career counselors, or community services.

What do you think?

Why do you think people with addictions resist seeking treatment, even when they may admit they have a problem? ✳ *What factors need to be considered in helping addicted individuals prevent relapse?*

Taking Charge

11 11 **11**

Confronting Addictive Behaviors

After reading this chapter, you know that addictions can be devastating not only to addicts, but to their families and friends as well. Addictions usually progress gradually, and it is difficult to know for certain when a person crosses the line from habit to addiction. Keep in mind that a behavior or chemical is problematic when it causes a person to incur negative consequences. If a person continues to perform the behavior or use the chemical despite these negative consequences, chances are that he or she is addicted.

Stop and think about your own behaviors for a minute. Do you have any of the habits discussed in this chapter? If you or someone you know lives with an addiction or is heading in that direction, the following checklists may provide some constructive strategies to help.

Checklist for Change

Making Personal Choices

☐ Are you ready to change or modify your behavior or substance use? Who can help support your decision?

☐ Have you thought about what impact your decision will have on your lifestyle? Are you ready to give up friends, activities, and environments that do not support your efforts?

☐ Rehearse things you may say or do if you find yourself in a situation that makes it difficult to stick with your behavior change.

☐ Remember that your motivation will decrease. During the times you are tempted, think about the reasons you decided to give up the behavior or substance.

☐ Realize that relapses happen. If you relapse, do not let the relapse serve as an excuse to slip back into old patterns of addiction.

Talk with someone you trust, and start again. Recovery is difficult—give yourself a break.

☐ Join a self-help group. There are lots of 12-step groups that are free and confidential. Your university or college counseling service is another place to seek help.

Making Community Choices

☐ Do you sometimes participate or look the other way when someone you know engages in a behavior that may lead to addiction?

☐ Do you support policies, such as laws against drunk driving, that protect the community from the effects of addictive behaviors?

☐ Are you aware of what's happening in your own environment regarding identification of and help for addicts? Do you discuss alternatives or solutions to unhealthy behavior?

Summary

✳ Addiction is the continued involvement with a substance or activity despite ongoing negative consequences.

✳ Habits are repeated behaviors whereas addiction is behavior resulting from compulsion; without the behavior, the addict experiences withdrawal. All addictions share four common symptoms: compulsion, loss of control, negative consequences, and denial.

✳ Addiction is a process, evolving over time through a pattern known as nurturing through avoidance. Mood-altering substances and experiences produce biochemical reactions that make the body feel good; when absent, the per-

son feels a withdrawal effect. The biopsychosocial model of addiction takes into account biological (genetic) factors as well as psychological and environmental influences in understanding the addiction process.

✳ Addictions include money addictions (compulsive gambling, spending, and borrowing), work addiction, exercise addiction, sexual addiction, Internet addiction, and codependence. Codependents are "addicted to the addict." These behaviors are all addictive because they are mood-altering.

* Treatment begins with abstinence from the addictive behavior or substance, usually instituted through intervention by significant others. Treatment programs may include individual, group, or family therapy, as well as 12-step programs.

Questions for Discussion and Reflection

1. What factors distinguish a habit from an addiction? Is it possible for you to tell whether someone else is really addicted?
2. Explain why the biopsychosocial model is a more effective model for treatment than a single-factor model.
3. Explain the potential genetic, environmental, and psychological risk factors for addiction.
4. Discuss how addiction affects family and friends. What role do family and friends play in helping the addict get help and maintain recovery?
5. What are some key components of an effective treatment program? Do the components vary for men and women? Why or why not?

Application Exercises

Reread the What Do You Think? scenarios at the beginning of the chapter and answer the following questions.

1. If Evan decides to cut down on gambling, what will he need to do to ensure he doesn't relapse? Knowing he will still be in an environment with many gambling opportunities, what would you suggest he include in a relapse prevention plan?
2. How can Evan's roommate support him in dealing with his gambling problem? What steps should his roommate take to confront Evan effectively? What might his roommate try if his intervention fails?
3. How can Kelly approach her father and mother about her father's drinking?
4. What risk factors for developing addiction does Kelly face because of her family history and environment? How can she prevent such problems?

Accessing Your Health on the Internet

Visit the following Internet sites to explore further topics and issues related to various forms of addiction and treatment. Many offer self-assessment profiles designed to give you more information about your own health practices. To visit an organization's website, go to the Companion Website for *Access to Health, Eighth Edition* at www.aw.com/donatelle, click on the book image, and select "Accessing Your Health on the Internet" from the navigation menu on the left.

1. **Behavioral Health Online.** A comprehensive addiction site with information on Internet, gambling, eating, and other addiction issues. Includes news briefs, features, and Ask an Expert.
2. **Center for Online Addiction.** Information and assistance for those dealing with Internet addiction.
3. **The Wager.** A weekly research report on compulsive gambling. Summarizes current research and resources pertaining to gambling.
4. **Web of Addiction.** A comprehensive listing of various resources related to self-help, treatment, and policy.

Further Reading

Elster, J. (ed.). *Addiction: Entries and Exits.* New York: Russell Sage Foundation, 2000.

Addresses current addiction controversies from an international perspective, with authors from the United States and Norway. Topics include whether addicts have a choice in their behavior and current addiction theories.

Hurley, J. (ed.). *Addiction: Opposing Viewpoints.* San Diego: Greenhaven Press, 2000.

Part of the Opposing Viewpoints series; addresses addiction theories, treatment approaches, and risk factors, among other topics.

Nakken, C. *The Addictive Personality.* Center City, MN: Hazelden, 1996.

A very down-to-earth overview of addiction, including nonsubstance addictions.

Peele, S. *The Meaning of Addiction: An Unconventional View.* San Francisco: Jossey-Bass, 1998.

One of the leading critics of the disease-view of addictions provides an alternative model of addiction.

Stevens, S., and H. Wexler (eds.). *Women and Substance Abuse: Gender Transparency.* New York: Haworth, 1998.

A collection of the most current research pertaining to women and substance abuse.

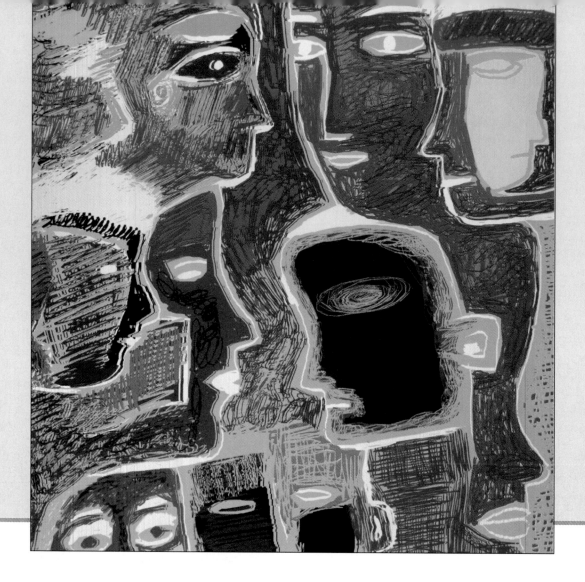

Objectives

* Summarize the alcohol use patterns of college students, and discuss overall trends in consumption.

* Explain the physiological and behavioral effects of alcohol, including blood alcohol concentration, absorption, metabolism, and immediate and long-term effects of alcohol consumption.

* Explain the symptoms and causes of alcoholism, its cost to society, and its effects on the family.

* Explain the treatment of alcoholism, including the family's role, varied treatment methods, and whether or not alcoholics can be cured.

Drinking Responsibly

A Lifestyle Challenge on Campus

What do you think?

Jean's 21st birthday had arrived, and she planned to live it up. She and a group of friends decided to go barhopping. Wherever Jean went, friends and acquaintances would buy her a drink. At 11:30, Jean was already intoxicated. As she clumsily made her way onto the dance floor, a young man caught her eye. Within the hour, this man was leading Jean toward the door. One of Jean's friends saw this and wanted to stop him, but another friend, also quite intoxicated, said, "Let her do what she wants. It's her birthday!" The next morning, Jean's friends found out that she had been beaten and raped.

Do you believe Jean's friends had an obligation to watch out for her? ✳ Do you believe her friends are partly responsible for her intoxication? ✳ What can be done differently when celebrating the stereotypical 21st birthday to avoid the kind of consequences that Jean faced?

Mark and his friends were regulars at a local bar. Nearly every night that they met at this bar, they would play a drinking game. One favorite game was "quarters," which involved bouncing a quarter off a table into a glass. The losing team had to chug a beer. Mark wanted to introduce his younger, 19-year-old brother, Tim, to the game, so he and his buddies got Tim into the bar. During about two hours of play, Tim's team lost continuously. Tim consumed about 11 glasses of beer. Mark and his friends kept laughing at Tim and urging him on.

Do you encounter drinking games at bars or parties? ✳ Would you view these games as "drinking to get drunk"? ✳ Why would Mark sneak Tim into the bar and then urge him to drink more and more? ✳ What possible short-term and long-term consequences might Tim face?

341

Most of us think of alcohol the way it is portrayed in ads or in the movies: a way of having fun in social company and an important adjunct to a romantic dinner or a cozy evening in front of the fireplace. We don't think of it as a dangerous drug—in our society, illegal substances such as cocaine, heroin, LSD, and marijuana are considered dangerous. Alcohol, on the other hand, is legal and socially accepted. But the fact is, alcohol is a drug, and if it is not used responsibly, it becomes dangerous. Alcohol is a chemical substance that affects physical and mental behavior. The tragedies associated with alcohol addiction receive far less attention than cocaine-related deaths, drug busts, and efforts to eradicate marijuana crops. Nevertheless, alcohol-related problems are more common and may have devastating effects on people of all ages.

Responsible use of alcohol, however, can render it harmless. In fact, the drinking of alcoholic beverages is interwoven with many traditions. Moderate use of alcohol can enhance celebrations or special times. Research shows that very low levels of drinking may actually lower some health risks. We may also consume alcohol to help ease the pain caused by rejection or loss. We are certainly not unique in this regard; people all over the world and throughout history have used alcohol for everything from social gatherings to religious ceremonies.

Alcohol: An Overview

An estimated 65 percent of Americans consume alcoholic beverages regularly, though consumption patterns are unevenly distributed throughout the drinking population. Ten percent are heavy drinkers, and they account for half of all the alcohol consumed. The remaining 90 percent of the drinking population are infrequent, light, or moderate drinkers.

Alcohol and College Students

Alcohol is the most widely used (and abused) recreational drug in our society. It is also the most popular drug on college campuses, where approximately 84 percent of students consume alcoholic beverages.[1] About one-third of college students are classified as heavy drinkers, meaning that they consume large amounts of alcohol per drinking occasion. Therefore, students who might go out and drink only once a week are considered heavy drinkers if they consume a great deal of alcohol. In a new trend on college campuses, women's consumption of alcohol is close to equaling men's. (Exactly how much does a typical college student consume? See the Reality Check box.) Colleges and universities have been described as "alcohol-drenched institutions." Every year, America's 12 million undergraduates drink 4 billion cans of beer, averaging 55 six-packs apiece, and spend $446 each on alcoholic beverages—more than they spend on soft drinks and textbooks combined.[2]

Despite these figures, fewer students are drinking alcohol than in the past. In 1980, 9.5 percent of students nationwide said they abstained from alcohol; in 2001, 19 percent were abstainers.[3] According to the University of Michigan's Institute for Social Research, the percentage of students who report drinking daily also has declined, from 6.5 percent in 1980 to 4.7 percent in 2001.[4]

College is a critical time to become aware of and responsible for drinking. There is little doubt that drinking is a

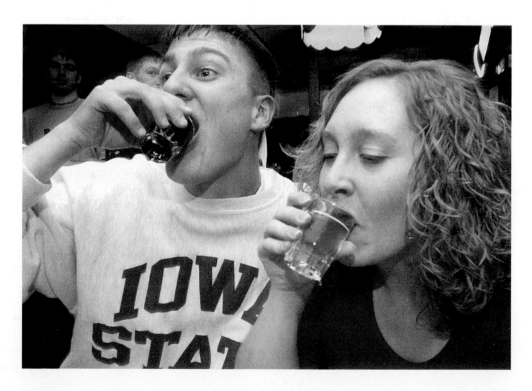

Deciding when to drink, and how much, is no small matter. Irresponsible consumption of alcohol can easily result in disaster.

The Facts about College Students and Drinking

Perhaps you've heard conflicting reports in the media about the prevalence and effects of drinking on campus. What are the facts? The following statistics reveal the scope of the problem.

✔ Alcohol kills more people below age 21 than cocaine, marijuana, and heroin combined.

✔ One night of heavy drinking can impair the ability to think abstractly for up to 30 days, limiting a student's ability to relate textbook reading to a professor's lecture, or to think through a football play.

✔ College administrators estimate that alcohol is involved with 29 percent of dropouts, 38 percent of academic failures, 64 percent of violent behaviors, and 6 percent of unsafe sexual practices.

✔ All-women colleges saw a 135 percent increase in frequent binge drinking between 1993 and 2001.

✔ An estimated 259,000 students think that wine coolers or beer cannot get a person drunk.

✔ There has been a threefold increase since 1993 in the number of college women who report having been drunk on 10 or more occasions in the previous month.

✔ The National Bureau of Economic Research found that areas of a college campus offering cheap beer prices had more violent and nonviolent crime, including trouble between students and police or other campus authorities, arguments, physical fighting, property damage, false fire alarms, and sexual misconduct.

✔ Alcohol is involved in more than two-thirds of suicides among college students, one-third of all emotional and academic problems, 90 percent of campus rapes and sexual assaults, and 95 percent of violent crime on campus.

✔ Close to 40 percent of students surveyed reported binge drinking in high school.

✔ Women who drink heavily are 40 percent more likely to experience unwanted sexual advances than are those who drink less.

✔ Seventy-five percent of male students and 55 percent of female students involved in acquaintance rape had been drinking or using drugs at the time.

✔ College binge drinking occurs more frequently among male students, students who reside on campus, intercollegiate athletes, and members of fraternities and sororities.

✔ Approximately 40 percent of fraternity and sorority members report being frequent binge drinkers.

✔ As many as 360,000 of the nation's 12 million undergraduates will die from alcohol-related causes while in school. This is more than the number who will receive M.A. and Ph.D. degrees.

✔ College students under the age of 21 are more prone to binge drinking and pay less for their alcohol than their older classmates do, according to researchers at the Harvard University School of Public Health.

✔ Though underage students are likely to drink less often, they consume more per occasion than students age 21 and older who are allowed to drink legally.

✔ College students who have serious alcohol problems and engage in dangerous behaviors are more likely than other students to have guns with them at school.

Source: Data were compiled from the numerous studies cited throughout this chapter and from: Center for Science in the Public Interest, "Booze News" 2002 (see http://www.cspi.prg/booze); L. D. Johnson, P. M. O'Malley, and J. G. Bachman, "The Monitoring the Future Study, 1975–1999," Vol. II (Rockville, MD: NIDA, 2000); H. Wechsler et al., "College Binge Drinking in the 1990s: A Continuing Problem," *Journal of American College Health* 48 (2000); A. Cohen, "Battle of the Binge," *Time*, September 8, 1997.

part of campus culture and tradition. Students are away from home, often for the first time, and many are excited by their newfound independence. For some students, this independence and the rite of passage into the college culture are symbolized by the use of alcohol. It provides the answer to one of the most commonly heard statements on any college campus: "There is nothing to do." Additionally, many students suggest they drink "to have fun." Having fun, which often means drinking simply to get drunk, may really be a way of coping with stress, boredom, anxiety, or pressures created by academic and social demands.

Statistics about college students' drinking may not always reflect the actual incidence of alcohol consumption. Students consistently report that their friends drink much more than they do and that average drinking within their own social living group is higher than actual self-reports.

Such misinformation may promote or be used to excuse excessive drinking practices among college students. In a survey of students at a large midwestern university, 42 percent reported not having a hangover in the past six months. Yet that same group of surveyed students believed that only 3 percent of their peers had not had a hangover in the past month. Efforts to reduce misperceptions concerning normal drinking behavior among college students have begun on many college campuses. It is hoped that providing students with accurate information about their peers' drinking behavior will reduce the pressure on students who feel as though they need to drink, or to drink in excess.

An example of such a "social norms" campaign is Oregon State University's "Just the Facts" program. It seeks to publicize the fact that the majority of the university's students are responsible and moderate drinkers. Students are often surprised to learn that 87 percent of their peers have never driven a car while under the influence of alcohol, and 89 percent have never passed out due to their alcohol use. Almost 90 percent have never performed poorly on a test or important project due to their alcohol use and 77 percent have never missed a class due to their alcohol use. Almost 75 percent have zero to four drinks per week, and 60 percent had four or fewer drinks the last time they went to a party. Clearly there are many students who use alcohol responsibly and in moderation.

Table 12.1
College Students' Patterns of Alcohol Use, 2001

CATEGORY	TOTAL (%)	MEN (%)	WOMEN (%)
Abstainer (past year)	19.3	20.1	18.7
Non–binge drinker	36.3	31.3	40.4
Occasional binge drinker	21.6	23.4	20.0
Frequent binge drinker	22.8	25.2	20.9

Source: H. Wechsler et al., "Trends in College Binge Drinking during a Period of Increased Prevention Efforts: Findings from four Harvard School of Public Health College Study Surveys: 1993–2001," *Journal of American College Health* 50 (5) (2002): 207.

Table 12.2
Alcohol-Related Problems among Students in Different Binge-Drinking Categories

PROBLEM REPORTED	NON–BINGE DRINKERS (%)	FREQUENT BINGE DRINKERS (%)
Did something regrettable	18	62
Missed a class	9	63
Forgot where they were or what they did	10	54
Got behind in schoolwork	10	46
Argued with friends	10	43
Got hurt or injured	4	27
Damaged property	2	23
Engaged in unplanned sexual activities	8	42
Drove after drinking	19	57

Source: H. Wechsler et al., "College Binge Drinking in the 1990s: A Continuing Problem," *Journal of American College Health* 48, (2002): 207.

Table 12.3
Secondhand Effects of Binge Drinking

SECONDARY EFFECT	PERCENTAGE
Been insulted or humiliated	29
Had your studying/sleeping interrupted	60
Had to take care of a drunken fellow student	48
Experienced unwanted sexual advances	19.5

Source: H. Wechsler et al., "Trends in College Binge Drinking during a Period of Increased Prevention Efforts: Findings from four Harvard School of Public Health College Study Surveys: 1993–2001," *Journal of American College Health* 50 (5) (2002): 211.

Should Colleges Call Parents without Student Consent?

Students' right to privacy versus parents' right to know is at the heart of a debate over a federal law that allows school administrators to disclose a student's academic or probationary record to parents without the student's consent. In 1999, Congress amended the Family Educational Rights and Privacy Act of 1974 as a means of reducing drug and alcohol abuse on college campuses. The revised law gives universities the option of telling a student's parents about underage drinking and illicit drug violations. Some college officials are taking a wait-and-see approach whereas others are embracing the law, saying it gives them a chance to respond to early warning signs to curb alcohol and drug abuse on campus.

What is your campus's policy on parental notification? What are some of the issues surrounding this amendment? Do you think this is a good idea? Why or why not?

"Binge" Drinking and College Students

There are, however, some students who indulge in heavy episodic or **binge drinking.** This is defined as having five drinks in a row for men or four in a row for women on a single occasion. The stakes of binge drinking are high because of the increased risk for alcohol-related injuries and death. An estimated 50 students die annually from alcohol poisonings. In a single month, November 1997, five college students died in alcohol-related accidents in the state of Virginia alone.

According to a 2001 study by the Harvard School of Public Health, 44.8 percent of students were found to be binge drinkers, and of those, 22.8 percent were reported as frequent bingers (people who binge drink three times or more in a two-week period).[5] (See Table 12.1.) Compared with nonbingers, frequent bingers were more likely to have an array of problems on campus (see Table 12.2.) For example, frequent binge drinkers are 16 times more likely to miss class, 8 times more likely to fall behind in their school work, and more apt to get into trouble with campus or local police.[6] Unfortunately, recent studies confirm what students have been experiencing for a long time—binge drinkers cause problems not only for themselves but also for those around them (see Table 12.3).

Although everyone is at some risk for alcohol-related problems, college students seem to be particularly vulnerable for the following reasons:

- Alcohol exacerbates their already high risk for suicide, automobile crashes, and falls.
- Many college and university customs, norms, traditions, and mores encourage certain dangerous practices and patterns of alcohol use.
- University campuses are heavily targeted by advertising and promotions from the alcoholic beverage industry.
- It is more common for college students than their noncollegiate peers to drink recklessly and to engage in drinking games and other dangerous drinking practices.
- College students are particularly vulnerable to peer influences and have a strong need to be accepted by their peers.

- There is institutional denial by college administrators that alcohol problems exist on their campuses.

A recent study shows that 6 percent of college students meet the criteria for a diagnosis of alcohol dependence (also referred to as alcoholism) and 31 percent meet the criteria for alcohol abuse. Students who attend colleges with heavy drinking environments are more likely to be diagnosed with abuse or dependence. Those students at most risk are the frequent bingers, and male students are generally at greater risk than females. Nearly one in 10 college men under 24 meet the criteria for alcohol dependence, compared to one in 20 college women. Despite the prevalence of alcohol disorders on campus, very few students seek treatment.[7]

To prevent alcohol abuse, many colleges and universities are instituting strong policies against drinking. University presidents have formed a leadership group to help curb the problem of alcohol abuse. Many fraternities have elected to have dry houses. At the same time, colleges and universities are making more help available to students with drinking problems. Today, both individual and group counseling are offered on most campuses, and more attention is being directed toward the prevention of alcohol abuse. See the Health Ethics box on another aspect of colleges' responses to alcohol.

Trends in Consumption

In general, alcohol consumption levels among Americans have been steadily declining since the late 1970s. In 1998, the estimated per capita consumption was the equivalent of 2.19 gallons of pure alcohol per person.[8] This represents a substantial decline from 2.64 gallons in 1977. (This measure indicates the amount of alcohol that a person would obtain

> **Binge drinking** Drinking for the express purpose of becoming intoxicated; five drinks in a single sitting for men and four drinks in a sitting for women.

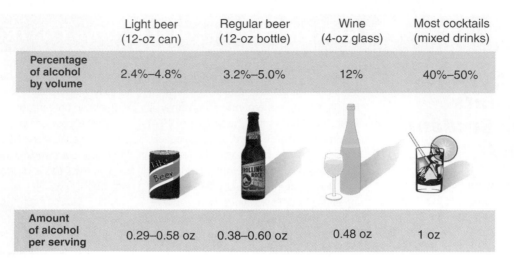

	Light beer (12-oz can)	Regular beer (12-oz bottle)	Wine (4-oz glass)	Most cocktails (mixed drinks)
Percentage of alcohol by volume	2.4%–4.8%	3.2%–5.0%	12%	40%–50%
Amount of alcohol per serving	0.29–0.58 oz	0.38–0.60 oz	0.48 oz	1 oz

Figure 12.1
Alcoholic Beverages and Their Alcohol Equivalencies

by drinking approximately 50 gallons of beer, 20 gallons of wine, or more than 4 gallons of distilled spirits.)

This downward trend has been tied to a growing attention to weight, personal health, and physical activity. The alcohol industry has responded by introducing beer and wines with fewer calories and reduced alcohol content.

> **What do you think?**
>
> *Why do college students drink excessive amounts of alcohol? ✳ Are there particular traditions or norms related to when and why students drink on your campus? ✳ Have you ever had your sleep or studies interrupted or have you had to baby-sit a roommate or friend because of drinking? ✳ Did you say anything about it to your friend or roommate? ✳ How did the person respond?*

Physiological and Behavioral Effects of Alcohol

The Chemical Makeup of Alcohol

The intoxicating substance found in beer, wine, liquor, and liqueurs is **ethyl alcohol,** or **ethanol.** It is produced during a process called **fermentation,** whereby plant sugars are broken down by yeast organisms, yielding ethanol and carbon dioxide. Fermentation continues until the solution of plant sugars (called mash) reaches a concentration of 14 percent alcohol. At this point, the alcohol kills the yeast and halts the chemical reactions that produce it.

For beers and ales, which are fermented from malt barley, the process stops when the alcohol concentration is 14 percent. Manufacturers then add other ingredients that dilute the alcohol content of the beverage. Other alcoholic beverages are produced through further processing called **distillation,** during which alcohol vapors are released from the mash at high temperatures. The vapors are then condensed and mixed with water to make the final product.

The **proof** of an alcoholic drink is a measure of the percentage of alcohol in the beverage. "Proof" comes from "gunpowder proof," a reference to the gunpowder test, whereby potential buyers would test the distiller's product by pouring it on gunpowder and attempting to light it. If the alcohol content was at least 50 percent, the gunpowder would burn; otherwise the water in the product would put out the flame. Thus, alcohol percentage is 50 percent of the given proof. For example, 80 proof whiskey or scotch is 40 percent alcohol by volume, and 100 proof vodka is 50 percent alcohol by volume. The proof of a beverage indicates its strength. Lower-proof drinks will produce fewer alcoholic effects than the same amount of higher-proof drinks.

Most wines are between 12 and 15 percent alcohol, and ales are between 6 and 8 percent. The alcoholic content of beers is between 2 and 6 percent, varying according to state laws and type of beer (see Figure 12.1).

Behavioral Effects

Blood alcohol concentration (BAC) is the ratio of alcohol to total blood volume. It is the factor used to measure the physiological and behavioral effects of alcohol. Despite individual differences, alcohol produces some general behavioral effects depending on BAC (see Table 12.4). At a BAC of 0.02, a person feels slightly relaxed and in a good mood. At 0.05, relaxation increases, there is some motor impairment, and a willingness to talk becomes apparent. At 0.08, the person feels euphoric and there is further motor impairment. At 0.10, the depressant effects of alcohol become apparent, drowsiness sets in, and motor skills are further impaired, followed by a loss of judgment. Thus, a driver may not be able

Table 12.4

Psychological and Physical Effects of Various Blood-Alcohol Concentration Levels*

NUMBER OF DRINKS†	BLOOD-ALCOHOL CONCENTRATION (%)	PSYCHOLOGICAL AND PHYSICAL EFFECTS
1	0.02–0.03	No overt effects, slight mood elevation
2	0.05–0.06	Feeling of relaxation, warmth; slight decrease in reaction time and in fine-muscle coordination
3	0.08–0.09	Balance, speech, vision, and hearing slightly impaired; feelings of euphoria, increased confidence; loss of motor coordination
	0.01	Legal intoxication in most states; some have lower limits
4	0.11–0.12	Coordination and balance becoming difficult; distinct impairment of mental faculties, judgment
5	0.14–0.15	Major impairment of mental and physical control; slurred speech, blurred vision, lack of motor skills
7	0.20	Loss of motor control—must have assistance in moving about; mental confusion
10	0.30	Severe intoxication; minimum conscious control of mind and body
14	0.40	Unconsciousness, threshold of coma
17	0.50	Deep coma
20	0.60	Death from respiratory failure

*For each hour elapsed since the last drink, subtract 0.015 percent blood-alcohol concentration, or approximately one drink.
†One drink = one beer (4 percent alcohol, 12 ounces), one highball (1 ounce whiskey), or one glass table wine (4 ounces).
Source: Modified from data given in Ohio State Police Driver Information Seminars and the National Clearinghouse for Alcohol and Alcoholism Information, Rockville, MD.

to estimate distances or speed, and some drinkers lose their ability to make value-related decisions and may do things they would not do when sober. As BAC increases, the drinker suffers increased physiological and psychological effects. All these changes are negative. Alcohol ingestion does not enhance any physical skills or mental functions.

People can acquire physical and psychological tolerance to the effects of alcohol through regular use. The nervous system adapts over time, so greater amounts of alcohol are required to produce the same physiological and psychological effects. Some people can learn to modify their behavior so that they appear to be sober even when their BAC is quite high. This ability is called **learned behavioral tolerance.**

Absorption and Metabolism

Unlike the molecules found in most other ingestible foods and drugs, alcohol molecules are sufficiently small and fat-soluble to be absorbed throughout the entire gastrointestinal system. A negligible amount of alcohol is absorbed through the lining of the mouth. Approximately 20 percent of ingested alcohol diffuses through the stomach lining into the bloodstream, and nearly 80 percent passes through the linings of the upper third of the small intestine. Absorption into the bloodstream is rapid and complete.

Several factors influence how quickly your body will absorb alcohol: the alcohol concentration in your drink, the amount of alcohol you consume, the amount of food in your stomach, pylorospasm (spasm of the pyloric valve in the digestive system), and your mood. The higher the concentration of alcohol in your drink, the more rapidly it will be absorbed in your digestive tract. As a rule, wine and beer are absorbed more slowly than distilled beverages. Carbonated

Ethyl alcohol (ethanol) An addictive drug produced by fermentation and found in many beverages.

Fermentation The process whereby yeast organisms break down plant sugars to yield ethanol.

Distillation The process whereby mash is subjected to high temperatures to release alcohol vapors, which are then condensed and mixed with water to make the final product.

Proof A measure of the percentage of alcohol in a beverage.

Blood alcohol concentration (BAC) The ratio of alcohol to total blood volume; the factor used to measure the physiological and behavioral effects of alcohol.

Learned behavioral tolerance The ability of heavy drinkers to modify behavior so that they appear to be sober even when they have high BAC levels.

alcoholic beverages—such as champagne and carbonated wines—are absorbed more rapidly than those containing no sparkling additives, or fizz. Carbonated beverages and drinks served with mixers cause the pyloric valve—the opening from the stomach into the small intestine—to relax, thereby emptying the contents of the stomach more rapidly into the small intestine. Since the small intestine is the site of the greatest absorption of alcohol, carbonated beverages increase the rate of absorption. On the other hand, if your stomach is full, absorption is slowed because the surface area exposed to alcohol is smaller. A full stomach also retards the emptying of alcoholic beverages into the small intestine.

In addition, the more alcohol you consume, the longer absorption takes. Alcohol can irritate the digestive system, causing a spasm in the pyloric valve (pylorospasm). When the pyloric valve is closed, nothing can move from the stomach to the upper third of the small intestine, which slows absorption. If the irritation continues, it can cause vomiting.

Mood is another factor, since emotions affect how long it takes for the contents of the stomach to empty into the intestine. Powerful moods, such as stress and tension, are likely to cause the stomach to "dump" its contents into the small intestine. That is why alcohol is absorbed much more rapidly when people are tense than when they are relaxed.

Alcohol is metabolized in the liver, where it is converted by the enzyme alcohol dehydrogenase to acetaldehyde. It is then rapidly oxidized to acetate, converted to carbon dioxide and water, and eventually excreted from the body. Acetaldehyde is a toxic chemical that can cause immediate symptoms such as nausea and vomiting as well as long-term effects such as liver damage. A very small portion of alcohol is excreted unchanged by the kidneys, lungs, and skin.

Like food, alcohol contains calories. Proteins and carbohydrates (starches and sugars) each contain 4 kilocalories (kcal) per gram. Fat contains 9 kcal per gram. Alcohol, although similar in structure to carbohydrates, contains 7 kcal per gram. The body uses the calories in alcohol in the same manner it uses those found in carbohydrates: for immediate energy or for storage as fat if not immediately needed.

When compared to the variable breakdown rates of foods and other beverages, the breakdown of alcohol occurs at a fairly constant rate of 0.5 ounces per hour. This amount of alcohol is equivalent to 12 ounces of 5 percent beer, 8 ounces of malt liquor, 4 ounces of 12 percent wine, or 1.5 ounces of 40 percent (80 proof) liquor. Legal limits of BAC for operating motor vehicles vary from state to state. Most states set the legal limit at 0.08 to 0.10 percent. A driver whose level of BAC exceeds the state's legal limit is considered legally intoxicated.

A drinker's BAC depends on weight and body fat, the water content in body tissues, the concentration of alcohol in the beverage consumed, the rate of consumption, and the volume of alcohol consumed. Heavier people have larger body surfaces through which to diffuse alcohol; therefore, they have lower concentrations of alcohol in their blood than do thin people after drinking the same amount. Because alcohol does not diffuse as rapidly into body fat as into water, alcohol concentration is higher in a person with more body fat. Because a woman is likely to have more body fat and less water in her body tissues than a man of the same weight, she will be more intoxicated than a man after drinking the same amount of alcohol.

Alcohol Poisoning Alcohol poisoning occurs much more frequently than people realize, and all too often it can be fatal. Drinking large amounts of alcohol in a short period of time can cause the blood alcohol level to reach the lethal range relatively quickly. Alcohol, used either alone or in combination with other drugs, is probably responsible for more toxic overdose deaths than any other substance.

Death from alcohol poisoning can be caused by either central nervous system (CNS) and respiratory depression or the inhalation of vomit or fluid into the lungs. The amount of alcohol it takes for a person to become unconscious is dangerously close to the lethal dose. Signs of alcohol poisoning include the following: being unable to be aroused; a weak, rapid pulse; an unusual or irregular breathing pattern; and cool (possibly damp), pale, or bluish skin. If you are with someone who has been drinking heavily and who exhibits these conditions, or if you are unsure about the person's condition, call 911 for emergency help right away.

What do you think?

Have you noticed that some types of alcoholic beverages affect people more quickly than others? ✳ *What factors affect BAC levels?* ✳ *Are these factors different for men and women?* ✳ *If so, how?*

Women and Alcohol Body fat is not the only contributor to the differences in alcohol's effects on men and women. Compared to men, women appear to have half as much alcohol hydrogenase, the enzyme that breaks down alcohol in the stomach before it has a chance to get to the bloodstream and the brain. Therefore, if a man and a woman drink the same amount of alcohol, the woman's BAC will be approximately 30 percent higher than the man's, leaving her more vulnerable to slurred speech, careless driving, and other drinking-related impairments. In addition to differences in stomach enzymes and body fat in men and women, there are also hormonal differences that can affect a woman's BAC. Specifically, one week prior to menstruating, women maintain the peak level of intoxication for longer periods of time than menstruating or postmenstruating women do. Women who are using oral contraceptives are also likely to maintain peak intoxication for longer periods of time than they would otherwise. This prolonged peak appears to be related to estrogen levels.

Women who consume alcohol need to pay close attention to how much they consume. It is possible that a woman matching her male friend drink per drink could become twice as intoxicated. For example, if a 180-pound college-age male and a 120-pound college-age female each have three drinks, the BAC for the male would be .06 and for the

Table 12.5
Calculation of Estimated Blood Alcohol Concentration for Women and Men

DRINKS*	90	100	120	140	160	180	200	220	240	
WOMEN										
0	.00	.00	.00	.00	.00	.00	.00	.00	.00	Only safe driving limit
1	**.05**	**.05**	**.04**	.03	.03	.03	.02	.02	.02	Impairment begins
2	.10	**.09**	**.08**	**.07**	**.06**	**.05**	**.05**	**.04**	**.04**	**Driving skills**
3	.15	.14	.11	.10	**.09**	**.08**	**.07**	**.06**	**.06**	**significantly affected**
4	.20	.18	.15	.13	.11	.10	.09	**.08**	**.08**	**Possible criminal**
5	.25	.23	.19	.16	.14	.13	.11	.10	**.09**	**penalties**
6	.30	.27	.23	.19	.17	.15	.14	.12	.11	
7	.35	.32	.27	.23	.20	.18	.16	.14	.13	Legally intoxicated
8	.40	.36	.30	.26	.23	.20	.18	.17	.15	
9	.45	.41	.34	.29	.26	.23	.20	.19	.17	Criminal penalties
10	.51	.45	.38	.32	.28	.25	.23	.21	.19	
MEN										
0		.00	.00	.00	.00	.00	.00	.00	.00	Only safe driving limit
1		**.04**	.03	.03	.02	.02	.02	.02	.02	Impairment begins
2		**.08**	**.06**	**.05**	**.05**	**.04**	**.04**	**.03**	**.03**	**Driving skills**
3		.11	**.09**	**.08**	**.07**	**.06**	**.06**	**.05**	**.05**	**significantly affected**
4		.15	.12	.11	**.09**	**.08**	**.08**	**.07**	**.06**	
5		.19	.16	.13	.12	.11	**.09**	**.09**	**.08**	**Possible criminal**
6		.23	.19	.16	.14	.13	.11	.10	**.09**	**penalties**
7		.26	.22	.19	.16	.15	.13	.12	.11	Legally intoxicated
8		.30	.25	.21	.19	.17	.15	.14	.13	
9		.34	.28	.24	.21	.19	.17	.15	.14	Criminal penalties
10		.38	.31	.27	.23	.21	.19	.17	.16	

Note: Blood alcohol percentages above bold values indicate beginning impairment; all percentages below bold values indicate legal intoxication with criminal penalty.
Subtract 0.01% for each 40 minutes of drinking.
*One drink is 1.25 oz. of 80-proof liquor, 12 oz. of beer, or 4 oz. of table wine.
Source: Data supplied by the Pennsylvania Liquor Control Board.

female .11, almost double that of her male friend. Table 12.5 compares blood-alcohol levels by sex, weight, and consumption. Although this table can provide an estimate of probable BAC levels, many additional factors may cause considerable variation in these rates.

Breathalyzer and Other Tests The Breathalyzer tests used by law enforcement officers determine BAC based on the amount of alcohol exhaled in the breath. Urinalysis can also yield a BAC based on the concentration of unmetabolized alcohol in the urine. Both breath analysis and urinalysis are used to determine whether a driver is legally intoxicated, but blood tests are more accurate measures. An increasing number of states are requiring blood tests for people suspected of driving under the influence of alcohol. In some states, refusal to take the breath or urine test results in immediate revocation of the person's driver's license.

Immediate Effects

The most dramatic effects produced by ethanol occur within the central nervous system (CNS). The primary action of the drug is to reduce the frequency of nerve transmissions and impulses at synaptic junctions. This depresses CNS functions, with resulting decreases in respiratory rate, pulse rate, and blood pressure. As CNS depression deepens, vital functions become noticeably depressed. In extreme cases, coma and death can result.

Alcohol is a diuretic, causing increased urinary output. Although this effect might be expected to lead to automatic **dehydration** (loss of water), the body actually retains water,

Dehydration	Loss of fluids from body tissues.

Table 12.6
Drugs and Alcohol: Actions and Interactions

DRUG CLASS/TRADE NAME(S)	EFFECTS WITH ALCOHOL
Antialcohol: Antabuse	Severe reactions to even small amounts: headache, nausea, blurred vision, convulsions, coma, possible death.
Antibiotics: Penicillin, Cyantin	Reduced therapeutic effectiveness.
Antidepressants: Elavil, Sinequan, Tofranil, Nardil	Increased central nervous system (CNS) depression, blood pressure changes. Combined use of alcohol and MAO inhibitors, a specific type of antidepressant, can trigger massive increases in blood pressure, even brain hemorrhage and death.
Antihistamines: Allerest, Dristan	Drowsiness and CNS depression. Driving ability impaired.
Aspirin: Anacin, Excedrin, Bayer	Irritates stomach lining. May cause gastrointestinal pain, bleeding.
Depressants: Valium, Ativan, Placidyl	Dangerous CNS depression, loss of coordination, coma. High risk of overdose and death.
Narcotics: heroin, codeine, Darvon	Serious CNS depression. Possible respiratory arrest and death.
Stimulants: caffeine, cocaine	Masks depressant action of alcohol. May increase blood pressure, physical tension.

Source: Reprinted by permission from *Drugs and Alcohol: Simple Facts about Alcohol and Drug Combinations* (Phoenix: DIN Publications, 1988), no. 121.

most of it in the muscles or in cerebral tissues. This is because water is usually pulled out of the **cerebrospinal fluid** (fluid within the brain and spinal cord), leading to what is known as mitochondrial dehydration at the cell level within the nervous system. Mitochondria are miniature organs within cells that are responsible for specific functions, and they rely heavily upon fluid balance. When mitochondrial dehydration occurs from drinking, the mitochondria cannot carry out their normal functions, resulting in symptoms that include the "morning-after" headaches suffered by some drinkers.

Alcohol irritates the gastrointestinal system and may cause indigestion and heartburn if taken on an empty stomach. Long-term use of alcohol causes repeated irritation that has been linked to cancers of the esophagus and stomach. In addition, people who engage in brief drinking sprees during which they consume unusually high amounts of alcohol put themselves at risk for irregular heartbeat or even total loss of heart rhythm, which can disrupt blood flow and damage the heart muscle.

A **hangover** is often experienced the morning after a drinking spree. The symptoms of a hangover are familiar to most people who drink: headache, muscle aches, upset stomach, anxiety, depression, and thirst. **Congeners** are thought to play a role in the development of a hangover. Congeners are forms of alcohol that are metabolized more slowly than ethanol and are more toxic. The body metabolizes the congeners after the ethanol is gone from the system, and their toxic by-products may contribute to the hangover. In addition, alcohol upsets the water balance in the body, resulting in excess urination and thirst the next day. Increased production of hydrochloric acid can irritate the stomach lining

and cause nausea. It usually takes 12 hours to recover from a hangover. Bed rest, solid food, and aspirin may help relieve its discomforts, but unfortunately, nothing cures it but time.

Drug Interactions When you use any drug (and alcohol is a drug), you need to be aware of the possible interactions with any other drugs, whether prescription or over-the-counter. Table 12.6 summarizes possible interactions. Note that alcohol may cause a negative interaction even with aspirin.

Long-Term Effects

Alcohol is distributed throughout most of the body and may affect many different organs and tissues. Problems associated with long-term, habitual use of alcohol include diseases of the cardiovascular system, nervous system, and liver, and some cancers.

Effects on the Nervous System The nervous system is especially sensitive to alcohol. Even people who drink moderately experience shrinkage in brain size and weight and a loss of some degree of intellectual ability. The damage that results from alcohol use is localized primarily in the left side of the brain, which is responsible for written and spoken language, logic, and mathematical skills. The degree of shrinkage appears to be directly related to the amount of alcohol consumed. In terms of memory loss, the evidence suggests that having one drink every day is better than saving up for a binge and consuming seven or eight drinks in a night. The amount of alcohol consumed at one time is critical. Alcohol-related brain damage can be partially reversed with good nutrition and sobriety.

Cardiovascular Effects Alcohol affects the cardiovascular system in a number of ways. Numerous studies have associated light-to-moderate alcohol consumption (no more than two drinks a day) with a reduced risk of coronary artery disease. Several mechanisms have been proposed to explain how this might happen. The strongest evidence favors an increase in high-density lipoprotein (HDL) cholesterol, which is known as the "good" cholesterol. Studies have shown that drinkers have higher levels of HDL. Another factor that might help is an *antithrombotic effect*. Alcohol consumption is associated with a decrease in clotting factors that contribute to the development of atherosclerosis.

However, alcohol consumption is not recommended as a preventive measure against heart disease because it causes many more cardiovascular health hazards than benefits. Alcohol contributes to high blood pressure and slightly increased heart rate and cardiac output. Those who report drinking three to five drinks a day, regardless of race or sex, have higher blood pressure than those who drink less.

Liver Disease One of the most common diseases related to alcohol abuse is **cirrhosis** of the liver. It is among the top 10 causes of death in the United States. One result of heavy drinking is that the liver begins to store fat—a condition known as fatty liver. If there is insufficient time between drinking episodes, this fat cannot be transported to storage sites, and the fat-filled liver cells stop functioning. Continued drinking can cause a further stage of liver deterioration called fibrosis, in which the damaged area of the liver develops fibrous scar tissue. Cell function can be partially restored at this stage with proper nutrition and abstinence from alcohol. If the person continues to drink, however, cirrhosis results. At this point, the liver cells die and the damage becomes permanent. **Alcoholic hepatitis** is a serious condition resulting from prolonged use of alcohol. A chronic inflammation of the liver develops, which may be fatal in itself or progress to cirrhosis.

Cancer The repeated irritation caused by long-term use of alcohol has been linked to cancers of the esophagus, stomach, mouth, tongue, and liver. Research has also shown a link between breast cancer and moderate levels of alcohol consumption in women. One compelling report has demonstrated that "drinkers of three or more glasses of alcoholic beverages per day appear to be at greater risk for breast cancer."[9] A 1994 study of male drinkers by the Harvard Medical School showed a 12 percent increased risk for cancer for those who had only one drink a day and 123 percent for those who had two drinks a day. It is unclear how alcohol exerts its carcinogenic effects, though it is thought that it inhibits the absorption of carcinogenic substances, permitting them to be taken to sensitive organs.

Other Effects An irritant to the gastrointestinal system, alcohol may cause indigestion and heartburn if ingested on an empty stomach. It also damages the mucous membranes and can cause inflammation of the esophagus, chronic stomach irritation, problems with intestinal absorption, and chronic diarrhea.

Alcohol abuse is a major cause of chronic inflammation of the pancreas, the organ that produces digestive enzymes and insulin. Chronic abuse of alcohol inhibits enzyme production, which further inhibits the absorption of nutrients. Drinking alcohol can block the absorption of calcium, a nutrient that strengthens bones. This should be of particular concern to women, for as women age their risk for osteoporosis (bone thinning and calcium loss) increases. Heavy consumption of alcohol worsens this condition.

Evidence also suggests that alcohol impairs the body's ability to recognize and fight foreign bodies such as bacteria and viruses. The relationship between alcohol and AIDS is unclear, especially since some of the populations at risk for AIDS are also at risk for alcohol abuse. But any stressor like alcohol, with a known effect on the immune system, would probably contribute to the development of the disease.

Alcohol and Pregnancy

Of the 30 known teratogens in the environment, alcohol is one of the most dangerous and common. Alcohol can harm fetal development.

More than 10 percent of all children have been exposed to high levels of alcohol in utero. All will suffer varying degrees of effects, ranging from mild learning disabilities to major physical, mental, and intellectual impairment. It takes very little alcohol to cause serious damage. Research has shown that even a single exposure to high levels of alcohol can cause significant brain damage in the infant.[10] A disorder called **fetal alcohol syndrome (FAS)** is associated with alcohol consumption during pregnancy. Alcohol consumed during the first trimester poses the greatest threat to organ

---

Cerebrospinal fluid Fluid within and surrounding the brain and spinal cord tissues.

Hangover The physiological reaction to excessive drinking, including symptoms such as headache, upset stomach, anxiety, depression, diarrhea, and thirst.

Congeners Forms of alcohol that are metabolized more slowly than ethanol and produce toxic by-products.

Cirrhosis The last stage of liver disease associated with chronic heavy use of alcohol during which liver cells die and damage becomes permanent.

Alcoholic hepatitis Condition resulting from prolonged use of alcohol in which the liver is inflamed. It can result in death.

Fetal alcohol syndrome (FAS) A disorder that may affect the fetus when the mother consumes alcohol during pregnancy. Among its effects are mental retardation, small head, tremors, and abnormalities of the face, limbs, heart, and brain.

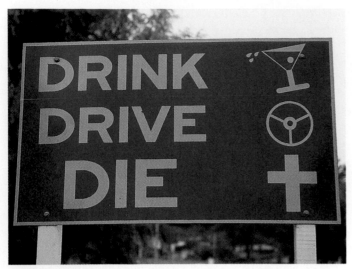

All too often, drinking and driving make a deadly combination. Approximately 40 percent of U.S. traffic fatalities are alcohol-related.

development; exposure during the last trimester, when the brain is developing rapidly, is most likely to affect CNS development. FAS is the third most common birth defect and the second leading cause of mental retardation in the United States. The incidence of FAS is estimated to be 1 to 2 of every 1,000 live births. It is the most common preventable cause of mental impairments in the Western world.

FAS occurs when alcohol ingested by the mother passes through the placenta into the infant's bloodstream. Because the fetus is so small, its BAC will be much higher than that of the mother. Among the symptoms of FAS are mental retardation, small head, tremors, and abnormalities of the face, limbs, heart, and brain. Problems that children with FAS experience may include the following:

- Difficulty in structuring work time.
- Impaired rates of learning.
- Poor memory.
- Trouble in generalizing behaviors and information.
- Impulsive behaviors.
- Reduced attention span or distractible behavior.
- Fearlessness and unresponsive reactions to verbal cautions.
- Poor social judgment.
- Inability to handle money in an age-appropriate manner.
- Trouble with internalizing modeled behaviors.
- Differences in sensory awareness (hyposensitive or hypersensitive).
- Language production higher than comprehension.
- Poor problem-solving strategies.[11]

Children with a history of prenatal alcohol exposure but with fewer than the full physical or behavioral symptoms of FAS may be categorized as having **fetal alcohol effects (FAE)**. FAE is estimated to occur three to four times as often as FAS, although it is much less recognized. The signs of FAE in newborns are low birthweight and irritability, and there may be permanent mental impairment. Infants whose moth-

ers habitually consumed more than three ounces of alcohol (approximately six drinks) in a short time period when pregnant are at high risk for FAS. Risk levels for babies whose mothers consume smaller amounts are uncertain.

Alcohol can also be passed to a nursing baby through breast milk. For this reason, most doctors advise nursing mothers not to drink for at least four hours before nursing their babies and preferably to abstain altogether.

> **What do you think?**
>
> *Why do we hear so little about FAS in this country when it is the third most common birth defect and second leading cause of mental retardation?*
> ✳ *Is this a reflection of our society's denial of alcohol as a dangerous drug?*

Drinking and Driving

The leading cause of death for all age groups from 5 to 45 years old (including college students) is traffic accidents. Approximately 40 percent of all traffic fatalities are alcohol-related.[12] Unfortunately, college students are overrepresented in alcohol-related crashes. The College Alcohol Study findings indicated that 20 percent of nonbingers, 43 percent of occasional bingers, and 59 percent of frequent bingers reported driving while intoxicated.[13] Furthermore, it is estimated that three out of every ten Americans will be involved in an alcohol-related accident at some time in their lives.[14] Studies show that those involved in car crashes after drinking have a 40 to 50 percent higher chance of dying than nondrinkers involved in car crashes.

In 2000, there were 16,653 alcohol-related traffic fatalities (ARTFs), a 30 percent reduction from the ARTF reported in 1990. This number represents an average of one alcohol-related fatality every 32 minutes.[15] From 1990 to 2000, intoxication rates (BAC of 0.10 percent or greater) decreased for drivers of all age groups involved in fatal crashes (see Figure 12.2). The highest intoxication rates in fatal crashes in 2000 were recorded for drivers 21 to 24 years old (27.0 percent), followed by ages 25 to 34 (24.0 percent) and 35 to 44 (22.0 percent). Approximately 1.5 million drivers were arrested in 1999 for driving under the influence of alcohol. This is an arrest rate of 1 for every 121 licensed drivers in the United States.[16]

Several factors probably contributed to these reductions in ARTFs: laws that raised the drinking age to 21; stricter law enforcement; increased emphasis on zero tolerance (laws prohibiting those under 21 from driving with *any* detectable BAC); and the educational and other prevention programs designed to discourage drinking and driving. Most states have set 0.10 percent as the BAC at which drivers are considered to be legally drunk (refer to Table 12.5). However, several states have lowered the standard to 0.08 percent, and others are likely to follow.

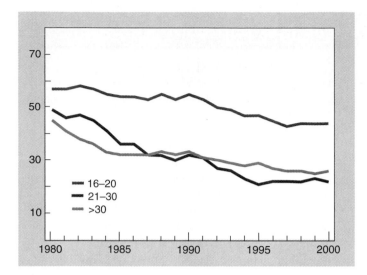

Figure 12.2
Percentage of Fatally Injured Passenger Vehicle Drivers with BACs > 0.10 Percent, by Driver Age

Laboratory and test track research shows that the vast majority of drivers, even experienced drinkers, are impaired at 0.08 with regard to critical driving tasks. Braking, steering, lane changing, judgment, and divided attention, among other measures, are all affected significantly at 0.08 BAC. National groups such as MADD (Mothers Against Drunk Driving), started by a mother whose child was killed by a drunk driver, go as far as tracking drunk driving cases through the court systems to ensure that drunk drivers are punished. Members of the high school group SADD (Students Against Destructive Decisions) educate their peers about the dangers of drinking and driving.

Despite all these measures, the risk of being involved in an alcohol-related automobile crash remains substantial. Researchers have shown a direct relationship between the amount of alcohol in a driver's bloodstream and the likelihood of a crash. A driver with a BAC level of 0.10 percent is approximately 10 times more likely to be involved in a car accident than a driver who has not been drinking. At a BAC of 0.15 on weekend nights, the likelihood of dying in a single-vehicle crash is more than 380 times higher than for nondrinkers. Alcohol involvement is highest during nighttime (9 P.M. to 6 A.M.) single-vehicle crashes, in which 53 percent of fatally injured passenger vehicle drivers in 2000 had BACs at or over 0.10 percent. Only 27 percent of fatally injured drivers involved in nighttime single-vehicle crashes had no alcohol in their blood.

Not only does the time of day increase risk of being involved in an alcohol-related crash, but it also makes a difference whether it is a weekday or weekend. In 2000, 30 percent of all fatal crashes during the week were alcohol-related, compared with 53 percent on weekends.[17]

What do you think?

What do you think the legal BAC for drivers should be? ✳ *Why do you think that many states have not lowered the legal limit to 0.08?* ✳ *What should the penalty be for people arrested for driving under the influence of alcohol (DUI) for the first offense?* ✳ *The second offense?* ✳ *The third offense?*

Alcohol Abuse and Alcoholism

Alcohol use becomes **alcohol abuse** or **alcoholism** when it interferes with work, school, or social and family relationships or when it entails any violation of the law, including driving under the influence (DUI).

Identifying a Problem Drinker

As in other drug addictions, tolerance, psychological dependence, and withdrawal symptoms must be present to qualify a drinker as an addict. Addiction results from chronic use over a period of time that may vary from person to person. Problem drinkers or irresponsible users are not necessarily alcoholics. The stereotype of the alcoholic on skid row applies to only 5 percent of the alcoholic population. The remaining 95 percent of alcoholics live in some type of extended family unit. They can be found at all socioeconomic levels and in all professions, ethnic groups, geographical locations, religions, and races.

Studies suggest that the lifetime risk of alcoholism in the United States is about 10 percent for men and 3 percent for women. Moreover, 25 percent of the American population (50 million people) is affected by the alcoholism of a friend or family member. The 2001 National Household Survey on Drug Abuse found that 5.7 percent of Americans were heavy drinkers and 20.7 percent were binge drinkers.

Recognizing and admitting the existence of an alcohol problem are often extremely difficult. Alcoholics themselves deny their problem, often making statements such as "I can stop any time I want to. I just don't want to right now." Their families also tend to deny the existence of a problem, saying things like "He really has been under a lot of stress lately. Besides, he only drinks beer." The fear of being labeled a "problem drinker" often prevents people from seeking help. The Skills for Behavior Change box describes strategies to cut down on drinking.

Fetal alcohol effects (FAE) A syndrome describing children with a history of prenatal alcohol exposure but without all the physical or behavioral symptoms of FAS. Among its symptoms are low birthweight, irritability, and possible permanent mental impairment.

Alcohol abuse (alcoholism) Use of alcohol that interferes with work, school, or personal relationships or that entails violations of the law.

How to Cut Down on Your Drinking

If you think you are drinking too much, you can improve your life and health by cutting down. Start with these steps:

1. Write your reasons for cutting down or stopping.
2. Set a drinking goal.
   - Choose a limit for how much you will drink each day.
3. Keep a diary of your drinking for a month.
   - This will show you how much you drink and when, also how much money you spend. Realizing how much money you spend per month could be surprising.

If you want to know how to keep your drinking under control, use these tips.

1. Watch it at home.
   - Keep a small amount of alcohol or no alcohol in your house or apartment. Don't keep temptations around.

2. Drink slowly.
   - When you drink, don't get involved in drinking games or use beer bongs or other methods of guzzling alcohol quickly.
   - Take a break of one hour between drinks, and alternate with nonalcoholic drinks such as soda.
3. Take a break from alcohol.
   - Limit your alcohol intake to no more than a couple of days a week. Think about how you feel physically and emotionally on these days. When you feel better, you may find it easier to cut down for good.
4. Learn how to say NO.
   - You do not have to drink when other people drink. Stay away from others who give you a hard time about not drinking and from places where you will feel awkward if you don't have a drink in your hand.
5. Stay active!
   - Ask yourself what you would like to do other than go out drinking. Go out to eat, see a movie, go to the Recreation Center, or do something fun with friends.

6. Get support.
   - Cutting down on your drinking may be difficult at times. Surround yourself with friends who are interested in helping you, not people who are interested in getting you to drink with them.
7. Watch out for temptations.
   - Be careful about places, people, or times that make you drink, even if you do not want to. Stay away from friends who drink a lot or bars where you used to go. Plan ahead to avoid drinking when you are tempted.
   - Do not drink when you are angry or upset or have had a bad day. These are habits you need to break if you are going to drink less.

Source: Adapted from: National Institute on Alcohol Abuse and Alcoholism, NIH Publication no. 96-3770, "How to Cut Down on Your Drinking," 1996.

Alcoholics tend to have a number of symptoms in common. The Assess Yourself box lists several. People who recognize one or more of these behaviors in themselves may wish to seek professional help to determine whether alcohol has become a controlling factor in their lives.

Women are the fastest-growing population of alcohol abusers. They tend to become alcoholic at a later age and after fewer years of heavy drinking than do male alcoholics. Women at highest risk for alcohol-related problems are those who are unmarried but living with a partner, are in their 20s or early 30s, or have a husband or partner who drinks heavily.

The Causes of Alcohol Abuse and Alcoholism

We know that alcoholism is a disease with biological and social/environmental components, but we do not know what role each component plays in the disease.

Biological and Family Factors Research into the hereditary and environmental causes of alcoholism has found higher rates of alcoholism among family members of alcoholics. In

fact, according to researchers, alcoholism is four to five times more common among children of alcoholics than in the general population.

Male alcoholics, especially, are more likely than non-alcoholics to have alcoholic parents and siblings. Two distinct subtypes of alcoholism have provided important information about the inheritance of alcoholism. *Type 1 alcoholics* are drinkers who had at least one parent of either sex who was a problem drinker and who grew up in an environment that encouraged heavy drinking. Their drinking is reinforced by environmental events during which there is heavy drinking. Type 1 alcohol abusers share certain personality characteristics. They avoid novelty and harmful situations and are concerned about the thoughts and feelings of others. *Type 2 alcoholism* is seen in males only. These alcoholics are typically the biological sons of alcoholic fathers who have a history of both violence and drug use. Type 2 alcoholics display the opposite characteristics of Type 1 alcoholics. They do not seek social approval, they lack inhibition, and they are prone to novelty-seeking behavior.[18]

One study found a strong relationship between alcoholism and alcoholic patterns within the family.[19] Children

Alcohol Abuse and Alcoholism: Common Questions

Although many people think that they have a clear understanding of the disease called alcoholism, much remains in question. Answering the following questions may indicate your own level of knowledge about the disease. For further information, particularly as it relates to alcohol use on college campuses, check out the National Institute of Alcohol Abuse and Alcoholism's website (www.niaaa.nih.gov).

1. Alcoholism is a disease characterized by what four symptoms?

   a.

   b.

   c.

   d.

2. Is alcoholism an inherited trait?   Yes   Probably   No

3. Do you have to be an alcoholic to experience alcohol-related problems?   Yes   No

4. What groups of individuals tend to have the most problems with alcoholism?

ANSWERS:

1. The four symptoms of alcoholism include

   Craving (a strong need or urge to drink alcohol).
   Loss of control (not being able to stop drinking once drinking begins).
   Physical dependence (withdrawal symptoms, such as nausea, sweating, shakiness, and anxiety after stopping drinking).
   Tolerance (the need to drink greater amounts of alcohol to achieve the same effect).

   (See the *Diagnostic Statistical Manual IV* of the American Psychological Association for further information.)

2. Probably yes. The risk of developing alcoholism does indeed run in families. While part of this may be explained by genetics, lifestyle is a major factor. Currently, researchers are trying to locate the actual genes that put you at risk. Your friends, the amount of stress in your life, and how readily available alcohol is are also factors that increase risk. Remember that risk is not destiny. A child of an alcoholic won't automatically become an alcoholic. Others develop alcoholism even though no one in their family is an alcoholic. If you know you are at risk, you can take steps to protect yourself.

3. No. Alcoholism is only one type of alcohol problem. Alcohol abuse can be just as harmful. A person can abuse alcohol without being an alcoholic—that is, he or she may drink too much, too often, and still not be dependent on alcohol. Some of the problems of alcohol abuse include not being able to meet work, school, or family responsibilities; drunk driving arrests and car crashes; and drinking-related medical conditions. Under some circumstances, even social or moderate drinking is dangerous—for example, when driving, during pregnancy, or when taking certain medications.

4. Alcohol abuse and alcoholism cut across gender, race, and nationality. Nearly one in three adults abuse alcohol in the United States today. In general, more men than women are alcohol dependent or have alcohol problems. Alcohol problems are most common among young adults, ages 18–29, and rarest among adults ages 65 and older. We also know that the younger you start, the more likely that you will have a problem.

Source: National Institute on Alcohol Abuse and Alcoholism, "College Drinking: FAQ's on Alcohol Abuse and Alcoholism", 2002 (see http://www.collegedrinkingprevention.gov/facts/faq.aspx).

---

with one alcoholic parent had a 52 percent chance of becoming alcoholics themselves. With two alcoholic parents, the chances of becoming alcoholic jumped to 71 percent. The researchers felt that both heredity and environment were significant factors in the development of alcoholism but were reluctant to specify precisely how these factors worked.

Because the effects of heredity and environment are so difficult to separate, some scientists have chosen to examine the problem through twin and adoption studies.[20] So far, these studies have produced inconclusive results, although a slightly higher rate of similar drinking behaviors has been demonstrated among identical twins. Moreover, sons living away from their alcoholic parents tend to more closely resemble them in drinking behavior than they do their adoptive or foster parents.

Social and Cultural Factors   Although a family history of alcoholism may predispose a person to problems with alcohol, numerous other factors may mitigate or exacerbate that tendency. Social and cultural factors may trigger the affliction for many people who are not genetically predisposed to alcoholism. Some people begin drinking as a way to dull the pain of an acute loss or an emotional or social problem. For example, college students may drink to escape the stress of college life, disappointment over unfulfilled expectations, difficulties in forming relationships, or loss of the security of home, loved ones, and close friends. Involvement in a painful relationship, death of a family member, and other problems may trigger a search for an anesthetic. Unfortunately, the emotional discomfort that causes many people to turn to alcohol also ultimately causes them to become even more uncomfortable as the depressant effect of the drug begins to take its toll. Thus, the person who is already depressed may become even more depressed, antagonizing friends and other social supports until they begin to turn away. Eventually, the drinker becomes physically dependent on the drug.

Family attitudes toward alcohol also seem to influence whether or not a person will develop a drinking problem. It has been clearly demonstrated that people who are raised in cultures in which drinking is a part of religious or ceremonial activities or in which alcohol is a traditional part of the family meal are less prone to alcohol dependency. In contrast, in societies in which alcohol purchase is carefully controlled and drinking is regarded as a rite of passage to adulthood, the tendency for abuse appears to be greater.

Certain social factors have been linked with alcoholism as well. These include urbanization, the weakening of links to the extended family and a general loosening of kinship ties, increased mobility, and changing religious and philosophical values. Apparently, then, some combination of heredity and environment plays a decisive role in the development of alcoholism. Certain ethnic and racial groups also have special alcohol abuse problems.

What do you think?

How was alcohol used in your family when you were growing up? ✳ *Was alcohol used only on special occasions or not at all?* ✳ *How much do you think your family's attitudes and behaviors toward alcohol have shaped your behavior?*

Effects of Alcoholism on the Family

Only recently have people begun to recognize that it is not only the alcoholic but the alcoholic's entire family that suffers. Although most research focuses on family effects during the late stages of alcoholism, the family unit actually begins to react early on as the person starts to show symptoms of the disease.

An estimated 76 million Americans (about 43 percent of the U.S. adult population) have been exposed to alcoholism in the family.[21] Twenty-two million members of alcoholic families are age 18 or older, and many have carried childhood emotional scars into adulthood. Approximately one in four children under age 18 lives in an atmosphere of anxiety, tension, confusion, and denial.[22]

In dysfunctional families, children learn certain rules from a very early age: Don't talk, don't trust, and don't feel. These unspoken rules allow the family to avoid dealing with

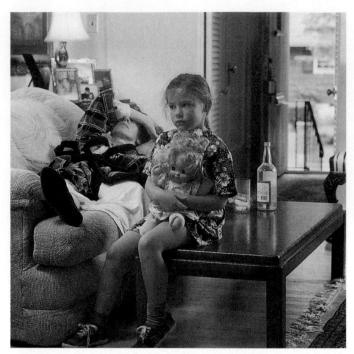

Health officials suspect that a person's attitudes about alcohol use may be influenced by the behavior patterns witnessed while growing up.

real problems and real issues. Family members unconsciously adapt to the alcoholic's behavior by adjusting their own behavior. Unfortunately, these behaviors actually help keep the alcoholic drinking. Children in such dysfunctional families generally assume at least one of the following roles:

- *Family hero.* Tries to divert attention from the problem by being too good to be true.
- *Scapegoat.* Draws attention away from the family's primary problem through delinquency or misbehavior.
- *Lost child.* Becomes passive and quietly withdraws from upsetting situations.
- *Mascot.* Disrupts tense situations by providing comic relief.

For children in alcoholic homes, life is a struggle. They have to deal with constant stress, anxiety, and embarrassment. Because the alcoholic is the center of attention, the children's wants and needs are often ignored. It is not uncommon for these children to be victims of violence, abuse, neglect, or incest. As we have seen, when such children grow up, they are much more prone to alcoholic behaviors themselves than are children from nonalcoholic families.

In the past decade, we have come to recognize the unique problems of adult children of alcoholics whose difficulties in life stem from a lack of parental nurturing during childhood. Among these problems are an inability to develop social attachments, a need to be in control of all emotions and situations, low self-esteem, and depression. Fortunately, not all individuals who have grown up in alcoholic families are doomed to have lifelong problems. As many of these people mature, they develop a resiliency in response to their families' problems. They thus enter adulthood armed with positive strengths and valuable career-oriented skills, such as the ability to assume responsibility, strong organizational skills, and realistic expectations of their jobs and others.

Costs to Society

The entire society suffers the consequences of individuals' alcohol abuse. Close to half of all traffic fatalities are attributable to alcohol. According to the National Institute on Alcohol Abuse and Alcoholism, in 1998, alcohol-related costs to society were at least $184.6 billion when health insurance, criminal justice, treatment costs, and lost productivity were factored in. Reportedly, alcoholism is directly and indirectly responsible for over 25 percent of the nation's medical expenses and lost earnings. Well over 50 percent of all child abuse cases are the result of alcohol-related problems. Finally, the costs in emotional health are impossible to measure.[23]

Women and Alcoholism

In the past, women have consumed less alcohol and have had fewer alcohol-related problems than have men. But now, greater percentages of women, especially college-age women, are choosing to drink and are drinking more heavily.

Studies indicate that there are now almost as many female as male alcoholics. Risk factors for drinking problems among *all women* include the following:

- A family history of drinking problems.
- Pressure to drink from a peer or spouse.
- Depression.
- Stress.

Risk factors among young women include the following:

- College attendance: Women in college drink more, and more frequently, than they do after they graduate.
- Nontraditional, low-status, and part-time jobs, and unemployment.
- Being single, divorced, or separated.

Risk factors among *middle-aged women* include the following:

- Loss of social roles (e.g., through divorce or children growing up and leaving the home).
- Abuse of prescription drugs.
- Heavy drinking by spouse.
- Presence of other disorders, such as depression.

Risk factors among *older women* include the following:

- Heavy- or problem-drinking spouse.
- Retirement, with a loss of social networks centered on the workplace.

Drinking patterns among *different age groups* also differ in these ways:

- Younger women drink more overall, drink more often, and experience more alcohol-related problems, such as drinking and driving, assaults, suicide attempts, and difficulties at work.

- Middle-aged women are more likely to develop drinking problems in response to a traumatic or life-changing event, such as divorce, surgery, or death of a significant other.
- Older women are more likely than older men to have developed drinking problems within the past 10 years.[24]

It is estimated that only 14 percent of women who need treatment get it. In one study, women cite potential loss of income, not wanting others to know they may have a problem, inability to pay for treatment, and fear that treatment would not be confidential as reasons for not seeking treatment.[25] Another major obstacle is child care. Most residential treatment centers do not allow women to bring their children with them.

Despite growing recognition of our national alcohol problem, fewer than 10 percent of alcoholics in the United States receive any care. Factors contributing to this low figure include an inability or unwillingness to admit to an alcohol problem; the social stigma attached to alcoholism; breakdowns in referral and delivery systems (failure of physicians or psychotherapists to follow up on referrals, client failure to follow through with recommended treatments, or failure of rehabilitation facilities to give quality care); and failure of the professional medical establishment to recognize and diagnose alcoholic symptoms among patients. Certain minority groups have unique drinking profiles. See the Health in a Diverse World box.

Most alcoholics and problem drinkers who seek help have experienced a turning point or dramatic occurrence: A spouse walks out, taking children and possessions; the boss issues an ultimatum to dry out or ship out. The alcoholic ready for treatment has, in most cases, reached a low point. Devoid of hope, physically depleted, and spiritually despairing, the alcoholic has finally recognized that alcohol controls his or her life. The first step on the road to recovery is to regain that control and assume responsibility for personal actions.

> ### What do you think?
>
> *Why do you think women appear to be drinking more heavily today than they did in the past?* ✳ *Does society look at men's and women's drinking habits in the same way?* ✳ *Can you think of ways to increase support for women in their recovery process?*

Recovery

The Family's Role

Members of an alcoholic's family sometimes take action before the alcoholic does. They may go to an organization or a treatment facility to seek help for themselves and their relative. As we saw in Chapter 11, *intervention* is an effective method of helping an alcoholic to confront the disease.

Alcohol Availability and Diverse Populations

Most of the available literature on the effects of alcohol in ethnic populations divides the communities into the following five groups: African American, American Indian/Alaska Native, Asian/Pacific Islander, Latino or Hispanic, and white. It should be noted that within these communities, there are often other sociocultural factors involved as well. This box focuses on alcohol availability and advertising in these particular ethnic communities.

Alcohol Availability

On average, low-income Latino and African American communities have more alcohol outlets (liquor stores, package stores, grocery stores, or any establishment that can sell alcohol in the bottle or can for take-out) than do wealthy white communities. An overconcentration of alcohol outlets may adversely affect the economic and physical health of the community. For example, adding a single outlet in the average Los Angeles County city is estimated to result in about 2.7 more traffic injuries and 3.4 more assaults. In a study of three northern California cities, alcohol outlet density (the number of outlets in a given geographical area) was associated with youth violence.

Alcohol outlets often display advertisements, which increase the blight associated with alcohol billboards. One California study found that Latino communities have five times more advertisements than predominantly white communities. Children walking home from school in the Mexican American communities studied are exposed to 10 to 61 advertisements, depending on the route they take. Many of these advertisements are on the walls of alcohol outlets. Such concentrated advertising of alcohol is particularly problematic because alcohol advertising is associated with increased use of alcohol, and alcohol use has been linked with injuries and violence.

African Americans

While African Americans use less alcohol overall than do whites and Latinos, the African American community as a whole suffers a disproportionate level of alcohol problems. For example, in California, African Americans are more likely to die from alcohol-related homicide than those categorized as whites, Latinos, or "Asian/Others." Also, African American women suffer more social consequences (abuse, isolation, and poverty) from alcohol than do white women. Alcoholism is one of the most significant problems in the African American community. Malt liquor advertisements are targeted almost exclusively at African Americans. Nearly every inner-city neighborhood is plastered with malt liquor ads projecting images meant to appeal to blacks.

Latinos

Latino men consume more alcohol than do white and African American men. The rates of alcohol-related injuries and death are higher for Latinos than for whites in California. Among Latinos, 10.15 per 100,000 died in alcohol-related homicides as compared to 2.9 per 100,000 whites. The circumstances may differ somewhat for women. While 48 percent of Latinas abstained from alcohol, they suffered nearly three times as many social consequences related to alcohol use (abuse, isolation, and poverty) as did white women.

Asians/Pacific Islanders

Research regarding Asians/Pacific Islanders in the United States is sparse; however, studies that have been done generally show that Asians/Pacific Islanders have lower alcohol-related death rates than do other ethnic groups. As a group, Asian Americans and Pacific Islanders also have lower than average rates of alcohol abuse. Asian taboos and community sanctions against excessive drinking are thought to protect against alcohol abuse.

American Indians/Alaska Natives

Alcohol abuse is one of the most widespread and severe health problems for American Indians and Alaska Natives, especially adolescents and young adults. Excessive drinking varies from tribe to tribe but is generally high among both men and women. The rate of alcoholism among American Indians is two to three times that of the general population, and the death rate from alcohol-related causes is about eight times higher.

As we look toward the future, the answer to reducing this nation's alcohol-related problems may lie in the availability of alcohol, its pricing, and how it is marketed. State and local officials may need to limit the overconcentration of alcohol outlets in communities and work with the alcohol beverage industry to eliminate promotions that encourage heavy consumption among all ethnic groups.

Source: The Trauma Foundation, "Alcohol-Related Injury and Violence" (see http://www.traumafdn.org/alcohol/ariv/index.html); and E. Hernandez, "The Effects of Alcohol on Latinos in California: A Report for Alcohol Awareness Month," CalPartners Coalition, April 1998.

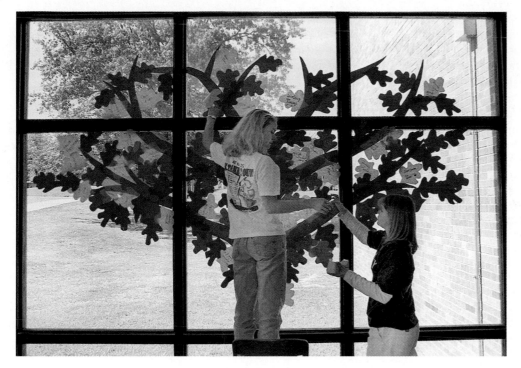

After two of their classmates were killed in a high-speed car accident, students at William Chrisman High in Independence, MO, started their own chapter of SADD—Students Against Destructive Decisions, formerly Students Against Drunk Driving. Students and teachers donated 50 cents for each tree leaf, and the money went to resources and activities that help students say no to all forms of destructive behavior.

Family members express their love and concern, telling the alcoholic that they will no longer refrain from acknowledging the problem and affirming their support for appropriate treatment. A family intervention is the turning point for a growing number of alcoholics.

Treatment Programs

The alcoholic who is ready for help has several avenues of treatment: psychologists and psychiatrists specializing in the treatment of alcoholism, private treatment centers, hospitals specifically designed to treat alcoholics, community mental health facilities, and support groups such as Alcoholics Anonymous.

Private Treatment Facilities Private treatment facilities have been making concerted efforts to attract patients through radio and television advertising. Upon admission to the treatment facility, the patient is given a complete physical exam to determine whether underlying medical problems will interfere with treatment. Alcoholics who decide to quit drinking will experience withdrawal symptoms, including the following:

- Hyperexcitability.
- Confusion.
- Sleep disorders.
- Convulsions.
- Agitation.
- Tremors of the hands.
- Brief hallucinations.
- Depression.
- Headache.
- Seizures.

For a small percentage of people, alcohol withdrawal results in a severe syndrome known as **delirium tremens (DTs)**. Delirium tremens is characterized by confusion, delusions, agitated behavior, and hallucinations.

For any long-term addict, medical supervision is usually necessary. *Detoxification,* the process by which addicts end their dependence on a drug, is commonly carried out in a medical facility, where patients can be monitored to prevent fatal withdrawal reactions. Withdrawal takes from 7 to 21 days. Shortly after detoxification, alcoholics begin their treatment for psychological addiction. Most treatment facilities keep their patients from three to six weeks. Treatment at private treatment centers costs several thousand dollars, but some insurance programs or employers will assume most of this expense.

Family Therapy, Individual Therapy, and Group Therapy

In family therapy, the person and family members gradually examine the psychological reasons underlying the addiction. In individual and group therapy with fellow addicts, alcoholics learn positive coping skills for situations that have regularly caused them to turn to alcohol. On some college campuses, the problems associated with alcohol abuse are so great that student health centers are opening their own treatment programs.

> **Delirium tremens (DTs)** A state of confusion brought on by withdrawal from alcohol. Symptoms include hallucinations, anxiety, and trembling.

Other Types of Treatment   Two other treatments are drug and aversion therapy. Disulfiram (trade name: Antabuse) is the drug of choice for treating alcoholics. If alcohol is consumed, the drug causes unpleasant effects such as headache, nausea, vomiting, drowsiness, and hangover. These symptoms discourage the alcoholic from drinking.

Aversion therapy is based on conditioning therapy. It works on the premise that the sight, smell, and taste of alcohol will acquire aversive properties if repeatedly paired with a noxious stimulus. For a period of 10 days, the alcoholic takes drugs that induce vomiting when combined with several drinks. These treatments work best in conjunction with some type of counseling.

Alcoholics Anonymous (AA) is a private, nonprofit, self-help organization founded in 1935. The organization, which relies upon group support to help people stop drinking, currently has over 1 million members and has branches all over the world. At meetings, last names are never used and no one is forced to speak. Members are taught to believe that their alcoholism is a lifetime problem and they may never use alcohol again. They share their struggles with each other and talk about the devastating effects alcoholism has had on their personal and professional lives. All members are asked to place their faith and control of the habit into the hands of a "higher power." The road to recovery is taken one step at a time. AA offers specialized meetings for gay, atheist, HIV-positive, and professional individuals with alcohol problems.

Alcoholics Anonymous also has auxiliary groups to help spouses or partners, friends, and children of alcoholics. *Al-Anon* is the group dedicated to helping adult relatives and friends of alcoholics understand the disease and how they can contribute to the recovery process. Spouses and other adult loved ones often play an unwitting role in perpetuating the alcoholic's problems. For example, the adult relative may call the alcoholic's boss and lie about why the alcoholic missed work. At Al-Anon, these people's roles in their loved one's alcoholism are examined and explored, and alternative behaviors are suggested.

The support gained from talking with others who have similar problems is one of the greatest benefits derived from participation in Al-Anon. Many members learn how to exert greater control over their own lives and rid themselves of the guilt they feel about their participation in their loved one's alcoholism.

Alcoholics Anonymous (AA)   An organization whose goal is to help alcoholics stop drinking; includes auxiliary branches such as Al-Anon and Alateen.

Alateen, another AA-related organization, helps adolescents live with alcoholic parents. They are taught that they are not at fault for their parents' problems. They develop their self-esteem to overcome their guilt and function better socially.

Other self-help groups include Women for Sobriety and Secular Organizations for Sobriety (SOS). Women for Sobriety addresses the differing needs of female alcoholics, who often have more severe problems than males. Unlike AA meetings, where attendance can be quite large, each group has no more than 10 members. Secular Organizations for Sobriety was founded to help people who are uncomfortable with AA's spiritual emphasis.

Relapse

Success in recovery from alcoholism varies with the individual. A return to alcoholic habits often follows what appears to be a successful recovery. Some alcoholics never recover. Some partially recover and improve other parts of their lives, but remain dependent on alcohol. Many alcoholics refer to themselves as "recovering" throughout their lifetime; they never use the word *cured.*

Roughly 60 percent of alcoholics relapse (resume drinking) within the first three months of treatment. Why is the relapse rate so high? Treating an addiction requires more than getting the addict to stop using a substance; it also requires getting the person to break a pattern of behavior that has dominated his or her life.

People who are seeking to regain a healthy lifestyle must not only confront their addiction, but must also guard against the tendency to relapse. Drinkers with compulsive personalities need to learn to understand themselves and take control. Others need to view treatment as a long-term process that takes a lot of effort beyond attending a weekly self-help group meeting. In order to work, a recovery program must offer the alcoholic ways to increase self-esteem and resume personal growth.

Can Recovering Alcoholics Take a Drink?   During the mid-1970s, some scientists believed that recovering alcoholics could return to drinking on a limited social basis. Several studies supported this notion, but they have since been refuted. Research conducted over a period of 5 to 10 years has shown that fewer than 1 percent of recovering alcoholics are able to resume drinking on a limited basis. To prevent the return to the bottle, abstinence is the safest and sanest path.

A comprehensive approach that includes drug therapy, group support, family therapy, and personal counseling designed to improve living and coping skills is usually the most effective course of treatment. The alcoholics most likely to recover completely are those who developed their dependencies after the age of 20, those with intact and supportive family units, and those who have reached a high level of personal disgust coupled with strong motivation to recover.

Managing Your Drinking Behaviors

After reading this chapter, you probably realize that the use of alcohol affects many aspects of life. Assuming your religion doesn't forbid it, there is nothing wrong with using alcohol as long as you use it responsibly. But in order to make informed decisions, you must understand the possible problems and options regarding the use of alcohol and how it affects those around you. Societal pressure to drink is everywhere and alcohol is easily available. Take time to decide how you want to behave in situations in which alcohol is being served. Have you ever felt you or someone you know might have a drinking problem?

Checklist for Change

Compare your drinking habits with the following to gauge how appropriately you use alcohol. Remember, though, that it is not necessary for a person to have every symptom to fit into one of these categories. Also, social drinkers do not ordinarily become problem drinkers, and problem drinkers do not have to become alcoholics. Do you have an appropriate relationship with alcohol?

A social drinker typically
- [ ] Drinks slowly (no fast gulping).
- [ ] Knows when to stop drinking (does not drink to get drunk).
- [ ] Eats before or while drinking.
- [ ] Never drives after drinking.
- [ ] Respects nondrinkers.
- [ ] Knows and obeys laws related to drinking.

A problem drinker
- [ ] Drinks to get drunk.
- [ ] Tries to solve problems by drinking alcohol.
- [ ] Experiences changes in personality and may become loud, angry, or violent, or silent, remote, and reclusive.
- [ ] Drinks when he or she should not—before driving or going to class or work.
- [ ] Causes other problems—harms himself or herself, family, friends, and strangers.
- [ ] Needs "liquid courage" before parties or dates.

An alcoholic typically
- [ ] Spends lots of time thinking about drinking and planning when and where to get the next drink.
- [ ] Keeps bottles hidden for quick pick-me-ups.
- [ ] Starts drinking without conscious planning and loses awareness of the amount consumed.
- [ ] Denies drinking.
- [ ] Drinks alone.
- [ ] Needs to drink before facing a stressful situation.
- [ ] May have blackouts—cannot remember what he or she did while drinking, although he or she may have appeared normal to people at the time.
- [ ] Goes from having hangovers to more dangerous withdrawal symptoms, such as delirium tremens (DTs), which can be fatal.
- [ ] Has or causes major problems—with police, an employer, professor, friends, or family.

Summary

- Alcohol is a central nervous system depressant used by 70 percent of all Americans and 83 percent of all college students; 44 percent of college students are binge drinkers. While consumption trends are slowly creeping downward, college students are under extreme pressure to consume alcohol.
- Alcohol's effect on the body is measured by the blood alcohol concentration (BAC), the ratio of alcohol to total blood volume. The higher the BAC, the greater the impaired judgment and coordination and drowsiness.
- Some negative consequences associated with alcohol use and college students are lower grade-point averages, academic problems, dropping out of school, unplanned sex, hangovers, and injury. Long-term effects of alcohol overuse include damage to the nervous system, cardiovascular damage, liver disease, and increased risk for cancer.

Use during pregnancy can cause fetal alcohol effects (FAE) or fetal alcohol syndrome (FAS). Alcohol is also a causative factor in traffic accidents.

✳ Alcohol use becomes alcoholism when it interferes with school, work, or social and family relationships or entails violations of the law. Causes of alcoholism include biological and family factors and social and cultural factors. Alcoholism has far-reaching effects on families, especially on children. Children of alcoholics have problematic childhoods and generally take those problems into adulthood.

✳ Recovery is problematic for alcoholics. Most alcoholics do not admit to a problem until reaching a major life crisis or having their families intervene. Treatment options include detoxification at private medical facilities, therapy (family, individual, or group), and programs like Alcoholics Anonymous. Most alcoholics relapse (60 percent within three months) because alcoholism is a behavioral addiction as well as a chemical addiction.

Questions for Discussion and Reflection

1. When it comes to drinking alcohol, how much is too much? How can you avoid drinking amounts that will affect your judgment? When you see a friend having "too many" drinks at a party, what actions do you normally take? What actions could you take?

2. What are some of the most common negative consequences college students experience as a result of drinking? What are secondhand effects of binge drinking? Why do students tolerate negative behaviors of students who have been drinking?

3. Determine what your BAC would be if you drank four beers in two hours (assume they are spaced at equal intervals). What physiological effects will you feel after each drink? Would a person of similar weight show greater

effects after having four gin and tonics instead of beer? Why or why not? At what point in your life should you start worrying about the long-term effects of alcohol abuse?

4. Describe the difference between a problem drinker and an alcoholic. What factors can cause someone to slide from responsibly consuming alcohol to becoming an alcoholic? What effect does alcoholism have on an alcoholic's family?

5. Does anyone ever recover from alcoholism? Why or why not? Do you think society's views on drinking have changed over the years? Explain your answer.

Application Exercises

Reread the What Do You Think? scenarios at the beginning of the chapter and answer the following questions.

1. What is it about a college environment that encourages such excessive celebrations on one's 21st birthday?

2. What precautions might Jean and her friends have taken prior to going out and celebrating? What have you said to friends who were about to make similar mistakes? What resources are available on your campus to help someone like Jean and her friends in the aftermath of rape?

3. What dangers are associated with drinking games? What signs show that someone might be developing alcohol poisoning?

4. What do you think the legal drinking age should be? What responsibility does Mark have for his brother's safety? In what ways do people "learn how to drink"?

Accessing Your Health on the Internet

Visit the following Internet sites to explore further topics and issues related to personal health. To visit an organization's website, go to the Companion Website for *Access to Health, Eighth Edition* at www.aw.com/donatelle, click on the book image, and select "Accessing Your Health on the Internet" from the navigation menu on the left.

1. *College Drinking: Changing the Culture.* This online resource center is based on a series of reports published by the Task Force of the National Advisory Council on Alcohol Abuse and Alcoholism. It advocates a three-in-one framework that targets three audiences: the student population as a whole; the college and its surrounding environment; and the individual at-risk or alcohol-dependent drinker.

2. ***Had Enough.*** This entertaining website is designed for college students who have suffered the secondhand effects (baby-sitting a roommate who has been drinking, having sleep interrupted, etc.) of other students' drinking. It offers suggestions for taking action and being proactive about policy issues on your campus.

3. ***Higher Education Center for Alcohol and Other Drug Prevention.*** This website is funded through the U.S. Department of Education and provides information relevant to colleges and universities. A specific site exists for students who are seeking information regarding alcohol.

Further Reading

Jersild, Devon. *Happy Hours: Alcohol in a Woman's Life.* New York: HarperCollins, 2001.

This book, a combination of cutting-edge research and personal stories of women who have struggled with alcohol problems, examines the role that alcohol plays in women's lives.

Kuhn, C., S. Swartzwelder, W. Wilson, J. Foster, and L. Wilson. *Buzzed: The Straight Facts about the Most Used and Abused Drugs from Alcohol to Ecstasy.* New York: Norton, 1998.

A straightforward, informative book. The first part consists of chapters on each of 12 kinds of drugs: alcohol, caffeine, enactogens, hallucinogens, herbal drugs, inhalants, marijuana, nicotine, opiates, sedatives, steroids, and stimulants. The second part of the book describes the complex neurochemistry with great clarity.

National Institute on Alcohol Abuse and Alcoholism (NIAAA). *Research Monographs.* Washington, DC: U.S. Department of Health and Human Services.

A series of publications containing the results of a number of studies conducted by research scientists under the auspices of NIAAA through 2002. These monographs address issues such as alcohol use among the elderly, occupational alcoholism, social drinking, and the relationship between heredity and alcoholism.

Nuwer, H. *Wrongs of Passage: Fraternities, Sororities, Hazing, and Binge Drinking.* Bloomington: Indiana University Press, 1999.

A comprehensive exposé on the continuing crisis of death and injury among fraternity and sorority pledges. The book provides an overview of Greek customs and demands that encouraged hazing as well as the recent deaths of students at some of the nation's most prestigious universities. The author argues that we need to control the Greek system as well as other organizations that employ similar, sometimes deadly, hazing practices.

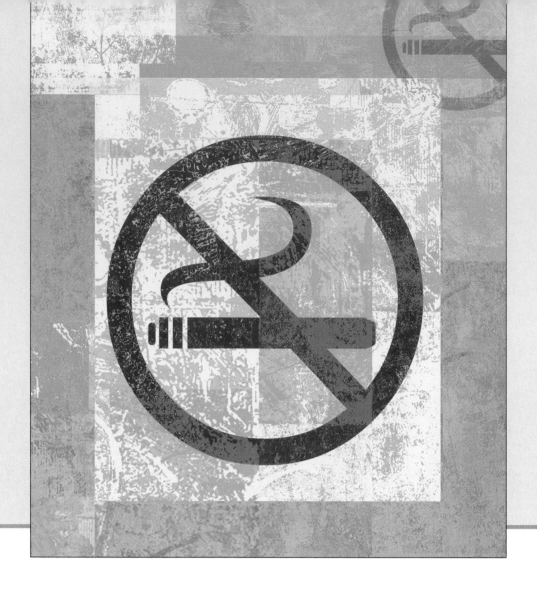

Objectives

❋ Discuss the social issues involved in tobacco use, including advertising and the medical costs.

❋ Discuss how the chemicals in tobacco products affect a smoker's body.

❋ Review how smoking affects a smoker's risk for cancer, cardiovascular disease, and respiratory diseases and how it adversely affects a fetus's health.

❋ Discuss the risks associated with using smokeless tobacco.

❋ Evaluate the risks to nonsmokers associated with environmental tobacco smoke.

❋ Discuss the role of politics in regulating tobacco products.

❋ Describe strategies people adopt to quit using tobacco products, including strategies aimed at breaking the nicotine addiction as well as habit.

❋ Compare the benefits and risks associated with caffeine, and summarize the health consequences of long-term caffeine use.

13 Tobacco and Caffeine

Daily Pleasures, Daily Challenges

What do you think?

Sarah and Evan are sophomores at a large midwestern university. During their freshman year, both of these students, along with some of their friends, began smoking when they went to bars. Neither Evan nor Sarah smokes daily, and both strongly believe that they will be able to stop smoking whenever they choose.

How common is this scenario on your campus? ✸ Given that most students already know the dangers of smoking, what are some of the reasons why students begin smoking once they get to college? ✸ Are Evan and Sarah really occasional smokers, or are they just fooling themselves?

Although Jonathan is not a cigarette smoker, he has begun to smoke bidis. He found that bidis taste much better than regular cigarettes, as they come in a variety of flavors. Bidis are also pretty cheap and easy to buy. Jonathan and his best friend, A. J., first began buying bidis over the Internet when they were seniors in high school. Now, as bidis are becoming more popular, they are easy to buy in convenience stores and gas stations.

Why do people who smoke bidis think they are safer than cigarettes? ✸ What makes bidis attractive to younger adults? ✸ Do bidis appeal to a certain subculture of students? ✸ If so, why? ✸ Would it be more difficult to get smoking cessation information to this group of smokers?

T obacco use is the single most preventable cause of death in the United States.[1] While tobacco companies continue to publish full-page advertisements refuting the dangers of smoking, nearly 440,000 Americans die each year of tobacco-related diseases[2] (see Figure 13.1). This is 50 times as many as will die from all illegal drugs combined. In addition, 10 million will suffer from diseases caused by tobacco. To date, tobacco is known to be the probable cause of about 25 diseases. One in every five deaths in the United States is smoking related. New studies estimate that about half of all regular smokers die of smoking-related diseases. Therefore, any contention by the tobacco industry that tobacco use is not dangerous is irresponsible and ignores the scientific evidence.

Our Smoking Society

In 1991, the Youth Risk Assessment Survey (YRAS), which includes only middle and high school students, indicated that 27.5 percent of teenagers smoked; by 2001, 28.5 percent were current smokers. The most recent survey of adolescent smokers has shown a downward trend from the 1999 survey (see Figure 13.2). Currently, the percentage of teenage males and females who smoke is equal, at approximately 28.5 percent.[3] The number of teenagers who become daily smokers before the age of 18 is estimated to be more than 3,000 per day. Every day another 6,000 teens under the age of 18

Table 13.1
Percentage of Population That Smokes (age 18 and older) among Select Groups in the United States

	PERCENTAGE
United States overall	24.7
RACE	
American Indian/Alaska Native	34.1
Asian/Pacific Islander	16.9
Black	26.7
Hispanic	20.4
White	25.3
AGE	
18–24	28.7
25–44	28.6
45–64	24.4
>64	12.0
SEX	
Male	27.6
Female	22.1
EDUCATION	
>12 years	18.4
12 years	29.5
<12 years	30.4
INCOME LEVEL	
Below poverty level	33.3
At or above poverty level	24.6

Source: Centers for Disease Control, *Morbidity and Mortality Weekly* 48, p. 994.

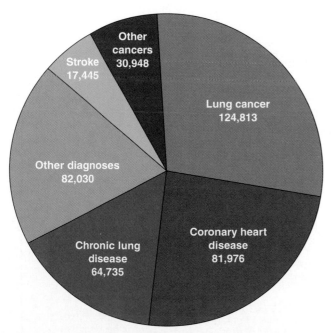

Figure 13.1
Annual Deaths Attributable to Smoking: United States, 1995–1999
Source: Centers for Disease Control, 2002, *Morbidity and Mortality Weekly* 51 (14), pp. 300–303.

smoke their first cigarette. The increase in cigarette use is attributed in part to the ready availability of tobacco products through vending machines and the aggressive drive by tobacco companies to entice young people to smoke.

Cigarette smoking in the United States results in untold loss of human potential, with thousands of Americans dying prematurely each year. As you can see in Table 13.1, the age groups with almost identical rates of smoking are the 18- to 24- year-old age group and the 25- to 44-year-old age group. While the 18- to 24-year-old age group has been heavily targeted by cigarette promotions and advertising, the 25- to 44-year-olds developed their habits as adolescents 10 to 20 years ago, when the practice of smoking was more common.

Tobacco and Social Issues

The production and distribution of tobacco products in the United States and abroad involve many political and economic issues. During the 1980s, tobacco products were one of the top five U.S. exports. Tobacco-growing states derive substantial income from tobacco production, and federal, state, and local governments benefit enormously from cigarette taxes.

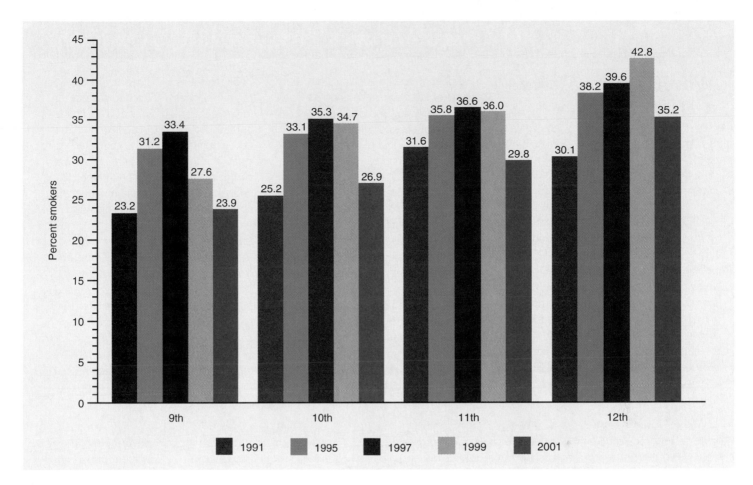

Figure 13.2
Cigarette Smoking by Grade Level: 1991–2001
Source: Centers for Disease Control, "Youth Risk Behavior Survey," 2002, *Morbidity and Mortality Weekly* 51 (19).

More recently, nationwide health awareness has led to a decrease in the use of tobacco products among U.S. adults. To compensate for revenue losses, many major tobacco companies have merged with or purchased other corporations that market food or beverage products.

Advertising According to estimates, the tobacco industry spends $18 million per day on advertising and promotional materials. With the number of smokers declining by about 1 million each year, the industry must actively recruit new smokers. Campaigns are directed at all age, social, and ethnic groups, but because children and teenagers constitute 90 percent of all new smokers, much of the advertising has been directed toward them. Evidence of product recognition among underage smokers is clear: eighty-six percent of underage smokers prefer one of the three most heavily advertised brands—Marlboro, Newport, or Camel. One of the most blatant campaigns aimed at young adults was the popular Joe Camel ad campaign. After R. J. Reynolds introduced the cartoon figure, Camel's market share among underage smokers jumped from 3 to 13.3 percent in three years.

Advertisements in women's magazines imply that smoking is the key to financial success, independence, and social acceptance. Many brands also have thin spokeswomen pushing "slim" and "light" cigarettes to cash in on women's fear of gaining weight. These ads have apparently been working. From the mid-1970s through the late 1990s, cigarette sales to women increased dramatically. By 1987, cigarette-induced lung cancer had surpassed breast cancer as the leading form of cancer death among women.

Women are not the only targets of gender-based cigarette advertisements. Males are depicted changing clothes in a locker room, charging over rugged terrain in off-road vehicles, or riding bay stallions into the sunset in blatant appeals to a need to feel and appear masculine. In addition, minorities are often targeted.

Apparently, 18- to 24-year-olds have become the new target for tobacco advertisers. The tobacco industry has set up very aggressive marketing promotions in bars and at music festivals and the like, specifically targeted to this age group. Additionally, modeling and peer influence have an impact on smoking initiation. This potential impact is

Working to Make a Difference

Philip Morris is the world's largest producer and marketer of consumer packaged goods and the largest food company in the nation. It is also the world's largest and most profitable tobacco corporation. To many Americans, Philip Morris, which owns Kraft Foods, is firmly linked to the more than 400,000 people in the United States and 3.4 million worldwide who die each year from smoking-related illnesses. This company has also led the way, in the United States and internationally, in spreading the tobacco epidemic, in particular to girls and women in regions where they traditionally have not smoked. In addition, Philip Morris and other tobacco companies have been charged with lying and deliberately deceiving the public regarding the safety of tobacco and creating and marketing a chemical addiction for profit.

However, a visit to the Philip Morris headquarters in New York paints a different picture. The company is aggressively promoting its charitable work, in particular its youth smoking-prevention program. It houses the Whitney Museum exhibit of an Indian artist and sponsors the "Thurgood Marshall Scholars." Furthermore, Philip Morris employees are involved in efforts to fight hunger and combat domestic violence. The company donates $60 million a year to charity and spends another $100 million in advertising to inform the public about its good deeds. The advertising campaign is a concerted strategy to improve Philip Morris's corporate image and build credibility. In addition to the advertising campaign, the company has established a speakers' bureau where top company executives go on the road to address PTA meetings and other groups about the company's charitable work.

Is there an ethical dilemma associated with this corporation? What is the tobacco company's ethical obligation to society? Do you think Philip Morris is attempting to do the right thing, or are these initiatives merely a public relations effort? Since smokers choose to start smoking, is it fair to blame Philip Morris if they develop tobacco-related health problems?

heightened by the fact that, although over half of campuses are considered smoke-free, they do permit smoking in residence hall rooms, student centers, and cafeterias, and many sell tobacco products in campus stores and student lounges. See the Health Ethics box for more on the tobacco industry.

Financial Costs to Society The use of tobacco products is costly to all of us in terms of lost productivity and lost lives. Estimates show that tobacco use caused over $150 billion in annual health-related economic losses from 1995 to 1999. The economic burden of tobacco use was more than $75.5 billion in medical expenditures (these costs include hospital, physician, and nursing home expenditures; prescription drugs; and home health care expenditures) and $89.1 billion in indirect costs (absenteeism, added cost of fire insurance, training costs to replace employees who die prematurely, disability payments, and so on). The economic costs of smoking are estimated to be about $3,391 per smoker per year. Another way of thinking about this is that for each pack of cigarettes sold in the United States, it costs the nation $7.18 in medical costs and lost productivity.[4]

College Students and Smoking

College and university students are especially vulnerable when they are placed in a new, often stressful social and academic environment. For many, the college years are their initial taste of freedom from parental supervision. Smoking may begin earlier, but most college students are a part of the significant age group in which people initiate smoking and become hooked.

A recent study found that cigarette smoking among U.S. college students increased by 32 percent between 1991 and 1999. In 1999, researchers surveyed more than 14,000 students from 119 U.S. colleges. This poll took into account all types of tobacco use, including cigars, smokeless tobacco, and pipe smoking, rather than just cigarettes. Researchers found that more than 60 percent of college students had tried some tobacco product. One-third of students had used tobacco in the month before the study, and just under half

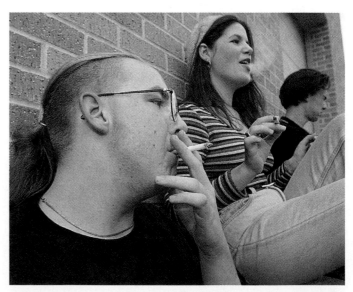

Despite all that we know about the long-term effects of smoking, young people continue to put their health at risk. Why?

Are You Nicotine Dependent?

It's probably safe to say that no one who starts out smoking intends to become hooked. Imagine making a conscious decision to reduce your oxygen intake and deposit gooey tar on your lungs. It wouldn't be a very wise decision, would it?

Smoking usually begins innocently enough, as an experiment or a dare or perhaps an attempt to fit in. Is it an innocent habit that you could give up right now without any problem? Or do you have a dependency? Take the following test to see.

	0 Points	1 Point	2 Points	3 Points
1. How soon after you wake up do you smoke your first cigarette?	After 60 minutes	31–60 minutes	6–30 minutes	Within 5 minutes
2. Do you find it difficult to refrain from smoking in places where it is forbidden?	No	Yes	–	–
3. Which cigarette would you hate most to give up?	The first one in the morning	Any other	–	–
4. How many cigarettes a day do you smoke?	10 or less	11–20	21–30	31 or more
5. Do you smoke more frequently during the first hours after awakening than during the rest of the day?	No	Yes	–	–
6. Do you smoke if you are so ill that you are in bed most of the day?	No	Yes	–	–

Scoring:

If you scored over 7 points, your level of nicotine dependence is high. You and your doctor should consider various medications to help you stop smoking.

If you scored under 4 points, you probably will be able to succeed in stopping smoking without medication.

Source: T. F. Heatherton, L. T. Kozlowski, R. C. Frecker, K. O. Fagerstrom, "The Fagerstrom Test for Nicotine Dependence: A Revision of the Fagerstrom Tolerance Questionnaire," *British Journal of Addictions* 86 (1991): 1119–1127. Reprinted by permission of Dr. Karl Fagerstrom.

had used tobacco in the past year, however, they did not consider themselves "smokers." Among current smokers, the survey found a wide range of smoking behaviors: Thirty-two percent smoked less than a cigarette a day, while 13 percent smoked a pack or more per day. Furthermore, the study found students who used tobacco products were more likely to smoke marijuana, binge drink, have multiple sex partners, earn lower grades, rate parties as more important than academic activities, and spend more time socializing with friends.[5]

A common perception is that students are not interested in smoking cessation efforts. However, a recent study reported that 70 percent of cigarette smokers had tried to quit smoking. Unfortunately, three out of four were still smokers.[6] It is important that colleges and universities engage in antismoking efforts, strictly control tobacco advertising, provide smoke-free residence halls, and offer greater access to smoking cessation programs. See the Assess Yourself box to determine whether you are dependent on tobacco.

What do you think?

Have you noticed an increase in the number of your friends who have become smokers or occasional smokers? ✹ How many of them smoked prior to coming to college, and how many picked up the habit at college? ✹ What are their reasons for smoking? ✹ What barriers keep your friends from quitting?

Table 13.2
What's in Cigarette Smoke?

More than 4,000 chemicals, including these:

CANCER-CAUSING AGENTS	METALS	OTHER CHEMICALS	
Benzo(a)pyrene	Aluminum	Acetic acid (vinegar)	Hexamine (barbecue lighter)
B-Napthylamine	Copper	Acetone (nail polish remover)	Hydrogen cyanide (gas
Cadmium	Gold	Ammonia (floor/toilet cleaner)	chamber poison)
Crysenes	Lead	Arsenic (poison)	Methane (swamp gas)
Diberiz acidine	Magnesium	Butane (cigarette lighter fluid)	Methanol (rocket fuel)
Nickel	Mercury	Cadmium (rechargeable	Napthalene (mothballs)
Nitrosamines	Silicon	batteries)	Nicotine (insecticide/addictive
N. nitrosonornicotine	Silver	Carbon monoxide (car	drug)
P.A.H.'s	Titanium	exhaust fumes)	Nitrobenzene (gasoline additive)
Polonium 210	Zinc	DDT/dieldrin (insecticides)	Nitrous oxide phenols (disinfectant)
Toluidine		Ethanol (alcohol)	Stearic acid (candle wax)
		Formaldehyde (preserver of	Toluene (industrial solvent)
		body tissue and fabric)	Vinyl chloride (makes PVC)

Tobacco and Its Effects

The chemical stimulant **nicotine** is the major psychoactive substance in all tobacco products. In its natural form, nicotine is a colorless liquid that turns brown upon oxidation (exposure to oxygen). When tobacco leaves are burned in a cigarette, pipe, or cigar, nicotine is released and inhaled into the lungs. Sucking or chewing a quid (a pinch of snuff typically tucked between the gum and lower lip) of tobacco releases nicotine into the saliva, and the nicotine is then absorbed through the mucous membranes in the mouth.

Smoking is the most common form of tobacco use. Smoking delivers a strong dose of nicotine to the user, along with an additional 4,000 chemical substances (see Table 13.2). Among these chemicals are various gases and vapors that carry particulate matter in concentrations that are 500,000 times greater than those of the most air-polluted cities in the world.[7]

Particulate matter condenses in the lungs to form a thick, brownish sludge called **tar.** Tar contains various carcinogenic (cancer-causing) agents such as benzo(a)pyrene and chemical irritants such as phenol. Phenol has the potential to combine with other chemicals to contribute to the development of lung cancer.

In healthy lungs, millions of tiny hairlike tissues called cilia sweep away foreign matter, to be expelled from the lungs by coughing. Nicotine impairs the cleansing function of the cilia by paralyzing them for up to one hour following the smoking of a single cigarette. This allows tars and other solids in tobacco smoke to accumulate and irritate sensitive lung tissue.

Tar and nicotine are not the only harmful chemicals in cigarettes. In fact, tars account for only 8 percent of tobacco smoke. The remaining 92 percent consists of various gases,

the most dangerous of which is **carbon monoxide.** In tobacco smoke, the concentration of carbon monoxide is 800 times higher than the level considered safe by the U.S. Environmental Protection Agency (EPA). In the human body, carbon monoxide reduces the oxygen-carrying capacity of the red blood cells by binding with the receptor sites for oxygen. This causes oxygen deprivation in many body tissues.

The heat from tobacco smoke, which can reach 1,616 degrees Fahrenheit, is also harmful. Inhaling hot gases exposes sensitive mucous membranes to irritating chemicals that weaken the tissues and contribute to cancers of the mouth, larynx, and throat.

Tobacco Products

Tobacco comes in several forms. Cigarettes, cigars, pipes, and bidis are used for burning and inhaling tobacco. Smokeless tobacco is sniffed or placed in the mouth.

Filtered cigarettes designed to reduce levels of gases such as hydrogen cyanide and hydrocarbons may actually deliver more hazardous carbon monoxide to the user than do nonfiltered brands. Some smokers use low-tar and low-nicotine products as an excuse to smoke more cigarettes. This practice is self-defeating because they wind up exposing themselves to more harmful substances than they would with regular-strength cigarettes. People smoking low-tar cigarettes also tend to inhale more often and more deeply than people smoking regular cigarettes.

Clove cigarettes contain about 40 percent ground cloves (a spice) and about 60 percent tobacco. Many users mistakenly believe that these products are made entirely of ground cloves and that smoking them eliminates the risks associated with tobacco. In fact, clove cigarettes contain higher levels of tar, nicotine, and carbon monoxide than do regular cigarettes.

Table 13.3

A Comparison Between Filter Cigarettes and Cigars Shows a Marked Difference in Quantities

	FILTER CIGARETTE	REGULAR CIGAR
Weight	Approx. 0.68 g	Approx. 0.8 g
Nicotine	0.5–1.4 mg	1.7–5.2 mg
Tar	0.5–18 mg	16–110 mg
Carbon monoxide	0.5–18 mg	90–120 mg

Source: Downloaded from www.ymn.org, "No Such Thing as a Safe Smoke!" (1998). Reprinted by permission of Youth Media Network.

In addition, the numbing effect of eugenol, the active ingredient in cloves, allows smokers to inhale the smoke more deeply.

Cigars Those big stogies that we see celebrities and government figures puffing on these days are nothing more than tobacco fillers wrapped in more tobacco. Since 1991, cigar sales in the United States have increased by 250 percent. This growing fad is especially popular among young men and women, fueled in part by the willingness of celebrities to be photographed puffing on a cigar. Among some women, cigar smoking symbolizes an impulse to be slightly outrageous and liberated. Many people believe that cigars are safer than cigarettes, when in fact nothing could be further from the truth.[8] Cigar smoke contains 23 poisons and 43 carcinogens. As shown in Table 13.3, any argument about the safety of cigars is, well, a smokescreen.

Smoking as little as one cigar per day can increase the risk of several cancers, including cancer of the oral cavity (lip, tongue, mouth, and throat), esophagus, larynx, and lungs. Daily cigar smoking, especially for people who inhale, also increases the risk of heart disease (cigar smokers double their risk of heart attack and stroke) and a type of lung disease known as chronic obstructive pulmonary disease (COPD). Smoking one or two cigars daily doubles the risk for oral cancers and esophageal cancer, compared with the risk for someone who has never smoked. The risks increase with the number of cigars smoked per day.

A common question asked is whether cigars are addictive. Most cigars have as much nicotine as several cigarettes, and nicotine is highly addictive. When cigar smokers inhale, nicotine is absorbed as rapidly as it is with cigarettes. For those who don't inhale, nicotine is still absorbed through the mucous membranes in the mouth.

Bidis Bidis are small hand-rolled, flavored cigarettes, generally made in India or Southeast Asia. They come in a variety of flavors, such as vanilla, chocolate, and cherry, and cost $2–$4 for a pack of 20. Bidis look similar to a marijuana joint or a clove cigarette and have become increasingly popular with college students, who view them as safer, cheaper, and

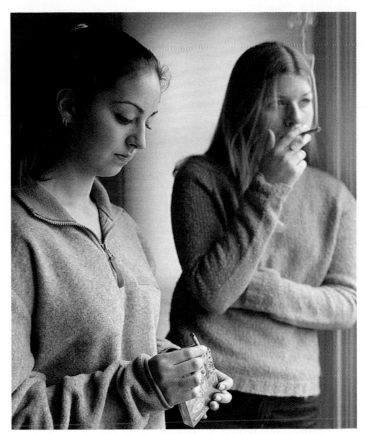

Bidis are becoming increasingly popular among teens and college students. But though they are cheaper and easier to obtain than cigarettes, bidis pose an equal or greater risk to health.

easier to obtain than cigarettes. However, they are far more toxic than cigarettes. A study by the Massachusetts Department of Health found that bidis produced three times more carbon monoxide and nicotine and five times more tar than cigarettes. The tendu leaf wrappers are nonporous, meaning that smokers have to pull harder to inhale and inhale more to keep the bidi lit. During testing, it took an average of 28 puffs to smoke a bidi, compared to only 9 puffs for a regular cigarette. This results in much more exposure to the higher amounts of tar, nicotine, and carbon monoxide, and bidis lack any sort of filter to lessen the levels. Research clearly indicates that bidi smokers are at the same, if not higher, risk for coronary heart disease and cancer due to smoking.[9]

Nicotine The stimulant chemical in tobacco products.

Tar A thick, brownish substance condensed from particulate matter in smoked tobacco.

Carbon monoxide A gas found in cigarette smoke that binds at oxygen receptor sites in the blood.

Bidis Hand-rolled flavored cigarettes.

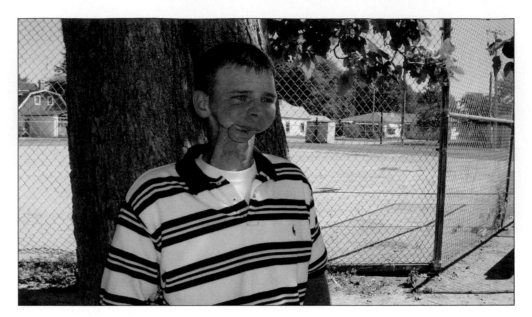

This 25-year-old cancer survivor has undergone almost 30 disfiguring surgeries. One operation removed half his neck muscles and lymph nodes and half of his tongue. He first tried smokeless tobacco at age 13; by age 17, he was diagnosed with squamous cell carcinoma. He now speaks out about the dangers of smokeless tobacco.

Smokeless Tobacco Approximately 5 million U.S. adults use smokeless tobacco. Most of them are teenage (20 percent of male high school students) and young adult males, who are often emulating a professional sports figure or family member. There are two types of smokeless tobacco—chewing tobacco and snuff.

Chewing tobacco is placed between the gums and teeth for sucking or chewing. It comes in three forms: loose leaf, plug, or twist. Chewing tobacco contains tobacco leaves treated with molasses and other flavorings. The user places a "quid" of tobacco in the mouth between the teeth and gums and then sucks or chews the quid to release the nicotine. Once the quid becomes ineffective, the user spits it out and inserts another. **Dipping** is another method of using chewing tobacco. The dipper takes a small amount of tobacco and places it between the lower lip and teeth to stimulate the flow of saliva and release the nicotine. Dipping rapidly releases nicotine into the bloodstream.

Snuff is a finely ground form of tobacco that can be inhaled, chewed, or placed against the gums. It comes in dry or moist powdered form or sachets (tea bag–like pouches).

Usually snuff is placed inside the cheek. Inhaling dry snuff is more common in Europe than in the United States.[10]

Smokeless tobacco is just as addictive as cigarettes because of its nicotine content. There is nicotine in all tobacco products, but smokeless tobacco contains even more than cigarettes. Holding an average-sized dip or chew in the mouth for 30 minutes delivers as much nicotine as smoking four cigarettes. A two-can-a-week snuff dipper gets as much nicotine as a one-and-a-half-pack-a-day smoker.

A major risk of chewing tobacco is **leukoplakia,** a condition characterized by leathery white patches inside the mouth produced by contact with irritants in tobacco juice. Smokeless tobacco contains 10 times the amount of cancer-producing substances found in cigarettes and 100 times more than the Food and Drug Administration allows in foods and other substances used by the public. Between 3 and 17 percent of diagnosed leukoplakia cases develop into oral cancer. It is estimated that 75 percent of the 28,900 oral cancer cases in 2002 resulted from either smokeless tobacco or cigarettes.[11] Users of smokeless tobacco are 50 times more likely to develop oral cancers than are nonusers. Warning signs of oral cancers include lumps in the jaw or neck; color changes or lumps inside the lips; white, smooth, or scaly patches in the mouth or on the neck, lips, or tongue; a red spot or sore on the lips or gums or inside the mouth that does not heal in two weeks; repeated bleeding in the mouth; and difficulty or abnormality in speaking or swallowing.

The lag time between first use and contracting cancer is shorter for smokeless tobacco users than for smokers because absorption through the gums is the most efficient route of nicotine administration. A growing body of evidence suggests that long-term use of smokeless tobacco also increases the risk of cancer of the larynx, esophagus, nasal cavity, pancreas, kidney, and bladder. Moreover, many smokeless tobacco users eventually "graduate" to cigarettes.

The stimulant effects of nicotine may create the same circulatory and respiratory problems for chewers as for

---

Chewing tobacco A stringy type of tobacco that is placed in the mouth and then sucked or chewed.

Dipping Placing a small amount of chewing tobacco between the front lip and teeth for rapid nicotine absorption.

Snuff A powdered form of tobacco that is sniffed and absorbed through the mucous membranes in the nose or placed inside the cheek and sucked.

Leukoplakia A condition characterized by leathery white patches inside the mouth produced by contact with irritants in tobacco juice.

A Sweet but Deadly Addiction in India

Promoted by a slick and many-tentacled advertising campaign, *gutka,* an indigenous form of smokeless tobacco, has become a fixture in the mouths of millions of Indians over the last two decades. It has spread through the subcontinent, and even to South Asians in England. But what has prompted particular concern is the way that in the last 10 years, gutka—as portable as chewing gum and sometimes as sweet as candy—has found its way into the mouths of Indian children.

Young people have become gutka consumers in large numbers, and they have become an alarming avant-garde in what doctors say is an oral cancer epidemic.

That, among other factors, has prompted the state of Maharashtra, which includes Bombay, to take an unusual step. It enacted a five-year ban, the longest permitted by law, on the production, sale, transport, and possession of gutka, a $30 million business in the state, that started in August 2002. Several other states have undertaken similar bans, although some have been stayed by the courts.

It is easy, on the streets of Bombay, to find young men like Raga Vendra, now 19, a railway worker who began taking gutka at age 11. It is also easy to find gutka sellers, like Ahmed Maqsood, who say they have had customers as young as 6.

Dr. Surendra Shastri, the head of preventive oncology at Tata Memorial Hospital, noticed about five years ago that his patients were getting younger, by about eight to ten years. "High school and college students were coming in with precancerous lesions," he said. "Usage was starting much earlier."

India has 75,000 to 80,000 new cases of oral cancers a year—the world's highest incidence, and about 2,000 deaths a day are tobacco related.

A 1998 survey of 1,800 boys ages 13 to 15 from a wide range of socioeconomic groups found that up to 20 percent were already using three to five packets of gutka daily. The price is low: sometimes less than two cents a packet. The contents, a mixture of ingredients including tobacco, are usually placed in the cheek lining, savored, then expelled.

Gutka was the product of a packaging revolution that made an Indian tradition portable and cheap. Many Indians have long chewed paan, a betel leaf wrapped around a mixture of lime paste, spices, areca nut, and often tobacco. But obtaining paan required a visit to a paanwallah—it was too messy to be transported.

All of that changed with gutka, a dried version of the concoction, but without the betel leaf, preserved and perfumed with chemicals and sealed in a plastic or foil pack. Gutka could be used at will, at work or at home or at school, and it was used, in very large quantities. Sales of gutka and its tobaccoless counterpart, paan masala, are now more than $1 billion a year, having quintupled during the 1990s.

"What caused this boom of oral cancers was this packaging of tobacco," said Dr. A. K. D'Cruz, the lead head-and-neck surgeon at Tata Memorial Hospital. "Convenience got them hooked."

Many consumers say they welcome the ban, because they see no other way to curb their addiction. Even some vendors like Mr. Maqsood have embraced it, saying they felt they were trading in toxins. "The chemicals used in gutka were poisonous," he said. "I have seen some customers who can't open their mouth."

Gutka is seen by doctors as particularly insidious because it contains many unhealthful additives, like magnesium carbonate, and is cheap. For children and teenagers, smoking cigarettes remains taboo. Gutka has no social stigma among peers, and it is easy to hide from parents.

Padmini Samini, who started an anti-tobacco advocacy group after her father got oral cancer, said she had found cases in which gutka makers had given free samples to children after school. Some of it was sweetened so much to mask the harsh tobacco taste, she said, that children considered it candy.

About 30 percent of the cancers in India are in the head and neck, compared with 4.5 percent in the West. Furthermore, Dr. D'Cruz added, "most of our cancers come a decade earlier than the West." They come in the cheek and jaw, often preceded by submucosal fibrosis, a hardening of the palate that can make it almost impossible to open the mouth.

Source: A. Waldman, "Sweet but Deadly Addiction Is Seizing the Young in India," *The New York Times,* August 13, 2002. Copyright 2002 by The New York Times Co. Reprinted by permission.

smokers. Chronic smokeless tobacco use also results in delayed wound healing and peptic ulcer disease.

Like smoked tobacco, smokeless tobacco also impairs the senses of taste and smell, causing the user to add salt and sugar to food, which may contribute to high blood pressure and obesity. Some smokeless tobacco products contain high levels of sodium (salt), which also contributes to high blood pressure. In addition, dental problems are common among users of smokeless tobacco. Contact with tobacco juice causes receding gums, tooth decay, bad breath, and discolored teeth. Damage to both the teeth and jawbone can contribute to early loss of teeth. Users of all tobacco products may not be able to absorb the vitamins and other nutrients in food effectively.

Smokeless tobacco users have the same problems that smokers do when trying to quit. Withdrawal symptoms are almost universal; relapse is common. Symptoms that often accompany nicotine withdrawal include headache, gastrointestinal discomfort, sleeping problems, irritability, anxiety, aggressiveness, craving for tobacco, and a reduction in heart rate, blood pressure, and hormone secretions. See the Health in a Diverse World Box for a new threat from the smokeless world.

Table 13.4
Pairings with "Hits" of Nicotine over Time

	PAIRINGS PER DAY	PAIRINGS PER MONTH	PAIRINGS PER YEAR
¼ pack (5 cigarettes)	50	1,500	18,250
½ pack (10 cigarettes)	100	3,000	36,500
1 pack (20 cigarettes)	200	6,000	73,000

Based on an average of 10 drags (or hits) per cigarette

What do you think?

Should smokeless tobacco be banned in all venues that also ban smoking? ✳ What is attractive about the use of smokeless tobacco? ✳ Why do you think that it is popular with many athletes and males?

Physiological Effects of Nicotine

Nicotine is a powerful central nervous system stimulant that produces a variety of physiological effects. Its stimulant action in the cerebral cortex produces an aroused, alert mental state. Nicotine also stimulates the adrenal glands, increasing the production of adrenaline. The physical effects of nicotine stimulation include increased heart and respiratory rate, constricted blood vessels, and subsequent increased blood pressure because the heart must work harder to pump blood through the narrowed vessels.

Nicotine decreases blood sugar levels and the stomach contractions that signal hunger. These factors, along with decreased sensation in the taste buds, reduce appetite. For this reason, many smokers eat less than nonsmokers do and weigh, on average, seven pounds less than nonsmokers.

Beginning smokers usually feel the effects of nicotine with their first puff. These symptoms, called **nicotine poisoning,** include dizziness, lightheadedness, rapid and erratic pulse, clammy skin, nausea, vomiting, and diarrhea. The effects of nicotine poisoning cease as soon as tolerance to the chemical develops. Medical research indicates that tolerance develops almost immediately in new users, perhaps after the second or third cigarette. In contrast, tolerance to most other drugs, such as alcohol, develops over a period of months or years. Regular smokers often do not experience the "buzz" of smoking. They continue to smoke simply because stopping is too difficult.

Tobacco Addiction

Smoking is a complicated behavior. Somewhere between 60 and 80 percent of people have tried or taken at least a "puff" on a cigarette. Why is it that some walk away from cigarettes and others get hooked? For one thing, smoking is a very efficient drug delivery system. It gets the drug to the brain in just a few seconds, much faster than it would travel if injected. A pack-a-day smoker experiences 70,000 "hits," or **pairings,** per

year (see Table 13.4). In pairing, an environmental cue triggers a craving for nicotine.[12] Simple pairings, such as drinking a cup of coffee, sitting in a car, finishing a meal, or sipping a beer, induce nicotine craving. Some college students, who "only smoke occasionally," find it hard to quit because of these paired associations. For example, when an occasional smoker goes through a half pack of cigarettes while out drinking, this smoker experiences 100 "hits," or chemical pairings between alcohol and tobacco, in one evening, and within a month, this reaches 800 pairings. The brain gets used to that pairing and cries out in displeasure when the association is missing. It is easy to see how stopping even occasional use can be very difficult.

Why does this association occur? One explanation might lie in a person's genes. Two different twin studies found genetic factors to be more influential than environmental factors in smoking initiation and nicotine dependence. Two specific genes may influence smoking behavior by affecting the action of the brain chemical dopamine.[13] Understanding the influence of genetics on nicotine addiction will be crucial to developing more effective treatments for smoking cessation.

What do you think?

Because nicotine is highly addictive, should it be regulated as a controlled substance? ✳ How could tobacco be regulated effectively? ✳ Should more resources be used for research into nicotine addiction? ✳ Why or why not?

Health Hazards of Smoking

Cigarette smoking adversely affects the health of every person who smokes. Each day cigarettes contribute to over 1,000 deaths from cancer, cardiovascular disease, and respiratory disorders.

Cancer

The American Cancer Society estimates that tobacco smoking causes more than 85 to 90 percent of all cases of lung cancer—fewer than 10 percent of cases occur among nonsmokers.[14] Lung cancer is the leading cause of cancer deaths in the United States. It is estimated that there were 169,500 *new*

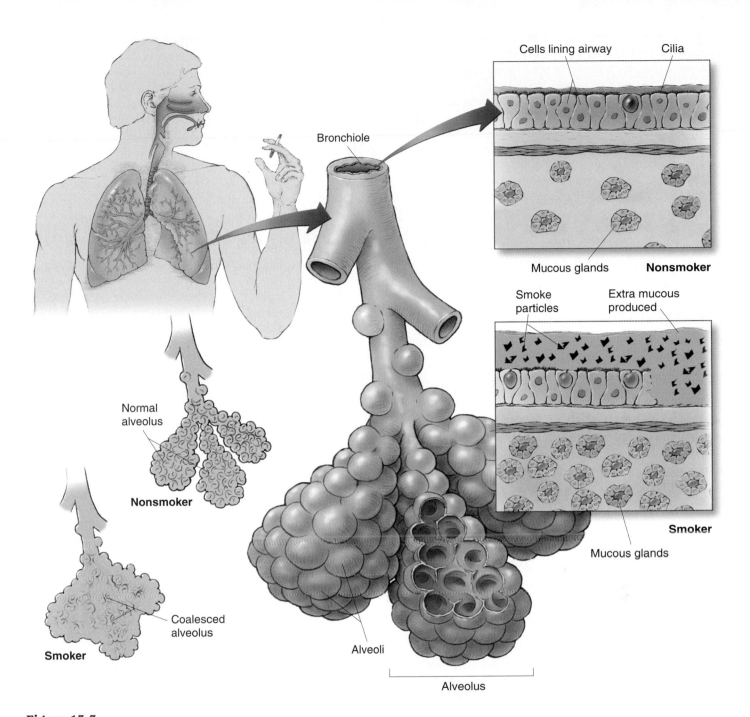

Figure 13.3
How Cigarette Smoking Damages the Lungs
Smoke particles irritate the lung airways, causing excess mucous production. They also indirectly destroy the walls of the lungs' alveoli, which coalesce. Both factors reduce lung efficiency. In addition, tar in tobacco smoke has a direct cancer-causing action.

cases of lung cancer in the United States in 2001 alone, and an estimated 154,900 Americans died of the disease in 2002. Figure 13.3 illustrates how tobacco smoke damages the lungs.

Lung cancer can take 10 to 30 years to develop. The outlook for victims of this disease is poor. Most lung cancer is not diagnosed until it is fairly widespread in the body; at that point, the five-year survival rate is only 13 percent. When a malignancy is diagnosed and recognized while still localized, the five-year survival rate rises to 47 percent.

Nicotine poisoning   Symptoms often experienced by beginning smokers, including dizziness, diarrhea, light-headedness, rapid and erratic pulse, clammy skin, nausea, and vomiting.

Pairings   Paired associations (e.g., coffee and a cigarette) that trigger cravings.

If you are a smoker, your risk of developing lung cancer depends on several factors. First, the number of cigarettes you smoke per day is important. Someone who smokes two packs a day is 15 to 25 times more likely to develop lung cancer than a nonsmoker. If you started smoking in your teens, you have a greater chance of developing lung cancer than people who started later. If you inhale deeply when you smoke, you also increase your chances. So will occupational or domestic exposure to other irritants, such as asbestos and radon.[15]

Tobacco is linked to other cancers as well. Cigarette smoking increases the risk of pancreatic cancer by 70 percent. Smokers can reduce those odds by 30 percent if they quit for 11 years or more.[16] Cancers of the lip, tongue, salivary glands, and esophagus are five times more likely to occur among smokers than among nonsmokers. Smokers are also more likely to develop kidney, bladder, and larynx cancers.

Cardiovascular Disease

Half of all tobacco-related deaths occur as a result of some form of heart disease.[17] Smokers have a 70 percent higher death rate from heart disease than nonsmokers do, and heavy smokers have a 200 percent higher death rate than moderate smokers. In fact, smoking cigarettes poses as great a risk for developing heart disease as high blood pressure and high cholesterol levels do.

Smoking contributes to heart disease by adding the equivalent of 10 years of aging to the arteries.[18] One explanation is that smoking encourages atherosclerosis, the buildup of fatty deposits in the heart and major blood vessels. For unknown reasons, smoking decreases blood levels of HDLs (high-density lipoproteins), which help protect against heart attacks. Smoking also contributes to **platelet adhesiveness,** the sticking together of red blood cells that is associated with blood clots. The oxygen deprivation associated with smoking decreases the oxygen supplied to the heart and can weaken tissues. Smoking also contributes to irregular heart rhythms, which can trigger a heart attack. Both carbon monoxide and nicotine in cigarette smoke can precipitate angina attacks (pain spasms in the chest when the heart muscle does not get the blood supply it needs).

The number of years a person has smoked does not seem to bear much relation to cardiovascular risk. If a person quits smoking, the risk of dying from a heart attack is reduced by half after only one year without smoking and declines gradually thereafter. After about 15 years without smoking, the ex-smoker's risk of cardiovascular disease is similar to that of people who have never smoked.

Platelet adhesiveness Stickiness of red blood cells associated with blood clots.

Emphysema A chronic lung disease in which the tiny air sacs in the lungs are destroyed, making breathing difficult.

Stroke Smokers are twice as likely to suffer strokes as nonsmokers are. A stroke occurs when a small blood vessel in the brain bursts or is blocked by a blood clot, denying oxygen and nourishment to vital portions of the brain. Depending on the area of the brain supplied by the vessel, stroke can result in paralysis, loss of mental functioning, or death. Smoking contributes to strokes by raising blood pressure, thereby increasing the stress on vessel walls. Platelet adhesiveness contributes to clotting. Five to 15 years after they stop smoking, the risk of stroke for ex-smokers is the same as that for people who have never smoked.

Respiratory Disorders

Smoking quickly impairs the respiratory system. Smokers can feel its impact in a relatively short period of time—they are more prone to breathlessness, chronic cough, and excess phlegm production than nonsmokers their age. Smokers tend to miss work one-third more often than nonsmokers do, primarily because of respiratory diseases, and they are up to 18 times more likely to die of lung disease.

Chronic bronchitis is the presence of a productive cough that persists or reoccurs frequently. It may develop in smokers because their inflamed lungs produce more mucous and constantly try to rid themselves of this mucous and foreign particles. The effort to do so results in "smoker's hack," the persistent cough experienced by most smokers. Smokers are more prone than nonsmokers to respiratory ailments such as influenza, pneumonia, and colds.

Emphysema is a chronic disease in which the alveoli (the tiny air sacs in the lungs) are destroyed, impairing the lungs' ability to obtain oxygen and remove carbon dioxide. As a result, breathing becomes difficult. Whereas healthy people expend only about 5 percent of their energy in breathing, people with advanced emphysema expend nearly 80 percent of their energy. A simple movement such as rising from a seated position becomes painful and difficult for the emphysema patient. Since the heart has to work harder to do even the simplest tasks, it may become enlarged, and the person may die from heart damage. There is no known cure for emphysema. Approximately 80 percent of all cases are related to cigarette smoking.

Sexual Dysfunction

Despite attempts by tobacco advertisers to make smoking appear sexy, research shows just the opposite: It can cause impotence in men. A number of recent studies have found that male smokers are about two times more likely than nonsmokers to suffer from some form of impotence. Toxins in cigarette smoke damage blood vessels, reducing blood flow to the penis and leading to an inadequate erection. It is thought that impotence could indicate oncoming cardiovascular disease.

Other Health Effects of Smoking

Gum disease is three times more common among smokers than among nonsmokers, and smokers lose significantly more

Women and Smoking

For more than 50 years, tobacco company advertisements have enticed women to smoke cigarettes. Though their messages have glamorized smoking, the real results are not very glamorous: Women who smoke have an increased risk of developing cancer, heart disease, and problems associated with the reproductive organs. The risk of cervical cancer, for instance, is higher among women who smoke than among those who don't. A woman reduces her risk dramatically when she quits.

According to a recent study, cigarettes are even more dangerous for women than for men; women are more likely to develop lung cancer and to do so with fewer cigarettes. Already lung cancer deaths have surpassed breast cancer deaths for women. The risk of heart disease for women smokers who smoke more than 25 cigarettes per day is 500 percent higher than it is for nonsmokers. Even smoking one to four cigarettes per day doubles a woman's risk for heart attack. It makes no difference if she smokes low- or high-nicotine cigarettes.

Smoking appears to send women into menopause one to two years early. (Smokers who quit start menopause at about the same age as women who have never smoked.) Smoking also contributes to osteoporosis, a condition involving bone loss that particularly afflicts women. Current female smokers age 35 and older are more than 10 times as likely to die of emphysema or chronic bronchitis than male smokers.

Women smokers who take oral contraceptives (birth control pills) greatly increase their risk of heart attack. In a recent study, the risk for a heart attack was shown to be 20 times higher for pill users who smoked 10 or more cigarettes per day than it was for women who did not smoke and did not use the pill. Oral contraceptives increase the risk of developing blood clots, which can block the already narrowing arteries of women with atherosclerosis, another disease with an increased risk for smokers. For these reasons, smoking while taking oral contraceptives also increases the risk of peripheral vascular disease and stroke.

Although cigarette smoking is dangerous for all women, it presents special risks for pregnant women and their fetuses. Each year in the United States, approximately 50,000 miscarriages are attributed to smoking during pregnancy. On average, babies born to mothers who smoke weigh less than those born to nonsmokers, and low birthweight is correlated with many developmental problems. Pregnant women who stop smoking in the first three or four months of their pregnancies give birth to higher-birthweight babies than do women who smoke throughout their pregnancies. Prenatal exposure to smoking has also been linked with impairments in memory, learning, cognition, and perception in the growing child. Infant mortality rates are also higher among babies born to smokers.

Maternal smoking has long been linked to increased risk of sudden infant death syndrome (SIDS). SIDS, or "crib death," occurs when an infant, usually less than one year of age, dies during its sleep for no apparent reason. The more the mother smokes, the greater the risk. Passive smoke has also been associated with SIDS. This risk is increased in normal-weight infants, about twofold with passive smoke exposure, and about threefold when the mother smokes both during the pregnancy and after the baby is born. Infants who are born to mothers who smoke during pregnancy have more episodes of apnea and excessive sweating. It has been suggested that smoking may influence the development of the infant's nervous system.

One study found that daughters of women who smoked during pregnancy are four times more likely to begin smoking during adolescence and to continue smoking than the daughters of nonsmoking women. The study suggests that nicotine, which crosses the placental barrier, may affect the female fetus during an important period of development so as to predispose the brain to the addictive influence of nicotine more than a decade later.

Sources: Harvard Women's Health Watch, "Tobacco Smoke and Women: A Special Vulnerability?" May 2000, p. 1; WHO Collaborative Study of Cardiovascular Disease and Steroid Hormone Contraception, "Acute Myocardial Infarction and Combined Oral Contraceptives: Results of an International Multicentre Case-Control Study," *The Lancet* April 26, 1997, pp. 1202–1209; NIDA Notes, "Nicotine Conference Highlights Research Accomplishments and Challenges," September/October 1995, pp. 11–12; "Women and Smoking: A Report of the Surgeon General, Executive Summary, " *Morbidity and Mortality Weekly,* August 30, 2002, vol. 57.

teeth.[19] Smokers are also likely to use more medications. Nicotine and the other ingredients in cigarettes interfere with the metabolism of drugs: Nicotine speeds up the process by which the body uses and eliminates drugs, so that medications become less effective. The smoker may therefore have to take a higher dosage of a drug or take it more frequently. There are also tobacco-related health issues of special concern to women (see the Women's Health/Men's Health box).

What do you think?

Most people are very aware of the long-term hazards associated with tobacco use, yet despite prevention efforts, people continue to smoke. ✸ Why do you think this is so? ✸ What strategies to reduce the number of people who begin smoking might be effective?

Environmental Tobacco Smoke (ETS)

Although fewer than 30 percent of Americans are smokers, air pollution from smoking in public places continues to be a problem. **Environmental tobacco smoke (ETS)** is divided into two categories: mainstream and sidestream smoke (also called secondhand smoke). **Mainstream smoke** refers to smoke drawn through tobacco while inhaling; **sidestream smoke** refers to smoke from the burning end of a cigarette or smoke exhaled by a smoker. People who breathe smoke from someone else's smoking product are said to be *involuntary* or *passive* smokers. Nearly 9 out of 10 nonsmoking Americans are exposed to environmental tobacco smoke.

Risks from ETS

Although involuntary smokers breathe less tobacco than active smokers do, they still face risks from exposure to tobacco smoke. Sidestream smoke actually contains more carcinogenic substances than the smoke that a smoker inhales. According to the American Lung Association, sidestream smoke has about 2 times more tar and nicotine, 5 times more carbon monoxide, and 50 times more ammonia than mainstream smoke. ETS is estimated to be responsible for approximately 3,000 lung cancer deaths, 37,000 cardiovascular disease deaths, and 13,000 deaths from other cancers each year in the U.S.[20] The Environmental Protection Agency (EPA) has designated secondhand tobacco smoke a *group A cancer-causing agent* that is even worse than other group A threats such as benzene, arsenic, and radon. There is also evidence that sidestream smoke poses an even greater risk for death due to heart disease than for death due to lung cancer.[21]

Sidestream smoke is estimated to cause more deaths per year than any other environmental pollutant. The risk of dying because of exposure to passive smoking is 100 times greater than the risk that requires the EPA to label a pollutant as carcinogenic and 10,000 times greater than the risk that requires the labeling of a food as carcinogenic.[22]

Lung cancer and heart disease are not the only risks involuntary smokers face. Exposure to ETS among children increases their risk of lower respiratory tract infections. An estimated 300,000 children are at greater risk of pneumonia and bronchitis as a result.[23] Children exposed to sidestream smoke have a greater chance of developing other respiratory problems, such as cough, wheezing, asthma, and chest colds, along with a decrease in lung function. The greatest effects of sidestream smoke are seen in children under the age of five. Children exposed to sidestream smoke daily in the home miss 33 percent more school days and have 10 percent more colds and acute respiratory infections than those not exposed. A recent study found that 31.2 percent of children are exposed to cigarette smoke daily in the home. This study found wide regional, income, and education differences: Children of high-income, high-education-level parents in California are exposed far less than are children of low-income, low-education-level parents in the Midwest.[24]

Cigarette, cigar, and pipe smoke in enclosed areas presents other hazards. Ten to 15 percent of nonsmokers are extremely sensitive (hypersensitive) to cigarette smoke. These people experience itchy eyes, difficulty in breathing, painful headaches, nausea, and dizziness in response to minute amounts of smoke. The level of carbon monoxide in cigarette smoke contained in enclosed places is 4,000 times higher than that allowed in the clean air standard recommended by the EPA.

Efforts to reduce the hazards associated with passive smoking have been gaining momentum in recent years. Groups such as GASP (Group Against Smokers' Pollution) and ASH (Action on Smoking and Health) have been working since the early 1970s to reduce smoking in public places. In response to their efforts, some 44 states have enacted laws restricting smoking in public places such as restaurants, theaters, and airports. The federal government has restricted smoking in all government buildings. Hotels and motels now set aside rooms for nonsmokers, and car rental agencies designate certain vehicles for nonsmokers. Since 1990, smoking has been banned on all domestic airline flights.

> **What do you think?**
>
> *What rights, if any, should smokers have with regard to smoking in public places? ✳ Does your campus allow smoking in residence halls? ✳ Does your community have nonsmoking restaurants, or does it only have nonsmoking sections? ✳ Do you think your community would support nonsmoking restaurants and bars? ✳ Why or why not?*

Tobacco and Politics

It has been at least 30 years since the government began warning that tobacco use was hazardous to the health of the nation. Today the tobacco industry is under fire—46 states have sued to recover health care costs related to treating smokers.

Environmental tobacco smoke (ETS)   Smoke from tobacco products, including sidestream and mainstream smoke.

Mainstream smoke   Smoke that is drawn through tobacco while inhaling.

Sidestream smoke   The cigarette, pipe, or cigar smoke breathed by nonsmokers; also called secondhand smoke.

Nicotine withdrawal   Symptoms, including nausea, headaches, and irritability, suffered by smokers who cease using tobacco.

In 1998, the tobacco industry reached a Master's Settlement Agreement with these states. Key provisions include the following:

- The tobacco payments will total approximately $206 billion to be paid over 25 years nationwide.
- The industry will pay $1.5 billion over 10 years to support antismoking measures, including education and advertising. An additional $250 million will fund research to determine the most effective ways to stop kids from smoking.
- The industry is barred from billboard advertising, including advertisements on transit systems. In-store ads are still permitted but will be limited in size.
- All outdoor advertising is banned, including billboards, signs, and placards larger than a poster in arenas, stadiums, shopping malls, and video arcades.
- The agreement bans youth access to free samples, proof-of-purchase gifts, and sale and distribution of "branded" merchandise, such as T-shirts, hats, and other items bearing tobacco brand names or logos.
- There is a ban on the use of cartoon characters, such as Joe Camel, in advertising. (Such advertising is considered particularly appealing to young children.)
- Tobacco company sponsorship of concerts, athletic events, or any event in which a significant portion of the audience is comprised of youth is forbidden.
- The industry agreed not to market cigarettes to children and not to misrepresent the health effects of cigarettes.[25]

Other states and communities are advocating stricter tobacco control. A number of states have imposed extra taxes on cigarette sales in an effort to discourage use. The monies are then used for various purposes, including prevention and cessation programs and school health programs. Two community-based programs, ASSIST (American Stop Smoking Intervention Study) and IMPACT (Initiatives to Mobilize for the Prevention and Control of Tobacco Use), are tobacco control initiatives focused on creating legislation to prohibit the sale of tobacco to minors and assist with enforcement.

Quitting

Quitting smoking isn't easy. Smokers must break the physical addiction to nicotine. And they must break the habit of lighting up at certain times of the day.

From what we know about successful quitters, quitting is often a lengthy process involving several unsuccessful attempts before success is finally achieved. Even successful quitters suffer occasional slips, emphasizing the fact that stopping smoking is a dynamic process that occurs over time.

Approximately one-third of smokers attempt to quit each year. Unfortunately, 90 percent or more of those attempts fail. The person who wishes to quit smoking has several options. Most try to quit "cold turkey"—that is, they decide simply not to smoke again. Others resort to short-term programs, such as those offered by the American Cancer Society, which are based on behavior modification and

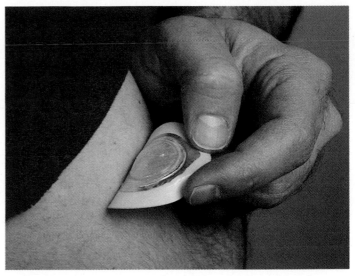

The unpleasant symptoms of nicotine withdrawal can be lessened by a nicotine patch that delivers nicotine through the skin. Success rates for quitting are highest when the patch is combined with counseling or a behavior modification program.

a system of self-rewards. Still others turn to treatment centers that are part of large franchises or a local medical clinic's community outreach plan. Finally, some people work privately with their physicians to reach their goal.

Prospective quitters must decide which method or combination of methods will work best for them. Programs that combine several approaches have shown the most promise. Financial considerations, personality characteristics, and level of addiction are all factors to consider.

Breaking the Nicotine Addiction

Nicotine addiction may be one of the toughest addictions to overcome. Smokers' attempts to quit lead to withdrawal symptoms. Symptoms of **nicotine withdrawal** include irritability, restlessness, nausea, vomiting, and intense cravings for tobacco.

Nicotine Replacement Products Nontobacco products that replace depleted levels of nicotine in the bloodstream have helped some people stop using tobacco. The two most common are nicotine chewing gum and the nicotine patch, both of which are available over the counter. The FDA has also approved a nicotine nasal spray, a nicotine inhaler, and a nicotine pill.

Some patients use Nicorette, a prescription chewing gum containing nicotine, to reduce nicotine consumption over time. Under the guidance of a physician, the user chews between 12 and 24 pieces of gum per day for up to six months. Nicorette delivers about as much nicotine as a cigarette does, but because it is absorbed through the mucous membrane of the mouth, it doesn't produce the same rush. Users experience no withdrawal symptoms and fewer cravings for nicotine as the dosage is reduced until they are completely weaned.

Some controversy surrounds the use of nicotine replacement gum. Opponents believe that it substitutes one addiction for another. Successful users counter that it is a valid way to help break a deadly habit without suffering the unpleasant cravings that often lead to relapse.

The nicotine patch, first marketed in 1991, is generally used in conjunction with a comprehensive smoking-behavior cessation program. A small, thin, 24-hour patch placed on the smoker's upper body delivers a continuous flow of nicotine through the skin, helping to relieve cravings. The patch is worn for 8 to 12 weeks under the guidance of a physician. During this time, the dose of nicotine is gradually reduced until the smoker is fully weaned from nicotine. Occasional side effects include mild skin irritation, insomnia, dry mouth, and nervousness. The patch costs less than a pack of cigarettes—about four dollars—and some insurance plans will pay for it.

How effective is the nicotine patch? According to an analysis of 17 studies involving 5,098 people, the nicotine patch was at least twice as effective as placebo (fake) patches. At the end of treatment periods lasting at least four weeks, 27 percent of nicotine patch wearers were free of cigarettes versus 13 percent of placebo patch users. Six months later, 22 percent of the nicotine patch users were abstinent compared with only 9 percent of the placebo users. The study also showed that the patch was effective with or without intensive counseling.[26]

The nasal spray, which requires a prescription, is much more powerful and delivers nicotine to the bloodstream faster than gum or the patch. Patients are warned to be careful not to overdose; as little as 40 milligrams of nicotine taken at once could be lethal. The spray is somewhat unpleasant to use. The FDA has advised that it should be used for no more than three months and never for more

---

SKILLS FOR BEHAVIOR CHANGE

Developing a Plan to Kick the Habit

There is no magic cure that can help you stop. Take the first step by answering this question: Why do I want to stop smoking?

Write your reasons in the space below. Once you have prepared your list, carry a copy of it with you. Memorize it. Every time you are tempted to smoke, go over your reasons for stopping.

My Reasons for Stopping

1. _____
2. _____
3. _____
4. _____
5. _____

Develop a Plan; Change Some Habits

Over time, smoking becomes a strong habit. Daily events such as finishing a meal, talking on the phone, drinking coffee, and chatting with friends trigger the urge to smoke. Breaking the link between the trigger and the smoking will help you stop. Think about the times and places you usually smoke. What could you do instead of smoking at those times?

Things to Do Instead of Smoking

1. _____
2. _____
3. _____

The Bottom Line: Commit Yourself

There comes a time when you have to say good-bye to your cigarettes.

- Pick a day to stop smoking.
- Fill out the Behavior Change Contract.
- Have a family member or friend sign the contract.

THEN

- Throw away all your cigarettes, lighters, and ashtrays at home and at work. You will not need them again.
- Be prepared to feel the urge to smoke. The urge will pass whether or not you smoke. Use the four Ds to fight the urge:

Delay
Deep breathing
Drink water
Do something else

- Keep "mouth toys" handy: lifesavers, gum, straws, and carrot sticks can help.
- If you've had trouble stopping before, ask your doctor about nicotine chewing gum, patches, nasal sprays, inhalers, or pills.
- Tell your family and friends that you've stopped smoking.

- Put "no smoking" signs in your car, work area, and house.
- Give yourself a treat for stopping. Go to a movie, go out to dinner, or buy yourself a gift.

Focus on the Positives

Now that you have stopped smoking, your mind and your body will begin to feel better. Think of the good things that have happened since you stopped. Can you breathe more easily? Do you have more energy? Do you feel good about what you've done?

Use the space below to list the good things about not smoking. Carry a copy with you, and look at it when you have the urge to smoke.

_____
_____
_____
_____
_____
_____
_____
_____
_____
_____

Source: Reprinted by permission from *Smart Move! A Stop Smoking Guide.* © 1996, American Cancer Society, Inc.

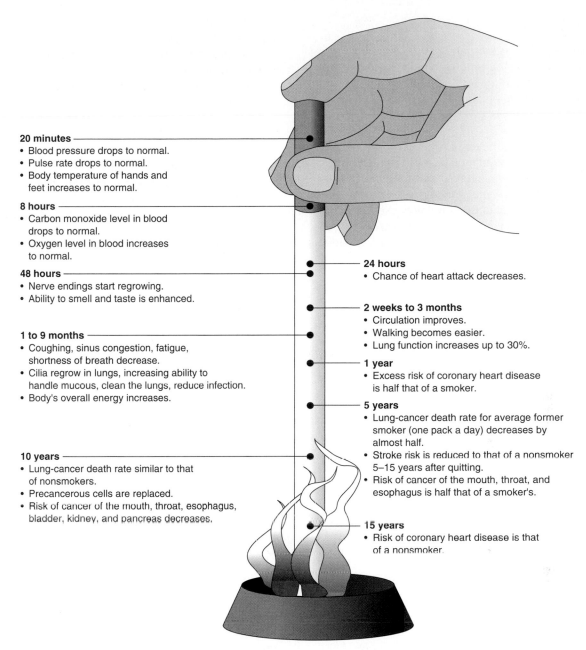

20 minutes
- Blood pressure drops to normal.
- Pulse rate drops to normal.
- Body temperature of hands and feet increases to normal.

8 hours
- Carbon monoxide level in blood drops to normal.
- Oxygen level in blood increases to normal.

48 hours
- Nerve endings start regrowing.
- Ability to smell and taste is enhanced.

1 to 9 months
- Coughing, sinus congestion, fatigue, shortness of breath decrease.
- Cilia regrow in lungs, increasing ability to handle mucous, clean the lungs, reduce infection.
- Body's overall energy increases.

10 years
- Lung-cancer death rate similar to that of nonsmokers.
- Precancerous cells are replaced.
- Risk of cancer of the mouth, throat, esophagus, bladder, kidney, and pancreas decreases.

24 hours
- Chance of heart attack decreases.

2 weeks to 3 months
- Circulation improves.
- Walking becomes easier.
- Lung function increases up to 30%.

1 year
- Excess risk of coronary heart disease is half that of a smoker.

5 years
- Lung-cancer death rate for average former smoker (one pack a day) decreases by almost half.
- Stroke risk is reduced to that of a nonsmoker 5–15 years after quitting.
- Risk of cancer of the mouth, throat, and esophagus is half that of a smoker's.

15 years
- Risk of coronary heart disease is that of a nonsmoker.

Figure 13.4
When Smokers Quit
Within 20 minutes of smoking that last cigarette, the body begins a series of positive changes that continues for years. All benefits are lost by smoking just one cigarette a day, according to the American Cancer Society.
Source: *Drugs and Society* (5th ed.) by G. Hanson and P. Venturelli (Sudbury, MA: Jones and Bartlett, 1998). www.jbpum.com.

than six months, so that smokers don't find themselves as dependent on nicotine in spray form as they were on cigarettes. The FDA also advises that no one who experiences nasal or sinus problems, allergies, or asthma should use it.

The nicotine inhaler, which also requires a prescription, consists of a mouthpiece and cartridge. By puffing on the mouthpiece, the smoker inhales air saturated with nicotine, which is absorbed through the lining of the mouth, not the lungs. This nicotine enters the body much more slowly than the nicotine in cigarettes does. Using the inhaler mimics the hand-to-mouth actions used in smoking and causes the back of the throat to feel as it would when inhaling tobacco smoke. Each cartridge lasts for 80 long puffs, and each cartridge is designed for 20 minutes of use.

Approved in 1997 by the FDA, Zyban, the smoking cessation pill, offers new hope to many who thought they could never quit. Zyban is thought to work on dopamine and norepinephrine receptors in the brain to decrease craving and withdrawal symptoms. Because of the way this prescription medication works, it is important to start the pills 10 to 14 days before the targeted quit date; it requires planning ahead.

Breaking the Habit

For many smokers, the road to quitting includes antismoking therapy. Among the more common techniques are aversion therapy, operant conditioning, and self-control therapy. The Skills for Behavior Change box presents one of the American Cancer Society's approaches.

Aversion Therapy Aversion techniques attempt to reduce smoking by pairing the act of smoking with a noxious stimulus so that smoking itself is perceived as unpleasant. For example, the technique of rapid smoking instructs patients to smoke rapidly and continuously until they exceed their tolerance for cigarette smoke, producing unpleasant sensations. Short-term rates of success are high, but many patients relapse over time.

Operant Strategies Pairing the act of smoking with an external stimulus is a typical example of this method. For example, one technique requires smokers to carry a timer that sounds a buzzer at different intervals. When the buzzer sounds, the patient is required to smoke a cigarette. Once the smoker is conditioned to associate the buzzer with smoking, the buzzer is eliminated, and, one hopes, so is the smoking.

Self-Control Self-control strategies view smoking as a learned habit associated with specific situations. Therapy is aimed at identifying these situations and teaching smokers the skills necessary to resist smoking.

Benefits of Quitting

According to the American Cancer Society, many tissues damaged by smoking can repair themselves. As soon as smokers stop, the body begins the repair process (see Figure 13.4). Within eight hours, carbon monoxide and oxygen levels return to normal, and "smoker's breath" disappears. Often, within a month of quitting, the mucous that clogs airways is broken up and eliminated. Circulation and the senses of taste and smell improve within weeks. Many ex-smokers say they have more energy, sleep better, and feel more alert. By the end of one year, the risk for lung cancer and stroke decreases. In addition, ex-smokers reduce considerably their risks of developing cancers of the mouth, throat, esophagus, larynx, pancreas, bladder, and cervix. They also cut their risk of peripheral artery

disease, chronic obstructive lung disease, coronary heart disease, and ulcers. Women are less likely to bear babies with low birthweight. Within two years, the risk for heart attack drops to near normal. At the end of 10 smoke-free years, the ex-smoker can expect to live out his or her normal life span.

> **What do you think?**
>
> *Do you know people who have tried to quit smoking?* ✳ *What was this experience like for them?* ✳ *Were they successful?* ✳ *If not, what factors contributed to relapse?*

Caffeine

Caffeine is the most popular and widely consumed drug in the United States. Almost half of all Americans drink coffee every day, and many others use caffeine in some other form, mainly for its well-known "wake-up" effect. Drinking coffee is legal, even socially encouraged. Many people believe caffeine is not a drug and not really addictive. Coffee, soft drinks, and other caffeine-containing products seem harmless; with no cream or sugar added, they are calorie-free and therefore a good way to fill up if you are dieting. If you share these attitudes, you should think again because research in the past decade has linked caffeine to certain health problems.

Caffeine is a drug derived from the chemical family called **xanthines**. Two related chemicals, *theophylline* and *theobromine,* are found in tea and chocolate, respectively. The xanthines are mild central nervous system stimulants that enhance mental alertness and reduce feelings of fatigue. Other stimulant effects include increases in heart muscle contractions, oxygen consumption, metabolism, and urinary output. These effects are felt within 15 to 45 minutes of ingesting a product that contains caffeine.

Side effects of the xanthines include wakefulness, insomnia, irregular heartbeat, dizziness, nausea, indigestion, and sometimes mild delirium. Some people also experience heartburn. As with some other drugs, the user's psychological outlook and expectations will influence the effects.

Different products contain different concentrations of caffeine. A five-ounce cup of coffee contains anywhere from 25 to 105 milligrams of caffeine. Caffeine concentrations vary with the brand of the beverage and the strength of the brew. Small chocolate bars contain up to 15 milligrams of caffeine and theobromine. Table 13.5 compares various caffeine-containing products.

Caffeine Addiction

As the effects of caffeine wear off, users may feel let down—mentally or physically depressed, exhausted, and weak. To counteract this, people commonly choose to drink another cup of coffee. Habitually engaging in this practice leads to tolerance and psychological dependency. Until the mid-

---

Caffeine A stimulant found in coffee, tea, chocolate, and some soft drinks.

Xanthines The chemical family of stimulants to which caffeine belongs.

Caffeinism Caffeine intoxication brought on by excessive use; symptoms include chronic insomnia, irritability, anxiety, muscle twitches, and headaches.

1970s, caffeine was not medically recognized as addictive. Chronic caffeine use and its attendant behaviors were called "coffee nerves." This syndrome is now recognized as *caffeine intoxication,* or **caffeinism.**

Symptoms of caffeinism include chronic insomnia, jitters, irritability, nervousness, anxiety, and involuntary muscle twitches. Withdrawing the caffeine may compound the effects and produce severe headaches. (Some physicians ask their patients to take a simple test for caffeine addiction: Don't consume anything containing caffeine, and if you get a severe headache within four hours, you are addicted.) Because caffeine meets the requirements for addiction—tolerance, psychological dependency, and withdrawal symptoms—it can be classified as addictive.

Although you would have to drink between 67 and 100 cups of coffee in a day to produce a fatal overdose of caffeine, you may experience sensory disturbances after consuming only 10 cups of coffee within a 24-hour period. These symptoms include tinnitus (ringing in the ears), spots before the eyes, numbness in arms and legs, poor circulation, and visual hallucinations. Because 10 cups of coffee is not an extraordinary amount to drink in one day, caffeine use clearly poses health threats.

The Health Consequences of Long-Term Caffeine Use

Long-term caffeine use has been suspected of being linked to a number of serious health problems, ranging from heart disease and cancer to mental dysfunction and birth defects. However, no strong evidence exists to suggest that moderate caffeine use (less than 500 milligrams daily, approximately five cups of coffee) produces harmful effects in healthy, non-pregnant people.

It appears that caffeine does not cause long-term high blood pressure and it has not been linked to strokes. Nor is there any evidence of a relationship between coffee and heart disease.[27] However, people who suffer from irregular heartbeat are cautioned against using caffeine because the resultant increase in heart rate might be life-threatening. Both decaffeinated and caffeinated coffee products contain ingredients that can irritate the stomach lining and be harmful to people with stomach ulcers.

For years, caffeine consumption was linked with fibrocystic breast disease, a condition characterized by painful, noncancerous lumps in the breast. Reports claim that caffeine promotes cyst formation in female breasts. Although these conclusions have been challenged, many clinicians advise patients with mammillary cysts to avoid caffeine. In addition, some reports indicate that very high doses of caffeine given to pregnant laboratory animals can cause stillbirths or offspring with low birthweights or limb deformations. Studies

have found that moderate consumption of caffeine (less than 300 milligrams per day) did not significantly affect human fetal development.[28] Mothers are usually advised to avoid or at least reduce caffeine use during pregnancy.

Table 13.5
Caffeine Content of Various Products

PRODUCT	CAFFEINE CONTENT (AVERAGE MG PER SERVING)
COFFEE (5-OZ. CUP)	
Regular Brewed	65–115
Decaffeinated Brewed	3
Decaffeinated instant	2
TEA (6-OZ. CUP)	
Hot steeped	36
Iced	31
Bottled (12 oz.)	15
SOFT DRINKS (12-OZ. SERVINGS)	
Jolt Cola	100
Dr. Pepper	61
Mountain Dew	54
Coca-Cola	46
Pepsi-Cola	36–38
CHOCOLATE	
1 oz. baking chocolate	25
1 oz. chocolate candy bar	15
½ cup chocolate pudding	4–12
OVER-THE-COUNTER DRUGS	
No Doz (2 tablets)	200
Excedrin (2 tablets)	130
Midol (2 tablets)	65
Anacin (2 tablets)	64

What do you think?

*How much caffeine do you consume? * What is your pattern of caffeine consumption for the day? * Why do you consume it? * Have you ever experienced any ill effects after avoiding caffeine consumption for a period of time?*

Managing the Use of Tobacco and Caffeine

A common mistake people make when they try to stop any bad habit, particularly smoking, is picking a stressful time to quit. This is likely to result in failure. It is best to start any cessation plan when you are relatively free of stress (note the word *relatively!*). The following guidelines will help you or someone you know who is trying to quit smoking or cut back on caffeine.

Checklist for Change

Making Personal Choices
To quit smoking, do the following:

☐ Identify your smoking habits. Keep a daily journal and record when and where you smoked and whom you were with at the time. Write down how you felt, and note how important that cigarette was to you at the time on a scale of one to five. Maintain your diary for one or two weeks.

☐ Get support. It can be extremely difficult to go it alone when you are trying to quit smoking. Phone your local chapter of the American Cancer Society or community hospital to find out about programs and support groups.

☐ Begin by tapering off. For a period of one to two weeks, either aim at cutting down or change to a lower-nicotine brand (in the latter case, be careful not to increase the number of cigarettes you smoke). Stop carrying matches.

Don't buy a new pack until you finish the one you're smoking, and never buy a carton. Cut back on those cigarettes you smoke automatically (e.g., when you get into your car or every time you have a cup of coffee).

☐ Set a quit date. At some point, announce to family and friends when you are going to stop.

☐ Stop. A week before you quit, cut your cigarette consumption down to a few cigarettes per day. Smoke these in the late day or evening. By this time, you may be able to notice some of the negative effects of smoking. On the day you quit, treat yourself to something nice.

☐ Continue to seek support from your support group. Increase your physical activity. Avoid situations you associate most closely with smoking.

☐ If you fail to stop despite your best efforts, don't beat yourself up. Try again soon.

To reduce caffeine consumption, follow these steps:

☐ Cut back gradually. Going cold turkey can result in severe headaches and other unpleasant symptoms, such as irritability and insomnia.

☐ Mix caffeinated products with decaffeinated products, gradually increasing the proportion of the latter until the former is eliminated.

☐ Caffeine is metabolized faster in smokers than in nonsmokers, so smokers need more caffeine to feel its effects. If you try to quit

smoking, the caffeine you ingest will have very potent effects. Therefore, you may want to cut down on caffeine before you give up the nicotine habit.

☐ Caffeinated products often play a central role in social customs ("Let's get together over a cup of coffee"). Finding satisfying alternatives will help you in this process.

Making Community Choices

☐ What policies exist regarding smoke-free environments on your campus and in your community? What issues still need to be resolved?

☐ How do you counter the messages of advertisements targeted at your age group to promote unhealthy products?

☐ Do you participate in community or nationwide activities, such as the Great American Smokeout, that encourage the adoption or maintenance of healthy behaviors?

☐ When you vote in local, state, or national elections, do you support legislation aimed to foster healthy lifestyles (such as laws that ban the sale of cigarettes to those under age)?

☐ Have you done anything on your campus, in your community, or at work to promote policies protecting nonsmokers?

Summary

* The use of tobacco involves many social issues, including advertising targeted at youth and women, the largest growing populations of smokers. Health care and lost productivity resulting from smoking cost the nation as much as $150 billion per year.

* Tobacco is available in smoking and smokeless forms, both containing addictive nicotine (a psychoactive substance). Smoking also delivers 4,000 other chemicals to the lungs of smokers.

* The health hazards of smoking include markedly higher rates of cancer, heart and circulatory disorders, respiratory diseases, and gum diseases. Smoking while pregnant presents risks for the fetus, including miscarriage and low birthweight.

* Smokeless tobacco contains more nicotine than do cigarettes and dramatically increases risks for oral cancer and other oral problems.

* Environmental tobacco smoke (sidestream smoke) puts nonsmokers at risk for elevated rates of cancer and heart disease, according to an EPA study.

* For over 30 years the government has been warning consumers of the dangers associated with tobacco use. In 1997, 46 states sued the tobacco industry for health care recovery costs to treat smokers' illnesses. In a landmark 1998 legal settlement, the tobacco industry agreed to reimburse states for health care costs related to smoking and finance various antismoking initiatives. Further legal battles are pending.

* Quitting is complicated by the dual nature of smoking: Smokers must kick a chemical addiction as well as a habit. Nicotine replacement products (gum and the patch) can help wean smokers off nicotine. Several therapy methods can help smokers break the habit.

* Caffeine is a widely used central nervous system stimulant. No long-term ill-health effects have been proved, although caffeine may produce withdrawal symptoms for chronic users who try to quit.

Questions for Discussion and Reflection

1. New research suggests that genetic factors might be more influential than environmental factors in smoking initiation and nicotine dependency. How might this information change current prevention efforts? How would you design smoking prevention strategies targeted at adolescents?

2. Discuss the varied ways in which tobacco is used. Is any method less addictive or hazardous to health than another?

3. List short-term and long-term health hazards associated with smoking. How will increased tobacco use among adolescents and college students impact the medical system in the future? Who should be responsible for the medical expenses of smokers? Insurance companies? Smokers?

4. Do you believe that the tobacco companies will develop a "safe" cigarette? What would it take for you to consider a cigarette "safe"? Consider the claims for safety previously made by tobacco companies as you give your answer.

5. Discuss the various risks of smokeless tobacco use.

6. Restrictions on smoking are increasing in our society. Do you think these restrictions are fair? Do they infringe on people's rights? Are the restrictions too strict or not strict enough?

7. Describe the pros and cons of each method of quitting smoking. Which would be most effective for you? Explain why?

8. Discuss problems related to the ingestion of caffeine. How much caffeine do you consume? Why?

Application Exercises

Reread the What Do You Think? scenarios at the beginning of this chapter and answer the following questions.

1. What immediate health problems might Sarah and Evan experience from smoking? Is Evan at greater risk than Sarah for particular health problems?

2. Why is it likely that both Evan and Sarah are more addicted to smoking than they believe themselves to be?

3. Is Jonathan being honest with himself by claiming not to be a cigarette smoker? Explain your answer.

4. What are the chances that Jonathan and A. J. will become addicted to bidis? Explain your answer.

5. Are bidis safer than cigarettes? Why or why not?

Accessing Your Health on the Internet

Visit the following Internet sites to explore further topics and issues related to tobacco and health. To visit an organization's website, go to the Companion Website for *Access to Health, Eighth Edition* at www.aw.com/donatelle, click on the book image, and select "Accessing Your Health on the Internet" from the navigation menu on the left.

1. *American Lung Association.* This site offers a wealth of information regarding smoking trends, environmental smoke, and advice on smoking cessation.
2. *ASH (Action on Smoking and Health).* The nation's oldest and largest antismoking organization, ASH regularly takes hard-hitting legal actions and does other work to fight smoking and protect the rights of nonsmokers. ASH provides nonsmokers with legal forms and valuable information about protecting their rights and about the problems and costs of smoking to nonsmokers. ASH's actions have helped prohibit cigarette commercials; ban smoking on planes, buses, and in many public places; and lower insurance premiums for nonsmokers.
3. *TIPS (Tobacco Information and Prevention Source).* This website provides access to a variety of information regarding tobacco use in the United States, with specific information for and about young people.

Further Reading

Glantz, S. A., and E. D. Balbach. *The Tobacco War: Inside the California Battles.* Berkeley: University of California Press, 2000.

Charts the dramatic and complex history of tobacco politics in California over the past quarter century. Shows how the accomplishments of tobacco-control advocates have changed how people view the tobacco industry and its behavior.

Kluger, R. *Ashes to Ashes: America's Hundred-Year Cigarette War, the Public Health, and the Unabashed Triumph of Philip Morris.* New York: Vintage Books, 1997.

A definitive history of America's controversial tobacco industry, focusing on Philip Morris. Traces the development of the cigarette, revelations of its toxicity, and the impact of political and corporate shenanigans on the battle over smoking.

Whelan, E. *Cigarettes: What the Warning Label Doesn't Tell You—The First Comprehensive Guide to the Health Consequences of Smoking.* New York: Prometheus Books, 1997.

From impotence to diabetes, cataracts to psoriasis, the proven dangers of smoking go well beyond heart and lung disease. This book details all the known health threats of smoking. Twenty-one experts explain how smoking can affect the body.

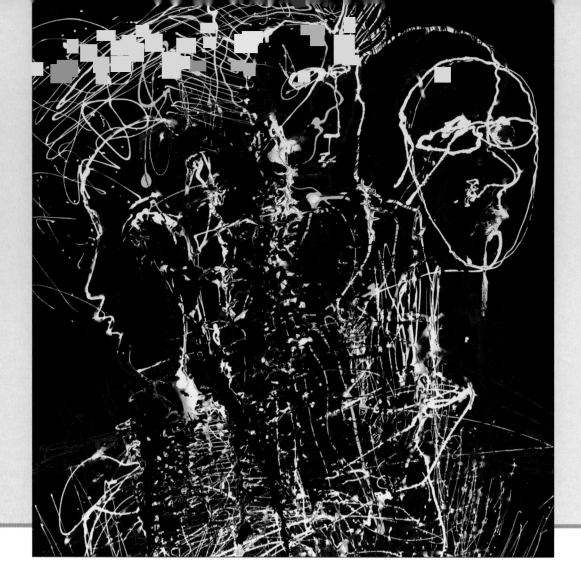

Objectives

* List the six categories of drugs, and explain their routes of administration.

* Discuss patterns of illicit drug use, including who uses illicit drugs and why they use them.

* Describe the use and abuse of controlled substances, including cocaine, amphetamines, marijuana, opiates, hallucinogens, designer drugs, inhalants, and steroids.

* Profile overall illegal drug use in the United States, including frequency, financial impact, arrests for drug offenses, and impact on the workplace.

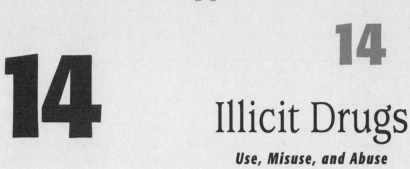

Illicit Drugs

Use, Misuse, and Abuse

14 14 14 14 14 14 14 14 14

What do you think?

Greg and some of his friends were smoking marijuana in Greg's residence hall room. They used fans to blow the smoke out the window, air freshener candles to mask the smell, and a towel at the bottom of the door to prevent the smoke from escaping. However, the residence hall assistant smelled the scent and immediately called security. Greg and his friends were arrested and eventually kicked out of the residence hall. Greg felt this measure was extremely unfair because students caught drinking alcohol in their rooms were rarely written up.

Do you think Greg has a valid point? ✳ How common is marijuana use on your campus? ✳ Do you know the penalty for smoking marijuana on campus? ✳ What are the substance abuse policies on your campus? ✳ Do you think your school's substance abuse policies are enough to deter students from using controlled substances?

Sean and his friends regularly popped an Ecstasy pill before heading to the clubs downtown. Tonight was no exception. An hour after arriving at the club, however, Sean was complaining that he must have gotten an impostor pill because he wasn't feeling any effects. He'd just bombed a big test that day and wanted to forget about it, so he swallowed another pill with a shot of whiskey.

Are you aware of the prevalence of Ecstasy on your campus? ✳ Are you familiar with the substances often contained in impostor pills? ✳ What are some possible risks associated with Sean's decision to take another pill, along with alcohol?

lllicit drug abuse is a problem of staggering proportions in our society. It is important to understand how these drugs work and why people use them. Human beings appear to have a need to alter their consciousness, or mental state. We like to feel good. Sometimes we like to change our awareness of things and feel different. Consciousness can be altered in many ways. Children spinning until they become dizzy and adults enjoying thrilling high-speed activities are examples. Many of us listen to music, skydive, ski, skate, read, daydream, meditate, pray, or have sexual relations to change our awareness. For others, illicit drugs offer ways to alter consciousness.

Drug Dynamics

Drugs work because they physically resemble the chemicals produced naturally within the body (see Figure 14.1). For example, many painkillers resemble the endorphins ("mor-phine within") that are manufactured in the body. Most bodily processes result from chemical reactions or from changes in electrical charge. Because drugs possess an electrical charge and a chemical structure similar to those of chemicals that occur naturally in the body, they can affect physical functions in many different ways.

A current explanation of drug actions is the *receptor site theory,* which states that drugs bind to specific **receptor sites** in the body. These sites are specialized cells to which, because of their size, shape, electrical charge, and chemical properties, drugs can attach themselves. Most drugs attach to multiple receptor sites located throughout the body in places such as the heart and blood system and the lungs, liver, kidneys, brain, and gonads (testicles or ovaries).

Types of Drugs

Scientists divide drugs into six categories: prescription, over-the-counter (OTC), recreational, herbal, illicit, and commercial drugs. These classifications are based primarily upon drug action, although some are based on the source of the

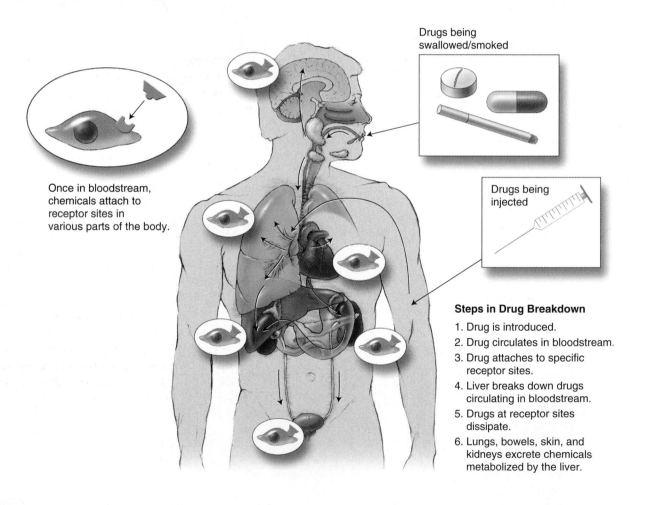

Once in bloodstream, chemicals attach to receptor sites in various parts of the body.

Drugs being swallowed/smoked

Drugs being injected

Steps in Drug Breakdown

1. Drug is introduced.
2. Drug circulates in bloodstream.
3. Drug attaches to specific receptor sites.
4. Liver breaks down drugs circulating in bloodstream.
5. Drugs at receptor sites dissipate.
6. Lungs, bowels, skin, and kidneys excrete chemicals metabolized by the liver.

Figure 14.1
How the Body Metabolizes Drugs

chemical in question. Each category includes some drugs that stimulate the body, some that depress body functions, and others that produce hallucinations. Each category also includes **psychoactive drugs,** which have the potential to alter a person's mood or behavior.

- **Prescription drugs** are those substances that can be obtained only with the written prescription of a licensed physician. More than 10,000 types of prescription drugs are sold in the United States.
- **Over-the-counter (OTC) drugs** can be purchased without a prescription. Each year, Americans spend over $14 billion on OTC products, and the market is increasing at the rate of 20 percent annually. More than 300,000 OTC products are available through stores, pharmacies, and the Internet. An estimated three out of four people routinely self-medicate with these products.
- **Recreational drugs** belong to a somewhat vague category whose boundaries depend upon how people define *recreation*. Generally, these substances contain chemicals used to help people relax or socialize. Most of them are legally sanctioned even though they are psychoactive. Alcohol, tobacco, coffee, tea, and chocolate products are usually included in this category.
- **Herbal preparations** form another vague category. Included among these approximately 750 substances are herbal teas and other products of botanical origin that are believed to have medicinal properties.
- **Illicit (illegal) drugs** are the most notorious type of drug. Although laws governing their use, possession, cultivation, manufacture, and sale differ from state to state, illicit drugs are generally recognized as harmful. All of them are psychoactive.
- **Commercial preparations** are the most universally used yet least commonly recognized chemical substances having drug action. More than 1,000 of these substances exist, including seemingly benign items such as perfumes, cosmetics, household cleansers, paints, glues, inks, dyes, gardening chemicals, pesticides, and industrial by-products.

Routes of Administration of Drugs

Route of administration refers to the way in which a given drug is taken into the body. Common routes are oral ingestion, injection, inhalation, inunction, and suppository.

Oral ingestion is the most common route of administration. Drugs that are swallowed include tablets, capsules, and liquids. Oral ingestion generally results in relatively slow absorption compared to other methods of administration because the drug must pass through the stomach, where digestive juices act upon it, and then move on to the small intestine before it enters the bloodstream.

Many oral preparations are coated to keep them from being dissolved by corrosive stomach acids before they reach the intestine as well as to protect the stomach lining from irritating chemicals in the drugs. A stomach that contains food slows the absorption of drugs. Some drugs must not be taken with certain foods because the food will inhibit their action. Others must be taken with food to prevent stomach irritation.

Depending on the drug and the amount of food in the stomach, drugs taken orally produce their effects within 20 minutes to 1 hour after ingestion. The only exception is alcohol, which takes effect sooner because some of it is absorbed directly into the bloodstream from the stomach.

Injection, another common form of drug administration, involves using a hypodermic syringe to introduce a drug into the body. **Intravenous injection,** or injection directly into a vein, puts the chemical in its most concentrated form directly into the bloodstream. Effects will be felt within three minutes, making this route extremely effective, particularly in medical emergencies. But injection of many substances into the bloodstream may cause serious or even fatal reactions. In addition, some serious diseases, such as hepatitis and AIDS, can be transferred in this way. For this reason, intravenous injection can be one of the most dangerous routes of administration.

Receptor sites Specialized cells to which drugs can attach themselves.

Psychoactive drugs Drugs that have the potential to alter mood or behavior.

Prescription drugs Medications that can be obtained only with the written prescription of a licensed physician.

Over-the-counter (OTC) drugs Medications that can be purchased without a physician's prescription.

Recreational drugs Legal drugs that contain chemicals that help people relax or socialize.

Herbal preparations Substances of plant origin that are believed to have medicinal properties.

Illicit (illegal) drugs Drugs whose use, possession, cultivation, manufacture, and/or sale are against the law because they are generally recognized as harmful.

Commercial preparations Commonly used chemical substances including cosmetics, household cleaning products, and industrial by-products.

Route of administration The manner in which a drug is taken into the body.

Oral ingestion Intake of drugs through the mouth.

Injection The introduction of drugs into the body via a hypodermic needle.

Intravenous injection The introduction of drugs directly into a vein.

Intramuscular injection places the hypodermic needle into muscular tissue, usually in the buttocks or the back of the upper arm. Normally used to administer antibiotics and vaccinations, this route of administration results in much slower absorption than intravenous injection, but ensures slow and consistent dispersion of the drug into body tissues.

Subcutaneous injection puts the drug into the layer of fat directly beneath the skin. Its common medical uses include administration of local anesthetics and insulin replacement therapy. A drug injected subcutaneously will circulate even more slowly than an intramuscularly injected drug because it takes longer to be absorbed into the bloodstream.

Inhalation refers to administration of drugs through the nostrils or mouth. This method transfers the drug rapidly into the bloodstream through the alveoli (air sacs) in the lungs. Examples of illicit inhalation include cocaine sniffing, inhaling aerosol sprays, gases, or fumes from solvents, or smoking marijuana. Effects are frequently immediate but do not last as long as effects associated with slower routes of administration because only small amounts of a drug can be absorbed and metabolized in the lungs.

Inunction introduces chemicals into the body through the skin. A common example is the small adhesive patches that are used to alleviate motion sickness. These patches, which contain a prescription medicine, are applied to the skin behind one ear, where they slowly release their chemicals to provide relief for nauseated travelers. Another example is the nicotine patch.

Suppositories are drugs that are mixed with a waxy medium designed to melt at body temperature. The most common type is inserted into the anus past the rectal sphincter muscles, which hold it in place. As the wax melts, the drug is released and absorbed through the rectal walls into the bloodstream. Since this area of the anatomy contains many blood vessels, the effects are usually felt within 15 minutes. Other types of suppositories are for use in the vagina. Vaginal suppositories usually release drugs, such as antifungal agents, that treat problems in the vagina itself rather than drugs meant to travel in the bloodstream.

Using, Misusing, and Abusing Drugs

Although drug abuse is usually referred to in connection with illicit psychoactive drugs, many people abuse and misuse prescription and OTC medications. **Drug misuse** involves the use of a drug for a purpose for which it was not intended. For example, taking a friend's high-powered prescription painkiller for your headache is a misuse of that drug. This is not too far removed from **drug abuse,** or the excessive use of any drug. The misuse and abuse of drugs may lead to *addiction,* the habitual reliance on a substance or behavior to produce a desired mood.

Both risks and benefits are involved in the use of any type of chemical substance. Intelligent decision making requires a clear-headed evaluation of these risks and benefits. If, after considering all the facts, you feel that the benefits outweigh the potential problems associated with a particular drug, you may decide to use it. But sometimes unforeseeable reactions or problems arise even after the most careful deliberation.

Illicit Drugs

Whereas some people become addicted to prescription drugs and painkillers, others use **illicit drugs**—those drugs that are illegal to possess, produce, or sell. The problem of illicit drug use touches us all. We may use illicit substances ourselves, watch someone we love struggle with drug abuse, or become the victim of a drug-related crime. At the very least, we are forced to pay increasing taxes for law enforcement and drug rehabilitation. An estimated 9.4 percent of full-time employees in the U.S. workforce is under the influence of illicit substances or alcohol on any given day.[1] When our coworkers use drugs, the effectiveness of our own work is diminished. If the car we drive was assembled by drug-using workers at the plant, we are in danger. A drug-using bus driver, train engineer, or pilot jeopardizes our safety.

The good news is that the use of illicit drugs has declined significantly in recent years in most segments of society. Use of most drugs increased from the early 1970s to the late 1970s, peaked between 1979 and 1986, and declined until 1992, from which point it has not changed. In 2001, an estimated 15.9 million Americans were illicit drug users, about half the 1979 peak level of 25 million users. Among youth, however, illicit drug use, notably of marijuana, has been increasing in recent years.[2]

Intramuscular injection   The introduction of drugs into muscles.

Subcutaneous injection   The introduction of drugs into the layer of fat directly beneath the skin.

Inhalation   The introduction of drugs through the nostrils.

Inunction   The introduction of drugs through the skin.

Suppositories   Mixtures of drugs and a waxy medium designed to melt at body temperature that are inserted into the anus or vagina.

Drug misuse   The use of a drug for a purpose for which it was not intended.

Drug abuse   The excessive use of a drug.

Illicit drugs   Drugs that are illegal to possess, produce, or sell.

Addiction across Cultures

Like the United States, many countries are struggling with epidemic rates of drug addiction. In fact, demand for addiction treatment services is increasing in many nations. Here's a look at current drug addiction treatment data from around the world:

- In India, more people are seeking treatment for heroin addiction, based on estimates that up to 1 million people became addicted to the substance during the 1980s.
- Political upheaval and the resulting disintegration of the family appear to be strongly related to rising drug abuse. A study in Ireland found that as many as 10 percent of young people (ages 15–20) in Dublin were addicted to heroin.
- In the Americas as a whole, cocaine and cocaine derivatives account for almost 60 percent of the demand for drug treatment.
- In contrast, in European nations, opiates, primarily heroin, are the drug of choice for nearly three-quarters of individuals seeking treatment.
- Opiates are also the leading drug of choice for about two-thirds of addicted individuals in Asian nations.
- Amphetamine use is higher in Nordic nations such as Sweden and Finland, where it accounts for 20 percent and 40 percent of treatment needs, respectively.
- Treatment for cannabis (marijuana, hashish) issues is much higher in the Caribbean, including Jamaica, where it accounts for over 50 percent of treatment demand.

Sources: From "The Social Impact of Drug Abuse," 1995, United Nations Office for Drug Control and Crime Prevention, New York; and "Global Illicit Drug Trends," 1999, United Nations Office for Drug Control and Crime Prevention, New York.

Who Uses Illicit Drugs?

Illicit drug users come from all walks of life. While many of us have stereotypes in our minds of who uses illicit drugs, it is difficult to generalize. Illicit drug users span all age groups, ethnicities, occupations, and socioeconomic groups. What can be said is that in the United States as in many other countries illicit drug use has a devastating effect on those who use and their families. (See the Health in a Diverse World box.)

After more than a decade of declining use on American college campuses, illicit drugs have reappeared. In 2001, the number of college students nationwide who had tried any drug stood at almost 54 percent; over a third had smoked pot in the past year, and 20 percent had done so in the past month; daily use of marijuana was at its highest point since 1989.[3] Cocaine use is down sharply, but LSD use has more than doubled. These figures vary from school to school.

The reasons for using drugs vary. Age, gender, genetic background, physiology, personality, experiences, and expectations are all factors.

Patterns of drug use vary considerably by age. For example, a nationwide study of college campuses reported that approximately 35.6 percent of students had tried marijuana during the previous year[4] (see Table 14.1). In contrast, only 9 percent of all Americans used marijuana during that time. Approximately 4.7 percent of college students surveyed reported using cocaine in the past year, whereas only 2.2 percent of all Americans said they had used cocaine during the previous year.

Table 14.1

Prevalence of Use for Various Types of Drugs, 2001: Full-Time College Students versus Respondents 1–4 Years beyond High School

	Total	
	FULL-TIME COLLEGE (%)	**OTHERS (%)**
Any illicit drug	37.9	41.3
Any illicit drug other than marijuana	16.4	22.8
Marijuana	35.6	37.6
Inhalants	2.8	3.1
Halllucinogens	7.5	10.3
LSD	4.0	8.0
Cocaine	4.7	9.6
Crack	0.9	2.5
MDMA (Ecstasy)	9.2	13.6
Heroin	0.4	1.3
Other narcotics	4.5	8.5
Amphetamines, adjusted	5.7	9.9
Ice	0.6	2.7
Barbiturates	3.8	6.7
Tranquilizers	5.1	8.6
Alcohol	83.0	80.9
Cigarettes	39.0	54.9
Approximate Weighted N =	*1,340*	*960*

Source: The Monitoring the Future Study, the University of Michigan, 2002.

Table 14.2
Selected Drugs and Risk of Dependence

DRUG	RISK OF DEPENDENCE
Cocaine	Psychological: high Physical (especially crack): moderate
Amphetamines	Psychological: high Physical: high
Marijuana	Psychological: moderate Physical: varies
Opiates	Psychological: high Physical: high
Hallucinogens	Psychological: low Physical: varies
Inhalants	Psychological: high Physical: moderate

Source: American College Health Association, "Alcohol and Other Drugs: Risky Business," 1999.

Most anti-drug programs have not been effective because they have focused on only one aspect of drug abuse, rather than examining all factors that contribute to the problem. The pressures to take drugs are often tremendous, and the reasons for using them are complex.

People who develop drug problems generally begin with the belief that they can control their drug use. Initially, they often view taking drugs as a fun and controllable pastime. Peer influence is a strong motivator, especially among adolescents, who greatly fear not being accepted as part of the group. Other people use drugs to cope with feelings of worthlessness and despair or to battle depression and anxiety. Since most illegal drugs produce physical and psychological dependency, it is unrealistic to think that a person can use them regularly without becoming addicted. See Table 14.2 for a summary of the risk of dependence of selected illicit drugs. Consider whether you are controlled by drugs or a drug user by answering the questions in the Assess Yourself box.

What do you think?

*What factors do you believe influence trends of illicit drug use in the United States? * What is the attitude toward drug use on your college campus? * Are some drugs considered more acceptable than others? * Is drug use considered more acceptable at certain times or occasions? * Explain your answer.*

Cocaine A powerful stimulant drug made from the leaves of the South American coca shrub.

Controlled Substances

To counteract the increased use of illegal drugs and the overuse of certain prescription drugs, Congress passed the Controlled Substances Act of 1970 (Public Law 91-513). This law created categories for both prescription and illegal substances that the federal government felt required strict regulation. The Drug Enforcement Agency (DEA) was founded within the Department of Justice to administer the law.

The law classified drugs into five "schedules," or categories, based on their potential for abuse, their medical uses, and accepted standards of safe use (see Table 14.3 on page 396). Schedule I drugs, those with the highest potential for abuse, are considered to have no valid medical uses. Although Schedule II, III, IV, and V drugs have known and accepted medical applications, many of them present serious threats to health when abused or misused. Penalties for illegal use are tied to the drugs' schedule level. Despite the 1970 law, however, manufacturing of and trafficking in illegal drugs in the United States have not diminished.

In 1986, the Drug Free America Act expanded penalties for the sale, manufacture, possession, and trafficking of illicit drugs. The goal of the new act was to eliminate drug abuse in schools and communities and to focus efforts on drug rehabilitation, medical treatment, and education.

Hundreds of illegal drugs exist. For general purposes, they can be divided into the following categories: stimulants such as cocaine; marijuana and its derivatives; depressants such as the opiates; psychedelics/hallucinogens; designer drugs; inhalants; and steroids.

Stimulants

Cocaine A white crystalline powder derived from the leaves of the South American coca shrub (not related to cocoa plants), **cocaine** ("coke") has been described as one of the most powerful naturally occurring stimulants.

Methods of Cocaine Use Cocaine can be taken in several ways. The powdered form of the drug is "snorted" through the nose. When cocaine is snorted, it can damage mucous membranes in the nose and cause sinusitis. It can destroy the user's sense of smell, and occasionally it even eats a hole through the septum.

Smoking (known as *freebasing*) and intravenous injections are even more dangerous means of taking cocaine. Freebasing has become more popular than injecting in recent years because people fear contracting diseases such as AIDS and hepatitis by sharing contaminated needles. But freebasing involves other dangers as well. Because the volatile mixes it requires are very explosive, some people have been killed or seriously burned. Smoking cocaine can also cause lung and liver damage.

Many cocaine users still occasionally "shoot up," which introduces large amounts into the body rapidly. Within

Recognizing a Drug Problem

Are You Controlled by Drugs?

How do you know whether you are chemically dependent? A dependent person can't stop using drugs. This abuse hurts the user and everyone around him or her. Take the following assessment. The more "yes" checks you make, the more likely you have a problem.

YES NO
☐ ☐ Do you use drugs to handle stress or escape from life's problems?
☐ ☐ Have you unsuccessfully tried to cut down on or quit using your drug?
☐ ☐ Have you ever been in trouble with the law or been arrested because of your drug use?
☐ ☐ Do you think a party or social gathering isn't fun unless drugs are available?
☐ ☐ Do you avoid people or places that do not support your usage?
☐ ☐ Do you neglect your responsibilities because you'd rather use your drug?
☐ ☐ Have your friends, family, or employer expressed concern about your drug use?
☐ ☐ Do you do things under the influence of drugs that you would not normally do?
☐ ☐ Have you seriously thought that you might have a chemical dependency problem?

Are You Controlled by a Drug User?

Is your life controlled by a chemical abuser? Your love and care (codependence) may actually be enabling the person to continue the abuse, hurting you and others. Try this assessment; the more "yes" checks you make, the more likely there's a problem.

YES NO
☐ ☐ Do you often have to lie or cover up for the chemical abuser?
☐ ☐ Do you spend time counseling the person about the problem?
☐ ☐ Have you taken on additional financial or family responsibilities?
☐ ☐ Do you feel that you have to control the chemical abuser's behavior?
☐ ☐ At the office, have you done work or attended meetings for the abuser?
☐ ☐ Do you often put your own needs and desires after the user's?
☐ ☐ Do you spend time each day worrying about your situation?
☐ ☐ Do you analyze your behavior to find clues to how it might affect the chemical abuser?
☐ ☐ Do you feel powerless and at your wit's end about the abuser's problem?

Source: Reprinted by permission of Krames Communications, 1100 Grundy Lane, San Bruno, CA 94066-3030. (www.krames.com).

seconds, a sense of euphoria sets in. This intense high lasts for 15 to 20 minutes, and then the user heads into a "crash." To prevent the unpleasant effects of the crash, users must shoot up frequently, which can severely damage veins. Injecting users place themselves at risk not only for AIDS and hepatitis but also for skin infections, inflamed arteries, and infection of the lining of the heart.

Physical Effects of Cocaine The effects of cocaine are felt rapidly. Snorted cocaine enters the bloodstream through the lungs in less than one minute and reaches the brain in less than three minutes. When cocaine binds at its receptor sites in the central nervous system, it produces intense pleasure. The euphoria quickly abates, however, and the desire to regain the pleasurable feelings makes the user want more cocaine (see Figure 14.2).

Cocaine is both an anesthetic and a central nervous system stimulant. In tiny doses, it can slow heart rate. In larger doses, the physical effects are dramatic: increased heart rate and blood pressure, loss of appetite that can lead to dramatic weight loss, convulsions, muscle twitching, irregular heartbeat, and even eventual death due to overdose. Other effects of cocaine include temporary relief of depression, decreased fatigue, talkativeness, increased alertness, and heightened self-confidence. Again, however, as the dose increases, users become irritable and apprehensive, and their behavior may turn paranoid or violent.

Cocaine-Affected Babies Because cocaine rapidly crosses the placenta (as virtually all drugs do), the fetus is vulnerable when a pregnant woman snorts, freebases, or shoots up. It is estimated that 2.4 to 3.5 percent of pregnant women

Table 14.3
How Drugs Are Scheduled

SCHEDULE	CHARACTERISTICS	EXAMPLES
Schedule I	High potential for abuse and addiction; no accepted medical use	Amphetimine (DMA, STP) Heroin Phencyclidine (PCP) LSD Marijuana Methaqualone
Schedule II	High potential for abuse and addiction; restricted medical use	Cocaine Codeine* Methadone Opium Secorbarbital (Seconal) Pentobarbital (Nembutal)
Schedule III	Some potential for abuse and addiction; currently accepted medical use	Butalbital combinations (Fiorinal) Nalorphine Noludar
Schedule IV	Low potential for abuse and addiction; currently accepted medical use	Chlorpromazine (Thorazine) Phenobarbital Minor tranquilizers
Schedule V	Lowest potential for abuse; accepted medical use	Robitussin A-C OTC preparations

*Can also be Schedule III or Schedule IV, depending on use.
Source: Information from *Drug Enforcement,* July 1979; National Institute on Drug Abuse, Statistical Series, Annual Data Report, 1989 (Rockville, MD: US. OHHS, 1989), 228–236.

between the ages of 12 and 34 abuse cocaine. It is difficult to gauge how many newborns have been exposed to cocaine because pregnant users are reluctant to discuss their drug habit with health care providers for fear of prosecution. The most threatening problem during pregnancy is the increased risk of a miscarriage. (See the Women's Health/Men's Health box.)

Fetuses exposed to cocaine or crack in the womb are more likely to suffer a small head, premature delivery, reduced birthweight, increased irritability, and subtle learning and cognitive deficits. Recent research suggests that a significant number of these children develop problems with learning and language skills that require remedial attention.[5] It is critical that these children are identified early and receive immediate intervention. For both financial and humane reasons, developing prenatal care and education programs for mothers at risk should be a priority for state and local government.[6]

Freebase Cocaine Freebase is a form of cocaine that is more powerful and costly than the powder or chip (crack) form. Street cocaine (cocaine hydrochloride) is converted to pure base by removing the hydrochloride salt and many of the "cutting agents." The end product, freebase, is smoked through a water pipe.

Because freebase cocaine reaches the brain within seconds, it is more dangerous than snorted cocaine. It produces a quick, intense high that disappears quickly, leaving an intense craving for more. Freebasers typically increase the amount and frequency of the dose. They often become severely addicted and experience serious health problems.

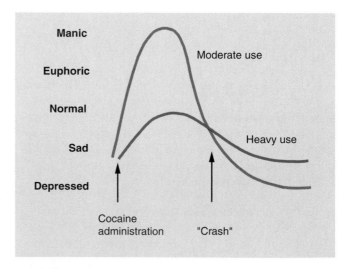

Figure 14.2
Ups and Downs of a Typical Dose of Cocaine
Source: C. Levinthal, *Drugs, Behavior, and Modern Society,* 2nd ed. (Boston: Allyn & Bacon, 1999). © Pearson Education.

Women and Drug Abuse

Approximately 3.8 million U.S. women of all ages, races, and cultures use drugs. It is estimated that 31 percent of U.S. women (over age 17) have used an illicit drug at least once in their lives. Today, approximately 28,000 (66 percent) of AIDS cases among U.S. women are related either to injecting drugs or to having sex with a man who injects drugs; consequently, AIDS is now the fourth leading cause of death among women of childbearing age.

Many women who use drugs have had troubled lives. Studies show that at least 70 percent of them have been sexually abused by the age of 16. Most of these women had at least one parent who abused alcohol or drugs. Furthermore, they often have low self-esteem, little self-confidence, and a sense of powerlessness. They frequently feel lonely and are isolated from support networks.

Unfortunately, many female drug users are unable to seek help. Whereas some may not be able to find or afford child care during a course of treatment, others worry that the courts may take away their children once the drug problem is known.

Others may fear violence from their husbands, boyfriends, or partners.

Research has shown that female drug abusers have a better chance of recovery when treatment takes care of their basic needs. Some women need the basic services of food, shelter, and clothing. Others also need transportation, child care, and training in parenting. The most successful treatments also teach reading, basic education, and the skills needed to find a job. As a woman's self-esteem increases, so do her chances of remaining drug-free.

Source: "Monitoring the Future: Women and Drug Abuse," by the National Institute on Drug Abuse, *NIDA Capsules,* 1997.

Side effects of freebasing cocaine include weight loss, increased heart rate and blood pressure, depression, paranoia, and hallucinations. Freebase is an extremely dangerous drug and is responsible for a large number of cocaine-related hospital emergency-room visits and deaths.

Crack Crack is the street name given to freebase cocaine processed from cocaine hydrochloride by using ammonia or sodium bicarbonate (baking soda), water, and heat to remove the hydrochloride. (Crack can also be processed with ether, but this is much riskier because ether is flammable.) The mixture (90 percent pure cocaine) is then dried. The soapy-looking substance that results can be broken into "rocks" and smoked. These rocks are approximately five times as strong as cocaine. Crack gets its name from the popping noises it makes when burned. Crack is also sometimes called "rock," an alias that should not be confused with rock cocaine.

Rock cocaine is a cocaine hydrochloride substance that is primarily sold in California. White in color, it is about the shape of a pencil eraser and is typically snorted.

Because crack is such a pure drug, it takes much less time to achieve the desired high. One puff of a pebble-size rock produces an intense high that lasts for approximately 20 minutes. The user can usually get three or four hits off a rock before it is used up. Crack is typically sold in small vials, folding papers, or heavy tinfoil containing two or three rocks, and costing between $10 and $20.

A crack user may quickly become addicted. Addiction is accelerated by the speed at which crack is absorbed through the lungs (it hits the brain within seconds after use) and by the intensity of the high. It is not uncommon for crack addicts to spend over $1,000 a day on the habit.

Cocaine Addiction and Society Cocaine addicts often suffer both physiological damage and serious disruption in lifestyle, including loss of employment and self-esteem. It is estimated that the annual cost of cocaine addiction in the United States exceeds $3.8 billion. However, there is no way to measure the cost in wasted lives. An estimated 5 million Americans from all socioeconomic groups are addicted, and 5,000 new users try cocaine or crack every day. Federal agencies estimate that 3 to 4 million people used the drug at least once in the past year. Experts suggest that 10 percent of recreational users will go on to heavy use.[7]

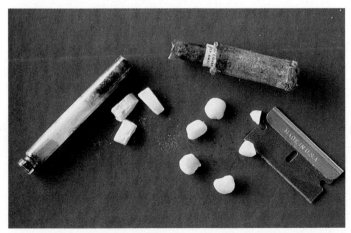

Although new "drugs of choice" make the news frequently, the availability of crack cocaine continues to be a problem.

Freebase The most powerful distillate of cocaine

Crack A distillate of powdered cocaine that comes in small, hard "chips" or "rocks."

Table 14.4
Effects of Amphetamines on the Body and Mind

	BODY	MIND
Low Dose	Increased heartbeat	Decreased fatigue
	Increased blood pressure	Increased confidence
	Decreased appetite	Increased feeling of alertness
	Increased breathing rate	Restlessness, talkativeness
	Inability to sleep	Increased irritability
	Sweating	Fearfulness, apprehension
	Dry mouth	Distrust of people
	Muscle twitching	Repetitive behaviors
	Convulsions	Hallucinations
	Fever	Psychosis
	Chest pain	
	Irregular heartbeat	
	Death due to overdose	
High Dose		

Source: G. Hanson and P. Venturelli, *Drugs and Society* (Sudbury, MA: Jones and Bartlett, 1998), 259.

The DEA has to date found no successful method to fight cocaine and crack use in the United States. Cocaine has been called unpredictable by drug experts, deadly by coroners, dangerous by former users, and disastrous by the media. Apparently, the risks associated with the use of the drug do not override users' desire to experience the euphoria it produces.

Because cocaine is illegal, a complex underground network has developed to manufacture and sell the drug. Buyers may not always get the product they think they are purchasing. Cocaine marketed for snorting may be only 60 percent pure. Usually, it is mixed, or "cut," with other white powdery substances such as mannitol or sugar, though occasionally it is cut with arsenic or other cocainelike powders that may themselves be highly dangerous.

What do you think?

Have all segments of society been affected by crack use? ✳ If not, which segments of the U.S. population experience the greatest impact from crack use? ✳ Why might this be the case? ✳ Is there a difference in the profile of a person who uses crack rather than cocaine? ✳ Explain your answer.

Amphetamines The **amphetamines** include a large and varied group of synthetic agents that stimulate the central nervous system. Small doses of amphetamines improve alertness, lessen fatigue, and generally elevate mood. With repeated use, however, physical and psychological dependency develops. Sleep patterns are affected (insomnia); heart

rate, breathing rate, and blood pressure increase; restlessness, anxiety, appetite suppression, and vision problems are common. High doses over long time periods can produce hallucinations, delusions, and disorganized behavior. Abusers become paranoid, fearing everything and everyone. Some become aggressive or antisocial (see Table 14.4).

Amphetamines for recreational use are sold under a variety of names: "Bennies" (amphetamine/Benzedrine), "dex" (dextroamphetamine/Dexedrine), and "meth" or "speed" (methamphetamine/Methedrine). Other street terms for amphetamines are "cross tops," "uppers," "wake-ups," "lid poppers," "cartwheels," and "blackies." Amphetamines do have therapeutic uses (see Chapter 22) in the treatment of attention deficit/hyperactivity disorder in children (Ritalin, Cylert) and of obesity (Pondimin).

Newer-Generation Stimulants Methamphetamine, a form of amphetamine, is a powerfully addictive drug that strongly activates certain areas of the brain and affects the central nervous system in general. Methamphetamine is closely related chemically to amphetamine, but its central nervous system effects are greater.

Methamphetamine is relatively easy to make. People nicknamed "cookers" produce methamphetamine batches using cookbook-style recipes that often include common over-the-counter ingredients such as ephedrine and pseudoephedrine. Laws have strengthened the penalties associated with manufacturing methamphetamine.

The effects of methamphetamine last six to eight hours, considerably longer than those produced by crack and cocaine. The immediate effects can include irritability and anxiety; increased body temperature, heart rate, and blood pressure; and possible death. The high state of irritability and agitation has been associated with violent behavior among some users.

Ice is a potent methamphetamine that is imported primarily from Asia, particularly from South Korea and Taiwan. It is purer and more crystalline than the version manufactured in many large U.S. cities. Because it is odorless, public use of ice often goes unnoticed.

Typically, ice quickly becomes addictive. Some users have reported severe cravings after using it only once. The effects of ice are long lasting. They include wakefulness, mood elevation, and excitability, all of which appeal to work-addicted young adults, particularly those who must put in long hours in high-stress jobs. Because the drug is inexpensive and produces such an intense high (lasting from 4 to 14 hours), it has become popular among young people looking for a quick high. However, as is true of other methamphetamines, the "down" side of this drug is devastating. Prolonged use can cause fatal lung and kidney damage as well as long-lasting psychological damage. In some instances, major psychological dysfunction has lasted as long as two and a half years after last use.

Marijuana

Although archaeological evidence documents the use of **marijuana** ("grass," "weed," "pot") as far back as 6,000 years, the drug did not become popular in the United States until the 1960s. Marijuana receives less media attention today than it did then, but it still is the illicit drug used most frequently by far. Nearly one of every three Americans over the age of 12 has tried marijuana at least once. Some 12 million Americans have used it; more than 1 million cannot control their use.

Physical Effects of Marijuana Marijuana is derived from either the *Cannabis sativa* or *Cannabis indica* (hemp) plants. Current American-grown marijuana is a turbocharged version of the hippie weed of the late 1960s. Developed using cross-breeding, genetic engineering, and American farming ingenuity, top-grade cannabis packs a punch very similar to that of hashish. **Tetrahydrocannabinol (THC)** is the psychoactive substance in marijuana and the key to determining how powerful a high it will produce. Whereas a marijuana cigarette three decades ago averaged 10 mg of THC, a current cigarette may contain around 150 mg of THC. Thus the modern-day marijuana user may be exposed to doses of THC many times greater than were users in the 1960s and 1970s.[8]

Hashish, a potent cannabis preparation derived mainly from the thick, sticky resin of the plant, contains high concentrations of THC. Hash oil, a substance produced by percolating a solvent such as ether through dried marijuana to extract the THC, is a tarlike liquid that may contain up to 300 mg of THC in a dose.

Most of the time, marijuana is rolled into cigarettes (joints) or smoked in a pipe or water pipe (bong). Effects are generally felt within 10 to 30 minutes and usually wear off within three hours.

The most noticeable effect of THC is the dilation of the eyes' blood vessels, which produces the characteristic blood-shot eyes. Smokers of the drug also exhibit coughing, dry mouth and throat ("cotton mouth"), increased thirst and appetite, lowered blood pressure, and mild muscular weakness, primarily exhibited in drooping eyelids. Users can also experience severe anxiety, panic, paranoia, and psychosis.

Users can experience intensified reactions to various stimuli. Colors and sounds, as well as the speed at which things move, may seem magnified. High doses of hashish may produce vivid visual hallucinations.

Effects of Chronic Marijuana Use Because marijuana is illegal in most parts of the United States and has been widely used only since the 1960s, long-term studies of its effects have been difficult to conduct. Also, studies conducted in the 1960s involved marijuana with THC levels constituting only a fraction of today's plant levels, so their results may not apply to the stronger forms available today. Most current information about chronic marijuana use comes from countries such as Jamaica and Costa Rica, where the drug is not illegal. These studies of long-term users (for 10 or more years) indicate that it causes lung damage comparable to that caused by tobacco smoking. Indeed, smoking a single joint may be as bad for the lungs as smoking three tobacco cigarettes. The chemicals themselves do not injure the heart, but the effects of inhaling burning material do.

Inhalation of marijuana transfers carbon monoxide to the bloodstream. Because the blood has a greater affinity for carbon monoxide than it does for oxygen, this diminishes the oxygen-carrying capacity of the blood. The heart must work harder to pump the vital element to oxygen-starved tissues. As well, the tar from cannabis contains higher levels of carcinogens than does tobacco smoke. Smoking marijuana results in three times as much tar inhalation and retention in the respiratory tract as does tobacco use.

Amphetamines A large and and varied group of synthetic agents that stimulate the central nervous system.

Methamphetamine A powerfully addictive drug that strongly activates certain areas of the brain and affects the central nervous system.

Ice A potent, inexpensive stimulant that has long-lasting effects.

Marijuana Chopped leaves and flowers of the *Cannabis indica* or *Cannabis sativa* plant (hemp); a psychoactive stimulant that intensifies reactions to environmental stimuli.

Tetrahydrocannabinol (THC) The chemical name for the active ingredient in marijuana.

Hashish The sticky resin of the cannabis plant, which is high in THC.

Medicinal Use of Marijuana: Legal Challenges Continue

For a number of years, marijuana's legal status for use for medicinal purposes has been hotly debated. So far, 30 states and the District of Columbia have laws on the books that recognize marijuana's medical value. Twelve states with "Therapeutic Research Program" laws are nevertheless unable to give patients legal access to medical marijuana because of the federal laws. Ten states and the District of Columbia have symbolic laws that recognize marijuana's medical value but fail to provide patients with protection from arrest for possession of an illegal drug. Voters in Alaska, California, Colorado, Hawaii, Maine, Oregon, Nevada, and Washington state have chosen to legalize marijuana for medicinal uses (see the accompanying figures). These new state laws, however, conflict with federal laws against the possession of marijuana and have led to new, as yet unresolved, battles in courts.

Source: R. Schmitz and C. Thomas, "State by State Medical Marijuana Laws: How to Remove the Threat of Arrest," 2002 (see http://mpp.org/statelaw/index.html). Copyright Marijuana Policy Project; used by permission.

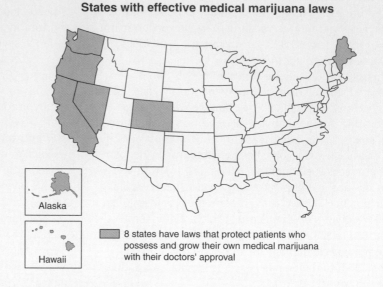

States with effective medical marijuana laws

8 states have laws that protect patients who possess and grow their own medical marijuana with their doctors' approval

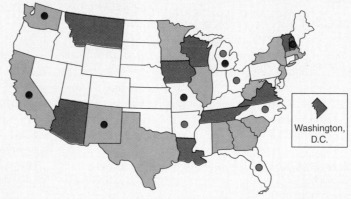

States with other medical marijuana laws

These states have laws to allow therapeutic research programs, provided that the federal government cooperates (California and Washington also have effective laws)

These states and the District of Columbia have symbolic medical marijuana laws

States that used to have favorable laws, which have expired or been repealed

States where legislatures have passed favorable non-binding resolutions

Other risks associated with marijuana include suppression of the immune system, blood pressure changes, and impaired memory function. Recent studies suggest that pregnant women who smoke marijuana are at a higher risk for stillbirth or miscarriage and for delivering low-birthweight babies and babies with abnormalities of the nervous system. Babies born to marijuana smokers are five times more likely to have features similar to those exhibited by children with fetal alcohol syndrome.

Debates concerning the effects of marijuana on the reproductive system have yet to be resolved. Studies conducted in the mid-1970s suggested that marijuana inhibited testosterone (and thus sperm) production in males and caused chromosomal breakage in both ova and sperm. Subsequent research in these areas is inconclusive. The question of whether the high-level THC plants currently available will increase the risks associated with this drug is, as yet, unanswered.

Marijuana and Medicine Although recognized as a dangerous drug by the U.S. government, marijuana has several medical purposes. It helps control the side effects (such as severe nausea and vomiting) produced by chemotherapy (chemical treatment for cancer). It improves appetite and

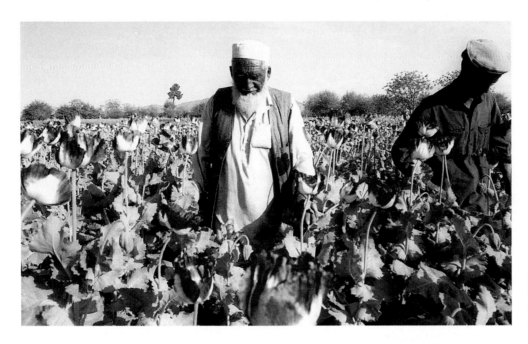

Despite its beautiful flower and innocent appearance, the poppy is the source of opium, a powerful narcotic.

forestalls the loss of lean muscle mass associated with AIDS-related wasting syndrome. Marijuana reduces the muscle pain and spasticity caused by diseases such as multiple sclerosis. It also temporarily relieves the eye pressure of glaucoma, although it is unclear whether it is more effective than legal glaucoma drugs.[9] Marijuana's legal status for medicinal purposes continues to be hotly debated (see the New Horizons in Health box).

Marijuana and Driving   Marijuana use presents clear hazards for drivers of motor vehicles as well as others on the road. The drug substantially reduces a driver's ability to react and to make quick decisions. Studies reveal that 60 to 80 percent of marijuana users sometimes drive while high.[10] Studies of automobile accident victims show that 6 to 12 percent of nonfatally injured drivers and 4 to 16 percent of fatally injured drivers had THC in their bloodstreams. Perceptual and other performance deficits resulting from marijuana use may persist for some time after the high subsides, though users often fail to recognize their impairment.

What do you think?

Why do you think that marijuana is the most popular illicit drug on college campuses? ✳ How widespread is marijuana use on your campus?

Opiates

Among the oldest analgesics (pain relievers) known to humans, opiates cause drowsiness, reduce pain, and induce euphoria. Also called **narcotics,** they are derived from the parent drug **opium,** a dark, resinous substance made from the milky juice of the opium poppy. Other opiates include *morphine, codeine, heroin,* and *black tar heroin.*

The word *narcotic* comes from the Greek word for "stupor" and is generally used to describe sleep-inducing substances. For many years, opiates were widely used by the medical community and until the early twentieth century, many patent medicines contained them. Suppliers advertised these concoctions as cures for everything from menstrual cramps to teething pains. More powerful than opium, **morphine** (named after Morpheus, the Greek god of sleep) was widely used as a painkiller during the Civil War. **Codeine,** a less powerful analgesic derived from morphine, also became popular. As opiates became more common, physicians noted that patients tended to become dependent on them. Contrary to earlier belief, all of the opiates are highly addictive. Growing concern about addiction led to government controls of narcotic use. The Harrison Act of 1914 prohibited the production, dispensation, and sale of opiate products unless prescribed by a physician. Subsequent legislation required physicians prescribing opiates to keep careful records. Physicians are still subject to audits of their prescriptions.

Narcotics   Drugs that induce sleep and relieve pain; primarily the opiates.

Opium   The parent drug of the opiates; made from the seedpod resin of the opium poppy.

Morphine   A derivative of opium; sometimes used by medical practitioners to relieve pain.

Codeine   A drug derived from morphine; used in cough syrups and certain painkillers.

OxyContin: A New and Dangerous Opioid Threat

OxyContin, a prescription central nervous system depressant in the opioid drug family, has catapulted to the top of the drug abuse scene in America. Since its 1995 approval as a painkiller by the FDA, it has become a major contributor to young adult drug abuse, causing the diversion of pills and theft of prescriptions in many regions of the country. According to a National Drug and Intelligence Center (NDIC) national drug threat survey in 2000 and DEA reporting, OxyContin had become the drug of choice in many eastern states and has now hit the midwestern and western states at an epidemic pace.

Why the popularity? OxyContin is the brand name for *oxycodone hydrochloride,* one of a larger group of pain relief products commonly prescribed for persons in chronic pain. Painkillers such Percocet, Percodan, Vicodan, and other high strength painkillers are in this category and most are highly addictive if taken for prolonged periods of time. Most of these painkillers only contain 2.5–5 mg. of oxycodone. In contrast, OxyContin was marketed in doses of 10, 20, 40, 80 and even 160 mg. tablets. The strength, duration, and known dosage of Oxycontin make it a very powerful painkiller, and also make it extremely

attractive to abusers. OxyContin abuse has become a substitute for heroin for some addicts who find pharmaceutical drugs to be purer and cheaper than street drugs.

Due to OxyContin's widespread availability, the crimes, addictions, and fatal overdoses associated with this drug have skyrocketed—many people have no idea of the risks they take when abusing Oxy. Although exact numbers of deaths are unavailable, it is likely that there are hundreds every year among unsuspecting young adults. Formulated as a 12-hour time release pill, OxyContin has a low addiction rate among those who take it as prescribed for the most acute pain of cancer or injury. However, abusers actually "disable" the time release structure of the pill by chewing it, crushing it, or dissolving the pill into liquid form and then eating, snorting, or injecting the solution. When taken orally or injected in this form, the user experiences a rush similar to heroin. The mind and body easily become obsessed with this pleasurable rush and a physical craving can develop causing addiction. Chronic use results in increasing tolerance so that more of the drug is needed to feel the same effects that smaller doses once provided. Often the user is unaware this is happening and goes from using 2 pills a day, to 2 pills an hour, to 2 pills every fifteen minutes as drug tolerance builds rapidly. Self-control in using the drug is lost as the brain becomes dependent.

Because many Oxy users do not know of the dangers of the drug, they may make the situation even more risky by using sleeping pills, over-the-counter pain medications, or drinking alcohol while taking Oxy. These drug interactions many times have caused serious side effects, even coma or death.

The good news is that complete recovery from Oxy addiction is possible, but addicted users can not do it on their own. Medical supervision and appropriate therapeutic techniques must be utilized to ensure recovery.

Source: Center for Drug Education and Research (CDER). Drug Information. OxyContin. 2002. http://www.fda.gov/cder/drug/infopage/oxycontin/oxycontin-qa.htm.

Some opiates are still used today for medical purposes. Doctors sometimes prescribe morphine for severe pain. Codeine is found in prescription cough syrups and other painkillers. Several prescription drugs, including Percodan, Demerol, and Dilaudid, contain synthetic opiates. All opiate use is strictly regulated.

Physical Effects of Opiates Opiates are powerful depressants of the central nervous system. In addition to relieving pain, these drugs lower heart rate, respiration, and blood pressure. Side effects include weakness, dizziness, nausea, vomiting, euphoria, decreased sex drive, visual disturbances, and lack of coordination. Of all the opiates, heroin has the greatest notoriety as an addictive drug. The following section

discusses the progression of heroin addiction; addiction to any opiate follows a similar path. (See the Reality Check box on OxyContin.)

Heroin Addiction Heroin is a white powder derived from morphine. **Black tar heroin** is a sticky, dark brown, foul-smelling form of heroin that is relatively pure and inexpensive. It is estimated that 600,000 Americans are addicted to heroin, with men outnumbering women addicts by three to one.[11] Authorities believe that the United States is at the beginning of a new heroin epidemic. There is concern that this epidemic will be worse than previous ones because the drug is now two to three times more available than ever before.

The contemporary version of heroin is so potent that users can get high by snorting or smoking the drug rather than by injecting it and putting themselves at risk for AIDS (see Chapter 17), although many addicts continue to inject the drug. Once an inner-city drug, heroin is now becoming more widely used by middle-class people who tend to try whatever drug is new and trendy. Many people have switched from cocaine to heroin because heroin is less stimulating and less expensive.

Once considered a cure for morphine dependency, heroin was later discovered to be even more addictive and potent than morphine. Today, heroin has no medical use.

Heroin is a depressant that produces drowsiness and a dreamy, mentally slow feeling. It can cause drastic mood swings, with euphoric highs followed by depressive lows. Heroin also slows respiration and urinary output and constricts the pupils of the eyes. In fact, pupil constriction is a classic sign of narcotic intoxication; hence, the stereotype of the drug user hiding behind a pair of dark sunglasses. Symptoms of tolerance and withdrawal can appear within three weeks of first use.

The most common route of administration for heroin addicts is "mainlining"—intravenous injection of powdered heroin mixed in a solution. Many users describe the "rush" they feel when injecting themselves as intensely pleasurable, whereas others report unpredictable and unpleasant side effects. The temporary nature of the rush contributes to the drug's high potential for addiction—many addicts shoot up four or five times a day. Mainlining can cause veins to scar and eventually collapse. Once a vein has collapsed, it can no longer be used to introduce heroin into the bloodstream. Addicts become expert at locating new veins to use: in the feet, the legs, even the temples. When they do not want their needle tracks (scars) to show, they inject themselves under the tongue or in the groin.

The physiology of the human body could be said to encourage opiate addiction. Opiate-like substances called **endorphins** are manufactured in the body and have multiple receptor sites, particularly in the central nervous system. When endorphins attach themselves at these points, they create feelings of painless well-being. Medical researchers have referred to endorphins as "the body's own opiates." When endorphin levels are high, people feel euphoric. The same euphoria occurs when opiates or related chemicals are active at the endorphin receptor sites.

Treatment for Heroin Addiction   Programs to help heroin addicts kick the habit have not been very successful. The rate of *recidivism* (tendency to return to previous behaviors) is high. Some addicts resume drug use even after years of drug-free living because the craving for the injection rush is very strong. It takes a great deal of discipline to seek alternative, nondrug highs.

Heroin addicts experience a distinct pattern of withdrawal. They begin to crave another dose four to six hours after their last dose. Symptoms of withdrawal include intense desire for the drug, yawning, a runny nose, sweating, and crying. About 12 hours after the last dose, addicts experience sleep disturbance, dilated pupils, loss of appetite, irritability, goose bumps, and muscle tremors. The most difficult time in the withdrawal process occurs 24 to 72 hours following last use. All of the preceding symptoms continue, along with nausea, abdominal cramps, restlessness, insomnia, vomiting, diarrhea, extreme anxiety, hot and cold flashes, elevated blood pressure, and rapid heartbeat and respiration. Once the peak of withdrawal has passed, all these symptoms begin to subside. Still, the recovering addict has many hurdles to jump.

Methadone maintenance is one treatment available for people addicted to heroin or other opiates. Methadone is a synthetic narcotic that blocks the effects of opiate withdrawal. It is chemically similar enough to the opiates to control the tremors, chills, vomiting, diarrhea, and severe abdominal pains of withdrawal. Methadone dosage is decreased over a period of time until the addict is weaned off the drug.

Methadone maintenance is controversial because of the drug's own potential for addiction. Critics contend that the program merely substitutes one addiction for another. Proponents argue that people on methadone maintenance are less likely to engage in criminal activities to support their habits than heroin addicts are. For this reason, many methadone maintenance programs are financed by the state or federal government and are available to clients free of charge or at reduced costs.

A number of new drug therapies for opiate dependence are emerging. Naltrexone (Trexan), an opiate antagonist, has been approved as a treatment. While on Naltrexone, recovering addicts do not have the compulsion to use heroin, and if they do use, they don't get high, so there is no point in using the drug. More recently, researchers have reported promising results with Temgesic (buprenorphine) a mild, nonaddicting synthetic opiate, which, like heroin and methadone, bonds to certain receptors in the brain, blocks pain messages, and persuades the brain that its cravings for heroin have been satisfied. Junkies report that while they are taking buprenorphine, they do not crave heroin anymore.

Heroin   An illegally manufactured derivative of morphine, usually injected into the bloodstream.

Black tar heroin   A dark brown, sticky form of heroin.

Endorphins   Opiate-like hormones that are manufactured in the human body and contribute to natural feelings of well-being.

Methadone maintenance   A treatment for people addicted to opiates that substitutes methadone, a synthetic narcotic, for the opiate of addiction.

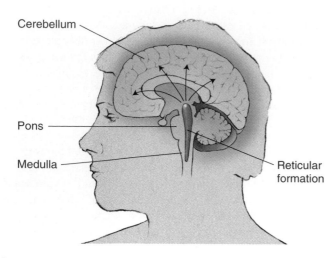

Cerebellum

Pons

Medulla

Reticular
formation

Figure 14.3
Reticular Formation

Hallucinogens (Psychedelics)

Hallucinogens are substances that are capable of creating auditory or visual hallucinations, or images that are perceived but are not real. These types of drugs are also known as **psychedelics,** which was adapted from the Greek phrase meaning "mind manifesting." Hallucinogens are a group of drugs whose primary pharmacological effect is to alter feelings, perceptions, and thoughts in a user. The major receptor sites for most of these drugs are in the part of the brain that is responsible for interpreting outside stimuli before allowing these signals to travel to other parts of the brain. This area, the **reticular formation,** is located in the brain stem at the upper end of the spinal cord (see Figure 14.3). When a hallucinogen is present at a reticular formation site, messages become scrambled, and the user may see wavy walls instead of straight ones or may smell colors and hear tastes. This mixing of sensory messages is known as **synesthesia.**

In addition to synesthetic effects, users may recall events long buried in the subconscious mind or become less inhibited than they are in a non-drug-use state. The most widely recognized hallucinogenics are LSD, mescaline, psilocybin, psilocin, and PCP. All are illegal and carry severe penalties for manufacture, possession, transportation, or sale.

LSD Of all the psychedelics, **lysergic acid diethylamide (LSD)** is the most notorious. First synthesized in the late 1930s by Swiss chemist Albert Hoffman, LSD resulted from experiments to derive medically useful drugs from the ergot fungus found on rye and other cereal grains. Because LSD seemed capable of unlocking the secrets of the mind, psychiatrists initially felt it could be beneficial to patients unable to remember suppressed traumas. From 1950 through 1968, the drug was used for such purposes.

Media attention focused on LSD in the late 1960s. Young people were using the drug to "turn on" and "tune out" the world that gave them the war in Vietnam, race riots, and political assassinations. In 1970, federal authorities, under intense pressure from the public, placed LSD on the list of controlled substances (Schedule I). LSD's popularity peaked in 1972, then tapered off, primarily because of users' inability to control dosages accurately.

Because of the recent wave of nostalgia for the 1960s, this dangerous psychedelic drug has been making a comeback. Known on the street as "acid," LSD is now available in virtually every state. Over 11 million Americans, most of them under age 35, have tried LSD at least once. LSD especially attracts younger users. Approximately 10 percent of high school seniors report having tried it at least once. A national survey of college students showed that 4 percent had used the drug.[12]

An odorless, tasteless, white crystalline powder, LSD is most frequently dissolved in water to make a solution that can then be used to manufacture the street forms of the drug: tablets, blotter acid, and windowpane. What the LSD consumer usually buys is blotter acid—small squares of blotterlike paper that have been impregnated with the liquid. The blotter is swallowed or chewed briefly. LSD also comes in tiny, thin squares of gelatin called windowpane and in tablets called microdots, which are less than an eighth of an inch across (it would take 10 or more to add up to the size of an aspirin tablet). Microdots and windowpane are just a sideshow; blotter is the medium of choice. It comes decorated with a mind-boggling array of designs, some of them copied from characters created by Disney and other cartoon studios. As with any illegal drug, purchasers run the risk of buying an impure product.

LSD is one of the most powerful drugs known to science and can produce strong effects in doses as low as 20 micrograms. (To give you an idea of how small a dose this is, the average postage stamp weighs approximately 60,000 micrograms.) The potency of the typical dose of LSD currently ranges from 20 to 80 micrograms, compared to 150 to 300 micrograms commonly used in the 1960s.

Despite its reputation for being primarily a psychedelic, LSD produces a number of physical effects, including slightly increased heart rate, elevated blood pressure and temperature, goose flesh (roughened skin), increased reflex speeds, muscle tremors and twitches, perspiration, increased salivation, chills, headaches, and mild nausea. Since the drug also stimulates uterine muscle contractions, it can lead to premature labor and miscarriage in pregnant women. Research into long-term effects has been inconclusive.

The psychological effects of LSD vary. The mindset of the user and setting in which the drug is used are very influential factors. Euphoria is the common psychological state produced by the drug, but *dysphoria* (a sense of evil and foreboding) may also be experienced. The drug also shortens attention span, causing the mind to wander. Thoughts may be interposed and juxtaposed, so the user experiences several different thoughts simultaneously. Synesthesia occurs occasionally. Users become introspective, and suppressed memories may surface, often taking on bizarre symbolism. Many more effects are possible, including decreased aggressiveness and enhanced sensory experiences.

Although LSD rarely produces hallucinations, it can create illusions. These distortions of ordinary perceptions may include movement of stationary objects. "Bad trips," the most publicized risk of LSD, are commonly related to set or setting. The user, for example, may interpret increased heart rate as a heart attack (a "bad body trip"). Often bad trips result when a user confronts a suppressed emotional experience or memory (a "bad head trip").

While there is no evidence that LSD creates physical dependency, it may well create psychological dependency. Many LSD users become depressed for one or two days following a trip and turn to the drug to relieve this depression. The result is a cycle of LSD use to relieve post-LSD depression, which often leads to psychological addiction.

> ### What do you think?
> *Are people today using LSD for the same reasons it was used in the 1960s?* ✳ *What are the perceived attractions and the real dangers of LSD use?*

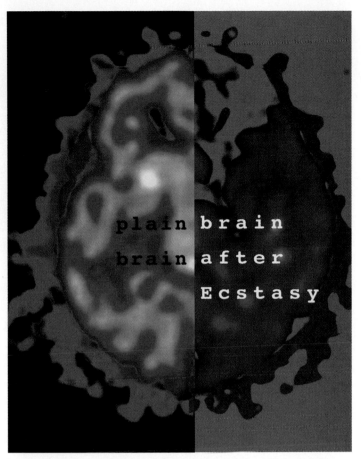

This composite brain scan shows some of the effects of the drug Ecstasy. The left side shows healthy serotonin sites. The dark sections on the right are serotonin sites no longer present even after three weeks without Ecstasy. Serotonin helps regulate mood, learning, and sleep.

Mescaline Mescaline is one of hundreds of chemicals derived from the **peyote** cactus, a small, buttonlike cactus that grows in the southwestern United States and Latin America. Natives of these regions have long used the dried peyote buttons for religious purposes. In fact, members of the Native American Church (a religion practiced by thousands of North American Indians) have been granted special permission to use the drug during religious ceremonies in some states. Users normally swallow 10 to 12 dried peyote buttons. These buttons taste bitter and generally induce immediate nausea or vomiting. Longtime users claim that the nausea becomes less noticeable with frequent use.

Those who are able to keep the drug down begin to feel the effects within 30 to 90 minutes, when mescaline reaches maximum concentration in the brain. (It may persist for up to 9 or 10 hours.) Unlike LSD, mescaline is a powerful hallucinogen. It is also a central nervous system stimulant.

Products sold on the street as mescaline are likely to be synthetic chemical relatives of the true drug. Street names of these products include DOM, STP, TMA, and MDMA. Any of these can be toxic in small quantities.

Psilocybin Psilocybin and psilocin are the active chemicals in a group of mushrooms sometimes called "magic mushrooms." Psilocybe mushrooms, which grow throughout the world, can be cultivated from spores or harvested wild. Because many mushrooms resemble the psilocybe variety, people who use wild mushrooms for any purpose should be certain of what they are doing. Mushroom varieties can

Hallucinogens Substances capable of creating auditory or visual hallucinations.

Psychedelics Drugs that distort the processing of sensory information in the brain.

Reticular formation An area in the brain stem that is responsible for relaying messages to other areas in the brain.

Synesthesia A (usually) drug-created effect in which sensory messages are incorrectly assigned—for example, the user hears a taste or smells a sound.

Lysergic acid diethylamide (LSD) Psychedelic drug causing sensory disruptions; also called *acid*.

Mescaline A hallucinogenic drug derived from the peyote cactus.

Peyote A cactus with small "buttons" that, when ingested, produce hallucinogenic effects.

Psilocybin The active chemical found in psilocybe mushrooms; it produces hallucinations.

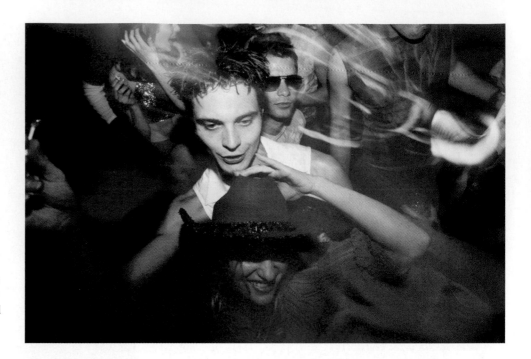

Beware of claims that the latest club drugs, often distributed at parties or dances, are "totally harmless" or "all natural." Such substances can be hazardous.

easily be misidentified, and mistakes can be fatal. Psilocybin is similar to LSD in its physical effects, which generally wear off within 4 to 6 hours.

PCP   Phencyclidine, or **PCP,** is a synthetic substance that became a black-market drug in the early 1970s. PCP was originally developed as a "dissociative anesthetic," which means that patients administered this drug could keep their eyes open, apparently remain conscious, and feel no pain during a medical procedure. Patients would afterward experience amnesia for the time the drug was in their system. Such a drug had obvious advantages as an anesthetic, but its unpredictability and drastic effects (postoperative delirium, confusion, and agitation) made doctors abandon it, and it was withdrawn from the legal market.

On the illegal market, PCP is a white, crystalline powder that users often sprinkle onto marijuana cigarettes. It is dangerous and unpredictable regardless of the method of administration. Common street names for PCP are "angel dust" for the crystalline powdered form and "peace pill" and "horse tranquilizer" for the tablet form.

Phencyclidine (PCP)   A deliriant commonly called "angel dust."

Designer drug   A synthetic analog (a drug that produces similar effects) of an existing illicit drug.

Ecstasy   A "club drug" that creates feelings of openness and warmth but also raises heart rate and blood pressure.

Inhalants   Products that are sniffed or inhaled in order to produce highs.

The effects of PCP depend on the dosage. A dose as small as 5 mg will produce effects similar to those of strong central nervous system depressants—slurred speech, impaired coordination, reduced sensitivity to pain, and reduced heart and respiratory rate. Doses between 5 and 10 mg cause fever, salivation, nausea, vomiting, and total loss of sensitivity to pain. Doses greater than 10 mg result in a drastic drop in blood pressure, coma, muscular rigidity, violent outbursts, and possible convulsions and death.

Psychologically, PCP may produce either euphoria or dysphoria. It is also known to produce hallucinations as well as delusions and overall delirium. Some users experience a prolonged state of "nothingness." The long-term effects of PCP use are unknown.

Designer Drugs (Club Drugs)

Designer drugs are produced in chemical laboratories, often manufactured in homes, and sold illegally. These drugs are easy to produce from available raw materials. The drugs themselves were once technically legal because the law had to specify the exact chemical structure of an illicit substance. However, there is now a law in place that bans all chemical cousins of illegal drugs.

Collectively known as *club drugs,* these dangerous substances include Ecstasy, GHB, Special K, and Rohypnol. Although users may think them harmless, research has shown that club drugs can produce a range of unwanted effects, including hallucinations, paranoia, amnesia, and in some cases, death. Some club drugs work on the same brain mechanisms as alcohol and can dangerously boost the effects of both substances. Since the drugs are odorless and tasteless, people can easily slip them into drinks. Some of them have been associated with sexual assaults and for that reason are referred to as "date rape drugs" (see the Reality Check box).

Club Drugs on Campus

Every era seems to have its hot drug. At one point it was Valium, then LSD, and then crack. The late 1990s, however, saw more than its share. The so-called club drugs had their greatest popularity on college campuses. Three of note include Rohypnol (flunitrazepam), also called "ropies" or "roofies"; GHB (gamma hydroxybutyrate), or as it is known on the street, "grievous bodily harm"; and Special K (ketamine).

Rohypnol is a very potent tranquilizer similar in nature to Valium, but many times stronger. The drug produces a sedative effect, amnesia, muscle relaxation, and a slowing of psychomotor responses. Commonly known as the "date rape" drug, Rohypnol gained notoriety a few years ago when it was reported as a growing problem on college campuses, especially in fraternities. The drug has been added to punch and other drinks at fraternity parties and college social gatherings, where it is reportedly given to female partiers in hopes of lowering their inhibitions and facilitating potential sexual conquests. To make matters worse, roofies are inexpensive and have been reported to sell for as little as $3 to $5 a pill. While "ropie" fervor has subsided somewhat, it continues to be of concern to campus officials.

No sooner had the immediate threat of Rohypnol died down when it was replaced by the lust for a newer, liquid substance called GHB, or gamma hydroxybutyrate. GHB has a variety of uses, which include being taken as an aphrodisiac to increase one's sense of touch and sexual prowess, as a muscle builder, and as a tranquilizer. Some people also use it as a substitute for alcohol, obtaining the high without the hangover. GHB is an odorless, tasteless fluid that can be made easily at home in a chemistry lab. Like Rohypnol, GHB has been slipped into drinks without being detected, resulting in loss of memory, unconsciousness, amnesia, and even death. Side effects of GHB include nausea, vomiting, seizures, memory loss, hallucinations, coma, and respiratory distress. During the 1980s, GHB was available in U.S. health food stores. Concerns about its use led the FDA to ban OTC sales in 1990 and push for further controls in 1997.

The Special K we're referring to is not the breakfast cereal, but rather an analog of phencyclidine, used as an anesthetic in many hospital and veterinary clinics. On the street, Special K is most often diverted in liquid form from veterinary offices or medical suppliers. Dealers dry the liquid (usually by cooking it) and grind the residue into powder. Special K causes hallucinations as it inhibits the relay of sensory input; the brain fills the resulting void with visions, dreams, memories, and sensory distortions. The effects of Special K are not as severe as those of Ecstasy, so it has grown in popularity among people who have to go to work or school after a night of partying.

Sources: J. Cloud, "Is Your Kid on K?" *Time,* October 20, 1997, 90–91; D. Rosenberg, "Death of the Party," *Time,* October 27, 1997, 55; S. A. Lyman, C. Hugher-McLain, and G. Thompson, "Date-Rape Drugs: A Growing Concern," *Journal of Health Education* 29: 271–274; Information from Emergencynet NEWS Service, 1996; and Kit Lively, "The 'Date-Rape Drug,'" *Chronicle of Higher Education,* June 28, 1996, A29.

Ecstasy (methylenedioxymethylamphetamine, or *MDMA*), once dubbed the "LSD of the 80s," has had a resurgence of popularity on many college campuses. Almost one of every four students at some universities report having used it. Ecstasy creates feelings of openness and warmth, combined with the mind-expanding characteristics of hallucinogens. Effects begin within 30 minutes and can last for four to six hours. Young people may use Ecstasy initially to improve mood or get energized so they can keep dancing; it also raises heart rate and blood pressure and may lead to an elevated body temperature that can cause kidney and/or cardiovascular failure. Chronic use appears to damage the brain's ability to think and regulate emotion, memory, sleep, and pain. Combined with alcohol, Ecstasy can be extremely dangerous and sometimes fatal. Recent studies indicate that Ecstasy may cause long-lasting neurotoxic effects by damaging brain cells that produce serotonin, and it is unknown whether these brain cells will regenerate.[13] (See the Health Ethics box on page 408.)

Inhalants

Inhalants are chemicals that produce vapors that, when inhaled, can cause hallucinations and create intoxicating and euphoric effects. Not commonly recognized as drugs, inhalants are legal to purchase and universally available, but dangerous when used incorrectly. These drugs generally appeal to young people who can't afford illicit substances.

Some of these agents are organic solvents representing the chemical by-products of the distillation of petroleum products. Rubber cement, model glue, paint thinner, lighter fluid, varnish, wax, spot removers, and gasoline belong to

Should We "Protect" Illicit Drug Users?

In the spring of 2000, three young people died in Chicago after taking tablets they thought contained Ecstasy. One young woman ingested what she thought was a potent brand of Ecstasy; she had apparently taken Ecstasy for the first time a couple of months earlier, and the pills she had taken were supposed to be "Mitsubishi," the hottest version of Ecstasy around. Within a few hours, she was rushed to the hospital. There she lapsed into a coma, and her body temperature rose quickly to 108 degrees. She was bleeding from her mouth and stomach and began having seizures. By the following afternoon, she was dead. Instead of taking Ecstasy (methylenedioxymethamphetamine or MDMA, the chemical found in unadulterated Ecstasy), she had unknowingly swallowed paramethoxymethamphetamine (PMA). PMA is cheaper and easier to manufacture than Ecstasy, but far more dangerous.

Contaminated illegal drugs have never been a big issue in the United States. But if the use of Ecstasy continues to rise, as some researchers speculate it will, more and more dealers may start substituting deadly substances like PMA for less potent substances like MDMA, or speed, cocaine, caffeine, PCP, Valium, ketamine, or a variety of other drugs. To deal with this potential danger, on-site pill testing has become available at some raves run by Dance Safe (a nonprofit organization promoting health and safety within the rave and nightclub community). Also available are pill-testing kits, which can be purchased on the web, so that people can test their own Ecstasy pills. Alternatively, pills may be sent to a laboratory for testing.

Do you believe that such pill-testing services should be readily available? Why or why not? What ethical issues do such harm-reduction services raise? What benefits do they offer? Would you advocate an increase in such services? What other programs are you familiar with that aim to reduce the harm caused by drug use and abuse?

Source: "Ecstasy: The Poisoning of Suburbia," by T. Oehmke, *Icon,* July 27, 2000, pp. 7–8.

---

this group. Most of these substances are sniffed by users in search of a quick, cheap high.

Because they are inhaled, the volatile chemicals in these products reach the bloodstream within seconds. An inhaled substance is not diluted or buffered by stomach acids or other body fluids and thus is more potent than it would be if swallowed. This characteristic, along with the fact that dosages are extremely difficult to control because everyone has unique lung and breathing capacities, makes inhalants particularly dangerous.

The effects of inhalants usually last for less than 15 minutes. Users may experience dizziness, disorientation, impaired coordination, reduced judgment, and slowed reaction times. Signs of inhalant use include the following: unjustifiable collection of glues, paints, lacquer thinner, cleaning fluid, and ether; sniffles similar to those produced by a cold; and a smell on the breath similar to the inhaled substance. The effects of inhalants resemble those of central nervous system depressants, and combining inhalants with alcohol produces a synergistic effect. In addition, these substances in combination can cause severe liver damage that may be fatal.

An overdose of fumes from inhalants can cause unconsciousness. If the user's oxygen intake is reduced during the inhaling process, death can result within five minutes. Whether a user is a first-time or chronic user, sudden sniffing death (SSD) syndrome can be a fatal consequence. This syndrome can occur if a user inhales deeply and then participates in physical activity or is startled.

Amyl Nitrite Sometimes called "poppers" or "rush," **amyl nitrite** is packaged in small, cloth-covered glass capsules that can be crushed to release the active chemical. The drug is often prescribed to alleviate chest pain in heart patients because it dilates small blood vessels and reduces blood pressure. Dilation of blood vessels in the genital area is thought to enhance sensations or perceptions of orgasm. It also produces fainting, dizziness, warmth, and skin flushing.

Nitrous Oxide **Nitrous oxide** is sometimes used as an adjunct to dental anesthesia or minor surgical anesthesia. It is also a propellant chemical in aerosol products such as whipped toppings. Users experience a state of euphoria, floating sensations, and illusions. Effects also include pain relief and a "silly" feeling, demonstrated by laughing and giggling (hence its nickname "laughing gas"). Regulating dosages of this drug can be difficult. Sustained inhalation can lead to unconsciousness, coma, and death.

Amyl nitrite A drug that dilates blood vessels and is properly used to relieve chest pain.

Nitrous oxide The chemical name for "laughing gas," a substance properly used for surgical or dental anesthesia.

Anabolic steroids Artificial forms of the hormone testosterone that promote muscle growth and strength.

Ergogenic drug Substance that enhances athletic performance.

Steroids

Public awareness of **anabolic steroids** has recently been heightened by media stories about their use by amateur and professional athletes, including Arnold Schwarzenegger during his competitive bodybuilding days. Anabolic steroids are artificial forms of the male hormone testosterone that promote muscle growth and strength. These **ergogenic drugs** are used primarily by young men who believe the drugs will increase their strength, power, bulk (weight), speed, and athletic performance.

Most steroids are obtained through the black market. It was once estimated that approximately 17 to 20 percent of college athletes used them. Now that stricter drug-testing policies have been instituted by the NCAA, reported use of anabolic steroids among intercollegiate athletes has dropped to 1.1 percent. However, a recent survey among high school students found a significant increase in the use of anabolic steroids since 1991. Few data exist on the extent of steroid abuse by adults. It has been estimated that hundreds of thousands of people age 18 and older abuse anabolic steroids at least once a year. Among both adolescents and adults, steroid abuse is higher among males than females. However, steroid abuse is growing most rapidly among young women.[14]

Steroids are available in two forms: injectable solution and pills. Anabolic steroids produce a state of euphoria, diminished fatigue, and increased bulk and power in both sexes. These qualities give steroids an addictive quality. When users stop, they most commonly experience a psychological withdrawal, mainly caused by the disappearance of the physique they have become accustomed to. Some users experience severe depression, in some cases leading to suicide attempts. If untreated, such depression associated with steroid withdrawal has been known to last for a year or more after steroid use stops.

Adverse effects occur in both men and women who use steroids. These drugs cause mood swings (aggression and violence), sometimes known as "roid rage"; acne; liver tumors; elevated cholesterol levels; hypertension; kidney disease; and immune system disturbances. There is also a danger of AIDS transmission through shared needles. In women, large doses of anabolic steroids may trigger the development of masculine attributes such as lowered voice, increased facial and body hair, and male pattern baldness; they may also result in an enlarged clitoris, smaller breasts, and changes in or absence of menstruation. When taken by healthy males, anabolic steroids shut down the body's production of testosterone, causing men's breasts to grow and testicles to atrophy.

To combat the growing problem of steroid use, Congress passed the Anabolic Steroids Control Act (ASCA) of 1990. This law makes it a crime to possess, prescribe, or distribute anabolic steroids for any use other than the treatment of specific diseases. Anabolic steroids are now classified as a Schedule III drug. Penalties for their illegal use include up to five years' imprisonment and a $250,000 fine for the first offense, and up to 10 years' imprisonment and a $500,000 fine for subsequent offenses.

A new and alarming trend is the use of other drugs to achieve the supposed "performance-enhancing" effects of steroids. The two most common steroid alternatives are gamma hydroxybutyrate (GHB) and clenbuterol. GHB is a deadly, illegal drug that is a primary ingredient in many "performance-enhancing" formulas. GHB does not produce a high. It does, however, cause headaches, nausea, vomiting, diarrhea, seizures, and other central nervous system disorders, and possibly death. Clenbuterol is used in some countries for veterinary treatments, but is not approved for any use—in animals or humans—in the United States.

In 1998 new attention was drawn to the issue of steroids and related substances when St. Louis Cardinals' slugger Mark McGwire admitted to using a supplement containing androstenedione (andro), an adrenal hormone that is produced naturally in both men and women. Andro raises levels of the male hormone testosterone, which helps build lean muscle mass and promotes quicker recovery after injury. McGwire had done nothing illegal, as the supplement can be purchased over the counter (with sales estimated at up to $800 million a year) and its use is legal in baseball, although banned by the NFL, NCAA, and International Olympic Committee. A recent study found that when men take 100 milligrams of andro three times daily, it increases estrogen levels by up to 80 percent, enlarges the prostate gland, and increases heart disease risk by 10 to 15 percent. This finding may or may not affect its use in major league baseball—no decision has yet been made.

Other muscle-building supplements are also common. Though andro has been banned by many sports organizations, visits to the locker rooms of many teams belonging to these organizations would disclose large containers of other supplements, such as creatine, intended to help athletes build muscle mass. Although they are legal, questions remain whether enough research has been done concerning the safety of these supplements. Some people worry that they may bring consequences similar to those of steroids, such as liver damage and heart problems.

What do you think?

Do you think androstenedione should be declared illegal? ✳ Would you consider using supplements for the sole purpose of increasing your body build and potentially your athletic performance? ✳ Are steroid users stigmatized in our society in the same way as users of other illicit drugs? ✳ Do you think they should be? ✳ Why or why not?

Illegal Drug Use in the United States

Stories of people who have tried illegal drugs, enjoyed them, and suffered no consequences may tempt you to try them yourself. You may tell yourself it's "just this once," convincing yourself that onetime use is harmless. Given the dangers surrounding these substances, however, you should think twice. The risks associated with drug use extend beyond the personal. The decision to try any illicit substance encourages illicit drug manufacture and transport, thus contributing to the national drug problem. The financial burden of illegal drug use on the U.S. economy is staggering, with an estimated economic cost of around $160 billion.[15] This estimate includes substance abuse treatment and prevention costs, other health care costs, costs associated with reduced job productivity or lost earnings, and social costs such as crime and social welfare. Related health care costs alone are thought to total over $14.9 billion annually.

In addition, roughly one-half of all expenditures to combat crime are related to illegal drugs. The burden of these costs is absorbed primarily by the government (46 percent), followed by those who abuse drugs and members of their households (44 percent). In a study to determine how much money is spent on illegal drugs, the White House Office of National Drug Control Policy (ONDCP) found that Americans spent $64 billion on illicit drugs annually. These numbers broke down as follows: $35 billion on cocaine, $10 billion each on marijuana and heroin, and $5 billion on methamphetamines. This is eight times the total the federal government spends on research on HIV/AIDS, cancer, and heart disease put together.[16]

Drugs in the Workplace

Tne National Institute of Drug Abuse (NIDA) estimates that 8.5 percent of all U.S. workers use dangerous drugs on the job at some time. With approximately 70 to 75 percent of drug users in the United States employed to some degree, the cost to American businesses soars into the billions of dollars annually.[17] These costs reflect reduced work performance and efficiency, lost productivity, absenteeism and turnover, increased use of health benefits, accidents, and indirect losses stemming from impaired judgment.

The highest rates of illicit drug use among workers exist in the construction, food preparation, restaurant, transportation, and material-moving industries. Workers who require a considerable amount of public trust, such as police officers, teachers, and child-care workers, report the lowest use. In addition, younger employees (18–24 years old) are more likely to report drug use than employees aged 25 and older. Drug users are 1.6 times more likely than nonusers to quit their jobs or be fired, and 1.5 times more likely to be disciplined by their supervisor.[18]

Many companies have instituted drug testing for their employees. Mandatory drug urinalysis is controversial. Critics argue that such testing violates Fourth Amendment rights of protection from unreasonable search and seizure. Proponents believe the personal inconvenience entailed in testing pales in comparison to the problems caused by drug use in the workplace. Several court decisions have affirmed the right of employers to test their employees for drug use. They contend that Fourth Amendment rights pertain only to

employees of government agencies, not to those of private businesses. Most Americans apparently support drug testing for certain types of job categories.

Drug testing is expensive, with costs running as high as $100 per individual test. Moreover, some critics question the accuracy and reliability of the results. Both false positives and false negatives can occur. As drug testing becomes more common in the work environment, it is gaining greater acceptance by employees, who see testing as a step to improving safety and productivity.

What do you think?

What do you believe are the moral and ethical issues surrounding drug testing? ☀ *Are you in favor of drug testing?* ☀ *Should all employees be subjected to drug tests or just those in high-risk jobs? Is it the employer's right to conduct drug testing at the work site?* ☀ *Explain your answer.*

Solutions to the Problem

Americans are alarmed by the increasing use of illegal drugs, particularly crack and other forms of cocaine. In recent years, we have been constantly warned through the media about this "chemical menace" to our society. Respondents in a poll felt that the most important strategy for fighting drug abuse was educating young people; they also endorsed strategies such as working with foreign governments to stop drug trafficking, making a concerted effort to arrest dealers, providing treatment assistance, and arresting drug users.

The most popular antidrug strategies for many years were total prohibition and "scare tactics." Both approaches proved ineffective. Prohibition of alcohol during the 1920s created more problems than it solved, as did prohibition of opiates in 1914. Outlawing other illicit drugs has neither eliminated them nor curtailed their traffic across U.S. borders.

In general, researchers in the field of drug education agree that a multimodal approach is best. Students should be taught the difference between drug use and abuse. Factual information that is free of scare tactics must be presented; lecturing and moralizing about drug use and abuse do not work. Emphasis should be placed on things that are important to young people. Telling adolescent males that girls will find them disgusting if their breath stinks of cigarettes or pot will get their attention. Likewise, lecturing on the negative effects of drug use is a much less effective deterrent than teaching young people how to negotiate the social scene. D.A.R.E., one program intended to educate students, has been largely ineffective. Education efforts need to be focused on achieving better drug use prevention outcomes.

We must target at-risk groups for study so we can better understand the circumstances that make them susceptible to drug use. Time, money, and effort by educators, parents, and policy makers are needed to ensure that today's youth are given the love and security essential for building productive and meaningful lives.

Among the strategies suggested for combating drug abuse are stricter border surveillance to reduce drug trafficking, longer prison sentences for drug pushers, increased government spending on prevention and enforcement of antidrug laws, and greater cooperation between government agencies and private groups and individuals. All of these approaches will probably help up to a point, but neither alone nor in combination do they offer a total solution to the problem. Drug abuse has been a part of human behavior for thousands of years, and it is not likely to disappear in the near future. For this reason, it is necessary to educate ourselves and develop the self-discipline necessary to avoid dangerous drug dependencies.

> **What do you think?**
>
> *Do you feel the public has a social responsibility to fight drug abuse? ✳ What is the cost society pays for drug use? ✳ Have you ever personally known someone who has suffered because of addiction to drugs? ✳ How did you respond?*

Taking Charge

14 14 **14**

Managing Drug Use Behavior

A college environment offers many opportunities for a young person, most of which are good. Unfortunately, others can be dangerous, including the availability of illegal drugs. Are you aware of the drug culture on your campus? Have drugs had an effect on your life? Before you try a new drug, take a moment to think about what you're doing. Think about what you want to experience or why you want to change your mental state. Then ask yourself whether the drug will really achieve that. Are there alternatives for reaching the desired change? What are the potential side effects? Are the risks worth the momentary high? Are you willing to risk potential addiction?

Checklist for Change

Making Personal Choices

☐ What drugs are most popular among your peers? What is it about these drugs that makes them popular?

☐ How do you and your peers feel about illicit drug use? Is it condoned or condemned? Has this viewpoint changed in the past few years? What has led to these feelings?

☐ Are you prepared for the challenge of refusing to use illicit drugs that you may be offered and for dealing with the consequences associated with that decision?

☐ Do you practice assertiveness? Do you practice speaking up and voicing your opinion regardless of the subject?

☐ Do you have strategies for coping with stress? Do you use exercise, meditation, or some other healthy activity to reduce stress?

☐ Do you take the time to find out about the current drug problems on your campus and in your community?

☐ Would you be willing to assist friends in combating a substance abuse problem? Would you take them or accompany them to support groups?

Making Community Choices

☐ Would you be willing to be a role model in community programs such as Big Brothers or Big Sisters?

☐ Do you volunteer your time for any campus or community organizations that provide opportunities for high-risk youth?

☐ Would you be willing to volunteer to help out at an addiction hotline or community center?

Summary

✳ The six categories of drugs are prescription drugs, OTC drugs, recreational drugs, herbal preparations, illicit drugs, and commercial preparations. Routes of administration include oral ingestion, injection (intravenous, intramuscular, and subcutaneous), inhalation, inunction, and suppositories.

✳ People from all walks of life use illicit drugs, although college students report higher usage rates than does the general population. Drug use has declined since the mid-1980s.

* Controlled substances include cocaine and its derivatives, amphetamines, newer-generation stimulants, marijuana, the opiates, hallucinogens, designer drugs, inhalants, and steroids. Users tend to become addicted quickly to such drugs.

* The drug problem reaches everyone through crime and elevated health care costs. Drugs are a major problem in the workplace; workplace drug testing is one proposed solution to this problem.

Questions for Discussion and Reflection

1. What is the name of the current theory that explains how drugs work in the body? Explain this theory.
2. Do you think there is such a thing as responsible use of illicit drugs? Would you change any of the current laws governing drugs? How would you determine what is legitimate use and illegitimate use?
3. Why do you think that many people today feel that marijuana use is not dangerous? What are the arguments in favor of legalizing marijuana? What are the arguments against legalization? How common is the use of marijuana on your campus?
4. How do you and your peers feel about illicit drug use? How and why has your opinion changed in recent years, if it has?
5. Debate the issue of workplace drug testing. Would you apply for a job that had drug testing as an interview requirement? As a continuing requirement?

6. What could you do to help a friend who is fighting a substance abuse problem? What resources on your campus could help you?
7. Why are drugs such as Rohypnol and Ecstasy of great concern these days? If someone has "consensual" sex with another person after lacing his or her drink with one of these drugs, do you think it's a case of rape and should be prosecuted as such? Why or why not?
8. How do you think reports in the media about the use of stimulants and/or steroids by athletes affect the popularity of these drugs? Would you consider taking such a drug to improve your appearance or your athletic performance? Explain your answer.
9. What types of programs do you think would be effective in preventing drug abuse among high school and college students? How would programs for high school differ from those for college students?

Application Exercises

Reread the What Do You Think? scenarios at the beginning of the chapter and answer the following questions.

1. What are some of the health risks associated with smoking marijuana? How frequently do you think marijuana use contributes to students' academic problems?
2. Do you think that Greg and his friends were treated fairly? Why or why not? Do you think more students come to your campus having used marijuana in the past, or do you

think they more typically begin using marijuana when they get to campus? Do you think marijuana should continue to be a Schedule I drug? Why or why not?
3. What possible health risks might Sean be taking by mixing alcohol and Ecstasy? Is there any way to determine whether the Ecstasy was pure or not? What potential problems are associated with chronic use of Ecstasy?

Accessing Your Health on the Internet

Visit the following Internet sites to explore further topics and issues related to personal health. To visit an organization's website, go to the Companion Website for *Access to Health, Eighth Edition* at www.aw.com/donatelle, click on the book image, and select "Accessing Your Health on the Internet" from the navigation menu on the left.

1. *Club Drugs.* A website designed to disseminate science-based information about club drugs.

2. *Join Together.* An excellent site for the most current information related to substance abuse. This site also includes information on gun violence and provides advice on organizing and taking political action.
3. *National Institute on Drug Abuse.* The homepage of this U.S. government agency has information on the latest statistics and findings in drug research.

Further Reading

Elster, J. (ed.). *Addiction: Entries and Exits*. New York: Russell Sage Foundation, 2000.
Addresses current addiction controversies from an international perspective, with authors from the United States and Norway. Topics include whether addicts have a choice in their behavior and current addiction theories.

Goldstein, A. *Addiction: From Biology to Drug Policy*. New York: Oxford University Press, 2001.
This book discusses how drugs impact the brain, how each drug causes addiction, and how addictive drugs impact society. The author offers an explanation of what we know about drug addiction, how we know what we know, and what we can and cannot do about the drug problem.

Hales, D., and R. E. Hales. *Caring for the Mind: The Comprehensive Guide to Mental Health*. New York: Bantam, 1995.
An easy-to-understand reference that includes chapters on substance abuse problems and impulse control–related disorders, including compulsive gambling and compulsive shopping.

James, W. H., and S. L. Johnson. *Doin' Drugs: Patterns of African American Addiction*. Austin: University of Texas Press, 1997.
A concise examination of historical and current patterns of drug use in the African American community; begins with a historical overview and then proceeds to specific drugs, such as alcohol and cocaine; includes an exploration of the involvement of the church in dealing with drugs and addiction.

Reinarman, C., and H. G. Levine (eds.). *Crack in America: Demon Drugs and Social Justice*. Berkeley: University of California Press, 1997.
Examines the myths and realities of crack cocaine and how government policies toward crack may reflect racism and classism. Also explores the failure of drug prohibition.

West, J. W. *The Betty Ford Center Book of Answers: Help for Those Struggling with Substance Abuse and the People Who Love Them*. New York: Pocket Books, 1997.
Written by the former director of the Betty Ford Center, one of the leading alcohol and drug treatment centers in the United States. Provides answers to the most frequently asked questions about treatment and recovery; includes comprehensive coverage of drug abuse issues for addicts and their families.

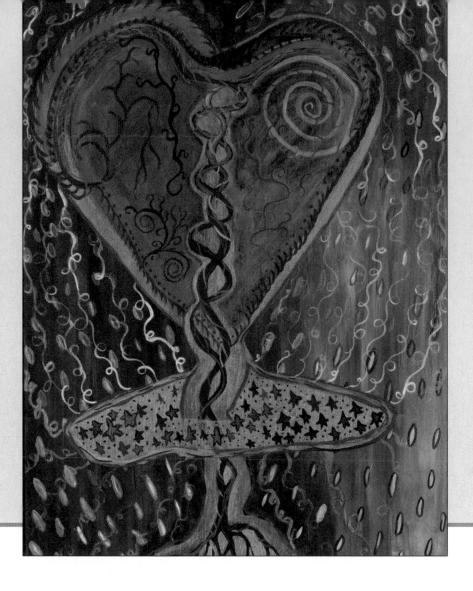

Objectives

* Discuss the incidence, prevalence, and outcomes of cardiovascular disease in America, including its impact on society.

* Describe the anatomy and physiology of the heart and circulatory system and the importance of healthy heart functioning.

* Review the various types of heart disease, factors that contribute to their development, current diagnostic and treatment options, and the importance of fundamental lifestyle modifications aimed at prevention.

* Discuss the controllable risk factors for cardiovascular disease, including smoking, cholesterol and triglycerides, certain infectious organisms, diet and obesity, exercise, hypertension, diabetes mellitus, and stress. Examine your own risk profile and determine those risk factors you can and cannot control.

* Discuss the issues surrounding cardiovascular disease risk and disease burden from the perspective of women.

* Discuss some of the newer methods of diagnosing and treating cardiovascular disease, and the importance of being a wise health care consumer.

15 Cardiovascular Disease

Reducing Your Risk

What do you think?

Jim is a wrestler with a Division I collegiate team in the Pacific Northwest. Because he tends to be a bit heavy, he routinely loses large amounts of weight to "make weight" for the next lower weight class. He wears rubberized suits, starves himself, and exercises to exhaustion in the days prior to a meet. His coaches ignore this high-risk behavior until Jim begins passing out from serious dehydration and an elevated heart rate.

Jennifer, a gymnast at a large public university, routinely binges and purges to keep her weight down for improved performance in floor exercise, bars, and vaulting. During a routine checkup, the team physician notes that Jennifer has several significant heart irregularities.

Sam, a basketball player for a large public university in the South, finds out that he has an irregular heartbeat. But because he is the top gun on the team and the NCAA tournaments are coming up, he gets clearance to play from his physician, who argues that the heart irregularity is not significant and that Sam has had it for many years without incurring any problems.

Why are young college athletes often at increased risk to their physical health during the competitive season? ✳ *Is cardiovascular risk a significant issue for athletes such as those discussed here?* ✳ *Why or why not?* ✳ *What actions could university administrators, students, and parents take to ensure that students avoid unnecessary risks when confronted with the win-at-any-cost mentality that dominates some athletic programs?* ✳ *Which sports seem particularly associated with this mentality?* ✳ *Do you know anyone who has participated in athletic competition under such risky conditions?*

An Epidemiological Overview

Despite the many medical advances we enjoy, diseases of the heart/cardiovascular system continue to be a significant health threat in the United States (see Figure 15.1). In fact, **cardiovascular disease (CVD)** remains the leading single cause of death around the world.

In 2000, CVD accounted for approximately 41 percent of all deaths in the United States, nearly 1 out of every 2.5. This is nearly three times the rate of the second leading killer, cancer, and more than the number of deaths caused by all other diseases combined. Of the nearly 2 million deaths per year in the United States, CVD was listed as a primary or contributing cause of death on about 1.4 million death certificates.[1] CVD has been the number one killer in the United States since 1900 in every year but one—1918, when another killer, a particularly virulent strain of influenza (the flu), struck with blinding force. Since 1900, the number of deaths from heart disease has risen steadily (see Figure 15.2). To clarify just how serious CVD is, consider the following points:[2]

- More than 2,600 Americans die of CVD each day, an average of 1 every 33 seconds. That was 958,775 people in 2000.
- Many of these fatalities are **sudden cardiac deaths,** meaning that these Americans die from sudden, abrupt loss of heart function (cardiac arrest), either instantly or shortly after symptoms occur. Most of these deaths result from coronary heart disease (CHD); in fact, over 220,000 people, nearly half of all victims of heart attack, die from CHD before they get to a hospital. People who attempt to save such victims through cardiac resuscitation are sometimes riddled with guilt when they fail to save a life. However, many such deaths are due to sudden heart stoppage or slowing that even the most heroic efforts cannot prevent.
- CVD claims more lives each year than the next seven leading causes of death combined.
- More than 150,000 Americans killed each year by CVD are under age 65.
- The 1998 death rates from CVD were 419.3 for white males and 532.0 for black males; 294.9 for white females and 400.7 for black females (rate is per 110,000 of population).
- From 1988 to 1998, death rates from CVD declined by 20.4 percent. However, due to increases in the total population, the decline in actual numbers of deaths was only about 3 percent.
- If all forms of major CVD were eliminated, life expectancy would rise by almost seven years. If all forms of cancer were eliminated, the gain would be three years.
- The probability at birth of eventually dying of CVD is 47 percent; of dying from cancer, 22 percent; from accidents, 3 percent; from diabetes, 2 percent; and from HIV, 0.7 percent.

Though these statistics seem grave enough, they do not include the effects of CVD experienced by the untold numbers who live with the ravages of the disease. Today, nearly 62 million Americans live with one of the major categories of CVD. Of these, nearly 30 million are male and 32 million are female. This is particularly noteworthy in that up until the last decade, CVD was considered a "man's" disease and research, treatment, and surgical instruments and devices were largely designed for males. Many people with CVD do not know they have a serious problem.[3] Nearly 13 million of

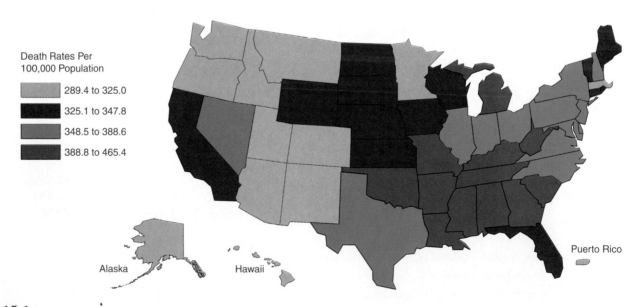

Figure 15.1

1996–1998 Total Cardiovascular Disease Age-Adjusted Death Rates (2001 Standard) by State

Note: Each state's death rate for CVD, CHD, and stroke and the percentage change over 10 years are available online in the full "2002 Heart and Stroke Statistical Update" at www.americanheart.org.

Source: "2002 Heart and Stroke Statistical Update." © 2002, Copyright American Heart Association. Reproduced by permission.

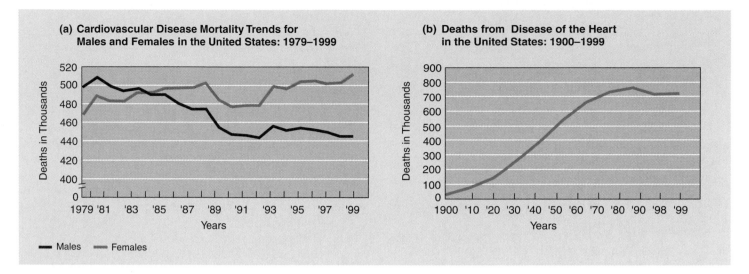

Figure 15.2
Trends in Deaths from CVD
Total cardiovascular disease data are not available for much of the time period covered by this chart.
Source: Centers for Disease Control/National Center for Health Statistics; American Heart Association, "2002 Heart and Stroke Statistical Update."

them have a history of heart attack, angina pectoris (chest pain), or both.[4] In spite of major improvements in medication, surgery, and other health care procedures, the prognosis for many of these individuals is not good:[5]

- Twenty-five percent of men and 38 percent of women will die within one year after having an initial heart attack. In part because women have heart attacks at an older age than men do, women are more likely to die from heart attacks within just a few weeks.
- People who survive the acute stages of a heart attack have a chance of illness and death that is 1.5–15 times higher than that of the general population, depending on their sex and clinical outcomes. The risk of another heart attack, sudden death, angina pectoris, heart failure, and stroke—for both men and women—is substantial.
- Coronary heart disease is a major cause of death among adults at the peak of their reproductive lives.[6]
- Within six years after a recognized heart attack, 18 percent of men and 35 percent of women will have another heart attack, 7 percent of men and 6 percent of women will experience sudden death, and about 22 percent of men and 46 percent of women will be disabled with heart failure. About two-thirds of heart attack patients won't make a complete recovery, but 88 percent of those under age 65 will be able to return to their usual work.
- CHD will permanently disable 19 percent of the U.S. labor force.
- CVD death rates are highest in the southeastern regions of the United States and lowest in the Northwest and Southwest (see Figure 15.1).

Although it is impossible to place a monetary value on human life, the economic burden of cardiovascular disease on our society is staggering—more than an estimated $329.2 billion in 2002.[7] This figure includes the cost of physician

and nursing services, hospital and nursing home services, medications, and lost productivity resulting from disability. (By comparison, in 2001 the estimated cost of all cancers was $156.7 billion and in 1999, the estimated costs of HIV infections were approximately $29 billion.) To keep this in perspective, between 1979 and 1998, the number of cardiovascular operations and procedures increased nearly 400 percent.[8] As Americans live longer, these numbers will continue to increase, resulting in a tremendous burden on the health care system. The many Americans who think that CVD can be cured with a bypass or other surgical procedure, after which life simply returns to normal, are wrong. The effects of CVD are far reaching and take a toll on quality of life.

The best line of defense against CVD is to prevent it from developing in the first place. How can you cut your risk? Take steps now to change certain behaviors. For example, controlling high blood pressure and reducing intake of saturated fats and cholesterol are two things you can do to lower your chances of heart attack. By maintaining your weight, exercising, decreasing your intake of sodium, not smoking, and changing your lifestyle to reduce stress, you can lower your blood pressure. You can also monitor the levels of fat and cholesterol in your blood and adjust your diet to prevent arteries from becoming clogged. Having combinations of risk factors seems to increase overall risk by a factor greater than those of the combined risks. Happily, the converse is also true: Reducing several risk factors can have a dramatic effect

Cardiovascular disease (CVD) Disease of the heart and blood vessels.

Sudden cardiac death Death that occurs as a result of sudden, abrupt loss of heart function.

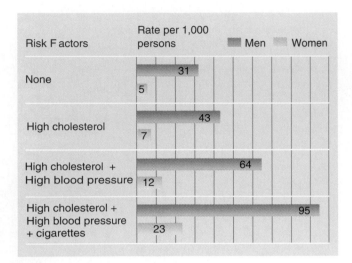

Figure 15.3

Heart Attacks: Compounded Risks
This graph shows how the risk of heart disease rises dramatically in people who have high cholesterol, high blood pressure, and/or smoke cigarettes. In the graph, "high cholesterol" is 260 or above and "high blood pressure" is 150 or above (that's systolic pressure—the higher number).
Source: Copyright 1995, Center for Science in the Public Interest. Reprinted from *Nutrition Action Healthletter* 4 (October 1995), by Stephen B. Schmidt; data from Framingham Heart Study; personal communication, Thomas Thorn, National Heart, Lung and Blood Institute.

(see Figure 15.3). Answer the questions in the Assess Yourself box on page 420 to determine your overall coronary risk and any need to treat your cholesterol levels.

Understanding how your cardiovascular system works will help you understand risks to cardiovascular health and reduce them.

What do you think?

*Consider what happens when people who suffer a heart attack survive. What unique challenges do they face? * What difficulties might they encounter at home, at work, and in leisure time? * What might it be like to live in fear that your heart might give out or a problem could crop up at any time? * What support services are available for coping with the unique fears and anxieties faced by CVD survivors and their families?*

Understanding the Cardiovascular System

The **cardiovascular system** is the network of organs and elastic tubes through which blood flows as it carries oxygen and nutrients to all parts of the body. It includes the *heart, arteries, arterioles* (small arteries), and *capillaries* (minute

blood vessels). It also includes *venules* (small veins) and *veins,* the blood vessels though which blood flows as it returns to the heart and lungs.

The Heart: A Mighty Machine

The heart is a muscular, four-chambered pump, roughly the size of your fist. It is a highly efficient, extremely flexible organ that manages to contract 100,000 times each day, pumping the equivalent of 2,000 gallons of blood to all areas of the body. In a 70-year lifetime, an average human heart beats 2.5 billion times. This number is significantly higher for hearts that must fight to keep people moving who are out of shape and overweight.

Under normal circumstances, the human body contains approximately 6 quarts of blood. This blood transports nutrients, oxygen, waste products, hormones, and enzymes throughout the body. It also regulates body temperature, cellular water levels, and acidity levels of body components and aids in bodily defense against toxins and harmful microorganisms. An adequate blood supply is essential to health and well-being.

The heart has four chambers that work together to constantly recirculate blood throughout the body (see Figure 15.4). The two upper chambers of the heart, called **atria,** or auricles, are large collecting chambers that receive blood from the rest of the body. The two lower chambers, known as **ventricles,** pump the blood out again. Small valves regulate the steady, rhythmic flow of blood between chambers and prevent inappropriate backwash. The *tricuspid valve* (located between the right atrium and the right ventricle), the *pulmonary (pulmonic) valve* (between the right ventricle and the pulmonary artery), the *mitral valve* (between the left atrium and left ventricle), and the *aortic valve* (between the left ventricle and the aorta) permit blood to flow in only one direction.[9]

Heart Function Heart activity depends on a complex interaction of biochemical, physical, and neurological signals. The following is a simplified version of the steps involved in heart function:

1. Deoxygenated blood enters the right atrium after having been circulated through the body.
2. From the right atrium, blood moves to the right ventricle and is pumped through the pulmonary artery to the lungs, where it receives oxygen.
3. Oxygenated blood from the lungs then returns to the left atrium of the heart.
4. Blood from the left atrium is forced into the left ventricle.
5. The left ventricle pumps blood through the aorta to all body parts.

Different types of blood vessels are required for different parts of this process. **Arteries** carry blood away from the heart—except for pulmonary arteries, which carry deoxygenated blood to the lungs, where it picks up oxygen and gives off carbon dioxide. As they branch off from the heart, the arteries divide into smaller blood vessels called

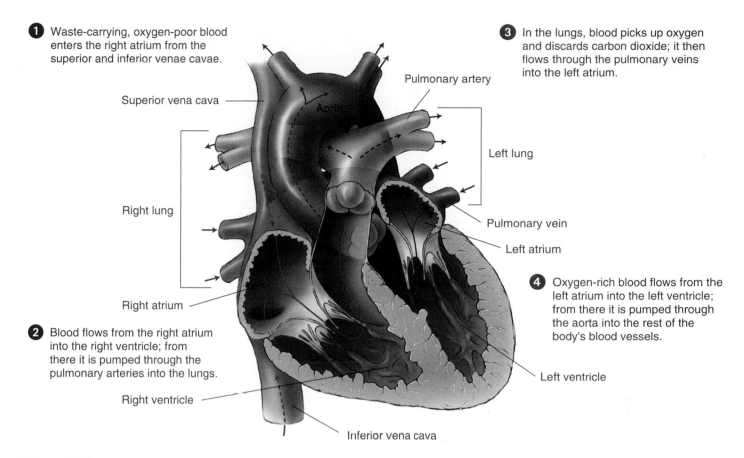

① Waste-carrying, oxygen-poor blood enters the right atrium from the superior and inferior venae cavae.

③ In the lungs, blood picks up oxygen and discards carbon dioxide; it then flows through the pulmonary veins into the left atrium.

Superior vena cava

Aorta

Pulmonary artery

Left lung

Right lung

Pulmonary vein

Left atrium

Right atrium

② Blood flows from the right atrium into the right ventricle; from there it is pumped through the pulmonary arteries into the lungs.

④ Oxygen-rich blood flows from the left atrium into the left ventricle; from there it is pumped through the aorta into the rest of the body's blood vessels.

Left ventricle

Right ventricle

Inferior vena cava

Figure 15.4
Anatomy of the Heart

arterioles, and then into even smaller blood vessels called **capillaries.** Capillaries have thin walls that permit the exchange of oxygen, carbon dioxide, nutrients, and waste products with body cells. The carbon dioxide and waste products are transported to the lungs and kidneys through **veins** and venules (small veins).

For the heart to function properly, the four chambers must beat in an organized manner. Your heartbeat is governed by an electrical impulse that directs the heart muscle to move when the impulse moves across it, which results in a sequential contraction of the four chambers. This signal starts in a small bundle of highly specialized cells, the **sino-atrial node (SA node),** located in the right atrium. The SA node serves as a form of natural pacemaker for the heart.[10] People with a damaged SA node (either a congenital defect or one injured by disease) must often have a mechanical pacemaker implanted to ensure the smooth passage of blood through the sequential phases of the heartbeat.

The average adult heart at rest beats 70 to 80 times per minute, although a well-conditioned heart may beat only 50 to 60 times per minute to achieve the same results. When overly stressed, a heart may beat over 200 times per minute, particularly in an individual who is overweight or out of shape. A healthy heart functions more efficiently and is less likely to suffer damage from overwork.

Cardiovascular system A complex system consisting of the heart and blood vessels that transports nutrients, oxygen, hormones, and enzymes throughout the body and regulates temperature, the water levels of cells, and the acidity levels of body components.

Atria The two upper chambers of the heart, which receive blood.

Ventricles The two lower chambers of the heart, which pump blood through the blood vessels.

Arteries Vessels that carry blood away from the heart to other regions of the body.

Arterioles Branches of the arteries.

Capillaries Minute blood vessels that branch out from the arterioles; their thin walls allow for the exchange of oxygen, carbon dioxide, nutrients, and waste products among body cells.

Veins Vessels that carry blood back to the heart from other regions of the body.

Sinoatrial node (SA node) Node serving as a form of natural pacemaker for the heart.

Find Your Cholesterol Plan

The following two-step program will guide you through the National Cholesterol Education Program's new treatment guidelines. The first step helps you establish your overall coronary risk; the second uses that information to determine your LDL treatment goals and how to reach them.

You'll need to know your blood pressure, your total LDL and HDL cholesterol levels, and your triglyceride and fasting glucose levels. If you're not sure of those numbers, ask your doctor and, if necessary, schedule an exam to get them. (Everyone should have a complete lipid profile every five years, starting at age 20.)

STEP 1: TAKE THE HEART-ATTACK RISK TEST

This test will identify your chance of having a heart attack or dying of coronary disease in the next 10 years. (People with previously diagnosed coronary disease, diabetes, aortic aneurysm, or symptomatic carotid- or peripheral-artery disease already face more than a 20 percent risk; they can skip the test and go straight to Step 2.) The test uses data from the Framingham Heart Study, the world's longest-running study of cardiovascular risk factors. The test is limited to established, major factors that are easily measured.

Circle the point value for each of the risk factors shown at right and below.

1 AGE

YEARS	WOMEN	MEN
20–34	–7	–9
35–39	–3	–4
40–44	0	0
45–49	3	3
50–54	6	6
55–59	8	8
60–64	10	10
65–69	12	11
70–74	14	12
75–79	16	13

2 TOTAL CHOLESTEROL

MG/DL	AGE 20–39 WOMEN	AGE 20–39 MEN	AGE 40–49 WOMEN	AGE 40–49 MEN	AGE 50–59 WOMEN	AGE 50–59 MEN	AGE 60–69 WOMEN	AGE 60–69 MEN	AGE 70–79 WOMEN	AGE 70–79 MEN
<160	0	0	0	0	0	0	0	0	0	0
160–199	4	4	3	3	2	2	1	1	1	0
200–239	8	7	6	5	4	3	2	1	1	0
240–279	11	9	8	6	5	4	3	2	2	1
280+	13	11	10	8	7	5	4	3	2	1

3 HIGH-DENSITY LIPOPROTEIN (HDL) CHOLESTEROL

MG/DL	WOMEN AND MEN
60+	-1
50–59	0
40–49	1
<40	2

4 SYSTOLIC BLOOD PRESSURE (THE HIGHER NUMBER)

MM/HG	UNTREATED WOMEN	UNTREATED MEN	TREATED WOMEN	TREATED MEN
<120	0	0	0	0
120–129	1	0	3	1
130–139	2	1	4	2
140–159	3	1	5	2
>159	4	2	6	3

5 SMOKING

AGE 20–39 WOMEN	AGE 20–39 MEN	AGE 40–49 WOMEN	AGE 40–49 MEN	AGE 50–59 WOMEN	AGE 50–59 MEN	AGE 60–69 WOMEN	AGE 60–69 MEN	AGE 70–79 WOMEN	AGE 70–79 MEN
9	8	7	5	4	3	2	1	1	1

TOTAL YOUR POINTS

Now find your total point score in the men's or women's column at right, then locate your 10-year risk in the far-right column.

WOMEN'S SCORE	MEN'S SCORE	YOUR 10-YEAR RISK
Less than 20	Less than 12	Less than 10%
20–22	12–15	10%–20%
Greater than 22	Greater than 15	Greater than 20%

STEP 2: FIND YOUR LOW-DENSITY LIPOPROTEIN (LDL) TREATMENT PLAN

Consult the table below to learn how your overall coronary risk affects whether you need to lower your LDL cholesterol level and, if you do, by how much. First, locate your coronary risk in the left-hand column. (That's based on the 10-year heart-attack risk that you just calculated as well as your coronary risk factors and any heart-threatening diseases you may have.) Then look across that row to see whether you should make lifestyle changes and take cholesterol-lowering medication, based on your current LDL level.

CORONARY-RISK GROUP	START LIFESTYLE CHANGES IF YOUR LDL LEVEL IS . . . [1]	ADD DRUGS IF YOUR LDL LEVEL IS . . .
Very High 1. Ten-year heart-attack risk of 20% or more or 2. history of coronary heart disease, diabetes, peripheral-artery disease, carotid-artery disease, or aortic aneurysm.	100 mg/dl or higher. (Aim for an LDL under 100.) Get retested after three months.	130 or higher. (Drugs are optional if your LDL is between 100 and 130.)
High 1. Ten-year heart-attack risk of 10% to 20% and 2. two or more major coronary risk factors.[2]	130 or higher. (Aim for an LDL under 130.) Get retested after three months.	130 or higher and lifestyle changes don't achieve your LDL goal in three months.
Moderately High 1. Ten-year heart-attack risk under 10% and 2. two or more major coronary risk factors.[2]	Same as above.	160 or higher, and lifestyle changes don't achieve your LDL goal in three months.[3]
Low to Moderate 1. One or no major coronary risk factors.[2, 4]	160 or higher. (Aim for an LDL under 160.) Get retested after three months.	190 or higher, and lifestyle changes don't achieve your LDL goal in three months. (Drugs are optional if your LDL is between 160 and 189.)

1. People who have the metabolic syndrome should make lifestyle changes, even if their LDL level alone doesn't warrant it. You have the metabolic syndrome if you have three or more of these risk factors: HDL under 40 in men, 50 in women; systolic blood pressure of 130 or more or diastolic pressure of 85 or more; fasting glucose level of 110 to 125; triglyceride level of 150 or more; and waist circumference over 40 inches in men, 35 inches in women. People with the syndrome should limit their carbohydrate intake, get up to 30 to 35 percent of their calories from total fat (more than usually recommended), and make the other lifestyle changes, including restriction of saturated fat.
2. The major coronary risk factors are cigarette smoking; coronary disease in a father or brother before age 55 or a mother or sister before age 65; systolic blood pressure of 140 or more, a diastolic pressure of 90 or more, or being on drugs for hypertension; and an HDL level under 40. If your HDL is 60 or more, subtract one risk factor. (High LDL is a major factor, of course, but it's already figured into the table.)
3. While the goal is to get LDL under 130, the use of drugs in these people usually isn't worthwhile, even if lifestyle steps fail to achieve that goal.
4. People in this group usually have less than 10 percent 10-year risk. Those who have higher risk should ask their doctor whether they need more aggressive treatment than shown here.

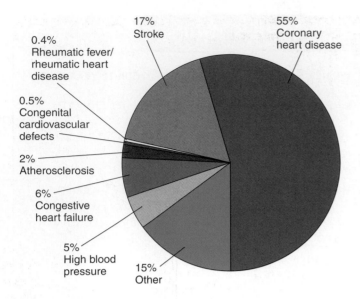

Figure 15.5
Percentage Breakdown of Deaths from Cardiovascular Disease
United States: 1999

Source: Centers for Disease Control/National Center for Health Statistics; American Heart Association, "2002 Heart and Stroke Statistical Update."

Types of Cardiovascular Disease

There are several different types of cardiovascular disease (see Figure 15.5):

- Atherosclerosis (fatty plaque buildup in arteries).
- Coronary heart disease (CHD).

Atherosclerosis   A general term for thickening and hardening of the arteries.

Hyperlipidemia   Elevated levels of lipids in the blood.

Plaque   Buildup of deposits in the arteries.

Arteriosclerosis   Condition characterized by deposits of fatty substances, cholesterol, cellular waste products, calcium, and fibrin in the inner lining of an artery.

Myocardial infarction (MI)   Heart attack.

Heart attack   A blockage of normal blood supply to an area in the heart.

Coronary thrombosis   A blood clot occurring in the coronary artery.

Embolus   A blood clot that becomes dislodged and moves through the circulatory system.

Collateral circulation   Adaptation of the heart to partial damage accomplished by rerouting needed blood through unused or underused blood vessels while the damaged heart muscle heals.

Ischemia   Reduced oxygen supply to the heart.

- Chest pain (angina pectoris).
- Irregular heartbeat (arrhythmia).
- Congestive heart failure (CHF).
- Congenital and rheumatic heart disease.
- Stroke (cerebrovascular accident).

Prevention and treatment of these diseases range from changes in diet and lifestyle to medications and surgery.

Atherosclerosis

Atherosclerosis is a process that leads to a group of diseases characterized by a thickening of the artery walls.[11] **Hyperlipidemia** (an abnormally high blood lipid level) is a key factor in its development,[12] as is the deposit of fatty substances, cholesterol, cellular waste products, calcium, and *fibrin* (a clotting material in the blood) in the inner lining of the artery. The resulting buildup is referred to as **plaque.** Atherosclerosis is actually a form of **arteriosclerosis,** or hardening and thickening of vessel walls that leads to loss of elasticity and general inability to circulate blood efficiently.[13] Often, atherosclerosis is called *coronary artery disease (CAD)* because of the resultant damage done to coronary arteries.

Atherosclerotic plaque appears primarily in large and medium-size elastic and muscular arteries and can block blood flow to the heart, brain, or extremities. Plaque may be present throughout a person's lifetime, with the earliest formation, known as a "fatty streak," being fairly common in infants and young children.[14]

Early Theories   Initially, it was thought that plaque developed in response to injury and tended to collect at sites of injury. Many scientists believed that the process of plaque buildup begins because the protective inner lining of the artery *(endothelium)* became damaged, and fats, cholesterol, and other substances in the blood tend to aggregate in these damaged areas. High blood pressure surges, elevated cholesterol and triglyceride levels in the blood, and cigarette smoking were the main suspects in having caused this injury to artery walls. As a result of national campaigns aimed at reducing dietary fats, millions of people cut down on animal fat and dairy products. However, despite massive lifestyle changes and the use of cholesterol-lowering drugs, cardiovascular diseases continue to be the leading cause of death in the United States, Europe, and most of Asia.[15]

Inflammatory Risks   Today, scientists are beginning to view the formation of atherosclerotic lesions in a new way, with a vastly expanded list of possible causes. Many experts believe that atherosclerosis is an inflammatory disease, with numerous factors contributing to plaque formation.[16] Among these culprits are elevated and modified low-density lipoprotein, free radicals caused by cigarette smoking, high blood pressure, diabetes mellitus, and certain infectious microorganisms, such as *herpesviruses* or *Chlamydia pneumoniae,* and a combination of these and other factors.[17] (See the New Horizons in Health box on page 424 about the role of homocysteine for another factor.) The bottom line is that while elevated

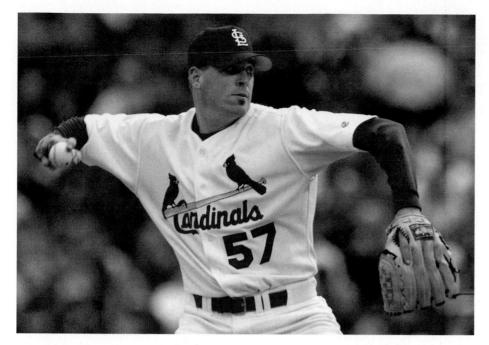

Cardiovascular disease can affect even the youngest and most fit people. Daryl Kile, a 33-year-old professional baseball player, died suddenly from atherosclerosis. It was discovered after his death that two of the main arteries in his heart were 80 to 90 percent blocked. His heart was also enlarged, weighing 20 percent more than normal.

cholesterol continues to be important in approximately 50 percent of patients with cardiovascular disease,[18] other factors also need to be considered, particularly those that inflame and injure the interior of artery walls.[19]

Syndrome X According to Gerald Reaven, endocrinologist and doctor at Stanford University, when people consume too many calories, particularly carbohydrates, their bodies eventually become insulin resistant, meaning that their cells resist, or don't work properly in, handling blood glucose levels. Consequently, insulin and blood sugar levels remain high over time. According to Reaven's book, *Syndrome X: Overcoming the Silent Killer That Can Give You a Heart Attack,* these dynamics can cause a cluster of metabolic problems such as high blood pressure and glucose intolerance that raise the risk of heart disease.[20]

Coronary Heart Disease (CHD)

Of all the major cardiovascular diseases, coronary heart disease (CHD) is the greatest killer. In fact, this year well over 1,100,000 people will suffer a heart attack, and over 40 percent of them will die.[21] Those of you raised on a weekly dose of TV doctor programs will recognize *Code Blue* as the term for a **myocardial infarction (MI),** or **heart attack.** A heart attack involves an area of the heart that suffers permanent damage because its normal blood supply has been blocked. This condition is often brought on by a **coronary thrombosis,** or blood clot in the coronary artery, or through an atherosclerotic narrowing that blocks an artery. When a blood clot or thrombus becomes dislodged and moves through the circulatory system, it is called an **embolus.** When blood does not flow readily, there is a corresponding decrease in oxygen flow. If the blockage is extremely minor, the otherwise healthy heart will adapt over time by utilizing small unused or underused blood vessels

to reroute needed blood through other areas. This system, known as **collateral circulation,** is a form of self-preservation that allows an affected heart muscle to cope with the damage.

When heart blockage is more severe, however, the body is unable to adapt on its own, and outside lifesaving support is critical. The hour following a heart attack is the most critical period—over 40 percent of heart attack victims die within this time. See the Skills for Behavior Change box on page 425 to learn what to do in case of a heart attack.

The sudden death from cardiac arrest can occur within minutes, when the heart's electrical impulses become rapid (*ventricular tachycardia*) and then chaotic (*ventricular fibrillation* or VF). Portable defibrillators, CPR, and other emergency techniques may save lives.

Although young adults can also succumb to cardiac arrest, abnormalities of the heart are the most likely cause. Under certain conditions, various heart medications, other prescription drugs, or illegal drug abuse can lead to abnormal heart rhythms that cause cardiac arrest or death. Respiratory arrest caused by asthma, electrocution, high blood pressure, drowning, choking, and trauma are other potential causes.

What do you think?

What risk factors might typical college-age students have for plaque formation? ✳ *What information should new CVD prevention guidelines include if the new theories discussed in this section prove true?*

Angina Pectoris

As a result of atherosclerosis and other circulatory impairments, the heart's oxygen supply is often reduced, a condition known as **ischemia.** Individuals with ischemia often

More than Just Cholesterol: New Research Targets Homocysteine in CVD Risk

The autopsy of an eight-year-old boy who died of a stroke in 1969 revealed that not only did his arteries have the sclerotic look of the blood vessels of an elderly man, but his blood contained excess levels of the amino acid *homocysteine.* In subsequent years, numerous studies have shown an apparently strong and direct relationship between elevated homocysteine levels and heart attacks in both men and women. In fact, in cases where other risks such as smoking are present, there appears to be almost a synergistic increase in heart attack risk for those with elevated homocysteine levels. Excess homocysteine is believed to damage vessel walls and contribute to heart attack risk in the following ways:

- By injuring arterial walls and stimulating growth of smooth muscle cells.
- By initiating blood platelet activation (clumping) and thrombus (clot) formation and possibly causing spasms in coronary arteries.
- By modifying adhesive properties of the endothelium (making it more susceptible to sticky plaque/fatty deposits).
- By impairing the way vessels respond to various substances such as L-arginine.

The reasons for elevated homocysteine levels in some people remain unclear; however, what is clear is that nearly 30 percent of CHD patients and 40 percent of patients with CVD do have abnormally high levels. Theories often point to a deficiency of B vitamins (B$_6$, B$_{12}$, and particularly *folate*). Lifestyle factors such as cigarette smoking and high coffee intake, as well as high meat intake, also appear to increase homocysteine levels.

Many researchers are cautiously optimistic about the potential for the B vitamins and folate, or its synthetic counterpart, *folic acid,* in future prevention efforts. Even small amounts of this vitamin, which is plentiful in nuts and seeds; dark green, leafy vegetables; beans and peas; and orange juice, lower homocysteine levels. Making it easier for consumers, flours, breads, cereals, and pastas have been fortified with folic acid since 1999.

Researchers at a recent Diet and Optimal Health conference in Oregon gave an enthusiastic "thumbs up" for future folic acid trials based on preliminary results of several well-designed studies. More research must be conducted to describe the exact mechanisms at work and to determine optimum amounts of folic acid that will prevent homocysteine-related CVD risks.

Sources: W. McArdle, F. Katch, and V. Katch, *Exercise Physiology,* 5th ed. (Boston: Lippincott, Williams and Wilkins, 2001), p. 900; J. W. Eikelboom et al., "Homocysteine and Cardiovascular Disease: A Critical Review of Epidemiological Evidence," *Annals of Internal Medicine* 131 (1999): 362; P. M. Ridker, et al. "Homocysteine and Risk of Cardiovascular Disease among Postmenopausal Women." *Journal of the American Medical Association* 281 (1999): 1817.

---

suffer from varying degrees of **angina pectoris,** or chest pain. In fact, an estimated 2.3 million men and 4 million women suffer mild to crushing forms of chest pain each day.[22] Many people experience short episodes of angina whenever they exert themselves physically. Symptoms may range from slight indigestion to a feeling that the heart is being crushed. Generally, the more serious the oxygen deprivation, the more severe the pain. Although angina pectoris is not a heart attack, it does indicate underlying heart disease.

Currently, there are several methods of treating angina. In mild cases, rest is critical. The most common treatments for more severe cases involve using drugs that affect (1) the supply of blood to the heart muscle or (2) the heart's demand for oxygen. Pain and discomfort are often relieved with *nitroglycerin,* a drug used to relax (dilate) veins, thereby reducing the amount of blood returning to the heart and thus lessening its workload. Patients whose angina is caused by spasms of the coronary arteries are often given drugs called *calcium channel blockers.* These drugs prevent calcium atoms from passing through coronary arteries and causing heart contractions. They also appear to reduce blood pressure and slow heart rates. *Beta blockers,* the other major type of drugs used to treat angina, control potential overactivity of the heart muscle.

Arrhythmias

Over 4 million Americans experience some type of **arrhythmia,** an irregularity in heart rhythm. A person who complains of a racing heart in the absence of exercise or anxiety may be experiencing *tachycardia,* the medical term for abnormally fast heartbeat. On the other end of the continuum is *bradycardia,* or abnormally slow heartbeat. When a heart goes into **fibrillation,** it beats in a sporadic, quivering pattern resulting in extreme inefficiency in moving blood through the cardiovascular system. If untreated, fibrillation may be fatal.

Not all arrhythmias are life threatening. In many instances, excessive caffeine or nicotine consumption can trigger an arrhythmia episode. However, severe cases may require drug therapy or external electrical stimulus to prevent serious complications.

Congestive Heart Failure (CHF)

When the heart muscle is damaged or overworked and lacks the strength to keep blood circulating normally through the body, its chambers are often taxed to the limit. **Congestive heart failure (CHF)** affects over 5 million Americans and dramatically increases risk of premature death.[23] The heart

What to Do in the Event of a Heart Attack

Because heart attacks are so serious and frightening, we would prefer not to think about them. However, knowing how to act in an emergency could save your life or that of somebody else.

KNOW THE WARNING SIGNS OF A HEART ATTACK

- Uncomfortable pressure, fullness, squeezing, or pain in the center of the chest, lasting two minutes or longer.
- Jaw pain and/or shortness of breath.
- Pain spreading to the shoulders, neck, or arms.
- Dizziness, fatigue, fainting, sweating, and/or nausea.

Not all these warning signs occur in every heart attack. If some of these symptoms do appear, however, don't wait. Get help immediately!

KNOW WHAT TO DO IN AN EMERGENCY

- Find out which hospitals in your area have 24-hour emergency cardiac care.
- Determine (in advance) the hospital or medical facility that's nearest your home and office, and tell your family and friends to call this facility in an emergency.
- Keep a list of emergency rescue service numbers next to your telephone and in your pocket, wallet, or purse.
- If you have chest or jaw discomfort that lasts more than two minutes, call the emergency rescue service.
- If you can get to a hospital faster by not waiting for an ambulance, have someone drive you there. Do not drive yourself.

BE A HEART SAVER

- If you're with someone who is showing signs of a heart attack and the warning signs last for two minutes or longer, act immediately.
- Expect a denial. It's normal for a person with chest discomfort to deny the possibility of anything as serious as a heart attack. Don't take no for an answer, however. Insist on taking prompt action.
- Call the emergency rescue service, or get to the nearest hospital emergency room that offers 24-hour emergency cardiac care.
- Give CPR (mouth-to-mouth breathing and chest compression) if it's necessary and if you're properly trained.

Source: American Heart Association, "Heart and Stroke Facts," 2002.

---

muscle may be injured by a number of health conditions, including rheumatic fever, pneumonia, heart attack, or other cardiovascular problems. In some cases, the damage is due to radiation or chemotherapy treatments for cancer. These weakened muscles respond poorly, impairing blood flow out of the heart through the arteries. The return flow of blood through the veins begins to back up, causing congestion in body tissues. This pooling of blood causes the heart to enlarge and decreases the amount of blood that can be circulated. Fluid begins to accumulate in other body areas, such as the vessels in the legs, ankles, or lungs, causing swelling or difficulty in breathing. Today, CHF is the single most frequent cause of hospitalization in the United States.[24] If untreated, congestive heart failure can be fatal. However, most cases respond well to treatment that includes *diuretics* (water pills) for relief of fluid accumulation; drugs, such as *digitalis,* that increase the pumping action of the heart; and drugs called *vasodilators* that expand blood vessels and decrease resistance, allowing blood to flow more easily and making the heart's work easier.

Congenital and Rheumatic Heart Disease

Approximately 1 out of every 125 children is born with some form of **congenital heart disease** (disease present at birth).[25] These forms may be relatively minor, such as slight *murmurs* (low-pitched sounds caused by turbulent blood flow through the heart or problematic heart valve action), resulting from valve irregularities which some children outgrow.

Other congenital problems involve serious complications in heart function that can be corrected only with surgery. Their underlying causes are unknown but may be related to hereditary factors, maternal diseases, such as rubella, occurring during fetal development; or chemical intake (particularly alcohol) by the mother during pregnancy. Because of advances in pediatric cardiology, the prognosis for children with congenital heart defects is better than ever before.

Rheumatic heart disease can cause similar heart problems in children. It is attributed to rheumatic fever, an

Angina pectoris Chest pain occurring as a result of reduced oxygen flow to the heart.

Arrhythmia An irregularity in heartbeat.

Fibrillation A sporadic, quivering pattern of heartbeat resulting in extreme inefficiency in moving blood through the cardiovascular system.

Congestive heart failure (CHF) An abnormal cardiovascular condition that reflects impaired cardiac pumping and blood flow; pooling blood leads to congestion in body tissues.

Congenital heart disease Heart disease that is present at birth.

Rheumatic heart disease A heart disease caused by untreated streptococcal infection of the throat.

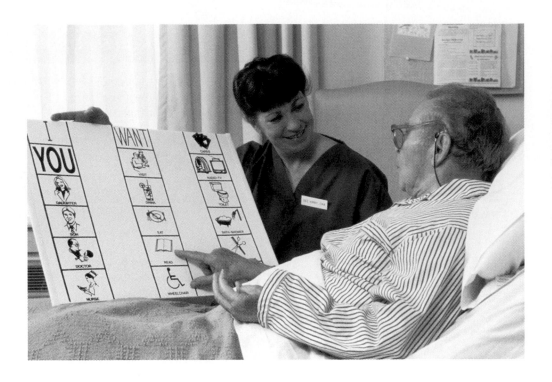

Recovery after a stroke can be a long process, often requiring therapy to improve speech and mobility.

inflammatory disease that may affect many connective tissues of the body, especially those of the heart, joints, brain, or skin, and which is caused by an unresolved *streptococcal infection* of the throat (strep throat). In a small number of cases, this infection can lead to an immune response in which antibodies attack the heart as well as the bacteria. Many of the 96,000 annual operations on heart valves in the United States are related to rheumatic heart disease.[26]

Stroke

Like heart muscle, brain cells must have a continuous adequate supply of oxygen in order to survive. A **stroke** (also called a cerebrovascular accident) occurs when the blood supply to the brain is interrupted. Strokes may be caused by a **thrombus** (a clot in a blood vessel), an **embolus** (a clot that

has broken off a vessel and is floating in the bloodstream), or an **aneurysm** (a weakening in a blood vessel that causes it to bulge and, in severe cases, burst). Figure 15.6 illustrates these blood vessel disorders. When any of these events occurs, the result is the death of brain cells, which do not have the capacity to heal or regenerate. Some strokes are mild and cause only temporary dizziness or slight weakness or numbness. More serious interruptions in blood flow may cause speech impairments, memory problems, and loss of motor control.

Other strokes affect parts of the brain that regulate heart and lung function and kill within minutes. Stroke killed 167,366 Americans in 2000 and accounted for 1 in 14.3 of our total deaths, surpassed only by CHD and cancer.[27] On average, someone suffers a stroke every 53 seconds, with someone dying every 3 minutes.[28] About one in ten major strokes is preceded (days, weeks, or months before) by **transient ischemic attacks (TIAs),** brief interruptions of the blood supply to the brain that cause only temporary impairment. Symptoms of TIAs include dizziness, particularly at first rising in the morning, weakness, temporary paralysis or numbness in the face or other regions, temporary memory loss, blurred vision, nausea, headache, slurred speech, or other unusual physiological reactions. TIAs are often indications of an impending major stroke.

The warning signs of stroke include the following:

- Sudden weakness or numbness of the face, arm, or leg on one side of the body.
- Sudden dimness or loss of vision, particularly in only one eye.
- Loss of speech, or trouble talking or understanding speech.
- Sudden, severe headaches with no known cause.
- Unexplained dizziness, unsteadiness, or sudden falls, especially with any of the previously listed symptoms.

Stroke   A condition occurring when the brain is damaged by disrupted blood supply.

Thrombus   Blood clot.

Embolus   Blood clot that is forced through the circulatory system.

Aneurysm   A weakened blood vessel that may bulge under pressure and, in severe cases, burst.

Transient ischemic attacks (TIAs)   Brief interruptions of the blood supply to the brain that cause only temporary impairment; often an indicator of impending major stroke.

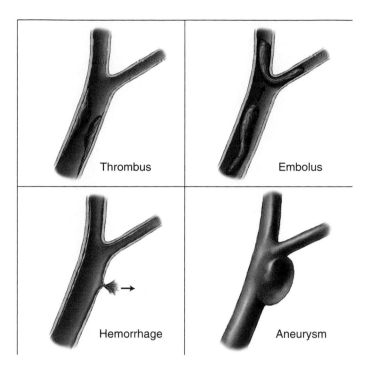

Figure 15.6
Common Blood Vessel Disorders

If you experience any of these symptoms, or if you are with someone who does, seek medical help immediately. The earlier treatment starts, the more effective it will be.

One of the greatest medical successes in recent years has been the decline in the fatality rates from strokes, a rate that has dropped by one third in the United States since the 1980s and continues to decline. Improved diagnostic procedures, better surgical options, clot-busting drugs injected early after a stroke has occurred, and acute care centers specializing in stroke treatment and rehabilitation have all been factors. Increased awareness of risk factors for stroke, especially high blood pressure, knowledge of warning signals, and an emphasis on prevention also have contributed. It is estimated that more than half of all remaining strokes could be avoided if more people followed the recommended preventive standards.

Unfortunately, those who survive a stroke do not always make a full recovery. Some 50 to 70 percent of stroke survivors regain functional independence, while 15 to 40 percent are permanently disabled and require assistance. Today stroke is a leading cause of serious long-term disability and contributes a significant amount to Medicaid and Medicare expenses for older Americans.[29]

Reducing Your Risk For Cardiovascular Diseases

What is your own risk for heart disease? Factors that increase the risk for cardiovascular problems fall into two categories: those we can control and those we cannot. Fortunately, we can take steps to minimize many risk factors.

Risks You Can Control

Avoid Tobacco   As early as 1984, the Surgeon General of the United States asserted that smoking was the greatest risk factor for heart disease. Today, one in five deaths from CVD are directly related to smoking.[30] Generally, the more a person smokes, the greater the risk for heart attack or stroke. The risk for cardiovascular disease is 70 percent greater for smokers than for nonsmokers. Smokers who have a heart attack are more likely to die suddenly (within one hour) than are nonsmokers. Evidence also indicates that chronic exposure to environmental tobacco smoke (ETS or passive smoking) increases the risk of heart disease by as much as 30 percent.[31]

How does smoking damage the heart? There are two plausible explanations. One theory states that nicotine increases heart rate, heart output, blood pressure, and oxygen use by heart muscles. Because the carbon monoxide in cigarette smoke displaces oxygen in heart tissue, the heart is forced to work harder to obtain sufficient oxygen. The other theory states that chemicals in smoke damage the lining of the coronary arteries, allowing cholesterol and plaque to accumulate more easily. This additional buildup constricts the vessels, increasing blood pressure and causing the heart to work harder.

When people stop smoking, regardless of how long or how much they've smoked, their risk of heart disease declines rapidly.[32] Three years after quitting, the risk of death from heart disease and stroke for people who smoked a pack a day or less is almost the same as for people who never smoked. Quitting today will also raise your HDL levels, reducing your risks even further (see the next section).[33]

Cut Back on Fats and Cholesterol   How concerned should you be about the amount of fat and cholesterol in your diet? Very concerned. According to recent evidence, cholesterol risks may be greater than ever for Americans. In their *Third Report on Detection, Evaluation, and Treatment of Cholesterol National Guidelines,* dietary experts at the National Heart, Lung and Blood Institute (NHLBI) gave Americans a wake-up call by slashing the levels of cholesterol that are considered acceptable. These guidelines not only provide evidence that cholesterol levels are out of control in the United States but also indicate that the number of people needing cholesterol-cutting drugs may be three times higher than originally thought. In fact, nearly 36 million people in the United States—one-fifth of all adults—may require medications to avoid cardiovascular problems.[34]

Why all the fuss about fats and cholesterol? Diets high in saturated fats are known to raise cholesterol levels, send the body's blood-clotting system into high gear, and make the blood sludgy in just a few hours, increasing the risk of heart attack or stroke. Studies indicate that fatty foods apparently trigger production of *factor VII,* a blood-clotting substance. Switching to a low-fat diet lowers the risk of clotting.

A fatty diet also increases the amount of cholesterol in the blood, contributing to atherosclerosis. In past years, cholesterol levels between 200 to 240 milligrams per 100 milliliters of blood (mg/dL) were considered normal. Recent research indicates that levels between 180 and 200 mg/dL are more desirable and that 150 mg/dL levels would be even better to reduce CVD risks.[35] See Table 15.1.

However, it isn't just the total cholesterol level that you should be concerned about. It is important to know that cholesterol comes in two main varieties: **low-density lipoprotein (LDL)** and **high-density lipoprotein (HDL).** Low-density lipoprotein, often referred to as "bad" cholesterol, is believed to build up on artery walls. In contrast, high-density lipoprotein, or "good" cholesterol, appears to remove cholesterol from artery walls, thus serving as a protector. In theory, if LDL levels get too high or HDL levels too low, largely because of too much saturated fat in the diet, a lack of physical exercise, high stress levels, or genetic predisposition, cholesterol will accumulate inside arteries and lead to cardiovascular problems. Scientists now believe that there are other factors that may increase CVD risk. A component of HDL known

as LP(a) may be the most important element of the HDL makeup. The more of this protective protein a person has, the lower the risk for CVD seems to be.[36]

The goal is to control the ratio of HDL to total cholesterol, by lowering LDL levels, raising HDL, or both. Regular exercise and a healthy diet low in saturated fat continue to be the best methods for maintaining healthy ratios. However, if dietary efforts and exercise do not reduce total cholesterol or LDL, several medications are available that may help.

Triglycerides, another type of fat in the blood, also appear to promote atherosclerosis. As people get older, heavier, or both, their triglycerides and cholesterol levels tend to rise. Although some CVD patients have elevated triglyceride levels, a causal link between high triglyceride levels and CVD has yet to be established. It may be that high triglyceride levels do not directly cause atherosclerosis but, rather, are among the abnormalities that speed its development.

While it is wise to cut back on saturated fat, be aware that some fat is necessary to overall health. Ironically, the consumption of too many low-fat or fat-free foods, such as salad dressings and other products, may actually contribute to the escalating problem of obesity in America. According to top researchers, it is better to eat foods with olive oil, canola oil, and other monounsaturated fats than to consume low-fat or no-fat products. (For a complete discussion of this topic, see Chapter 8.) Of course, all fat intake should be in moderation.

Monitor Your Cholesterol Levels   To get an accurate assessment of your total cholesterol and LDL and HDL levels, consider a lipoprotein analysis. This analysis requires that you not eat or drink anything for 12 hours prior to the test and that a reputable health provider do the analysis. The LDL level is derived using a standard formula:

$$LDL = total\ cholesterol - HDL - (triglycerides \div 5)$$

For example, if the level of total cholesterol is 200, the level of HDL 45, and the level of triglycerides 150, the LDL level would be 125 (200 – 45 – 30).

In general, LDL is more closely associated with cardiovascular risk than is total cholesterol. However, most authorities agree that looking only at LDLs ignores the positive effects of HDL. Perhaps the best method of evaluating risk is to examine the ratio of HDL to total cholesterol or the percentage of HDL in total cholesterol. If the level of HDL is lower than 35, the risk increases dramatically.

Change Lifestyle to Reduce Your Risk   Of the more than 100 million Americans who need to worry about their cholesterol levels, almost half, particularly those at the low-to-moderate risk levels, should be able to reach their LDL and HDL goals through lifestyle changes alone. People who are at higher risk or those for whom lifestyle modifications make no difference may need to take cholesterol-lowering drugs while they continue modifying their lifestyle. See Table 15.2 for a list of current cholesterol-fighting drugs, their side effects, and factors to consider.

Table 15.2
Common Cholesterol-Lowering Drugs

DRUG*	COST†	TYPICAL BENEFIT	SIDE EFFECTS	COMMENTS
Statins				
Alorvastatin (Lipitor)	$57 to $98	LDL ↓ 20%–60%	Mild stomach or muscle pain fairly common; severe muscle pain rare, though more common when taken with gemfibrozil, niacin, or certain antifungals and antibiotics. Abnormal liver function in 1% to 2% of patients; to prevent liver damage, liver tests must be done for first 3 months, periodically thereafter.	Best choice for most people with high LDL since it's by far the most effective and generally the best tolerated. However, users must be sure to undergo periodic liver testing.
Cerivastatin (Baycol)	$46 to $68	HDL ↑ 5%–15%		
Fluvastatin (Lescol)	$41 to $83	Triglycerides ↓ 15%–30%		
Lovastatin (Mevacor)	$70 to $248			Proven to reduce total mortality in people with coronary disease; almost certainly has some effect on others as well. In addition to lipid effects, may protect heart by reducing inflammation and stabilizing plaque deposits. May also reduce risk of osteoporosis, stroke, Alzheimer's disease.
Pravastatin (Pravachol)	$70 to $113			
Simvastatin (Zocor)	$113			
Folic acids				
Gemfibrozil (generic, Lopid)	$29 to $85	LDL ↓ 5%–20%	Heartburn and stomach pain common; diarrhea, nausea, skin rash, gallstones, and muscle pain less common. Both drugs may increase effect of anticoagulants and certain oral antidiabetic drugs.	Good choice in people who have low HDL, high triglycerides, or both, especially when LDL isn't particularly high.
Fenofibrate (Tricor)	$71	HDL ↑10%–70%		
		Triglycerides ↓ 20%–50%		Gemfibrozil proven to reduce mortality in people who have coronary disease and low HDL, elevated triglycerides, and low LDL (including those with the metabolic syndrome). Fenofibrate has larger effect on LDL and triglycerides but not yet proven to reduce coronary risk.
Niacin				
Immediate release (generic Niacor)	$13 to $49	LDL ↓ 5%–25%	Skin flushing and itching common; gastrointestinal problems, blurred vision, fatigue, glucose intolerance, gout less common. Niaspan may be better tolerated.	Can also be good choice in people with low HDL and high triglycerides.
Extented release (generic Niaspan)	$11 to $65	HDL ↑ 15%–35%		
		Triglycerides ↓ 20%–50%		Proven to reduce mortality in people with coronary disease. People with diabetes or stomach ulcers should generally avoid niacin. Starting with low dose and pretreating with aspirin or ibuprofen can lessen skin side effects.

*A fourth class of drugs not included in the table—bile-acid resins such as cholestyramine (Questran), colestipol (Colestid), and colesevelam (Welchol)—can also be added when LDL levels don't fall enough.
†Average cost to consumer for 30 days of treatment based on data from retail pharmacies nationwide, provided by Scott-Levin's Source Prescription Audit May 2000 to April 2001. Lower price for statins is initial dose, higher price is maximum dose; lower price for others is generic, higher price is brand. Costs rounded off to nearest whole dollar.

Reduce Intake of Saturated Fats   Current guidelines suggest that you should reduce intake of saturated fat (obtained mostly from animal products) to *less than 7 percent of your total daily caloric expenditures*. Also, minimize your consumption of *trans*-fat (see Chapter 8), found in partially hydrogenated foods such as margarine, many fast foods, and many packaged products. According to the NHLBI, cutting back on saturated fats and *trans*-fats could reduce LDL levels by as much as 10 percent.[37] In addition, NHLBI experts advocate consuming fewer than 200 milligrams per day of cholesterol, which is found mainly in eggs and meat. Doing so may reduce LDL by as much as 5 percent.[38]

Maintain a Healthy Weight No question about it—body weight plays a role in CVD. Researchers are not sure whether high-fat, high-sugar, high-calorie diets are a direct risk for CVD or whether they invite risk by causing obesity, which strains the heart, forcing it to push blood through the many miles of capillaries that supply each pound of fat. A heart that has to continuously move blood through an overabundance of vessels may become damaged. Overweight people are more likely to develop heart disease and stroke even if they have no other risk factors. If you're overweight, losing even 5 to 10 pounds can make a significant difference of as much as 5 percent LDL reduction,[39] especially if you're an "apple" (thicker around your upper body and waist) rather than a "pear" (thicker around your hips and thighs). Your waist measurement divided by your hip measurement should be less than 0.9 (for men) and less than 0.8 (for women). (See Chapter 9 for more tips on weight control.)[40]

Modify Other Dietary Habits The NHLBI guidelines recommend the following dietary changes to reduce CVD risk:

• Consume 5 to 10 milligrams per day of soluble fiber from sources such as psyllium seeds, oat bran, fruits, vegetables, and legumes. (See Chapter 8.) Even this small dietary modification may result in another 5 percent drop in LDL levels.

• Consume about 2 grams per day of plant sterols or sterol derivatives, substances that reduce LDL cholesterol. They are available in products sich as Benecol or Take Control margarine. These are the first widely available sources of sterols, but more will be on the market soon. This has the potential to reduce LDL by another 5 percent.

• Although less widely supported by rigorous research findings, many experts believe that consuming at least 25 grams of soy protein from various soy foods, instead of dairy sources, could reduce LDL by 5 percent.

Exercise Regularly According to all available evidence, inactivity is a definite risk factor for CVD.[41] The good news is that you do not have to be an exercise junkie or fanatic to reduce your risk. Even modest levels of low-intensity physical activity—walking, gardening, housework, dancing—are beneficial if done regularly and over the long term. Exercise can increase HDL, lower triglycerides, and reduce coronary risks in several ways. For more information, see Chapter 10.

Making the above modifications could reduce LDL levels by as much as 35 percent—similar to taking any of the statin drugs typically prescribed.

Control Diabetes The recent NHLBI guidelines underscore the unique risks for CVD for people with diabetes. Diabetics who have taken insulin for a number of years have a greater chance of developing CVD. In fact, CVD is the leading cause of death among diabetic patients. Because overweight people have a higher risk for diabetes, distinguishing between the effects of the two conditions is difficult. Diabetics also tend to have elevated blood fat levels, increased atherosclerosis, and a tendency toward deterioration of small blood vessels, particularly in the eyes and extremities. However, through a prescribed regimen of diet, exercise, and medication, diabetics can control much of their increased risk for CVD (see Chapter 18).

Control Your Blood Pressure **Hypertension** refers to sustained high blood pressure. If it cannot be attributed to any specific cause, it is known as **essential hypertension.** Approximately 90 percent of all cases of hypertension fit this category. **Secondary hypertension** refers to hypertension caused by specific factors, such as kidney disease, obesity, or tumors of the adrenal glands. In general, the higher your blood pressure, the greater your risk for CVD.

Hypertension is known as the "silent killer" because it usually has no symptoms. Although it affects more than 50 million Americans over the age of 6, 20 percent of them don't know they have the condition, and only one-third of those who are aware of it have it under control.[42] Common forms of treatment are dietary changes (reducing salt and calorie intake), weight loss (when appropriate), the use of diuretics and other medications (only when prescribed by a physician), regular exercise, and the practice of relaxation techniques and effective coping and communication skills.

Blood pressure is measured in two parts and is expressed as a fraction—for example, 110/80, or 110 over 80. Both values are measured in *millimeters of mercury* (mm Hg). The first number refers to **systolic pressure,** or the pressure being applied to the walls of the arteries when the heart *contracts,* pumping blood to the rest of the body. The second value is **diastolic pressure,** or the pressure applied to the walls of the arteries during the heart's *relaxation* phase. During this phase, blood is reentering the chambers of the heart, preparing for the next heartbeat.

Normal blood pressure varies depending on weight, age, and physical condition, and for different groups of people, such as women and minorities. Systolic blood pressure tends to increase with age, while diastolic blood pressure increases until age 55 and then declines. As a rule, men have a greater risk for high blood pressure than women have until

Hypertension Sustained elevated blood pressure.

Essential hypertension Hypertension that cannot be attributed to any cause.

Secondary hypertension Hypertension caused by specific factors, such as kidney disease, obesity, or tumors of the adrenal glands.

Systolic pressure The upper number in the fraction that measures blood pressure, indicating pressure on the walls of the arteries when the heart contracts.

Diastolic pressure The lower number in the fraction that measures blood pressure, indicating pressure on the walls of the arteries during the relaxation phase of heart activity.

Table 15.3
Blood Pressure Values and What They Mean

CLASSIFICATION	SYSTOLIC READING	DIASTOLIC READING	ACTIONS
Normal	Below 130	Below 85	Recheck in two years.
High normal	130–139	85–89	Recheck in one year.
Mild hypertension	140–159	90–99	Check in two months.
Moderate hypertension	160–179	100–109	See physician within a month.
Severe hypertension	180 or above	110 or above	See physician immediately.

Note: If systolic and diastolic readings fall into different categories, follow recommendations for earlier follow-up.
Source: Adapted from "Sixth Report of the Joint National Committee on Detection, Evaluation, and Treatment of High Blood Pressure," National Heart, Lung, and Blood Institute, 1997, NIH Publication No. 98-4080 (see http://www.nhlbi.nih.gov/guidelines/hypertension/jnc6.pdf).

age 55, when their risks become about equal. At age 75 and over, women are more likely to have high blood pressure than men.[43] For the average person, 110 over 80 is a healthy blood pressure level. If your blood pressure exceeds 140 over 90, you probably need to take steps to lower it. See Table 15.3 for a summary of blood pressure values and what they mean.

High blood pressure (HBP) is usually diagnosed when systolic pressure is 140 or above. Diastolic pressure does not have to be high to indicate high blood pressure. When only systolic pressure is high, the condition is known as isolated systolic hypertension (ISH), the most common form of high blood pressure for older Americans.[44] Causes of HBP include narrowing of the arteries and the heart beating more quickly or more forcefully than it should. However, many times the underlying cause is not known.

Manage Stress Some scientists have noted a relationship between CVD risk and a person's stress level, behavior habits, and socioeconomic status. These factors may affect established risk factors. For example, people under stress may start smoking or smoke more than they otherwise would.[45] Other studies have challenged the apparent link between emotional stress and heart disease. Although it was once widely assumed that the Type A personality who suffered from high stress levels was a time bomb ticking toward a heart attack, this theory has not been proven clinically.

Researcher-physician Robert S. Eliot demonstrated that approximately one out of five people has an extreme cardiovascular reaction to stressful stimulation. These people experience alarm and resistance so strongly that, when under stress, their bodies produce large amounts of stress chemicals, which in turn cause tremendous changes in the cardiovascular system, including remarkable increases in blood pressure. These people are called *hot reactors*. Although their blood pressure may be normal when they are not under stress—for example, in a doctor's office—it increases dramatically in response to even small amounts of everyday stress.

Cold reactors are those who are able to experience stress (even to live as Type A's) without showing harmful cardiovascular responses. Cold reactors may internalize stress, but their self-talk and perceptions about the stressful events

lead them to a nonresponse state in which their cardiovascular system remains virtually unaffected.[46] Some research indicates that people who have an underlying predisposition toward a toxic core personality (in other words, who are chronically hostile and hateful) may be at greatest risk for a CVD event. See Chapter 3 for tips on managing your stress, whether you are a hot or cold reactor.

What do you think?

What is your resting heart rate? ✳ *You can find out by taking your pulse. Gently press the pads of your first two fingers against the inside of your wrist, just below the base of your thumb. Sit quietly, and count the number of beats that occur during a 10-second period. Multiply the number of beats by 6. Repeat the process.* ✳ *How does your heart rate compare to that of your friends?*

Risks You Cannot Control

There are, unfortunately, some risk factors for CVD that we cannot prevent or control. The most important are these:

- *Heredity.* Having a family history of heart disease appears to increase the risk significantly. Whether this is because of genetics or environment is an unresolved question.
- *Age.* Seventy-five percent of all heart attacks occur in people over age 65. The rate of CVD increases with age for both sexes.
- *Gender.* Men are at much greater risk for CVD until old age. Women under 35 have a fairly low risk unless they have high blood pressure, kidney problems, or diabetes. Using oral contraceptives and smoking also increase the odds. Hormonal factors appear to reduce risk for women, although after menopause or after estrogen levels are otherwise reduced (e.g., by hysterectomy), women's LDL levels tend to go up, increasing their chances for CVD. (For more on the gender factor, see the next section.)

Disparity in CVD Risks

Cardiovascular disease is not an "equal opportunity" disease. In fact, when it comes to risk of attack and eventual mortality, there are huge disparities based on gender, race, and age. Consider the following:

- Higher CVD risks exist among black and Mexican American women than among white women of comparable socioeconomic status (SES). The striking differences by both ethnicity and SES underscore the critical need to improve screening, early detection, and treatment of CVD-related conditions for black and Mexican American women, as well as for women of lower SES in all ethnic groups.

- Among American Indians/Alaskan Natives age 18 and older, 63.7 percent of men and 61.4 percent of women have one or more CVD risk factors (hypertension, current cigarette smoking, high blood cholesterol, obesity, or diabetes). If data on physical activity had been included in this analysis, the prevalence of risk factors would have been much higher.

- In 1999, CHD death rates were 225.4 per 100,000 for white males and 216.4 for black males (7 percent higher) at all ages and stages of life.

- In 1999, CHD death rates were 135.0 per 100,000 for white females and 154.7 for black females.

- Blacks are 60 percent more likely to suffer a stroke than are whites, and two and a half times more likely to die from a stroke.

- A family history of diabetes, gout, high blood pressure, or high cholesterol increases one's risk of heart disease. Blacks are more likely to have these familial risk factors, increasing their overall chances for CVD.

- Cholesterol levels higher than 200 mg/dL in those age 20 and over are found in the following:

  53% of non-Hispanic white females
  47% of non-Hispanic black females
  43% of Mexican Americans
  28% of American Indians/Alaskan Natives
  27% of Asian/Pacific Islanders

Source: American Heart Association, "Heart and Stroke Facts," 2001.

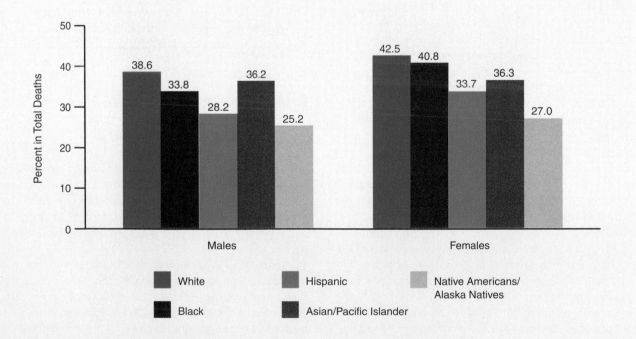

Deaths from Cardiovascular Disease in the United States: 2000 Mortality, Final Data
Source: American Heart Association. "2002 Heart and Stroke Statistical Update."

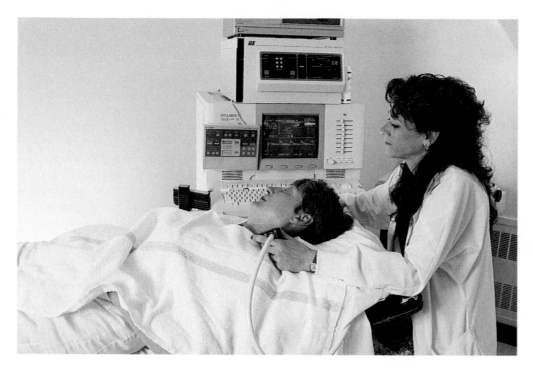

Heart attack symptoms experienced by women often differ from those of men. Shortness of breath, fatigue, and persistent jaw pain are more common symptoms among women.

• *Race.* Blacks are at 45 percent greater risk for hypertension and thus at greater risk for CVD than are whites. In addition, African Americans have less chance of surviving heart attacks, as discussed in the Health in a Diverse World box.

What do you think?

What risk factors for heart disease do you currently have? ✳ *What is your current resting heart rate?* ✳ *Do you know what your cholesterol level is?* ✳ *Which of your risk factors are the most critical?* ✳ *What actions can you start taking today to reduce your risk?*

Women and Cardiovascular Disease

While men tend to have more heart attacks and to have them earlier in life than do women, some interesting trends in survivability have emerged. In 1999, CVD claimed the lives of 445,692 men and a surprising 503,927 women in the United States. Why do more men have heart attacks and more women die of them? Why do some studies say that women have about the same mortality rates after myocardial infarction and others indicate there are vast differences, supported by actual numbers?[47] Although we understand the mechanisms that cause heart disease in men and women (or at least we think we do!), their experiences in the health care system, their reactions to life-threatening diseases, and a host of other technological and environmental factors may play a role in these statistics.

Risk Factors for Heart Disease in Women

Premenopausal women are unlikely candidates for heart attacks, except for those who suffer from diabetes, high blood pressure, or kidney disease or who have a genetic predisposition to high cholesterol levels. Family history and smoking can also increase the risk.

The Role of Estrogen   Once her estrogen production drops with menopause, a woman's chance of developing CVD rises rapidly. A 60-year-old woman has the same heart attack risk as a 50-year-old man. By her late 70s, a woman has the same heart attack risk as a man her age. To date, much of this changing risk has been attributed to the aging process, but the role of estrogen remains unclear. Early studies of various **hormone replacement therapies (HRTs)** indicated that HRT might reduce the risk of CVD by as much as 12 to 25 percent. However, newer findings throw a huge wrench in what was previously believed to be the CVD-risk-reducing powers of HRT (see the Women's Health/Men's Health box on CVD and hormones). Even when their total blood cholesterol levels are higher than men's, however, women may be at less risk because they typically have a higher percentage of HDL.[48]

But that's only part of the story. It's true that women age 25 and over tend to have lower cholesterol levels than men of the same age. But when they reach 45, things change. Most men's cholesterol levels become more stable, while both LDL and total cholesterol levels in women start to rise. And the gap widens further beyond age 55.[49]

Hormone replacement therapies (HRTs)   Therapies that replace estrogen in postmenopausal women.

CVD Protection or Increased Risk? The Hormone Controversy

For decades, the prevailing wisdom was that taking hormones during and after menopause would not only reduce hot flashes, it would provide protection against cardiovascular disease in women. The rate of CVD increases in women only after menopause, leading experts to believe that by keeping hormone levels high after menopause, CVD risk would be controlled. Although scientists didn't really know why this apparent relationship existed, doctors began to prescribe hormones to millions of women. The results of a major study in the mid-1990s, the Postmenopausal Estrogen/Progestin Intervention (PEPI) Trial, seemed to give doctors the proof they needed that hormone replacement therapy (HRT) lowered CVD risk by raising levels of HDL and decreasing LDL. This led to widespread promotion of HRT as a panacea for CVD risk by professional organizations, doctors, educators, and the community at large. Other studies seemed to confirm these facts, and women moved to take HRT in unprecedented numbers—some 38 percent of all post-menopausal women in the most recent data.

Women choose to take HRT for various reasons. Although reduction of CVD risk has been one of the factors, most women take HRT because it is the most effective treatment for menopausal symptoms such as hot flashes, night sweats, sexual dysfunction and vaginal dryness, insomnia, and hair loss. For women experiencing these problems, short-term use of HRT to get them through the years when the symptoms are most disruptive may seem worth any small risk. Other women took HRT because it has been shown to reduce the risk of bone fractures and osteoporosis, another major threat to older women's health.

NEW FINDINGS RAISE QUESTIONS

Today, results from several new studies provide growing evidence that the advice to take HRT to prevent CVD was not only inaccurate, it may have been deadly for some of those who followed it. Consider the following:

- The 1998 Heart and Estrogen/Progestin Replacement Study (HERS), a large-scale, randomized, controlled clinical trial, showed that after four years on HRT, there was no difference in heart attack rates but higher rates of coronary death for those on HRT compared to those taking a placebo. Perhaps the most alarming results of HERS indicated a 52 percent increase in cardiovascular events in the first year for those taking HRT.
- The 2000 Estrogen Replacement and Atherosclerosis (ERA) Trial, the first study to use angiographic images to assess the effects of HRT and estrogen replacement therapy (ERT) on women with pre-existing coronary disease, showed no effect on disease progression with hormone replacement.
- In the spring of 2000, investigators conducting the huge (over 26,000 participants) Women's Health Initiative (WHI) study stirred up even more controversy. Researchers announced that they had noted an alarming trend in their data that suggested that women on HRT in the study were experiencing a small but unacceptable increase in heart attacks, blood clots in the lungs (pulmonary embolism) and legs (deep vein thrombosis), and stroke. Although the study was scheduled to continue until 2005, these results caused the researchers to stop this portion of the study and send warning letters to women in the trial informing them of the possible risk. One version of HRT, known as Prempro, appeared to pose a greater risk than others.

WHAT ARE THE IMPLICATIONS FOR CONSUMERS?

Should a woman toss out her hormones based on the WHI results? Generally, experts recommend that if you are overweight, have high cholesterol, or have a family history of heart disease, you may already be at increased risk for cardiovascular disease, and it may be prudent to look for alternatives.

How great *is* the risk? Scientists indicate that if 10,000 women took HRT for one year:

The number of women with	Would increase by	Would decrease by
Breast cancer	8[*]	
Heart attack	7	
Stroke	8	
Pulmonary embolism	8[**]	
Venous thrombosis	10[**]	
Colorectal cancer		6[***]
Hip fracture		5

[*]Risk appears after four years of use.

[**]Risk is greatest in first two years of use.

[***]Benefit appears after three years of use.

It should be noted that these increased risks apply to women on HRT, not on estrogen alone. They also do not apply to women who had had hysterectomies and were on HRT. The decision to use ERT or HRT is complex and should be made in consultation with knowledgeable health care providers and after reviewing the latest information from reputable sources. The most important thing to take away from the WHI findings is that HRT does not seem to prevent or improve cardiovascular risks, so no woman should take it to protect against heart attacks or stroke.

New information about the effects of estrogen alone, or various levels of HRT, may become available soon. If you have questions about the exact findings of the studies or where you might get additional information, the references below are valuable sources of information.

Sources: The Postmenopausal Estrogen/Progestin Intervention (PEPI) Trial: The Writing Group for the PEPI Trial, "Effects of Estrogen or Estrogen/Progestin regimens on Heart Disease Risk Factors in Menopausal Women," *JAMA* 273 (1995): 199–208; L. Mosca, D. Herrington, R. Pasternak, K. Schenck-Gustafsson, S. Smith, and N. Wenger, "Hormone Replacement Therapy and Cardiovascular Disease," *Circulation* 104 (2001): 499 (see http://circ.ahajournals.or/cgi/content/full/104/4/4 99); S. Hulley, D. Grady, T. Bust, et al.,

"Randomized Trial of Estrogen Plus Progestin for Secondary Prevention of Coronary Heart Disease in Postmenopausal Women," Heart and Estrogen/Progestin Replacement Study (HERS) Research Group, *JAMA* 280 (1998): 605–613; Writing Group for the Women's Health Initiative Investigators, "Risks and Benefits of Estrogen Plus Progestin in Healthy Postmenopausal Women," *JAMA* 288 (3) (2002); U.S. Preventive Services Task Force, "Hormone Replacement Therapy for Primary Prevention of Chronic Conditions: Recommendations and Rationale," October 2002, Agency for Healthcare Research and Quality, Rockville, MD (see http://www.ahrq.gov/clinic/3rduspstf/hrt/hrtrr.htm); C. Runowics, "A Clearer Picture of HRT," *Health News* 8 (9) (September 2002): 1–4.

Before age 45, women's total blood cholesterol levels average below 220 mg/dL. By the time she is 45 to 55, the average woman's blood cholesterol rises to between 223 and 246 mg/dL. Studies of men have shown that for every 1 percent drop in cholesterol, there is a 2 percent decrease in CVD risk.[50] If this holds true for women, prevention efforts focusing on dietary interventions and exercise may significantly help postmenopausal women.

Neglect of Heart Disease Symptoms in Women

During the past decade, research has suggested three main reasons for the widespread neglect of the signs of heart disease in women: (1) Physicians may be gender-biased in their delivery of health care, tending to concentrate on women's reproductive organs rather than on the whole woman; (2) physicians tend to view male heart disease as a more severe problem because men have traditionally had a higher incidence of the disease; and (3) women decline major procedures more often than men do. Other explanations for diagnostic and therapeutic difficulties encountered by women with heart disease include the following:[51]

- Delay in diagnosing a possible heart attack.
- The complexity involved in interpreting chest pain in women.
- Typically less aggressive treatment of women who are heart attack victims.
- Their older age, on average, and greater frequency of other health problems.
- The fact that women's coronary arteries are often smaller than men's, making surgical or diagnostic procedures more difficult technically.
- Their increased incidence of postinfarction angina and heart failure.

In addition, symptoms of heart attack often differ for women and men, making it more difficult for women to determine whether to go to the doctor. See the Women's Health/Men's Health box on page 436 for more information on disparities in treatment of CVD between men and women. While there is considerable debate over whether inequities exist in treatment of CVD in men compared to women, at least one study suggests that any disparities may reflect overtreatment of men rather than undertreatment of women.[52]

Gender Bias in CVD Research?

The traditional view that heart disease is primarily a male problem has carried over into research as well. A well-publicized example was a study suggesting that aspirin could help prevent heart attacks—based entirely on its effects in 22,000 male doctors. To address such concerns, the National Institutes of Health has launched a 15-year, $625 million study of 140,000 postmenopausal women (known as the Women's Health Initiative), focusing on the leading causes of death and disease. Researchers hope to determine how a healthy lifestyle and increased medical attention can help prevent women's heart disease, as well as cancer and osteoporosis.

> **What do you think?**
>
> *How do men and women differ in their experiences related to CVD? ✳ Why do you think women's risks were largely ignored until fairly recently? ✳ What actions do you think individuals can take to help improve the situation for both men and women? ✳ What actions can communities and medical practitioners take?*

Differences Between the Sexes: Key Factors in Early Detection and Prognosis

As more research is done concerning diagnosis and treatment of CVD, it is clear that women sometimes experience different symptoms and benefit from different treatments than men do. For example, consider the following:

FEELING PAIN

Several studies have documented that women experience pain more acutely and more frequently than men, indicating that the sexes may detect and react to pain differently. In a study of dental patients, women responded more favorably than men to a class of pain relievers known as kappa opioids, including pentazocine. This finding suggests that receptors for inhibiting pain may vary by sex. Also, women appear to be less responsive than men to non-steroidal anti-inflammatory drugs, such as ibuprofen. Women typically need slightly lower doses of aspirin and should be warned that taking 325 mg of aspirin per day may result in anticoagulation levels that exceed those of men. Surgical risks, accidents that lead to excessive bleeding, and so on, may be greater for aspirin-using women.

NOTING HEART ATTACK SYMPTOMS

Although we are taught that the classic symptom of a heart attack is chest-crushing pain, this type of pain is not that common in women. Women's heart attacks, by contrast, tend to show up as shortness of breath, fatigue, and jaw pain, stretched out over hours rather than minutes. Women tend to suffer their first heart attack 10 years later than men, and in part because they are older when they have these attacks, they are more likely to die. Because women have the benefits of estrogen for so many years and because estrogen helps keep blood vessels elastic and free of plaque formation, they have a decreased risk of heart disease compared to men during their early years. Estrogen also is believed to signal the liver to produce more HDL, or good cholesterol.

TREATING CVD

Interestingly, drugs used to break up clots and stabilize erratic heartbeats are less effective in women than in men. Beta blockers, one common form of treatment for reducing blood pressure and migraines, take longer to metabolize in women than in men, meaning that women often have more difficulty regulating dosage and preventing side effects. Until recently, hormone replacement therapy—estrogen and progestin—had been believed to help. Now that beneficial effect has been shown to be nonexistent (see the Women's Health/Men's Health box on hormonal protection). Recent studies have shown that angioplasty, a technique in which a small, flexible catheter is inserted in coronary vessels to break up plaque and clear blocked arteries, is one of the best techniques for reducing risk of heart attack.

New Weapons Against Heart Disease

The victim of a heart attack today has a variety of options that were not available a generation ago. Medications can strengthen heartbeat, control arrhythmias, remove fluids in case of congestive heart failure, and relieve pain. New surgical procedures are saving many lives.

Techniques of Diagnosing Heart Disease

Several techniques are used to diagnose heart disease, including electrocardiogram, angiography, and positron emission tomography scans. An **electrocardiogram (ECG)** is a record of the electrical activity of the heart, measured during a stress test. Patients walk or run on treadmills while their hearts are monitored. A more accurate method of testing for heart disease is **angiography** (often referred to as *cardiac catheterization*), in which a needle-thin tube called a *catheter* is threaded through heart arteries, a dye is injected, and an x-ray is taken to discover which areas are blocked. (See New Horizons in Health box on page 438.) A more recent and even more effective method of measuring heart activity is **positron emission tomography (PET scan),** which produces three-dimensional images of the heart as blood flows through it. During a PET scan, a patient receives an intravenous injection of a radioactive tracer. As the tracer decays, it emits positrons that are picked up by the scanner and transformed by a computer into color images of the heart. Other tests include the following:

- *Radionuclide imaging* (includes tests such as thallium test, MUGA scan, and acute infarct scintigraphy). These procedures involve injecting substances called radionuclides into the bloodstream. Computer-generated pictures can then show them in the heart. These tests can show how well the heart muscle is supplied with blood, how well the heart's chambers are functioning, and which part of the heart has been damaged by a heart attack.
- *Magnetic resonance imaging* (also called MRI or NMR). This test uses powerful magnets to look inside the body. Computer-generated pictures can reveal the heart muscle and help physicians identify damage from a heart attack, diagnose congenital heart defects, and evaluate disease of larger blood vessels such as the aorta.

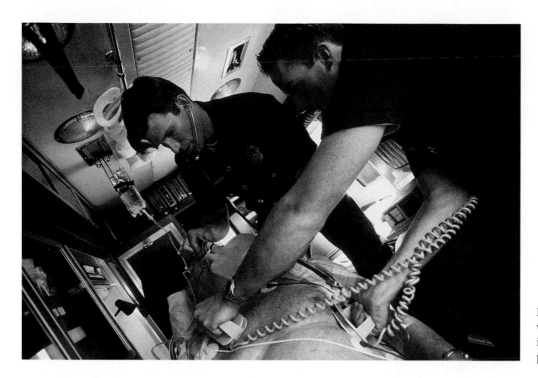

Because 40 percent of heart attack victims die within the first hour, immediate attention is vital to the patient's survival.

• *Digital cardiac angiography* (also called DCA or DSA). This modified form of computer-aided imaging records pictures of the heart and its blood vessels.

Angioplasty versus Bypass Surgery

Coronary bypass surgery has helped many patients who had coronary blockages or suffered heart attacks. In coronary bypass surgery, a blood vessel taken from another site in the patient's body (usually the *saphenous vein* in the leg or the *internal mammary artery*) is implanted to transport blood by bypassing blocked arteries. Bypass patients typically spend four to seven days in the hospital to recuperate. The average cost of the procedure itself is well over $50,000, and the additional intensive care treatments and follow-ups often result in total medical bills of $125,000. Death rates are generally much lower at medical centers where surgical teams and intensive care teams see large numbers of patients.[53]

Another procedure, called **angioplasty** (sometimes called *balloon angioplasty*), carries fewer risks and may be more effective than bypass surgery in selected cases. As in angiography, a needle-thin catheter is threaded through blocked heart arteries. The catheter has a balloon at the tip, which is inflated to flatten fatty deposits against the artery walls, allowing blood to flow more freely. Angioplasty patients are generally awake but sedated during the procedure and spend only one or two days in the hospital after treatment. Most people can return to work within five days. In about 30 percent of patients, the treated arteries become clogged again within six months. Some patients may undergo the procedure as many as three times within a five-year period. Some surgeons argue that given angioplasty's high rate of recurrence, bypass may be a more effective treatment.

Research suggests that in many instances, drug treatments may be just as effective in prolonging life as the invasive surgical techniques, but it is critical that doctors follow an aggressive drug treatment program and that patients comply with it.

Aspirin for Heart Disease: Can It Help?

Research indicates that low-dose aspirin (80 milligrams daily or every other day) is beneficial to heart patients due to its blood-thinning properties. It has even been advised as a

Electrocardiogram (ECG) A record of the electrical activity of the heart measured during a stress test.

Angiography A technique for examining blockages in heart arteries. A catheter is inserted into the arteries, a dye is injected, and an x-ray is taken to find the blocked areas. Also called *cardiac catheterization*.

Positron emission tomography (PET scan) Method for measuring heart activity by injecting a patient with a radioactive tracer that is scanned electronically to produce a three-dimensional image of the heart and arteries.

Coronary bypass surgery A surgical technique whereby a blood vessel is implanted to bypass a clogged coronary artery.

Angioplasty A technique in which a catheter with a balloon at the tip is inserted into a clogged artery; the balloon is inflated to flatten fatty deposits against artery walls, allowing blood to flow more freely.

Advances against Heart Disease and Stroke

Although heart disease continues to be the leading cause of death in the United States, actual rates of heart disease have declined substantially in recent decades. Every year we learn more about the functioning of the heart, and this knowledge has helped promote preventive behaviors as well as increases in longevity among those who have experienced a heart or stroke event. As we begin the new millennium, health officials cite major strides in preventing and treating cardiovascular health problems:

- *High blood pressure gene.* Discovery of a gene that produces a special protein receptor that appears to serve as a "master regulator of the body's handling of salt" provides researchers with greater insight into an inherited form of high blood pressure in children. A defective gene makes the receptor stick in the "on" position, which causes the kidneys to retain salt, leading to increases in blood pressure.
- *Congenital heart defects.* A genetic defect has been identified as the cause of DiGeorge syndrome, a condition marked by malformations of the heart and face. Identification of this missing gene, called UFD1, may provide clues to the prevention and treatment of congenital heart defects.

- *New diagnostic testing.* A special process called microarray analysis can detect missing or defective genes more quickly than ever before. Using this process, researchers found a genetic defect in people with Tangier disease, a blood-fat disorder caused by a shortage of HDL, the good cholesterol that carries fat from tissues. This knowledge may help researchers learn more about raising HDL levels for millions of individuals.
- *Reducing "stunning."* Scientists have found the cause of "stunning," a condition in which the heart's pumping action is severely weakened and that often strikes after heart attacks or heart surgery. The problem has been traced to a genetic flaw that affects a protein, troponin I, needed for normal heart contractions.
- *Tissue growth.* Remarkable advances in tissue engineering have enabled scientists to successfully grow heart valves in the laboratory. These new valves may eventually replace the mechanical valves and preserved pig valves commonly used now.
- *Diabetes link.* A link between diabetes and CVD has resulted in diabetes joining smoking, high blood pressure, high cholesterol, and lack of exercise as a risk factor for heart disease and stroke. It is now believed that diabetes increases the risk of dying of heart attack, stroke, heart failure, or kidney failure threefold.
- *New uses for an old drug.* A study of 10,000 heart and diabetes patients

found that a standard high blood pressure drug, ramipril, can reduce the risk of death from a wide range of circulatory problems and may help prevent atherosclerosis.
- *New clot busters.* Experimental blood clot busters were shown to prevent brain damage and disability from stroke if given within three to six hours after the attack.
- *New imaging procedures.* New ultrafast CT imaging and magnetic resonance angiography (MRA), which uses magnets and radio waves to view the inside of arteries, offer exciting new means of noninvasive diagnosis of artery blockage.
- *Robotic surgery.* Preliminary studies on the use of robotics in bypass surgery provide hope for safer options. Operating through three small holes in the chest, robotic arms mimic the actions of a surgeon working the controls. The use of robotics provides greater steadiness, eliminates human error, and increases the potential for microsurgery.

Sources: National Institutes of Health, National Heart, Lung, and Blood Institute; "Heart Memo," 1999; Dr. Claude Lenfant and Dr. Phillip Gorden, "Diabetes Mellitus: A Major Risk Factor for Cardiovascular Disease," National Institutes of Health, National Heart, Lung, and Blood Institute, News Release, September 1, 1999; Live Healthier, Live Longer website at http://rover.nhlbi.nih.chd; American Heart Association, "Gene Discoveries among Top 10 Research Advances in Heart Disease and Stroke for 1999," AHA News Release, December 30, 1999.

preventive strategy for individuals with no current heart disease symptoms. However, major problems associated with aspirin use are gastrointestinal intolerance and a tendency for some people to have difficulty with blood clotting, and these factors may outweigh its benefits in these cases. Although the findings concerning aspirin and heart disease are inconclusive, the research seems promising.[54]

Thrombolysis Injection of an agent to dissolve clots and restore some blood flow, thereby reducing the amount of tissue that dies from ischemia.

Thrombolysis

Whenever a heart attack occurs, prompt action is vital. When a coronary artery is blocked, the heart muscle doesn't die immediately, but time determines how much damage occurs. If a victim reaches an emergency room and is diagnosed fast enough, a form of reperfusion therapy called **thrombolysis** can be performed. Thrombolysis involves injecting an agent such as TPA (tissue plasminogen activator) to dissolve the clot and restore some blood flow, thereby reducing the amount of tissue that dies from ischemia.[55] These drugs must be used within one to three hours after a heart attack for best results.

Cardiac Rehabilitation

Every year, nearly 1 million people survive heart attacks. Over 7 million more have unstable angina and about 650,000 undergo bypass surgery or angioplasty. Heart failure is the most common discharge diagnosis for hospitalized Medicare patients and the fourth most common diagnosis among all patients hospitalized in the United States. Most of these patients are eligible for cardiac rehabilitation (including exercise training and health education classes on good nutrition and CVD risk management), needing only a doctor's prescription for these services. However, many Americans do not have access to these programs, and many find them difficult to afford in light of skyrocketing costs for prescription drugs. While some patients must choose between home health care and cardiac rehabilitation, others stay away from such programs due to cost, transportation, or other factors. Perhaps the biggest deterrent is fear of having another attack due to exercise exertion. The benefits of cardiac rehabilitation (including increased stamina and strength and faster recovery), however, far outweigh the risks when these programs are run by certified health professionals.

Personal Advocacy and Heart-Smart Behaviors

People who suspect they have cardiovascular disease are often overwhelmed and frightened. Where should they go for diagnosis? What are the best treatments? Answering these questions becomes even more difficult if they are upset, scared, or tend to listen unquestioningly to doctors' orders. If you or a loved one must face a CVD crisis, it is important to act with knowledge, strength, and assertiveness. The following suggestions will help you deal with hospitals and health care providers in the wake of a cardiac event or any major health problem (see Chapter 22 for more on being a smart consumer of health care services):

1. *Know your rights as a patient.* Ask about the risks and costs of various diagnostic tests. Some procedures, particularly angiography, may pose significant risks for people who are elderly, who have a history of minor strokes, or who have had chemotherapy or other treatments that could have dam-

aged their blood vessels. Ask for test results and an explanation of any abnormalities.

2. *Find out about informed consent procedures, living wills, durable power of attorney, organ donation, and other legal issues before you become sick.* Having someone shove a clipboard in your face and ask you if life support can be terminated in case of a problem is one of the great horrors of many people's hospital experiences. Be prepared.

3. *Ask about alternative procedures.* If possible, seek a second opinion at a different health care facility (in other words, get at least two opinions from doctors who are not in the same group and who cannot read each other's diagnoses). New research indicates that doctors may not use drug treatments as aggressively as they could and that medications may be as effective as major bypass or open heart surgeries. Ask, ask, and ask again. Remember, it is your life, and there is always the possibility that another treatment will be better for you.

4. *Remain with your loved one as a "personal advocate."* If your loved one is weak and unable to ask questions, ask the questions yourself. Inquire about new medications, new tests, and other potentially risky procedures that may be undertaken during the course of treatment or recovery. If you feel your loved one is being removed from intensive care or other closely monitored areas prematurely, ask if the hospital is taking this action to comply with DRGs (established limits of treatment for certain conditions) and if this action is warranted. Most hospitals have waiting areas or special rooms so family members can stay close to a patient. Exercise your right to this option.

5. *Monitor the actions of health care providers.* To control costs, some hospitals are hiring nursing aides and other untrained personnel to handle duties previously performed by registered nurses. Ask about the patient-to-nurse ratio, and make sure that people monitoring you or your loved ones have appropriate credentials.

6. *Be considerate of your care provider.* One of the most stressful jobs any person can be entrusted with is care of a critically ill person after a major cardiac event. Although questions are appropriate and your emotions are running high, be as tactful and considerate as possible. Nurses often carry a disproportionate responsibility for the care of patients during critical times. They are often forced to carry a higher than necessary patient load. Try to remain out of their way, ask questions as necessary, and report any irregularities in care to the supervisor.

7. *Be patient with the patient.* The pain, suffering, and fears associated with a cardiac event often cause otherwise nice people to act in not-so-nice ways. Be patient and helpful, and allow time for the person to rest. Talk with the patient about his or her feelings, concerns, and fears. Do not ignore these concerns to ease your own anxieties.

We still have much to learn about CVD and its causes, treatments, and risk factors. Staying informed is an important part of staying healthy. Overall, choices in dietary habits, exercise patterns, management of stress, prompt attention to suspicious symptoms, and other behaviors can greatly enhance your chances of remaining CVD-free. Other factors that influence risk include how much emphasis our health care systems place on access to health care for all underserved populations,

education about risks, and other community-based interventions for those at high risk. Action on both community and individual levels can help address the challenge of CVD.

Taking Charge

15 15 **15**

Reducing the Risk of Cardiovascular Disease

Although it is easy to read about what we should be doing to keep our hearts and circulatory systems healthy, few of us ever really make a healthy heart one of our priorities. Other issues often take precedence over long-term commitment to cardiovascular wellness. Cardiovascular disease rarely occurs overnight; in some cases, a person is predisposed to it, but in most cases, it is the result of poor health behaviors.

What is your risk? Are you taking precautions to prevent the development of CVD? Although cardiovascular disease continues to plague persons of all ages, races, and socioeconomic statuses, many believe that we are winning the war against this dreaded killer. Medical advances in technology, pharmaceutical agents that control symptoms and lower risk, as well as major lifestyle adjustments can help you remain healthy well into your later

years. Are you motivated to change your health behaviors and help your cardiovascular system?

Checklist for Change

Making Personal Choices

☐ Determine your hereditary risk. If it is high, outline the steps that you can take to reduce your overall risk.

☐ Become familiar with the normal changes in CVD risk that occur with age. Take the extra steps needed to minimize your risks as you age.

☐ If you smoke, quit. If you don't smoke, don't start.

☐ Find out what your cholesterol level is, including your HDL and LDL levels.

☐ Reduce saturated fat in your diet, and take steps to reduce your triglyceride and cholesterol levels.

☐ Get out and exercise. Even a relaxing walk every day is a good

CVD risk reducer. Nobody says you have to run and exercise until you drop. Take it easy, but keep it up.

☐ Control your blood pressure. Monitor it regularly and see your doctor if you are hypertensive.

☐ Lose weight if you are overweight. Obesity is a significant risk factor for both men and women.

☐ Control your stress levels.

Making Community Choices

☐ Take a class in CPR. Your local Red Cross likely offers them; even your college may. Be prepared to offer bystander CPR.

☐ Consider becoming an emergency medical technician (EMT). You don't have to make a career of it. But you could be prepared to save people in your dorm, your office building, and your community.

☐ Volunteer for the local chapter of the American Heart Association. Give a few hours of your time answering phone calls and mailing information.

Summary

* Cardiovascular disease incidence and prevalence rates have changed considerably in the past 50 years. Certain segments of the population have disproportionate levels of risk.
* The cardiovascular system consists of the heart and circulatory system and is a carefully regulated, integrated network of vessels that supply the body with the nutrients and oxygen necessary to perform daily functions.
* Cardiovascular diseases include atherosclerosis (hardening of the arteries), heart attack, angina pectoris, arrhythmias, congestive heart failure, congenital and rheumatic heart disease, and stroke. These combine to be the leading cause of death in the United States today.
* Many risk factors for cardiovascular disease can be controlled, such as cigarette smoking, high blood fat and cho-

lesterol levels, hypertension, lack of exercise, high-fat diet, obesity, diabetes, and emotional stress. Some risk factors, such as age, gender, and heredity, cannot be controlled. Many of these factors have a compounded effect when combined. Dietary changes, exercise, weight reduction, and attention to lifestyle risks can greatly reduce susceptibility to cardiovascular disease.
* Women have a unique challenge in controlling their risk for CVD, particularly after menopause, when estrogen levels are no longer sufficient to be protective.
* New methods developed for treating heart blockages include coronary bypass surgery and angioplasty. Also, drugs such as beta blockers and calcium channel blockers can reduce high blood pressure and treat other

symptoms. Research has provided important clues on how best to prevent or reduce risk of CVD today. Recognizing your own risks and acting now to reduce risk are important elements of lifelong cardiovascular health.

Questions for Discussion and Reflection

1. Trace the path of a drop of blood from the time it enters the heart until it reaches the extremities.
2. List the different types of CVDs. Compare and contrast their symptoms, risk factors, prevention, and treatment.
3. What are the major indicators that CVD poses a particularly significant risk to people of your age? To the elderly? To people from selected minority groups?
4. Discuss the role that exercise, stress management, dietary changes, checkups, sodium reduction, and other factors can play in reducing risk for CVD. What role may chronic infections play in CVD risk?
5. Discuss why age is such an important factor in women's risk for CVD. What can be done to decrease women's risks in later life?
6. Describe some of the diagnostic and treatment alternatives for CVD. If you had a heart attack today, which treatment would you prefer? Explain why.

Application Exercises

Reread the What Do You Think? scenarios at the beginning of the chapter and answer the following questions.

1. Are the situations of Jim, Jennifer, and Sam typical of college athletes you know? Explain your answer. Why do you think so many young Americans deny their risk for CVD?
2. As a friend of one of these three athletes, what advice might you give?
3. Consider the behavior of coaches and doctors in the scenarios. What suggestions would you have for them? What role should colleges have in such situations?
4. What kinds of community support would help Jim, Jennifer, and Sam?

Accessing Your Health on the Internet

Visit the following Internet sites to explore further topics and issues related to personal health. To visit an organization's website, go to the Companion Website for *Access to Health, Eighth Edition* at www.aw.com/donatelle, click on the book image, and select "Accessing Your Health on the Internet" from the navigation menu on the left.

1. *American Heart Association.* Homepage for the leading private organization dedicated to heart health. This site provides information, statistics, and resources regarding cardiovascular care, including an opportunity to test your own risk for CVD.
2. *Johns Hopkins Cardiac Rehabilitation Homepage.* Information about prevention of heart disease and rehabilitation from CVDs from one of the best cardiac care centers in the United States, including information about programs available to help individuals stop smoking, lose weight, lower blood pressure and blood cholesterol, and reduce emotional stress.
3. *National Heart, Lung, and Blood Institute.* A valuable resource for information on all aspects of cardiovascular health and wellness.
4. *U.S. National Library of Medicine: Health Services/Technology Assessment Text.* Access to numerous databases of health care documents outlining procedures for clinicians and patients. Choose the database for the Agency for Health Care Policy and Research (AHCPR) to review various guidelines regarding all forms of cardiac care.

Further Reading

American Heart Association. *Heart and Stroke Facts*. Dallas, TX: American Heart Association.
   An annual overview providing facts and figures concerning cardiovascular disease in the United States. Supplement provides key statistics about current trends and future directions in treatment and prevention.

McCrum, Robert. *My Year Off: Recovering after a Stroke*. New York: Broadway Books, 1999.
   The chronicle of a young man's recovery from a severe stroke.

Pashkow, Frederic, and Charlotte Libov. *The Women's Heart Book*. New York: Hyperion, 2001.

Gersh, Bernard, and Michael Wood (eds.). *The Mayo Clinic Heart Book*. New York: William Morrow, 2000.
   These books provide an overview of heart disease in America, including risk factors, trends, and options for heart patients.

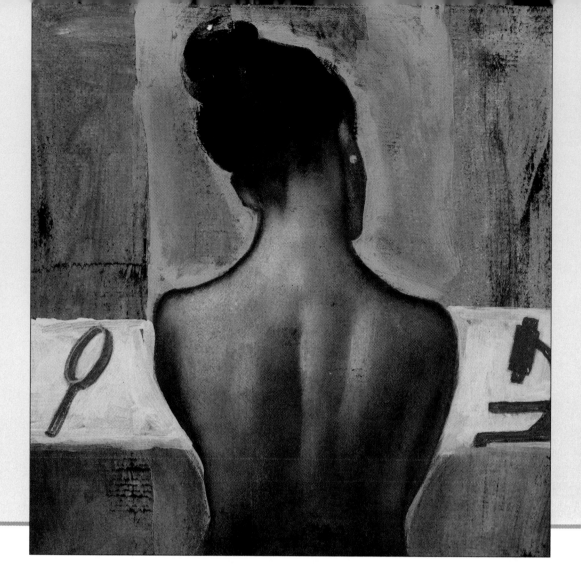

Objectives

* Define cancer and discuss how it develops.

* Discuss the causes of cancer, including biological causes, occupational and environmental hazards, lifestyle, psychological factors, chemicals in foods, viruses, medical causes, and combined causes.

* Describe the different types of cancer and the risks they pose to people at different ages and stages of life.

* Explain the importance of understanding and responding appropriately to self-exams, medical exams, and symptoms related to different types of cancer. Note how appropriate responses affect cancer survival rates.

* Discuss ways of preventing cancer and the implications of behavioral risks.

* Discuss cancer detection and treatment, including radiation therapy, chemotherapy, immunotherapy, and other common methods of detection and treatment in use today.

Cancer

Reducing Your Risk

What do you think?

Jeanie, a 20-year-old sophomore at a large Midwestern university, has just learned that her 26-year-old sister has advanced breast cancer. This news came a month after Jeannie learned that her grandmother had been diagnosed with breast cancer at age 78. Distraught, Jeanie decided to go to her doctor and ask for genetic tests to determine if she is at risk for breast cancer herself. She tells her friends that if she gets the test and finds that she has the "breast cancer gene," she has decided to have both breasts removed immediately to reduce her own risk.

Are Jeanie's concerns about possible increased risk for breast cancer legitimate? ✳ Why or why not? ✳ What actions would you recommend for someone in Jeanie's situation? ✳ Are such decisions for radical elective surgery ever warranted? ✳ Why or why not?

Nick, an avid sunbather, lives in Phoenix. He routinely "suns" himself for one to two hours a day. In bad weather, he goes to the health spa for tanning sessions to maintain his rugged, dark tan. When his girlfriend tells him that all that sun isn't good for him, he says that it helps his complexion and the tanning booths filter out all the bad ultraviolet light. He believes that because he has naturally dark hair and skin, he isn't at risk for any form of skin cancer. Anyway, he says, it's no big deal. Even if he does get skin cancer, he'll just go in and get it taken care of.

Is Nick's information about skin cancer correct? ✳ What are the risks associated with sunbathing in artificial and natural environments? ✳ If Nick insists on getting his tan, what actions can he take to reduce cancer risks?

As few as 50 years ago, a diagnosis of cancer was usually a death sentence. Health professionals could only guess at the cause, and treatments were often as deadly as the disease itself. Because we had no idea how a person "got" cancer, fears about possible infection led to ostracism and bigotry aimed at people who desperately needed support.

Fortunately, we've come a long way since then. Today we know that there are multiple causes of cancer and very few are linked to any type of infectious agent. Early detection and vast improvements in technology have dramatically improved the prognosis for most cancer patients. We also know that there are many actions we can take individually and as a society to prevent cancer. Knowing the facts about cancer, recognizing your own risk, and taking action to reduce your risk are important steps in the battle.

An Overview of Cancer

During 2003, approximately 556,500 Americans died of cancer and nearly 1.3 million new cases were diagnosed. Cancer is the second leading cause of death, exceeded only by heart disease, in the United States.[1] Put into perspective, this means that each day of the year more than 1,500 people die of some form of cancer. One of four deaths in the United States is from cancer; over 5 million lives have been lost since 1990. However, it is important to note that although more than 2.5 million people will be diagnosed with cancer in a year, nearly 4 in 10 will be alive five years after diagnosis. Many will be considered "cured," meaning that they have no subsequent cancer in their bodies five years after diagnosis and can expect to live a long and productive life.[2]

When adjusted for normal life expectancy (factors such as dying of heart disease, accidents, etc.), a relative five-year survival of 62 percent is seen for all cancers. Some cancers that only a few decades ago presented a very poor outlook are often cured today: acute lymphocytic leukemia in children, Hodgkin's disease, Burkitt's lymphoma, Ewing's sarcoma (a form of bone cancer), Wilms' tumor (a kidney cancer in children), testicular cancer, and osteogenic (bone) sarcoma are among the most remarkable indicators of progress.

Cancer   A large group of diseases characterized by the uncontrolled growth and spread of abnormal cells.

Neoplasm   A new growth of tissue that serves no physiological function and results from uncontrolled, abnormal cellular development.

Tumor   A neoplasmic mass that grows more rapidly than surrounding tissue.

Malignant   Very dangerous or harmful; refers to a cancerous tumor.

Benign   Harmless; refers to a noncancerous tumor.

Variations in Rates

While cancer strikes people of all ages, races, cultures, and socioeconomic levels, some Americans are at greater risk (see the Health in a Diverse World box). Overall, blacks are more likely to develop cancer than persons of any other racial and ethnic group. In 2002, incidence rates were 445.3 per 100,000 blacks and 401.4 per 100,000 whites; 270.0 per 100,000 Hispanics; 283.4 per 100,000 Asians/Pacific Islanders; and 202.7 per 100,000 Alaska Natives and American Indians.[3] Cancer sites for which blacks have significantly higher incidence and mortality rates include the esophagus, uterus, cervix, stomach, liver, prostate, and larynx. Blacks are 33 percent more likely to die of cancer than whites and more than twice as likely to die of cancer than Hispanics, Asians/Pacific Islanders, and American Indians. Researchers at the National Cancer Institute (NCI) believe that these differences are due more to blacks' lower average socioeconomic status and generally more limited access to health care than to any inherent physical characteristics.[4] Some findings indicate that certain cancers are simply more common in different races.

Cancer incidence and mortality rates within other minority groups, such as Hispanics, are often lower (sometimes by as much as 25 percent or more) than those of white or black Americans. Due to Hispanics' low average socioeconomic status, we might expect that they would have cancer rates similar to those of blacks. But Hispanics seem to be "protected" from high rates. Why? No one knows for sure, but the answer may lie in differences in diet, exercise patterns, or other culturally influenced behaviors. Because cancer risk is strongly associated with lifestyle and behavior, differences in ethnic and cultural groups can provide clues to factors involved in its development. Culturally influenced values and belief systems can also affect whether a person seeks care, participates in screenings, or follows recommended treatments. Socioeconomic factors such as lack of health insurance or lack of transportation to treatment centers can lead to late diagnosis and poor survival.

What Is Cancer?

Cancer is the name given to a large group of diseases characterized by the uncontrolled growth and spread of abnormal cells.[5] Think of a healthy cell as a small computer, programmed to operate in a particular fashion. Under normal conditions, healthy cells are protected by a powerful overseer, the immune system, as they perform their daily functions of growing, replicating, and repairing body organs. When something interrupts normal cell programming, however, uncontrolled growth and abnormal cellular development result in a new growth of tissue serving no physiologic function, which is called a **neoplasm.** This neoplasmic mass often forms a clumping of cells known as a **tumor.**

Not all tumors are **malignant** (cancerous); in fact, most are **benign** (noncancerous). Benign tumors are generally harmless unless they grow in such a fashion as to obstruct or crowd out normal tissues. A benign tumor of the brain, for

Cancer, Sex, and Race: Disparities in Incidence and Death

There's no question about it: If you are a black American, you are more likely to develop and die from cancer than persons of any other racial and ethnic group. Likewise, if you are a male, you have a much greater overall chance of dying of cancer than your female counterpart. While overall rates of cancer have decreased between 1992 and 1999 by 1.6 percent per year among Hispanics, by 0.9 percent among whites, and by 1.3 percent among blacks, rates among American Indians/Alaskan Natives and Asians/Pacific Islanders have remained fairly constant. Access to health care, diet, hormones, exposures to toxic chemicals in homes and on the job, and other factors contribute to these differences.

Incidence and Mortality Rates* by Site, Race, and Ethnicity, United States, 1992–1999

INCIDENCE	WHITE	BLACK	ASIAN/ PACIFIC ISLANDER	AMERICAN INDIAN/ ALASKAN NATIVE	HISPANIC†
All sites					
Males	568.2	703.6	408.9	277.7	393.1
Females	424.4	404.8	306.5	224.2	290.5
Total	480.4	526.6	348.6	244.6	329.6
Breast (female)	137.0	120.7	93.4	59.4	82.6
Colon and rectum					
Males	64.4	70.7	58.7	40.7	43.9
Females	46.1	55.8	39.5	30.8	29.7
Total	53.9	61.9	47.9	35.2	35.7
Lung and bronchus					
Males	82.9	124.1	63.8	51.4	44.1
Females	51.1	53.2	28.5	23.3	22.8
Total	64.3	82.6	44.0	35.4	31.5
Prostate	172.9	275.3	107.2	60.7	127.6

MORTALITY	WHITE	BLACK	ASIAN/ PACIFIC ISLANDER	AMERICAN INDIAN/ ALASKAN NATIVE	HISPANIC†
All sites					
Males	258.1	369.0	160.6	154.5	163.7
Females	171.2	204.5	104.4	110.4	105.7
Total	205.1	267.3	128.6	128.6	129.2
Breast (female)	29.3	37.3	13.1	14.8	17.5
Colon and rectum					
Males	26.7	34.8	16.5	14.6	16.6
Females	18.4	25.4	11.6	11.3	10.6
Total	21.9	29.1	13.7	12.8	13.2
Lung and bronchus					
Males	81.7	113.0	42.3	49.3	38.2
Females	41.1	39.6	19.3	24.9	13.8
Total	57.9	68.9	29.3	35.5	24.1
Prostate	32.9	75.1	15.1	18.8	22.6

*Per 100,000, age-adjusted to the 2000 U.S. standard population. Incidence rates obtained from SEER registries covering 10%-15% of the U.S. population. Mortality data are from all states.
†Hispanics are not mutually exclusive from whites, African American, Asian/Pacific Islanders, and American Indian/Alaskan Natives.
Source: Surveillance, Epidemiology, and End Results Program, 1973–99, Division of Cancer Control and Population Sciences, National Cancer Institute, Bethesda, MD, 2002. American Cancer Society Surveillance Research, 2003.

instance, is life threatening when it grows enough to restrict blood flow and cause a stroke. The only way to determine whether a tumor is malignant is through **biopsy,** or microscopic examination of cell development.

Benign and malignant tumors differ in several key ways. Benign tumors generally consist of ordinary-looking cells enclosed in a fibrous shell or capsule that prevents their spreading to other body areas. Malignant tumors are usually not enclosed in a protective capsule and can therefore spread to other organs. This process, known as **metastasis,** makes some forms of cancer particularly aggressive in their ability to overcome bodily defenses. By the time they are diagnosed, malignant tumors have frequently metastasized throughout the body, making treatment extremely difficult. Unlike benign tumors, which merely expand to take over a given space, malignant cells invade surrounding tissue, emitting clawlike protrusions that disturb the ribonucleic acid (RNA) and deoxyribonucleic acid (DNA) within normal cells. Disrupting these substances, which control cellular metabolism and reproduction, produces **mutant cells** that differ in form, quality, and function from normal cells. Assess your own cancer risk by completing the Assess Yourself box.

What Causes Cancer?

After decades of research, most cancer epidemiologists believe that cancers are, at least in theory, preventable, and many could be avoided by suitable choices in lifestyle and environment.[6] Many specific causes of cancer are believed to be known, the most important of which are smoking, obesity, and a few organic viruses; however, wide global variations in common cancers, such as those of the breast, prostate, colon, and rectum, remain unexplained. (See Figure 16.1.) Most research supports the idea that cancer is caused by both *external* (chemicals, radiation, viruses, and lifestyle) and *internal* (hormones, immune conditions, and inherited mutations) factors. Causal factors may act together or in sequence to promote cancer development.[7] We do not know why some people have malignant cells in their body and never develop cancer, while others may take 10 years or more to develop the disease.

Cellular Change/Mutation Theories

One theory of cancer development proposes that cancer results from a spontaneous error that occurs during cell reproduction. Perhaps cells that are overworked or aged are more likely to break down, causing genetic errors that result in mutant cells.

Another theory suggests that cancer is caused by some external agent or agents that enter a normal cell and initiate the cancerous process. Numerous environmental factors, such as radiation, chemicals, hormonal drugs, immunosuppressant drugs (drugs that suppress the normal activity of the immune system), and other toxins, are considered possible **carcinogens** (cancer-causing agents); perhaps the most com-

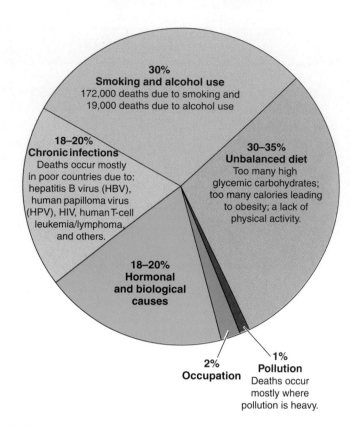

Figure 16.1

Factors Believed to Contribute to Global Causes of Cancer

Sources: Public session/panel discussion, Diet and Optimal Health International Conference, Linus Pauling Institute, May 2001 (panel participants: Steve Hecht, Bruce Ames, Jeffrey Blumberg, Barry Halliwall, Baley Irei); American Cancer Society, *Cancer Facts & Figures 2001.*

mon carcinogen is the tar in cigarettes. The greater the dose or exposure to environmental hazards, the greater the risk of disease. People who are forced to work, live, and pass through areas that have high levels of environmental toxins may be at greater risk for several types of cancers.[8]

A third theory came out of research on certain viruses that are believed to cause tumors in animals. This research led to the discovery of **oncogenes,** suspected cancer-causing genes that are present on chromosomes. Although oncogenes are typically dormant, scientists theorize that certain conditions such as age, stress, and exposure to carcinogens, viruses, and radiation may activate them. Once activated, they grow and reproduce in an out-of-control manner.

Scientists are uncertain whether only people who develop cancer have oncogenes or whether we all have **proto-oncogenes,** genes that can become oncogenes under certain conditions. Many **oncologists** (physicians who specialize in the treatment of malignancies) believe that the oncogene theory may lead to a greater understanding of how individual cells function and bring us closer to developing effective treatments.

Many factors are believed to contribute to cancer development. Combining risk factors can dramatically increase a person's risk for cancer.

Risks for Cancer—Lifestyle

Over the years, researchers have found that people who engage in certain behaviors show a higher incidence of cancer. In particular, diet, sedentary lifestyle (and resultant obesity), consumption of alcohol or cigarettes, stress, and other lifestyle factors seem to play a role. Likewise, colon and rectal cancer occur more frequently among persons with a high-fat, low-fiber diet; in those who don't eat enough fruits and vegetables; and in those who are inactive. See Chapter 8 on nutrition for information about certain dietary risks related to cancer and the role of supplements in prevention. More research is needed to pinpoint the mechanisms that act in the body to increase the odds of cancer. For now, there is compelling evidence that certain actions are clearly associated with a greater than average risk of developing the disease.

Relative risk is a measure of the strength of the relationship between risk factors and particular cancers. It compares the risk of developing cancer in persons with a certain exposure or trait to the risk in persons who do not have this exposure or trait. For example, male smokers have a 20-fold relative risk of developing lung cancer when compared with nonsmokers. This means that they are about 20 times more likely to develop lung cancer than nonsmokers. Most relative risks are not this large. Keep in mind that when there is a high relative risk for some exposure, it does not guarantee cause and effect; it merely indicates the likelihood of a particular risk factor being related to a particular outcome.

Smoking and Cancer Risk   Of all the potential risk factors for cancer, smoking is among the greatest. Over the five decades since British and American epidemiologists singled out tobacco as a culprit in lung cancer and other diseases, tar levels in British cigarettes have declined dramatically, as has the prevalence of smoking in general. As a result, the lung cancer rate for British men under age 55 has fallen by two-thirds since 1955, placing it among the lowest in the developed world. In the last 20 years, America's rates have shown a similar decline. Lung cancer rates among men are still increasing in most developing countries and in Eastern Europe, however, where consumption of cigarettes remains high and is still increasing in some areas.

Most authorities have believed that cigarettes cause only cancers of the lung, pancreas, bladder and kidney, and (synergistically with alcohol) the larynx, mouth, pharynx, and esophagus. However, more recent evidence indicates that several other types of cancer are also related to tobacco. Most notably, cancer of the stomach, liver, and cervix seem to be directly related to long-term smoking.

Obesity and Cancer Risk   It is extremely difficult to sort through the accumulated evidence about the role of certain nutrients, obesity, sedentary lifestyle, and related variables. Nevertheless, a body of research has emerged that seems to point (albeit not with absolute certainty) to a cancer link. What is clear is this: Cancer is more common among people who are overweight, and risk increases as obesity increases.

This evidence for a link is strongest for postmenopausal breast cancer and cancers of the endometrium, gallbladder, and kidney, but obesity is also implicated in other cancers. For women, the cervix and ovaries are added to this list; for men, cancers of the colon and prostate seem to be related to obesity and/or diet. The following facts provide evidence for this obesity/cancer link:

- The relative risk of breast cancer in postmenopausal women is 50 percent higher for obese women.
- The relative risk of colon cancer in men is 40 percent higher for obese men.
- The relative risks of gallbladder and endometrial cancer are five times higher in obese individuals compared to individuals with "healthy" weight.
- Some studies show a positive association between obesity and cancers of the kidney, pancreas, rectum, esophagus, and liver.
- Obesity is believed to alter complex interactions among diet, metabolism, physical activity, hormones, and growth factors.

Biological Factors

Early theorists believed that we inherit a genetic predisposition toward certain forms of cancer.[9] Cancers of the breast, stomach, colon, prostate, uterus, ovaries, and lungs appear to run in families. For example, a woman runs a much higher risk of breast cancer if her mother or sisters (primary relatives) have had the disease, particularly at a young age. Hodgkin's disease and certain leukemias show similar familial patterns. Can we attribute these familial patterns to genetic susceptibility, or to the fact that people in the same

---

Biopsy   Microscopic examination of tissue to determine if a cancer is present.

Metastasis   Process by which cancer spreads from one area to different areas of the body.

Mutant cells   Cells that differ in form, quality, or function from normal cells.

Carcinogens   Cancer-causing agents.

Oncogenes   Suspected cancer-causing genes present on chromosomes.

Protooncogenes   Genes that can become oncogenes under certain conditions.

Oncologists   Physicians who specialize in the treatment of malignancies.

Relative risk   A measure of the strength of the relationship between risk factors and the condition being studied, such as a particular cancer.

Cancer: Assessing Your Personal Risks

Although the evidence is pretty clear that there are some types of cancer that you may be predisposed to due to genetic, biological, and/or environmental causes, there are many more that may be, at least in part, prevented through lifestyle behavior changes and risk reduction strategies. If you carefully assess your individual risks, you can then make behavior changes that may make you less susceptible to the various cancers. By answering each of the following questions, you will have an indicator of your susceptibility. Of course, no single instrument can serve as a complete risk assessment or diagnostic guide. These questions merely serve as the basis for personal introspection and thoughtful planning about ways to reduce your risk.

Read each question and circle the number in parentheses next to your response. Be honest and accurate in order to get the most complete understanding of your cancer risks. Individual scores for specific questions should not be interpreted as a precise measure of relative risk, but the totals in each section give a general indication of your risk.

SECTION 1: BREAST CANCER

1. Do you check your breasts at least monthly using BSE procedures?   Yes (1)   No (2)

2. Do you look at your breasts in the mirror regularly, checking for any irregular indentations/lumps, discharge from the nipples, or other noticeable changes?   Yes (1)   No (2)

3. Has your mother, sister, or daughter been diagnosed with breast cancer?   Yes (2)   No (1)

4. Have you ever been pregnant?   Yes (1)   No (2)

5. Have you had a history of lumps or cysts in your breasts or underarm?   Yes (2)   No (1)

Total Points _____

SECTION 2: SKIN CANCER

1. Do you spend a lot of time in the sun, either at work or at play?   Yes (2)   No (1)

2. Do you use sunscreens with an SPF rating of 15 or more when you are in the sun?   Yes (1)   No(2)

3. Do you use tanning beds or sun booths regularly to maintain a tan?   Yes (2)   No (1)

4. Do you examine your skin once a month, checking any moles or other irregularities, particularly in hard-to-see areas such as your back, genitals, neck, and under your hair?   Yes (1)   No (2)

5. Do you purchase and wear sunglasses that adequately filter out harmful sun rays?   Yes (1)   No (2)

Total Points _____

SECTION 3: CANCERS OF THE REPRODUCTIVE SYSTEM

(Men)

1. Do you examine your penis regularly for unusual bumps or growths?   Yes (1)   No (2)

2. Do you perform regular testicular self-examination?   Yes (1)   No (2)

3. Do you have a family history of prostate or testicular cancer?   Yes (2)   No (1)

4. Do you practice safer sex and wear condoms with every sexual encounter? Yes (1) No (2)

5. Do you avoid exposure to harmful environmental hazards such as mercury, coal tars, benzene, chromate, and vinyl chloride? Yes (1) No (2)

Total Points _____

(Women)

1. Do you have a regularly scheduled Pap test? Yes (1) No (2)

2. Have you been infected with the human papillomaviruses, Epstein-Barr virus, or other viruses believed to increase cancer risk? Yes (2) No (1)

3. Has your mother, sister, or daughter been diagnosed with breast, cervical, uterine, or ovarian cancer (particularly at a young age)? Yes (2) No (1)

4. Do you practice safer sex and use condoms with every sexual encounter? Yes (1) No (2)

5. Are you obese, taking estrogen, and/or consuming a diet that is very high in saturated fats? Yes (2) No (1)

Total Points _____

SECTION 4: CANCERS IN GENERAL

1. Do you smoke cigarettes on most days of the week? Yes (2) No (1)
2. Do you consume a diet that is rich in fruits and vegetables? Yes (1) No (2)
3. Are you obese and/or do you lead a primarily sedentary lifestyle? Yes (2) No (1)
4. Do you live in an area with high air pollution levels and/or work in a job where you are exposed to several chemicals on a regular basis? Yes (2) No (1)
5. Are you careful about the amount of animal fat in your diet, substituting olive oil or canola oil for animal fat whenever possible? Yes (1) No (2)
6. Do you limit your overall consumption of alcohol? Yes (1) No (2)
7. Do you eat foods rich in lycopene (such as tomatoes) and antioxidants? Yes (1) No (2)
8. Are you "body aware" and alert for changes in your body? Yes (1) No (2)
9. Do you have a family history of ulcers or of colorectal, stomach cancer, or other digestive system cancers? Yes (2) No (1)
10. Do you try to avoid unnecessary exposure to radiation, cell phone emissions, and microwave emissions? Yes (1) No (2)

Total Points _____

Analyzing Your Scores

Take a careful look at each question for which you received a "2" score. Are there any areas in which you received mostly "2's"? Did you receive total points of 6 or higher in Sections 1-3? Did you receive total points of 11 or higher in Section 4? If so, you have at least one identifiable risk. The higher the score, the more risks you may have. However, rather than focusing just on your score, focus on which items you might change. Review the suggestions throughout this chapter and list actions that you could take right now that might help you reduce your risk for these cancers. Plan a course of action that you can continue in the months ahead and use the Behavior Change Contract to put these plans into action.

families experience similar environmental risks? To date, the research in this area is inconclusive. Recent research conducted by the University of Utah indicates that a gene for breast cancer exists. A rare form of eye cancer does appear to be passed genetically from mother to child. It is possible that we can inherit a tendency toward a cancer-prone, weak immune system or, conversely, that we can inherit a cancer-fighting potential. But the complex interaction of hereditary predisposition, lifestyle, and environment on the development of cancer makes it a challenge to determine a single cause.

Biological sex also affects the likelihood of developing certain forms of cancer. For example, breast cancer occurs primarily among females, although men do occasionally get breast cancer. Obviously, factors other than heredity and familial relationships affect which sex develops a particular cancer. In the 1950s, for example, women rarely contracted lung cancer. But with increases in the number of women who smoke and the length of time they have smoked, lung cancer rates have soared to become the leading cause of cancer death in women. However, while gender plays a role in certain cases of cancer, other variables such as lifestyle are probably more significant.

Reproductive and Hormonal Risks for Cancer   The effects of reproductive factors on breast and cervical cancer have been well-documented. Pregnancy and estrogen supplementation in the form of oral contraceptives or hormone replacement therapy increase a woman's chances of breast cancer. Late menarche, early menopause, early first childbirth, and high parity (having many children) have been shown to reduce a woman's risk of breast cancer. A higher risk of endometrial cancer is also associated with hormone replacement therapy.

Breast cancer incidence is much higher in most Western countries than in developing countries. This is partly— and perhaps largely—accounted for by dietary effects (consuming a diet high in calories and fat), combined with later first childbirth, lower parity (having fewer children), shorter breastfeeding, and higher obesity rates.

Occupational and Environmental Factors

Overall, workplace hazards account for only a small percentage of all cancers. However, various substances are known to cause cancer when exposure levels are high or exposure is prolonged. One of the most common occupational carcinogens is asbestos, a fibrous material once widely used in the construction, insulation, and automobile industries. Nickel, chromate, and chemicals such as benzene, arsenic, and vinyl chloride have definitively been shown to be carcinogens for humans. Also, people who routinely work with certain dyes and radioactive substances may have increased risks for cancer. Working with coal tars, as in the mining profession, or working near inhalants, as in the auto-painting business, is hazardous. So is working with herbicides and pesticides, although the evidence is inconclusive for low-dose exposures.

Several federal and state agencies are responsible for monitoring such exposures and ensuring that businesses comply with standards designed to protect workers.

Radiation: Ionizing and Nonionizing   Ionizing radiation (IR)—radiation from x-rays, radon, cosmic rays, and ultraviolet radiation (primarily UVB radiation)—is the only form of radiation proven to cause human cancer. (See the section on skin cancer.) Incidents such as the Chernobyl accident in the 1980s focused attention on the potential risks of ionizing radiation. Evidence that high-dose IR (x-rays, radon, etc.) causes cancer comes from studies of atomic bomb survivors, patients receiving radiotherapy, and certain occupational groups (for example, uranium miners). Virtually any part of the body can be affected by IR, but bone marrow and the thyroid are particularly susceptible. Radon exposures in homes can increase lung cancer risk, especially in cigarette smokers. To reduce the risk of harmful effects, diagnostic medical and dental x-rays are set at the lowest dose levels possible.[10]

Although nonionizing radiation produced by radio waves, cell phones, microwaves, computer screens, televisions, electric blankets, and other products has been a topic of great concern in recent years, research has not proven excess risk to date.

Social and Psychological Factors

Many researchers claim that social and psychological factors play a major role in determining whether a person gets cancer. Stress has been implicated in increased susceptibility to several types of cancers. By reducing stress levels in your daily life, you may, in fact, lower your risk for cancer. A number of therapists have even established preventive treatment centers where the primary focus is on "being happy" and "thinking positive thoughts." Is it possible to laugh away cancer?

Although medical personnel are skeptical of overly simplistic solutions, we cannot rule out the possibility that negative emotional states contribute to disease. People who are under chronic, severe stress or who suffer from depression or other persistent emotional problems show higher rates of cancer than their healthy counterparts. Whether due to sleep disturbances, diet, or a combination of factors, the body's immune system may become weakened, increasing the susceptibility to cancer. The "Type C" personality described in Chapter 2 is just one example of psychological characteristics that may make a person more vulnerable to cancer.

Although psychological factors may play a part in cancer development, exposure to substances such as tobacco and alcohol is far more important. The American Cancer Society states that cigarette smoking is responsible for 30 percent of all cancer deaths—87 percent of all lung cancer deaths. Heavy consumption of alcohol has been related to cancers of the mouth, larynx, throat, esophagus, and liver. These cancers show up even more frequently in people whose heavy drinking is accompanied by smoking. The negative effects of smoking are not just concerns for the active smoker. Environmental (passive) tobacco smoke (ETS) causes

Table 16.1
Preventing Cancer through Diet and Lifestyle

TYPE	DECREASES RISK	INCREASES RISK	PREVENTABLE BY DIET
Lung	Vegetables, fruits	Smoking; some occupations	33–50%
Stomach	Vegetables, fruits; food refrigeration	Salt; salted foods	66–75%
Breast	Vegetables, fruits	Obesity; alcohol	33–50%
Colon/rectum	Vegetables; physical activity	Meat; alcohol; smoking	66–75%
Mouth/throat	Vegetables, fruits; physical activity	Salted fish; alcohol; smoking	33–50%
Liver	Vegetables	Alcohol; contaminated food	33–66%
Cervix	Vegetables, fruits	Smoking	10–20%
Esophagus	Vegetables, fruits	Deficient diet; smoking; alcohol	50–75%
Prostate	Vegetables	Meat or meat fat; dairy fat	10–20%
Bladder	Vegetables, fruits	Smoking; coffee	10–20%

HERE ARE SOME TIPS ISSUED BY A PANEL OF CANCER RESEARCHERS:

- Avoid being underweight or overweight, and limit weight gain during adulthood to less than 11 pounds.
- If you don't get much exercise at work, take an hour's brisk walk or similar exercise daily, and exercise vigorously for at least one hour a week.
- Eat eight or more servings a day of cereals and grains (such as rice, corn, breads, and pasta), legumes (such as peas), roots (such as beets, radishes, and carrots), tubers (such as potatoes), and plantains (including bananas).
- Eat five or more servings a day of a variety of other vegetables and fruits.
- Limit consumption of refined sugar.
- Limit alcoholic drinks to less than two a day for men and one for women.
- Limit intake of red meat to less than three ounces a day, if eaten at all.
- Limit consumption of salted foods and use of cooking and table salt. Use herbs and spices to season foods.

Sources: World Cancer Research Fund, American Institute for Cancer Research.

an estimated 3,000 deaths each year from lung cancer, 10,000 deaths from heart disease, up to 300,000 respiratory problems, and countless deaths among nonsmokers. Cancers of the mouth and throat pose significant risks for smokers.[11]

Chemicals in Foods

Among the food additives suspected of causing cancer is *sodium nitrate,* a chemical used to preserve and give color to red meat. Research indicates that the actual carcinogen is not sodium nitrate but *nitrosamines,* substances formed when the body digests the sodium nitrates. Sodium nitrate has not been banned, primarily because it kills *Clostridium botulinum,* the bacterium that causes the highly virulent food-borne disease botulism. It should also be noted that the bacteria found in the human intestinal tract may contain more nitrates than a person could ever take in from eating cured meats or other nitrate-containing food products. Nonetheless, concern about the carcinogenic properties of nitrates has led to the introduction of meats that are nitrate-free or contain reduced levels of the substance.

Much of the concern about chemicals in foods centers on the possible harm caused by pesticide and herbicide residues. While some of these chemicals cause cancer at high doses in experimental animals, the very low concentrations found in some foods are well within established govern-

ment safety levels. Continued research regarding pesticide and herbicide use is essential, and the continuous monitoring of agricultural practices is necessary to ensure a safe food supply. Scientists and consumer groups stress the importance of a balance between chemical use and the production of high-quality food products. Prevention efforts should focus on policies to protect consumers, develop low-chemical pesticides and herbicides, and reduce environmental pollution. See Table 16.1 for more information on cancer prevention through diet and lifestyle.

Viral Factors

The chances of becoming infected with a "cancer virus" are very remote. However, several forms of virus-induced cancers have been observed in laboratory animals and there is some indication that human beings display a similar tendency toward virally transmitted cancers. For example, the *herpes-related viruses* may be involved in the development of some forms of leukemia, Hodgkin's disease, cervical cancer, and Burkitt's lymphoma. The *Epstein-Barr virus,* associated with mononucleosis, may also contribute to cancer, and cervical cancer has been linked to *human papillomavirus,* the virus that causes genital warts.[12] *Helicobacter pylori,* a chronic gastric bacterium that causes ulcers, is a major factor in the development of stomach cancer.[13]

Many scientists believe that selected viruses help to provide an *opportunistic* environment for subsequent cancer development. It is likely that a combination of immunological bombardment by viral or chemical invaders and other risk factors substantially increases the risk of cancer.

Medical Factors

Some medical treatments increase a person's risk for cancer. One famous example is the prescription drug *diethylstilbestrol (DES),* widely used from 1940 to 1960 to control problems with bleeding during pregnancy and reduce the risk of miscarriage. Not until the 1970s did the dangers of this drug became apparent. Although DES caused few side effects in the millions of women who took it, their daughters were found to have an increased risk for cancers of the reproductive organs. Some scientists claim that estrogen replacement therapy in postmenopausal women is dangerous because it increases the risks for uterine cancer. Others believe that the benefits of estrogen outweigh its risks. Chemotherapy to treat one cancer may increase the risks of the patient developing other forms of cancer.

> ### What do you think?
>
> *How do we determine whether a given factor is a "risk factor" for a disease?* ❊ *Although a direct causal relationship between lung cancer and smoking has not been proved, the evidence supporting such a relationship is strong. Must a clearly established "causal" link exist before consumers are warned about risk?* ❊ *Can you think of apparent dietary risks for cancer that seemed conclusive but have since been refuted?* ❊ *How does the consumer know whom or what to believe?*

Types of Cancers

As mentioned earlier, the term *cancer* refers not to a single disease but to hundreds of different diseases. They are grouped into four broad categories based on the type of tissue from which the cancer arises.

Classifications of Cancer

• *Carcinomas.* Epithelial tissues (tissues covering body surfaces and lining most body cavities) are the most common sites for cancers. Carcinomas of the breast, lung, intestines, skin, and mouth are examples. These cancers affect the outer layer of the skin and mouth as well as the mucous membranes. They metastasize through the circulatory or lymphatic system initially and form solid tumors.
• *Sarcomas.* Sarcomas occur in the mesodermal, or middle, layers of tissue—for example, in bones, muscles, and general connective tissue. They metastasize primarily via the blood in the early stages of disease. These cancers are less common but generally more virulent than carcinomas. They also form solid tumors.
• *Lymphomas.* Lymphomas develop in the lymphatic system—the infection-fighting regions of the body—and metastasize through the lymph system. Hodgkin's disease is an example. Lymphomas also form solid tumors.
• *Leukemias.* Cancer of the blood-forming parts of the body, particularly the bone marrow and spleen, is called leukemia. A nonsolid tumor, leukemia is characterized by an abnormal increase in the number of white blood cells.

Trained oncologists determine the seriousness and general prognosis of a particular cancer. Once laboratory results and clinical observations have been made, cancers are rated by level and stage of development. Those diagnosed as "carcinoma in situ" are localized and often curable. Cancers with higher level or stage ratings have spread farther and are less likely to be cured. Figure 16.2 shows the most common sites of cancer and the number of deaths annually from each type.

Lung Cancer

Although lung cancer rates have dropped among white males during the past decade, the rate among white females and black males and females continues to be a pervasive threat. Lung cancer killed an estimated 171,900 people in 2003. Since 1987, more women have died from lung cancer than from breast cancer, which for over 40 years had been the major cause of cancer deaths in women. Today, lung cancer continues to be the leading cancer killer for both men and women.[14] As smoking rates have declined over the past 30 years, however, we have seen significant declines in male lung cancer. But these rates are not dropping as quickly among women. Another cause for concern is that although fewer adults are smoking, tobacco use among youth is again on the rise.

Symptoms of lung cancer include a persistent cough, blood-streaked sputum, chest pain, and recurrent attacks of pneumonia or bronchitis. Treatment depends on the type and stage of the cancer. Surgery, radiation therapy, and chemotherapy are all options. If the cancer is localized, surgery is usually the treatment of choice. If it has spread, surgery is combined with radiation and chemotherapy. Unfortunately, despite advances in medical technology, survival rates for lung cancer have improved only slightly over the past decade. Just 13 percent of lung cancer patients live five or more years after diagnosis. These rates improve to 47 percent with early detection, but only 15 percent of lung cancers are discovered in their early stages.[15]

Prevention Smokers, especially those who have smoked for over 20 years, and people who have been exposed to industrial substances such as arsenic and asbestos or to radiation from occupational, medical, or environmental sources are at

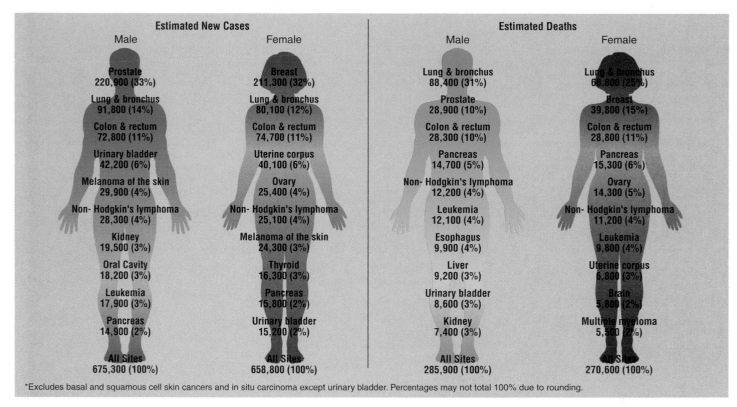

Estimated New Cases

Male

Prostate
220,900 (33%)

Lung & bronchus
91,800 (14%)

Colon & rectum
72,800 (11%)

Urinary bladder
42,200 (6%)

Melanoma of the skin
29,900 (4%)

Non-Hodgkin's lymphoma
28,300 (4%)

Kidney
19,500 (3%)

Oral Cavity
18,200 (3%)

Leukemia
17,900 (3%)

Pancreas
14,900 (2%)

All Sites
675,300 (100%)

Female

Breast
211,300 (32%)

Lung & bronchus
80,100 (12%)

Colon & rectum
74,700 (11%)

Uterine corpus
40,100 (6%)

Ovary
25,400 (4%)

Non-Hodgkin's lymphoma
25,100 (4%)

Melanoma of the skin
24,300 (3%)

Thyroid
16,300 (3%)

Pancreas
15,800 (2%)

Urinary bladder
15,200 (2%)

All Sites
658,800 (100%)

Estimated Deaths

Male

Lung & bronchus
88,400 (31%)

Prostate
28,900 (10%)

Colon & rectum
28,300 (10%)

Pancreas
14,700 (5%)

Non-Hodgkin's lymphoma
12,200 (4%)

Leukemia
12,100 (4%)

Esophagus
9,900 (4%)

Liver
9,200 (3%)

Urinary bladder
8,600 (3%)

Kidney
7,400 (3%)

All Sites
285,900 (100%)

Female

Lung & bronchus
68,800 (25%)

Breast
39,800 (15%)

Colon & rectum
28,800 (11%)

Pancreas
15,300 (6%)

Ovary
14,300 (5%)

Non-Hodgkin's lymphoma
11,200 (4%)

Leukemia
9,800 (4%)

Uterine corpus
6,800 (3%)

Brain
5,800 (2%)

Multiple myeloma
5,500 (2%)

All Sites
270,600 (100%)

*Excludes basal and squamous cell skin cancers and in situ carcinoma except urinary bladder. Percentages may not total 100% due to rounding.

Figure 16.2

Leading Sites of New Cancer Cases and Deaths, by Sex—2003 Estimates

Source: Reprinted by permission of the American Cancer Society, Inc., from *Cancer Facts and Figures 2002.*

the highest risk for lung cancer. The American Cancer Society estimated that in 2002, over 440,000 cancer deaths were caused by tobacco use and an additional 20,000 cancer deaths were related to alcohol use, frequently in combination with tobacco use.[16] Exposure to sidestream cigarette smoke, known as *environmental tobacco smoke* or *ETS,* increases the risk for nonsmokers. Researchers theorize that 90 percent of all lung cancers could be avoided if people did not smoke. Substantial improvements in overall prognosis have been noted in smokers who quit at the first signs of precancerous cellular changes and allow their bronchial linings to return to normal.

Breast Cancer

About 1 out of 8 women will develop breast cancer at some time in her life. Although this oft-repeated ratio has frightened many women, it represents lifetime risk. Thus, not until the age of 80 does a woman's risk of breast cancer rise to 1 in 8.[17] Here is the risk at earlier ages:

- Birth to age 39: 1 in 227
- Ages 40–59: 1 in 25
- Ages 60–79: 1 in 15
- Birth to death: 1 in 8

In 2003, approximately 211,300 women in the United States were diagnosed with invasive breast cancer for the first time.

In addition, 55,700 new cases of *in situ* breast cancer, typically ductal carcinoma in situ (DCIS), a more localized cancer, were diagnosed. The increase in detection of DCIS is a direct result of earlier detection through mammographies.[18] In the same year, about 1,500 new cases of breast cancer were diagnosed in men. About 39,600 women (and 400 men) died, making breast cancer the second leading cause of cancer death for women.[19] According to the most recent data, mortality rates went down dramatically from 1990 to 2000, with the largest decrease in younger women, both white and black.[20] The decline in rates may be due to earlier diagnosis and improved treatment, as numerous studies have shown that early detection increases survival and treatment options.

The earliest signs of breast cancer are usually observable on mammograms, often before lumps can be felt. However, it is important to note that mammograms are not foolproof. Reports of errors in reading mammograms (resulting in false positives and false negatives) occur every year. Hence, vigilance in breast self-examination and careful attention to subtle body changes are important. If a suspicious mass or lump is detected by a mammogram, a biopsy is performed to provide a more definitive assessment of the type of cancer and the treatment options.

Once breast cancer has grown to where it can be palpated, symptoms may include persistent breast changes such as a lump in the breast or surrounding lymph nodes—particularly in the underarm region; thickening, swelling, dimpling,

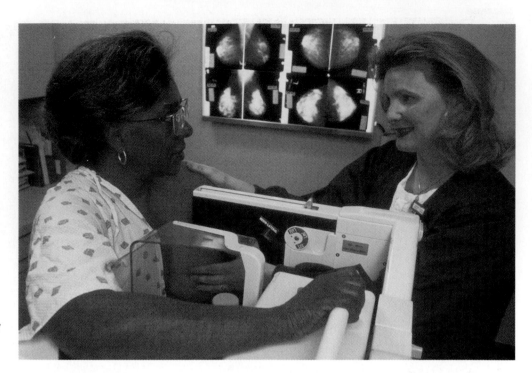

Early detection through mammography and other techniques greatly increases a woman's chance of surviving breast cancer.

skin irritation, distortion, retraction, or scaliness of the nipple; nipple discharge; possible pain; or tenderness. Breast pain is commonly due to noncancerous conditions, such as fibrocystic breasts, and is not usually a first symptom. However, any time pain or tenderness persists in the breast or surrounding area, it is a good idea to seek medical attention. Women who have ignored this symptom have been shocked to find out later that it was, for them, a symptom of cancer.

Risk Factors The incidence of breast cancer increases with age. Although there are many possible risk factors, those that are supported by research include the following:[21]

- Personal or family history of breast cancer (primary relatives such as mother, daughter, sister); the younger the relative was when diagnosed, the greater the family risk.
- Biopsy-confirmed atypical hyperplasia (excessive increase in the number of cells or tissue growth).
- Long menstrual history (menstrual periods that started early and ended late in life).
- Obesity after menopause.
- Recent use of oral contraceptives or postmenopausal estrogens or progestin (see the Women's Health/Men's Health box on hormones in Chapter 15).
- Never having children, or having a first child after age 30.
- Consuming two or more drinks of alcohol per day.
- Higher education and socioeconomic status.

Risk factors that need more rigorous research before being firmly established as risks include these:[22]

- Consuming a diet high in saturated fats.
- Exposure to pesticides and other chemicals.
- Weight gain, particularly after menopause.

- Physical inactivity.
- Genetic predisposition through BRCA1 and BRCA2 genes (genes appear to account for over 5 percent of all cases of breast cancer).

Although risk factors are useful indicators, they do not always predict individual susceptibility. However, because of increased awareness, better diagnostic techniques, and improved treatments, breast cancer patients have a better chance of surviving today. The five-year survival rate for people with localized breast cancer (which includes all women living five years after diagnosis, whether the patient is in remission, disease-free, or under treatment) has risen from 72 percent in the 1940s to 96 percent today. These statistics vary dramatically, however, based on the stage of the cancer when it is first detected. If the cancer has spread to surrounding tissue, the five-year survival rate is 78 percent; if it has spread to distant parts of the body, these rates fall to 21 percent; and, if the breast cancer has not spread at all, the survival rate approaches 100 percent. Survival after a diagnosis of breast cancer continues to decline beyond five years. Seventy-three percent of women diagnosed with breast cancer survive 10 years, and 59 percent survive 15 years.[23] Those with early stage cancers such as DCIS appear to have the best prognosis.

As with other cancers, patients who become actively involved in treatment decision making, who seek out the best oncologists with the most experience with their type of cancer, and who become knowledgeable about options and treatments often fare best. Of course, this takes time, access to health care providers, supportive family members, and attention to health-promoting lifestyles before, during, and after treatment.

Prevention A study of the role of exercise in reducing the risk for breast cancer generated much excitement in the scientific community. The study, involving 1,090 women who were 40 or younger (545 with breast cancer and 545 without) analyzed subjects' exercise patterns since they began menstruating. The risk of those who averaged four hours of exercise a week since menstruation was 58 percent lower than that of women who did no exercise at all. More good news: Subjects did not have to be avid joggers to have reduced risk. Their exercise included team sports, individual sports, dance, exercise classes, swimming, walking, and a variety of other activities. Researchers speculate that exercise may protect women by altering the production of the ovarian hormones estrogen and progesterone during menstrual cycles.

Other research has shown that vigorous athletics can delay the onset of menstruation and halt ovulation in some women. A woman's cumulative exposure to the sex hormones is associated with breast cancer risk.[24] Exercise can increase muscle mass and decrease body fat, which also lowers risk.[25]

Regular self-examination (see Figure 16.3) and mammography are the best ways to detect breast cancer early. The American Cancer Society offers guidelines for how often women should get mammograms and checkups (see Table 16.2). All women, no matter their age, should be in the habit of breast self-examination every month. International differences in breast cancer incidence correlate with variations in diet, especially fat intake, although a causal role for these dietary factors has not been firmly established. Sudden weight gain has also been implicated. Exciting new research about the BRCA1 and BRCA2 susceptibility genes for breast cancer offers new hope for early detection.

Treatment Today, people with breast cancer (like people with nearly any type of cancer) have many treatment options to choose from. It is important to thoroughly check out a physician's track record and his or her philosophy on the best treatment. Is the physician's recommendation consistent with that of major cancer centers in the country? Check out the doctor's credentials and the experiences of patients who have seen this doctor as well as the surgeon who will perform your biopsy and other surgical techniques. If possible, seek a facility that has a significant number of breast cancer patients, does many surgeries, is regarded as a "teaching facility" for new oncologists, has the "latest and greatest" in terms of technology, and is highly regarded by past patients. Often, cancer support groups can provide invaluable information and advice. Treatments range from a lumpectomy to radical mastectomy to various combinations of radiation or chemotherapy. Figure 16.4 on page 457 reviews these options. Among nonsurgical options, promising

Figure 16.3
Breast Self-Examination
The illustration demonstrates breast self-examination—the 10-minute habit that could save your life.

How to Examine Your Breasts

Do you know that 95% of breast cancers are discovered first by women themselves? And that the earlier the breast cancer is detected, the better the chance for a complete cure? Of course, most lumps or changes are not cancer. But you can safeguard your health by making a habit of examining your breasts once a month — a day or two after your period, or, if you're no longer menstruating, on any given day. And, if you notice anything changed or unusual — a lump, thickening, or discharge — contact your doctor right away.

How to Look for Changes

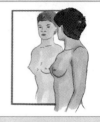

Step 1
Sit or stand in front of a mirror with your arms at your side. Turning slowly from side to side, check your breasts for
- changes in size or shape
- puckering or dimpling of the skin
- changes in size or position of one nipple compared to the other

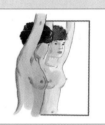

Step 2
Raise your arms above your head and repeat the examination in Step 1.

Step 3
Gently press each nipple with your fingertips to see if there is any discharge.

How to Feel for Changes

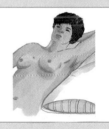

Step 1
Lie down and put a pillow or folded bath towel under your left shoulder. Then place your left hand under your head. (From now on you will be feeling for a lump or thickening in your breasts.)

Step 2
Imagine that your breast is divided into quarters.

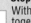

Step 3
With the fingers of your right hand held together, press firmly but gently, using small circular motions to feel the inner, upper quarter of your left breast. Start at your breastbone and work toward the nipple. Also examine the area around the nipple. Now do the same for the lower, inner portion of your breast.

Step 4
Next, bring your arm to your side and feel under your left armpit for swelling.

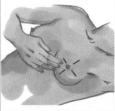

Step 5
With your arm still down, feel the upper, outer part of your breast, starting with your nipple and working outwards. Examine the lower, outer quarter in the same way.

Step 6
Now place the pillow under your right shoulder and repeat all the steps, using your left hand to examine your right breast.

Table 16.2
Recommendations for the Early Detection of Cancer in Asymptomatic People

SITE	RECOMMENDATION
CANCER-RELATED CHECKUP	A cancer-related checkup is recommended every 3 years for people ages 20–39 and every year for people age 40 and older. This exam should include health counseling and, depending on a person's age, might include examination for cancers of the thyroid, oral cavity, skin, lymph nodes, testes, and ovaries, as well as for some nonmalignant diseases.
BREAST	Women 40 and older should have an annual mammogram and an annual clinical breast exam (CBE) performed by a health care professional, and should perform monthly breast self-examination. Ideally, the CBE should occur before the scheduled mammogram.
	Women ages 20–39 should have a clinical breast exam performed by a health care professional every 3 years and should perform monthly breast self-examination.
COLON AND RECTUM	Beginning at age 50, men and women should follow one of the examination schedules below: • A fecal occult blood (FOBT) test every year, or • A flexible sigmoidoscopy (FSIG) every five years, or • Annual fecal occult blood test and flexible sigmoidoscopy every five years.* • A double-contrast barium enema every 5 to 10 years. • A colonoscopy every 10 years.
PROSTATE	The ACS recommends that both the prostate-specific antigen (PSA) blood test and the digital rectal examination be offered annually, beginning at age 50, to men who have a life expectancy of at least 10 years. Men at high risk (African-American men and men with a strong family history of one or more first-degree relatives diagnosed with prostate cancer at an early age) should begin testing at age 45. Information should be provided to patients about what is known and what is uncertain about the benefits and limitations of early detection and treatment of prostate cancer, so that they can make an informed decision.
UTERUS	**Cervix:** All women who are or have been sexually active or who are 18 and older should have an annual Pap test and pelvic examination. After three or more consecutive satisfactory examinations with normal findings, the Pap test may be performed less frequently. Discuss the matter with your physician. **Endometrium:** The American Cancer Society recommends that all women should be informed about the risks and symptoms of endometrial cancer, and strongly encouraged to report any unexpected bleeding or spotting to their physicians. Annual screening for endometrial cancer with endometrial biopsy beginning at age 35 should be offered to women with or at risk for hereditary nonpolyposis colon cancer (HNPCC).

*Combined testing is preferred over either annual FOBT or FSIG every 5 years alone. People who are at moderate or high risk for colorectal cancer should talk with a doctor about a different testing schedule.
Source: American Cancer Society, *Cancer Facts and Figures 2003.* Reprinted with permission.

results have been noted among women using selective estrogen-receptor modulators (SERMs) such as tamoxifen and raloxifen, particularly among women whose cancers appear to grow in response to estrogen.[26] Remember that it is always a good idea to seek more than one opinion before making a treatment decision.

Colon and Rectum Cancers

Colorectal cancers (cancers of the colon and rectum) continue to be the third most common cancers in men and women today, with over 148,500 cases diagnosed in 2003.[27] Although colon cancer rates have increased steadily in recent decades, many people are unaware of their risk. Bleeding

from the rectum, blood in the stool, and changes in bowel habits are the major warning signals. Anyone can get colorectal cancer, but people who are over age 40, who are obese, who have a family history of colon and rectum cancer, a personal or family history of polyps (benign growths) in the colon or rectum, or inflammatory bowel problems such as colitis run an increased risk. Other possible risk factors include diets high in fats or low in fiber, smoking, physical inactivity, high alcohol consumption, and low intake of fruits and vegetables. Approximately 90 percent of all colorectal cancers are preventable.[28] Recent studies have suggested that estrogen replacement therapy and aspirin may reduce colorectal risk.[29] See Table 16.3 for an overview of relative risks from these and other factors.

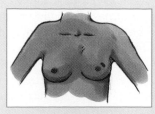

Lumpectomy
Performed when tumor is in earliest localized stages. Prognosis for recovery is better than 95 percent. Only tumor itself is removed. Some physicians may also remove normal tissue in surrounding area.

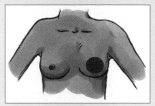

Simple mastectomy
Removal of breast and underling tissue. Prognosis for full recovery better than 80 percent.

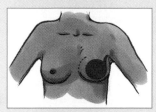

Modified radical mastectomy
Breast and lymph nodes in immediate area removed. Prognosis for full recovery dependent on level of spread.

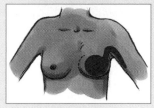

Radical mastectomy
Removal of breast, lymph nodes, pectoral muscles, all fat and underlying tissue. Prognosis for full recovery may be as low as 60 percent dependent on level of spread.

Figure 16.4
Surgical Procedures for Diagnosed Breast Cancer
These surgeries are typically followed by radiation treatment and/or chemotherapy.

Because colorectal cancer tends to spread slowly, the prognosis is quite good if it is caught in the early stages. Early screening can detect and remove precancerous polyps and diagnose disease at early, more treatable stages.[30] However, in spite of major educational campaigns, only 21 percent of all Americans over age 50 have had the most basic screening test—the fecal occult blood test—in the last five years, and 33 percent have had a colonoscopy during that same time period.[31] Colonoscopy or barium enemas are recommended screening tests for at-risk populations and everybody over age 50. Treatment often consists of radiation or surgery. Chemotherapy, although not used extensively in the past, is today a possibility. A permanent *colostomy,* the creation of an abdominal opening to eliminate body wastes, is seldom required for people with colon cancer and even less frequently for those with rectum cancer.

As with many cancers, African Americans appear to have the highest risk of colorectal cancer, followed by whites, Asians/Pacific Islanders, American Indians/Alaska Natives, and Hispanics.[32]

Prevention and Screening Regular exercise, a diet with lots of fruits and plant-origin foods, a healthy weight, and moderation in alcohol consumption appear to be among the most promising prevention strategies. New research also suggests that aspirin-like drugs, postmenopausal hormones, folic acid, calcium supplements, selenium, and vitamin E may also contribute to prevention; however, more research must be conducted to conclusively determine if and how these substances appear to reduce risk.[33]

The most commonly recommended screenings, particularly for those over the age of 50, include the following:[34]

- *Fecal occult blood tests (FOBT):* Cancers and large polyps often bleed sporadically into the intestine. The FOBT detects "hidden" or "occult" blood in a stool sample. You take samples of your own stool in the privacy of your home, place them in a preservative medium, and take them to the lab for evaluation. This is a relatively inexpensive test (less than $20 in most cases), and it has been proven to play a significant role in early detection.
- *Digital rectal exam:* In this test, a physician inserts his/her finger into the rectum to feel for irregularities. This is often part of a routine examination, but used alone it is not sufficient to rule out possible colon problems.
- *Flexible sigmoidoscopy:* In this test, a two-foot-long, slender, flexible, hollow, lighted tube is inserted into the rectum and up into the lower region of the colon. This test requires less preparation, is safer than a colonoscopy, and is a significant early screening exam. However, any polyps or other irregularities require a colonoscopy to assess the entire bowel and further ensure that all is well. The cost is $150 or more.

Table 16.3
Risk Factors for Colorectal Cancer

	RELATIVE RISK
Family history (first-degree relative)	1.8
Physical inactivity (less than 3 hours per week)	1.7
Inflammatory bowel disease (physician-diagnosed Crohn's disease, ulcerative colitis, or pancolitis)	1.5
Obesity	1.5
Red meat	1.5
Smoking	1.5
Alcohol (more than 1 drink/day)	1.4
High vegetable consumption (5 or more servings per day)	0.7
Oral contraceptive use (5 or more years of use)	0.7
Estrogen replacement (5 or more years of use)	0.8
Multivitamins containing folic acid	0.5

Modifiable factors are in **bold** text.
Source: Adapted, with permission, from Colditz et al. (2000).

- *Barium enema with air contrast:* For this test, the bowel must be completely clean and a white, chalky substance known as barium sulfate is introduced into the colon and allowed to spread, while air is pumped into the colon. X-rays monitor irregular outcroppings and deviations that might indicate tumor invasion. The cost is from $300 to $500 or more. If abnormalities are found, the colonoscopy may still need to be performed.
- *Colonoscopy:* Like the sigmoidoscopy, this test allows for direct visual examination of the colon and rectum, but it includes a much larger portion of the colon itself. Polyps can be removed via the colonoscope; cost is $1,000 or more.
- *Newer tests.* In the future, genetic-based fecal screening and other techniques may be widely available. It is currently possible to swallow a small camera and have a form of virtual examination of the colon as the camera passes through. However, this technique is more time-consuming and the optics are not yet as clear and reliable as those in the regular colonoscopic techniques. For many people—particularly older adults—the preparation for any of these tests, which may include distasteful fluids to induce bowel movements, self-enemas, long fasting, and other techniques, is an obstacle that must be reduced to ensure better participation.

Prostate Cancer

Cancer of the prostate gland is the most common type of cancer in males today, after skin cancer, and the second leading cause of cancer death in men after lung cancer.[35] In 2003, 220,900 new cases of prostate cancer were diagnosed, and from these, about 28,300 men would die.

From 1980 to 1990, prostate cancer incidence rates increased by 65 percent, largely due to earlier diagnosis in men without symptoms. This was accomplished by increased use of *prostate-specific antigen (PSA)* blood-test screenings and increased public awareness.[36] Today, prostate cancer rates are declining, although rates remain more than twice as high among black men than white men.

Most signs of prostate cancer are nonspecific—that is, they mimic the signs of infection or enlarged prostate. Symptoms include weak or interrupted urine flow; difficulty starting or stopping the urine flow; the need to urinate frequently; pain or difficulty in urinating; blood in the urine; and continued pain in the lower back, pelvis, or upper thighs. Many males mistake these symptoms for infections, normal changes associated with aging, or other conditions and delay treatment.

Incidence of prostate cancer increases with age; over 70 percent of all cases are diagnosed in men over age 65, although increasing numbers of young men seem to be affected. Black Americans have the highest prostate cancer rates in the world. The disease is most common in northwestern Europe and North America, but rare in the Near East, Africa, Central America, and South America. There seems to be a slightly increased risk if a family member has the disease, but it is unclear whether this is due to genetic or environmental factors. Recent genetic studies suggest that strong familial predisposition may be responsible for 5–10 percent of prostate cancers.[37] International studies suggest that dietary fat may also be a factor.

Fortunately, even with so many generalized symptoms, 83 percent of all prostate cancers are detected while they are still in the local or regional stages and tend to progress slowly. The five-year survival rate in these early stages is 100 percent. Because most men develop the disease in their late 60s and early 70s, it is likely that they will die of other causes first. For this reason, some health care groups question the cost effectiveness and necessity of prostate surgeries and other costly procedures that may have little real effect on life

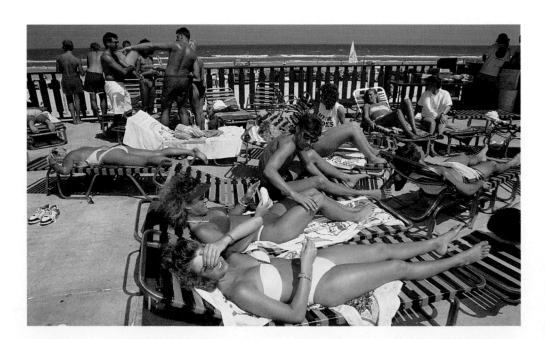

During spring break, thousands of college students try to achieve "the perfect tan," risking overexposure to sunlight and inviting skin cancer in later years.

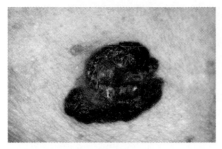 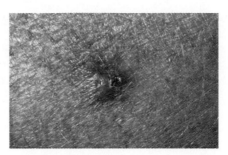 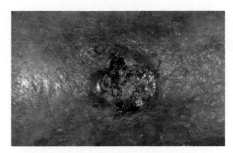

Prevention of skin cancer includes keeping a careful watch for any new pigmented growths and for changes to any moles. Melanoma symptoms, as shown in the left photo, include scalloped edges, asymmetrical shapes, discoloration, and an increase in size. Basal cell carcinoma and squamous cell carcinoma (middle and right photos) should be brought to your physician's attention but are not as deadly as melanoma.

expectancy. Over the past 20 years, the survival rate for all stages combined has increased from 67 percent to 96 percent, largely due to earlier diagnosis and improved treatment.

Because the incidence of prostate cancer increases with age, every man over age 40 should have an annual digital rectal prostate examination. In addition, the American Cancer Society recommends that men age 50 and older have an annual prostate-specific antigen (PSA) test. Men at high risk (African American men and men with a close relative who was diagnosed with prostate cancer at a young age) should begin testing at 45. If either result is suspicious, further evaluation in the form of transrectal ultrasound is recommended.[38]

Skin Cancer: Sun Worshippers Beware

If you are one of the millions of people each year who are trying to get a "healthy tan," you should think again. In fact, that phrase isn't just an oxymoron; it stands for premature aging and wrinkling at the very least, and life-threatening illness at its worst. The damage to your skin from a single bad sunburn lasts the rest of your life! What is worse is that such damage is cumulative. Early signs of sun damage (photodamage) include sunburn, tanning, and increased freckling. Later, these "cute" freckles are followed by wrinkling, premature aging and age spots, cataracts and other forms of eye damage, sagging of the skin and, the most serious consequence: skin cancer. If you are an avid sunbather, compare areas such as the front of your hands and your face to areas that are almost always covered from the sun's rays, such as your buttocks or breasts. The differences that you note are almost always the result of sun exposure over time.[39]

The long-term effects of sun exposure may be devastating:

• Skin cancer is the most common form of cancer in the United States today, affecting over 1.3 million people in 2003. Most of these were *basal* or *squamous cell* skin cancers, but 54,200 were malignant melanomas.[40]

• Today, one in five adults develops skin cancer, accounting for one-third of all reported malignancies.[41]

• **Malignant melanoma,** the deadliest form of skin cancer, is beginning to occur at a much higher rate in women under age 40. In fact, while relatively few people die from the

highly treatable basal or squamous cell skin cancer, the highly virulent malignant melanoma has become the most frequent cancer in women aged 25–29 and runs second only to breast cancer in women ages 30–34. If you think skin cancer is something that only older people get, think again![42]

• Rates of melanoma are 10 times higher among whites than blacks.

• In 2003, 9,800 people died of skin cancer. Of those, 7,600 died of melanoma and 2,200 died of other forms of skin cancer.

The sun gives off three types of harmful ultraviolet rays:

1. *UVA (ultraviolet A):* These longer wavelengths penetrate deeply into the skin, damaging the skin's collagens. They result in premature aging and help prime the skin for cancers.
2. *UVB (ultraviolet B):* These are short wavelengths and are believed to be the primary rays causing sunburns and ultimately resulting in cancers.
3. *UVC (ultraviolet C):* These very short rays are deadly to plants and animals. The ozone layer protects us by absorbing UVC rays. As the ozone layer becomes depleted, we are exposed to more UVC rays, which contribute to skin cancers and eye damage. Interestingly, as the global ozone layer has become progressively depleted over the last decade, the incidence of skin cancer has risen dramatically, as have cases of sun-related eye damage. (See Chapter 21 for more on the effects of damage to the ozone layer.)[43]

What happens when you expose yourself to too much sun? Biologically, the skin responds to photodamage by increasing its thickness and the number of pigment cells (melanocytes), which produce the "tan" look. An important part of the skin's immune system (the Langerhans cell) is reduced by photodamage, lowering the normal immune protection of our skin and priming it for cancer.[44] In addition, wrinkling occurs due to photodamage to the "elastic substances" (collagens) that keep skin soft and pliable.

Malignant melanoma A virulent cancer of the melanin (pigment-producing portion) of the skin.

Tips for Sun Worshippers

Planning on working on your suntan? Before heading out, consider these facts.

TIME OF DAY

How long you're in the sun matters, but so does time of day. Burning is more likely between 10:00 A.M. and 3:00 P.M., when the atmosphere filters out less ultraviolet energy.

CLOUD COVER

Clouds let 80 percent of UV rays through and increase exposure by scattering the rays. It's important to use good protection on cloudy days too.

PEAK PROTECTION

At high altitudes more UV rays get through, and snow reflects 80 percent of sunlight. Wear protective clothing and a high-SPF sunscreen.

IN THE WATER

UV rays can burn parts of your body that are underwater, so use waterproof sunscreen. Wearing a shirt while swimming and wading is advisable, because UV rays reflected off water and sand intensify exposure.

SUNGLASSES

Shades not only cut glare but also reduce the risk of UV-caused cataracts.

WHAT TO WEAR

An ordinary T-shirt has an effective SPF of only 6 to 8, dropping to 4 or 5 when wet. The more opaque the material, the fewer UV rays get through. Color doesn't matter. Special sun-blocking clothing has an SPF of 30 or more.

SUNSCREEN TIPS

Apply an SPF 15 or higher sunscreen to the entire body 15 to 30 minutes before going out. Use at least a full ounce. Re-apply even "waterproof" sunscreen if you're in the water longer than 80 min-utes, towel off, or perspire heavily. Recent reports have highlighted the potential harmful effects of some active ingredients in sunscreens (such as oxybenzone), particularly after repeated applications. The concern is over the fact that this chemical is absorbed in the body and may have long-term negative effects.

STAY ALERT

Avoid alcohol use on hot, sunny days. It can make you so sleepy that you doze off in the sun or it can numb the first warning signs of a sunburn.

Sources: Adapted by permission from "A Sun Worshiper's Guide," *U.S. News & World Report,* June 24, 1996. Basic data from the American Academy of Dermatology, American Optometric Association, and Sun Precautions, Inc., "The Active Ingredients in Sunscreen: Is It Safe?" *Healthfacts* 23 (1998): 5.

Although sun exposure risks have been widely reported, over 60 percent of Americans 25 years and under report that they are "working on a tan" at any given time. These numbers spike dramatically just prior to spring break as tanning booths fill with students and others trying to get "starter tans" before heading out to tropical climates for spring vacations. Are these tanning booths safer than natural sunlight, as many people believe? No. Tanning lamps emit large amounts of ultraviolet radiation that are at least two to three times more powerful than the natural UVA rays emitted from the sun. However, the most important difference between the booths and the sun and the reason the booths produce tans so quickly is that users are in the tanning bed right next to those bulbs, rather than millions of miles away. The newer the bulbs, the faster the tan, the faster the potential burn, and the greater the risk of damage. In fact, just a single 15–30 minute salon session exposes the body to the same amount of harmful UV light as an entire day at the beach, according to experts at the American Academy of Dermatology.[45]

Who's at risk for skin cancer? Anyone who overexposes himself or herself without adequate protection. The risk is greatest for people who fit the following categories:

- Have fair skin.
- Have blonde, red, or light brown hair.
- Have blue, green, or gray eyes.
- Always burn before tanning.
- Burn easily and peel readily.
- Don't tan easily, but spend lots of time outdoors.
- Have previously been treated for skin cancer or have a family history of skin cancer (if you have a family history of melanoma, see your physician for regular skin exams).
- Live in or take regular vacations to high altitudes (UV exposure increases with altitude).
- Work indoors all week and try to play tanning "catch-up" on weekends.
- Use no or low-SPF sunscreens.

Preventing skin cancer is a matter of limiting exposure to harmful UV rays. See the Skills for Behavior Change box for strategies on safely spending time in the sun. If you do get sunburned, be careful about treating it.

- Drink more fluids than usual.
- Apply cool compresses gently, without rubbing the area. If you shower or bathe, use a mild soap.

- Moisturize the skin with aquaphor petroleum jelly, plain Calamine lotion, or Sarna lotion. Some forms of aloe work well, but make sure you read the ingredients on the label.
- Avoid "caine" products such as benzocaine.
- Take aspirin or ibuprofen to help reduce inflammation.
- For severe symptoms, including nausea, vomiting, chills, malaise, weakness, and blistering, stay awake and see a doctor.

Many people do not know what to look for when they are concerned about skin cancer. Basal and squamous cell carcinomas can be a recurrent annoyance, showing up most commonly on the face, ears, neck, arms, hands, and legs as warty bumps, colored spots, or scaly patches. Surgery may be necessary to remove them, but they are seldom life threatening.

In striking contrast is the insidious melanoma, an invasive killer that quickly spreads to regional organs and throughout the body, accounting for over 75 percent of all skin cancer deaths. Risks increase dramatically among whites after age 20.[46] Often, these moles start as normal-looking growths, but quickly develop abnormal characteristics. A simple *ABCD* rule outlines the warning signs of melanoma:

- *Asymmetry* —One half of the mole does not match the other half.
- *Border irregularity*—The edges are uneven, notched, or scalloped.
- *Color*—The pigmentation is not uniform. Melanoma may vary in color from tan to deeper brown, reddish black, black, or deep bluish black.
- *Diameter*— Greater than 6 millimeters (about the size of a pea).

If you notice any of these symptoms, consult a physician promptly.

Treatment of skin cancer depends on its seriousness. Surgery is used in 90 percent of all cases. Radiation therapy, *electrodesiccation* (tissue destruction by heat), and *cryo-surgery* (tissue destruction by freezing) are also common forms of treatment. For melanoma, treatment may involve surgical removal of the regional lymph nodes, radiation, or chemotherapy.

Testicular Cancer

Testicular cancer is one of the most common types of solid tumors found in young adult males. Those between the ages of 17 and 34 are at greatest risk. There has been a steady increase in tumor frequency over the past several years in this age group.[47] Although the cause of testicular cancer is unknown, several risk factors have been identified. Males with undescended testicles appear to be at greatest risk, and some studies indicate a genetic influence.

In general, testicular tumors first appear as a painless enlargement of the testis or thickening in testicular tissue.

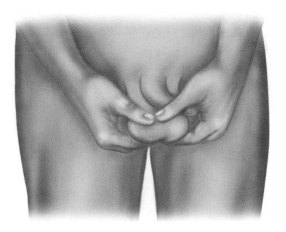

Figure 16.5
Testicular Self-Examination
Examine each testicle by placing the index and middle fingers of both hands on the underside of the testicle and the thumbs on top. Gently roll the testicle between your thumb and fingers. If a suspicious lump or thickening is found, consult a doctor immediately. Perform the exam after a bath or shower, as the heat causes the testicles to descend and the scrotal skin to relax.

Because this enlargement is often painless, it is extremely important that all young males practice regular testicular self-examination (see Figure 16.5).

Ovarian Cancer

Ovarian cancer is the fourth leading cause of cancer death for women, diagnosed in almost 25,200 of them in 2003 and killing over 14,000.[48] The most common sign is enlargement of the abdomen (or a feeling of bloating) in women over age 40. (Abnormal vaginal bleeding is rarely a symptom.) Other symptoms include vague digestive disturbances, such as gas and stomachaches that persist and cannot be explained, fatigue, pain during intercourse, unexplained weight loss, unexplained changes in bowel or bladder habits, urinary frequency, and incontinence.[49] Because its symptoms are often non-specific, ovarian cancer frequently goes undiagnosed in its early stages.

The risk for ovarian cancer increases with age, with the highest rates found in women in their 70s. Women who have never had children are twice as likely to develop ovarian cancer as are those who have. This is because the main risk factor appears to be exposure to the reproductive hormone estrogen. Women who have multiple pregnancies or use oral contraceptives, both of which inhibit estrogen, are at lower risk. In addition, having one or more primary relatives (mother, sisters, grandmothers) who have had the disease appears to increase individual risk. With the exception of Japan, the highest incidence rates are reported in the industrialized countries of the world. Research indicates that mutations in the BRCA1 and BRCA2 genes may increase risks.[50]

Prevention An early Yale University study indicated that diet may played a role in ovarian cancer.[51] When comparing 450 Canadian women with newly diagnosed ovarian cancer with 564 demographically similar, healthy women, the researchers found that the women without ovarian cancer had a diet lower in saturated fat. For every 10 grams of saturated fat a woman ate per day, her risk of ovarian cancer rose 20 percent. Conversely, women who lowered their saturated fat consumption by 10 grams a day experienced a 20 percent drop in risk. Every 10 grams of vegetable fiber (but not fruit or cereal fiber) added to a woman's daily menu lowered her risk by 37 percent. The study also found that each full-term pregnancy lowered risk by about 20 percent and each year of oral contraceptive use lowered it by 5 to 10 percent. So, should you go out and get pregnant or start taking birth control pills to reduce risk? No. However, these results, particularly when combined with cardiovascular risks and other health information, provide yet another reason to eat plenty of vegetables and cut down on your fat intake. General prevention strategies focusing on diet, exercise, sleep, stress management, and weight control are good ideas for this and any of the cancers discussed in this chapter.

To protect yourself, annual thorough pelvic examinations are important. Pap tests, although useful in detecting cervical cancer, do not reveal ovarian cancer. Women over the age of 40 should have a cancer-related checkup every year. Transvaginal ultrasound and a tumor marker, CA125, may assist in diagnosis but are not recommended for routine screening.[52] If you have any symptoms of ovarian cancer and they persist, see your doctor promptly.

Cervical and Endometrium (Uterine) Cancer

In 2003, an estimated 40,100 new cases of uterine cancer were diagnosed in the United States. Most uterine cancers develop in the body of the uterus, usually in the endometrium (lining). The rest develop in the cervix, located at the base of the uterus. The overall incidence of early-stage uterine cancer—that is, cervical cancer—has increased slightly in recent years in women under the age of 50.[53] In contrast, invasive, later-stage forms of the disease appear to be decreasing. This may be due to more regular screenings of younger women using the **Pap test,** a procedure in which cells taken from the cervical region are examined for abnormal cellular activity. Although these tests are very effective for detecting early stage cervical cancer, they are less effective for detecting cancers of the uterine lining and not effective at all for detecting cancers of the fallopian tubes or ovaries.[54]

Risk factors for cervical cancer include early age of first intercourse, multiple sex partners, cigarette smoking, and certain sexually transmitted diseases, such as the herpes virus and the human papillomavirus. For endometrial cancer, a history of infertility, failure to ovulate, obesity, and treatment with tamoxifen or unopposed estrogen therapy appear to be major risk factors.[55]

Early warning signs of uterine cancer include bleeding outside the normal menstrual period or after menopause or persistent unusual vaginal discharge. These symptoms should be checked by a physician immediately.[56]

Cancer of the Pancreas

The incidence of cancer of the pancreas, known as a "silent" disease, has increased substantially during the last 25 years to 30,700 cases in 2003.[57] Chronic inflammation of the pancreas, obesity, physical inactivity, diabetes, cirrhosis, and a high-fat diet may contribute to its development. Smokers have double the risk of nonsmokers.[58] Unfortunately, pancreatic cancer is one of the worst cancers to get, with only 5 percent of patients living more than five years after diagnosis, usually because the disease is well advanced by the time there are any symptoms.

Leukemia

Leukemia is a cancer of the blood-forming tissues that leads to proliferation of millions of immature white blood cells. These abnormal cells crowd out normal white blood cells (which fight infection), platelets (which control hemorrhaging), and red blood cells (which prevent anemia). As a result, symptoms such as fatigue, paleness, weight loss, easy bruising, repeated infections, nosebleeds, and other forms of hemorrhaging occur. In children, these symptoms can appear suddenly.[59]

Leukemia can be acute or chronic in nature and can strike both sexes and all age groups. Although many people think of it as a childhood disease, leukemia struck many more adults (30,600) than children (2,000) in 2003.[60] Chronic leukemia can develop over several months and have few symptoms. The five-year survival rate for patients with leukemia had increased to 60 percent by the late 1990s.

> ### What do you think?
>
> *What types of cancers do you think you and your friends are at greatest risk for right now?* ❋ *Do you practice regular breast or testicular self-exams?* ❋ *Do you think it's important for a man to know how to do a breast self-exam or a woman to do a testicular self-exam—or are these individual responsibilities only?* ❋ *Would you be able to help your partner with his or her exam?*

Facing Cancer

While heart disease mortality rates have declined steadily over the past 50 years, cancer mortality has increased consistently in the same period. Based on current rates, about 83 million—or one in three of us now living—will eventually develop cancer. Many factors have contributed to the rise in cancer mortality, but the increased incidence of lung cancer

What's New in Cancer Research, Prevention, and Treatment?

THE LATEST ON FIBER

Although fiber has been downplayed in the past year as a protective agent against colon and other forms of cancer, don't throw out that bran muffin just yet. A recent study of more than 68,000 women found that dietary fiber—particularly from breakfast cereals—can significantly decrease the risk of heart attacks by improving cholesterol levels, lowering blood sugar, boosting sensitivity to insulin, and lowering the risk of blood clotting. A previous study of men showed similar results. Also, while some recent studies questioned fiber's benefits for cancer prevention, many experts doubt that these findings should outweigh all the previous studies that indicate it does indeed reduce risk. In short, the scientific community is unsure of the fiber–cancer link but quite sure that the benefits in other areas more than justify a healthy high-fiber, low-fat diet.

ALCOHOL AND CANCER

Heavy drinking is associated with an increased risk for several cancers—notably, cancer of the mouth, esophagus, pharynx, larynx, liver, and pancreas. An analysis of multiple studies found that having two alcoholic drinks per day (any type of alcohol) increased a woman's chances of developing breast cancer by nearly 25 percent. The reasons for this are unclear, but researchers speculate that alcohol influences the metabolism of estrogen and that prolonged exposure to high levels of estrogen increases breast cancer risk, particularly for women on hormone replacement therapy (HRT). The effect of one drink per day is controversial, although most experts feel that one daily drink does not increase risk. But, before you toss out all of your alcohol, you should know that there is increasing evidence that a glass of red wine, with its antioxidant potential and HDL-boosting potential, seems to protect against heart disease.

NEW METHODS OF DETECTION

Several new methods of breast cancer detection are on the horizon:

- *Blood tests.* Researchers from the John Wayne Cancer Center in Santa Monica are developing biological markers that would identify microscopic tumors as they travel through the blood, before they are large enough to be picked up on conventional tests.
- *"Pap smear for the breast."* Similar to the Pap smear, which checks fluids from the cervix for abnormal cells, this newer test analyzes fluids from the breasts' milk ducts (where most tumors originate). It may be widely available soon. This test would pick up cancerous cells in their earliest, most treatable stages.
- *Better breast scans.* Researchers at the University of Chicago and elsewhere are developing better computer programs to point out questionable spots on mammograms and better, more reliable machines such as MRIs.

Sources: "High-Fiber Diet and Decreased Risk of Heart Disease in Women," by J. Manson, 1999, *Journal of the American Medical Association,* June 23; "The Facts about Drinking and Your Health," *Johns Hopkins Medical Health Letter—Health after 50* 12 (5) (2000): 4–6; "The Search for Smaller Tumors," by C. Gorman, *Time* (June 26, 2000): 50.

—a largely preventable disease—is probably the most important. Despite these gloomy predictions, recent advancements in the diagnosis and treatment of many forms of cancer have reduced much of the fear and mystery that once surrounded this disease.

Detecting Cancer

The earlier cancer is diagnosed, the better the prospect for survival. Several new, high-tech tools to detect cancer have been developed:

- New high-technology diagnostic imaging techniques have replaced exploratory surgery for some cancer patients. In **magnetic resonance imaging (MRI),** a huge electromagnet detects hidden tumors by mapping the vibrations of the various atoms in the body on a computer screen. The **computerized axial tomography scan (CAT scan)** uses x-rays to examine parts of the body. In both of these painless, noninvasive procedures, cross-sectioned pictures can reveal a tumor's shape and location more accurately than can conventional x-rays. (See New Horizons in Health box.)

- *Prostatic ultrasound* (a rectal probe using ultrasonic waves to produce an image of the prostate) is currently being investigated as a means to increase the early detection of prostate cancer. Recently, prostatic ultrasound has been combined with a blood test for **prostate-specific antigen (PSA),** an antigen found in prostate cancer patients.

Pap test A procedure in which cells taken from the cervical region are examined for abnormal cellular activity.

Magnetic resonance imaging (MRI) A device that uses magnetic fields, radio waves, and computers to generate an image of internal tissues of the body for diagnostic purposes without the use of radiation.

Computerized axial tomography scan (CAT scan) A machine that uses radiation to view internal organs not normally visible on x-rays.

Prostate-specific antigen (PSA) An antigen found in prostate cancer patients.

Table 16.4
Cancer's Seven Warning Signals

1. Changes in bowel or bladder habits
2. A sore that does not heal
3. Unusual bleeding or discharge
4. Thickening or lump in breast or elsewhere
5. Indigestion or difficulty in swallowing
6. Obvious change in a wart or mole
7. Nagging cough or hoarseness

If you have a warning signal, see your doctor.

Such medical techniques, along with regular self-examinations and checkups, play an important role in the early detection and secondary prevention of cancer.

Most of the sites that pose the highest risk for cancer have screening tests available for early detection. Other common forms of cancer have readily identifiable symptoms. The key seems to be whether people have the financial resources (insurance) to seek medical diagnosis and early treatment. A health care reform package that focuses on payment for regular checkups and preventive services would help many poor and middle-class Americans seek medical care early, when the chances of a cure are best.

Regardless of insurance status, the best way to detect cancer early is to stay actively involved in your own health care. Table 16.4 lists the seven warning signals of cancer. If you notice any of these signals, and they don't appear to be related to anything else, see a doctor immediately. For example, difficulty swallowing may be due to a cold or flu. But if you are otherwise symptomless and the difficulty continues, consult your physician. Make sure you receive all appropriate diagnostic tests.

Also, make a realistic assessment of your own risk factors and avoid the ones that you can control. Do you have a family history of cancer? If so, what types? Make sure you know which symptoms to watch for, and follow the recommendations for self-exams and medical checkups in Table 16.2. Avoid known carcinogens—such as tobacco—and other environmental hazards. Eat a nutritious diet. Heeding the suggestions for primary prevention can significantly decrease your own risk for cancer.

Radiotherapy   The use of radiation to kill cancerous cells.

Chemotherapy   The use of drugs to kill cancerous cells.

Immunotherapy   A process that stimulates the body's own immune system to combat cancer cells.

New Hope in Cancer Treatments

Although cancer treatments have changed dramatically over the past 20 years, surgery, in which the tumor and surrounding tissue are removed, is still common. Today's surgeons tend to remove less surrounding tissue than previously and to combine surgery with either **radiotherapy** (the use of radiation) or **chemotherapy** (the use of drugs) to kill cancerous cells.

Radiation works by destroying malignant cells or stopping cell growth. It is most effective in treating localized cancer masses. Unfortunately, in the process of destroying malignant cells, radiotherapy also destroys some healthy cells. It may also increase the risks for other types of cancers. Despite these qualifications, radiation continues to be one of the most common and effective forms of treatment.

When cancer has spread throughout the body, it is necessary to use some form of chemotherapy. Currently, over 50 different anticancer drugs are in use, some of which have excellent records of success. A chemotherapeutic regimen of four anticancer drugs combined with radiotherapy has resulted in remarkable survival rates for some cancers, including Hodgkin's disease. Ongoing research will result in new drugs that are less toxic to normal cells and more potent against tumor cells. Current research indicates that some tumors may actually be resistant to certain forms of chemotherapy and that the treatment drugs do not reach the core of the tumor. Scientists are working to circumvent resistance and make tumor cells more vulnerable.

Whether used alone or in combination, radiotherapy and chemotherapy have side effects, including extreme nausea, nutritional deficiencies, hair loss, and general fatigue. Long-term damage to the cardiovascular system and other body systems can be significant. It is important to discuss these matters fully with doctors when making treatment plans.

Substances found in nature, such as taxol (originally found in Pacific yew trees), are being synthesized in laboratories and tested on a variety of cancers. Other compounds, including those derived from sea urchins, are rich in resources for anticancer drugs.

Today, researchers are targeting cancer as a genetic disease that is brought on by some form of mutation, either inherited or acquired. Promising treatments focus on stopping the cycle of these mutant cells, targeting toxins through monoclonal antibodies, and rousing the immune system to be more effective. Others include the following:[61]

- An estrogen-blocking drug called *tamoxifen* is used to treat women who have breast cancer that is estrogen positive, or grows more rapidly when estrogen levels are high. This drug is often an alternative to chemotherapy.
- **Immunotherapy** enhances the body's own disease-fighting systems to help control cancer. Interferon (a naturally occurring body protein that protects healthy cells and kills cancer cells), interleukin 2 (a growth factor that stimulates cells of the immune system to find cancer), and other biologic response modifiers are under study.

• One of the most exciting new approaches for spurring the immune system to ward off cancer is the use of *cancer-fighting vaccines*. Cancer vaccines are not to be confused with the vaccines for measles and other infectious diseases, which prime the body to keep bacteria and viruses from taking hold. They essentially keep people healthy, but they don't cure anything. Cancer vaccines alert the body's immune defenses, but instead of warning of germs, they provide indicators of good cells that have gone bad. Consequently, rather than preventing disease, they help people who are already ill. Today, hundreds of studies are examining the effectiveness of possible cancer vaccines. These vaccines may be the next generation of cancer treatment.

• Research on the effectiveness of *gene therapy* has moved into early clinical trials. Scientists have found hopeful signs of a virus carrying genetic information that makes the cells it infects susceptible to an antiviral drug. Findings from human trials are expected soon. Scientists also are looking at ways of transferring genes that increase the patient's immune response to the cancerous tumor, or that confer drug resistance to the bone marrow so that higher doses of chemotherapeutic drugs can be given.

• In other studies, researchers are testing compounds that may stop tumors from forming new blood vessels, a process known as *angiogenesis*. By inhibiting angiogenesis, scientists hope to inhibit the flow of nutrient- and oxygen-rich blood to the cancerous tumors and slow their growth.

• In recent years, scientists have identified various steps in what is termed the *cancer pathway*. These include oncogene actions, hormone receptors, growth factors, metastasis, and angiogenesis. Preliminary studies are under way to "design"

compounds (*rational drug design*) aimed at specific molecules along the cancer pathway with the intent of inhibiting actions at these various steps.

• Cell mutations can trigger increased production of destructive enzymes that allow them to invade surrounding tissues and penetrate blood vessels to travel to other parts of the body. A powerful enzyme inhibitor, *TIMP-2,* shows promise for slowing the metastasis of tumor cells. A metastasis suppressor gene, NM23, has also been identified.

• *Neoadjuvant chemotherapy* (giving chemotherapy to shrink the cancer and then removing it surgically) has been tried against various types of cancers. This is a promising new approach.

In addition, psychosocial and behavioral research has become increasingly important as health professionals learn more about lifestyle factors that influence risk and survivability. Health care practitioners have become more aware of the psychological needs of patients and families and have begun to tailor treatment programs to meet their diverse needs.

Talking with Your Doctor about Cancer

Any time the presence of cancer is suspected, people react with great anxiety, fear, and anger. Emotional distress is sometimes so intense that they are unable to make critical health care decisions. If you find it difficult to know what to ask your doctor during a routine exam, imagine how hard it would be to discuss life-or-death options for yourself or a loved one. Before you arrive at the doctor's office, prepare a

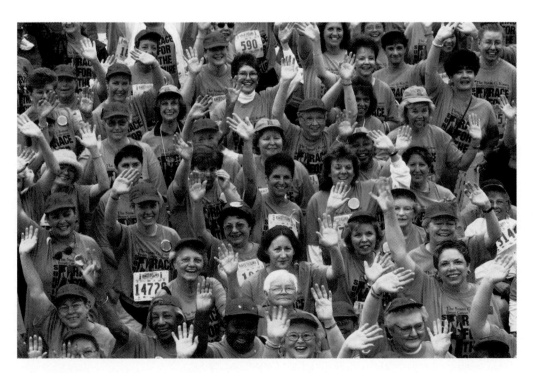

Cancer survivors can live long and healthy lives. Some, such as these breast cancer survivors and their supporters, take part in walk-athons, races, and other activities to raise money for cancer research and treatment and to raise public awareness about prevention.

list of important questions to discuss. Remember, your health care provider should be your partner and help you make the best decisions for you.

If the diagnosis is cancer, here are some suggestions for questions to ask:

- What kind of cancer do I have? What stage is it in? Based on my age and stage, what prognosis do I have?
- What are my treatment choices? Which do you recommend? Why?
- What are the benefits of each kind of treatment?
- What are the long- and short-term risks and possible side effects?
- Would a clinical trial be appropriate for me? (Clinical trials are research studies designed to answer specific questions and to find better ways to prevent or treat cancer. Often new cancer-fighting treatments are used.)

If surgery is recommended, you may want to ask:

- What kind of operation will it be, and how long will it take? What form of anesthesia will be used? How many similar procedures has this surgeon done in the past month? What is his or her success rate?
- How will I feel after surgery? If I have pain, how will you help me?
- Where will the scars be? What will they look like? Will they cause disability?

- Will I have any activity limitations after surgery? What kind of physical therapy, if any, will I have? When will I get back to normal activities?

If radiation is recommended, you may want to know:

- Why do you think this treatment is better than my other options?
- How long will I need to have treatments, and what will the side effects be in the short and long term? What body organs or systems may be damaged?
- What can I do to take care of myself during therapy? Are there services available to help me?
- What is the long-term prognosis for people of my age with my type of cancer who are using this treatment?

Questions to ask about chemotherapy include the following:

- Why do you think this treatment is better than my other options?
- Which drug combinations pose the fewest risks and most benefits?
- What will be the short- and long-term side effects on my body?
- What are my options?

Before beginning any form of cancer therapy, it is imperative to be a vigilant and vocal consumer. Read and seek information from cancer support groups. Check the skills of your

Table 16.5
Five-Year Relative Survival Rates by Stage at Diagnosis*

SITE	ALL STAGES %	LOCAL %	REGIONAL %	DISTANT %
Breast (female)	86	96	78	21
Cervix (uterus)	70	92	49	15
Colon and rectum	61	90	64	8
Endometrium (uterus)	84	96	63	26
Esophagus	14	27	13	2
Kidney	62	89	61	9
Larynx	65	83	50	38
Liver	6	14	6	2
Lung	15	48	21	3
Melanoma	89	96	61	12
Oral cavity	56	82	46	21
Ovary	52	95	81	29
Pancreas	4	16	7	2
Prostate	96	100	—**	34
Stomach	22	59	22	2
Testis	95	99	94	76
Thyroid	95	99	94	42
Urinary bladder	81	94	48	6

*Adjusted for normal life expectancy. This chart is based on cases diagnosed from 1992–1997; followed through 1997.
**Rate for local stage represents local and regional stages combined.
Source: NCI Surveillance, Epidemiology, and End Results Program, 1998. (c) 2002, American Cancer Society, Inc.

surgeon, your radiation therapist, and your doctor in terms of clinical experience and interpersonal interactions.

Life after Cancer

Heightened public awareness and an improved prognosis have made the cancer experience less threatening and isolating than it once was (see Table 16.5). While you may hear stories of recovering cancer patients experiencing job discrimination and being unable to obtain health or life insurance, these cases are decreasing. Several states have even enacted legislation to prevent insurance companies from canceling policies or instituting other forms of discrimination. Health insurance can be obtained through large employers.

Because large companies spread the insurance risk among many employees, insurance companies accept new employees without underwriting.

In fact, assistance for the cancer patient is more readily available than ever before. Cancer support groups, cancer information workshops, and low-cost medical consultation are just a few of the forms of assistance now offered in many communities. The national breast cancer coalition and other groups have successfully lobbied Congress to increase cancer research dollars. As a result, government funding has increased substantially over the past decade. The battle for funds continues. Increasing efforts in cancer research, improvements in diagnostic equipment, and advances in treatment provide hope for the future.

Taking Charge **16** 16 **16**

Managing Cancer Risks

Cancer is no longer an automatic death sentence. Oncologists continually increase our chances of surviving cancer with new and improved medical care as well as better early detection tests. But we each hold the key to fulfilling our own hopes by doing what we can to prevent cancer. Regular checkups and monthly self-exams improve the odds of survival by providing early diagnosis. Proper diet, regular exercise, and staying clear of carcinogens improve the odds. From the self-assessment that you completed earlier in this chapter, which factors put you at risk for cancer? What actions can you take today to reduce your risk?

Checklist for Change

Making Personal Choices

☐ *Don't smoke.* Smoking accounts for about 30 percent of all cancer deaths and 90 percent of all lung cancer deaths. Those who smoke two or more packs of cigarettes a day have lung cancer mortality rates 17 to 25 times greater than those of nonsmokers.

☐ *Avoid excessive sunlight.* Almost 600,000 cases of nonmelanoma skin cancer diagnosed each year in the United States are considered to be sun related.

☐ *Avoid excessive alcohol consumption.* Oral cancer and cancers of the larynx, throat, esophagus, breast, and liver occur more frequently among heavy drinkers.

☐ *Do not use smokeless tobacco.* Use of chewing tobacco or snuff increases risk for cancer of the mouth, larynx, throat, and esophagus and is highly habit forming.

☐ *Monitor estrogen use.* Estrogen treatment to control menopausal symptoms may increase risk for endometrial cancer. While estrogen therapy does seem to lower women's risk for osteoporosis, it should not be undertaken without careful discussion between a woman and her physician.

☐ *Avoid occupational carcinogens.* Exposure to several different industrial agents increases risk for various cancers. Risk from asbestos is greatly increased when combined with cigarette smoking.

☐ *Avoid obesity.* Risk for colon, breast, ovarian, endometrial, and uterine cancers increases in obese people.

☐ *Eat your fruits and vegetables.* Eat at least five servings of fruits and vegetables every day to reduce your risk.

☐ *Cut back on fats.* Reduce fat consumption, especially saturated fats and red meats, to reduce risk for colon, breast, prostate, pancreatic, and ovarian cancers.

Making Community Choices

☐ Does your community have any major sources of carcinogens (toxic waste dumps, chemical factories, etc.)? What precautions are taken to ensure that environmental risks are reduced?

☐ Does your community have cancer support groups that you could join if you developed cancer? Where would you find out about such support groups?

Summary

* Cancer is a group of diseases characterized by uncontrolled growth and spread of abnormal cells. These cells may create tumors. Benign (noncancerous) tumors grow in size but do not spread; malignant (cancerous) tumors spread to other parts of the body.
* Several causes of cancer have been identified. Lifestyle factors include smoking and obesity. Biological factors include inherited genes and gender. Occupational and environmental hazards are carcinogens present in people's home or work environments. Chemicals in foods that may act as carcinogens include preservatives and pesticides. Viral diseases that may lead to cancer include herpes, mononucleosis, and human papillomavirus (which causes genital warts). Medical factors include certain drug therapies given for other conditions that may elevate the chance of cancer. Combined risk refers to a combination of the above factors, which tends to compound the risk for cancer.
* There are many different types of cancer, each of which poses different risks, depending on a number of factors. Common cancers include lung, breast, colon and rectum, prostate, skin, testicular, ovarian, uterine, and pancreatic cancers, as well as leukemia.
* Early diagnosis improves survival rate. Self-exams for breast, testicular, and skin cancer, and knowledge of the seven warning signals of cancer aid early diagnosis.
* New types of cancer treatments include various combinations of radiotherapy, chemotherapy, and immunotherapy.

Questions for Discussion and Reflection

1. What is cancer? How does it spread? What is the difference between a benign and a malignant tumor?
2. List the likely causes of cancer. Do any of them put you at greater risk? What can you do to reduce this risk? What risk factors do you share with family members? Friends?
3. What are the symptoms of lung, breast, prostate, and testicular cancer? What can you do to reduce your risk of developing these cancers or increase your chances of surviving them?
4. What are the differences between carcinomas, sarcomas, lymphomas, and leukemia? Which is the most common? Least common?
5. Why are breast and testicular self-exams important for women and men? What could be the consequences of not doing these exams regularly?
6. Discuss the seven warning signals of cancer. What could indicate that you have cancer instead of a minor illness? How soon should you seek treatment for any of the warning signs?

Application Exercises

Reread the What Do You Think? scenarios at the beginning of this chapter and answer the following questions.

1. What factors should a young woman like Jeanie consider before making such a decision about her breasts? Does a grandparent's diagnosis of breast cancer in her late 70s really signal an increased risk for Jeanie? How would you go about gathering information about such choices?
2. Why is a tan so important to young Americans? What are the risks of tanning? What actions could be taken to reduce the risk of developing skin cancer?

Accessing Your Health on the Internet

Visit the following Internet sites to explore further topics and issues related to personal health. To visit an organization's website, go to the Companion Website for *Access to Health, Eighth Edition* at www.aw.com/donatelle, click on the book image, and select "Accessing Your Health on the Internet" from the navigation menu on the left.

1. ***American Cancer Society.*** Homepage for the leading private organization dedicated to cancer prevention. This site provides information, statistics, and resources regarding cancer.
2. ***International Cancer Information Center.*** Sponsored by the National Cancer Institute, this site is designed to be a comprehensive information resource on cancer for patients and health professionals.
3. ***National Cancer Institute.*** Check here for valuable information on clinical trials and the Physician Data Query (PDQ), a comprehensive database of cancer treatment information.
4. ***National Women's Health Information Center (NWHIC).*** Provides a wealth of information about cancer in women. Cosponsored by the National Cancer Institute.

5. *Oncolink.* Sponsored by the University of Pennsylvania Cancer Center, this site seeks to educate cancer patients and their families by offering information on support services, cancer causes, screening, prevention, and common questions.

Further Reading

American Cancer Institute Journal, published monthly.

Focuses on current risk factors, prevention, and treatment research in the area of cancer.

American Cancer Society. *Cancer Facts and Figures.* Atlanta, GA: published annually.

A summary of major facts relating to cancer. Provides information on incidence, prevalence, symptomology, prevention, and treatment. Available through local divisions of the American Cancer Society.

American Cancer Society. *Colorectal Cancer: A Thorough and Compassionate Resource for Patients and Their Families.* New York: Random House, 2000.

Contains up-to-date information about the disease, medical options, and emotional support.

Nutrition and Cancer Journal, published monthly.

Focuses on etiological aspects of various dietary factors and research on risks for cancer development. Also includes current research on dietary factors and prevention.

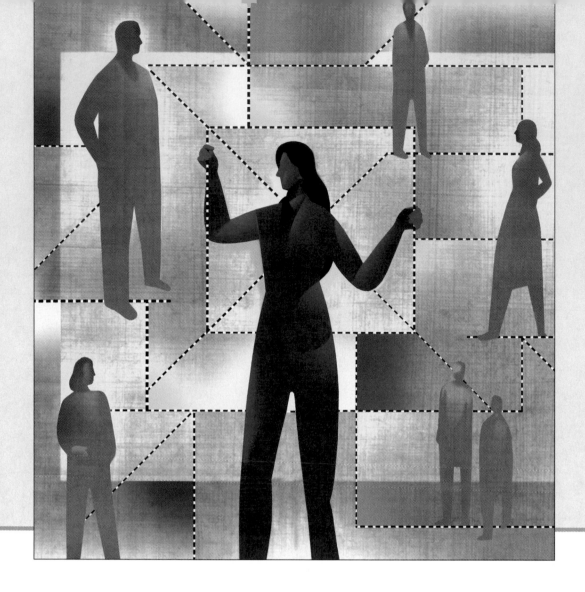

Objectives

* Discuss the risk factors for infectious diseases, including those you can control and those you cannot.

* Describe the most common pathogens infecting humans today, and summarize the major characteristics of each pathogen as well as the typical diseases caused by each.

* Describe your immune system and how it works to protect you, as well as factors that may make your immune system less effective.

* Explain the major emerging and resurgent diseases affecting humans today; discuss why they are increasing in incidence and what actions are being taken to reduce risks.

* Discuss the various sexually transmitted infections, their means of transmission, and actions that can be taken to prevent their spread.

* Discuss human immunodeficiency virus (HIV) and acquired immune deficiency syndrome, trends in infection and treatment, and the impact on special populations, such as women and members of the international community.

17 Infectious Diseases and Sexually Transmitted Infections

Risks and Responsibilities

What do you think?

Heather is a member of a sorority on a campus on the East Coast. Fun-loving and wild, she likes to burn the candle on both ends and routinely parties several nights of the week. Because she also is involved in several organizations on campus and is working hard to maintain the high GPA necessary to get into a physical therapy program, she sleeps very little and has little time for eating regular meals. She notes that she doesn't feel well a lot of the time, her hair is falling out, and the cold she got two weeks ago is still hanging on.

Does Heather sound like anyone whom you know? ✻ What actions might Heather take to build the stamina necessary to maintain her busy work schedule and enjoy her social life? ✻ What factors about living in a group housing situation might increase the risk of contracting infectious diseases?

Susan and Perry have been involved in a committed relationship for the past two years. During a medical checkup, Susan questions the doctor about some burning blisters that she has noticed on her genitals. The doctor tells her that she has genital herpes. Upon hearing this, Susan is devastated. She believes that Perry has been cheating on her and she has picked up this infection from him.

Do you think that Susan is justified in her suspicions? ✻ What possible scenarios for infection might exist here? ✻ If Perry had, in fact, experienced a previous herpes outbreak, should he have told Susan before having sex with her, even if he didn't have any active herpes sores? ✻ Can Susan be certain that Perry infected her?

Every moment of every day, you are in contact with microscopic organisms that have the ability to make you ill or even kill you. These disease-causing agents, known as **pathogens,** are found in air and food and on nearly every object or person with whom you come in contact. Although new varieties of pathogens arise all the time, many have existed for as long as there has been life on the planet. Fossil evidence shows that infections afflicted the earliest human beings. At times, infectious diseases wiped out whole groups of people through **epidemics** such as the Black Death, or bubonic plague, that killed more than half of the population of Europe and Asia in the 1300s. **Pandemics,** or global epidemics of diseases such as influenza, killed more than 20 million people in 1918, while unrelenting strains of tuberculosis and cholera continue to cause premature death among populations throughout the world.

In spite of our best efforts to eradicate these diseases, they are a continuing menace to all of us. While vaccines, pasteurization, improvements in sanitation, and other public health measures have slowed or stopped the spread of many diseases, some infections that were once held in check by antibiotics have begun to resurge, or emerge, in new, more deadly resistant forms. If we are unable to replace antibiotics as they lose their effectiveness and to limit the emergence and spread of resistance, some diseases may simply become untreatable in the next decade, much as they were in the *preantibiotic* era, when deaths from bacterial diseases were routine.

The news isn't all bad, however. Even though we are bombarded by potential pathogenic threats, our immune systems are remarkably adept at protecting us. *Endogenous microorganisms* are those that live in peaceful coexistence with

their human host most of the time. For people in good health and whose immune systems are functioning properly, endogenous organisms are usually harmless. But in sick people, or those with weakened immune systems, these normally harmless pathogenic organisms can cause serious health problems. *Exogenous microorganisms* are organisms that do not normally inhabit the body. When they do, however, they are apt to produce an infection and/or illness. The more easily these pathogens can gain a foothold in the body and sustain themselves, the more **virulent** or aggressive, they may be in causing disease. However, if your immune system is strong, you will often be able to fight off even the most virulent attacker. Just because you inhale a flu virus does not mean that you will get the flu. Just because your hands are teeming with bacteria does not mean that you will become ill. Several factors influence your susceptibility to disease.

Assessing Your Disease Risks

Most diseases are **multifactorial,** or caused by the interaction of several factors from inside and outside the person. For a disease to occur, the *host* must be *susceptible,* meaning that the immune system must be in a weakened condition; an *agent* capable of transmitting a disease must be present; and the *environment* must be hospitable to the pathogen in terms of temperature, light, moisture, and other requirements. Other risk factors also apparently increase or decrease levels of susceptibility. Figure 17.1 summarizes the body's defenses against invasion.

Risk Factors You Can't Control

Unfortunately, some risk factors are beyond our control. Here are some of the most common:

Heredity Perhaps the single greatest factor influencing longevity is the longevity of a person's parents. Being born into a family in which heart disease, cancer, or other illnesses are prevalent seems to increase a person's risk. Still other diseases are caused by direct chromosomal inheritance. **Sickle-cell anemia,** an inherited blood disease that primarily affects African Americans, is frequently transmitted to the fetus if both parents carry the sickle-cell trait.

It is often unclear whether hereditary diseases occur as a result of inherited chromosomal traits or inherited insufficiencies in the immune system.

Aging After age 40, we become more vulnerable to most of the chronic diseases. Moreover, as we age, our immune systems respond less efficiently to invading organisms, increasing the risk for infection and illness. The same flu that produces an afternoon of nausea and diarrhea in a younger person may cause days of illness or even death in an older person. The very young are also at risk for many diseases, particularly if they are not vaccinated against them.

Pathogen   A disease-causing agent.

Epidemic   Disease outbreak that affects many people in a community or region at the same time.

Pandemics   Global epidemics of diseases.

Virulent   Strong enough to overcome host resistance and cause disease.

Multifactorial disease   Disease caused by interactions of several factors.

Sickle-cell anemia   Genetic disease commonly found among African Americans; results in organ damage and premature death.

Immunological competence   Ability of the immune system to defend the body from pathogens.

Botulism   A resistant food-borne organism that is extremely virulent.

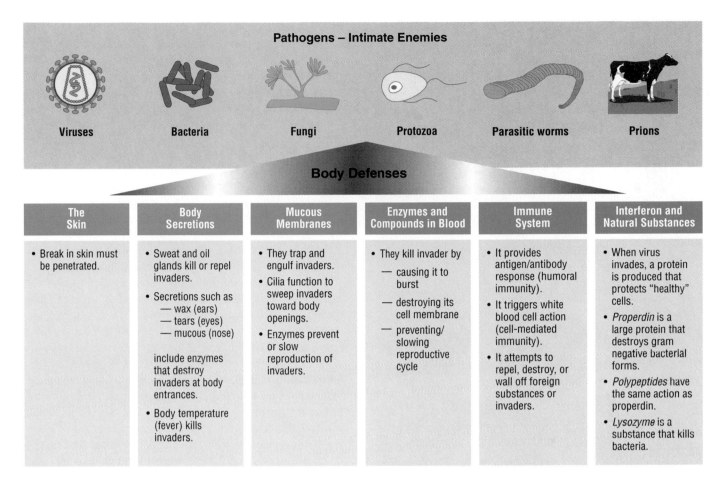

Figure 17.1
The Body's Defenses against Disease-Causing Pathogens

Environmental Conditions Unsanitary conditions and the presence of drugs, chemicals, and hazardous pollutants and wastes in food and water probably have a great effect on our immune systems. It is well documented that poor environmental conditions can weaken **immunological competence**—the body's ability to defend itself against pathogens.

Organism Resistance Some organisms, such as the food-borne organism **botulism,** are particularly virulent, and even tiny amounts may make the most hardy of us ill. Other organisms have mutated and are resistant to the body's defenses as well as other conventional treatments designed to protect against them. Still other, newer pathogens pose unique challenges for our immune systems—ones that our bodily defenses are ill-adapted to fight.

Risk Factors You Can Control

Every minute of every day, we come in contact with agents that could make us sick. Some of these agents are difficult to avoid. However, the good news is that we all have some degree of personal control over many risk factors for disease.

Too much stress, inadequate nutrition, a low physical fitness level, lack of sleep, misuse or abuse of legal and illegal substances, poor personal hygiene, high-risk behaviors, and other variables significantly increase the risk for a number of diseases. Various chapters of this text discuss these variables. Several factors influence our individual susceptibility to various diseases. Those we have the most control over, via lifestyle decisions and behaviors, are noted on the following list with an asterisk (*):[1]

- Personal habits: smoking, alcohol use, sleep, exercise, stress levels, drug use/abuse.*
- Dosage, virulence, and portal of entry of agent.
- Age at time of infection.
- Preexisting level of immunity.*
- Health and vigor of immune system response.*
- Genetic factors controlling immune response.
- Nutritional status of host.*
- Comorbidities: the number of battles your immune system is fighting at the same time.*
- Environmental surroundings, such as temperature, humidity, and sanitary conditions.*
- Psychological factors (e.g., motivation, emotional status, and so on).*

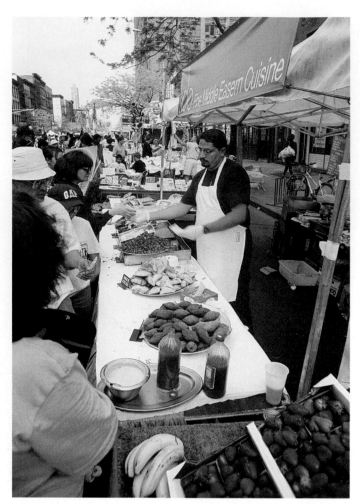

Airborne pathogens can be transmitted easily and unknowingly, which is why special precautions must be taken to ensure the health and safety of patrons of food markets and other public places.

that was just touched by someone whose hands were contaminated by a recent sneeze or failure to wash after using the toilet. You may also **autoinoculate** yourself, or transmit a pathogen from one part of your body to another. For example, you may touch a sore on your lip that is teeming with viral herpes, then transmit the virus to your eye when you scratch your itchy eyelid.

Pathogens are also transmitted by *airborne contact*—you can breathe in air that carries a particular pathogen—or by *food-borne infection* if you eat something contaminated by microorganisms. Recent episodes of food poisoning from *salmonella* bacteria in certain foods and *E. coli* bacteria in undercooked beef have raised concerns about the safety of the U.S. food supply. As a direct result of these concerns, food labels caution consumers to cook meats thoroughly, wash utensils, and take other food-handling precautions.

Your best friend may be the source of *animal-borne pathogens.* Dogs, cats, livestock, and wild animals can spread numerous diseases through their bites or feces or by carrying infected insects into living areas and transmitting diseases either directly or indirectly. Although **interspecies transmission** of diseases (the passing of diseases from humans to animals and vice versa) is rare, it does occur. *Water-borne diseases* are transmitted directly from drinking water and indirectly from foods washed or sprayed with contaminated water. These pathogens can also invade your body if you wade or swim in contaminated streams, lakes, and reservoirs. Pathogens may also be transmitted via insects such as mosquitoes, ticks, and other hosts that carry pathogens in their saliva or other body fluids. They spread *insect-borne diseases* through sucking or biting other animals or humans. Mothers may transmit diseases *perinatally* to an infant in the womb or as the baby passes through the vagina during birth.

What do you think?

If you were to list your own risk factors for infectious diseases, what would they be? ✳ What actions can you take to reduce your risks? ✳ Are your risks greater today than before you entered college? ✳ Why or why not?

Types of Pathogens and Routes of Transmission

Pathogens enter the body in several ways (see Table 17.1). They may be transmitted by *direct contact* between infected persons, such as during sexual relations, kissing, or touching, or by *indirect contact,* such as by touching an object the infected person has had contact with. The hands are probably the greatest source of infectious disease transmission. For example, you may touch the handle of a drinking fountain

Table 17.1
Routes of Disease Transmission

MODE OF TRANSMISSION	ASPECTS OF TRANSMISSION
1. Contact	Either *direct* (e.g., skin or sexual contact) or *indirect* (e.g., infected blood or body fluid)
2. Food- or water-borne	Eating or coming in contact with contaminated food or water or products passed through them
3. Airborne	Inhalation; droplet spread as through sneezing, coughing, or talking
4. Vector-borne	Vector-transmitted via secretions, biting, egg-laying, as done by mosquitoes, ticks, snails, avians, etc; depends on how infectious the organism is
5. Perinatal	Similar to contact infection; happens in the uterus or as the baby passes through the birth canal

We can categorize pathogens into six major types: bacteria, viruses, fungi, protozoa, parasitic worms, and prions. Each has a particular route of transmission and characteristic elements that make it unique. In the following pages we discuss each of these categories and give an overview of diseases they cause that have a significant impact on public health. Some are particularly *virulent,* meaning that they are able to successfully invade a host and sustain themselves in a potentially hostile environment. Others are weak and die before they even penetrate the body because of the far-reaching body defense system.

Bacteria

Bacteria are single-celled organisms that are plantlike in nature but lack chlorophyll (the pigment that gives plants their green coloring). There are three major types of bacteria: cocci, bacilli, and spirilla. Each type is distinguished by its shape, size, and other unique characteristics. Bacteria can be viewed under a standard light microscope.

Although there are several thousand species of bacteria, only approximately 100 cause diseases in humans. In many cases, it is not the bacteria themselves that cause disease but rather the poisonous substances, called **toxins,** that they produce. The following are the most common bacterial infections.

Staphylococcal Infections Staphylococci are normally present on our skin at all times and usually cause few problems. But when there is a cut or break in the **epidermis,** or outer layer of the skin, staphylococci may enter and cause a localized infection. If you have ever suffered from acne, boils, styes (infections of the eyelids), or infected wounds, you have probably had a staph infection.

At least one staph-caused disorder, **toxic shock syndrome,** is potentially fatal. Media reports in the 1980s indicated that the disorder was exclusive to menstruating women, particularly those who used high-absorbency tampons and left them inserted for prolonged periods of time. Although most cases of toxic shock syndrome have occurred in menstruating women, the disease was first reported in 1978 in a group of children and continues to appear in people recovering from wounds, surgery, or other injury.

To reduce the likelihood of toxic shock syndrome, take the following precautions: (1) avoid superabsorbent tampons except during the heaviest menstrual flow; (2) change tampons at least every four hours; and (3) use pads at night instead of tampons. Call your doctor immediately if you experience any of the following symptoms: high fever, headache, vomiting, diarrhea and chills, stomach pains, or shocklike symptoms such as faintness, rapid pulse, pallor (which can be caused by a drop in blood pressure), or a sunburnlike rash, particularly on fingers and toes.

Streptococcal Infections At least five types of the **streptococcus** microorganism are known to cause bacterial infections. While most strep infections are of the type A strep variety, you should be aware that there are actually five known types that cause problems: groups A, B, C, D, and G. Group A causes the bacterial diseases that are the most common, such as:[2]

- Streptococcal pharyngitis, or "strep throat."
- Scarlet fever, which is often preceded by a sore throat.
- Skin infections (impetigo, etc.).
- Localized infections limited to a particular body site.
- Toxic shock and blood infections.

Most of these infections respond readily to antibiotics. However, resistant forms of streptococcal infections are emerging and pose threats for the future.

The second most common form of strep infection is the group B streptococcus (GBS), a type of bacterium that causes illness in newborn babies, pregnant women, the elderly, and adults with other illnesses such as diabetes or liver disease. GBS is the most common cause of life-threatening infections in newborns. In pregnant women, GBS can cause bladder infections, womb infections, and stillbirth. Among men and nonpregnant women, it can cause blood infections and pneumonia. Approximately 20 percent of men and nonpregnant women with GBS die of the disease. This has caused increasing concern among health professionals today.[3]

Pneumonia In the early twentieth century, **pneumonia** was one of the leading causes of death in the United States. This disease is characterized by chronic cough, chest pain, chills, high fever, fluid accumulation, and eventual respiratory failure. One of the most common forms of pneumonia is caused by bacterial infection and responds readily to antibiotic treatment in the early stages. Other forms are caused by viruses, chemicals, or other substances in the lungs and

---

Autoinoculation Transmission of a pathogen from one part of the body to another.

Interspecies transmission Transmission of disease from humans to animals or from animals to humans.

Bacteria Single-celled organisms that may cause disease.

Toxins Poisonous substances produced by certain microorganisms that cause various diseases.

Staphylococci Round, gram-positive bacteria, usually found in clusters.

Epidermis The outermost layer of the skin.

Toxic shock syndrome A potentially life-threatening bacterial infection that is most common in menstruating women who use tampons.

Streptococus A round bacterium, usually found in chain formation.

Pneumonia Bacterially caused disease of the lungs.

Table 17.2
Tuberculosis Cases by Age and Race/Ethnicity, 2001

AGE	NUMBER OF CASES	PERCENT	RATE PER 100,000 POPULATION
0–14	931	6	1.5
15–24	1,594	10	4.0
25–44	5,630	35	6.6
45–64	4,534	28	7.2
65 and over	3,295	21	9.1
RACE/ETHNICITY			
White, non-Hispanic	3,357	21	1.6
Black, non-Hispanic	4,796	30	13.8
Hispanic	4,001	25	11.9
American Indian/Alaskan Native	233	1	11.0
Asian/Pacific Islander	3,552	22	32.7

Source: Centers for Disease Control and Prevention, National Center for HIV, STD, and TB Prevention, "Reported TB in the U.S.—2001," 2001 (see http://www.cdc.gov/nchstp/tb/surv/surv2001/default.htm).

are more difficult to treat. Although medical advances have reduced the overall incidence and severity of pneumonia, it continues to be a major threat in the United States and throughout the world. Vulnerable populations include the poor, the elderly, and those already suffering from other illnesses such as AIDS.[4]

Legionnaire's Disease This bacterial disorder gained widespread publicity in 1976, when several Legionnaires at the American Legion convention in Philadelphia contracted it and died before the invading organism was isolated and effective treatment devised. Although one of the lesser-known diseases, its water-borne nature has led to several recent outbreaks in the United States.[5] The symptoms are similar to those for pneumonia, which sometimes makes identification difficult. In people whose resistance is lowered, particularly the elderly, delayed identification can have serious consequences.

Tuberculosis One of the leading fatal diseases in the United States in the early twentieth century, **tuberculosis (TB),** or "consumption" or "white death" as it was once known, was largely controlled in America by 1950 due to improved sanitation, isolation of infected persons, and treatment with drugs such as *rifampin* or *isoniazid*. In fact, the number of reported cases in 1985 reached an all-time low of about 22,000. Many health professionals assumed that TB had been conquered, but today it is on the increase in many regions of the world. During the past 20 years, deteriorating social conditions, including overcrowding and poor sanitation, failure to isolate active cases of TB, a weakening of the public health infrastructure that led to less funding for screening, and migration of TB to the United States through international travel have led to an epidemic rise in the disease. By 1992, there were nearly 27,000 cases of TB in the United States.[6] Although rapid public health intervention stopped the increase, TB still infected nearly

16,000 Americans in 2001.[7] Newer strains of multiple-drug-resistant tuberculosis (MDR-TB) make this epidemic potentially more devastating than previous outbreaks. See Table 17.2 for a breakdown of cases by age and ethnic group.

People residing in overcrowded prisons and homeless shelters with poor ventilation (which means that people continuously inhale the same contaminated air) are at special risk. Early release programs for infected prisoners and the migratory patterns of infected homeless people make the spread of tuberculosis difficult to control. The poor, especially children and the chronically ill, seem to be among those at greatest risk. As the HIV/AIDS epidemic has evolved, persons with compromised immune systems are also at high risk for TB infection. In the United States during 1997–2001, the top five countries of origin for foreign-born persons with TB were Mexico, the Philippines, Vietnam, India, and China. Fully one-half of all TB cases in the United States in 2001 occurred in foreign-born individuals.[8]

Although tuberculosis increases in the United States are troubling, U.S. statistics pale by comparison to the staggering tuberculosis burden in the global population. The World Health Organization (WHO) ranks tuberculosis among the most serious health threats in the world. It is estimated that one-third of the world's inhabitants (over 1.9 billion humans) are latently infected with the TB bacterium, *M. tuberculosis*. In addition, 7–8 million new cases of tuberculosis occur each year, and approximately 2 million people die of the disease. Ninety-five percent of these deaths occur in developing nations. Tuberculosis causes 25 percent of all preventable adult deaths in the developing world, and 75 percent of cases and 80 percent of deaths in these areas occur among adults ages 15–55.[9] Assuming no significant improvements in prevention and control between now and 2020, WHO estimates that in the first two decades of the twenty-first century, 1 billion people will acquire a new tuberculosis infection,

200 million will develop active disease, and 70 million will die.[10] New, highly virulent drug-resistant forms of the disease pose a potentially devastating threat in certain countries, such as India and Pakistan.[11] "Hot spot" areas of the world for tuberculosis include Latvia, Russia, the Dominican Republic, China, India, and Argentina.[12] Rates in Southeast Asia, Central and South America, the Caribbean, and Africa increased dramatically between 1997 and 2001.[13]

Tuberculosis is caused by bacterial infiltration of the respiratory system that results in a chronic inflammatory reaction in the lungs. Airborne transmission via the respiratory tract is the primary and most efficient mode of transmitting TB. People with active cases can transmit the disease while talking, coughing, sneezing, or singing. Fortunately, it is fairly difficult to catch, and prolonged exposure, rather than single exposure, is the typical mode of infection. Only about 20–30 percent of those exposed to an active case will become infected.[14] In some regions of the world, bovine tuberculosis, which is found in unpasteurized milk and dairy products from tuberculous cattle, is more common. A rare mode of transmission is by infected urine, especially for young children using the same toilet facilities. Many people infected with TB are contagious without actually showing any symptoms themselves. Fortunately, the average healthy person is not at high risk; however, those who may be fighting other diseases may be at increased risk. Symptoms include persistent coughing, weight loss, fever, and spitting up blood. If you or someone you know has these symptoms, check with a doctor. A simple skin test can indicate infection, to be followed by chest x-rays and other confirmatory tests. Treatments are effective for most nonresistant cases. Treatment includes rest, careful infection-control procedures, and drugs to combat the infection.

Periodontal Diseases   Diseases of the tissue around the teeth, called **periodontal diseases,** affect three out of four adults over age 35. Improper tooth care, including lack of flossing and poor brushing habits, and the failure to obtain professional dental care regularly lead to increased bacterial growth, caries (tooth decay), and gum infections. If left untreated, permanent tooth loss may result.

Rickettsia-Caused Diseases   Once believed to be closely related to viruses, **rickettsia** are now considered to be a small form of bacteria. They produce toxins and multiply within small blood vessels, causing vascular blockage and tissue death.

Rickettsia require an insect vector (carrier) for transmission to humans. Two common forms of human rickettsia disease are Rocky Mountain spotted fever (RMSF), carried by a tick, and typhus, carried by a louse, flea, or tick. These diseases produce similar symptoms, including high fever, weakness, rash, and coma, and both can be life threatening. You do not actually have to be bitten by a vector to contract these diseases. Because the vectors themselves harbor the developing rickettsia in their intestinal tracts, insect excrement deposited on the skin and entering the body through abrasions and scratches may be a common source of infection.

Although the name Rocky Mountain spotted fever seems to imply a specific geographic risk, RMSF is found throughout the United States as well as southern Canada, Mexico, Central America, and parts of South America. Between 1981 and 1997, the disease was reported in every U.S. state except Hawaii, Vermont, Maine, and Alaska.[15]

What do you think?

Why do you think we are experiencing global increases in diseases such as tuberculosis today? ✴ *Should we be concerned about diseases in other countries?* ✴ *Do we have an obligation to help the world's population in its struggle against these diseases?* ✴ *What policies, programs, and services might help?*

Viruses

Viruses are the smallest pathogens, approximately 1/500th the size of bacteria. Because of their tiny size, they are visible only under an electron microscope and were not identified until this century.[16]

Over 150 viruses are known to cause diseases in humans, although their role in the development of various cancers and chronic diseases remains unclear. In fact, we still have much to learn about viruses, perhaps the most unusual microorganisms that infect humans.

Essentially, a virus consists of a protein structure that contains either *ribonucleic acid (RNA)* or *deoxyribonucleic acid (DNA)*. Incapable of carrying out the normal cell functions of respiration and metabolism, a virus cannot reproduce on its own and can exist only in a parasitic relationship with the cell it invades. In fact, some scientists question whether viruses should even be considered living organisms.

When viruses attach themselves to host cells, they inject their own RNA or DNA, causing the host cells to begin reproducing new viruses. Once they take control of a cell, these new viruses overrun it until, filled to capacity, the cell bursts, putting thousands of new viruses into circulation to begin the process of cell invasion and reproduction all over again.

Because viruses cannot reproduce outside living cells, they are especially difficult to culture in a laboratory, making their detection and study extremely time-consuming. Viral

---

Tuberculosis (TB)   A disease caused by bacterial infiltration of the respiratory system.

Periodontal diseases   Diseases of the tissue around the teeth.

Rickettsia   A small form of bacteria that live inside other living cells.

Viruses   Minute parasitic microbes that live inside another cell.

diseases can be difficult to treat because many viruses can withstand heat, formaldehyde, and large doses of radiation with little effect on their structure. In addition, some viruses may have **incubation periods** (the length of time required to develop fully and therefore cause symptoms in their hosts) that are measured in years rather than hours or days. Termed **slow-acting viruses,** these viruses infect the host and remain in a semidormant state for years, causing a slowly developing illness. HIV is the most recent deadly example of a slow-acting virus.

Drug treatment for viral infections is also limited. Drugs powerful enough to kill viruses generally kill the host cells, too, although some medications block stages in viral reproduction without damaging the host cells.

When exposed to certain viruses, the body produces a protein substance known as **interferon.** Interferon does not destroy the invading microorganisms but sets up a protective mechanism to aid healthy cells in their struggle against the invaders. Although interferon research is promising, it should be noted that not all viruses stimulate interferon production.

The Common Cold   In everyday life, perhaps no ailment is as bothersome as the common cold, with its irritating symptoms of runny nose, itchy eyes, and generally uncomfortable sensations. Colds are responsible for more days lost from work and more uncomfortable days spent at work than any other ailment.

Caused by any number of viruses (some experts claim there may be over 100 different viruses responsible for the common cold), colds are **endemic** (always present to some degree) among peoples throughout the world. Current research indicates that otherwise healthy people carry cold viruses in their noses and throats most of the time. These viruses are held in check until the host's resistance is lowered. In the true sense of the word, it is possible to "catch" a cold—from the airborne droplets of another person's sneeze or from skin-to-skin or mucous membrane contact—though recent studies indicate that the hands are the greatest avenue for transmitting colds and other viruses.

Obviously, then, covering your mouth with a tissue or hand-kerchief when sneezing is better than covering it with your bare hand, particularly if you next use your hand to touch food, shake your friend's hand, or open a door.

Although numerous theories exist concerning how to "cure" the common cold, including taking megadoses of vitamin C, little hard evidence supports any of them. The best rule of thumb is to keep your resistance level high. Sound nutrition, adequate rest, stress reduction, and regular exercise appear to be the best bets in fighting off infection. Avoid people with newly developed colds (colds appear to be most contagious during the first 24 hours of onset). If you contract a cold, bed rest, plenty of fluids, and aspirin to relieve pain and discomfort are the tried-and-true remedies for adults. Children should not be given aspirin for colds or the flu because this could lead to *Reye's syndrome,* a potentially fatal disease. Several over-the-counter preparations are effective for alleviating certain cold symptoms.

Influenza   In otherwise healthy people, **influenza,** or flu, is usually not life-threatening today. Influenza pandemics in 1918–1919 and other eras have wiped out nearly one-third the population of Europe. Today, vaccines provide significant protection for vulnerable populations. Symptoms, including aches and pains, nausea, diarrhea, fever, and coldlike ailments, generally pass quickly. (Figure 17.2 compares cold and flu symptoms.) However, in combination with other disorders or among the elderly (people over the age of 65), those with respiratory or heart disease, or the very young (children under age 5), the flu can be very serious. Thus, these individuals receive the highest priority for annual flu shots.

To date, three major varieties of flu virus have been discovered, with many different strains existing within each variety. The "A" form of the virus is generally the most virulent, followed by the "B" and "C" varieties. If you contract one form of influenza you may develop immunity to it, but you will not necessarily be immune to other forms of the disease. Little can be done to treat flu patients once the infection has become established.

Some vaccines have proved effective against certain strains of flu virus, but they are totally ineffective against others. In spite of minor risks, it is recommended that people over age 65, pregnant women, people with heart or lung disease, and those with certain other illnesses be vaccinated. Because flu shots take two to three weeks to become effective, you should get these shots in the fall, before the flu season begins.

Infectious Mononucleosis   Initial symptoms of mononucleosis, or "mono," include sore throat, fever, headache, nausea, chills, and pervasive weakness or fatigue. As the disease progresses, lymph nodes may enlarge and jaundice, and spleen enlargement, aching joints, and body rashes may occur.

Theories on the transmission and treatment of mononucleosis are highly controversial. Caused by the *Epstein-Barr virus,* mononucleosis is readily detected through a *monospot test,* a blood test that measures the percentage of

---

Incubation period   The time between exposure to a disease and the appearance of the symptoms.

Slow-acting viruses   Viruses having long incubation periods and causing slowly progressive symptoms.

Interferon   A protein substance produced by the body that aids the immune system by protecting healthy cells.

Endemic   Describing a disease that is always present to some degree.

Influenza   A common viral disease of the respiratory tract.

Hepatitis   A virally caused disease in which the liver becomes inflamed, producing symptoms such as fever, headache, and jaundice.

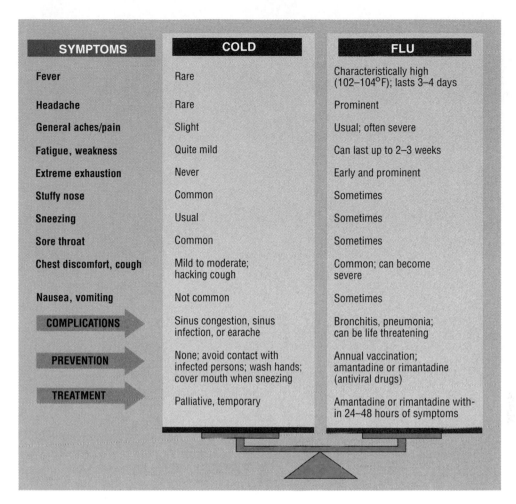

SYMPTOMS	COLD	FLU
Fever	Rare	Characteristically high (102–104°F); lasts 3–4 days
Headache	Rare	Prominent
General aches/pain	Slight	Usual; often severe
Fatigue, weakness	Quite mild	Can last up to 2–3 weeks
Extreme exhaustion	Never	Early and prominent
Stuffy nose	Common	Sometimes
Sneezing	Usual	Sometimes
Sore throat	Common	Sometimes
Chest discomfort, cough	Mild to moderate; hacking cough	Common; can become severe
Nausea, vomiting	Not common	Sometimes
COMPLICATIONS	Sinus congestion, sinus infection, or earache	Bronchitis, pneumonia; can be life threatening
PREVENTION	None; avoid contact with infected persons; wash hands; cover mouth when sneezing	Annual vaccination; amantadine or rimantadine (antiviral drugs)
TREATMENT	Palliative, temporary	Amantadine or rimantadine within 24–48 hours of symptoms

Figure 17.2
Is It a Cold or the Flu?
Adapted from "Is It a Cold or Is It the Flu?" by the National Institute of Allergy and Infectious Diseases, 2000.

specific forms of white blood cells. Because many viruses are caused by transmission of body fluids, many people once believed that young people passed the disease on by kissing (hence its nickname, "the kissing disease"). Although this is still considered a possible cause, mononucleosis is not believed to be highly contagious. It does not appear to be easily contracted through normal, everyday personal contact. Multiple cases among family members are rare, as are cases between intimate partners.

Treatment of mononucleosis is often a lengthy process that involves bed rest, balanced nutrition, and medications. Gradually, the body develops immunity to the disease and the person returns to normal activity.

Hepatitis   One of the most highly publicized viral diseases is **hepatitis,** a virally caused inflammation of the liver. Hepatitis symptoms include fever, headache, nausea, loss of appetite, skin rashes, pain in the upper right abdomen, dark yellow (with brownish tinge) urine, and the possibility of jaundice (yellowing of the whites of the eyes and the skin). In some regions of the United States and among certain

segments of the population, hepatitis has reached epidemic proportions. Internationally, viral hepatitis is one of the most frequently reported diseases and a major contributor to acute and chronic liver disease, accounting for high morbidity and mortality. Currently, there are seven known forms of hepatitis, with the following three having the highest rate of incidence (see Figure 17.3):

• *Hepatitis A (HAV).* HAV is contracted from eating food or drinking water contaminated with human excrement. Each year, over 35,000 people in the United States are infected, typically through something in the household, sexual contact, day care attendance, or recent international travel.[17] Infected food handlers, people who ingest seafood from contaminated water, and those who use contaminated needles are also at risk. Fortunately, individuals infected with hepatitis A do not become chronic carriers.[18]

• *Hepatitis B (HBV).* This disease, one of the more virulent forms of hepatitis, is spread primarily via body fluids being shared through unprotected sex. However, it is also contracted via sharing needles when injecting drugs, through needlesticks or sharps exposure on the job, or, in the case of

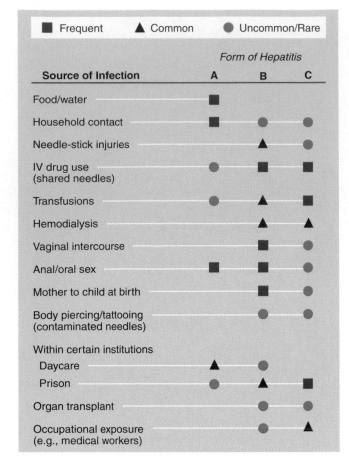

| | Form of Hepatitis | | |
Source of Infection	A	B	C
Food/water	■		
Household contact	■	●	●
Needle-stick injuries		▲	●
IV drug use (shared needles)	●	■	■
Transfusions	●	▲	■
Hemodialysis		▲	▲
Vaginal intercourse		■	●
Anal/oral sex	■	■	●
Mother to child at birth		■	●
Body piercing/tattooing (contaminated needles)		●	●
Within certain institutions Daycare	▲	●	
Prison	●	▲	■
Organ transplant		●	●
Occupational exposure (e.g., medical workers)		●	▲

Legend: ■ Frequent   ▲ Common   ● Uncommon/Rare

Figure 17.3

Ways in Which the Various Forms of Hepatitis May Be Contracted

Source: "Getting Hip to Hep: What You Should Know about Hepatitis A, B, and C," 2002 by the American Liver Foundation, 75 Maiden Lane, Suite 603, New York, NY 10038, 1-800-GO-LIVER, www. liverfoundation.org.

a newborn baby, from an infected mother. Although 30 percent of those who are infected have no symptoms, symptoms can include jaundice, fatigue, abdominal pain, loss of appetite, nausea and vomiting, and joint pain. One of the significant issues with HBV is that it is possible to become a chronic carrier and infect others. Approximately 90 percent of infants infected at birth, 30 percent of children infected at age 1–5, and 6 percent of persons infected after age 5 develop chronic infections.[19] Death from chronic liver disease occurs in 15–25 percent of all chronically infected persons. Although the number of new infections per year has declined from an average of 260,000 in the 1980s to 78,000 in 2001, an estimated 1.25 million Americans are chronically infected. Between 20 and 30 percent acquired their infection in childhood.[20]

Fortunately, a vaccine for HBV has been available since 1982 and is now available on most college campuses for a modest cost. This vaccine means that HBV is one of the only vaccine-preventable sexually transmitted infections in society today. Other than the vaccine, ways of preventing HBV infection include the following:[21]

- Use latex condoms correctly every time you have sex. (Note: The efficacy of latex condoms in preventing infection with HBV is unknown, but their proper use may reduce transmission.)
- If you are pregnant, get a blood test for HBV; infants born to HBV-infected mothers should be given HBIG (hepatitis B immune globulin) and vaccine within 12 hours of birth
- Do not shoot drugs and never share needles.
- Consider the risks of tattoos and body piercings. Only go to reputable artists or piercers who follow established sterilization and infection control protocols.
- If you have had HBV, do not donate blood, organs, or tissues.
- If you are a health care or public safety worker, get vaccinated and follow routine barrier precautions.

- *Hepatitis C (HCV).* This disease was spread primarily through blood transfusion or organ transplant prior to mass screenings that began in 1992, and, more recently, when blood or body fluids from an infected person enter the body of a person who is not infected. HCV infections are on an epidemic rise in many regions of the world today. Resistant forms of HCV are also on the rise. Although overall numbers of cases have declined since the 1980s, an estimated 3.9 million Americans (1.8 percent) have been infected with HCV, of whom 2.7 million are chronically infected.[22]

Symptoms of HCV are similar to those of HBV, with jaundice, fatigue, abdominal pain, loss of appetite, and nausea occurring frequently. In addition, dark urine is a hallmark symptom. The prognosis for a cure is bleak when compared to other forms of hepatitis. About 75–85 percent of those infected develop chronic HCV and 70 percent of those who become chronic carriers also develop chronic liver disease.[23] Today, HCV is one of the leading indicators for liver transplant in the United States.

Although there is no vaccine for HCV, one is currently being tested and may be available shortly. In the absence of a vaccine, other prevention strategies include the following:

- Don't shoot drugs or share needles.
- Don't share personal care items that might have blood on them, such as razors or toothbrushes.
- If you are a health care worker or public safety worker, follow barrier precautions and sharps protocols.
- Avoid tattoos or piercings, or follow the precautions described for HBV.
- Although rare, HCV can be spread by sex. Use latex condoms.
- If you are HCV positive, don't donate blood, organs, or tissue.

In the United States, hepatitis continues to be a major threat in spite of a safe blood supply and massive efforts at education about hand washing (hepatitis A) and safer sex (primarily hepatitis B). Treatment of all the forms of viral hepatitis is somewhat limited. A proper diet, bed rest, and antibiotics that combat bacterial invaders, which may cause additional problems, are recommended. Although tattoos and piercings may increase risk, exact numbers of infections from these procedures are not known. Vaccines for hepatitis A and B are available. Treatment for hepatitis C has been less successful, with only about 25 to 30 percent of those infected responding. Ongoing research, however, is promising.

Mumps Until 1968, mumps was a common viral disorder among children. That year a vaccine became available and the disease seemed to be largely under control, with reported cases declining from 80 per 100,000 people in 1968 to less than 2 per 100,000 people in 1984. Since then, mumps rates have continued to rise steadily. Failure to vaccinate children due to public apathy, misinformation, and social and economic conditions is responsible for the rise. Approximately one-half of all mumps infections are not apparent because they produce only minor symptoms. Large numbers of mumps cases are never reported, so actual incidence rates may be higher than indicated. Typically, there is an incubation period of 16 to 18 days, followed by symptoms caused by the lodging of the virus in the glands of the neck. The most common symptom is the swelling of the parotid (salivary) glands; however, about one-third of all infected people never have this symptom. One of the greatest dangers associated with mumps is the potential for sterility in men who contract the disease in young adulthood. Also, some victims suffer hearing loss.

Chicken Pox (HVZV) and Shingles Caused by the *herpes zoster varicella* virus (HVZV), chicken pox produces characteristic symptoms of fever and tiredness 13 to 17 days after exposure, followed by skin eruptions that itch, blister, and produce a clear fluid. The virus is present in these blisters for approximately one week. Symptoms are generally mild, and immunity to subsequent infection appears to be lifelong. (Some children experience more serious side effects, such as scarring, high fever, and other complications.) Although a vaccine for chicken pox is available, and all children should receive it, many parents incorrectly assume that the vaccine is not necessary. The failure to vaccinate means that many children still contract the disease. Scientists believe that after the initial infection, the virus goes into permanent hibernation and, for most people, there are no further complications. For a small segment of the population, however, the zoster virus may become reactivated. Blisters will develop, usually on only one side of the body and stopping abruptly at the midline. Cases in which the disease covers both sides of the body are far more serious. This disease, known as *shingles,* affects over 5 percent of the population each year. More than half the sufferers are over age 50.

Measles Technically referred to as *rubeola,* **measles** is a viral disorder that often affects young children. Symptoms, appearing about 10 days after exposure, include an itchy rash and a high fever. **German measles (rubella)** is a milder viral infection that is believed to be transmitted by inhalation, after which it multiplies in the upper respiratory tract and passes into the bloodstream. It causes a rash, especially on the upper extremities. It is not generally a serious health threat and usually runs its course in three to four days. The major exceptions to this rule are among newborns and pregnant women. Rubella can damage a fetus, particularly during the first trimester, creating a condition known as congenital rubella, in which the infant may be born blind, deaf, retarded, or with heart defects. Immunization has reduced the incidence of both measles and German measles. Infections in children not immunized against measles can lead to fever-induced problems such as rheumatic heart disease, kidney damage, and neurological disorders.

Rabies The **rabies** virus infects many warm-blooded animals. Bats are believed to be **asymptomatic** (symptom-free) carriers. Their urine, which they spray when flying, contains the virus, and even the air of densely populated bat caves may be infectious. In most other hosts, the disease is extremely virulent and usually fatal. A characteristic behavior of rabid animals is the frenzied biting of other animals and people. Not only does this behavior cause injury but it also spreads the virus through the infected animal's saliva. The most obvious symptoms of the disease are extreme cerebral excitement and rage, spasms in the pharynx (throat) muscles, especially at the sight of water, and the inability to drink water.

The incubation period for rabies is usually one to three months, yet it may range from one week to one year. The disease may be fatal if not treated immediately with the rabies vaccine. Anyone bitten by an animal that could carry rabies should seek immediate medical attention and try to bring the animal along for testing.

Other Pathogens

Although the pathogens discussed in this section are given less attention due to space constraints, the four other types of major pathogens also pose considerable risks to humans.

Fungi Hundreds of species of **fungi,** multi- or unicellular primitive plants, inhabit our environment. Many fungi are useful, providing such foodstuffs as edible mushrooms

---

Measles A viral disease that produces symptoms including an itchy rash and a high fever.

German measles (rubella) A milder form of measles that causes a rash and mild fever in children and may cause damage to a fetus or a newborn baby.

Rabies A viral disease of the central nervous system often transmitted through animal bites.

Asymptomatic Without symptoms, or symptom-free.

Fungi A group of plants that lack chlorophyll and do not produce flowers or seeds; several microscopic varieties are pathogenic.

and some cheeses. But some species of fungi can produce infections. *Candidiasis* (a vaginal yeast infection), athlete's foot, ringworm, and jock itch are examples of fungal diseases. Keeping the affected area clean and dry plus treatment with appropriate medications will generally bring prompt relief.

Protozoa Protozoa are microscopic, single-celled organisms that are generally associated with tropical diseases such as African sleeping sickness and malaria. Although these pathogens are prevalent in nonindustrialized countries, they are largely controlled in the United States. The most common protozoal disease in the United States is *trichomoniasis,* which we will discuss later in this chapter's section on sexually transmitted infections. A common water-borne protozoan disease in many regions of the country is *giardiasis.* Persons who drink or are exposed to the giardia pathogen may suffer intestinal pain and discomfort weeks after infection. Protection of water supplies is the key to prevention.

Parasitic Worms **Parasitic worms** are the largest of the pathogens. Ranging in size from the relatively small pinworms typically found in children to the large tapeworms found in all warm-blooded animals, most parasitic worms are more a nuisance than a threat. Of special note today are the worm infestations associated with eating raw fish in Japanese sushi restaurants. Cooking fish and other foods to temperatures sufficient to kill the worms and their eggs can prevent this.

Prions A **prion,** or unconventional virus, is a self-replicating, protein-based *agent* that can infect humans and other animals. Believed to be the underlying cause of spongiform diseases such as "mad cow disease," this agent systematically destroys brain cells. We will say more about prion-based diseases later in this chapter.

Protozoa   Microscopic, single-celled organisms.

Parasitic worms   The largest of the pathogens, most of which are more a nuisance than a threat.

Prions   One of the newest, more frightening pathogens to infect humans and animals in recent years; a self-replicating protein-based agent that systematically destroys brain cells.

Enzymes   Organic substances that cause bodily changes and destruction of microorganisms.

Antigen   Substance capable of triggering an immune response.

Antibodies   Substances produced by the body that are individually matched to specific antigens.

Your Body's Defenses: Keeping You Well

Although all the pathogens just described pose a threat if they take hold in your body, the chances that they will do so are actually quite small. First, they must overcome a number of effective barriers, many of which were established in your body before you were even born.

Physical and Chemical Defenses: Your Body Responds

Perhaps our single most critical early defense system is the skin. Layered to provide an intricate web of barriers, the skin allows few pathogens to enter. **Enzymes,** complex proteins manufactured by the body that appear in body secretions such as sweat, provide additional protection, destroying microorganisms on skin surfaces by producing inhospitable pH levels. Normal body pH is 7.0, but enzymatic or biochemical changes may cause the body chemistry to become more acidic (pH of less than 7.0) or more alkaline (pH of more than 7.0). In either case, microorganisms that flourish at a selected pH will be weakened or destroyed as these changes occur. A third protection is our frequent slight elevations in body temperature, which create an inhospitable environment for many pathogens. Only when cracks or breaks occur in the skin can pathogens gain easy access to the body.

The linings of the body provide yet another protection. Mucous membranes in the respiratory tract and other linings of the body trap and engulf invading organisms. *Cilia,* hairlike projections in the lungs and respiratory tract, sweep invaders toward body openings, where they are expelled. Tears, nasal secretions, ear wax, and other secretions found at body entrances contain enzymes designed to destroy or neutralize pathogens. Finally, any organism that manages to breach these initial lines of defense faces a formidable specialized network of defenses thrown up by the immune system (see Figure 17.4).

The Immune System: Your Body Fights Back

Immunity is a condition of being able to resist a particular disease by counteracting the substance that produces the disease. Any substance capable of triggering an immune response is called an **antigen.** An antigen can be a virus, a bacterium, a fungus, a parasite, or a tissue or cell from another individual. When invaded by an antigen, the body responds by forming substances called **antibodies** that are matched to the specific antigen much as a key is matched to a lock. Antibodies belong to a mass of large molecules known as *immunoglobulins,* a group of nine chemically distinct protein substances, each of which plays a role in neutralizing, setting up for destruction, or actually destroying antigens.

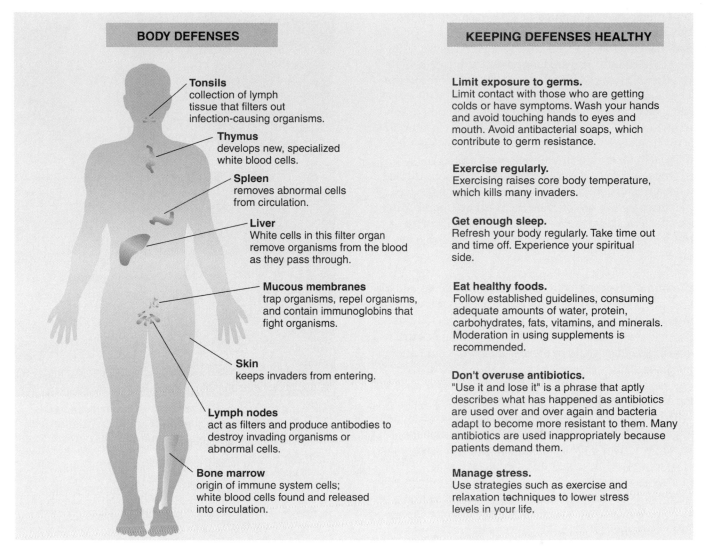

BODY DEFENSES

Tonsils
collection of lymph tissue that filters out infection-causing organisms.

Thymus
develops new, specialized white blood cells.

Spleen
removes abnormal cells from circulation.

Liver
White cells in this filter organ remove organisms from the blood as they pass through.

Mucous membranes
trap organisms, repel organisms, and contain immunoglobins that fight organisms.

Skin
keeps invaders from entering.

Lymph nodes
act as filters and produce antibodies to destroy invading organisms or abnormal cells.

Bone marrow
origin of immune system cells; white blood cells found and released into circulation.

KEEPING DEFENSES HEALTHY

Limit exposure to germs.
Limit contact with those who are getting colds or have symptoms. Wash your hands and avoid touching hands to eyes and mouth. Avoid antibacterial soaps, which contribute to germ resistance.

Exercise regularly.
Exercising raises core body temperature, which kills many invaders.

Get enough sleep.
Refresh your body regularly. Take time out and time off. Experience your spiritual side.

Eat healthy foods.
Follow established guidelines, consuming adequate amounts of water, protein, carbohydrates, fats, vitamins, and minerals. Moderation in using supplements is recommended.

Don't overuse antibiotics.
"Use it and lose it" is a phrase that aptly describes what has happened as antibiotics are used over and over again and bacteria adapt to become more resistant to them. Many antibiotics are used inappropriately because patients demand them.

Manage stress.
Use strategies such as exercise and relaxation techniques to lower stress levels in your life.

Figure 17.4

Bolstering Your Immune System

Adapted from "Make Your Immune System Invincible," by T. Mitchell, *USA Weekend* January 7–9, 2000. Reprinted by permission of T. L. Mitchell, M.D., *USA Weekend* Health Editor.

Once an antigen breaches the body's initial defenses, the body begins a process of antigen analysis. It considers the size and shape of the invader, verifies that the antigen is not part of the body itself, and then produces a specific antibody to destroy or weaken the antigen. This process, which is much more complex than described here, is part of a system called *humoral immune responses*. Humoral immunity is the body's major defense against many bacteria and bacterial toxins.

Cell-mediated immunity is characterized by the formation of a population of lymphocytes that can attack and destroy the foreign invader. These lymphocytes constitute the body's main defense against viruses, fungi, parasites, and some bacteria. Key players in this immune response are specialized groups of white blood cells known as *macrophages* (a type of phagocytic, or cell-eating, cell) and *lymphocytes,* other white blood cells in the blood, lymph nodes, bone marrow, and certain glands.

Two forms of lymphocytes in particular, the *B-lymphocytes* (B-cells) and *T-lymphocytes* (T-cells), are involved in the immune response. There are different types of B-cells, named according to the area of the body in which they develop. Most are manufactured in the soft tissue of the hollow shafts of the long bones. T-cells, in contrast, develop and multiply in the thymus, a multilobed organ that lies behind the breastbone. T-cells assist the immune system in several ways. *Regulatory T-cells* help direct the activities of the immune system and assist other cells, particularly B-cells, to produce antibodies. Dubbed "helper T's," these cells are essential for activating B-cells, other T-cells, and macrophages. Another form of T-cell, known as the "killer T's" or "cytotoxic T's," directly attacks infected or malignant cells. Killer T's enable the body to rid itself of cells that have been infected by viruses or transformed by cancer; they are also responsible for the rejection of tissue and organ grafts. The third type of T-cells, "suppressor T's," turns off or suppresses the activity of B-cells, killer

T's, and macrophages. Suppressor T's circulate in the blood-stream and lymphatic system, neutralizing or destroying antigens, enhancing the effects of the immune response, and helping to return the activated immune system to normal levels. After a successful attack on a pathogen, some of the attacker T- and B-cells are preserved as *memory T- and B-cells,* enabling the body to quickly recognize and respond to subsequent attacks by the same kind of organism at a later time. Thus macrophages, T- and B-cells, and antibodies are the key factors in mounting an immune response.

Once people have survived certain infectious diseases, they become immune to those diseases, meaning that in all probability they will not develop them again. Upon subsequent attack by the disease-causing microorganism, their memory T- and B-cells are quickly activated to come to their defense.

Autoimmune Diseases Although white blood cells and the antigen-antibody response generally work in our favor by neutralizing or destroying harmful antigens, the body sometimes makes a mistake and targets its own tissue as the enemy, builds up antibodies against that tissue, and attempts to destroy it. This is known as *autoimmune* disease (*auto* means "self"). Common autoimmune disorders are rheumatoid arthritis, lupus erythematosus, and myasthenia gravis.

In some cases, the antigen-antibody response completely fails to function. The result is a form of *immune deficiency syndrome.* Perhaps the most dramatic case of this syndrome was the "bubble boy," a youngster who died in 1984 after living his short life inside a sealed-off environment designed to protect him from all antigens. A much more common immune system disorder is *acquired immune deficiency syndrome (AIDS),* which we will discuss later in this chapter.

Fever If an infection is localized, pus formation, redness, swelling, and irritation often occur. These symptoms indicate that the invading organisms are being fought systematically. Another indication is the development of a fever, or a rise in body temperature above the norm of 98.6°F. Fever frequently results from toxins secreted by pathogens that interfere with the control of body temperature. Although this elevated temperature is often harmful to the body, it is also

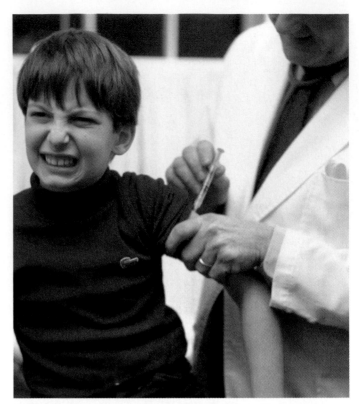

Following the recommended immunization schedule is an easy and effective way to protect a child from serious illnesses, while also helping to eradicate life-threatening disease.

believed to act as a form of protection. Raising body temperature by even one or two degrees provides an environment that destroys some disease-causing organisms. A fever also stimulates the body to produce more white blood cells, which destroy more invaders.

Pain

Although pain is not usually thought of as a defense mechanism, it is a response to injury, and it plays a valuable role in the body's response to invasion. Pain may be either direct, caused by the stimulation of nerve endings in an affected area, or referred, meaning it is present in one place although the source is elsewhere. An example of **referred pain** is the pain in the arm or jaw often experienced by someone having a heart attack. Most pain responses are accompanied by inflammation. Pain tends to be the earliest sign that an injury has occurred and often causes the person to slow down or stop the activity that was aggravating the injury, thereby protecting against further damage. Because it is often one of the first warnings of disease, persistent pain should not be overlooked or masked with short-term pain relievers.

Vaccines: Bolstering Your Immunity

Recall that once people have been exposed to a specific pathogen, subsequent attacks will activate their memory

Referred pain Pain that is present at one point, although the source of pain is elsewhere.

Vaccination Inoculation with killed or weakened pathogens or similar, less dangerous antigens in order to prevent or lessen the effects of some disease.

Acquired immunity Immunity developed during life in response to disease, vaccination, or exposure.

Natural immunity Immunity passed to a fetus by its mother.

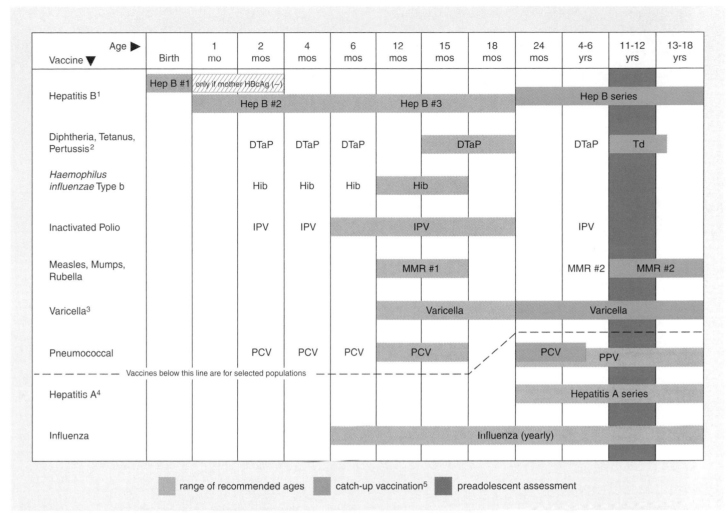

Age ▶ Vaccine ▼	Birth	1 mo	2 mos	4 mos	6 mos	12 mos	15 mos	18 mos	24 mos	4-6 yrs	11-12 yrs	13-18 yrs
Hepatitis B[1]	Hep B #1	only if mother HBcAg (–)									Hep B series	
		Hep B #2			Hep B #3							
Diphtheria, Tetanus, Pertussis[2]			DTaP	DTaP	DTaP		DTaP			DTaP	Td	
Haemophilus influenzae Type b			Hib	Hib	Hib	Hib						
Inactivated Polio			IPV	IPV	IPV					IPV		
Measles, Mumps, Rubella						MMR #1				MMR #2	MMR #2	
Varicella[3]						Varicella				Varicella		
Pneumococcal			PCV	PCV	PCV	PCV			PCV	PPV		
Hepatitis A[4]										Hepatitis A series		
Influenza					Influenza (yearly)							

Vaccines below this line are for selected populations

■ range of recommended ages ■ catch-up vaccination[5] ■ preadolescent assessment

Figure 17.5
Recommended Childhood Immunization Schedule

[1] Mothers who have tested positive for hepatitis B should consult their doctors about their infant's vaccinations.
[2] Tetanus and diphtheria toxoids (Td) are recommended at age 11–12 years if at least five years have elapsed since the last dose of tetanus and diphtheria vaccines. Subsequent routine Td boosters are recommended every 10 years.
[3] Varicella is recommended at any visit or after age 12 months for children who lack a reliable history of chicken pox. Susceptible persons over 13 years should receive two doses, given at least four weeks apart.
[4] Hepatitis A vaccine is recommended for use in selected states and regions and for certain high-risk groups; consult your physician.
[5] "Catch-up vaccination" indicates age groups that warrant special effort to administer any missed vaccines.
Source: American Academy of Pediatrics, "Recommended Childhood Immunization Schedule, United States, 2002" (see http://www.aap.org).

T- and B-cells, giving them immunity. This is the principle on which **vaccination** is based.

A vaccine consists of killed or attenuated (weakened) versions of a disease-causing microorganism, or an antigen that is similar to but less dangerous than the disease antigen. It is administered to stimulate the person's immune system to produce antibodies against future attacks—without actually causing the disease. Vaccines are given orally or by injection, and this form of artificial immunity is termed **acquired immunity,** in contrast to **natural immunity,** which a mother passes to her fetus via their shared blood supply.

Depending on the virulence of the organism, vaccines containing live, attenuated, or dead organisms are given for a variety of diseases. In some instances, if a person is already weakened by other health problems, vaccination may provoke an actual mild case of the disease. Figure 17.5 shows the recommended schedule for childhood vaccinations.

Active and Passive Immunity

If you are exposed to an organism, either during daily life or through vaccination, you will eventually develop an active acquired immunity to that organism. Your body will produce its own antibodies, and, in most cases, you will not have to worry about subsequent exposures to that disease.

Table 17.3
Factors Contributing to Emergent/Resurgent Disease Spread and Possible Solutions

CONTRIBUTING FACTORS	POSSIBLE SOLUTIONS
Hardier bugs: tiny size, adaptability, resistant strains, misuse of antibiotics	Increased pharmaceutical efforts, new drug development, selective use of new drugs; improved vaccination rates; funding of new research
Failure to prioritize public health initiatives on national level	Increased government funding; improved efforts aimed at prevention and intervention (less than 1 percent of the federal budget goes to prevention programs)
Explosive population growth: resource degradation, overcrowding, land used atrocities, increased urbanization	Population control, wise use of natural resources, environmental controls, reduced deforestation and increased pollution prevention efforts
International travel	Education or risk reduction; restrictions related to unvaccinated populations; improved air quality and venting on commercial airlines
Human behaviors, particularly IV drug use and risky sexual behavior	Education about risky behaviors; incentives for improved behaviors; increased personal motivation
Vector management failures: widespread overuse/misuse of pesticides and antimicrobial agents that hasten resistance	Management of pesticide use; focus on pollution prevention; regulation, enforcement of laws
Food and water contamination; globalization of food supply and centralized processing	Control of population growth; animal controls; food controls; improved environmental legislation; food safety; pollution prevention
Complacency and apathy	Education—develop "we" mentality rather than "me" mentality
Poverty	Government support; international aid for vaccination programs, early diagnosis, and treatment; care for disadvantaged
War and mass refugee migration, famine, disasters	Government intervention; international aid
Aging of population	Support for prevention/intervention against controllable age-related health problems
Irrigation, deforestation, and reforestation projects that alter habitats of disease-carrying insects and animals	Improved techniques for conservation; responsible use of resources; policies and programs that protect environment
Increased human contact with tropical rainforests and other wilderness habitats that are reservoirs for insects and animals that harbor unknown infectious agents	Increased regulation to reduce human impact; more research to improve interactions between humans and environment

Sources: Author, plus information found in "Preventing Emerging Infectious Diseases: A Strategy for the 21st Century," 1993 U.S. Department of Health and Human Services, Centers for Disease Control and Prevention, Atlanta, p. 3.

In some cases, however, the risks associated with contracting a disease are so severe that a person may not be able to wait the days or weeks that the body needs to produce antibodies. Also, in the event that resistance is terribly weakened as a result of cancer chemotherapy or other reasons, the body may be unable to produce its own antibodies. In this case, antibodies formed in another person or animal (called the donor) are often given. Termed **passive immunity,** this type of immunity is often short-lived but provides the necessary boost to get a person through a potentially critical period. Antibodies utilized for passive immunity are taken from *gammaglobulins,* proteins synthesized from a donor's blood. A mother also confers passive immunity on her newborn baby through breastfeeding.

Emerging and Resurgent Diseases

Although our immune systems are remarkably adept at responding to challenges, they are threatened by an army of microbes that is so diverse, virulent, and insidious that the invaders appear to be gaining ground. According to the World Health Organization's *World Health Report* issued in 2000, trends such as the aging of the population (the young and old are particularly vulnerable), the urbanization of developing countries, poverty, environmental pollution, globalization of the food supply, and crumbling health care systems bode very badly for the future. As international travel increases (over 1 million people per day cross international boundaries), with germs transported from remote regions to huge urban centers within hours, the likelihood of infection by microbes previously unknown on U.S. soil increases. Table 17.3 identifies major contributors to the emergence and resurgence of infectious diseases.

Tiny Microbes: Lethal Threats

Today's arsenal of antibiotics appears to be increasingly ineffective, with penicillin-resistant strains of diseases on the rise as microbes are able to outlast and outsmart even the best of our antibiotic weapons.[24] Old scourges are back, and new ones are emerging. See the New Horizons in Health box on increases in antibiotic resistance.

"Mad Cow Disease" Since 1998, when the first cases were documented, the British beef industry has been decimated by an attack of a life-threatening pathogen. Images of cows convulsing and foaming at the mouth and the potential for human infection from eating beef have sent millions of Europeans to the store for fish and tofu. Evidence has been increasing that there is a relationship between ongoing outbreaks in Europe of a disease in cattle known as *bovine spongiform encephalitis (BSE, or "mad cow disease")* and a disease in humans known as *new variant Creutzfeldt-Jacob Disease (NvCJD)*.[25] Both disorders are invariably fatal brain diseases with unusually long incubation periods measured in years, and both are caused by unconventional transmittable agents known as *prions*.

BSE is thought to have been transmitted when cows were fed a protein-based substance (slaughterhouse leftovers from sheep and other cows) to help them put on weight and grow faster. Failure to treat this protein by-product sufficiently to kill the BSE organism allowed it to infect the cows. The disease is believed to be transmitted to humans through the meat of these slaughtered cows. The resultant variant of BSE in humans, known as Creutzfeldt-Jakob disease and characterized by progressively worsening neurological damage and possible death, was noted in 10 people in England and linked by some studies to the BSE-diseased cows. With that, the mad-cow scare began.

As scientists continue to investigate this possible link, it should be noted that such a link has not yet been scientifically verified. In fact, the human form of BSE has not been detected in the United States despite active surveillance since 1990. It is extremely unlikely that BSE would be a food-borne hazard in the United States.[26]

Dengue and Dengue Hemorrhagic Fever Transmitted by mosquitoes, **dengue** viruses are the most widespread insect-borne viruses in the world. Today, dengue is found on most continents, and over one-half of all United Nations member states are threatened.[27] Dengue symptoms include flulike nausea, aches, and chronic fatigue and weakness. As urban areas become increasingly infected with mosquitoes, nearly 1.5 billion people, including about 600 million children, are at risk. Each year, it is estimated that more than 100 million people are infected, and over 8,000 die.[28] A more serious

form of the disease, **dengue hemorrhagic fever,** can kill children in 6 to 12 hours, as the virus causes capillaries to leak and spill fluid and blood into surrounding tissue. Dengue is on the rise in the United States, largely due to increased international travel.

Ebola Hemorrhagic Fever (Ebola HF) Another emerging disease, Ebola HF is a severe, often fatal disease in humans and nonhuman primates (monkeys, gorillas, and chimpanzees). Although much about Ebola is unknown, researchers believe that the virus is zoonotic (animal borne) and normally occurs in animal hosts that are native to the African continent.[29] The virus is spread via direct contact with blood and/or secretions, and may be aerosol (airborne) disseminated. With an incubation period of 2–21 days, the course of the disease is quick and characterized by fever, headache, joint and muscle aches, sore throat, and weakness, followed by diarrhea, vomiting, and stomach pain. A rash, red eyes, hiccups, and internal and external bleeding often occur in later phases.[30] Although there have been no known cases of human transmission in the United States, several outbreaks have occurred in various regions of Africa. In 1995, an Ebola outbreak in Zaire killed 245 of the 316 people infected, forcing strict government-enforced quarantine of the entire region. Subsequent infections in other regions of the world have caused increasing concern in the global community. Fortunately, Ebola is not as prevalent worldwide as dengue fever. See the New Horizons in Health box for information on another virus originating in Africa, West Nile virus.

Cryptosporidium In 1993, the intestinal parasite *Cryptosporidium* infected the municipal water supply of Milwaukee, Wisconsin. The result was the largest water-borne coccidian protozoan disease outbreak ever recognized in this country, causing many deaths and sickening hundreds of thousands of people. Exactly how the water supply became infected remains in question; however, the fact that humans, birds, and animals can carry the infective agent opens the door for many possible routes.

Escherichia Coli 0157:H7 *E. coli 0157:HF,* as it is most commonly referred to, is one of over 170 types of *E. coli* bacteria that can infect humans. While most *E. coli* organisms are harmless and live in the intestines of healthy animals and humans, *E. coli 0157:HF* produces a lethal toxin and can cause severe illness or death.

Passive immunity Antibodies formed in another person or animal, then given to someone with a weakened immune system.

Dengue A disease transmitted by mosquitoes, which causes flulike symptoms.

Dengue hemorrhagic fever A more serious form of dengue.

Antibiotic Resistance: What Doesn't Kill Them Makes Them Stronger

Imagine a world where people die from common colds, diarrhea, ear infections, and superficial cuts and infections. If this sounds like the stuff of science fiction or bioterrorism run amok, the facts indicate that such a scenario is not that outrageous. In fact, the 2000 annual report from the World Health Organization, *Overcoming Antimicrobial Resistance* , states that "people of the world may only have a decade or two to make use of many of the medicines presently available to stop infectious diseases before antimicrobial resistance begins to be a major threat to health." Either we develop entirely new antibiotic classes at a previously unheard-of rate, or we face the inevitable truth about the dwindling effectiveness of penicillin and other antibiotics. Our health care system has become increasingly dependent on the availability and efficacy of antibiotics as a part of a $24.5 million industry designed to quickly treat bacterial infections.

RESISTANT INFECTIONS

Drug-resistant infectious agents—those that are not killed or inhibited by antimicrobial compounds—are an increasingly important public health concern. Tuberculosis, gonorrhea, malaria, and childhood ear infections are just a few of the diseases that have become difficult, if not impossible, to treat due to the emergence of drug-resistant pathogens. The Institute of Medicine, part of the National Academy of Sciences, has estimated that the annual cost of treating antibiotic-resistant infections in the United States may be as high as $30 billion. How serious is the problem? Consider the following facts:

- Strains of *Staphylococcus aureus* resistant to most antibiotics are endemic in many hospitals today. In some cities

31 percent of staph infections are resistant, and in nursing homes as many as 71 percent of staph infections defy traditional antibiotic regimens.
- *Streptococcus pneumoniae* causes thousands of cases of meningitis and pneumonia and 7 million cases of ear infections in the United States each year. Currently, about 30 percent of these cases are resistant to penicillin, the primary drug for treatment. Many penicillin-resistant strains are also resistant to other antibiotics.
- An estimated 300 to 500 million people worldwide are infected with parasites that cause malaria. Resistance to chloroquine, once a widely used and highly effective treatment, is now found in most regions of the world, with other treatments losing their effectiveness at alarming rates.
- Strains of multidrug-resistant tuberculosis (MDR-TB) have emerged over the last decade and pose a particular threat to HIV-positive individuals.
- Diarrheal diseases cause almost 3 million deaths per year—mostly in developing countries where resistant forms of *Campylobacter, Shigella, Escherichia coli, Vibrio cholerae,* and *Salmonella* food poisoning have emerged. In some areas, as much as 50 percent of the *Campylobacter* cases are resistant to Cipro, the most effective treatment. A potentially deadly "superbug" known as *Salmonella typhimurium,* resistant to most antibiotics, has been found in Europe, Canada, and the United States.
- Resistant fungal diseases such as *Pneumocystis carinii* pneumonia are on the rise internationally.
- Viral resistance to HIV treatment has meant that many drugs quickly lose their effectiveness in treating HIV.

In the battle between drugs and bugs, the bugs are clearly scoring some big wins.

WHY IS ANTIMICROBIAL RESISTANCE GROWING?

Although the actual mechanisms are complex, antibiotics typically wipe out certain

bacteria that are susceptible to them. However, when used improperly, the antibiotics kill the weak bacteria and leave the "hardy" versions to thrive and replicate. Because bacteria can swap genes with one another under the right conditions, drug-resistant, hardy germs can share their resistance mechanisms with other germs. Eventually, an entire colony of resistant bugs grows and passes on its resistance traits to new generations of bacteria.

In developing countries, resistance commonly stems from underuse of drugs. For example, some patients may begin an antibiotic regimen, start to feel better, and stop taking the drug to save money by using the drug another time. The surviving bacteria then build immunity to the drugs used to treat them. In the United States, patients have historically failed to comply with their antibiotic regimens, leaving pills in the bottle that should have been used to kill all remnants of the bacteria. Also, doctors have overused antibiotics, prompting the CDC to estimate that one-third of the 150 million prescriptions written each year are unnecessary, resulting in bacterial strains that are tougher than the drugs used to fight them.

While patient noncompliance and doctor overuse are believed to be the most significant contributors to our epidemic of resistant bacteria, other factors are also cited as contributors.

- Overuse of antibiotics in food production has contributed to increased drug resistance. About 50 percent of antibiotic production today is used to treat sick animals and encourage growth in livestock and poultry. Although research is only in its infancy, many believe that ingesting meats and animal products that are rich in antibiotics may actually contribute to resistance in humans.
- Another area of concern is the American obsession with cleanliness. One need only look at the antibacterial soaps, cleaning products, and other products on the shelves to know that personal and home cleaning products

are the rage. Just how much these soaps and other products contribute to overall resistance is also in question; as with antibiotics, the germs these products do not kill may become stronger than before.

REDUCING THE RISK OF ANTIMICROBIAL RESISTANCE

What can be done to slow the growth of resistant organisms? Specific individual and community actions include the following:

- Enacting policies that severely restrict the use of antibiotics, growth hormones, and other products in our food supply, as well as buying foods and products that are antibiotic-free.
- Encouraging people to take medications as prescribed and to finish all medications: killing the bugs the first time, all the time.
- Encouraging doctors to prescribe antibiotics only when absolutely necessary and to educate patients about their use.
- Encouraging consumers not to pressure doctors to give them antibiotics for their ailments.
- Educating consumers about the fact that germs are not inherently bad and that exposure to many of them helps our immune systems develop arsenals capable of fighting pathogens.
- Educating people that washing the hands with a good flow of water and regular soap for a bit longer time than normal is better than using antibacterial soaps.
- Educating people that antibacterial dish detergents, cleaners, etc., are not recommended and are only designed to hook consumers by playing on unwarranted fears. It's a better choice to buy products with the least ingredients and not to buy antibacterial products.
- Encouraging pharmaceutical companies to develop, test, and market newer classes of antibiotics to keep up with growing resistance.

Sources: S. B. Levy, *The Antibiotic Paradox: How the Misuse of Antibiotics Destroys Their Curative Powers* (Cambridge, MA: Perseus Publishing, 2002); Harvard Health Letter (electronic source), "Overdoing Antibiotics," 2002. Retrieved November 19, 2002 (see http://www.health.harvard.edu); L. Bren, 2002 "Battle of the Bugs: Fighting Antibiotic Resistance." *FDA Consumer* 36 (4), 28–36, October 31, 2002, from EBSCOHost; National Institute of Allergy and Infectious Diseases, NIH, "Fact Sheet: Antimicrobial Resistance," 2002 (see http://www.niaid.nih.gov/factsheets/antimicro.htm).

E. coli 0157 can live in the intestines of healthy cattle and then contaminate food products at slaughterhouses. Eating ground beef that is rare or undercooked is a common way of becoming infected (see Chapter 8 for more information on safe food handling practices). Drinking unpasteurized milk or juices and drinking or swimming in sewage-contaminated water or public pools can also cause infection via ingestion of feces that contain *E. coli*.

A symptom of infection is nonbloody diarrhea, usually 2–8 days after exposure; however, asymptomatic cases have been noted. Children and the elderly are particularly vulnerable to serious side effects such as kidney failure, as are persons whose immune systems have been weakened by other diseases.

While *E. coli* organisms continue to pose threats to public health, strengthened regulations on the cooking of meat and regulation of chlorine levels in pools have helped. Recent findings indicate that simple changes in the way cattle are fed prior to slaughter may reduce the growth of *E. coli* in cattle stomachs; eliminating grains in the days prior to slaughter makes *E. coli* less likely to survive.

Cholera   Cholera, an infectious disease transmitted through fecal contamination of food or water supplies, has been rare in the United States for most of this century. Recent epidemic outbreaks in the Western Hemisphere (over 900,000 cases), however, have started to affect the United States. One theory of how cholera is introduced into distant regions of the world is that ships from endemic areas release contaminated bilge water into port towns, contaminating local shellfish.[31] Efforts to control cholera may be increasingly difficult as international travel and trade increase.

Hantavirus   Transmitted via rodent feces, this virus was responsible for many deaths in the desert southwestern United States in 1994 before experts were able to identify the culprit. Victims were believed to have come into contact with this organism through breathing the virus-laden dust created in rodent-infested homes. Within hours, victims showed serious symptoms as their lungs filled with fluid, they experienced respiratory collapse, and died. Today, cases of hantavirus have been noted in over 20 states, and vaccines are being developed to counteract it.

Listeriosis   Caused by a potent bacterium found in plants and animals, listeria has proved fatal in many cases in recent years. Early symptoms begin with mild or low fever and progress to headache and inflammation of the brain. Those who are immunocompromised are at greatest risk. Foods that are improperly cooked or that don't require cooking (such as luncheon meats) are particularly susceptible. New regulations that require strict monitoring of food processing plants should help reduce the risk of listeria infection.

Malaria   In the 1960s, after massive international efforts, malaria, a vector-borne disease transmitted by the anopheles mosquito, seemed to be on the decline. However, today there

New Scourge on the Land: West Nile Virus and Its Cousins

Until 1999, few Americans had heard of *West Nile Virus (WNV)*, a disease that was endemic in many other regions of the world. However, when thousands of birds (primarily crows) began to drop from the skies in the eastern part of the United States, scientists from the Centers for Disease Control and Prevention (CDC) were quick to note that it looked a lot like WNV was to blame. They weren't sure that it really was this disease; hence, the original designation of West Nile-*like* virus. Subsequent testing confirmed that the virus actually was the authentic disease and today, the "look-alike" designation has been dropped. Attention to the disease increased dramatically as horses, dogs, cats, and other birds throughout the eastern and central United States were stricken by the disease and peaked when the first human cases were confirmed. In 1999, 62 cases of severe disease were confirmed; 7 deaths resulted from this infection in New York state. Today, the disease has crossed the Mississippi and only a few states remained disease-free as of November 2002 (see map).

TRANSMISSION

West Nile virus is spread by the bite of an infected mosquito, one of the *Culex* species. The basic transmission cycle starts with the mosquitoes, which feed on infected birds. (Over 110 species of birds are known to be infected.) Although birds, particularly crows and jays, can die when infected, most survive, and the virus then circulates freely between the birds and mosquitoes in an ongoing cycle of infection. When a virus-free mosquito feeds on the bird, it contracts the virus. The virus is located in the mosquito's salivary glands, so when the insect bites a human or animal for a blood meal, it injects the virus

into its victim, where the virus multiplies and causes illness.

As of this date, there is no evidence to suggest that West Nile virus can be spread from person to person or from animal to person. However, the CDC just reported in 2002 a suspected case of a baby contracting the disease from breastfeeding. Cases where people may have become infected from organ donation or blood transfusion are currently under investigation.

SYMPTOMS AND TREATMENT

Most people who become infected with West Nile virus will have either no symptoms or only mild ones. However, on rare occasions, West Nile virus infection can result in severe and sometimes fatal illness. When symptoms appear, they include fever, headache, and body aches, often with skin rash and swollen lymph glands. More severe symptoms include a form of encephalitis, or inflammation of the brain, that can cause high fever, neck stiffness, stupor, disorientation, coma,

tremors, convulsions, muscle weakness, paralysis, and death.

Unfortunately, there is no vaccine on the horizon for WNV and no specific anti-viral medication. For severe symptoms, hospitalization with IV fluids, breathing management and respiratory support, and prevention of secondary infections are necessary.

If you think you have the disease, see your doctor as soon as possible.

PREVENTION

Avoiding WNV infection requires avoiding mosquito bites. Follow these strategies:

- Apply mosquito repellents containing DEET when you're outdoors. Note that supersprays with high percentages of DEET are generally not any more effective than milder forms and may cause side effects.
- When possible, wear long-sleeved clothing and long pants treated with repellents. Do not apply repellents containing permethrin directly to exposed skin.

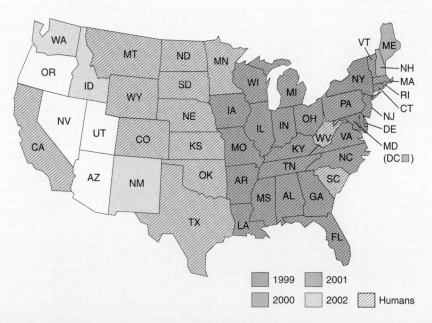

West Nile Virus in the United States, 1999–2002
Source: Centers for Disease Control and Prevention, "Surveillance and Control of West Nile Virus—Map 3," 2002 (see http://www.cdc.gov/ncidod/dvbid/westnile/surv&control.htm).

- Consider staying indoors at dawn, dusk, and in the early evening, which are peak mosquito feeding times.
- Limit mosquito egg laying areas by getting rid of any standing water sources around the home. One flower pot with water standing in it may be the home for thousands of mosquitoes.
- Work with your local government to ensure that some form of mosquito control program is in place in your neighborhood.

OTHER VIRUSES

Although West Nile virus has captured the media's attention for now, it is important to note that we are just in the early stages of being infected with several marauding viruses that may hop the world's oceans and infect America. Whether they arrive by bird, plane, ship, or food source, three noteworthy diseases are likely invaders and have public health officials worried:

Japanese Encephalitis (JE): Related to St. Louis encephalitis, JE is the leading cause of viral encephalitis in Asia, infecting 35,000–60,000 people each year and killing about 4,000. It is far more severe than West Nile virus. Symptoms include fever, headache, neck stiffness, and disorientation, with progression to convulsions and coma. Mosquitoes transmit it after feeding on infected birds or pigs and then biting humans or other animals. So far the mosquito that spreads this disease has not been noted in America, but experts fear that other mosquitoes can adapt and carry the virus if it comes to America. There is a preventive vaccine available.

Rift Valley Fever (RVF): Like West Nile virus, Rift Valley fever was first found in Africa. Mosquitoes help spread it both by biting people and animals and by laying infected eggs that are ingested by livestock. It has many varying symptoms, including severe headaches and eye pain. About 10 percent of victims have lasting eye damage, and about 1 percent die. There is no vaccine.

Ross River Fever (RRF): A relatively mild mosquito-borne virus that causes fever and joint pains, RRF has infected thousands in Australia and can cause lethargy that often lasts more than three months and sometimes more than two years. No vaccine is available.

Source: Centers for Disease Control, Division of Vector-Borne Infectious Diseases, "West Nile Virus," 2002 (see http://www.cdc.gov/ncidod/dvbid/westnile).

---

has been a major resurgence of malaria outbreaks, particularly in Africa, Asia, and Latin America. Currently, the malaria prevention effort is focused on personal protection against bites rather than elimination of mosquitoes.

Bioterrorism: The New Global Threat The idea of using infectious microorganisms as weapons is not new. In fact, during the English wars with Native Americans, blankets impregnated with scabs from smallpox patients were traded to Native Americans in hopes of causing disease.[32] In the 1980s, a large community outbreak of salmonellosis in Oregon was believed to originate from intentional contamination of salad bars in multiple restaurants, carried out by followers of an extremist religious group.[33]

The threat of delivering a lethal load of anthrax or other deadly microorganisms in the warheads of missiles is a topic of much discussion among today's world leaders, particularly after the cases of anthrax delivered via the mail following the September 11, 2001, terrorist attacks. For a complete listing of biological threats considered to pose the greatest risk, see the Health in a Diverse World box about bioterrorism in Chapter 4.

Flesh-Eating Strep The stuff of science fiction, this organism caused hysteria in the United States in 1994 as hospital patients fell prey to an illness that slowly invaded and killed tissue in healing wounds. The culprit? An otherwise treatable form of streptococcus that had suddenly become the victor

in the delicate war between antibiotics and microbes. In this case, our then-current arsenal of drugs was too weak to fight the microbe, until a newer antibiotic was found to stop it.

Sexually Transmitted Infections

Sexually transmitted infections (STIs) have been with us since our earliest recorded days on earth. Today, there are more than 20 known types of STIs. Once referred to as "venereal diseases" and then "sexually transmitted diseases," the most current terminology is more reflective of the number and types of these communicable diseases. More virulent strains and more antibiotic-resistant forms spell trouble for at-risk populations in the days ahead.

Sexually transmitted infections (STIs) affect men and women of all backgrounds and socioeconomic levels. In the United States alone, an estimated 15.3 million new cases of STIs are reported each year. Table 17.4 provides an overview of the prevalence and incidence of selected STIs. Additional facts to note include the following:[34]

> **Sexually transmitted infections (STIs)** Infectious diseases transmitted via some form of intimate, usually sexual, contact.

Table 17.4
Common Sexually Transmitted Infections

STI	INCIDENCE (ESTIMATED NUMBER OF NEW CASES PER YEAR)	PREVALENCE (ESTIMATED NUMBER OF PEOPLE CURRENTLY INFECTED)
Chlamydia	3 million	2 million
Gonorrhea	650,000	Not available*
Syphilis	70,000	Not available*
Herpes	1 million	45 million
Human papilloma virus (HPV)	5.5 million	20 million
Hepatitis B	120,000	417,000
Trichomoniasis	5 million	Not available*

*No recent surveys on national prevalence for gonorrhea, syphilis, or trichomoniasis have been conducted.
Source: Centers for Disease Control, "Tracking the Hidden Epidemics: Trends in STDs in the United States—2002" (see http://www.cdcnpin.org/std.start.htm).

- More than 65 million people are currently living with an incurable STI.
- Two-thirds of all STIs occur in people 25 years of age or younger.
- One in four new STI infections occurs in teenagers.
- One in five Americans has genital herpes, yet at least 80 percent of those are unaware of it.

According to Felicia Stewart of the Kaiser Family Health Foundation, "There is no indication that STIs are coming rapidly under control. In fact, people vastly underestimate risks and fail to take precautions. A Kaiser survey found that just 14 percent of men and 8 percent of women felt at risk for STIs, even though at least one-third will get one."[35]

Early symptoms of an STI are often mild and unrecognizable (see Figure 17.6). Left untreated, some of these infections can have grave consequences, such as sterility, blindness, central nervous system destruction, disfigurement, and even death. Infants born to mothers carrying the organisms for these infections are at risk for a variety of health problems.

As with many communicable diseases, much of the pain, suffering, and anguish associated with STIs can be eliminated through education, responsible action, simple preventive strategies, and prompt treatment. STIs can happen to anyone, but they won't if you take appropriate precautions when you decide to engage in a sexual relationship.

Possible Causes: Why Me?

Several reasons have been proposed to explain the present high rates of STIs. The first relates to the moral and social stigma associated with these infections. Shame and embarrassment often keep infected people from seeking treatment. Unfortunately, these people usually continue to be sexually active, thereby infecting unsuspecting partners. People who are uncomfortable discussing sexual issues may also be less likely to use and ask their partners to use condoms to protect against STIs and pregnancy.

Another reason proposed for the STI epidemic is our casual attitude about sex. Bombarded by media hype that glamorizes easy sex, many people take sexual partners without considering the consequences. Others are pressured into sexual relationships they don't really want. Generally, the more sexual partners a person has, the greater the risk for contracting an STI. Evaluate your own attitude about STIs by completing the Assess Yourself box.

Ignorance—about the infections, their symptoms, and the fact that someone can be asymptomatic but still be infected—is also a factor. A person who is infected but asymptomatic can unknowingly spread an STI to an unsuspecting partner, who may in turn ignore or misinterpret any symptoms. By the time either partner seeks medical help, he or she may have infected several others.

Modes of Transmission

Sexually transmitted infections are generally spread through some form of intimate sexual contact. Sexual intercourse, oral-genital contact, hand-genital contact, and anal intercourse are the most common modes of transmission. More rarely, pathogens for STIs are transmitted mouth to mouth or through contact with fluids from body sores. While each STI is a different infection caused by a different pathogen, all STI pathogens prefer dark, moist places, especially the mucous membranes lining the reproductive organs. Most of them are susceptible to light, excess heat, cold, and dryness, and many die quickly on exposure to air. (The toilet seat is not a likely breeding ground for most bacterial or viral STIs!) Although most STIs are passed on by sexual contact, other kinds of close contact, such as sleeping on sheets used by someone who has pubic lice, may also infect you.

Like other communicable infections, STIs have both pathogen-specific incubation periods and periods of time during which transmission is most likely, called periods of communicability.

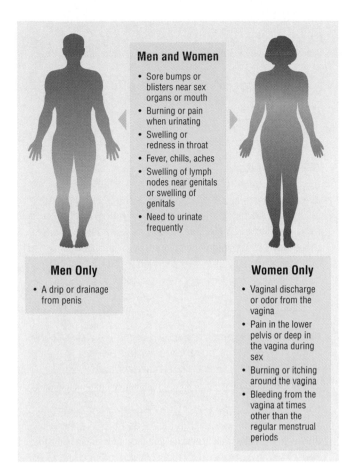

Men and Women

- Sore bumps or blisters near sex organs or mouth
- Burning or pain when urinating
- Swelling or redness in throat
- Fever, chills, aches
- Swelling of lymph nodes near genitals or swelling of genitals
- Need to urinate frequently

Men Only

- A drip or drainage from penis

Women Only

- Vaginal discharge or odor from the vagina
- Pain in the lower pelvis or deep in the vagina during sex
- Burning or itching around the vagina
- Bleeding from the vagina at times other than the regular menstrual periods

Figure 17.6

Signs or Symptoms of an STI

In their early stages, many STIs may be asymptomatic or have such mild symptoms that they are easy to overlook.

Chlamydia

Chlamydia, a disease that often presents no symptoms, tops the list of the most commonly reported infections in the United States. Chlamydia infects about 3 million people annually in the United States, the majority of them women.[36] Public health officials believe that the actual number of cases is probably higher because these figures represent only those cases reported. College students account for over 10 percent of infections, and these numbers seem to be increasing yearly.

The name of the disease is derived from the Greek verb *chlamys,* meaning "to cloak," because, unlike most bacteria, chlamydia can live and grow only inside other cells. Although many people classify chlamydia as either *nonspecific* or *nongonococcal urethritis (NGU),* a person may have NGU without having the organism for chlamydia.

In males, early symptoms may include painful and difficult urination, frequent urination, and a watery, puslike discharge from the penis. Symptoms in females may include a yellowish discharge, spotting between periods, and occasional spotting after intercourse. However, many chlamydia victims display no symptoms and therefore do not seek help until the disease has done secondary damage. Females are

especially likely to be asymptomatic; over 70 percent do not realize they have the disease until secondary damage occurs.

The secondary damage resulting from chlamydia is serious in both genders. Men can suffer damage to the prostate gland, seminal vesicles, and bulbourethral glands as well as arthritis-like symptoms and damage to the blood vessels and heart. In women, chlamydia-related inflammation can injure the cervix or fallopian tubes, causing sterility, and damage the inner pelvic structure, leading to pelvic inflammatory disease (PID). If an infected woman becomes pregnant, she has a high risk for miscarriage and stillbirth. Chlamydia may also be responsible for one type of **conjunctivitis,** an eye infection that affects not only adults but also infants, who can contract the disease from an infected mother during delivery. Untreated conjunctivitis can cause blindness.

If detected early, chlamydia is easily treatable with antibiotics such as tetracycline, doxycycline, or erythromycin. In most cases, treatment is successfully completed in two to three weeks. Unfortunately, chlamydia tests are not a routine part of many health clinics' testing procedures. Usually a person must specifically request a chlamydia check.

> **What do you think?**
>
> *Even though many college students have heard about the risks of STIs and AIDS, why do so many fail to use condoms and take other precautions?* ✳ *What actions could be taken to make more of your friends heed the warnings about STIs?*

Pelvic Inflammatory Disease (PID)

Pelvic inflammatory disease (PID) is a term used to describe a number of infections of the uterus, fallopian tubes, and ovaries. Although PID often results from an untreated sexually transmitted infection, especially chlamydia or gonorrhea, it is not actually an STI. Several nonsexual factors increase the risk of PID, particularly excessive vaginal douching, cigarette smoking, and substance abuse. In the United States, an estimated 500,000 to 1,000,000 cases of PID occur annually.[37] Symptoms of PID vary but generally include acute inflammation of the pelvic cavity, severe pain in the lower abdomen, menstrual irregularities, fever, nausea,

Chlamydia Bacterially caused STI of the urogenital tract.

Conjunctivitis Serious inflammation of the eye caused by any number of pathogens or irritants; can be caused by STDs such as chlamydia.

Pelvic inflammatory disease (PID) Term used to describe various infections of the female reproductive tract.

STI Attitude and Belief Scale

The following quiz will help you evaluate whether your beliefs and attitudes about STIs lead you to take risks that increase your risk of infection. Indicate that you believe the following items are true or false by circling the T or the F. Then consult the answer key that follows.

1. You can usually tell whether someone is infected with an STI, especially HIV infection. **T   F**

2. Chances are that if you haven't caught an STI by now, you probably have a natural immunity and won't get infected in the future. **T   F**

3. A person who is successfully treated for an STI needn't worry about getting it again. **T   F**

4. So long as you keep yourself fit and healthy, you needn't worry about STIs. **T   F**

5. The best way for sexually active people to protect themselves from STIs is to practice safer sex. **T   F**

6. The only way to catch an STI is to have sex with someone who has one. **T   F**

7. Talking about STIs with a partner is so embarrassing that it's better not to raise the subject and instead hope the other person will. **T   F**

8. STIs are mostly a problem for people who have numerous sex partners. **T   F**

9. You don't need to worry about contracting an STI so long as you wash yourself thoroughly with soap and hot water immediately after sex. **T   F**

10. You don't need to worry about AIDS if no one you know has ever come down with it. **T   F**

11. When it comes to STIs, it's all in the cards. Either you're lucky or you're not. **T   F**

12. The time to worry about STIs is when you come down with one. **T   F**

13. As long as you avoid risky sexual practices, such as anal intercourse, you're pretty safe from STIs. **T   F**

14. The time to talk about safer sex is before any sexual contact occurs. **T   F**

15. A person needn't be concerned about an STI if the symptoms clear up on their own in a few weeks. **T   F**

Scoring Key

1. *False.* While some STIs have telltale signs, such as the appearance of sores or blisters on the genitals or disagreeable genital odors, others do not. Several STIs, such as chlamydia, gonorrhea (especially in women), internal genital warts, and even HIV infection in its early stages, cause few if any obvious signs or symptoms. You often cannot tell whether your partner is infected with an STI. Many of the nicest-looking and well-groomed people carry STIs, often unknowingly. The only way to know whether a person is infected with HIV is by means of an HIV-antibody test.

2. *False.* If you practice unprotected sex and have not contracted an STI to this point, count your blessings. The thing about good luck is that it eventually runs out.

3. *False.* Sorry. Successful treatment does not render immunity against reinfection. You still need to take precautions to avoid reinfection, even if you have had an STI in the past and were successfully treated. If you answered true to this item, you're not alone. About one in five college students polled in a recent survey of more than 5,500 college students across Canada believed that a person who gets an STI cannot get it again.

4. *False.* Even people in prime physical condition can be felled by the tiniest of microbes that cause STIs. Physical fitness is no protection against these microscopic invaders.

5. *True.* If you are sexually active, practicing safer sex is the best protection against contracting an STI.

6. *False.* STIs can also be transmitted through nonsexual means, such as by sharing contaminated needles or, in some cases, through contact with disease-causing organisms on towels and bedsheets or even toilet seats.

7. *False.* Because of the social stigma attached to STIs, it's understandable that you may feel embarrassed about raising the subject with your partner. But don't let embarrassment prevent you from taking steps to protect your own and your partner's welfare.

8. *False.* While it stands to reason that people who are sexually active with numerous partners stand a greater chance that one of their sexual partners will carry an STI, all it takes is one infected partner to pass along an STI to you, even if he or she is the only partner you've had or even if the two of you had sex only once. STIs are a potential problem for anyone who is sexually active.

9. **False.** While washing your genitals immediately after sex may have some limited protective value, it is no substitute for practicing safer sex.

10. **False.** You can never know whether you may be the first among your friends and acquaintances to become infected. Moreover, symptoms of HIV infection may not appear for years after initial infection with the virus, so you may have sexual contacts with people who are infected but don't know it and who are capable of passing along the virus to you. You in turn may then pass it along to others, whether or not you are aware of any symptoms.

11. **False.** Nonsense. While luck may play a part in determining whether you have sexual contact with an infected partner, you can significantly reduce your risk of contracting an STI.

12. **False.** The time to start thinking about STIs (thinking helps, but worrying only makes you more anxious than you need be) is now, not after you have contracted an infection. Some STIs, like herpes and AIDS, cannot be cured. The only real protection you have against them is prevention.

13. **False.** Any sexual contact between the genitals, or between the genitals and the anus, or between the mouth and genitals, is risky if one of the partners is infected with an STI.

14. **True.** Unfortunately, too many couples wait until they have commenced sexual relations to have "a talk." By then it may

already be too late to prevent the transmission of an STI. The time to talk is before any intimate sexual contact occurs.

15. **False.** Several STIs, notably syphilis, HIV infection, and herpes, may produce initial symptoms that clear up in a few weeks. But while the early symptoms may subside, the infection is still at work within the body and requires medical attention. Also, as noted previously, the infected person is capable of passing along the infection to others, regardless of whether noticeable symptoms were ever present.

Interpreting Your Score

First, add up the number of items you got right. The higher your score, the lower your risk. The lower your score, the greater your risk. A score of 13 correct or better may indicate that your attitudes toward STIs would probably decrease your risk of contracting them. Yet even one wrong response on this test may increase your risk of contracting an STI. You should also recognize that attitudes have little effect on behavior unless they are carried into action. Knowledge alone isn't sufficient to protect yourself from STIs. You need to ask yourself how you are going to put knowledge into action by changing your behavior to reduce your chances of contracting an STI.

Source: From Jeffrey S. Nevid with Fern Gottfried, *Choices: Sex in the Age of STDs,* 10–13. © Copyright 1995 by Allyn & Bacon. Reprinted by permission.

---

painful intercourse, tubal pregnancies, and severe depression.[38] Major consequences of untreated PID are infertility, ectopic pregnancy, chronic pelvic pain, and recurrent upper genital infections. Risk factors include young age at first sexual intercourse, multiple sex partners, high frequency of sexual intercourse, and change of sexual partners within the past 30 days. Regular gynecological examinations and early treatment for STI symptoms reduce risk.

Gonorrhea

Gonorrhea is one of the most common STIs in the United States, surpassed only by chlamydia in number of cases. The Institute of Medicine estimates that there are over 800,000 cases per year, plus numbers that go unreported.[39] Health economists estimate that the annual cost of gonorrhea and its complications is over $1.1 billion.[40] Caused by the bacterial pathogen *Neisseria gonorrhoea,* this infection primarily infects the linings of the urethra, genital tract, pharynx, and rectum. It may spread to the eyes or other body regions via the hands or body fluids, typically during vaginal, oral, or anal sex. Most victims are males between the ages of 20 and 24, with sexually active females between the ages of 15 and 19 also at high risk.[41]

In males, a typical symptom is a white, milky discharge from the penis accompanied by painful, burning urination two to nine days after contact. This is usually enough to send most men to the physician for treatment. However, about 20 percent of all males with gonorrhea are asymptomatic.

In females, the situation is just the opposite: Only 20 percent experience any discharge, and few develop a burning sensation upon urinating until much later in the course of the infection (if ever). The organism can remain in the woman's vagina, cervix, uterus, or fallopian tubes for long periods with no apparent symptoms other than an occasional slight fever. Thus a woman can be unaware that she has been infected and that she is infecting her sexual partners.

If the infection is detected early, an antibiotic regimen using penicillin, tetracycline, spectiomycin, ceftriaxone, or other drugs is generally effective within a short period of time. If the infection goes undetected in a woman, it can spread throughout the genital-urinary tract to the fallopian

---

Gonorrhea Second most common STD in the United States; if untreated, may cause sterility.

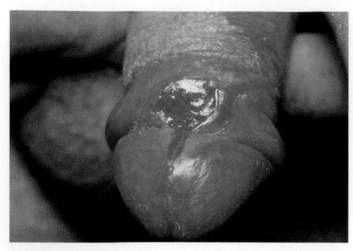

A chancre on the site of the initial infection is a symptom of primary syphilis.

tubes and ovaries, causing sterility, or at the very least, severe inflammation and PID. The bacteria can also spread up the reproductive tract, or more rarely, through the blood and infect the joints, heart valves, or brain. If an infected woman becomes pregnant, the infection can cause conjunctivitis in her infant. To prevent this, physicians routinely administer silver nitrate or penicillin preparations to the eyes of newborn babies.

In a man, untreated gonorrhea may spread to the prostate, testicles, urinary tract, kidney, and bladder. Blockage of the vasa deferentia due to scar tissue formation may cause sterility. In some cases, the penis develops a painful curvature during erection.

Syphilis

Syphilis is also caused by a bacterial organism, the *spirochete* known as *Treponema pallidum*. Because it is extremely delicate and dies readily upon exposure to air, dryness, or cold, the organism is generally transferred only through direct sexual contact. Typically, this means contact between sexual organs during intercourse, but in rare instances, the organism enters the body through a break in the skin, through deep

---

Syphilis   One of the most widespread STDs; characterized by distinct phases and potentially serious results.

Chancre   Sore often found at the site of syphilis infection.

Pubic lice   Parasites that can inhabit various body areas, especially the genitals; also called "crabs."

Genital warts   Warts that appear in the genital area or the anus; caused by the human papilloma viruses (HPVs).

Human papilloma viruses (HPVs)   A small group of viruses that cause genital warts.

---

kissing in which body fluids are exchanged, or through some other transmission of body fluids.

Syphilis is called the "great imitator" because its symptoms resemble those of several other infections. Left untreated, syphilis generally progresses through several distinct stages. It should be noted, however, that some people experience no symptoms at all.

Primary Syphilis   The first stage of syphilis, particularly for males, is often characterized by the development of a **chancre** (pronounced "shank-er"), a sore located most frequently at the site of the initial infection. Although painless, the dime-sized chancre is oozing with bacteria, ready to infect an unsuspecting partner. Usually it appears three to four weeks after contact.

In males, the site of the chancre tends to be the penis or scrotum because this is where the organism first enters the body. But, if the infection was contracted through oral sex, the sore can appear in the mouth, throat, or other "first contact" area. In females, the site of infection is often internal, on the vaginal wall or high on the cervix. Because the chancre is not readily apparent, the likelihood of detection is not great. In both males and females, the chancre will completely disappear in three to six weeks.

Secondary Syphilis   A month to a year after the chancre disappears, secondary symptoms may appear, including a rash or white patches on the skin or on the mucous membranes of the mouth, throat, or genitals. Hair loss may occur, lymph nodes may enlarge, and the victim may develop a slight fever or headache. In rare cases, sores develop around the mouth or genitals. As during the active chancre phase, these sores contain infectious bacteria, and contact with them can spread the infection. In a few cases, there may be arthritic pain in the joints. Because symptoms vary so much and appear so much later than the sexual contact that caused them, the victim seldom connects the two. The infection thus often goes undetected even at this second stage. Symptoms may persist for a few weeks or months and then disappear, leaving the person thinking that all is well.

Latent Syphilis   After the secondary stage, the syphilis spirochetes begin to invade body organs. Symptoms, including infectious lesions, may reappear periodically for two to four years after the secondary period. After this period, the infection is rarely transmitted to others, except during pregnancy, when it can be passed on to the fetus. The child will then be born with congenital syphilis, which can cause death or severe birth defects such as blindness, deafness, or disfigurement. Because in most cases the fetus does not become infected until after the first trimester, treatment of the mother during this period will usually prevent infection of the fetus.

In some instances, a child born to an infected mother will show no signs of the infection at birth but, within several weeks, will develop body rashes, a runny nose, and symptoms of paralysis. *Congenital syphilis* is usually detected before it progresses much further. But sometimes the child's immune system will ward off the invading organism, and further symptoms may not surface until the teenage years. One way that states protect against congenital syphilis is by requiring prospective marriage partners to be tested for syphilis prior to obtaining a marriage license.

In addition to causing congenital syphilis, latent syphilis, if untreated, will progress and infect more and more organs.

Late Syphilis   Years after syphilis has entered the body, its effects become all too evident. Late-stage syphilis indications include heart damage, central nervous system damage, blindness, deafness, paralysis, premature senility, and, ultimately, insanity.

Treatment for Syphilis   Because the organism is bacterial, it is treated with antibiotics, usually penicillin, benzathine penicillin G, or doxycycline. The major obstacle to treatment is misdiagnosis of this "imitator" infection.

Pubic Lice

Pubic lice, often called "crabs," are small parasites that are usually transmitted during sexual contact. More annoying than dangerous, they move easily from partner to partner during sex. They have an affinity for pubic hair, attaching themselves to the base of these hairs, where they deposit their eggs (nits). One to two weeks later, these nits develop into adults that lay eggs and migrate to other body parts, thus perpetuating the cycle.

Treatment includes washing clothing, furniture, and linens that may harbor the eggs. It usually takes two to three weeks to kill all larval forms. Although sexual contact is the most common mode of transmission, you can "catch" pubic lice from lying on sheets that an infected person has slept on. Sleeping in hotel and dormitory rooms in which sheets are not washed regularly, or sitting on toilet seats where the nits or larvae have been dropped and lie in wait for a new carrier, may put you at risk.

Genital HPV

Genital warts (also known as venereal warts or condylomas) are caused by a small group of viruses known as **human papilloma viruses (HPVs).** A person becomes infected when an HPV penetrates the skin and mucous membranes of the genitals or anus through sexual contact. HPV is among the most common forms of STI, infecting over 5.5 million Americans each year. The virus appears to be relatively easy to catch. The typical incubation period is from six to eight weeks after contact. Many people have no symptoms, particularly if the warts are located inside the reproductive tract. Others may develop a series of itchy bumps on the genitals, ranging in size from small pinheads to large cauliflower-like growths that can obstruct urination or sexual intercourse. On dry skin (such as the shaft of the penis), the warts are commonly small, hard, and yellowish gray, resembling warts that appear on other parts of the body.

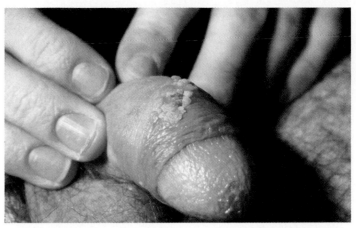

Genital warts are caused by the human papilloma virus and can be either full-blown or flat.

Genital warts can be one or both of two different types: (1) *full-blown genital warts* that are noticeable as tiny bumps or growths, and (2) the much more prevalent *flat warts* that are not usually visible to the naked eye. In females, these flat warts are often first detected by a doctor during a routine Pap test. Abnormal Pap results may prompt the physician to perform a procedure in which a vinegar-like solution is applied to the insides of the vaginal walls and cervix to bleach potential warts. The area is then viewed through a special magnifying instrument known as a colposcope. A relatively new photographic procedure known as a cerviscope can also detect genital warts. During a cerviscope, vinegar is applied to the vaginal and cervical areas, and an image of the area is projected onto a screen for a specialist to diagnose. This technique is relatively inexpensive and is believed to be five times more sensitive than standard colposcopy. An even newer method is the *DNA probe,* a technique that identifies the genetic makeup of possible warts.

Whereas women must see a physician for a diagnosis, a male can check for suspicious lesions by wrapping his penis in vinegar-soaked gauze or cloth, waiting for five minutes, and then checking for white bleached areas indicative of flat warts. However, genital warts of the rectum must be diagnosed by a physician.

Risks of Genital Warts   Many genital warts eventually disappear on their own. Others grow and generate unsightly flaps of irregular flesh on the external genitalia. If they grow large enough to obstruct urinary flow or become irritated by clothing or sexual intercourse, they can cause significant problems.

The greatest threat from genital warts may lie in the apparent relationship between them and a tendency for *dysplasia,* or changes in cells that may lead to a precancerous condition. Exactly how HPV infection leads to cervical cancer is uncertain. It is known that within five years after infection, 30 percent of all HPV cases will progress to the precancerous stage. Of those cases that become precancerous and are left untreated, 70 percent will eventually result in actual cancer. In addition, genital warts may pose a threat to a pregnant woman's unborn fetus if the fetus is exposed to the virus during birth. Cesarean deliveries may be considered in serious cases.

New research has also implicated HPV as a possible risk factor for coronary artery disease. It is hypothesized that HPV causes an inflammatory response in the artery walls, which makes cholesterol and plaque build up.

Treatment for Genital Warts   Treatment for genital warts may take several forms:

1. Warts may be painted with a medication called podophyllin during a visit to the doctor's office. The podophyllin is washed off after about four hours, and a few days later the warts begin to dry up and fall off. Sometimes more than one trip to the doctor is necessary. This procedure is relatively painless, but there are potential side effects. Because podophyllin may be absorbed through the skin, pregnant women should not use it. Some patients may experience skin reactions.
2. Warts may be removed by *cryosurgery*, a procedure in which an instrument treated with liquid nitrogen is held to the affected area, "freezing" the tissue. Within a few days, the warts fall off.
3. Depending on size and location, some warts are removed by *simple excision*.
4. For larger warts, *laser surgery* is often used. This is a major procedure that usually requires general anesthesia. The frequency of laser use for wart removal is currently being questioned by many health experts. (Precautions must also be taken during this procedure to shield medical staff from infection by viral spray.)
5. Creams containing 5-fluorouracil (an anticancer drug) are being used to prevent further precancerous cell development.
6. For warts located externally, injections of interferon are sometimes given to keep the virus from spreading to healthy tissue. This treatment shows promise, but it is expensive and, in large doses, may cause flulike symptoms.

Prevention is clearly the best approach. The same strategies that help protect you against AIDS can also protect you from genital warts and other STIs (see the section on AIDS prevention later in this chapter).

Candidiasis   Yeastlike fungal disease often transmitted sexually.

Vaginitis   Set of symptoms characterized by vaginal itching, swelling, and burning.

Trichomoniasis   Protozoan infection characterized by foamy, yellowish discharge and unpleasant odor.

Genital herpes   STI caused by the herpes simplex virus.

Candidiasis (Moniliasis)

Unlike many STIs, which are caused by pathogens that come from outside the body, the yeastlike fungus caused by the *Candida albicans* organism normally inhabits the vaginal tract in most women. Only under certain conditions, in which the normal chemical balance of the vagina is disturbed, will these organisms multiply to abnormal quantities and begin to cause problems. Factors affecting this balance include the following:

- Antibiotics.
- Changes in hormone levels brought on by pregnancy, breastfeeding, or menopause.
- Douches or spermicides.
- Sexual intercourse.
- Other sexually transmitted infections.

The likelihood of **candidiasis** (also known as moniliasis or a *yeast infection*) is greatest if a woman has diabetes, if her immune system is overtaxed or malfunctioning, if she is taking birth control pills or other hormones, or if she is taking broad-spectrum antibiotics. All of these factors decrease the acidity of the vagina and create favorable conditions for a yeastlike infection.

Symptoms of candidiasis include severe vaginal itching and burning of the vagina and vulva. A white, cheesy discharge and swelling of the vulva may also occur. These symptoms are often collectively called **vaginitis,** which means an inflammation of the vagina. When this microbe infects the mouth, whitish patches form, and the condition is referred to as *thrush*. This monilial infection also occurs in males and is easily transmitted between sexual partners.

Candidiasis strikes at least half a million American women a year. Antifungal drugs applied on the surface or by suppository usually cure it in just a few days. For approximately 1 out of 10 women, however, nothing seems to work, and the infection returns again and again. Symptoms can be aggravated by contact of the vagina with soaps, douches, perfumed toilet paper, chlorinated water, and spermicides. Tight-fitting jeans and pantyhose can provide the combination of moisture and irritant the organism thrives on.

Trichomoniasis

Unlike many STIs, **trichomoniasis** is caused by a protozoan. Although as many as half of the men and women in the United States may carry this organism, most remain free of symptoms until their bodily defenses are weakened. Both men and women may transmit the infection, but women are the more likely candidates for infection. Symptoms include a foamy, yellowish, unpleasant-smelling discharge accompanied by a burning sensation, itching, and painful urination. These symptoms are most likely to occur during or shortly after menstruation, but they can appear at any time or be absent altogether. Although usually transmitted by sexual contact, the "trich" organism can also be spread by toilet seats, wet towels, or other items that have discharged fluids on them. You can also contract trichomoniasis by sitting naked on the locker-room bench at your local health spa or gym. Treatment includes oral metronidazole, usually given to both sexual partners to avoid the possible "ping-pong" effect of repeated cross-infection so typical of STIs.

General Urinary Tract Infections (UTIs)

Although *general urinary tract infections (UTIs)* can be caused by various factors, particularly the insertion of catheters and other devices during hospitalization, some forms are sexually transmitted. Any time invading organisms enter the genital area, they can travel up the urethra and enter the bladder. Similarly, organisms normally living in the rectum, urethra, or bladder may travel to the sexual organs and eventually be transmitted to another person.

You can also get a UTI through autoinoculation, often during the simple task of wiping yourself after defecating. Wiping from the anus forward can transmit organisms found in feces to the vaginal opening or the urethra. Contact between the hands and the urethra and between the urethra and other objects are also common means of autoinoculation. Women, with their shorter urethras, are more likely to contract UTIs. Hand washing with soap and water prior to sexual intimacy, foreplay, and so on, is recommended.

Treatment depends on the nature and type of pathogen. For minor infections, some practitioners recommend drinking 8 to 10 glasses of fluids per day, particularly acidic liquids such as cranberry juice, to alter the acidity of the vagina and kill the pathogen. Other authorities consider this treatment worthless, however, since it has been estimated that a person would have to drink over four quarts of cranberry juice a day for several days to even begin to alter vaginal acidity. Considering the caloric intake, cost of the juice, and minimal effectiveness of this home treatment, you are better off visiting a doctor and obtaining proven medications from a pharmacy.

Herpes

Herpes is a general term for a family of infections characterized by sores or eruptions on the skin. Caused by herpes viruses, the herpes family of diseases is not transmitted exclusively sexually. Exchange of saliva and transmission by kissing or sharing eating utensils are other modes of herpes transmission. Herpes infections range from mildly uncomfortable to extremely serious. **Genital herpes** is an infection caused by the herpes simplex virus (HSV).

Historically, the herpes simplex type 2 virus was considered the primary culprit in genital herpes, and the herpes simplex type 1 virus was thought to affect the area of the lips and other body areas.[42] We now know that both type 1 and type 2 can infect any area of the body, producing lesions (sores) in and around the vaginal area, on the penis, around the anal opening, and on the buttocks or thighs. For example, you may have a type 1 infection on your lip and transmit the HSV-1 organism to your partner's genitals during oral sex. Practically speaking, the resulting symptoms would be virtually

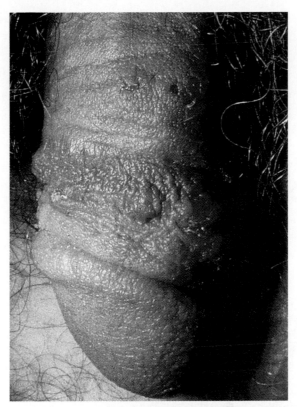

Genital herpes, a highly contagious sexually transmitted infection—for which no cure is currently available—is characterized by recurring cycles of painful blisters on the genitalia.

the same as if you had transmitted the type 2 virus. Occasionally, sores appear on other parts of the body. HSV remains in certain nerve cells for life and can flare up, or cause symptoms, when the body's ability to maintain itself is weakened.

The prodromal (precursor) phase of the infection is characterized by a burning sensation and redness at the site of infection. During this time prescription medicines such as acyclovir and over-the-counter medications such as Abreva will often keep the disease from spreading. However, this phase of the disease is quickly followed by the second phase, in which a blister filled with a clear fluid containing the virus forms. If you pick at this blister or otherwise touch the site and spread this fluid with fingers, lipstick, lip balm, or other products, you can autoinoculate other body parts. Particularly dangerous is the possibility of spreading the infection to your eyes, for a herpes lesion on the eye can cause blindness.

Over a period of days, the unsightly blister will crust over, dry up, and disappear, and the virus will travel to the base of an affected nerve supplying the area and become dormant. Only when the victim becomes overly stressed, when diet and sleep are inadequate, when the immune system is overworked, or when excessive exposure to sunlight or other stressors occurs will the virus become reactivated (at the same site every time) and begin the blistering cycle all over again. These sores cast off (shed) viruses that can be highly infectious. However, it is important to note that a herpes site can shed the virus even when no overt sore is present, particularly during the prodromal stages (the interval

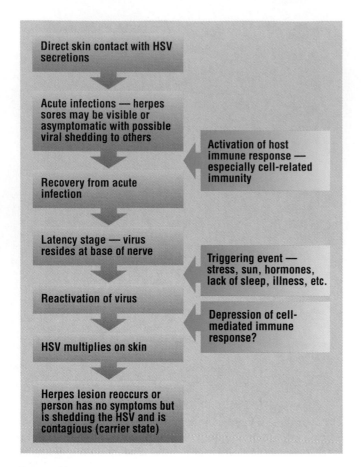

Figure 17.7
The Herpes Cycle
Source: Used by permission of Lippincott-Raven Publishers from "Sexually Transmitted Diseases in the 1990s," *STD Bulletin* 11 (1992): 485.

between the earliest symptoms and blistering). People may get genital herpes by having sexual contact with others who don't know they are infected or who are having outbreaks of herpes without any sores. A person with genital herpes can also infect a sexual partner during oral sex. The virus is spread only rarely, if at all, by touching objects such as a toilet seat or hot tub seat.[43] In fact, if you are seated on a toilet seat properly, the only thing in contact with your genitals should be air, and thus, the likelihood of contact exposure would be exceedingly rare! Figure 17.7 summarizes the herpes cycle.

Genital herpes is especially serious in pregnant women because the baby could be infected as it passes through the vagina during birth. Many physicians recommend cesarean deliveries for infected women. Additionally, women who have a history of genital herpes appear to have a greater risk of developing cervical cancer.

Although there is no cure for herpes at present, certain drugs can reduce symptoms. Unfortunately, they seem to work only if the infection is confirmed during the first few hours after contact. As you may guess, this is rather rare. The effectiveness of other treatments, such as L-lysine, is largely unsubstantiated. Newer over-the-counter medications seem to be moderately effective in reducing the severity of symp-toms. Although lip balms and cold-sore medications may provide temporary anesthetic relief, remember that rubbing anything on a herpes blister can spread herpes-laden fluids to other body parts.

Preventing Herpes You can take precautions to reduce your risk of herpes:

• Avoid any form of kissing if you notice a sore or blister on your partner's mouth. Kiss no one, not even a peck on the cheek, if you know that you have a herpes lesion or if you see one on a person you want to kiss. Although there is no set time period for safe kissing, the longer you refrain from deep kissing after a herpes sore has been present, the better. Keeping your lips healthy, moist, and crack-free will also reduce risk of infection.

• Be extremely cautious if you have casual sexual affairs. Not every partner will feel obligated to tell you that he or she has a problem. It's up to you to protect yourself.

• Wash your hands immediately with soap and water after any form of sexual contact.

• If you have questionable sores or lesions, seek medical help at once. Do not be afraid to name your contacts.

• If you have herpes, be responsible in your sexual contacts with others. If you have any suspicious lesions that might put your partner at risk, say so. Find an appropriate time and place, and hold a candid discussion.

• Reduce your risk of herpes outbreaks by avoiding excessive stress, sunlight, or whatever else appears to trigger an episode.

• Do not share lip balms or lipstick.

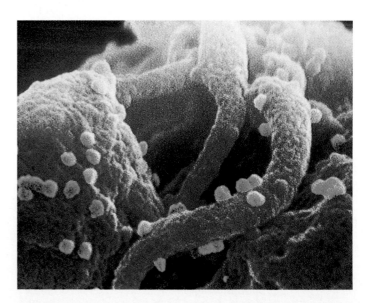

Viruses attach themselves to host cells and inject their own DNA or RNA in order to reproduce new cells. Some viruses run their course and expire. Others, such as HIV, shown here, are destructive over the long term.

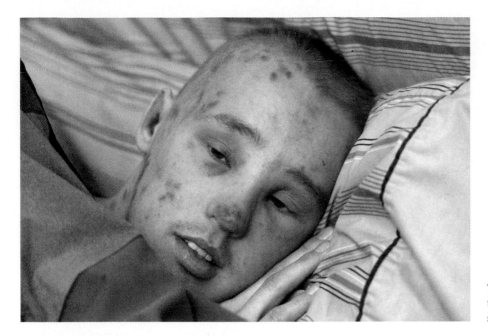

The effects of HIV/AIDS can be seen here in the form of Kaposi's sarcoma and wasting syndrome.

HIV/AIDS

Acquired immune deficiency syndrome (AIDS) is a significant global health threat. Since 1981, when AIDS was first recognized, over 60 million people in the world have become infected with **human immunodeficiency virus (HIV),** the virus that causes AIDS. Over 18 million of these people have died, and another 14 million struggle with the disease.[44] In the United States, as of December 2001, over 816,149 men, women, and children with AIDS have been reported to the Centers for Disease Control and Prevention (CDC), and at least 467,910 have died.[45] The CDC estimates that at least 40,000 new infections occur each year in the United States. See the Health in a Diverse World box for statistics on HIV worldwide.

The Onset of AIDS

Researchers believe that the AIDS virus may actually have been present in the United States since the early 1950s, although medical and government officials did not note problems related to the disease until the spring of 1981. Suddenly, federal officials began to receive an increasing number of requests for an experimental drug used to treat a rare disease called *Pneumocystis carinii pneumonia (PCP).* Caused by a protozoan, PCP appeared to be affecting significant numbers of previously healthy young homosexual males in New York and California.

At about the same time, increasing numbers of homosexual men in California were being diagnosed with a rare form of cancer known as *Kaposi's sarcoma.* These two groups of patients—those with PCP and those with Kaposi's sarcoma—tended to share many characteristics. They were typically white and homosexual, came from similar geographical regions, used specific types of drugs, and had generalized lymphadenopathy (chronic swelling of the lymph nodes) and general malfunctioning of the immune system. Because of the last problem, many of these people developed several diseases at the same time, making diagnosis of one underlying cause extremely difficult.

For many months, epidemiologists investigated possible causes of this apparent "gay plague," including the types of drugs used by many gay men and the water supplies in their communities. In 1984, two researchers, Robert C. Gallo at the National Cancer Institute in the United States and Luc Montagnier at the Pasteur Institute in Paris, independently isolated the retrovirus (a type of slow-acting virus) that causes AIDS. Initially called the human T-cell lymphotropic virus type III (HTLV-III) by most American researchers, this virus is today generally referred to as the human immunodeficiency virus (HIV).

Although during the early days of the epidemic it appeared that HIV infected only homosexuals, it quickly became apparent that the disease was not confined to groups of people but rather was related to high-risk behaviors such as unprotected sexual intercourse and sharing needles.

A Shifting Epidemic

Since 1981, when HIV infections were first noticed and the earliest victims began to die, the numbers of HIV-infected

---

Acquired immune deficiency syndrome (AIDS) Extremely virulent sexually transmitted disease that renders the immune system inoperative.

Human immunodeficiency virus (HIV) The slow-acting virus that causes AIDS.

The Staggering Toll of HIV/AIDS in the Global Community

In spite of noteworthy progress in stemming the tide of infectious diseases such as HIV/AIDS in the United States, epidemics of these diseases have had an increasingly devastating impact on other regions of the world. By 2002, over 42 million people from all regions of the world were infected with HIV, translating to nearly 1 out of every 100 men, women, and children. For many years, women,

children, and teenagers seemed to be on the periphery of the HIV/AIDS pandemic. However, by 2002, they were at the center of the epidemic. Consider the following:

AFRICA

- In Africa, 29.4 million people are HIV positive.
- In South Africa, one in every three people is now infected. In some regions, the rate is as high as one in two.
- In seven other African countries, at least one-fourth of the population is infected.
- According to UNAIDS and WHO estimates, more than 20 percent of the population in over 16 African countries

is infected, with more than 8,000 new cases every day among people 15–24 years old worldwide, and 10 million in 2002 alone.

- The AIDS epidemic is expected to wipe out about half the current population of teenagers in the worst-hit African nations, devastating economies and shattering societies. A child born in Botswana in 2010 can expect to live 29 years—the lowest life expectancy seen in a century. Men in several sub-Saharan countries will soon greatly outnumber women.
- Over two-thirds of the 42 million people worldwide who are infected with HIV live in sub-Saharan Africa. By 2002,

REGION	EPIDEMIC STARTED	ADULTS AND CHILDREN WITH HIV/AIDS	ADULTS AND CHILDREN NEWLY INFECTED WITH HIV	ADULT PREVALENCE RATE*	% OF HIV-POSITIVE ADULTS WHO ARE WOMEN	MAIN MODE(S) OF TRANSMISSION# FOR ADULTS LIVING WITH HIV/AIDS
SUB-SAHARAN AFRICA	Late '70s/ Early '80s	29.4 million	3.5 million	8.8%	58%	Hetero
NORTH AFRICA & MIDDLE EAST	Late '80s	550,000	83,000	0.3%	55%	Hetero, IDU
SOUTH & SOUTHEAST ASIA	Late '80s	6.0 million	700,000	0.6%	36%	Hetero, IDU
EAST ASIA & PACIFIC	Late '80s	1.2 million	270,000	0.1%	24%	IDU, hetero, MSM
LATIN AMERICA	Late '70s/ Early '80s	1.5 million	150,000	0.6%	30%	MSM, IDU, hetero
CARIBBEAN	Late '70s/ Early '80s	440,000	60,000	2.4%	50%	Hetero, MSM
EASTERN EUROPE & CENTRAL ASIA	Early '90s	1.2 million	250,000	0.6%	27%	IDU
WESTERN EUROPE	Late '70s/ Early '80s	570,000	30,000	0.3%	25%	MSM, IDU
NORTH AMERICA	Late '70s/ Early '80s	980,000	45,000	0.6%	20%	MSM, IDU, hetero
AUSTRALIA & NEW ZEALAND	Late '70s/ Early '80s	15,000	500	0.1%	7%	MSM
TOTAL		**42 million**	**5 million**	**1.2%**	**50%**	

*The proportion of adults (15 to 49 years of age) living with HIV/AIDS in 2002, using 2002 population numbers.
#Hetero (heterosexual transmission), IDU (transmission through injecting drug use), MSM (sexual transmission among men who have sex with men).

55 percent of all HIV infections were in women, primarily due to heterosexual contact with their infected male partners.

- Since the start of the HIV/AIDS pandemic, approximately 10 million children younger than age 15 have been orphaned worldwide due to the premature death of parents infected with HIV. Chilren under the age of 15 are among the fastest growing population of HIV-positive Africans.

NORTH AMERICA

- By 2002, there were an estimated 980,000 people living with AIDS. The United States has an infection rate of 0.60 percent of the adult population, and Canada has an infection rate of 0.32 percent.
- Public health workers were alarmed to note that there appears to be an increase in high-risk behavior among young homosexuals and a rise in gonorrhea, indicating that our AIDS numbers may begin to increase in the near future after a long downward trend.

LATIN AMERICA AND THE CARIBBEAN

- An estimated 2 million people were living with the AIDS virus by 2002, making it the second most infected region in the world based on rates per 100,000 population. The epidemic was mainly spread through heterosexual intercourse, injecting drug use, and men who have sex with men.
- Haiti was worst hit, with 6 percent of adults infected, followed by the Bahamas with 3.5 percent.

EUROPE

- An estimated 1.77 million people were living with the AIDS virus in 2002 in eastern and western Europe.
- Rates of infection are increasing among drug users sharing needles in eastern Europe and the former Soviet Union.

ASIA

- By 2002, an estimated 7.2 million people were living with AIDS in Southeast Asia, East Asia, and the Pacific region.
- Cambodia has the highest rate, with 5 percent infected, largely through heterosexual intercourse.
- Thailand has an infection rate of 2.75 percent, and good prevention campaigns have slowed the spread of disease through heterosexual intercourse.
- An estimated 5 million people in India live with the virus, the second highest national total behind South Africa, with an infection rate of 0.7 percent.

Source: UNAIDS and World Health Organization, "AIDS Epidemic Update," December 2002 (see http://www.unaids. org/worldaidsday/2002/press/update/ epiupdate_en.pdf).

persons and AIDS-diagnosed individuals have skyrocketed. Expansions in the definition of AIDS have caused these overall numbers to rise.

Under old definitions, people with HIV were diagnosed as having AIDS only when they developed blood infections, the cancer known as Kaposi's sarcoma, or any of 21 other indicator diseases, most of which were common in males. The CDC has expanded the indicator list to include pulmonary tuberculosis, recurrent pneumonia, and invasive cervical cancer. Perhaps the most significant new indicator is a drop in the level of the body's master immune cells, called CD4s, to 200 per cubic millimeter (one-fifth the level in a healthy person).

AIDS cases have been reported state by state throughout the United States since the early 1980s as a means of tracking the disease. While the numbers of actual reported cases have always been suspect, improved reporting and surveillance methods have helped increase accuracy. Today, the CDC recommends that all states report HIV infections as well as AIDS. Because of medical advances in treatment and increasing numbers of HIV-infected persons who do not progress to AIDS, it is believed that AIDS incidence statistics may not provide a true picture of the epidemic, the long-term costs of treating HIV-infected individuals, and other key information. HIV incidence data also provide a better picture of infection trends. Currently, most states mandate that those who test positive for the HIV antibody be reported. Although there is significant pressure to mandate reporting in all states, there is controversy over implementing such a mandate. Many believe that once we begin to mandate reporting of HIV-positive tests, many people will refuse to be tested, even though they may suspect that they are infected.

What do you think?

Do you favor mandatory reporting of HIV and AIDS cases? ✷ *If you knew that your name and vital statistics would be "on file" if you tested positive for HIV, would you be less likely to take the HIV test to begin with?* ✷ *On the other hand, do people who carry this contagious fatal disease have a responsibility to inform the general public and the health professionals who will provide their care?* ✷ *Explain your answer.*

Women and AIDS

HIV is an equal-opportunity pathogen that can attack anyone who engages in high-risk behaviors. This is true regardless of race, gender, sexual orientation, or socioeconomic status. Consider the following facts:[46]

- Women are 4 to 10 times more likely than men to contract HIV through unprotected sexual intercourse with an infected partner.[47]
- By the end of 2001, over 141,000 adult and adolescent women were reported to have AIDS in the United States;
- By the end of 2001, over 19.2 million women were living with HIV/AIDS worldwide, accounting for over 46 percent of the 42 million adults living with HIV/AIDS. Over 80 percent of all adolescent and adult transmission has been through heterosexual contact.
- HIV/AIDS due to heterosexual sexual transmission is increasing faster in rural America than in any other part of the country. Women most at risk are ethnic minorities and the economically disadvantaged. Among sexually active heterosexual teenagers, college students, and health care workers, nearly 60 percent of HIV cases are women.
- Thirteen- to 24-year-old females accounted for 44 percent of new HIV cases in 1997.
- Most women with AIDS were infected through heterosexual exposure to HIV, followed by injection drug use (sharing needles).
- Women of color are disproportionately affected by HIV; African American and Hispanic women together account for 76 percent of AIDS cases among women in the United States, though comprising less than 25 percent of all U.S. women.
- Of all AIDS cases among women, 61 percent were reported from five states: New York (26 percent), Florida (13 percent), New Jersey (10 percent), California (7 percent), and Texas (5 percent).
- AIDS is the leading cause of death among African American women ages 25 to 44, and the fourth leading cause of death among all American women in this age group.

Compounding the problems of women with HIV are serious deficiencies in our health and social service systems, including inadequate treatment for women addicts and lack of access to child care, health care, and social services for families headed by single women. Women with HIV/AIDS are of special interest because they are the major source of infection in infants. Virtually all new HIV infections among children in the United States are attributable to perinatal transmission of HIV.[48]

Special Concerns of Women with HIV/AIDS   Although contracting HIV is a serious problem for both males and females, women often have an even more difficult time protecting themselves from infection and taking care of themselves once they become ill. Irrefutable evidence indicates that HIV/AIDS disproportionately affects women, who, as mentioned earlier, are 4 to 10 times more likely than men to contract HIV through unprotected sexual intercourse with an infected partner. This discrepancy can be traced to both biological factors and socioeconomic factors.

Biological factors include the following:

- HIV can enter through mucous membrane surfaces of the genital tract; the vagina has a greater exposed mucous membrane area than does the urethra of the penis.

- The vaginal area is more likely to incur micro-tears during sexual intercourse, which facilitates entry of HIV.
- During intercourse, a woman is exposed to more semen than is the male to vaginal fluids.
- Semen is more likely to enter the vagina with force, whereas vaginal fluids do not enter the penis with force.
- Women who have STIs are more likely to be asymptomatic and therefore unaware they have a disease; STIs increase the risk of HIV transmission.

Socioeconomic factors include the following:

- Currently there are more HIV-infected men than HIV-infected women in the United States, which increases the likelihood that a woman would have an HIV-infected male partner.
- Women have been underrepresented in clinical trials for HIV treatment and prevention.
- Many cultural norms place women in subordination to men, especially in developing nations. This reduces women's decision-making power and ability to negotiate safer sex.
- Women are more vulnerable to sexual abuse from their male partners, and more likely to be involved in non-consensual sex or sex without condoms.
- Women are more likely to be economically dependent on men.
- Women may be less likely to seek medical treatment because of lack of money, caregiving burdens, and transportation problems.
- In the United States, HIV-positive women are more likely than are HIV-positive men to be younger and less educated.

Traditionally, women have played a relatively passive role in taking responsibility for protection during sexual intercourse and in general sexual decision making, particularly in third world countries. Efforts must be initiated to help women take control of their sexual health and participate actively in sexual decisions made with their partners.

In addition, women often carry the responsibility for caring for their children or caring for others who may be infected with HIV or suffering from AIDS. If the mother's role as caretaker must be abandoned due to illness, family members often suffer. As more and more women become infected with HIV, national efforts aimed at prevention, intervention, and treatment will undoubtedly increase.

What do you think?

Why do you think HIV/AIDS is increasing among women and minority groups in America? ✳ Why are some women particularly vulnerable to diseases such as AIDS? ✳ What actions can we take as a nation to reduce the spread of HIV/AIDS among women and minority groups? ✳ Should Americans be concerned about the global HIV/AIDS epidemic? ✳ Why or why not?

How HIV Is Transmitted

HIV typically enters one person's body when another person's infected body fluids (semen, vaginal secretions, blood, etc.) gain entry through a breach in body defenses. Mucous membranes of the genital organs and the anus provide the easiest route of entry. If there is a break in the mucous membranes (as can occur during sexual intercourse, particularly anal intercourse), the virus enters and begins to multiply.

After initial infection, the HIV multiplies rapidly, invading the bloodstream and cerebrospinal fluid. It progressively destroys helper T-lymphocytes, weakening the body's resistance to disease. The virus also changes the genetic structure of the cells it attacks. In response to this invasion, the body quickly begins to produce antibodies.

Despite some myths, HIV is not a highly contagious virus. Studies of people living in households with an AIDS patient have turned up no documented cases of HIV infection due to casual contact. Other investigations provide overwhelming evidence that insect bites do not transmit HIV.

Engaging in High-Risk Behaviors
AIDS is not a disease of gay people or minority groups. If you engage in high-risk behaviors, you increase your risk for the disease. If you do not practice these behaviors, your risk is minimal. It is as simple as that.

Unfortunately, the message has not gotten through to many Americans. They assume that because they are heterosexual, do not inject illegal drugs, and do not have sex with sex workers, they are not at risk. They couldn't be more wrong. Anyone who engages in unprotected sex is at risk, especially sex with a partner who has engaged in other high-risk behaviors. Sex with multiple partners is the greatest threat.

You can't determine the presence of HIV by looking at a person; you can't tell by questioning unless the person has been tested recently, is HIV negative, and is giving an honest answer. So what should you do?

Of course, the simplest answer is abstinence. If you don't exchange body fluids, you won't get the disease. As a second line of defense, if you decide to be intimate, the next best option is to use a condom. In spite of the message, in spite of all the educational campaigns, surveys consistently indicate that most college students throw caution to the wind if they think they "know" someone—they have unprotected sex. Even when they do not know the individual involved, most of them have unprotected sex.

Why do so many of us act so irresponsibly when the outcome is so deadly? The answer is probably a combination of ignorance, denial that it could be *you* who is HIV positive, a certain degree of apathy, and a bit of very real fear. People who are afraid often avoid testing. If they have symptoms, they may still avoid testing out of fear that they may be diagnosed positive and not have any real options for a cure.

Recognize the risk factors, and remember, if you do not engage in activities that are known to spread the virus, your chances of becoming infected are extremely small. The following activities are high-risk behaviors.

Exchange of Body Fluids
The greatest risk factor is the exchange of HIV-infected body fluids during vaginal or anal intercourse. Substantial research indicates that blood, semen, and vaginal secretions are the major fluids of concern. However, even though these risks are well documented, millions of Americans report inconsistent safer sex practices, particularly when drugs or alcohol affect rational thinking.

Although the virus was found in 1 person's saliva (out of 71 people in a study population), most health officials state that saliva is not a high-risk body fluid unless blood is present; saliva is a less significant risk than other shared body fluids (see the Reality Check box on tattoing and piercing for additional risks). The fact that the virus has been found in saliva does provide a good rationale for using caution when engaging in deep, wet kissing.

Initially, public health officials also included breast milk in the list of high-risk fluids because a few infants apparently contracted HIV while breastfeeding. Subsequent research has indicated that HIV transmission could have been caused by bleeding nipples as well as by actual consumption of breast milk and other fluids. Infection through contact with feces and urine is believed to be highly unlikely though technically possible.

Receiving a Blood Transfusion Prior to 1985
A small group of people have become infected after receiving blood transfusions. In 1985, the Red Cross and other blood donation programs implemented a stringent testing program for all donated blood. Today, because of these massive screening efforts, the risk of receiving HIV-infected blood is almost nonexistent.

Injecting Drugs
A significant percentage of AIDS cases in the United States result from sharing or using HIV-contaminated needles and syringes. Though users of illegal drugs are commonly considered the only members of this category, others may also share needles—for example, people with diabetes who inject insulin or athletes who inject steroids. People who share needles and also engage in sexual activities with members of high-risk groups, such as those who exchange sex for drugs, increase their risks dramatically.

Mother-to-Infant (Perinatal) Transmission
Approximately one in three of the children who has contracted AIDS received the virus from their infected mothers while in the womb or while passing through the vaginal tract during delivery.

Symptoms of HIV Disease

A person may go for months or years after infection by HIV before any significant symptoms appear. The incubation time varies greatly from person to person. Children have shorter incubation periods than adults. Newborns and infants are particularly vulnerable to AIDS because human beings do not become fully immunocompetent (that is, their immune

Body Piercing and Tattooing: Risks to Health

One look around college campuses reveals a trend that, while not necessarily new, has taken off in recent years. We're talking, of course, about body piercing and tattooing, also referred to as "body art."

For decades, tattoos appeared to be worn only by motorcyclists, military veterans, and general roughnecks; in many people's eyes, they represented the seedier part of society. Body piercing, on the other hand, was virtually nonexistent in our culture except for pierced ears, which were limited mostly to women. Various forms of body art, however, can be traced throughout human history as a means for people to "dress themselves up" to attract attention, be viewed as acceptable by their peers, or express themselves or their culture. Egyptian pharaohs underwent rites of passage by piercing their navels. Roman soldiers demonstrated manhood by piercing their nipples.

But why the surge in popularity of body art in current society? Today, people are getting their ears and bodies pierced in record numbers, in such places as the eyebrows, tongues, lips, noses, navels, nipples, genitals, and just about any place possible. Many view the trend as a fulfillment of a desire for self-expression, as one University of Wisconsin–Madison student points out: "The nipple [ring] was one of those things that I did as a kind of empowerment, claiming my body as my own and refuting the stereotypes that people have about me. . . . The tattoo was kind of a lark and came along the same lines and I like it, too. . . . [T]hey both give me a secret smile."

Whatever the reason, tattoo artists are doing a booming business in both tattooing and the "art" of body piercing. Amidst the "oohing" and "aahing" over the latest artistic creations, however, health officials and federal agencies are raising concerns over health risks. The most common

health-related problems associated with tattoos and body piercing include skin reactions, infections, and scarring. The average healing times for piercings depend on the size of the insert, location, and the person's overall health. Facial and tongue piercings tend to heal more quickly than areas not commonly exposed to open air or light and which are often teeming with bacteria, such as the genitals. Because the hands are great germ transmitters, "fingering" pierced areas poses a significant risk for infection.

Of even greater concern is the potential transmission of dangerous pathogens that any puncture of the human body exacerbates. The use of unsterile needles—which can cause serious infections and can transmit HIV, hepatitis B and C, tetanus, and a host of other diseases—poses a very real risk. Body piercing and tattooing are performed by body artists, unlicensed "professionals" who generally have learned their trade from other body artists. Laws and policies regulating body piercing and tattooing vary greatly by state. While some states don't allow tattoo and body-piercing parlors, others may regulate them carefully, and still others provide few regulations and standards by which parlors have to abide. Standards for safety usually include minimum age requirements, standards of sanitation, use of aseptic techniques, sterilization of equipment, informed risks, instructions for skin care, record keeping, and recommendations for dealing with adverse reactions. Because of the varying degree of standards regulating this business and the potential for transmission of dangerous pathogens, anyone who receives a tattoo, body piercing, or permanent makeup tattoo cannot donate blood for one year.

If you opt for tattooing or body piercing, remember the following points:

✔ Look for clean, well-lit work areas, and ask about sterilization procedures.
✔ Before having the work done, watch the artist at work. Tattoo removal is expensive and often impossible. Make sure the tattoo is one you can live with for years.

✔ Immediately before piercing or tattooing, the body area should be carefully sterilized. The artist should put on new latex gloves and touch nothing else while working.
✔ Packaged, sterilized needles should be used only once and then discarded. A piercing gun should not be used because it cannot be sterilized properly.
✔ Only jewelry made of noncorrosive metal, such as surgical stainless steel, niobium, or solid 14-karat gold, is safe for new piercings.
✔ Leftover tattoo ink should be discarded after each procedure. Do not allow the artist to reuse ink that has been used for other customers.
✔ If any signs of pus, swelling, redness, or discoloration persist, remove the piercing object and contact a physician.

How do you explain the popularity of tattoos and body piercings among young people today? What are the pros and cons of this trend?

Sources: M. L. Armstrong and K. P. Murphy, "Adolescent Tattooing and Body Piercing," *The Prevention Researcher,* Integrated Research Services, Eugene, OR 5 (3) (1998), p. 5; Center for Food Safety and Applied Nutrition, "Tattoos and Permanent Makeup," Office of Cosmetics Fact Sheet, U.S. Food and Drug Administration, February 1995 (see http://vm.cfsan.fda.gov/~dms/cos-204.html); M. Larkin, "Tattooing in the 90s: Ancient Art Requires Care and Caution," *FDA Consumer,* U.S. Food and Drug Administration, October 1993 (see http://vm.cfsan.fda.gov/~dms/cos-204.html).

system is not fully developed) until they are 6 to 15 months old. New information suggests that some very young children show the "adult" progression of AIDS.[49]

For adults who receive no medical treatment, it takes an average of 8 to 10 years for the virus to cause the slow, degenerative changes in the immune system that are characteristic of AIDS. During this time, the person may experience a large number of opportunistic infections (infections that gain a foothold when the immune system is not functioning effectively). Colds, sore throats, fever, tiredness, nausea, night sweats, and other generally non–life-threatening conditions commonly appear, and are described as pre-AIDS symptoms.

Testing for HIV Antibodies

Once antibodies have formed in reaction to the presence of HIV, a blood test known as the **ELISA** test may detect their presence. If sufficient antibodies are present, the ELISA test will be positive. When a person who previously tested *negative* (no HIV antibodies present) has a subsequent test that is *positive,* seroconversion is said to have occurred. In such a situation, the person would typically take another ELISA test, followed by a more expensive, precise test known as the **Western blot,** to confirm the presence of HIV antibodies.

Although the ELISA is viewed as quite accurate, it is a conservative test in that it errs on the side of caution, meaning it produces a large number of *false-positive results*. It was deliberately designed to do this because it was intended as a test for screening the nation's blood supply. There have also been instances of *false-negative results*. Some health professionals believe that there are chronic carriers of HIV who, for unknown reasons, continually show false-negative results on both the ELISA and Western blot tests. This, of course, raises serious concerns about risks for these people's sexual partners.

It should be noted that these tests are not AIDS tests per se. Rather, they detect antibodies for the disease, indicating the presence of HIV in the person's system. Whether the person will develop AIDS depends to some extent on the strength of the immune system. Although we have made remarkable progress in prolonging the relatively symptom-free period between infection, HIV-positive status, and progression to symptomatic AIDS, it is important to note that a cure does not yet exist. While many people have remained in good health , others find that drug treatments become less effective over time and AIDS symptoms eventually appear.

As testing for HIV antibodies has been perfected, scientists have explored various ways of making it easier for individuals to be tested. Health officials distinguish between *reported* and *actual* cases of HIV infection because it is believed that many HIV-positive people avoid being tested. One reason is fear of knowing the truth. Another is the fear of recrimination from employers, insurance companies, and medical staff if a positive test becomes known to others. (Even though it is illegal to discriminate against a person who is HIV positive or has AIDS, discrimination is not always an overt act that is easily punished. Subtle acts of discrimination and harassment continue to be reported.) Early detection and reporting are important, because immediate treatment for someone in the early stages of HIV disease is critical.

New Hope and Treatments

New drugs have slowed the progression from HIV to AIDS and have prolonged life expectancies for most AIDS patients. While these new therapies offer the promise of extended life for many, they may have inadvertently led to increases in risky behaviors and a noteworthy rise in cases in 2002. Although AIDS fell from the top 10 to the 14th leading cause of death in 1997 and has held steady at that ranking, many experts fear that we are taking steps backward. Advocates for AIDS patients believe the medications still cost too much money and cause too many side effects. Multidrug treatment for AIDS for one person now exceeds $20,000 per year. Medical costs for people with AIDS, from the time of diagnosis until death, exceed $102,000.[50] A new study, conducted by the Agency for Health Care Quality and Research (AHRQ), should provide an up-to-date estimate of HIV/AIDS costs sometime in 2003. Until then, the cost implications of improved treatments remain unclear.

Current treatments combine selected drugs, especially protease inhibitors and reverse transcriptase inhibitors. Protease inhibitors (for example, amprenavir, ritonavir, and saquinavir) resemble pieces of the protein chain that the HIV protease normally cuts. They block the HIV protease enzyme from cutting the protein chains needed to produce new viruses. Other drugs, including the nucleoside analogs, such as AZT, ddI, ddC, d4T, and 3TC, inhibit the HIV enzyme reverse transcriptase before the virus has invaded the cell. Protease inhibitors act to prevent the production of the virus in chronically infected cells that HIV has already invaded. In effect, the older drugs work by preventing the virus from infecting new cells, and the protease inhibitors work by preventing infected cells from reproducing new HIVs.

While protease inhibitors show promise, they have proved difficult to manufacture, and some have failed while others are successful. Side effects vary from person to person, and getting the right dose is critical for effectiveness. All of the protease drugs seem to work best in combination with other therapies. These combination treatments are still quite experimental, and no combination has proved to be absolute for all people as yet. Also, as with other antiviral treatments, resistance to the drugs can develop. Individuals who already show resistance to AZT may not be able to use

ELISA Blood test that detects presence of antibodies to the HIV virus.

Western blot A test more accurate than the ELISA to confirm presence of HIV antibodies.

Staying Safe in an Unsafe Sexual World

HIV transmission depends on specific behaviors; this is true of other STIs as well. You can do several things to protect yourself and reduce your risk:

- Avoid casual sexual partners. Ideally, have sex only if you are in a long-term, mutually monogamous relationship with someone who is equally committed to the relationship and whose HIV status is negative.
- Avoid unprotected sexual activity involving the exchange of blood, semen, or vaginal secretions with people whose present or past behaviors put them at risk for infection. Do not be afraid to ask intimate questions about your partner's sexual past. Remember, whenever you choose to have sexual relations, you expose yourself to your partner's history. Postpone sexual involvement until you are assured that he or she is not infected.
- All sexually active adults who are not in a lifelong monogamous relationship should practice safer sex by using latex condoms. Remember, however, that condoms still do not provide 100 percent safety.
- Never share injecting needles with anyone for any reason.
- Never share any devices through which the exchange of blood could occur, including needles, razors, tattoo instruments, body-piercing instruments, and any other sharp objects.
- Avoid injury to body tissue during sexual activity. HIV can enter the bloodstream through microscopic tears in anal or vaginal tissues.
- Avoid unprotected oral sex or any sexual activity in which semen, blood, or vaginal secretions could penetrate mucous membranes through breaks in the membrane. Always use a condom or a dental dam during oral sex.

- Avoid using drugs that may dull your senses and affect your ability to make decisions about responsible precautions with potential sex partners.
- Wash your hands before and after sexual encounters. Urinate after sexual relations and, if possible, wash your genitals.
- Although total abstinence is the only absolute means of preventing the sexual transmission of HIV, abstinence can be a difficult choice to make. If you have any doubt about the potential risks of having sex, consider other means of intimacy, at least until you can assure your safety. Enjoyable and safer alternatives include massage, dry kissing, hugging, holding and touching, and masturbation (alone or with a partner).
- When receiving care from medical professionals such as dentists or doctors, make sure they take appropriate precautions to prevent potential transmission, including washing their hands and wearing gloves and masks. Be sure that all equipment used for treatment is properly sterilized.
- If you are worried about your own HIV status, have yourself tested. Don't risk infecting others inadvertently.
- If you are a woman and HIV positive, you should take the steps necessary to ensure that you do not become pregnant.
- If you suspect that you may be infected or if you test positive for HIV antibodies, do not donate blood, semen, or body organs.

At no time in your life is it more important to communicate openly than when you are considering an intimate relationship. Do not be afraid to ask questions, so you can then make an informed decision about whether to get involved. Remember that you can't tell if someone has a sexually transmitted infection. Anyone who has ever had sex with anyone else or has injected drugs is at risk, and they may not even know it. The following tips can help you communicate about potential risks:

- Remember that you have a responsibility to your partner to disclose your own status. You also have a responsibility to yourself to stay healthy. Do not be afraid to ask about your partner's HIV status. If either person's status is unknown, suggest going through the testing together as a means of sharing something important.
- Be direct, honest, and determined in talking about sex before you become involved. Do not act silly or evasive. Get to the point, ask clear questions, and do not be put off in receiving a response. Remember, a person who does not care enough to talk about sex probably does not care enough to take responsibility for his or her actions.
- Discuss the issues without sounding defensive or accusatory. Develop a personal comfort level with the subject prior to raising the issue with your partner. Be prepared with complete information, and articulate your feelings clearly. Reassure your partner that your reasons for desiring abstinence or safer sex arise from respect and not distrust. Sharing feelings is easier in a calm, suspicion-free environment in which both people feel comfortable.
- Encourage your partner to be honest and to share feelings. This will not happen overnight. If you have never had a serious conversation with this person before you get into an intimate situation, you cannot expect honesty and openness when the lights go out.
- Analyze your own beliefs and values ahead of time. The worst thing you can do is to get into an awkward situation before you have had time to think about what is important to you. Know where you will draw the line on certain actions, and be very clear with your partner about what you expect. If you believe that using a condom is necessary, make sure you communicate this.
- Decide what you will do if your partner does not agree with you. Anticipate potential objections or excuses, and prepare your responses accordingly.

- Ask about your partner's history. Although it may seem as though you are prying into another person's business, your own health future depends upon knowing basic information about your partner's past. An idea of your partner's past sexual practices and use of injectable drugs is very valuable.

Again, it is important to let your partner know why you are concerned and that you are not inquiring due to jealousy or other ulterior motives.
- Ask about the significance of monogamy in your partner's relationships. A basic question to ask before becoming involved in a regular sexual relationship

is, "How important is a committed relationship to you?" You will need to decide early how important this relationship is to you and how much you are willing to work at arriving at an acceptable compromise on lifestyle.

---

a protease–AZT combination. This can pose a problem for many people who have been taking the common drugs and then find their options for combination therapy limited.

Although these drugs provide new hope and longer survival rates for people living with HIV, it is important to maintain caution. We are still a long way from a cure. Apathy and carelessness may abound if too much confidence is placed in these treatments. Furthermore, the number of people becoming HIV-infected each year has stabilized and even increased in some communities, meaning that we are still a long way from beating this disease. In fact, while AIDS death rates in America dropped nearly 66 percent during the 1995–1998 period, we are now seeing modest increases in the rate, as drug regimens lose effectiveness and rates of infection rise.[51]

Preventing HIV Infection

Although scientists have been searching for an HIV vaccine since 1983, they have had no success so far. The only way to prevent HIV infection is to avoid risky behaviors. HIV infection and AIDS are not uncontrollable conditions. You can

reduce your risk by the choices you make in sexual behaviors and by taking responsibility for your own health and the health of your loved ones. The Skills for Behavior Change box presents ways to reduce your risk for contracting HIV.

Because the status of your immune system is an important factor in your susceptibility to any of the STIs, it is important that you do everything possible to protect yourself. Adequate nutrition, sleep, stress management, vaccinations, and other preventive maintenance strategies can do a great deal to ensure your long term health.

Where to Go for Help If you are concerned about your own risk or the risk of a close friend, arrange a confidential meeting with the health educator or other health professional at your college health service. He or she will provide you with the information that you need to decide whether you should be tested for HIV antibodies. If the student health service is not an option for you, seek assistance through your local public health department or community STI clinic. Local physicians, members, counselors, professors, and other responsible people can often help you discover the answers you are looking for.

Taking Charge

Managing Risks from Infectious Diseases

Infectious diseases pose serious challenges in the United States as well as throughout the world. In particular, sexually transmitted infections, including HIV, present an increasing health risk to our nation's youth. Nearly all infectious diseases can be prevented by practicing safe and responsible behaviors. These are sensible steps you can take to avoid infectious diseases.

Checklist for Change

Making Personal Choices

☐ Be aware of factors that can threaten your health status. Assess your level of risk for acquiring an STI, including HIV infection.

☐ Know your disease and immunization history.

☐ Take the proper precautions to protect yourself from exposure to infectious pathogens.

☐ Know the health status of your intimate partners.

☐ Communicate openly and honestly with your partners about your feelings regarding sexual intimacy.

- If you have an infectious disease that can be spread through casual contact, remember to wash your hands frequently.
- Avoid traveling to places where outbreaks of infectious diseases have not been controlled.
- Follow a healthy routine of sleep, nutrition, and exercise.
- Follow safe measures when involved with someone with an infectious disease.
- Cook foods at their appropriate temperatures.
- Respect the symptoms that indicate a possible infection and seek treatment immediately.
- Recognize your responsibility for the health of others.

- Behave in sexually responsible ways.
- Limit your sexual partners.
- Avoid using alcohol or other drugs during intimate sexual encounters.
- Respect the rights and needs of individuals affected by an infectious disease.
- Follow your physician's instructions completely when seeking help.

Making Community Choices

- What services does your student health service offer for testing for STIs? for HIV?

- Name any local free clinics where you could be tested for STIs or HIV.
- What have you done to support government spending for HIV research and health promotion (education)? What else could you do?
- Have you written to your congressional representatives regarding your support of funding?
- Does your local school system offer a sex education curriculum including discussion about how to stop the spread of the HIV virus?

Summary

❋ The major uncontrollable risk factors for contracting infectious diseases are heredity, age, environmental conditions, and organism resistance. Major controllable risk factors include stress, nutrition, fitness level, sleep, hygiene, avoidance of high-risk behaviors, and drug use.

❋ The major pathogens are bacteria, viruses, fungi, protozoa, prions, and parasitic worms. Bacterial infections include staphylococcal infections, streptococcal infections, pneumonia, Legionnaire's disease, tuberculosis, periodontal diseases, and rickettsia. Major viral infections include the common cold, influenza, infectious mononucleosis, hepatitis, mumps, chicken pox and shingles, measles, and rabies.

❋ Your body uses a number of defense systems to keep pathogens from invading. The skin is our major protection, helped by enzymes. The immune system creates antibodies to destroy antigens. In addition, fever and pain play a role in defending the body. Vaccines bolster the body's immune system against specific diseases.

❋ Emerging and resurgent diseases pose significant threats for future generations. Many factors contribute to these risks. Possible solutions focus on a public health approach to prevention.

❋ Sexually transmitted infections are spread through intercourse, oral sex, anal sex, hand-genital contact, and sometimes mouth-to-mouth contact. Major STIs include chlamydia, pelvic inflammatory disease, gonorrhea, syphilis, pubic lice, genital warts, candidiasis, trichomoniasis, and herpes.

❋ Acquired immune deficiency syndrome (AIDS) is caused by the human immunodeficiency virus (HIV). HIV is not confined to certain high-risk groups. Globally, HIV/AIDS has become a major threat to the world's population. Anyone can get HIV by engaging in high-risk sexual activities that include exchange of body fluids, by having received a blood transfusion before 1985, or by injecting drugs (or having sex with someone who engages in any high-risk activities). Women appear to be particularly susceptible to infection. You can cut your risk for AIDS significantly by deciding not to engage in risky sexual activities.

Questions for Discussion and Reflection

1. What are the major controllable risk factors for contracting infectious diseases? Using this knowledge, how would you change your current lifestyle to prevent such infection?

2. What is a pathogen? What are the similarities and differences between pathogens and antigens? Discuss uncontrollable and controllable risk factors that can threaten your health. What can you do to limit the effects of either type of risk factor?

3. What are the six types of pathogens? What are the various means by which they can be transmitted? How have social conditions among the poor and homeless increased the risks for certain diseases, such as tuberculosis, influenza, and hepatitis? Why are these conditions a challenge to the efforts of public health officials?

4. What is the difference between active and passive immunity? How do they compare to natural and acquired

immunity? Explain why it is important to wash your hands often when you have a cold.

5. Identify possible reasons for the spread of emerging and resurgent diseases. Indicate public policies and programs that might reduce this trend.

6. Identify five sexually transmitted infections. What are their symptoms? How do they develop? What are their potential long-term effects?

7. Why are women more susceptible to HIV infection than men? What implication does this have for prevention, treatment, and research?

8. Should Americans be concerned about soaring HIV/AIDS rates elsewhere in the world? Explain your answer.

Application Exercises

Reread the What Do You Think? scenarios at the beginning of this chapter and answer the following questions:

1. Why are college students like Heather particularly vulnerable to infectious diseases?

2. At what point should Heather start paying attention to her symptoms? What should she do at the first signs of not feeling well? As a friend, what would you recommend to Heather?

3. Historically, public health practice has required reporting and contact tracing of people with certain contagious diseases. Which do you think should take precedence: the right to confidentiality or the duty to warn others of possible infection? Under what circumstances? What might Susan discover from such a tracing of contacts?

4. What obligations do health care workers have to tell patients and coworkers about health problems such as herpes or HIV? Do patients have the right to know if the doctor who is doing surgery is HIV infected? Do health care workers have the right to know if a patient is infected?

Accessing Your Health on the Internet

Visit the following Internet sites to explore further topics and issues related to personal health. To visit an organization's website, go to the Companion Website for *Access to Health, Eighth Edition,* at www.aw.com/donatelle, click on the book image, and select "Accessing Your Health on the Internet" from the navigation menu on the left.

1. *Centers for Disease Control and Prevention (CDC).* Homepage for the government agency dedicated to disease intervention and prevention, with links to all the latest data and publications put out by the CDC, including the MMWR, *HIV/AIDS Surveillance Report,* and the *Journal of Emerging Infectious Diseases,* and access to the CDC research database, Wonder.

2. *National Center for Infectious Disease.* Up-to-date perspectives on infectious diseases of significance to the global community.

3. *The New England Journal of Medicine Online.* Online version of a weekly journal reporting the results of important medical research worldwide; includes articles from current and past publications.

4. *World Health Organization.* Access to the latest information on world health issues as put out by WHO; direct access to publications and fact sheets; use keywords to find topics of interest.

Further Reading

Addressing Emerging Infectious Disease Threats: A Prevention Strategy for the U.S. Atlanta: Centers for Disease Control, 1998.

Useful slides and narrative addressing risks and threats of emerging diseases as well as a national strategy for prevention and control.

Benenson, A. *Control of Communicable Diseases in Man,* 16th ed. Washington, DC: American Public Health Association, 1998.

Outstanding pocket reference for information on infectious diseases. Published every three to five years in new editions.

Champeau, D., and R. Donatelle. *AIDS and STIs: A Global Perspective.* Englewood Cliffs, NJ: Prentice Hall, 2002.

An overview of issues, trends, and ethics surrounding the global pandemic of HIV/AIDS and sexually transmitted infections.

Levy, S. B. *The Antibiotic Paradox: How the Misuse of Antibiotics Destroys Their Curative Powers.* Cambridge, MA: Perseus Publishing, 2002.

A discussion of microbial resistance, history, progression, and implications for public health.

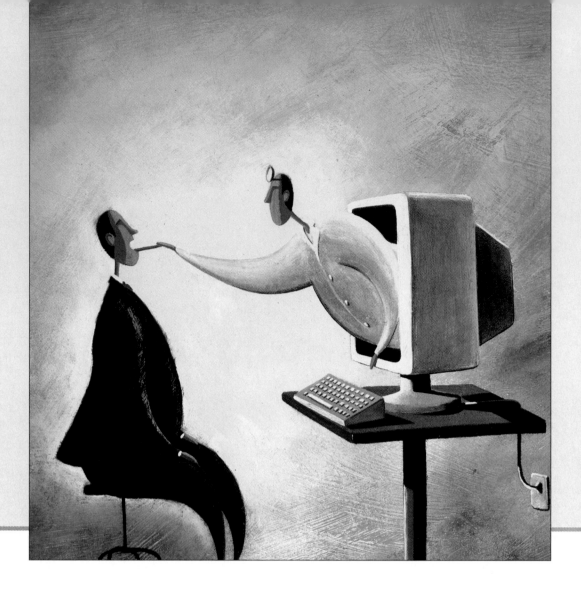

Objectives

* Discuss the chronic lung diseases, including allergies, hay fever, asthma, emphysema, and chronic bronchitis, as well as other problems.

* Explain common neurological disorders, including types of headaches and seizure disorders.

* Describe common gender-related disorders, risk factors for these conditions, their symptoms, and methods to control or prevent them.

* Discuss diabetes and other digestion-related disorders, including their symptoms, prevention, and control.

* Discuss the varied musculoskeletal diseases, including arthritis and other bone and joint problems, and their effects on the body.

* Describe chronic fatigue syndrome and job-related disorders.

18 Noninfectious Conditions

The Modern Maladies

What do you think?

Kate, a 38-year-old graduate student, has asthma and gets several respiratory infections each year. She also has smoked regularly for the past 20 years. Recently, she was diagnosed with an early stage of emphysema. She is defiant about her habit, insisting that because she doesn't smoke in her car, her friends' cars, or in her house, her smoking is nobody else's business. She says that several members of her family—even the nonsmokers—have a long history of respiratory problems. Kate believes that she would have developed asthma and emphysema anyway.

What part of Kate's argument about smoking is accurate? ✳ Inaccurate? ✳ If smokers don't harm others by their smoking, should nonsmokers try to motivate them to quit? ✳ What role does smoking play in asthma and emphysema? ✳ What strategies might you try to encourage Kate to quit smoking?

Jennifer, a 22-year-old college student, lost her father recently to colon cancer. Upon returning to classes, she finds that her steady boyfriend has been cheating on her with a good friend. Jennifer retreats into her studies and is hostile with anyone who talks to her. Recently, she blew up at an instructor over a small suggestion made on one of her papers. She is losing sleep, cries frequently, and can't concentrate on her classes. Jennifer wonders whether the stresses of the past months have caused her to develop chronic fatigue syndrome.

How is chronic fatigue similar to chronic depression? How is it different? ✳ Why might either diagnosis be appropriate in Jennifer's situation? ✳ Is any stigma associated with either condition? ✳ Why or why not? ✳ What services are available on your campus for someone with these problems?

Typically, when we think of the major ailments and diseases affecting Americans today, we think of "killer" diseases such as cancer and heart disease. Clearly, these diseases make up the major portion of life-threatening diseases—accounting for nearly two-thirds of all deaths. Yet although they capture much media attention, other forms of chronic disease often cause substantial pain, suffering, and disability. Fortunately, most of them can be prevented or their symptoms relieved.

Noninfectious conditions are usually not transmitted by a pathogen or by any form of personal contact. They often develop over a long period of time, and they cause progressive damage to human tissues. Although these conditions normally do not result in death, they do lead to illness and suffering for many people. Lifestyle and personal health habits are often implicated as underlying causes; however, a number of "newer" maladies seem to defy conventional wisdom about causation. For those known maladies and **idiopathic** (of unknown cause) disorders, education, reasonable changes in lifestyle, pharmacological agents, and public health efforts aimed at research, prevention, and control can minimize their effects. (See the Health Ethics box about funding priorities for research on selected diseases.) In this chapter, we will discuss common noninfectious conditions and the factors that contribute to them.

Chronic Lung Diseases

Chronic lung diseases pose a serious and significant threat to Americans today. Collectively, they have become the fourth leading cause of death, with most sufferers living with a condition known as chronic **dyspnea**, or chronic breathlessness. Depending on the situation, dyspnea may result in the inability to climb stairs, walk unassisted, or sleep without fear of stopping breathing. Chronic lung disease can result in major disability and lack of function as the lungs fill with mucous, become susceptible to bacterial or viral infections, and cause acute stress on the heart as they struggle to get valuable oxygen. Chronic cough, excessive phlegm, wheezing, or coughing up blood are frequent symptoms. Over time, many of these underlying conditions lead to hospitalization and possible death.

Among the more deadly chronic lung diseases are the **chronic obstructive pulmonary diseases (COPDs)**: asthma, emphysema, and chronic bronchitis. Other chronic

---

HEALTH IN A DIVERSE WORLD

Disparities in Disease Trends

In a review of the leading causes of death in the United States, marked gender, racial, and ethnic differences exist. African Americans, Hispanic Americans, Asian Americans, and white Americans display vastly different risk profiles. These differences are found not only among life-threatening diseases such as cardiovascular disease and cancer, but in many chronic conditions as well. Consider the following:

- Prevalence rates of asthma are consistently higher for blacks than for whites by approximately 50 percent. Among Hispanic Americans, death rates due to asthma are approximately 50 percent higher than among non-Hispanics.
- Females report approximately 50 percent more chronic bronchitis than males, and whites are 50 percent more likely to develop the condition than are blacks.
- Osteoarthritis is more common among males under age 45 than among their female counterparts. However, over the age of 54, osteoarthritis is more common among women than men.
- No significant racial differences in morbidity for rheumatoid arthritis are apparent; however, several Native American tribes have shown a high prevalence of the disease, including the Yakima of Central Washington and the Mille-Lac Band of Chippewa in Minnesota.
- Older Americans and minority populations suffer disproportionately high rates of diabetes and diabetes-related complications.
- The prevalence of type 1 diabetes is higher among whites than among people of other races (relative risk of 1.4). In contrast, the prevalence of type 2 diabetes is higher among races other than whites, including blacks (1.3), Hispanic Americans (3.1), and Native Americans (10.1).
- Parkinson's disease rates are higher among men than among women, and more common in whites than in blacks.

Source of statistics: Chronic Disease Epidemiology and Control by R. C. Brownson, P. L. Remington, and J. Davis (eds.), Washington, DC: American Public Health Association, 1998. Health: United States, 2002. Centers for Disease Control and Prevention. http://www.cdc.gov.

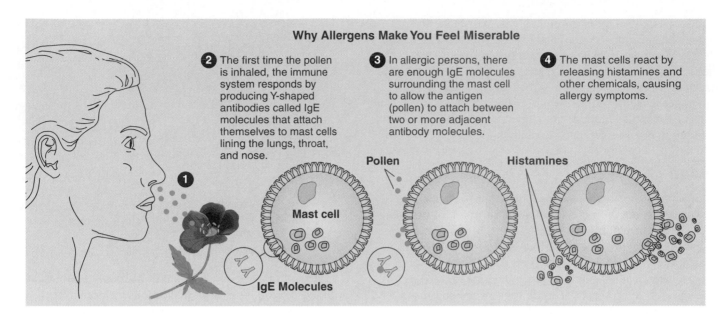

Why Allergens Make You Feel Miserable

2 The first time the pollen is inhaled, the immune system responds by producing Y-shaped antibodies called IgE molecules that attach themselves to mast cells lining the lungs, throat, and nose.

3 In allergic persons, there are enough IgE molecules surrounding the mast cell to allow the antigen (pollen) to attach between two or more adjacent antibody molecules.

4 The mast cells react by releasing histamines and other chemicals, causing allergy symptoms.

1

Pollen

Histamines

Mast cell

IgE Molecules

Figure 18.1
Steps of an Allergy Response

lung diseases also cause significant health risks, the most common of which are allergy-induced problems and hay fever. Each of these may exacerbate or contribute to the development of COPD.

Allergy-Induced Respiratory Problems

An **allergy** occurs as a part of the body's attempt to defend itself against a specific *antigen* or *allergen* by producing specific *antibodies*. When foreign pathogens such as bacteria or viruses invade the body, the body responds by producing antibodies to destroy these invading antigens. Under normal conditions, the production of antibodies is a positive element in the body's defense system. However, for unknown reasons, in some people the body overreacts by developing an overly elaborate protective mechanism against relatively harmless substances. The resultant *hypersensitivity reaction* to specific allergens or antigens in the environment is fairly common, as anyone who has awakened with a runny nose or itchy eyes will testify. Most commonly, these hypersensitivity, or allergic, responses occur as a reaction to environmental antigens such as molds, animal dander (hair and dead skin), pollen, ragweed, or dust. Once excessive antibodies to these antigens are produced, they trigger the release of **histamines**, chemical substances that dilate blood vessels, increase mucous secretions, cause tissues to swell, and produce other allergy-like symptoms, particularly in the respiratory system (see Figure 18.1).

Although many people think of allergies as childhood diseases, in reality allergies tend to become progressively worse with time and with increased exposure to allergens. In these circumstances, allergic responses become chronic in nature, and treatment becomes difficult. Many people take allergy shots to reduce the severity of their symptoms with

some success. In most cases, once the offending antigen has disappeared, allergy-prone people suffer few symptoms. Although allergies can cause numerous problems, one of the most significant effects is on the immune system.

Hay Fever

Perhaps the best example of a chronic respiratory disease is **hay fever**. Usually considered a seasonally related disease (most prevalent when ragweed and flowers are blooming), hay fever is common throughout the world. Hay fever attacks, which are characterized by sneezing and itchy, watery eyes and nose, cause a great deal of misery for countless people. The disorder appears to run in families, and research indicates that lifestyle is not as great a factor in developing

---

Idiopathic   Of unknown cause.

Dyspnea   Chronic breathlessness.

Chronic obstructive pulmonary diseases (COPDs) A collection of chronic lung diseases including asthma, emphysema, and chronic bronchitis.

Allergy   Hypersensitive reaction to a specific antigen or allergen in the environment in which the body produces excessive antibodies to that antigen or allergen.

Histamines   Chemical substances that dilate blood vessels, increase mucous secretions, and produce other symptoms of allergies.

Hay fever   A chronic respiratory disorder that is most prevalent when ragweed and flowers bloom.

hay fever as it is in other chronic diseases. Instead, an overzealous immune system and exposure to environmental allergens including pet dander, dust, pollen from various plants, and other substances appear to be the critical factors that determine vulnerability. For those people who are unable to get away from the cause of their hay fever response, medical assistance in the form of injections or antihistamines may provide the only possibility of relief.

Asthma

Unfortunately, for many persons who suffer from allergies such as hay fever, their condition often becomes complicated by the development of one of the major COPDs: asthma, emphysema, or bronchitis. **Asthma** is a long-term, chronic inflammatory disorder that blocks air flow in and out of the lungs. Asthma causes tiny airways in the lung to overreact with spasms in response to certain triggers. Symptoms include wheezing, difficulty in breathing, shortness of breath, and coughing spasms. Although most asthma attacks are mild and non–life-threatening, they can trigger bronchospasms (contractions of the bronchial tubes in the lungs) that are so severe that without rapid treatment, death may occur. Between attacks, most people have few symptoms.

A number of factors can trigger an asthma attack, including air pollutants; particulate matter, such as wood dust; indoor air pollutants, such as sidestream tobacco smoke; and allergens, such as dust mites, cockroach saliva, and pet dander. Stress is also believed to trigger attacks in some individuals.[1]

Asthma can occur at any age but is most likely in children between infancy and age 5 and in adults before age 40. In childhood, asthma strikes more boys than girls; in adulthood, it strikes more women than men. Also, the asthma rate is 50 percent higher among African Americans than whites, and four times as many African Americans die of asthma than do whites.[2] Midwesterners appear to be more prone to asthma than people from other areas of the country.

In recent years, concern over the rise in incidence of asthma has grown considerably. Consider these points:[3]

Asthma   A chronic respiratory disease characterized by attacks of wheezing, shortness of breath, and coughing spasms.

Emphysema   A respiratory disease in which the alveoli become distended or ruptured and are no longer functional.

Alveoli   Tiny air sacs of the lungs.

Bronchitis   An inflammation of the lining of the bronchial tubes.

Acute bronchitis   A form of bronchitis most often caused by viruses.

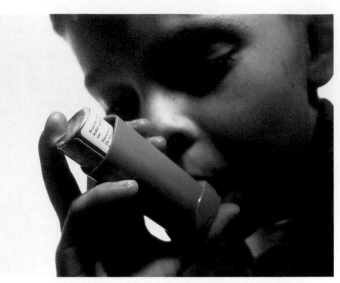

Although a number of new medications are available to relieve the symptoms of asthma, the marked increase of this respiratory problem among young children worries health officials.

- Asthma is the only chronic disease, besides AIDS and tuberculosis, with an increasing death rate. Each day 14 Americans die from asthma.
- Asthma has become the most common chronic disease of childhood, accounting for one-fourth of all school absences and affecting more than one child in 20.
- Asthma affects over 17 million Americans, including 5 million children; 13 percent of all students ages 5–19 have it.
- The annual direct costs of asthma are over $13 billion. Among adults, asthma is the fourth leading cause of work absence, resulting in over 9 million lost workdays per year.
- The number of asthma sufferers has increased by more than 65 percent since the 1980s; one in ten new cases is diagnosed in people over age 65.
- The death toll from asthma has nearly doubled since 1980, to more than 5,000 persons per year.

Ask a hundred experts what causes asthma and you might get a hundred different answers. Clearly, many factors contribute to increased risk. Although some studies have indicated a potential genetic link, much of this research is controversial, with critics pointing out that the gene pool hasn't changed much in the past few decades, yet asthma incidence has increased substantially. Most experts point to a potential allergenic cause, whereas others look to environmental, infectious, and familial links to explain the increases.

People with asthma fall into one of two distinctly different types of asthma development. The most common type, known as *extrinsic* (or *slow onset*) *asthma,* is most commonly associated with allergic triggers. This type tends to run in families and develop in childhood. Often, by adulthood, a person has few episodes, or the disorder completely goes away. *Intrinsic asthma* also may have allergic triggers, but the main difference is that any unpleasant event or stimulant

Keys to Asthma Prevention

Although asthma rates continue to increase internationally, there is much that individuals and communities can do to reduce risk:

- Work with local leaders to reduce air pollution in your communities. Scrutinize regulations on the burning of household and yard trash, field burning, wood-burning stoves, and sidestream smoke from cigarettes— all known triggers for asthma attacks. Revise them as necessary.
- Purchase a good air filter for your home and clean furnace filters regularly. Clean house often, using a high-suction vacuum rather than a broom to reduce dust particles in suspended air.

- Wash pillows regularly to avoid pesty mites and other debris inside the pillows. Use pillow protectors and mattress protectors, which keep dust mites and other critters out of your face and trapped inside the pillow or mattress. Don't purchase used mattresses, as they may be teeming with mites.
- Avoid having cats or dogs that are known for high dander production in the home. If you must have these pets, keep them off your bed and wash them and their bedding weekly. Vacuum their hair regularly.
- Have asthma medications handy and know where you keep them in case of an emergency.
- Keep your home clean and pest free; cockroaches and other vermin have enzymes in their saliva or particles on their bodies that may trigger allergic reactions.

- Keep mold concentrations low by using antimold cleaners or by running a dehumidifier to keep moisture levels down.
- Avoid mowing the lawn or excessive outdoor exposure to pollen during high-pollen times. Local news stations often provide pollen warnings. If you must be outdoors, wear a pollen mask.
- Exercise regularly to keep your lungs functioning well.
- Avoid cigarette and cigar smoke.
- If you have a fireplace or wood-burning stove, check it regularly to make sure that it is not spewing smoke and particulate matter.
- Let people close to you know that you are asthmatic, and educate them about what to do if you have an asthmatic attack. Understanding and knowledge are powerful tools for health consumers. Make sure your loved ones have access to information.

may trigger an attack. A common form of extrinsic asthma is *exercise-induced asthma (EIA)*, which may or may not have an allergic connection. Some athletes have no allergies yet live with asthma. Cold, dry air is believed to exacerbate EIA, thus, keeping the lungs moist and warming up prior to working out may help. The warm, moist air around a swimming pool is one of the best environments for people with asthma.

Relaxation techniques appear to help some asthma sufferers. Drugs may be necessary for serious cases. Determining whether a specific allergen provokes asthma attacks and then taking steps to reduce exposure to it, avoiding triggers such as certain types of exercise or stress, and finding the most effective medications are big steps in asthma prevention and control. Numerous new drugs are available that cause fewer side effects than older medications. It is critical to find a doctor who specializes in asthma and stays up to date on treatments and options. The Skills for Behavior Change box identifies important preventive measures.

Emphysema

If you have ever heard someone gasping for air for no apparent reason, or watched someone hooked up to an oxygen tank and struggling to breathe while climbing a flight of stairs, you have probably witnessed an emphysemic episode. **Emphysema** involves the gradual destruction of the **alveoli** (tiny air sacs) of the lungs. As the alveoli are destroyed, the affected person finds it more and more difficult to exhale. The victim struggles to take in a fresh supply of air before the

air held in the lungs has been expended. Over time the chest cavity gradually expands, producing the barrel-shaped chest characteristic of the chronic emphysema patient.

The exact cause of emphysema is uncertain. There is, however, a strong relationship between the development of emphysema and long-term cigarette smoking and exposure to air pollution. Victims of emphysema often suffer discomfort over many years. In fact, studies show that lung function decline may begin well before the age of 50 and the early morning "smoker's cough" may signal that the damage has already begun.[4] What most of us take for granted—the easy, rhythmic flow of air in and out of the lungs—becomes a continuous struggle for people with emphysema. Inadequate oxygen supply, combined with the stress of overexertion on the heart, eventually takes its toll on the cardiovascular system and leads to premature death.

Bronchitis

Bronchitis refers to an inflammation of the lining of the bronchial tubes. These tubes, the bronchi, connect the windpipe with the lungs. When the bronchi become inflamed or infected, less air is able to flow from the lungs, and heavy mucous begins to form. **Acute bronchitis** is the most common of the bronchial diseases, resulting in millions of visits to the doctor every year at a cost of over $300 million per year.[5] Over 95 percent of these acute cases are caused by viruses; however, they are often misdiagnosed and treated with antibiotics, even though little evidence supports this treatment. Typically, misdiagnosis occurs when a cluster of symptoms is labeled as bronchitis, despite the fact that there is no true laboratory diagnosis.

Chronic bronchitis, on the other hand, is defined by the presence of a productive (mucous-laden) cough most days of the month, over three months of a year for two successive years without underlying disease to explain the cough. Typically, cigarette smoking causes chronic bronchitis, and once bronchitis begins, secondary bacterial or viral infections often make the condition worse. Air pollution and industrial dusts and fumes are also risk factors. If you have either type of bronchitis, the following recommendations can help you reduce your risk of complications and lung damage:

- See your doctor or follow your doctor's instructions at the beginning of a cold or respiratory infection.
- Get a flu shot if you are at risk for COPDs.
- Don't smoke. If you do, quit.
- Follow a nutritious, well-balanced diet, get enough sleep, and maintain your ideal body weight.
- Get regular exercise.
- Do breathing exercises regularly to keep lungs healthy.
- Avoid exposure to colds and flu and to respiratory irritants such as secondhand smoke, dust, and air pollutants.

Sleep Apnea

Although not as life threatening as asthma and other COPDs, people who suffer from sleep apnea also puts people's health at risk. **Sleep apnea** is a condition characterized by periodic episodes when breathing stops completely for 10 seconds or longer at a time. The upper airway narrows or closes, initiating a sequence of events, including a decrease in arterial oxygen saturation, arousal from sleep, and subsequent relief of the obstruction. Episodes can occur several times during the course of a night, resulting in a restless night's sleep. Over time, repeated oxygen deprivation can raise blood pressure, trigger irregular heartbeats, and damage the cardiovascular system.

Sleep apnea affects about 5 percent of the general population and can be quite disconcerting to others when the sufferer stops breathing, even for a short time![6] Altering

sleeping position and schedules, using mechanical devices that increase air flow through the pharynx, and surgery are common methods of correction. Cutting back on alcohol can also reduce episodes.

> **What do you think?**
>
> *Which of the respiratory diseases described in this section do you or your family have problems with? ✷ How many of your college friends have these COPDs? ✷ What difficulties do they have in controlling their diseases? ✷ Why do you think the incidence of COPDs, as a group, is increasing? ✷ What actions can you or the people in your community take to reduce risks and problems from these diseases?*

Neurological Disorders

Headaches

Almost all of us have experienced the agony of at least one major headache. In fact, over 80 percent of women and 65 percent of men experience headaches on a regular basis.[7] Common types of headaches and their treatments include the following.

Tension Headache   Tension headaches, also referred to as *muscular contraction headaches,* are generally caused by muscle contractions or tension in the neck or head. This tension may be caused by actual strain placed on neck or head muscles due to overuse, static positions held for long periods of time, or tension triggered by stress. Recent research indicates that tension headaches may be a product of a more "generic mechanism" in which chemicals deep inside the brain may cause the muscular tension, pain, and suffering often associated with an attack. Possible triggers for this chemical assault include red wine, lack of sleep, fasting, menstruation, or other factors, and the same symptoms (sensitivity to light and sound, nausea, and/or throbbing pain) may characterize different types of headaches. Symptoms vary in intensity and duration. Relaxation, hot water treatment, and massage have surfaced as the new holistic treatments, while aspirin, Tylenol, Aleve, and Advil are the old standby forms of pain relief. Although such painkillers have brought temporary relief of symptoms for some people, it is believed that, over time, the drugs could dull the brain's own painkilling weapons and result in more headaches rather than fewer.

Migraine Headache   Migraine is not just a name for an unusually bad headache; it is a specific diagnosis, involving pain that begins on one side of the head, often accompanied by nausea and sensitivity to light and sounds. Many migraine sufferers experience the sensation of an "aura" in their visual

---

Chronic bronchitis   A serious respiratory disorder in which the bronchial tubes become so inflamed and swollen that respiratory function is impaired.

Sleep apnea   A condition of repetitive cessation of breathing during sleep.

Migraine   A condition characterized by localized headaches that possibly result from alternating dilation and constriction of blood vessels.

Epilepsy   A neurological disorder caused by abnormal electrical brain activity; can be accompanied by altered consciousness or convulsions.

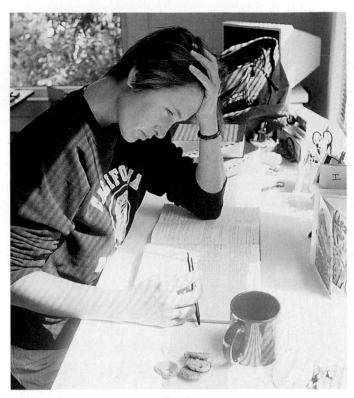

Tension headaches are triggered by many factors, including lack of sleep, stress, and strain on head and neck muscles.

field, typically some form of disturbance such as flashing lights or blind spots, along with numbness or weakness on one side of the body or slurred speech,[8] all signals of an ensuing bad headache. Most people report pain behind or around one eye and always on the same side of the head—a pain that can last for hours or days and then disappear. A migraine can strike at any time, although the hormonal changes around menstruation and ovulation often seem to set off migraines in women, who are three times more likely to get them than men. Migraines can occur in children as young as 2 years, with incidences peaking from the mid-20s through middle age and then trailing off around age 55.[9]

Patients report that migraines can be triggered by emotional stress, weather, certain foods, lack of sleep, and a litany of other causes. When tested under laboratory settings, however, much of this evidence is inconclusive. What is known is that migraines occur when blood vessels dilate in the membrane that surrounds the brain. Historically, treatments have centered on reversing or preventing this dilation, with the most common treatment derived from the rye fungus *ergot*. Today, fast-acting ergot compounds are available by nasal spray, vastly increasing the speed of relief. However, ergot drugs have many side effects, the least of which may be that they are habit forming, causing users to wake up with "rebound" headaches each morning after use.[10]

Critics of the blood vessel dilation theory question why only blood vessels of the head dilate in these situations. Furthermore, why aren't people who take hot baths or those who exercise more prone to migraine attacks? They suggest

that migraines originate in the cortex of the brain, where certain pain sensors are stimulated.

According to pioneering work by Harvard University neurology professor Michael Moskowitz, triggers, such as caffeine or wine, set off an electrical ripple on the surface of the cortex. Waves of nerve cells fire and then go quiet, creating an aura. This spurs a reaction in the meninges, the membranes above the cortex. The meninges contain endings of the brain's major nerve, the *trigeminus*, which release chemicals that inflame nearby tissues. The result is pain.[11]

Other doctors believe that pain signals begin deep in the brain in areas normally rich in the painkilling chemical serotonin. Migraines are started by disturbances that keep the pain-regulating chemicals from doing their job. Susceptibility to these disturbances may be hereditary. This theory would explain why drugs that interact with serotonin reduce headaches. (It must be said that there is no proof that serotonin irregularities cause headaches, only that serotonin drugs work.)[12]

When true migraines occur, relaxation is only minimally effective as a treatment. Often, strong pain-relieving drugs prescribed by a physician are necessary. In 1994, the FDA approved Imitrex, a drug tailor-made for migraines that works for about 80 percent of those who try it. But the cost of a single pill is a stunning $14, and second doses are often needed. In addition, its side effects make Imitrex inappropriate for anyone with uncontrolled high blood pressure or heart disease. Recently, treatment with lidocaine has also shown promising results, and newer drugs called triptans, such as Zomig, Amerge, and Maxalt, are now available. All triptans, however, are cleared from the body in a few hours, and the migraine sometimes returns.[13]

Secondary Headaches Secondary headaches arise as a result of some other underlying condition. Hypertension, blocked sinuses, allergies, low blood sugar, diseases of the spine, the common cold, poorly fitted dentures, problems with eyesight, and other types of pain or injury can trigger this condition. Relaxation and pain relievers such as aspirin are of little help in treating secondary headaches. Rather, medications or other therapies to relieve the underlying organic cause of the headache must be included in the treatment regimen.

Seizure Disorders

The word **epilepsy** is derived from the Greek *epilepsia,* meaning "seizure." Reports of epilepsy appeared in Greek medical records as early as 300 B.C. Ancient peoples interpreted seizures as invasions of the body by evil spirits or as punishments by the gods. Although much of the mystery surrounding epileptic seizures has been solved in recent years, the stigma and lack of understanding remain. Approximately 1 percent of all Americans suffer from some form of seizure-related disorder.

These disorders are generally caused by abnormal electrical activity in the brain and are characterized by loss of control of muscular activity and unconsciousness. Symptoms vary widely from person to person.

There are several forms of seizure disorders, such as narcolepsy, a condition in which the individual falls asleep at unpredictable times.[14] The most common forms of epilepsy are the following:

- *Grand mal, or major motor seizure.* These seizures are often preceded by a shrill cry or a seizure aura (body sensations such as ringing in the ears or a specific smell or taste). Convulsions and loss of consciousness generally occur and may last from 30 seconds to several minutes or more. Keeping track of the length of time elapsed is one aspect of first aid.
- *Petit mal, or minor seizure.* These seizures involve no convulsions. Rather, a minor loss of consciousness that may go unnoticed occurs. Minor twitching of muscles may take place, usually for a shorter time than grand mal convulsions.
- *Psychomotor seizure.* These seizures involve both mental processes and muscular activity. Symptoms include mental confusion and a listless state characterized by activities such as lip smacking, chewing, and repetitive movements.
- *Jacksonian seizure.* This is a progressive seizure that often begins in one part of the body, such as the fingers, and moves to other parts, such as the hand or arm. Usually only one side of the body is affected.

About half of all cases of seizure disorder are of unknown origin. Head injury or trauma is one possible cause; other causes include congenital abnormalities, injury or illness resulting in inflammation of the brain or spinal column, drug or chemical poisoning, tumors, nutritional deficiency, and heredity.

In most cases, people afflicted with seizure disorders can lead normal, seizure-free lives when under medical supervision. Public ignorance about these disorders is one of the most serious obstacles confronting them. Improvements in medication and surgical interventions to reduce some causes of seizures are among the most promising treatments today.

Providing First Aid for Seizures   There are several things you can do to help people during and after seizures.

1. *Note the length of the attack.* Seizures in which a person remains unconscious for long periods of time should be monitored closely. If medical help arrives, be sure to tell the medical personnel how long it has been since the person became unconscious.
2. *Remove obstacles that could harm the victim.* Because seizure victims may lose motor control during a convulsion, they inadvertently thrash around. To reduce the chances of serious injury, clear away any objects that could pose a threat.
3. *Loosen clothing and turn the victim's head to the side.* This procedure will ensure adequate ventilation and allow fluids or vomit to drain from the mouth.
4. *Do not force objects into the victim's mouth.* Although seizure victims may bite their tongues, causing possible damage, they will not swallow them. If the victim's mouth is clamped shut, forcing objects into the mouth may break teeth or cause damage more serious than what would have occurred if you had done nothing.
5. *Get help.* After you have completed steps 1–4, get help or send someone for help. This is particularly important if the victim does not regain consciousness within a few minutes.
6. *Reassure the victim.* In too many instances, the seizure victim regains consciousness only to face a crowd of staring people. When administering first aid, try to dissuade curious bystanders from hanging around. Calmly reassure the victim that everything is okay.
7. *Allow the victim to rest.* After a seizure, many victims will be exhausted. Allow them to sleep if possible.

What do you think?

Do you suffer from recurrent headaches or other neurological problems? ✳ *What might cause your problems?* ✳ *What actions could you take to reduce your risks and symptoms?*

Parkinson's disease   A chronic, progressive neurological condition that causes tremors and other symptoms.

Multiple sclerosis (MS)   A degenerative neurological disease in which myelin, an insulator of nerves, breaks down.

Fibrocystic breast condition   A common, noncancerous condition in which a woman's breasts contain fibrous or fluid-filled cysts.

Endometriosis   Abnormal development of endometrial tissue outside the uterus, resulting in serious side effects.

Hysterectomy   Surgical removal of the uterus.

Parkinson's Disease

Until recently, most people thought of Parkinson's disease as something that afflicted only older people. Many were surprised when one of the younger generation, Michael J. Fox, announced that he had to drop out of the popular television series *Spin City* due to persistent Parkinson's symptoms. Former U.S. attorney general Janet Reno further alerted the U.S. populace that Parkinson's could no longer be ignored when her tremors became so persistent that she could no longer keep them a secret. Although these two individuals are highly visible, they are not alone. Last year, over 1.5 million Americans were believed to have **Parkinson's disease**, a chronic, slowly progressive neurological condition that typically strikes after age 50. Rates of Parkinson's have quadrupled in the past 30 years and may increase even more dramatically as growing numbers of baby boomers pass age 60.[15] The hallmark of Parkinson's disease, and the symptom most commonly associated with it, is a tremor, or form of "shaking palsy." Tremors can become so severe that the simplest task, such as eating or brushing one's teeth, becomes difficult. These additional symptoms may also occur:

- Tremor of the hand when in a relaxed position or when under stress.
- Rigid or stiff muscles.
- Slowness in movement and a delay in initiating movements.
- Poor balance.
- Difficulty in walking, shuffling steps, and inability to take next steps.
- Slurred speech, slowness in thought, and small, cramped handwriting.

Although many theories exist concerning the causes of this disease, the most common appear to be these:[16]

- Familial predisposition (about 15–20 percent of those who have Parkinson's have a close relative with it).
- Acceleration of age-related changes.
- Exposure to environmental toxins such as pesticides.

Parkinson's is progressive and incurable; however, new drug therapies, including levodopa, dopamine antagonists, and MAO inhibitors, work to keep symptoms under control, possibly for years. Surgical options such as brain tissue transplants and the use of fetal tissue or genetically engineered cell transplants have also provided promising results.

Multiple Sclerosis (MS)

Multiple sclerosis (MS) is a degenerative neurological disease in which the myelin, a material composed of fats that serves as an insulator and conduit for transmission of nerve impulses, begins to break down and cause nerve malfunction, or short-circuiting. As the myelin degenerates, it scars; hence the sclerotic (scar) terminology. Typically MS appears between the ages of 15 and 50 and is often characterized by relapses in which symptoms flare up as well as symptom-free states known as remissions.

Actual symptoms of MS vary considerably from one person to the next. Some experience mild symptoms of episodic numbness, dizziness, fatigue, changes in gait, and temporary vision loss. Others face more severe symptoms, including loss of bladder control and severe muscle weakness, necessitating a wheelchair for mobility. Most MS patients lead fairly normal lives and have few disease flare-ups.

Though several theories hypothesize what causes MS, none has been proved conclusive. Allergies, viral exposure to an unknown pathogen, and environmental factors all have been considered as possible causes.

Those who have been diagnosed with MS should practice commonsense strategies for preventing flare-ups. As with most neurological problems, risk reduction includes practicing a healthy lifestyle—particularly getting adequate sleep, eating a well-balanced diet, and controlling stress.[17]

Gender-Related Disorders

Fibrocystic Breast Condition

A common, noncancerous problem among women in the United States is **fibrocystic breast condition.** Symptoms range in severity from a small, palpable lump to large masses of irregular tissue found in both breasts. The underlying causes of the condition are unknown. Although some experts believe it to be related to hormonal changes that occur during the normal menstrual cycle, many women report that their conditions neither worsen nor improve during their cycles. In fact, in most cases, the condition appears to run in families and to become progressively worse with age, irrespective of pregnancy or other hormonal disruptions. Although most cyst formations consist of fibrous tissue, some are filled with fluid. Treatment often involves removing fluid from the affected area or surgically removing the cyst itself.

Does fibrocystic breast condition predispose a woman to breast cancer? Experts believe that the risks for breast cancer among women with certain types of fibrocystic disease may be slightly higher than among the general populace, but it is likely that other factors, discussed in detail in Chapter 16, present much greater risks.

Endometriosis

Whether the incidence of **endometriosis** is on the rise in the United States or whether the disorder is simply attracting more attention is difficult to determine. Victims of endometriosis tend to be women between the ages of 20 and 40. Symptoms include severe cramping during and between menstrual cycles, irregular periods, unusually heavy or light menstrual flow, abdominal bloating, fatigue, painful bowel movements with periods, painful intercourse, constipation, diarrhea, menstrual pain, infertility, and low back pain.

Endometriosis is characterized by the abnormal growth and development of endometrial tissue (the tissue lining the uterus) in regions of the body other than the uterus. Among the most widely accepted theories concerning the causes of endometriosis are the transmission of endometrial tissue to other regions of the body during surgery or through the birthing process; the movement of menstrual fluid backward through the fallopian tubes during menstruation; and abnormal cell migration through body-fluid movement. Women with cycles shorter than 27 days or longer than a week are at increased risk. The more aerobic exercise a woman engages in and the earlier she starts it, the less likely she is to develop endometriosis.

Treatment ranges from bed rest and stress reduction to **hysterectomy** (the removal of the uterus) and/or the removal of one or both ovaries and the fallopian tubes. Physicians have

Uterine Fibroids

Severe abdominal cramps. Incontinence. Infertility. Excessive bleeding during the menstrual cycle. Back pain. If you are one of the many women who suffer from these symptoms but can't figure out what might be wrong, a trip to your gynecologist should be on your schedule. For the majority of women who have these symptoms, it isn't cancer that is stalking you; it is more likely to be the fairly common problem of uterine fibroids.

Uterine fibroids are benign (noncancerous) growths that can develop in a woman's uterine tissue and may range in size from pea-sized growths to the size of a football or larger, weighing in at over 20 pounds. It is not uncommon for a woman to have several at a time, ranging from the size of golf balls to tennis balls. Many fibroids grow in the thick inner walls of the uterus; others may grow from the outer walls of the uterus on stalks or as large masses.

Who is susceptible to fibroids? Although they are typically found in women between the ages of 35–50, fibroids can occur at any age. African American women are two to three times more likely to have fibroids and typically develop them at younger ages then other groups of women. Asian women have the lowest incidence.

Risk factors associated with fibroids include obesity and the consumption of red meat, pork, and ham. Green leafy vegetables, fruit, and fish seem to bestow some type of protective effect resulting in a reduced incidence of fibroids.

Fibroid symptoms include obvious changes in menstruation (excessive bleeding, longer periods, excessive cramps, bleeding between periods, anemia) and pain in the lower back or abdomen. Other symptoms include a feeling of pressure, abdominal cramping, the need to urinate more frequently, constipation, and/or pain during sex. However, some women have none of these symptoms. Fibroids may grow and obstruct the fallopian tubes, leading to infertility, or they may obstruct the bowel or other body parts, leading to dysfunction.

If symptoms become severe or persist, a woman must decide what options for treatment might be best for her. Because most fibroids grow in the presence of estrogen, if a woman is near menopause, the fibroids may begin to shrink on their own as a part of natural hormone depletion. Thus, if the pain or problems are tolerable, a woman can "wait them out," and the fibroids may shrivel and never cause further problems. Other women may opt for surgical removal of the fibroids. Women of childbearing age may choose to have a *myomectomy* (removal of the fibroids only, preserving the uterus), a *hysterectomy* (removal of the uterus and/or one or both ovaries), a *fibroid embolization* (a catheter is placed in an artery and guided to the uterus, where small particles are injected to block the blood supply feeding the fibroids, eventually killing them), or other techniques designed to destroy the fibroids' ability to grow.

It is estimated that between 30 percent and 80 percent of all women may have fibroids of varying size during their lives. Many never know they have them. Fibroids can be detected during an annual pelvic examination and verified by ultrasound, laparoscopy, magnetic resonance imaging (MRI), or computerized tomography (CT) scans. While little can be done to prevent fibroids, paying attention to changes or unusual events with the menstrual cycle and to general body health may lead to early detection of fibroids' presence. Regular check-ups are important for early detection and monitoring before the fibroids develop into more serious problems.

Source: National Uterine Fibroid Foundation. 2003. http://www.nuff.org/health_treatments.htm.

been criticized for being too quick to select hysterectomy as the treatment of choice. More conservative treatments that involve dilation and curettage, surgically scraping endometrial tissue off the fallopian tubes and other reproductive organs, and combinations of hormone therapy have become more acceptable. Hormonal treatments include gonadotropin-releasing hormone (GnRH) analogs, various synthetic progesterone-like drugs (Provera), and oral contraceptives. (See the Reality Check box for information about another problem of the female reproductive system: uterine fibroids.)

What do you think?

*Which of the preceding health problems do you think causes the most problems for women in the United States? * For college-age women? * Why might certain groups of women have more difficulties than others? * What actions could be taken to increase awareness and understanding of these conditions?*

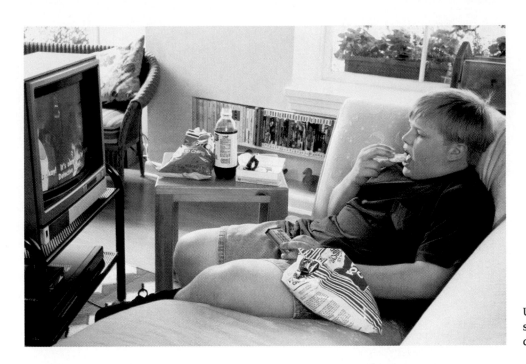

Unhealthy eating habits and a sedentary lifestyle can lead to type 2 diabetes even among children.

Digestion-Related Disorders

Diabetes: Disabling, Deadly, and on the Rise

Diabetes is a serious, widespread, and costly chronic disease, affecting not just the 17 million Americans who must live with it, but their families and communities. Between 1990 and 2000, diagnosed diabetes increased 49 percent among U.S. adults, giving it the rather dubious distinction of being the fastest growing chronic disease in American history.[18] (Figure 18.2 shows the rapid spread of diabetes since 1990.) A recent CDC study indicated that diabetes seems to be increasing even more dramatically among younger adults—it is up by almost 70 percent among those in their thirties.[19]

Over 2,200 people are diagnosed with diabetes each day in America and over 200,000 die each year of related complications, making diabetes the sixth leading cause of death in America today.[20] Diabetes has its greatest impact on the elderly and certain racial and ethnic groups. One in five adults over age 65 has diabetes. Among adults aged 20 and older, African Americans are twice as likely as whites to have diabetes and Native Americans and Alaska natives are 2.6 times more likely to develop it.[21]

What causes this serious disease? In healthy people, the *pancreas,* a powerful enzyme-producing organ, produces the hormone **insulin** in sufficient quantities to allow the body to use or store glucose (blood sugar). When this organ fails to produce enough insulin to regulate sugar metabolism or when the body fails to use insulin effectively, a disease known as **diabetes mellitus** occurs. Diabetics exhibit **hyperglycemia**, or elevated blood sugar levels, and high glucose levels in their urine. Other symptoms include excessive thirst, frequent urination, hunger, tendency to tire easily,

wounds that heal slowly, numbness or tingling in the extremities, changes in vision, skin eruptions, and, in women, a tendency toward vaginal yeast infections.

Of the 17 million people in the United States today who have diabetes, nearly 6 million are unaware of their condition until they begin to show symptoms (see Figure 18.3). How does a person become diabetic? The more serious form, known as *type 1 diabetes* (formerly known as insulin-dependent or juvenile diabetes), is an autoimmune disease in which the immune system destroys the insulin-making beta cells and most often appears during childhood or adolescence.[22] Type 1 diabetics typically must depend on insulin injections or oral medications for the rest of their lives because insulin is not present in their bodies. In *type 2 diabetes* (formerly known as noninsulin-dependent or adult-onset diabetes), insulin production is deficient or the body resists or is unable to utilize available insulin. Type 2 diabetes accounts for 90 to 95 percent of all diabetes cases and most often appears after age 40. However, it is no longer considered only an adult disease and is being diagnosed at younger ages and even among children and teens. This form of diabetes is typically linked to obesity and physical inactivity, both of which can be modified to control diabetes and

Insulin   A hormone produced by the pancreas; required by the body for the metabolism of carbohydrates.

Diabetes mellitus   A disease in which the pancreas fails to produce enough insulin or the body fails to use insulin effectively.

Hyperglycemia   Elevated blood sugar levels.

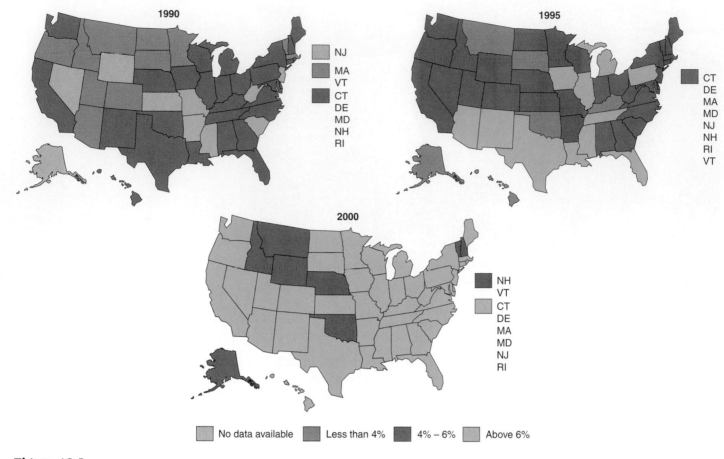

Figure 18.2

Percentage of Adults with Diagnosed Diabetes *
*Includes women with a history of gestational diabetes.

Source: Centers for Disease Control and Prevention. "Diabetes at a Glance" (data source: CDC, Behavioral Risk Factor Surveillance System, 2002). (see www.cdc.gov/diabetes/pubs/glance.htm).

improve health. If people with type 2 diabetes make lifestyle changes, they may be able to avoid oral medications or insulin indefinitely. A third type of diabetes, called *gestational diabetes,* can develop in a woman during pregnancy and affects 2–5 percent of all pregnant women. The condition usually disappears after childbirth, but it does leave the woman at greater risk of developing type 2 diabetes at some point. Other, even less common, forms of diabetes can result from genetic syndromes, surgery, drugs, malnutrition, infections, and other illnesses.[23]

Understanding Risk Factors   Diabetes tends to run in families. Being overweight, coupled with inactivity, dramatically increases the risk of type 2 diabetes. Older persons and mothers of babies weighing over 9 pounds also run an increased risk. Approximately 80 percent of all type 2 patients are overweight at the time of diagnosis. Weight loss, better nutrition, control of blood glucose levels, and exercise are important factors in lowering blood sugar and improving the efficiency of cellular use of insulin. Making these improvements can help to prevent overwork of the pancreas and the development of diabetes. In fact, recent findings

show that modest, consistent physical activity and a healthy diet can cut a person's risk of developing type 2 diabetes by nearly 60 percent.[24] African Americans, Hispanics, and Native Americans have the highest rates of type 2 diabetes in the world—much higher than that of Caucasians. The reasons for this increased risk are not clear.[25] See Figure 18.4 for a comparison of rates.

People who develop diabetes today have a much better prognosis than just 20 years ago. Recognize your own risk for this disease and take steps to reduce it. The Assess Yourself box on page 527 will help you determine if you are at risk for diabetes.

Controlling Diabetes   Most physicians attempt to control type 1 diabetes and later stages of type 2 with a variety of insulin-related drugs. Most of these drugs are taken orally, although self-administered hypodermic injections are prescribed when other treatments are inadequate. Recent breakthroughs in individual monitoring and the implanting of insulin monitors and insulin infusion pumps that regulate insulin intake "on demand" have provided many people with diabetes the opportunity to lead normal lives.

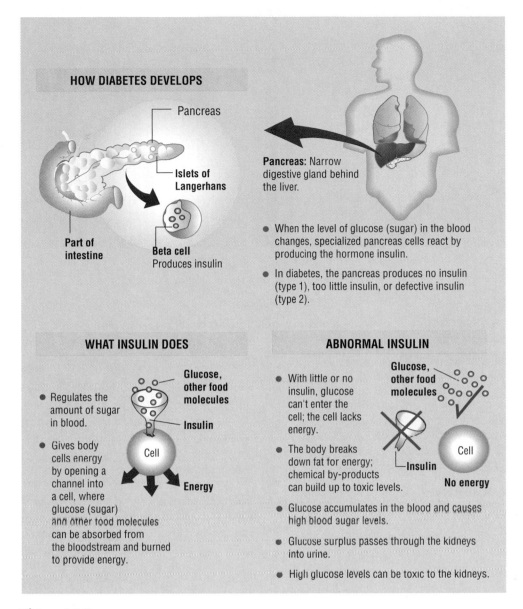

HOW DIABETES DEVELOPS

Pancreas

Islets of Langerhans

Part of intestine

Beta cell
Produces insulin

Pancreas: Narrow digestive gland behind the liver.

- When the level of glucose (sugar) in the blood changes, specialized pancreas cells react by producing the hormone insulin.

- In diabetes, the pancreas produces no insulin (type 1), too little insulin, or defective insulin (type 2).

WHAT INSULIN DOES

Glucose, other food molecules

Insulin

Cell

Energy

- Regulates the amount of sugar in blood.

- Gives body cells energy by opening a channel into a cell, where glucose (sugar) and other food molecules can be absorbed from the bloodstream and burned to provide energy.

ABNORMAL INSULIN

Glucose, other food molecules

Insulin

Cell

No energy

- With little or no insulin, glucose can't enter the cell; the cell lacks energy.

- The body breaks down fat for energy; chemical by-products can build up to toxic levels.

- Glucose accumulates in the blood and causes high blood sugar levels.

- Glucose surplus passes through the kidneys into urine.

- High glucose levels can be toxic to the kidneys.

Figure 18.3

Diabetes: Abnormal Sugar Metabolism

Sources: Adaptation based on *Oregonian,* September 5, 2000, A6; FDA *Consumer* magazine; *The Healing Handbook for Persons with Diabetes; The Bantam Medical Dictionary; Family Medical Guide;* research by Jutta Scheibe.

Newer forms of insulin that last longer in the body and have fewer side effects are now available. As we go to press, an insulin inhaler is being tested for possible widespread use. All of these treatments come at a price. On average, health care costs for diabetics are $10,000 to $20,000 higher per year than for healthy patients. The direct and indirect costs of treating diabetes in the United States total $100 billion per year.[26] However, the full burden of diabetes is hard to measure: Death records often do not reflect the role of diabetes in a person's death, and the costs related to undiagnosed diabetes are unknown.

Some people find that they can manage their diabetes more effectively by eating foods that are rich in complex carbohydrates, low in sodium, and high in fiber; by losing weight; and by getting regular exercise. Developing a routine for monitoring and controlling this disease can be stressful, particularly in the beginning. Some reports even suggest that diabetics may be at a greater-than-average risk for clinical depression.[27] Attention to psychosocial needs is often an important aspect of diabetic health.

Preventing Complications Depending on the type of diabetes diagnosed and the severity of the disease, diabetes affects people's lives by forcing them to use insulin, to modify their diets, and to make other lifestyle changes. In addition to these effects, diabetes can cause many complications and increase the severity of other existing conditions. If diabetes rates can be reduced, the real impact may be seen in

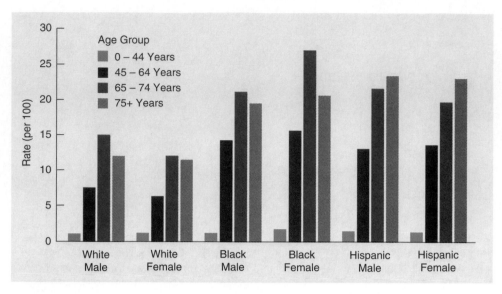

Figure 18.4

Age-Specific Prevalence of Diagnosed Diabetes, by Race/Ethnicity and Sex, 1999

Source: Centers for Disease Control and Prevention. "Diabetes Surveillance System," 2002 (see www.cdc.gov/diabetes/statistics/prev/national/fig51999.htm).

reductions in diabetes complications and prevention of diabetes-related diseases. Consider the following problems that diabetes causes or contributes to and actions that may help reduce their burden:[28]

- *Eye disease and blindness.* Each year, 12,000–24,000 people become blind because of diabetic eye disease. In fact, it is the leading cause of new blindness in America today. Screenings and care could prevent up to 90 percent of diabetes-related blindness but only 60 percent of people with diabetes receive annual dilated eye exams.
- *Kidney disease.* About 38,000 people with diabetes develop kidney failure each year and over 100,000 are in treatment for this condition. Better control of blood pressure and blood glucose levels could reduce diabetes-related kidney failure by about 50 percent.
- *Amputations.* About 82,000 people have diabetes-related leg and foot amputations each year. Foot care programs that include regular examinations and patient education could prevent up to 85 percent of these amputations.

Lactose intolerance The inability to produce lactase, an enzyme needed to convert milk sugar into glucose.

Ulcerative colitis An inflammatory disorder that affects the mucous membranes of the large intestine, producing bloody diarrhea.

Irritable bowel syndrome (IBS) Nausea, pain, gas, or diarrhea caused by certain foods or stress.

Diverticulosis A condition in which bulges form in the walls of the intestine; results in irritation and infection of the intestine.

- *Cardiovascular disease.* Heart disease and stroke cause about 65 percent of deaths among people with diabetes. These deaths could be reduced by 30 percent with improved care to control blood pressure and blood glucose and lipid levels.
- *Pregnancy complications.* About 18,000 women with pre-existing diabetes deliver babies each year, and an estimated 135,000 expectant mothers are diagnosed with gestational diabetes. These women and their babies have an increased risk for serious complications. Screenings and diabetes care before and after pregnancy can reduce the risk for complications such as stillbirths, congenital malformations, and the need for cesarean sections.
- *Flu- and pneumonia-related deaths.* Each year, 10,000–30,000 people with diabetes die of complications from flu or pneumonia. They are roughly three times more likely to die of these complications than people without diabetes, yet only 55 percent of people with diabetes get an annual flu shot.

Lactose Intolerance

As many as 50 million Americans are unable to eat dairy products such as milk, cheese, or ice cream. They suffer from **lactose intolerance**, meaning that they have lost the ability to produce the digestive enzyme lactase, which is necessary for the body to convert milk sugar (lactose) into glucose. That cold glass of milk becomes a source of stomach cramping, diarrhea, nausea, gas, and related symptoms. (See Chapter 8 for a discussion of other things we eat that may cause intolerances.) Lactose intolerance, however, need not be a death knell for future dairy product consumption. Once diagnosed, lactose intolerance can be treated by introducing low-lactose or lactose-free foods into the diet. Through trial and error, individuals usually find that they can tolerate one type of low-lactose food better than others. As an alternative

Are You at Risk for Diabetes?

Certain characteristics place people at greater risk for diabetes. Nevertheless, many people remain unaware of the symptoms of diabetes until after the disease has begun to progress. If you answer yes to three or more of the following questions, you should consider seeking medical advice. Talk to health professionals at your student health center, or make an appointment with your family physician.

1. Do you have a history of diabetes in your family?
2. Do any of your primary relatives (mother, father, sister, brother, grandparents) have diabetes?
3. Are you overweight or obese?
4. Are you typically sedentary (seldom, if ever, engage in vigorous aerobic exercise)?
5. Have you noticed an increase in your craving for water or other beverages?
6. Have you noticed that you have to urinate more frequently than you used to during a typical day?
7. Have you noticed any tingling or numbness in your hands and feet, which might indicate circulatory problems?
8. Do you often feel a gnawing hunger during the day, even though you usually eat regular meals?
9. Have you noticed that you are losing weight but don't seem to be doing anything in particular to make this happen?
10. Are you often so tired that you find it difficult to stay awake to study, watch television, or engage in other activities?
11. Have you noticed that you have skin irritations more frequently and that minor infections don't heal as quickly as they used to?
12. Have you noticed any unusual changes in your vision (blurring, difficulty in focusing, etc.)?
13. Have you noticed unusual pain or swelling in your joints?
14. If you are a woman, have you had several vaginal (yeast) infections during the past year?
15. Do you often feel weak or nauseated if you have to wait too long to eat a meal?

to learning to eat foods without lactose, some people purchase special products that supply the missing lactase and thus eat dairy foods without serious side effects. Most large grocery chains, food cooperatives, and drug stores have these products available in liquid or tablet form. It should be noted, however, that these products do not work for everyone and many people who think they are lactose intolerant actually are not. If you suspect that you are lactose intolerant, diagnostic tests can provide conclusive evidence.

Colitis and Irritable Bowel Syndrome (IBS)

Ulcerative colitis is a disease of the large intestine in which the mucous membranes of the intestinal walls become inflamed. Victims with severe cases may have as many as 20 bouts of bloody diarrhea a day. Colitis can also produce severe stomach cramps, weight loss, nausea, sweating, and fever. Although some experts believe that colitis occurs more frequently in people with high stress levels, this theory is controversial. Hypersensitivity reactions, particularly to milk and certain foods, have also been considered as a possible cause. It is difficult to determine the cause of colitis because the disease goes into unexplained remission and then recurs without apparent reason. This pattern often continues over periods of years and may be related to the later development of colorectal cancer. Because the cause of colitis remains unknown, treatment focuses exclusively on relieving the symptoms. Increasing fiber intake and taking anti-inflammatory drugs, steroids, and other medications

to reduce inflammation and soothe irritated intestinal walls can relieve symptoms.

Many people develop a condition related to colitis known as **irritable bowel syndrome (IBS)**, in which nausea, pain, gas, diarrhea attacks, or cramps occur after eating certain foods or when a person is under unusual stress. IBS symptoms commonly begin in early adulthood. Symptoms may vary from week to week and can fade for long periods of time, only to return.

The cause of IBS is unknown, but researchers suspect that people with IBS have digestive systems that are overly sensitive to what they eat and drink, to stress, and to certain hormonal changes. They may also be more sensitive to pain signals from the stomach. Stress management, relaxation techniques, regular activity, and diet can control IBS in the vast majority of cases. Problems with diarrhea can be reduced by cutting down on fat and avoiding caffeine and excessive amounts of sorbitol, a sweetener found in dietetic foods and chewing gum. Many IBS patients are lactose intolerant. Constipation can be relieved by a gradual increase in fiber. Some sufferers benefit from anticholinergic drugs, which relax the intestinal muscle, or from antidepressant drugs and psychological counseling. Medical advice should be sought whenever such conditions persist.

Diverticulosis

Diverticulosis occurs when the walls of the intestine become weakened for undetermined reasons and small pea-sized bulges develop. These bulges often fill with feces and, over

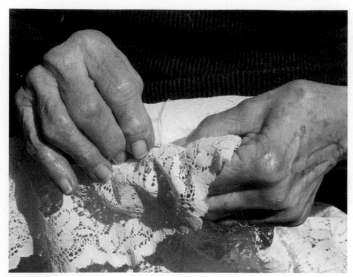

Arthritis can make simple tasks both painful and difficult to accomplish.

time, become irritated and infected, causing pain and discomfort. If this irritation persists, bleeding and chronic obstruction may occur, either of which can be life threatening.

Although diverticulosis may appear in any part of the intestinal wall, it most commonly occurs in the small intestine. Often the person affected may be unaware that the problem exists. However, in some cases, a person may actually have an attack similar to the pain of appendicitis except that the pain is on the left side of the body instead of the right, where the appendix is located. Although diverticulosis most frequently occurs during and after middle age, it can appear at any age. If you have persistent pain in the lower abdominal region, seek medical attention at once.

Peptic Ulcers

An ulcer is a lesion or wound that forms in body tissue as a result of some form of irritant. A **peptic ulcer** is a chronic ulcer that occurs in the lining of the stomach or the section of the small intestine known as the *duodenum*. It has been thought to be caused by the erosive effect of digestive juices on these tissues. The lining of these organs becomes irritated, the protective covering of mucous is reduced, and the gastric acid begins to digest the dying tissue, just as it would a piece of food. Typically, this irritation causes pain that disappears when the person eats, but returns about an hour later.

In 1994, after years of assuming that ulcers were caused by eating spicy foods, the National Institutes of Health (NIH) shocked the medical community by announcing that a common bacterium, *Helicobacter pylori,* appears to cause most ulcers. This means that antibiotics can effectively treat this disorder, which affects over 4 million Americans every year. This represents a dramatic departure from the traditional regimen of acid-reducing drugs and significantly reduces the risk of recurrence. People with ulcers should avoid high-fat foods, alcohol, and substances such as aspirin that may irritate organ linings or cause increased secretion of stomach acids and thereby exacerbate this condition. In extreme cases, surgery is necessary to relieve persistent symptoms.

Gallbladder Disease

Also known as *cholecystitis,* gallbladder disease occurs when the gallbladder has been repeatedly irritated by chemicals, infection, or overuse, thus reducing its ability to release bile used for the digestion of fats. Usually, gallstones, consisting of calcium, cholesterol, and other minerals, form in the gallbladder itself. When the patient eats foods that are high in fats, the gallbladder contracts to release bile and presses on the gallstones. One of the characteristic symptoms of gallbladder disease is acute pain in the upper right portion of the abdomen after eating fatty foods. This pain, which can last for several hours, may feel like a heart attack or an ulcer and is often accompanied by nausea.

Who gets gallbladder disease? The old adage about the "five f's" of risk factors frequently holds true. Anyone who is "female, fat, fair, forty, and flatulent" (prone to passing gas) appears to be at increased risk. However, people who don't fit this picture also get the disease.

Current treatment of gallbladder disease usually involves medication to reduce irritation, restriction of fat consumption, and surgery to remove the gallstones. New medications designed to dissolve small gallstones are currently being used in some patients. In addition, some doctors are using a new technique known as lithotripsy, in which a series of noninvasive shock waves breaks up small stones. Experiments are being done with lasers and various forms of laparoscopy to eliminate the risks associated with large surgical incisions.

> **What do you think?**
>
> *What role can a healthy diet play in reducing risks for and symptoms of the diseases discussed here?* ✳ *Are you or any of your family members at risk for these problems?* ✳ *What actions can you take today that will cut your risk?*

Musculoskeletal Diseases

Most of us will encounter chronic musculoskeletal disease during our lifetime. Some form of arthritis will afflict half of those over 65; low back pain hits 80 percent of us at some point. Arthritis and musculoskeletal diseases are the most common causes of physical disability in the United States.[29]

Arthritis: Many Types, Many Problems

Called "the nation's primary crippler," **arthritis** strikes one in seven Americans, or over 38 million people. Symptoms range from the occasional tendinitis of the weekend athlete to the horrific pain of rheumatoid arthritis. There are over 100 types of arthritis diagnosed today, accounting for over 30 million lost workdays annually. The cost to the U.S. economy is over $65 billion per year in lost wages and productivity and untold amounts in hospital and nursing home services, prescriptions, and over-the-counter pain relief.[30]

Osteoarthritis (OA), also known as degenerative joint disease, is a progressive deterioration of bones and joints that has been associated with the "wear and tear" theory of aging. More recent research indicates that as joints are used, they release enzymes that digest cartilage, while other cells in the cartilage try to repair the damage. When the enzymatic breakdown overpowers cellular repair, the cartilage is destroyed, causing bones to rub against each other. The pain, swelling, and lack of movement characteristic of arthritis is the result. Weather extremes, excessive strain, and injury often lead to osteoarthritis flare-ups. But a specific precipitating event does not seem to be necessary. Obesity, joint trauma, and repetitive joint usage all contribute to increased risk and thus are important targets for prevention.

Although age and injury are undoubtedly factors in osteoarthritis, heredity, abnormal use of the joint, diet, abnormalities in joint structure, and impaired blood supply to the joint may also contribute. Osteoarthritis of the hands seems to have a particularly strong genetic component. Over 80 percent of those with OA report an activity limitation; OA of the knee can be as disabling as any cardiovascular disease short of stroke.[31] When joints become so distorted that they impair activity, surgical intervention is often necessary. Joint replacement and bone fusion are common surgical repair techniques. For most people, anti-inflammatory drugs and pain relievers such as aspirin and cortisone-related agents ease discomfort. In some sufferers, applications of heat, mild exercise, and massage may also relieve the pain. Today 20.7 million Americans have osteoarthritis, the majority of them women.[32]

Rheumatoid arthritis is an autoimmune disease involving chronic inflammation that can appear at any age, but it most commonly appears between ages 20 and 45 and affects over 2.1 million Americans. It is three times more common among women than among men during early adulthood but equally common among men and women in the over-70 age group. Symptoms include stiffness, pain, redness, and swelling of multiple joints, often including the hands and wrists, and can be gradually progressive or sporadic, with occasional unexplained remissions. Other symptoms include loss of appetite, fever, loss of energy, anemia, and generalized aches.[33]

Rheumatoid arthritis typically attacks the synovial membrane, which produces the lubricating fluids for the joints. Advanced rheumatoid arthritis often involves destruction of the bony ends of joints. The remedy for this condition is typically bone fusion, which leaves the joint immobile. In some instances, joint replacement may be a viable alternative.

Although the exact cause of rheumatoid arthritis is unknown, some theorists believe it is caused by some form of invading microorganism that takes over the joint. Certain toxic chemicals and stress have also been mentioned as possible causes. Genetic predisposition is a strong predictor of risk, and a genetic marker called HLA-DR4 has been identified.[34]

Regardless of the cause, treatment of rheumatoid arthritis is similar to that for osteoarthritis. Emphasis is placed on pain relief and attempts to improve the functional mobility of the patient. In some instances, immunosuppressant drugs are given to reduce the inflammatory response.

Fibromyalgia

Fibromyalgia is a chronic, painful, rheumatoid-like disorder that affects 5 to 6 percent of the general population with bouts of muscle pain and extreme fatigue. Persons with fibromyalgia experience an array of other symptoms including headaches, dizziness, numbness and tingling, itching, fluid retention, chronic joint pain, abdominal or pelvic pain, and even occasional diarrhea. Suspected causes have ranged from sleep disturbances, stress, emotional distress, and viruses to autoimmune disorders; however, none has been proved in clinical trials. Because of fibromyalgia's multiple symptoms, it is usually diagnosed only after myriad tests have ruled out other disorders. The American College of Rheumatology identifies the major diagnostic criteria as the following:[35]

- History of widespread pain of at least three months' duration in the axial skeleton as well as in all four quadrants of the body.
- Pain in at least 11 of 18 paired tender points on digital palpation of about 4 kilograms of pressure.

The disease primarily affects women in their 30s and 40s, and it can be extremely debilitating due to the unrelieved pain, feelings of bloating or swelling, and fatigue that victims may suffer. Many people with fibromyalgia also become depressed and report chronic fatigue–like symptoms.

Treatment for fibromyalgia varies based on the severity of symptoms. Typically, adequate rest, stress management, relaxation techniques, dietary supplements and selected herbal remedies, and pain medications are prescribed. Patients are advised to avoid extreme temperatures, which can exacerbate symptoms.

Peptic ulcer   Damage to the stomach or intestinal lining, usually caused by digestive juices.

Arthritis   Painful inflammatory disease of the joints.

Osteoarthritis   A progressive deterioration of bones and joints that has been associated with the "wear and tear" theory of aging.

Rheumatoid arthritis   A serious inflammatory joint disease.

Fibromyalgia   A chronic, rheumatoid-like disorder that can be highly painful and difficult to diagnose.

Systemic Lupus Erythematosus (SLE)

Lupus is a disease in which the immune system attacks the body, producing antibodies that destroy or injure organs such as the kidneys, brain, and heart. The symptoms include sensitivity to sunlight, arthritis, kidney problems, anemia, and multiple infections; they vary from mild to severe and may disappear for periods of time. A butterfly-shaped rash covering the bridge of the nose and both cheeks is common. Nearly all SLE sufferers have aching joints and muscles, and 60 percent of them develop redness and swelling that move from joint to joint. The disease affects 1 in 700 Caucasians but 1 in 250 African Americans; 90 percent of all victims are females between the ages of 18 and 45. Extensive research has not yet found a cure for this sometimes fatal disease, although new studies suggest that there may be a genetic predisposition to it.

Scleroderma

Scleroderma (hardening of the skin) is a disease characterized by an increasing fibrous growth of connective tissue underlying the skin and body organs. These areas may form hard skin patches or a more generalized "ever-tightening case of steel," making movement difficult. Some cases of scleroderma are related to certain occupations, such as working with vibrating machines and exposure to chemicals in plastics or in mining. Others have an abrupt, unknown etiology. Scleroderma may cause swelling of the hands, face, or feet. Symptoms range from minor discomfort to severe pain. In some instances, scleroderma is life-threatening.

Raynaud's Syndrome

For most of us, a few minutes in the cold causes only minor discomfort. For people suffering from **Raynaud's syndrome**, fingers and toes go numb, then turn white, then deep purple; as fingers and toes warm, they throb. Raynaud's is caused by exaggerated constriction of small arteries in the extremities that shunts blood away from them and toward the vital organs. Why this disease occurs in people whose lives are not threatened by the cold (in which case vasoconstriction serves a vital function by sending blood to the body core) is unknown. It is believed that Raynaud's affects 5 to 10 per-

cent of the population, with women accounting for the majority of sufferers. In women, onset is usually between the ages of 15 and 40; men tend to develop Raynaud's later in life. Treatment for Raynaud's consists of trying to control body temperature by wearing warm gloves and boots, avoiding drugs that may alter blood flow (e.g., nicotine), taking drugs to regulate blood flow, and surgery to improve circulation or repair damaged areas.

Low Back Pain

Approximately 80 percent of all Americans will experience low back pain at some point. Some of these low back pain (LBP) episodes result from muscular damage and are short-lived and acute; others may involve dislocations, fractures, or other problems with spinal vertebrae or discs, resulting in chronic pain or requiring surgery. Low back pain is epidemic throughout the world. It is the major cause of disability for people age 20 to 45 in the United States, who suffer more frequently and severely from this problem than older people do.[36]

LBP causes more lost work time in the United States than any other illness except upper respiratory infections. In fact, costs associated with back injury exceed those associated with all other industrial injuries combined. Back injuries are the most frequently mentioned complaints in injury-related lawsuits and result in high medical and rehabilitation bills, costing businesses and industries in the United States over $50 billion annually in direct and indirect costs.[37] As a result, employers throughout the country have become increasingly interested in preventing these injuries. Note that these figures do not include the costs of human suffering, damaged self-worth, and other emotional problems that occur when a person becomes disabled. For more on funding allocations, see the Health Ethics box.

Risk Factors for Low Back Pain   Health experts believe that the following factors contribute to LBP:

- *Age.* People between the ages of 20 and 45 run the greatest risk of LBP. At age 50, the condition becomes less common. After age 65, the incidence again rises, apparently because of bone and joint deterioration.
- *Body type.* Many studies have indicated that people who are very tall, are overweight, or have lanky body types run an increased risk of LBP. However, much of this research is controversial.
- *Posture.* Poor posture may be one of the greatest contributors to LBP. If you routinely slouch, particularly during daily tasks, you run an increased risk.
- *Strength and fitness.* People with LBP tend to have less overall trunk strength than do other people. Weak abdominal muscles and weak back muscles also increase risk. In addition, total level of fitness and conditioning is a factor. The more fit you are, the lower your risk.
- *Psychological factors.* Numerous psychological factors appear to increase risk for LBP. Depression, apathy,

---

Lupus   A disease in which the immune system attacks the body, producing antibodies that destroy or injure organs such as the kidneys, brain, and heart.

Scleroderma   A disease in which fibrous growth of connective tissue underlying the skin and body organs hardens and makes movement difficult.

Raynaud's syndrome   A disease in which exposure to cold temperatures produces exaggerated constriction of the small arteries in the extremities, causing fingers and toes to go numb, turn white, and then turn deep purple.

Funding Allocations: What's Fair?

It seems logical that we should allocate research dollars to health problems based on the number of people affected and the risk for death and disability associated with a particular disease. However, that is not necessarily how money is distributed. Disability rankings are based on complex formulas and calculations in which numbers of persons affected, age, degree of functional capacity lost, and death are factored together to assess the level of disability that a condition represents in a population. For example, if many people die or are disabled at a very young age from a particular condition, it would be ranked as more severe than if it killed only the elderly (e.g., due to accounting for years of potential life lost).

Consider the expenditures and disability rankings for the conditions shown in the table. Although heart disease exacts the greatest human toll, its funding for research, prevention, and intervention is only a small percentage of funding alloca-tions for diseases such as AIDS, breast cancer, and diabetes.

For which other diseases do large discrepancies exist between societal impact and level of federal funding for battling the disease? Do the statistics for any disease surprise you? Why? What factors might influence the amount of funding allocated for fighting a given disease or disability? What factors should influence funding priorities? Does the concept of providing major research funding mainly for conditions that afflict numerous individuals disadvantage any groups of people? Explain your answer.

Disease Areas	NIH Funding in 2003: Millions of Dollars for Research (Estimates)	Disability Ranking
AIDS	2,770	15
Breast cancer	732	14
Diabetes	845	8
Heart disease	2,065	1
Schizophrenia	338	10
Stroke	283	4
Prostate cancer	408	19
Lung cancer	297	6
Asthma	256	17
Parkinson's	215	21
Multiple sclerosis	84	25

Source: National Institutes of Health. Research Initiatives/Programs of Interest. http://www4.od.nih.gov/officeofbudget/FundingResearchAreas.htm

inattentiveness, boredom, emotional upsets, drug abuse, and family and financial problems all heighten risk.
• *Occupational risks.* Evidence indicates that employees who are new to a particular job run the greatest risk of LBP problems. In addition, type of work and work conditions greatly affect risk. For example, truck drivers, who must endure the bumps and jolts of the road while in a sitting position, frequently suffer from back pain.

Preventing Back Pain and Injury What can you do to protect yourself from possible back injury? First, you need to know what area of the spinal column is most at risk and then protect that area as much as possible. Almost 90 percent of all back problems occur in the lumbar spine region (lower back). You can avoid many problems by consciously attempting to maintain good posture. Other preventive hints include the following:

• Purchase a supportive mattress, and avoid sleeping on your stomach.

• Avoid high-heeled shoes, which tilt the pelvis forward.
• Control your weight.
• Lift objects with your legs, not your back.
• Buy a good chair for doing your work, preferably one with lumbar support.
• Move your car seat forward so that your knees are elevated slightly.
• Warm up before exercising.
• Exercise—in particular do exercises that strengthen the abdominal muscles and stretch the back muscles.

Other Maladies

During the past 20 years, several afflictions have surfaced that seem to be products of our times. Some of these health problems relate to specific groups of people, some are due to technological advances, and others have not been explained (see Table 18.1).

Table 18.1
Other Modern Afflictions

DISEASE	DESCRIPTION	TREATMENT
Cystic fibrosis	Inherited disease occuring in 1 out of every 1,600 births. Characterized by pooling of large amounts of mucous in lungs, digestive disturbances, and excessive sodium excretion. Results in premature death.	Most treatments are geared toward relief of symptoms. Antibiotics are administered for infection. Recent strides in genetic research suggest better treatments and potential cure in the near future.
Sickle-cell anemia	Inherited disease affecting 8–10 percent of all African Americans, Disease affects hemoglobin, forming sickle-shaped red blood cells that interfere with oxygenation. Results in severe pain, anemia, and premature death.	Reduce stress, and attend to minor infections immediately. Seek genetic counseling.
Cerebral palsy	Disorder characterized by the loss of voluntary control over motor functioning. Believed to be caused by a lack of oxygen to the brain at birth, brain disorders, or an accident before or after birth, poisoning, or brain infections.	Follow preventive actions to reduce accident risks; improved neonatal and birthing techniques show promise.
Graves' disease	A thyroid disorder characterized by swelling of the eyes, staring gaze, and retraction of the eyelid. Can result in loss of sight. The cause is unknown and it can occur at any age.	Medication may help control symptoms. Radioactive iodine supplements also may be administered.

Chronic Fatigue Syndrome (CFS)

Fatigue is a subjective condition in which people feel tired before they begin activities, lack the energy to accomplish tasks that require sustained effort and attention, or become abnormally exhausted after normal activities. All of us experience fatigue occasionally. In the late 1980s, several U.S. clinics noted a characteristic set of symptoms including chronic fatigue, headaches, fever, sore throat, enlarged lymph nodes, depression, poor memory, general weakness, nausea, and symptoms remarkably similar to those of mononucleosis. Researchers initially believed these symptoms were caused by the same virus as mononucleosis, the Epstein-Barr virus. At first the disease was called *chronic Epstein-Barr disease,* or the "yuppie flu," because the pattern of symptoms appeared most commonly in baby boomers in their early 30s. Some cases were so severe that patients required hospitalization. Since those initial studies, however, researchers have all but ruled out the Epstein-Barr virus. Despite extensive testing, no viral cause has been found to date.[38]

Today, in the absence of a known pathogen, many researchers believe that the illness, now commonly referred to as chronic fatigue syndrome (CFS), may have strong psychosocial roots. Our heightened awareness of health makes some of us scrutinize our bodies so carefully that the slightest deviation becomes amplified. The more we focus on the body and on our perception of health, the worse we feel. In addition, the growing number of people who suffer from depression seem to be good candidates for chronic fatigue syndrome. Experts worry, however, that too many people approach CFS as something that is "in the person's head" and that such an attitude may prevent scientists from doing the serious research needed to find a cure.

The diagnosis of chronic fatigue syndrome depends on two major criteria and eight or more minor criteria. The major criteria are debilitating fatigue that persists for at least six months and the absence of other illnesses that could cause the symptoms. Minor criteria include headaches, fever, sore throat, painful lymph nodes, weakness, fatigue after exercise, sleep problems, and rapid onset of these symptoms. Because the cause is not apparent, treatment of CFS focuses on improved nutrition, rest, counseling for depression, judicious exercise, and development of a strong support network.

Repetitive Stress Injuries (RSIs)

It's the end of the term and you have dutifully typed the last of several papers. After hours of nonstop typing, you find that your hands are numb, and you feel an intense, burning pain that makes the thought of typing one more word almost

Repetitive stress injury (RSI) An injury to nerves, soft tissue, or joints due to the physical stress of repeated motions.

Carpal tunnel syndrome A common occupational injury in which the median nerve in the wrist becomes irritated, causing numbness, tingling, and pain in the fingers and hands.

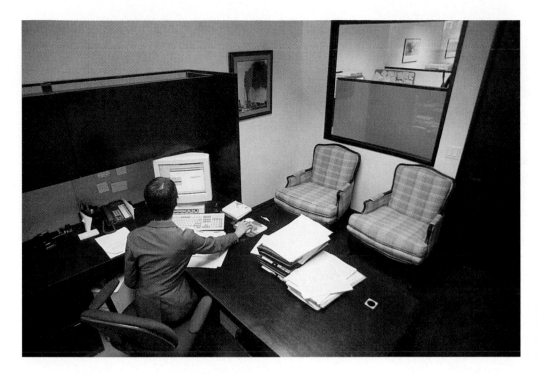

Poorly designed workspaces, long hours at a computer, and repetitive procedures are all potential causes of repetitive stress injuries.

unbearable. If you are like one of the thousands of students and workers who every year must quit a particular task due to pain, you may be suffering from a **repetitive stress injury (RSI)**. These are injuries to nerves, soft tissue, or joints that result from the physical stress of repeated motions.

While no good mechanism of reporting exists for students suffering from RSIs, the Bureau of Labor Statistics estimates that 25 percent of all injuries in the labor force that result in lost work time are due to repetitive motion or stress injuries. These injuries cost employers over $22 billion a year in workers' compensation and an additional $85 billion in related costs, such as absenteeism.

One of the most common RSIs is **carpal tunnel syndrome**, a product of both the information age and the age of technology in general. Hours spent typing at the computer, flipping groceries through computerized scanners, or other jobs "made simpler" by technology can irritate the median nerve in the wrist, causing numbness, tingling, and pain in the fingers and hands. Although carpal tunnel syndrome risk can be reduced by proper placement of the keyboard, mouse, wrist pads, and other techniques, RSIs are often overlooked until significant damage has been done. Better education and ergonomic workplace designs can eliminate many injuries of this nature.

Taking Charge

18 **18** **18**

Managing Chronic Ailments

Clearly, we have a long way to go before we are able to make a significant impact on some modern maladies. Many, however, can be prevented or their onset delayed, thereby improving quality of life and extending the life span. Personal health habits appear to be major contributing factors to the

rising incidence of chronic diseases. As with all diseases, we must work to reduce risks and avoid hazards that put individuals or groups at risk. An educated public, policies that protect the average citizen, and support for research that will provide answers to complex questions are key to reducing the impact of these disorders. What can you do now to reduce your risk of developing a chronic disease?

Checklist for Change

Making Personal Choices

☐ How much individual responsibility should we each accept for chronic diseases we could have prevented?

☐ Do you have any lifestyle or personal health habits that could cause a chronic disease? Do you smoke? Are you sedentary? Do you have poor eating habits? Are you overweight?

☐ If you have any of these habits, have you tried to change your habits? If so, what approaches have worked best? What approaches have not worked at all?

☐ What actions can you take today to reduce your own risks for the diseases and disorders discussed in this chapter? Which concern you most?

Making Community Choices

☐ If you worked for a government agency charged with helping people improve their personal health habits, what approaches would you take?

☐ Do you think the strategy of raising the cost of cigarettes is discouraging their use? With what other "habits" might this work?

☐ What role should businesses play in improving employee health? Should businesses be held liable for situations in which employees get carpal tunnel syndrome or experience low back problems?

Summary

✳ Chronic lung diseases include allergies, hay fever, asthma, emphysema, and chronic bronchitis. Allergies are part of the body's natural defense system. Chronic obstructive pulmonary diseases are the fifth leading cause of death in the United States.

✳ Neurological conditions include headaches and seizure disorders. Headaches may be caused by a variety of factors, the most common of which are tension, dilation and/or contraction of blood vessels in the brain, chemical influences on muscles and vessels that cause inflammation and pain, and underlying physiological and psychological disorders.

✳ Several modern maladies affect only women. Fibrocystic breast condition is a common, noncancerous buildup of irregular tissue. Endometriosis is the buildup of endometrial tissue in regions of the body other than the uterus.

✳ Diabetes occurs when the pancreas fails to produce enough insulin to regulate sugar metabolism. Other conditions, such as colitis, irritable bowel syndrome, gallbladder disease, and ulcers, are the direct result of functional problems in various digestion-related organs or systems. Pathogens, problems in enzyme or hormone production, anxiety or stress, functional abnormalities, and other problems are possible causes.

✳ Musculoskeletal diseases such as arthritis, lower back pain, repetitive stress injuries, and other problems cause significant pain and disability in millions of people. Age, occupation, gender, posture, abdominal strength, and psychological factors contribute to the development of lower back problems.

✳ Chronic fatigue syndrome (CFS) and repetitive stress injuries (such as carpal tunnel syndrome) have emerged as major chronic maladies. CFS is associated with depression. Repetitive stress injuries are preventable by proper equipment placement and usage.

Questions for Discussion and Reflection

1. What are some of the major noninfectious chronic diseases affecting Americans today? Do you think there is a pattern in the types of diseases that we get? What are the common risk factors?

2. List the common respiratory diseases affecting Americans. Which of these diseases has a genetic basis? An environmental basis? An individual basis? What, if anything, is being done to prevent, treat, or control each of these conditions?

3. Compare and contrast the different types of headaches, including their symptoms and treatments.

4. What are the medical risks of fibrocystic breast condition and endometriosis? How can they be treated?

5. Describe the risk factors for diabetes and its symptoms and treatment. What is the difference between type 1 diabetes and type 2 diabetes?

6. Compare the symptoms of colitis, diverticulosis, peptic ulcers, and gallbladder disease. How can you tell whether your stomach is reacting to final exams or telling you that you have a serious medical condition?

7. What are the major disorders of the musculoskeletal system? Why do you think there aren't any cures? Describe the difference between osteoarthritis and rheumatoid arthritis.

8. Chronic fatigue syndrome (CFS) is often associated with depression. Experts argue about whether depression precedes CFS or CFS causes depression. What do you think?

Application Exercises

Reread the What Do You Think? scenarios at the beginning of the chapter and answer the following questions.

1. Why do you think people like Kate persist in behaviors such as smoking, even though they know they are clearly

at risk for serious chronic diseases? What actions would you take if you were Kate's friend?

2. Do you think that chronic fatigue syndrome is a real physical disease? Or is it the physical manifestation of a mental disorder? Explain your answer. How many people that you know have experienced crises similar to Jennifer's?

Why are some able to get through them relatively easily while others suffer for a long time?

3. Do you think Jennifer has CFS? If not, how would you describe her problem? Where would you suggest she go for help?

Accessing Your Health on the Internet

Visit the following Internet sites to explore further topics and issues related to personal health. To visit an organization's website, go to the Companion Website for *Access to Health, Eighth Edition,* at www.aw.com/donatelle, click on the book image, and select "Accessing Your Health on the Internet" from the navigation menu on the left.

1. *American Academy of Allergy, Asthma, and Immunology.* Provides an overview of asthma information, particularly as it applies to children with allergies. Offers interactive quizzes to test your knowledge as well as an "ask the expert" section.
2. *American Diabetes Association.* Excellent resource for diabetes information.
3. *American Lung Association.* Includes the latest in asthma news, including a free monthly newsletter, *The Breathe Easy/Asthma Digest.*

4. *ChronicIllnet.* A multimedia information source dedicated to chronic illnesses, including AIDS, cancer, Gulf War syndrome, autoimmune diseases, chronic fatigue syndrome, heart disease, and neurological diseases.
5. *National Center for Chronic Disease Prevention and Health Promotion (NCCDPHP).* Access to a wide range of information from this CDC-linked organization dedicated to chronic diseases and health promotion.
6. *National Institute of Neurological Disorders and Stroke.* Many of the modern maladies result in chronic pain. This site provides up-to-date information to help you cope with pain-related difficulties.

Further Reading

Brownson, R., P. Remington, and J. Davis. *Chronic Disease Epidemiology and Control,* 2nd ed. American Public Health Association, 1998.

An excellent book covering the epidemiology of major human illnesses. Provides historical, pathological, and epidemiological perspectives on illness and infirmity.

National Center for Health Statistics. *Monthly Vital Statistics Report* and *Advance Data from Vital and Health Statistics.* Hyattsville, MD: Public Health Service.

Detailed government reports, usually published monthly, concerning mortality and morbidity data for the United

States, including changes occurring in the rates of particular diseases and in health practices so patterns and trends can be analyzed.

Public Health Services, Centers for Disease Control. *Chronic Disease News and Notes.* Washington, DC: U.S. Department of Health and Human Services.

Quarterly publication focusing on relevant chronic disease topics and issues.

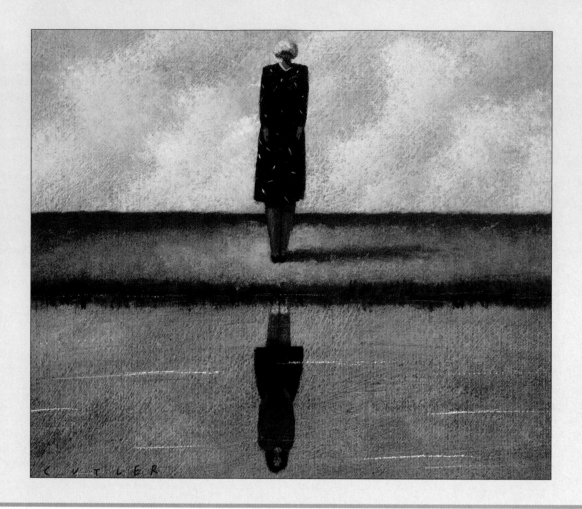

Objectives

* Review the definition of aging, and explain the related concepts of biological, psychological, social, legal, and functional age.

* Explain the impact on society of the growing population of older adults, including considerations of economics, health care, living arrangements, and ethical and moral issues.

* Discuss the biological and psychosocial theories of aging, and examine how knowledge of these theories may have an impact on your own aging process.

* Identify major physiological changes that occur as a result of the aging process.

* Discuss the unique health challenges faced by older adults, such as alcohol abuse, prescription medication and over-the-counter drug use, osteoporosis, urinary incontinence, depression, and Alzheimer's disease.

* Discuss strategies for healthy aging that can begin during young adulthood.

19

Healthy Aging

A Lifelong Process

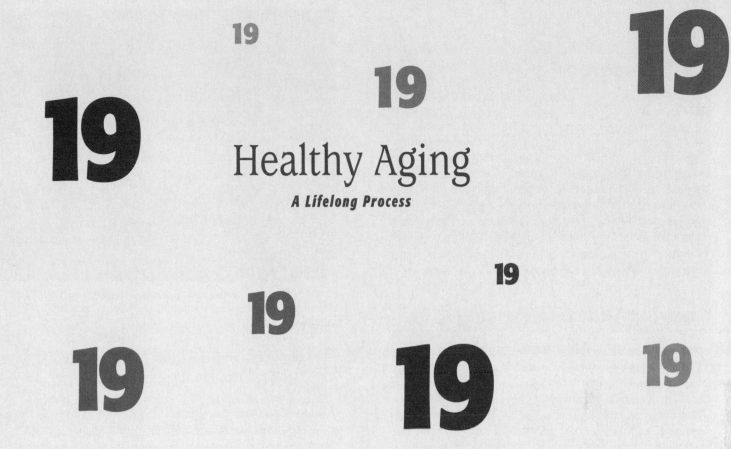

What do you think?

Juanita, age 55, has been smoking for nearly 25 years and has regular flare-ups of bronchitis and other respiratory problems. Fiercely independent, she has a large circle of friends. She also has several hobbies, such as gardening and traveling. Since her divorce seven years ago, she has not found time for a serious romantic relationship and is not worried about finding another person to make her "happy."

Susan, age 62, is a retired businesswoman who likes to play tennis. She has a large circle of friends but is not content to be alone. Although she is financially independent and in good health, she has few hobbies. Since her recent divorce, she is obsessed with finding another relationship. Her large family lives 2,000 miles away, and she has little interaction with them.

Rich, age 65, is a musician and an avid weight lifter. He spends hours every day working out to stay in shape. He has had two affairs with younger women, and although his wife has warned him that another affair will end their marriage, he is constantly looking for something to make him feel younger. He is dissatisfied with the choices he has made in life and wishes he could do things over.

John, age 68, is a college professor, overweight and out of shape, who has a hidden problem with alcohol. Divorced twice, he now lives alone in a small condominium. He has few friends, watches sports on TV for hours each day, and has long been estranged from his two sons. His work is his only source of satisfaction. He claims that people have been great disappointments in his life, and he can do without them.

Which of these people do you think is aging successfully? ☀ *What lifestyle choices has each person made that will help in coping effectively with aging?* ☀ *Which choices may cause significant risks and difficulties?*

Grow old along with me!

The best is yet to be,

The last of life, for which the first was made . . .

　　—Robert Browning, *Rabbi Ben Ezra*

In a society that seems to worship youth, researchers have finally begun to offer some good—even revolutionary—news about the aging process: Growing old doesn't have to mean a slow slide to disability, loneliness, and declining physical and mental health. Health promotion, disease prevention, and wellness-oriented activities can prolong vigor and productivity, even among those who haven't always led model lifestyles or made healthful habits a priority. In fact, getting older can mean getting better in many ways—particularly socially, psychologically, and intellectually.

Growing Old: Life Passages

Every moment of every day, we are involved in a steady aging process. Everything in the universe—animals, plants, mountain peaks, rivers, planets, even atoms—changes over time. This process is commonly referred to as *aging*. Aging is something that cannot be avoided, despite the perennial human quest for a fountain of youth. Since you can't stop the clock, why not resolve to have a positive aging experience by improving your understanding of this process, taking steps to maximize your potential, and developing strengths you can draw upon over a lifetime?

　　The manner in which you view aging (either as a natural part of living or an inevitable decline toward disease and death) is a crucial factor in how successfully you will adapt to life's transitions. If you view these transitions as periods of growth, as changes that will lead to improved mental, emotional, spiritual, and physical phases in your development as a human being, your journey through even the most difficult times will be easier. No doubt you have encountered vigorous 80-year-olds who wake up every morning looking forward to whatever challenges the day may bring. Such persons are socially active, have a zest for life, and seem much younger than their chronological age. In contrast, you have probably met 60-year-olds who lack energy and enthusiasm, who seem resigned to tread water for the rest of their lives. These people often appear much older than their chronologi-

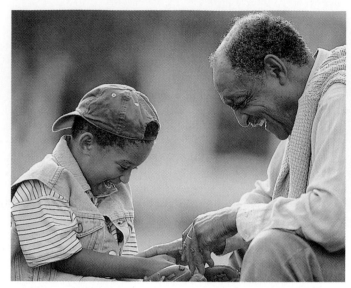

Learning to cope with challenges and changes early in life develops attitudes and skills that contribute to a full and satisfying old age.

cal age. In short, people experience the aging process in different ways. Explore your own notions about aging by reading the Assess Yourself box.

　　Aging has traditionally been described as the patterns of life changes that occur in members of all species as they grow older. Some believe that it begins at the moment of conception. Others contend that it starts at birth. Still others believe that true aging does not begin until we reach our 40s.

　　Typically, experts and laypersons alike have used chronological age to assign a person to a particular life-cycle stage. However, people of different chronological ages view age very differently. To the 4-year-old, a college freshman seems quite old. To the 20-year-old, parents in their 40s are over the hill. Have you ever heard your 65-year-old grandparents talking about "those old people down the street"? Views of aging are also colored by occupation. Most professional athletes are considering other careers by the time they reach 40. Airline pilots and police officers are often retired in their 50s, while actors, writers, musicians, and even college professors may work well into their 70s. Perhaps we need to reexamine our traditional definitions of aging.

Redefining Aging

Discrimination against people based on age is known as **ageism**. This type of discrimination carries with it social ostracism and negative portrayals of older people. A developmental task approach to life-span changes tends to reduce the potential for ageist or negatively biased perceptions about what occurs as a person ages chronologically.

　　The study of individual and collective aging processes, known as **gerontology**, explores the reasons for aging and the ways in which people cope with and adapt to this

Aging　The patterns of life changes that occur in members of all species as they grow older.

Ageism　Discrimination based on age.

Gerontology　The study of individual and collective aging processes.

Where Do You Want to Be?

When we are young, aging most likely is the furthest thing from our minds. As we reach the middle years, we are often too pre-occupied with work, career, finances, and ailing parents to really focus on our own aging. But at some point, maybe when the children are gone or our parents' failing health causes us to stop and take a look, the specter of old age stands on our own horizon. However, thinking about aging, what we expect from life, and our values and beliefs about life, death, and the passages we go through are important elements of a satisfying adult development process. Take a few minutes to answer the following questions. Your answers may tell you a great deal about yourself.

1. At this point in your life, what do you value most?
2. What do you think will be most important to you when you reach your 40s? Fifties? Sixties? What similarities and differences do you notice, and what causes these similarities and differences?

3. Do you think your parents are happy and content with the way their lives have turned out? If they could change anything, what do you think they might have done differently?
4. What about your own direction so far in life is similar to that of your parents? What have you done differently? Are the similarities and differences good? Why or why not?
5. What do you think are the keys to a happy and satisfying life?
6. What do you want to accomplish by the time you are 40? Fifty? Sixty?
7. Have you ever thought of retirement? Describe your retirement.
8. Describe the "you" that you would like to be at the age of 70. How is that "you" similar to or different from the "you" of today? What actions will you need to take to be that "you" in the future?

---

process. Gerontologists have identified several age-related characteristics that define where a person is in terms of biological, psychological, social, legal, and functional life-stage development:[1]

- *Biological age* refers to the relative age or condition of the person's organs and body systems. There are 70-year-old runners who have the cardiovascular system of a 40-year-old, and 40-year-olds who have less energy than their parents. Arthritis and other chronic conditions can accelerate the aging process.
- *Psychological age* refers to a person's adaptive capacities, such as coping abilities and intelligence, and to the person's awareness of his or her individual capabilities, self-efficacy, and general ability to adapt to new situations. Although chronic illness may render people physically handicapped, they may possess tremendous psychological reserves and remain alert and fully capable of making decisions.
- *Social age* refers to a person's habits and roles relative to society's expectations. People in a particular life stage usually share similar tastes in music, television shows, and politics.
- *Legal age* is probably the most common definition of age in the United States. Based on chronological years, legal age is used as a factor in determining voting rights, driving privileges, drinking age, eligibility for Social Security payments, and a host of other rights and obligations.
- *Functional age* refers to the ways—heart rate, hearing, etc.—in which people compare to others of a similar age. It is difficult to separate functional aging from many of the other types of aging, particularly chronological and biological aging.

What Is Successful Aging?

As people pass through critical periods in their lives, gerontologists discuss whether they are aging "successfully." Those who are successful usually develop positive coping skills that carry over into other areas of their lives they have realistic achievable goals that bring them pleasure and tend to think confidently and independently. In short, successful agers are more prepared to "experience" life. Those who are less successful in these rites of passage either develop a sense of learned helplessness and lose confidence in their ability to succeed or learn to cope by compensating for their failures in other ways.

Today, it is easier to find positive examples of aging than at any other time in our history. Many of today's "elderly" individuals lead active, productive lives. Typically, people who have aged successfully have the following characteristics:

- In general, they have managed to avoid serious, debilitating diseases and disability.
- They maintain a high level of physical functioning, live independently, and engage in most normal activities of daily living.
- They have maintained cognitive functioning and are actively engaged in mentally challenging and stimulating activities.
- They are actively engaged in social and productive activities.
- They are resilient and able to cope reasonably well with physical, social, and emotional changes.

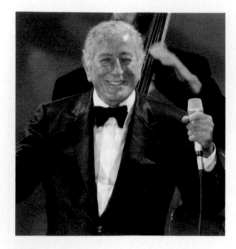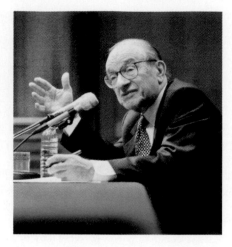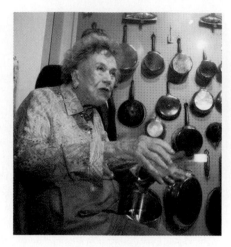

Singer Tony Bennett, economist Alan Greenspan, and chef Julia Child are examples of people who stay vigorous and active in their professions well into their 80s and 90s.

Although the process of aging has often been viewed with dread due to physical changes that inevitably occur, only in the past decade have we begun to fully appreciate the gains and positive aspects of normal adult development throughout the life span. According to gerontologist Dr. Karen Hooker, older adults as a population display much more differentiation in personalities, coping styles, and "possible selves" than any other age group. She states that "successful aging and development as individuals can be viewed as dynamic processes of adaptation between the self and the environment. Throughout our lives we make choices and respond to changes in vastly different ways. Each person is born with certain traits that stay reasonably stable throughout life, but character is deeply affected by personal action constructs that change with time and life history."[2] Thus, aging per se is not a static process, but one in which each of us changes and becomes someone uniquely fashioned by our life's story.

Gerontologists have devised several categories for specific age-related characteristics. People age 65 to 74 are viewed as the **young-old**; those aged 75 to 84 are the **middle-old** group; those 85 and over are classified as the **old-old**.

However, chronological age is not the only issue to be considered. The question is not how many years someone has lived, but how much life the person has packed into those years. This *quality-of-life index,* combined with the chronological process, appears to be the best indicator of the phenomenon of "aging gracefully." Most experts agree that the best way to experience a productive, full, and satisfying old age is to lead a productive, full, and satisfying life prior to old age. Essentially, older people are the product of their lifelong experiences and behaviors.

Older Adults: A Growing Population

The most recent census, in 2000, found that there were an estimated 35 million people aged 65 or older in the United States, nearly 13 percent of the total population. The number of older Americans has increased more than tenfold since 1900, when there were 3 million people age 65 or older (4 percent of the total population) and the numbers of those 65 and over is projected to double by 2040.[3] (See Figure 19.1.) Despite the growth of the older population, the United States is a relatively young country compared to many industrialized nations, where older persons account for 15 percent or more of the total population.[4] (See the Health in a Diverse World box.) According to researchers at the National Institute on Aging, "the aging of the 75 million–strong baby boomer generation could have an impact on our society of equal magnitude to that of immigration at the turn of the last century."[5]

By the year 2011, a whole generation of 1960s bead-wearing, tie-dye-flaunting "flower children," who once proclaimed that no one over 30 could be trusted, will be turning 65. The size of the older population is projected to double over the next 30 years, growing to 70 million in 2030.[6] What will this swelling of the aging population mean to the U.S. economy, our health care system, and the entire social structure of our country?

Leaders must take a proactive stance in developing programs and services to promote health and prevent premature disease and disability. In Utah, state officials are targeting 40-year-olds through their Healthy Aging program, encouraging regular checkups, exercise, healthy eating

Aging: The World's Oldest Countries

The growth of older populations around the world results from major achievements—reliable birth control that has decreased fertility rates, improvements in medical care and sanitation that have reduced infant and maternal mortality and infectious and parasitic diseases, and improvements in nutrition and education. Every month, the net increase in the world's population age 60 and over is more than 1 million; 70 percent of this increase occurs in developing countries and 30 percent in industrialized countries. Between 1991 and 2020, the world population over age 60 is projected to increase by 59 percent in industrialized nations and 159 percent in less developed countries. The world's older population—defined here as persons age 60 and over—numbers 495 million today and is expected to exceed 1 billion by the year 2020. Almost half of today's older adults live in just four nations: the People's Republic of China, India, the Commonwealth of Soviet States, and the United States. (The chart shows countries with the highest percentages of people over 60.) There is intense debate over issues—social security costs, health care, educational investments, and so on—that are directly linked to this changing age structure of societies.

Percent of Population Age 60 and Over — 2000

Country	%
Italy	24.1
Greece	23.4
Japan	23.2
Sweden	22.4
Switzerland	21.3
United Kingdom	20.6
France	20.5
Estonia	20.2
Denmark	20.0
Hungary	19.7
Czech Republic	18.4
Uruguay	17.2
United States	16.1

Source: United Nations Population Division, "World Population Prospects Population Database" (2002).(see http://esa.un.org/unpp).

Sources: United Nations, "International Plan of Action on Aging: Demographic Background" (March 2002) (see http://www.un.org/esa/socdev/ageing/ageipaa.htm) U.S. Department of Commerce, Bureau of the Census, Economics and Statistics Administration, *Global Aging: Comparative Indicators and Future Trends* (Washington, DC: Government Printing Office, 1991); U.S. Bureau of the Census, International Programs Center, International Data Base, 1998.

habits, and overall improved health behaviors. More health plans are considering ways to motivate clients to take more initiative, to work harder at health improvements that will save insurers money in the long run. Instead of focusing on only the negative aspects of aging, more health and social service leaders are focusing on "successful aging—what it means and what it will take to ensure that each of us can achieve it." By enhancing collective understanding of the aging process and the role of current behaviors in developing lifetime habits to inoculate us against the stresses and strains of living, our chances of achieving our "possible selves" will be improved.

Health Issues for an Aging Society

The concerns of government officials over the impending growth in the older population center around meeting their financial and medical needs. No doubt you have heard discussions on the potential bankruptcy of the Social Security system and the large increases in out-of-pocket costs for people on Medicare. With fewer people contributing to the system and greater numbers drawing on it, the likelihood of problems arising is great. According to the latest statistics,

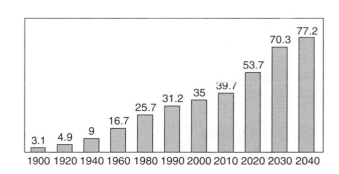

Figure 19.1
Number of Americans 65 and Older (in Millions)
Sources: U.S. Bureau of the Census, "Projections of the Total Resident Population by 5-Year Age Groups, Race, and Hispanic Origin with Special Age Categories: Middle Series, 1999 to 2000," U.S. Census Internet Release Date: January 13, 2000; "Population Projections of the United States by Age, Sex, Race, and Hispanic Origin: 1995–2050," *Current Population Reports*, pp. 25–1130. Data for 2000 are from the 2000 Census.

The Evolving Ratio of Women to Men

As in most countries of the world, there are more older women than older men in the United States, and the proportion of the population that is female increases with age. In 2000, women are estimated to account for 58 percent of the population age 65 and older and 70 percent of the population age 85 and older.

Although women suffer much more morbidity (numbers of illnesses), they tend to outlive their male counterparts by as much as five to seven years or more. Why? While the answers are not clear, several factors are known to account, at least in part, for some of these differences. Among them are marital status, living arrangements, and social activities.

MARITAL STATUS

Marital status can strongly affect a person's emotional and economic well-being by influencing living arrangements and availability of caregivers among the elderly who have an illness or disability. In 2001, 74 percent of men age 65–74 were married, compared with 44 percent of women in the same age group. Almost half of all older women in 2000 were widows. Among persons age 85 or older, about 50 percent of men were married, compared with only 13 percent of women. Those women who are still married tend to take on caretaker roles for ailing husbands. Many unmarried women in these age groups tend to live independently or with children, or they serve as surrogate parents for grandchildren.

LIVING ARRANGEMENTS

The living arrangements of America's older population are closely linked to income, health status, and the availability of caregivers. Older persons who live alone are more likely to be in poverty than older persons who live with spouses or other family members.

- In 1998, 73 percent of older men lived with their spouses, 7 percent lived with other relatives, 3 percent lived with nonrelatives, and 17 percent lived alone.
- In 1998, about 41 percent of older women lived with their spouses, 17 percent lived with other relatives, 2 percent lived with nonrelatives, and approximately 41 percent lived alone.
- In 1998, about 19 percent of white older women who lived alone were in poverty, and approximately half of the older black and Hispanic women who lived alone were also poor.

SOCIAL ACTIVITIES

Men and women benefit from social activity at older ages. Those who continue to interact with others tend to be healthier, both physically and mentally, than those who become socially isolated. Interactions with friends and family members can provide emotional and practical support that enables older persons to remain in the community and reduce the likelihood they will need formal health care services.

Sources: "Older Americans 2000: Key Indicators of Well-Being," by the Federal Interagency Forum on Aging-Related Statistics, December 27, 2000. Department of Health and Services, Administration on Aging, "A Profile of Older Americans: 2001," January 2002.

---

life expectancy for a person born in 2001 is 76.9 years, about 29 years longer than for a child born in 1900.[7] Whereas people age 65 and older made up 13 percent of the U.S. population in 1992, they are projected to make up over 21 percent of the population by 2030. Where will these older people live? How will they pay for their medical costs, and how long will they need to work to support themselves? These and other questions pose many challenges for all of us. (See the Women's Health/Men's Health box.)

Health Care Costs

Today, older Americans require approximately 38 percent of total national health care expenditures, with estimated costs in excess of $7500 per each year.[8] As people live longer, the chances of developing a costly chronic disease increase. As our technology improves, chronic illnesses that once were quickly fatal may now be treated successfully for years. Projected future costs are staggering. Health care expenditures rise with age, and 77 million baby boomers are now in middles age. Compared with people ages 18–44, people ages 45–64 are nearly three times more likely to have a disability,

six times more likely to have high blood pressure and 15 times more likely to die of cancer. Meeting the nations long term care needs will become even more challenging as the population ages and more people require constant help from outsiders. In 2000, 4 million Americans were age 85 and older, the segment most in need of long term care. By 2040, that number is projected to triple to more than 14 million.[9]

If Social Security goes bankrupt, large numbers of Americans will no longer have Medicare coverage. Even if they could afford to buy their own health insurance, most older individuals would face high out-of-pocket expenses and limited choices in treatments. Today, persons on medicare already pay over $3,000 each in out-of-pocket health care expenses. These numbers are certain to increase. Another large group of Americans falls into the category of "uninsured" or "underinsured"—those having only small levels of insurance, usually insufficient for their needs. It is important to note here that the highest rate of uninsured Americans today (22 percent) occurs in the 15- to 44-year-old age group; another 13 percent are in the 45- to 64-year-old age group. If insurance is too expensive or unavailable during the years when people are employed, is it likely that they will be able

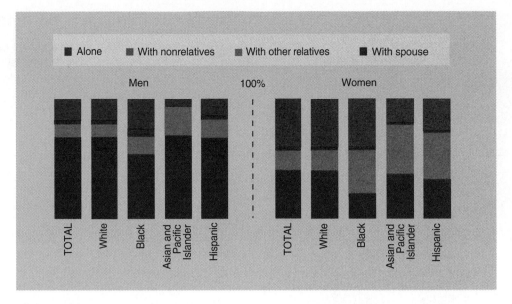

Figure 19.2

Living Arrangements of the U.S. Population Age 65 or Older, 1998

Source: Federal Interagency Forum on Aging-Related Statistics, "Older Americans 2000: Key Indicators of Well-Being" (December 2000) (see http://www.agingstats.gov/chartbook2000/population.html).

to afford insurance when they are retired or on a fixed income? Recent stock market downturns and company failures that resulted in the loss of retirement savings may make it even more difficult for older Americans to afford health insurance in the next decade.

Major questions loom: Will working Americans be willing to pay an increased share of the health care costs for people on fixed incomes who cannot pay for themselves? If not, what will become of these people? Perhaps most important, who will ultimately pay?

Housing and Living Arrangements Contrary to popular opinion, most older people (over 95 percent) never live in a nursing home. Community living, assisted living, skilled nursing care, and other options are new possibilities for those who have financial means or who have purchased some form of long-term care insurance (see Figure 19.2). However, housing problems for the low-income elderly

remain. Who will provide the necessary social services, and who will pay the bill? Will the family of the future be forced to coexist with several generations under one roof?

Ethical and Moral Considerations Difficult ethical questions arise when we consider the implications of an increasing population of older adults for an already overburdened health care system. Given the shortage of donor organs, will we be forced to decide whether a 50-year-old should receive a heart transplant instead of a 75-year-old? Questions have already surfaced regarding the efficacy of hooking up a terminally ill older person to costly machines that prolong life for a few weeks or months but overtax health care resources. Is the prolongation of life at all costs a moral imperative, or will future generations be forced to devise a set of criteria for deciding who will be helped and who will not? Understanding the process of aging and knowing what actions you can take to prolong your own healthy years are a part of our collective responsibility.

Theories on Aging

Biological Theories

Of the various theories about the biological causes of aging, the following are among the most commonly accepted.

- *The wear-and-tear theory* states that, like everything else in the universe, the human body wears out. Inherent in this theory is the idea that the more you abuse your body, the faster it will wear out. Fortunately, today's older adults can achieve

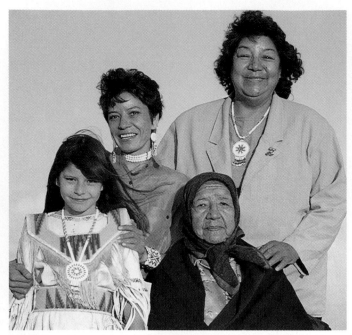

In most cases, you need look no further than your family tree to get an idea of the effects that aging will have on you.

Psychosocial Impacts on Aging

Numerous psychological and sociological factors also influence the manner in which people age. Psychologists Erik Erikson and Robert Peck have formulated theories of personality development that emphasize adaptation and adjustment. In his developmental model, Erikson states that people must progress through eight critical stages during a lifetime. If a person does not receive the proper stimulus or develop effective methods of coping with life's turmoil from infancy onward, problems are likely to develop later in life. According to this theory, maladjustments in old age are often a result of problems encountered in earlier stages of a person's life.

Peck argues that during middle and old age, people face a series of increasingly stressful tasks. Those who are poorly adjusted psychologically or who have not developed appropriate coping skills are likely to undergo a painful aging process.

Both Erikson and Peck suggest that a combination of psychosocial and biological factors and environmental "trigger mechanisms" causes each of us to age in a unique manner. But what is normal and what is unique in aging? How much change is inevitable and how much can be avoided?

Changes in the Body and Mind

Typical Physical Changes

Although the physiological consequences of aging can differ in severity and timing, certain standard changes occur as a result of the aging process.

The Skin As a normal consequence of aging, the skin becomes thinner and loses elasticity, particularly in the outer surfaces. Fat deposits, which add to the soft lines and shape of the skin, diminish. Starting at about age 30, lines develop on the forehead as a result of smiling, squinting, and other facial expressions. These lines become more pronounced, with added "crow's-feet" around the eyes, during the 40s. During a person's 50s and 60s, the skin begins to sag and lose color, leading to pallor in the 70s. Body fat in underlying layers of skin continues to be redistributed away from the limbs and extremities into the trunk region of the body. Age spots become more numerous because of excessive pigment accumulation under the skin, particularly in those with heavy sun exposure.

A common disorder of facial skin that affects millions of Americans is *rosacea* (pronounced roh-ZAY-sha). While the cause of rosacea is unknown and there is no cure, there are prescription medications that can treat symptoms and control signs. One symptom is redness on the cheeks, nose, chin, or forehead, particularly after exercise or alcohol ingestion. This redness looks like a blush or sunburn in the early stages and fades fairly quickly. However, as the condition worsens, the blush may deepen in color and last much longer. Other

high levels of fitness without having to be marathoners. Strength training, walking, gardening, and other activities allow even the most out of shape to improve. You don't have to feel "pain" to realize healthy gains.
- *The cellular theory* states that at birth we have only a certain number of usable cells, which are genetically programmed to divide or reproduce a limited number of times. Once these cells reach the end of their reproductive cycle, they die, and the organs they make up begin to deteriorate. The rate of deterioration varies from person to person, and its impact depends on the system involved.
- *The autoimmune theory* attributes aging to the decline of the body's immunological system. Studies indicate that as we age, our immune systems become less effective in fighting disease. Eventually, bodies that are subjected to too much stress, lack of sleep, and so on—especially if these factors are coupled with poor nutrition—show signs of disease and infirmity. In some instances, the immune system appears to lose control and turn its protective mechanisms inward, actually attacking the person's own body. Although autoimmune disorders may occur in all age groups, some gerontologists believe that they increase in frequency and severity with age.
- *The genetic mutation theory* proposes that the number of cells exhibiting unusual or different characteristics increases with age. Proponents of this theory believe that aging is related to the amount of mutational damage within the genes. The greater the mutation, the greater the chance that cells will not function properly, leading to eventual dysfunction of body organs and systems.

symptoms include small visible blood vessels on the nose or cheeks (these blood vessels look like thin red lines filled with red blood), small bumps and/or pimples on the skin surface, watery or itchy eyes along with a tendency for red eyes and stye development, enlargement of the nose after recurrent swelling of nasal tissue, and a puffy, red appearance of the face. Persons who suspect that they have rosacea should visit a reputable dermatologist who will treat the symptoms and help avoid more serious damage to facial tissue.

Bones and Joints   Throughout the life span, bones are continually changing because of the accumulation and loss of minerals. By the third or fourth decade of life, mineral loss from bones becomes more prevalent than mineral accumulation, resulting in a weakening and porosity (diminishing density) of bony tissue. This loss of minerals (particularly calcium) occurs in both sexes, although it is much more common in females. Loss of calcium can contribute to **osteoporosis**, a disease characterized by low bone density and structural deterioration of bone tissue. These porous, fragile bones are susceptible to fracture.[10] (See the Reality Check box.)

The Head   With age, features of the head enlarge and become more noticeable. Increased cartilage and fatty tissue cause the nose to grow a half inch wider and another half inch longer. Earlobes get fatter and longer, while overall head circumference increases one quarter of an inch per decade, even though the brain itself shrinks. The skull becomes thicker with age.

The Urinary Tract   At age 70, the kidneys can filter waste from the blood only half as fast as they could at age 30. The need to urinate more frequently occurs because the bladder's capacity declines from 2 cups of urine at age 30 to 1 cup at age 70.

One problem often associated with aging is **urinary incontinence**, which ranges from passing a few drops of urine while laughing or sneezing to having no control over urination. More than 13 million people in America—male and female, young and old—experience incontinence.[11] It is often temporary and results from an underlying medical condition. Women experience it at twice the rate of men, largely because pregnancy and childbirth, menopause, and the structure of the female urinary tract.

Incontinence can pose major social, physical, and emotional problems. Embarrassment and fear of wetting oneself may cause an older person to become isolated and avoid social functions. Caregivers may become frustrated with incontinent patients. Prolonged wetness and the inability to properly care for oneself can lead to irritation, infections, and other problems.

However, incontinence is not an inevitable part of aging. Most cases are caused by medications, highly treatable neurological problems that affect the central nervous system, infections of the pelvic muscles, weakness in the pelvic wall, or other problems. When the problem is treated, the incontinence usually vanishes.[12]

Drug therapy can slow bladder contractions, increase bladder capacity, contract or relax the bladder sphincter, and increase fluid output. Surgery to repair the pelvic floor is often successful in stress incontinence. Artificial devices that slow urine flow, improvements in access to toilet facilities, rigid schedules for urination, and many newer treatments have also shown promise. In addition, women can learn exercises to strengthen the pelvic floor and reduce their susceptibility to this problem later in life. Biofeedback to control urine flow and improve mind/body responses is another approach to prevention.

The Heart and Lungs   Resting heart rate stays about the same over the course of a person's life, but the stroke volume (the amount of blood the muscle pushes out per beat) diminishes as heart muscles deteriorate. Vital capacity, or the amount of air that moves when you inhale and exhale at maximum effort, also declines with age. Exercise can do a great deal to preserve heart and lung function.

Eyesight   By age 30, the lens of the eye begins to harden, causing problems by the early 40s. The lens begins to yellow and loses transparency, while the pupil of the eye shrinks, allowing less light to penetrate. Activities such as reading become more difficult, particularly in dim light. By age 60, depth perception declines and farsightedness often develops. A need for glasses usually develops in the 40s, and this evolves into a need for bifocals in the 50s and trifocals in the 60s. **Cataracts** (clouding of the lens) and **glaucoma** (elevated pressure within the eyeball) become more likely. Eventually a tendency toward color blindness may develop, especially for shades of blue and green.

Macular degeneration is the leading cause of blindness in the world and affects millions of Americans. Often called ARMD, or age-related macular degeneration, this disease breaks down the macula, the light-sensitive part of the retina responsible for the sharp, direct vision needed to read, watch television, or drive. Essentially, it causes permanent blindness in this central vision plane. Because it does not affect side vision, it does not lead to total blindness. However, because of central vision loss, its impact may be devastating.

Osteoporosis   A degenerative bone disorder characterized by increasingly porous bones.

Urinary incontinence   The inability to control urination.

Cataracts   Clouding of the lens that interrupts the focusing of light on the retina, resulting in blurred vision or eventual blindness.

Glaucoma   Elevation of pressure within the eyeball, leading to hardening of the eyeball, impaired vision, and possible blindness.

Osteoporosis: Preventing an Age-Old Problem

Although many people consider osteoporosis to be a disease only of older women, osteoporosis can occur at any age, and increasingly it poses a problem for men, too. When people hear that someone has osteoporosis, the image that comes to mind is a slumped-over individual with a characteristic "dowager's hump" in the upper back; however, this is a relatively rare, extreme version of the disease. Osteoporosis is progressive and occurs over many years, and without proper prevention in the form of diet, weight-bearing exercise, and overall fitness (see Chapter 10), each of us risks developing this condition. As awareness increases, millions of Americans are demanding "bone density" tests to determine just how far gone their bones and joints really may be. Health care providers, responding to the estimated $14 billion in direct and indirect costs that osteoporosis patients incur, are also motivated to focus on controlling risks.

EPIDEMIOLOGY OF THE DISEASE
Prevalence data indicate the following:

✔ The hips, wrists, and spine are most vulnerable to the ravages of osteoporosis.
✔ In the United States, osteoporosis affects over 44 million Americans, 68 percent of whom are women.
✔ Each year osteoporosis causes 1.5 million fractures: 300,000 at the hip, 700,000 in the vertebrae, 250,000 in the wrists, and more than 300,000 at other sites.
✔ One out of every two women and one in four men over age 50 will have an osteoporosis-related fracture sometime in life.
✔ More than 2 million American men have osteoporosis and millions more are at risk. Each year, 80,000 men

suffer a hip fracture, and one third of them die within a year.

RISK FACTORS
A number of factors may predispose a person to developing osteoporosis. Risk factors that we cannot control include the following:

✔ *Gender.* Chances of developing osteoporosis are greater if you are a woman. Women have less bone tissue and lose bone more rapidly than men because of the hormonal changes resulting from menopause.
✔ *Age.* The older you are, the greater your risk of osteoporosis. Your bones become less dense and weaker as you age.
✔ *Body size.* Small, thin-boned women are at greater risk.
✔ *Ethnicity.* Caucasian and Asian women are at highest risk; African American and Latino women have a lower but still significant risk.
✔ *Family history.* Susceptibility to fracture may be, in part, hereditary. People whose parents have a history of fractures also seem to have reduced bone mass.

However, we can modify the following risk factors by our choices in lifestyle behaviors, medication, and diet:

✔ *Levels of sex hormones*—abnormal absence of menstrual periods (amenorrhea), low estrogen levels (menopause), and low testosterone levels in men may signal potential problems
✔ *Anorexia.*
✔ A lifetime *diet low in calcium and vitamin D.*
✔ Use of *certain medications,* such as glucocorticoids or some anticonvulsants.
✔ An *inactive lifestyle* or extended bed rest.
✔ *Cigarette smoking*
✔ *Excessive use of alcohol.*

The following preventive measures can help everyone reduce the risk of osteoporosis.

INCREASE CALCIUM AND VITAMIN D INTAKE
Many studies support the notion that if you don't consume enough calcium, you will be at increased risk for osteoporosis. Calcium needs change over the course of a lifetime, with greater needs during childhood and adolescence when the skeleton is growing and during pregnancy and breastfeeding. Postmenopausal women and older men also need more calcium. Medications also may deplete calcium reserves. Because vitamin D helps with calcium absorption, taking adequate amounts of vitamin D will ensure that the body uses the calcium that it ingests.

EXERCISE
Like muscle, bone is living tissue that responds to exercise by becoming stronger. The best exercise for the bones is weight-bearing exercise that forces you to work against gravity. Examples include walking, hiking, jogging, weight training, tennis, and dancing.

Research conducted by Dr. Christine M. Snow, director of Oregon State University's bone research lab and internationally known exercise scientist, has shed interesting light on the importance of exercise for residents of nursing homes. Residents were given modest exercises to do while wearing weighted vests. Subjects not only improved bone density but also balance and strength, which together can reduce the risk of falling and fracturing bones. In addition, residents developed a faster gait, which made them less likely to fall to the side if they lost balance. In studies of young gymnasts, Snow has found that bone density can be increased through various types of exercise. She emphasizes that it is vitally important to begin exercising early in life to ensure bone health in later years.

Sources: National Institutes of Health, Osteoporosis and Related Bone Diseases National Resource Center, FAST FACTS: December 2002 (http://www.osteo.org/osteo.html).

Macular degeneration is diagnosed as either "dry" or "wet." The dry form is the most common type, affecting about 90 percent of those who have ARMD. The less common wet form can cause rapid and severe central vision deterioration. Both types occur most commonly in persons aged 65 and over, although it is found in persons in younger age groups.

The exact causes of age-related macular degeneration are unknown; however, having family members with ARMD, smoking, high blood pressure, farsightedness, and obesity tend to increase risks. Although many researchers and eye specialists believe that certain nutrients such as zinc, antioxidants such as vitamins A, C, and E, and lutein may reduce risks, these theories have not been proven in clinical trials. Efforts to treat ARMD are currently underway, but progress to date has been slow.

Hearing The ability to hear high-frequency consonants (for example, *s, t,* and *z*) diminishes with age. Much of the actual hearing loss lies in the ability to distinguish extreme ranges of sound rather than normal conversational tones.

Sexual Changes As men age, they experience notable alterations in sexual functioning. Whereas the degree and rate of change vary greatly from person to person, the following changes generally occur:

1. The ability to obtain an erection is slowed.
2. The ability to maintain an erection is diminished.
3. The length of the refractory period between orgasms increases.
4. The angle of the erection declines with age.
5. The orgasm itself grows shorter in duration.

Women also experience several changes:

1. Menopause usually occurs between the ages of 45 and 55. Women may experience hot flashes, mood swings, weight gain, development of facial hair, or other hormone-related symptoms.
2. The walls of the vagina become less elastic and the epithelium thins, possibly making intercourse painful.
3. Vaginal secretions, particularly during sexual activity, diminish.
4. The breasts become less firm. Loss of fat in various areas leads to fewer curves, with a decrease in the soft lines of the body contours.

While these physiological changes may seem somewhat discouraging, a study by the National Council on Aging indicated that older Americans continue to be sexually active. This study refutes long-held beliefs that sexual desire decreases as we age. Results indicated that nearly half of Americans over age 60 engage in sexual activity at least once a month and 4 out of 10 would like to have sex more frequently than they currently do.[13] With the advent of drugs designed to treat sexual dysfunction, such as Viagra, many older adults may get their wish.

Body Comfort Because of the loss of body fat, thinning of the epithelium, and diminished glandular activity, older adults experience greater difficulty regulating body temperature. This limits their ability to withstand extreme cold or heat, increasing the risks of hypothermia, heatstroke, and heat exhaustion.

> **What do you think?**
>
> *Of the health conditions discussed in this section, which ones can you prevent? ✹ Which ones can you delay? ✹ What actions can you take now to protect yourself from these problems?*

Mental Changes

Intelligence Recent research demonstrates that many of our previous beliefs about the intelligence of older adults were based on inappropriate testing procedures. Given an appropriate length of time, older people may learn and develop skills in a similar manner to younger people. Researchers have also determined that what many older adults lack in speed of learning they make up for in practical knowledge—that is, the "wisdom of age."

Memory Have you ever wondered why your grandfather seems unable to remember what he did last weekend even though he can graphically describe an event that occurred 40 years ago? This phenomenon is not unusual. Research indicates that although short-term memory may fluctuate on a daily basis, the ability to remember events from past decades seems to remain largely unchanged.

Flexibility versus Rigidity Although it is widely believed that people become more like one another as they age, nothing could be further from the truth. Having lived through a multitude of experiences and faced diverse joys, sorrows, and obstacles, the typical older person has developed unique methods of coping with life. These unique adaptive variations make for interesting differences in how they confront the many changes brought on by the aging process. As a group, the elderly are extremely heterogeneous. They flex and adapt and "make do" in ways that younger adults may not be able to duplicate. Labeling this highly flexible and resilient group as rigid or unmovable is inaccurate and misleading.

Depression Most adults continue to lead healthy, fulfilling lives as they grow older. However, some older people do suffer from mental and emotional disturbances. Some research indicates that depression may be the most common psychological problem facing older adults. However, the rate of major depression is actually lower among older people than among younger adults.

Regardless of age, those who have a poor perception of their health, who have multiple chronic illnesses, who take a lot of medications, abuse alcohol and other drugs, lack social support and who do not exercise have more challenges that require many emotional strengths to get through them. Strong coping skills and support systems will often lessen the duration and severity of the depression. However, those who are ill-equipped to deal with life's changes or who lack close ties may consider suicide as a means of solving their problems.

Senility: Getting Rid of Ageist Attitudes Over the years, older adults have often been victims of ageist attitudes. People who were chronologically old were often labeled "senile" whenever they displayed memory failure, errors in judgment, disorientation, or erratic behaviors. Today scientists recognize that these same symptoms can occur at any age and for various reasons, including disease or the use of over-the-counter and prescription drugs. When the underlying problems are corrected, the memory loss and disorientation also improve. Currently, the term **senility** is seldom used except to describe a very small group of organic disorders.

Alzheimer's Disease **Dementias** are progressive brain impairments that interfere with memory and normal intellectual functioning. Although there are many types of dementia, one of the most common forms is **Alzheimer's disease (AD).** Attacking over 4 million Americans and killing over 100,000 of them every year, this disease is one of the most painful and devastating conditions that families can endure. It kills its victims twice: first through a slow loss of personhood (memory loss, disorientation, personality changes, and eventual loss of the ability to function as a person), and then through the deterioration of bodily systems as they gradually succumb to the powerful impact of neurological problems.

Most recently, actor Charlton Heston revealed that he had developed what he described as "symptoms consistent with Alzheimer's." His August 2002 announcement brought more attention to the disease that has already affected former president Ronald Reagan and many other Americans. Currently, Alzheimer's afflicts an estimated 1 in 10 people over the age of 65 and 1 in 5 people over the age of 85. These numbers are certain to increase. It is estimated to cost society over $100 billion a year currently.[14] With the

U.S. population gradually aging, the economic burden of the future seems even more dismal. While the disease is associated in most people's minds strictly with the elderly, Alzheimer's has been diagnosed in people in their late 40s. In fact, about 5 percent of all cases occur before age 65.

Contrary to what many people think, Alzheimer's is not a new disease. Named after Alois Alzheimer, a German neuropathologist who recorded it as early as 1906, Alzheimer's refers to a degenerative disease of the brain in which nerve cells stop communicating with one another. Ordinarily, brain cells communicate by releasing chemicals that allow the cells to receive and transmit messages for various types of behavior. In Alzheimer's patients, the brain doesn't produce enough of these chemicals, cells can't communicate, and eventually the cells die.

This degeneration happens in the sections of the brain that affect memory, speech, and personality, leaving the parts that control other bodily functions, such as heartbeat and breathing, functioning at normal or near normal levels. Thus, the mind begins to go as the body lives on. It all happens in a slow, progressive manner, and it may be as long as 20 years before symptoms are noticed.

Alzheimer's is generally detected first by families, who note changes, particularly memory lapses and personality changes, in their loved ones. Medical tests rule out underlying causes, and certain neurological tests help confirm the diagnosis.

Alzheimer's disease characteristically progresses in three stages. During the *first stage,* symptoms include forgetfulness, memory loss, impaired judgment, increasing inability to handle routine tasks, disorientation, lack of interest in one's surroundings, and depression. These symptoms accelerate in the *second stage,* which also includes agitation and restlessness (especially at night), loss of sensory perceptions, muscle twitching, and repetitive actions. Many patients become depressed, combative, and aggressive. In the *final stage,* disorientation is often complete. The person becomes completely dependent on others for eating, dressing, and other activities. Identity loss and speech problems are common symptoms. Eventually, control of bodily functions may be lost.

Once Alzheimer's disease strikes, the victim's life expectancy is cut in half. Tragically, little can be done at present to treat the disorder, although scientists are experimenting with various drug regimens.

Researchers are investigating a number of possible causes, including genetic predisposition, malfunction of the immune system, a slow-acting virus, chromosomal or genetic defects, chronic inflammation, and neurotransmitter imbalance.

Preliminary research indicates that a defect in the chromosomes may be the most likely cause, partly because virtually everyone with Down syndrome eventually develops Alzheimer's. Treatment for Alzheimer's has focused on four drugs that have been approved by the Food and Drug Administration. Cognex, the first drug to be approved, is only used rarely because of side effects, including possible liver damage.

Senility   A term associated with the loss of memory and judgment and orientation problems occurring in a small percentage of the elderly.

Dementias   Progressive brain impairments that interfere with memory and normal intellectual functioning.

Alzheimer's disease   A chronic condition involving changes in nerve fibers of the brain that results in mental deterioration.

Table 19.1
Top Ten Health Problems of Older Americans

TOP TEN CAUSES OF DEATH	TOP TEN CHRONIC CONDITIONS
Diseases of the heart	Arthritis
Malignant neoplasms (cancer)	High blood pressure
Cerebrovascular diseases and stroke	Hearing impairment
Chronic obstructive pulmonary diseases/emphysema	Diseases of the heart
Pneumonia and influenza	Cataracts
Diabetes mellitus	Limb deformities or impairments
Unintentional injuries	Chronic sinusitis
Alzheimer's disease	Diabetes
Kidney disease	Tinnitus (ringing of the ears)
Bloodstream infections	Visual impairment

Source: "Healthy Aging/Healthy Living—START NOW," American Association for World Health, 1999.

Aricept (approved in 1996), Exelon (approved in 2000), and Reminyl (approved in 2001) are all cholinesterase inhibitors. They seem to slow the loss of memory by preventing the destruction of neurotransmitters. Although the drugs were associated with better results for users in memory and thinking tests than for patients taking a placebo, the differences were modest and more than half of the patients showed no improvement at all.[15]

Some researchers are looking at anti-inflammatory drugs, theorizing that Alzheimer's may develop in response to an inflammatory ailment. Others are focusing on estrogen as a possible preventive measure, noting that women who take estrogen during menopause have been found to develop Alzheimer's much later on average than women who don't. However, there may be additional risks associated with taking estrogen, as discussed in previous chapters. Still others are focusing on stimulating the brains of Alzheimer's-prone individuals, believing that as people learn, more connections between cells are formed that may offset those that are lost.

In general, medications to help patients with Alzheimer's have been designed to ease any discomfort and keep patients from becoming frustrated and combative. Although there is hope that pharmaceutical interventions may one day provide significant relief and improvements in the progression of the disease, until a definitive cause for the disease is isolated, effective treatment is unlikely.

Much attention has also focused on the family, as the family is often another victim when Alzheimer's occurs. Having to decide between tending to a loved one at home or seeking the assistance of a long-term care facility can be difficult. Caring for Alzheimer's patients is a challenge for even the most dedicated family members. And even the best preparation for the final days of a loved one with this disease does not make the process easy. Knowing what the options

are and being able to recognize the differences between normal physiological aging and the ravages of certain diseases can help make age-related problems easier to cope with for both older people themselves and their families.

Health Challenges of Older Adults

Some health problems common in older adults are brought on by failing health (see Table 19.1), others by society. Some result when people do not develop the ability to cope effectively with life's hurdles. Still other problems come from the older person's perceived loss of control over life's events—watching loved ones die, facing health problems, and confronting an uncertain economy on a fixed income. Developing life skills and a network of social support during earlier years can significantly reduce problems in old age.

Alcohol Use and Abuse

Early studies reported that 2 to 10 percent of older Americans were alcoholics, but the exact percentages are controversial today. However, a person who is prone to alcoholism during the younger and middle years is more likely to continue during later years. The older alcoholic is probably no more common in American society than the young alcoholic, despite the stereotype of the old, lost soul, hiding his or her sorrows in a bottle. Often, when many people think they see a drunken older person, they are really seeing a confused individual who has taken too many different prescription medications and is experiencing a form of drug interaction.

Men tend to have higher risks for alcoholism at all ages. Alcohol abuse is five times more common among older men than among older women. Yet as many as half of all older men and an even higher proportion of older women don't drink at all. Those who do drink do so less than younger persons, consuming only five to six drinks weekly.

If the more recent studies are accurate, the reason there aren't many heavy drinkers among older adults may be that very heavy drinkers tend either to die of alcoholic complications before they reach old age or to reform their drinking habits. Some older people reduce their consumption because they find they cannot process alcohol as readily as they did when they were younger or because they are afraid of combining it with the prescription drugs they must take. If the older reports are accurate, alcoholism among the elderly may be disguised by a tendency among health professionals and family members to associate forgetfulness, incontinence, poor grooming, dementia-like reactions, injuries, and so on with old age rather than with an alcohol problem. It is important to note that most older adults who consume alcohol are neither alcoholics nor people who drink to cope with their losses. Most drinking among older people is social and may, in fact, be much less of a problem than previously thought.

Prescription Drug Use

It is extremely rare for older people to use illicit drugs, but some do overuse and grow dependent upon prescription drugs. Some take four to six prescription drugs a day. Reported numbers of drugs taken are substantially higher for residents of health care institutions, but this may be because drugs that many of us purchase over the counter, such as aspirin, are counted in the total numbers.

Anyone who combines different drugs runs the risk of dangerous drug interactions. The risks of adverse effects are even greater for people with impaired circulation and declining kidney and liver function. Older people displaying symptoms of these drug-induced effects, which may include bizarre behavior patterns or disorientation, are all too often misdiagnosed as senile rather than examined for underlying causes and treated.

Currently there is not one system that tracks all of a patient's prescriptions. Pharmacists may not know about other drugs that a patient is taking and may not be able to warn patients of possible drug interactions. Illness or physiological abnormalities may affect the way drugs are metabolized, contributing to dose irregularities and other problems. In order to avoid drug interactions and other problems, older adults should try to use the same pharmacy consistently, ask questions about medicines and dosages, and have a family member or friend who can help interpret directions for taking medications.

Over-the-Counter Remedies

A substantial segment of the over-60 population avoids professional medical treatment, viewing it as only a last resort. This is becoming increasingly true as Medicare coverage becomes less adequate and older adults are forced to pay larger medical bills out of their own resources. The poor are particularly prone to turn to folk medicine and over-the-counter (OTC) preparations as cheaper, less intimidating alternatives. Aspirin and laxatives head the list of commonly used OTC medications for relief of arthritic pain and the irregular bowel activity sometimes experienced by older Americans.

Preventive Actions for Healthy Aging

As you know from reading this book, you can do many things to prolong your life and improve the quality of your life. Some factors, however, are especially important. To provide for healthy older years, make each of the following part of your younger years.

Develop and Maintain Healthy Relationships

Social bonds and relationships with others lend vigor and energy to life. Be willing to give to others, and seek variety in your relationships rather than befriending only people who agree with you. By experiencing diverse people and interacting with different points of view, we gain a new perspective on life.

Enrich the Spiritual Side of Life

Although we often take this for granted, cultivating a relationship with nature, the environment, a higher being, and yourself is a key factor in personal growth and development. Take time for thought and quiet contemplation, and enjoy the sunsets, sounds, and energy of life. These moments spent in

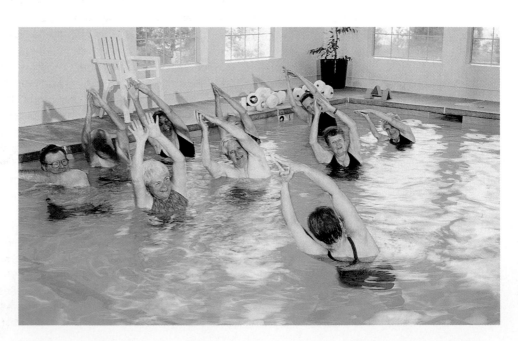

For many, the secret to aging well is to stay active and enjoy the company of good friends.

time prioritized for "you" will leave you invigorated and fresh—better able to cope with the ups and downs of life. If you don't take time for yourself now, it just may be that you won't have time in the later years.

Improve Fitness

If you're basically sedentary, just about any moderate-intensity exercise that gets your heart beating faster and increases strength and/or flexibility will maximize your physical health and functional years. The research presented in Chapter 10 shows that there is hope even for the most die-hard couch potato.

One of the inevitable physical changes that the body undergoes is **sarcopenia**, age-associated loss of muscle mass. The less muscle you have, the less energy you will burn even while resting. The lower your metabolic rate, the more likely weight gain. With regular strength training, you can increase your muscle mass, boost your metabolism, strengthen your bones, prevent osteoporosis, and, in general, feel better and function more efficiently. The Skills for Behavior Change box provides tips for exercise.

So, get moving and keep moving, no matter what the activity is. And remember, it is never too late to start. Even if you're in your 60s or 70s, exercise can increase life expectancy by improving circulation, reducing blood pressure, and reducing overall health risks. A lifetime of exercise and movement will pay dividends in later years.

Eat for Health

Although other chapters in this text provide detailed information about nutrition and weight control, certain nutrients are especially essential to healthy aging:

- *Calcium.* Bone loss tends to increase in women, particularly in the hip region, shortly before menopause. During perimenopause and menopause, this bone loss accelerates rapidly, with an average of about 3 percent skeletal mass lost per year over a five-year period. The result is an increased risk for fracture and disability. Few women actually consume the 1,000 milligrams of calcium recommended during the younger years, or the 1,500 milligrams recommended during and after menopause.
- *Vitamin D.* Vitamin D is necessary for adequate calcium absorption, yet as people age, particularly in their 50s and 60s, they do not absorb vitamin D from foods as readily as they did in their younger years. If vitamin D is unavailable, calcium levels are also likely to be lower.
- *Protein.* As older adults become more concerned about cholesterol and fatty foods, and as their budgets shrink, one nutrient that often takes the "hit" is protein. It costs more, takes longer to cook, and often has that "fat" stigma associated with animal products. Many older people cut back on protein to a point that is below the recommended daily amount. Large numbers of women in particular cut back so far that they get less than half of the daily amount necessary.

Because protein is necessary for muscle mass, protein insufficiencies can spell trouble.

Other nutrients, including vitamin E, folic acid (folate), iron, potassium, and vitamin B_{12}, are important to the aging process, and most of these are readily available in any diet that follows food pyramid recommendations.

In summary, aging is not just a static state that you suddenly achieve. You can feel old at a very young age or feel young at a very old age. You can have an engaging and active life full of challenges, friends, and fulfillment, or you can become socially isolated, bored, and unhappy. Many of these end products in life have to do with the path you choose to follow now.

Caring for Older Adults

Older women far outnumber older men in American society, and the discrepancy increases with age. Because women live seven years longer than men on average, older women are more likely to be living alone. Further, they are more likely to experience poverty and multiple chronic health problems, a situation referred to as **comorbidity**. Consequently, more elderly women than men are likely to need assistance from children, other relatives, friends, and neighbors.

Women have usually been the primary caregivers for older Americans, often for their ailing husbands. Research also indicates that women spend more hours than men (38 hours versus 27 hours per week) in caregiving activities and perform a wider range of activities. Regardless of the time spent, caregiving is a difficult and stressful experience for both women and men. **Respite care**, or care that is given by someone who relieves the primary caregiver, should be available to ease the burden. As the population ages and more older adults require care, it will become even more important to support caregivers' health and well-being.

What do you think?

Why are women often the primary caregivers for aging spouses and other family members? ✳ What problems can such caregiving cause? ✳ How can caregivers learn to cope with the stresses and strains of their situation?

Sarcopenia Age-related loss of muscle mass.

Comorbidity The presence of a number of diseases at the same time.

Respite care The care provided by substitute caregivers to relieve the principal caregiver from his or her continuous responsibility.

Aging and Exercise

Whether you're 20, 50, or 80 years old, you can exercise and improve your health. Physical activity is good for your heart, mood, and confidence. Exercising has even helped 90-year-olds living in nursing homes to grow stronger and more independent.

Staying physically active is a key to good health well into later years. Yet only about one in four older adults exercises regularly. Many think they are too old or too frail to exercise. Nothing could be further from the truth. Physical activity of any kind—from heavy-duty exercises such as jogging or bicycling to easier efforts like walking—is good for you. Vigorous exercise can help strengthen your heart and lungs. Taking a brisk walk regularly can help lower your risk of health problems like heart disease or depression. Climbing stairs, calisthenics, and housework can increase strength, stamina, and self-confidence. Weight lifting or strength training is a good way to slow down muscle and bone loss. Your daily activities will become easier as you feel better.

You can exercise at home alone, with a buddy, or as part of a group. Talk to your doctor before you begin, especially if you are over 60 or have a medical problem. Move at your own speed, and don't try to take on too much at first. A class can be a good idea if you haven't exercised for a long time or are just beginning. A qualified teacher will make sure you are doing the exercise in the right way.

Thirty minutes of moderate activity each day is a good goal. You don't have to exercise for 30 minutes all at once. Short bursts of activity, like taking the stairs instead of the elevator, or walking instead of driving, can add up to 30 minutes of exercise a day. Raking leaves, playing actively with children, gardening, and even doing household chores can count toward your daily total.

Include a mix of stretching, strength training, and aerobic or endurance exercise in your exercise plan. People who are weak or frail should start slowly. Begin with stretching and strength training; add aerobics later. Aerobics are safer and easier once you feel balanced and your muscles are stronger.

Stretching improves flexibility, eases movement, and lowers the risk of injury and muscle strain. It also increases blood flow and gets your body ready for exercise. A warm-up and cool-down period of 5 to 15 minutes should be done slowly and carefully, before and after all types of exercise. In addition to being relaxing, stretching can loosen muscles in the arms, shoulders, back, chest, stomach, buttocks, thighs, and calves.

Strength training (also called resistance training or weight lifting) builds muscle and bone, both of which decline with age. Lifting weights or working out with machines or an elastic band will strengthen the upper and lower body. It is very important to have an expert teach you how to work with weights; otherwise you could get hurt. With help, older adults can work their way up to many of the same weight-lifting routines as younger adults. Once you know what to do, simple strength training exercises can be done at home. Beginners can use household items, such as soup cans or milk jugs filled with water or sand, as weights. Strength training activities do not have to take a lot of time; 30 to 40 minutes at least two or three times each week are all that's needed. Try not to exercise the same muscles two days in a row.

Aerobic exercises (also called endurance exercises) strengthen the heart and improve overall fitness by increasing the body's ability to use oxygen. Swimming, walking, and dancing are "low-impact" aerobic activities. They avoid the muscle and joint pounding of more "high-impact" exercises like jogging and jumping rope. Aerobic exercises raise the number of heartbeats each minute (heart rate). It's best to get your heart rate to a certain point and keep it there for 20 minutes or more. If you have not exercised in a while, start slowly. As you get stronger, try to increase your heart rate. Aerobics should be done for 20 to 40 minutes at least three times each week.

Before starting any aerobics program, check with your doctor and ask about your own target heart rate. Some blood pressure medicines, for example, can affect how you calculate target heart rate.

Local gyms, universities, or hospitals can help you find a teacher or program that works for you. You can also check with local churches or synagogues, senior and civic centers, parks, recreation associations, YMCAs, YWCAs, and even local shopping malls for exercise and wellness programs. Many community centers also offer programs for older people who may be worried about special health problems like heart disease or falling. Look for books and tapes at your local library.

Source: Adapted from U.S. Department of Health and Human Services, National Institute on Aging, "Don't Take It Easy—Exercise!" (Gaithersburg, MD: National Institute on Aging, n.d.). Available at MedAccess Age Page, http://www.medaccess.com/seniors/agepg/ap41.htm.

Taking Charge

Reducing Age-Related Risks

There is no one right way to age. Most people who do age successfully, however, pay attention to their physical, spiritual, emotional, mental, and social well-being.

Revisit your answers to the Assess Yourself box and ask yourself what you can do now to ensure that you reach some of the goals you have set for yourself in retirement. Perhaps you haven't really given them that much thought. After all, you're still in college. You're still working at launching a career. But as you have read in this chapter, the aging process began the day you were born. Therefore, you can do many things now to ease the challenges of aging. The following also may help.

Checklist for Change

Making Personal Choices

☐ Keep active mentally. For some people, mentally active equals socially active. Take time as well for quiet reflection, concentrated thought, and idle musing.

☐ Schedule regular medical check-ups. One of the best ways to prevent major health problems is to take care of minor problems early.

☐ Develop a sense of self. Maintaining a sense of yourself as a worthwhile, productive member of society can be a challenge in the face of changes that appear to diminish individual prestige.

☐ Learn to accept help when you need it. Just as a healthy level of independence and personal control are important aspects of human development, so is the ability to ask questions and seek assistance without feeling foolish or intimidated.

☐ Make optimal use of your time and energy. Learn to maximize your energy potential.

☐ Make an honest evaluation of your personal weaknesses and strengths. Then make a conscious effort to improve in weak areas wherever possible and, where not, to give those areas less importance in your life.

☐ Take positive steps now to plan for a secure retirement. Living for the moment can result in financial problems that will seriously limit your options later in life.

☐ Become familiar with services that are available to assist older adults. Many communities offer services that help people remain independent.

☐ Do not allow yourself to stagnate. The willingness to encounter change and undertake new activities can add pleasure to life at any age. Aging is unavoidable, but the reaction to it is largely in your own hands.

Making Community Choices

☐ What community services are available to promote health at each of the different levels and stages of life?

☐ What services do you think are needed to help people achieve optimal health through the years?

☐ Do you keep up with the federal government's plans for Social Security and Medicare? Have you taken the time to learn how these programs will affect you in the future?

Summary

✻ Aging can be defined in terms of biological age, referring to a person's physical condition; psychological age, referring to a person's coping abilities and intelligence; social age, referring to a person's habits and roles relative to society's expectations; legal age, based on chronological years; or functional age, relative to how other people function at varied ages.

✻ The growing numbers of older adults (people age 65 and older) will have a growing impact on society in terms of the economy, health care, housing, and ethical considerations.

✻ Two broad groups of theories—biological and psychosocial—purport to explain the physiological and psychological changes that occur with aging. The biological theories include the wear-and-tear theory, the cellular theory, the autoimmune theory, and the genetic mutation theory. Psychosocial theories center on adaptation and adjustments related to self-development.

✻ Aging changes the body and mind in many ways. Physical changes occur in the skin, bones and joints, head, urinary tract, heart and lungs, senses, sexual functioning, and temperature regulation. Major physical concerns are osteoporosis and urinary incontinence. Most older people maintain a high level of intelligence and memory. Potential mental problems include depression and Alzheimer's disease.

* Special challenges for older adults include alcohol abuse, prescription drug and OTC interactions, questions about vitamin and mineral supplementation, and issues regarding caregiving.

* Lifestyle choices we make today will affect health status later in life. Choosing to exercise, eat a healthy diet, and foster lasting relationships will contribute to healthy aging. Decisions about caring for older adults and stresses related to caregiving are ongoing concerns as the number of older people increases in the United States.

Questions for Discussion and Reflection

1. Discuss the various definitions of aging. At what age would you place your parents for each category?
2. As the older population grows, how will it affect your life? Would you be willing to pay higher taxes to support government social programs for older adults? For example, do you believe that Social Security should continue its yearly increases in payments, which are pegged to inflation? Why or why not?
3. Which of the biological theories of aging do you think is most correct? Why?

4. List the major physiological changes that occur with aging. Which of these, if any, can you change?
5. Explain the major health challenges that older people may face. What advice would you give to your grandparents before they took a prescription or OTC drug?
6. Discuss actions you can start taking now to help ensure a healthier aging process.

Application Exercises

Reread the What Do You Think? scenarios at the beginning of the chapter and answer the following questions.

1. If you could change elements of each of these people to make them into someone you might like to be, which person would you change and how?
2. What one or two behaviors or attitudes characterizing each of these people would make them most likely to age successfully or unsuccessfully?

3. Which of these individuals is most typical of the older people you know?
4. What things would you need to change about yourself to help you achieve your vision of successful aging?

Accessing Your Health on the Internet

Visit the following Internet sites to explore further topics and issues related to personal health. To visit an organization's website, go to the Companion Website for *Access to Health, Eighth Edition* at www.aw.com/donatelle, click on the book image, and select "Accessing Your Health on the Internet" from the navigation menu on the left.

1. *Administration on Aging.* A link to the Health and Human Services agency dedicated to addressing the health needs of older Americans.

2. *Alzheimer's Association.* Archives of media releases and position statements, fact sheets on Alzheimer's disease, medical and research updates, and a brochure on how to recognize the 10 warning signs of Alzheimer's.
3. *SeniorCom.* Homepage to a link to numerous resources for senior citizens, including chatrooms, databases, and services dedicated to assisting the aging.
4. *Social Security Online.* Provides information about Social Security benefits and entitlements. Also offers links to related sites.

Further Reading

For more information about Alzheimer's disease, contact the National Alzheimer's Association at 1-800-272-3900 or http://www.alz.org for the newest readings and research studies focusing on this problem.

Gaby, A. R. *Preventing and Reversing Osteoporosis: Every Woman's Essential Guide.* Roseville, CA: Prima Publishing, 1995.

Excellent reference text focusing on osteoporosis risk factors and what you can do to reduce risks.

The Johns Hopkins Medical Letter—Health After 50.

Comprehensive, accurate overview of health topics relevant for this population.

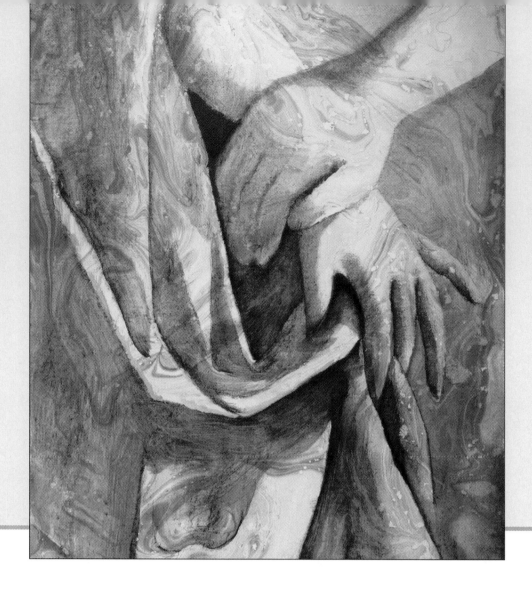

Objectives

* Define *death,* and analyze why people deny death in Western culture.

* Discuss the stages of the grieving process, and describe several strategies for coping more effectively with death.

* Describe the ethical concerns that arise from the concepts of the right to die and rational suicide.

* Review the decisions that need to be made when someone is dying or has died, including hospice care, funeral arrangements, wills, and organ donations.

Dying and Death
The Final Transition

20 20 20 20 20 20 20 20 20

What do you think?

Doug and Anthony have been domestic partners for over 15 years. Together they own a house and everything in it. Despite their attempts at discussing their relationship with their families, family members continue to disapprove. One night as Anthony is driving home from work, he is hit by a drunk driver and is taken to the hospital with severe head trauma. The prognosis for survival is not good. Doug knows that Anthony would not want to live with life-support measures keeping him alive. They have discussed these issues several times, but have never legally designated each other as primary medical decision maker. Anthony's family, not Doug, now has legal rights to make decisions about Anthony's care.

What can Doug do to make sure that Anthony gets the kind of care that Doug knows he wants?
❋ *What would you do if you faced a similar situation?*

Sheila has end-stage breast cancer. She is bedridden and experiences a great deal of pain. Her family does not want her to suffer, but they do not view physician-assisted death as an option. Sheila, however, has asked her doctor to assist her in dying when she is ready.

Do you think that Sheila has the right to end her own life? ❋ *Why or why not?* ❋ *If you were a family member, what would you do to support Sheila at this difficult time?* ❋ *What would you do in Sheila's position?*

Death eventually comes to everyone, but if you live life to the fullest and learn as much about end-of-life issues as you can, you will be better able to accept the inevitable. Distractions and denial may postpone the reality of death, but they cannot eliminate it. The acceptance of death helps shape attitudes about the importance of life. Throughout history, humans have attempted to determine the nature and meaning of death. This quest continues today. Although we will touch on moral and philosophical questions about death in this chapter, we will not explore such issues in depth. Rather, our primary focus is to present dying and death as normal components of life and to discuss how we can cope with these events.

Confrontations with death elicit different feelings depending on many factors, including age, religious beliefs, family orientation, health, personal experience with death, and the circumstances of the death itself. To cope effectively with dying, we must address the individual needs of those involved. We will identify some of these needs and offer information and suggestions that have been helpful to many people as they face this final transition. See the Assess Yourself box to evaluate your personal level of anxiety about death.

Understanding Death

Large-scale and impersonal death seems to surround us. Often sensationalized by the news media, it is regularly woven into our entertainment. In the context of this routine exposure, it seems paradoxical that Western society in the twenty-first century has been characterized as "death-denying." Why is it that we wish to deny, or even postpone, death? Let's begin by investigating what death means, at least in medical terms.

Defining Death

Dying is the process of decline in body functions resulting in the death of an organism. **Death** can be defined as the "final cessation of the vital functions" and also refers to a state in which these functions are "incapable of being restored."[1] This definition has become more significant as medical and scientific advances make it increasingly possible to postpone death.

Legal and ethical issues related to death and dying led to the Uniform Determination of Death Act in 1981, which was endorsed by the American Medical Association, the

American Bar Association, and the National Conference for Commissioners on Uniform State Laws. This act, which has been adopted by several states, reads as follows: "An individual who has sustained either (1) irreversible cessation of circulatory and respiratory functions, or (2) irreversible cessation of all functions of the entire brain, including the brain stem, is dead. A determination of death must be made in accordance with accepted medical standards."[2]

The concept of **brain death,** defined as the irreversible cessation of all functions of the entire brain stem, has gained increasing credence. As the Ad Hoc Committee of the Harvard Medical School defined it in 1968, brain death occurs when the following criteria are met:

- Unreceptivity and unresponsiveness—that is, no response even to painful stimuli.
- No movement for a continuous hour after observation by a physician and no breathing after three minutes off a respirator.
- No reflexes, including brain stem reflexes; fixed and dilated pupils.
- A "flat" EEG for at least 10 minutes.
- All of these tests repeated at least 24 hours later with no change.
- Certainty that hypothermia (extreme loss of body heat) and depression of the central nervous system caused by use of drugs such as barbiturates are not responsible for these conditions.[3]

The Harvard report provides useful guidelines; however, the definition of *death* and all its ramifications continues to concern us.

> ### What do you think?
> *Why is there so much concern over the definition of death?* ❋ *How does modern technology complicate the understanding of when death occurs?*

Denying Death

Attitudes toward death tend to fall on a continuum. At one end of the continuum, death is viewed as the mortal enemy of humankind. Both medical science and religion have promoted this idea of death. At the other end of the continuum, death is accepted and even welcomed.[4] For people whose attitudes fall at this end, death is a passage to a better state of being. But most of us perceive ourselves to be in the middle of this continuum. From this perspective, death is a bewildering mystery that elicits fear and apprehension while profoundly influencing attitudes, beliefs, and actions throughout life.

In the United States, a high level of discomfort is associated with death and dying. As a result, we may avoid speaking about death in an effort to limit our own discomfort. Those who deny death tend to do the following:

Dying The process of decline in body functions, resulting in the death of an organism.

Death The permanent ending of all vital functions.

Brain death The irreversible cessation of all functions of the entire brain stem.

Death-Related Anxiety Scale

How anxious or accepting are you about the prospect of your death? Indicate how well each statement describes your attitude.

Not true at all	0
Mainly not true	1
Not sure	2
Somewhat true	3
Very true	4

____ **1.** I tend not to be very brave in crisis situations.
____ **2.** I am an unusually anxious person.
____ **3.** I am something of a hypochondriac and am perhaps obsessively worried about infections.
____ **4.** I have never had a semimystical, spiritual, out-of-the-body, near-death, or "peak" experience.
____ **5.** I tend to be unusually frightened in planes at takeoff and landing.
____ **6.** I do not have a particular religion or philosophy that helps me to face dying.
____ **7.** I do not believe in any form of survival of the soul after death.
____ **8.** Personally, I would give a lot to be immortal in this body.
____ **9.** I am very much a city person and not really close to nature.
____ **10.** Anxiety about death spoils the quality of my life.
____ **11.** I am superstitious that preparing for dying might hasten my death.
____ **12.** I don't like the way some of my relatives died and fear that my death could be like theirs.
____ **13.** My actual experience of friends dying has been undilutedly negative.
____ **14.** I would feel easier being with a dying relative if he or she had not been told he or she was dying.
____ **15.** I have fears of dying alone without friends around me.
____ **16.** I have fears of dying slowly.
____ **17.** I have fears of dying suddenly.
____ **18.** I have fears of dying before my time or while my children are still young.
____ **19.** I have fears of dying before fulfilling my potential and fully using my talents.
____ **20.** I have fears of dying without adequately having expressed my love to those I am close to.
____ **21.** I have fears of dying before having really experienced much *joie de vivre*.
____ **22.** I have fears of what may or may not happen after death.
____ **23.** I have fears of what could happen to my family after my death.
____ **24.** I have fears of dying in a hospital or an institution.
____ **25.** I have fears of those caring for me feeling overwhelmed by the strain of it.
____ **26.** I have fears of not getting help with euthanasia when the time comes.
____ **27.** I have fears of being given unofficial and unwanted euthanasia.
____ **28.** I have fears of getting insufficient pain control while dying.
____ **29.** I have fears of being overmedicated and unconscious while dying.
____ **30.** I have fears of being declared dead when not really dead or being buried alive.
____ **31.** I have fears of getting confused at death or not being able to follow my spiritual practices.
____ **32.** I have fears of what may happen to my body after death.
____ **33.** I have fears of an Alzheimer's-type mental degeneration near death.
____ **34.** Overall I would say that I am unusually anxious about death and dying.

TOTAL

Add up your scores. If you are extremely anxious (scoring 65 or more), you might consider counseling or therapy; if you are unusually anxious (scoring between 40 and 64), you might want to find a method of meditation, philosophy, or spiritual practice to help experience, explore, and accept your feelings about death. Average anxiety is a score under 40. Continue to have a thoughtful and open ability to consider your own death in time.

Source: The New Natural Death Handbook (3rd ed., 2000). Copyright © 2000 The Natural Death Centre. Reprinted with permission.

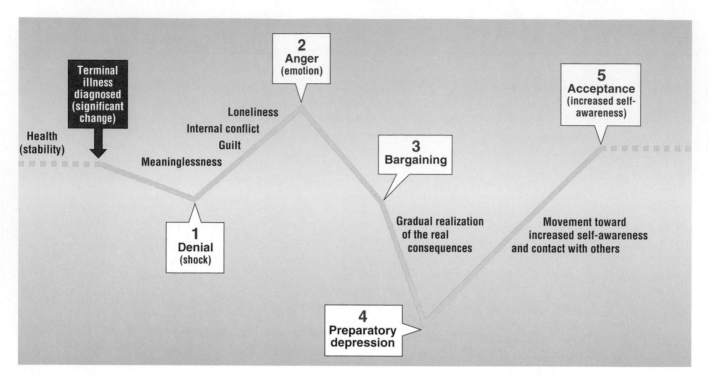

Figure 20.1
Kübler-Ross's Stages of Dying

- Avoid people who are grieving after the death of a loved one so they won't have to talk about it.
- Fail to validate a dying person's frightening situation by talking to the person as if nothing were wrong.
- Substitute euphemisms for the word *death* (a few examples are "passing away," "kicking the bucket," "no longer with us," "going to heaven," or "going to a better place").
- Give false reassurances to people who are dying by saying things like "everything is going to be okay."
- Shut off conversation about death by silencing people who are trying to talk about it.
- Avoid touching people who are dying.

Death denial has long been a predominant characteristic of our society, but we must keep in mind that social attitudes change over time. It is therefore important to understand the climate in which people developed their perceptions so we can understand their reactions to death.

Major changes in attitudes toward death accompanied the Industrial Revolution. An emphasis on autonomy and rejection of magic meant that, as a culture, Americans had to be independent and autonomous. Yet American rituals centered on connections to other people. Recent years have shown a greater effort on the part of the American public to mourn openly, as indicated by roadside crosses and memorials placed at the sites of violent or unexpected deaths. These types of impromptu memorials are a fairly new addition to the American landscape, though they have long been popular in other parts of the world, particularly in predominantly Catholic countries.[5]

The attitudes we develop about death are influenced by many factors. Modern technology, personal experiences, the environment, age, access to health care, and many other factors can influence attitudes about death and dying. The complex social environment we live in has added new experiences and sometimes confusion to the complexity of our own personal beliefs about death.

> **What do you think?**
>
> *"The art of living well and the art of dying well are one."* What do you think this quote from the Greek philosopher Epicurus means? ✳ Do you agree with it?

The Process of Dying

Dying is a complex process that includes physical, intellectual, social, spiritual, and emotional dimensions. Now that we have examined the physical indicators of death, we must consider the emotional aspects of dying and "social death."

Coping Emotionally with Death

Science and medicine have enabled us to understand changes associated with growth, development, aging, and social roles throughout the life span, but they have not fully explained the nature of death. This may partially explain why the transition from life to death evokes so much mystery and emotion. Although emotional reactions to dying vary, many people share similar experiences during this process.

Much of our knowledge about reactions to dying stems from the work of Elisabeth Kübler-Ross, a major figure in modern **thanatology,** the study of death and dying. In 1969, Kübler-Ross published *On Death and Dying,* a sensitive analysis of the reactions of terminally ill patients. This pioneering work encouraged the development of death education as a discipline and prompted efforts to improve the care of dying patients. Kübler-Ross identified five psychological stages (see Figure 20.1) that terminally ill patients often experience as they approach death:

1. *Denial.* ("Not me, there must be a mistake.") This is usually the first stage, experienced as a sensation of shock and disbelief. A person intellectually accepts the impending death but rejects it emotionally. The patient is too confused and stunned to comprehend "not being" and thus rejects the idea. Within a relatively short time, the anxiety level may diminish, enabling the patient to sort through the powerful web of emotions.
2. *Anger.* ("Why me?") Anger is another common reaction to the realization of imminent death. The person becomes angry at having to face death when others, including loved ones, are healthy and not threatened. The dying person perceives the situation as "unfair" or "senseless" and may be hostile to friends, family, physicians, or the world in general.
3. *Bargaining.* ("If I'm allowed to live, I promise...") This stage generally occurs at about the middle of the progression. The dying person may resolve to be a better person in return for an extension of life or may secretly pray for a short reprieve from death in order to experience a special event, such as a family wedding or birth.
4. *Depression.* ("It's really going to happen to me and I can't do anything about it.") Depression eventually sets in as vitality diminishes and the person begins to experience distressing symptoms with increasing frequency. The person's deteriorating condition becomes impossible for him or her to deny, and feelings of doom and tremendous loss may become unbearably pervasive. Feelings of worthlessness and guilt are also common in this depressed state because the dying person may feel responsible for the emotional suffering of loved ones and the arduous but seemingly futile efforts of caregivers.
5. *Acceptance.* ("I'm ready.") This is often the final stage. The patient stops battling with emotions and becomes tired and weak. The need to sleep increases, and wakeful periods become shorter and less frequent. With acceptance, the person does not "give up" and become sullen or resentfully resigned to death, but rather becomes passive. According to one dying person, the acceptance stage is "almost void of feelings . . . as if the pain had gone, the struggle is over, and there comes a time for the final rest before the long journey."[6] As he or she lets go, the dying person may no longer welcome visitors and may not wish to engage in conversation. Death usually occurs quietly and painlessly while the victim is unconscious.

The health care profession immediately embraced Kübler-Ross's "stage theory" and hastily applied it in clinical settings. However, some of Kübler-Ross's contemporaries consider her stage theory too neat and orderly. Subsequent research has indicated that the experiences of dying people do not fit easily into specific stages, and patterns vary from person to person. Research evidence supporting the concept of stages of grief is neither extensive nor convincing. Although it is normal to grieve when a severe loss has been sustained, some people never go through this process and instead remain emotionally calm. Others may pass back and forth between the stages. Even if it is not accurate in all its particulars, however, Kübler-Ross's theory offers valuable insights for those seeking to understand or deal with the process of dying.

> ### What do you think?
> *Do you agree with Elisabeth Kübler-Ross's stages of dying? ✷ Do you think it is important to help a person get through all the stages that Kübler-Ross has identified? ✷ Why or why not?*

Social Death

The need for recognition and appreciation within a social group is nearly universal. Although the size and nature of the social group may vary widely, the need to belong exists in all of us. Loss of being valued or appreciated by others can lead to **social death,** a seemingly irreversible situation in which a person is not treated like an active member of society. Dramatic examples of social death include the exile of nonconformists from their native countries or the excommunication of dissident members of religious groups. More often, however, social death is inflicted by denying a person normal social interaction. Numerous studies indicate that people are treated differently when they are dying. The following common behaviors contribute to the social death that often isolates people who are terminally ill:

- The dying person is referred to as if he or she were already dead.
- The dying person may be inadvertently excluded from conversations.
- Dying patients are often moved to terminal wards and are given minimal care.
- Bereaved family members are avoided, often for extended periods, because friends and neighbors are afraid of feeling uncomfortable in the presence of grief.
- Medical personnel may make degrading comments about patients in their presence.[7]

This decrease in meaningful social interaction often strips dying and bereaved people of their identity as valued members of society at a time when belonging is critical.

> **Thanatology** The study of death and dying.
>
> **Social death** A seemingly irreversible situation in which a person is not treated like an active member of society.

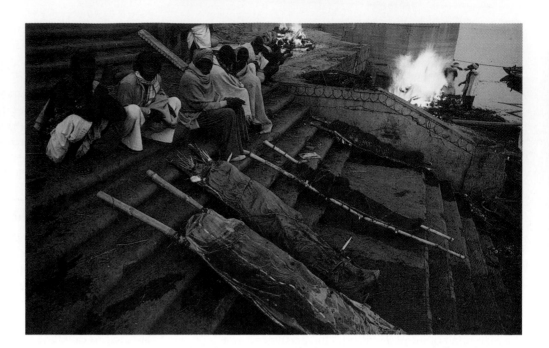

There is no single way to mourn. Each culture has its own unique ways of saying goodbye to the deceased.

Some dying people choose not to speak of their inevitable fate in an attempt to make others feel more comfortable and thus preserve vital relationships.

Coping with Loss

The losses resulting from the death of a loved one are extremely difficult to cope with. The dying person, as well as close family and friends, frequently suffers emotionally and physically from the impending loss of critical relationships and roles. Words used to describe feelings and behavior related to losses resulting from death include *bereavement, grief, grief work,* and *mourning.* These terms are related but not identical in meaning. Understanding them may help in comprehending the emotional processes associated with loss and the cultural constraints that often inhibit normal coping behavior (see Figure 20.2).

Bereavement is generally defined as the loss or deprivation experienced by a survivor when a loved one dies. Because relationships vary in type and intensity, reactions to

losses also vary. The death of a parent, spouse, sibling, child, friend, or pet will result in different kinds of feelings. In the lives of the bereaved or of close survivors, "holes" will be left by the loss of loved ones. We can think of bereavement as the awareness of these holes. Time and courage are necessary to fill these spaces.

A special case of bereavement occurs in old age. Loss is an intrinsic part of growing old. The longer we live, the more losses we are likely to experience. These losses include physical, social, and emotional losses as our bodies deteriorate and more and more of our loved ones die. The theory of *bereavement overload* has been proposed to explain the effects of multiple losses and the accumulation of sorrow in the lives of some elderly people. This theory suggests that the gloomy outlook, disturbing behavior patterns, and apparent apathy that characterize these people may be related more to bereavement overload than to intrinsic physiological degeneration in old age.[8]

Grief is a state of mental distress that occurs in reaction to significant loss, including one's own impending death, the death of a loved one, or a quasi-death experience (to be discussed later in this chapter). Grief reactions include any adjustments needed for one to "make it through the day" and may include changes in patterns of eating, sleeping, working, and even thinking.

When a person experiences a loss that cannot be openly acknowledged, publicly mourned, or socially supported, coping may be much more difficult. This type of grief is referred to as **disenfranchised grief.**[9] It may occur among those who miscarry, are developmentally disabled, or are close friends rather than relatives of the deceased. It may also include those relationships that are not socially approved, such as those between extramarital lovers or homosexual couples. When society does not assign significance to a high-grief death, grieving becomes more difficult for the bereaved.

Bereavement The loss or deprivation experienced by a survivor when a loved one dies.

Grief The state of mental distress that occurs in reaction to significant loss, including one's own impending death, the death of a loved one, or a quasi-death experience.

Disenfranchised grief Grief concerning a loss that cannot be openly acknowledged, publicly mourned, or socially supported.

Mourning The culturally prescribed behavior patterns for the expression of grief.

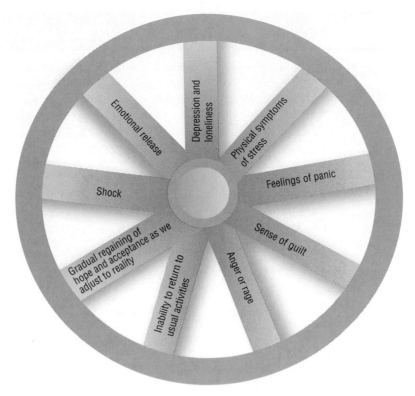

Figure 20.2
The Stages of Grief
People react differently to losses, but most eventually adjust. Generally, the stronger the social support system, the smoother the progression through the stages of grief.

The term *mourning* is often incorrectly equated with the term *grief*. As we have noted, *grief* refers to a wide variety of feelings and actions that occur in response to bereavement. **Mourning**, in contrast, refers to culturally prescribed and accepted time periods and behavior patterns for the expression of grief. In Judaism, for example, "sitting *shivah*" is a designated mourning period of seven days that involves prescribed rituals and prayers. Depending on a person's relationship with the deceased, various other rituals may continue for up to a year.

In some cases, people are so overwhelmed by grief that they do not return to normal daily living. Support and counseling should be sought when this occurs. Doctors, nurses, psychologists, psychiatrists, and clergy can be helpful in solving problems associated with the loss of a loved one.

Symptoms of grief vary in severity and duration, depending on the situation and the individual. However, the bereaved person can benefit from emotional and social support from family, friends, clergy, employers, and traditional support organizations, including the medical community and the funeral industry. The larger and stronger the support system, the easier readjustment is likely to be. See the Skills for Behavior Change box to learn about how you can best help a grieving friend.

Religion provides comfort to many dying and grieving people. Although some people question the existence of an afterlife, others gain support from religious beliefs that pro- vide a purpose and meaning to life. By accepting dying as a part of the continuum of life, many people are able to make necessary readjustments after the death of a loved one. This holistic concept, which accepts dying as a part of the total life experience, is shared by both believers and nonbelievers.

What Is "Normal" Grief?

This is a difficult question to answer. Grief responses vary widely from person to person. Despite these differences, a classic acute grief syndrome often occurs when a person acknowledges a loss. This common reaction can include the following symptoms:

- Periodic waves of physical distress lasting 20 minutes to an hour.
- A feeling of tightness in the throat.
- Choking and shortness of breath.
- A frequent need to sigh.
- A feeling of emptiness in the abdomen.
- A sensation of muscular weakness.
- Intense anxiety that is described as actually painful.

Other common symptoms of grief include insomnia, memory lapse, loss of appetite, difficulty concentrating, a tendency to engage in repetitive or purposeless behavior, an "observer" sensation or feeling of unreality, difficulty in making decisions, lack of organization, excessive speech, social

Talking to Friends When Someone Dies

I t's always hard to know just what to say, and how to say it, when talking with a grieving friend or relative. Sometimes, even though we mean well, what we say can hurt more than help. Here are some do's and don'ts:

1. Be honest. If you don't know what to say, don't be afraid to say so.
2. Respect your friend's need for privacy.
3. Send a card with a handwritten message, note, or letter expressing your sorrow.
4. Share your fond memories of the person who died.
5. Don't judge the way in which a person grieves.
6. Don't assume that the person thinks the death was "for the best."
7. Don't say "I know how you feel," no matter what your experience has been.
8. Don't ask for things that belonged to the person who passed away.
9. Don't make parallels with animals—don't compare a dog's death with a person's.

Source: Don't Ask for the Dead Man's Golf Clubs: What to Do and Say (And What Not To) When A Friend Loses a Loved One, by L. Kelly (New York: Workman, 2000).

withdrawal or hostility, guilt feelings, and preoccupation with the image of the deceased. Susceptibility to disease increases with grief and may even be life threatening in severe and enduring cases.

A bereaved person may suffer emotional pain and may exhibit a variety of grief responses for many months after the death of a loved one. The rate of the healing process depends on the amount and quality of grief work that a person does. **Grief work** is the process of integrating the reality of the loss into everyday life and learning to feel better. Often, the bereaved person must deliberately and systematically work at reducing denial and coping with the pain that results from memories of the deceased. This process takes time and requires emotional effort.

Not everyone grieves in the same way. For differences between how women and men grieve, see the Women's Health/Men's Health box.

What do you think?

Do you think men grieve differently than women do? ☀ What have you personally observed about these differences, if any?

When an Infant or a Child Dies

At the beginning of the twentieth century, children under the age of 15 made up 34 percent of the U.S. population but accounted for 53 percent of total deaths. Eighty years later, children made up only 22 percent of the population and merely 3 percent of total deaths.[10] Children are highly valued in our society, and their deaths are considered major tragedies. No matter what the cause of premature death— miscarriage, fatal birth defects, childhood illness, accident, suicide, homicide, or war injuries—the grief experienced when a child dies may be overwhelming.

The death of a child is terribly painful for the whole family. However, for several reasons, the siblings of the deceased

child have a particularly hard time with grief work. Bereaved children usually have limited experience with death and therefore have not yet learned how to deal with major loss. Children may feel uncomfortable talking about death, and they may also receive less social support and sympathy than do the parents of the deceased child. Because so much attention and energy are devoted to the deceased child, the surviving children may feel emotionally abandoned by their parents.

A Child's Response to Death

In the past, children were thought to be miniature adults and were expected to behave as adults. It is now understood that children and adults react to death quite differently. Often, when children suffer a loss, they will react in ways that seem "normal" to the adult observer. However, children often do not show their feelings as openly as adults do. Although their actions may not reveal what they are truly feeling, children tend to experience more prolonged mourning periods. They typically grapple with these questions: (1) Did I cause the death to happen? (2) Is it going to happen to me? (3) Who is

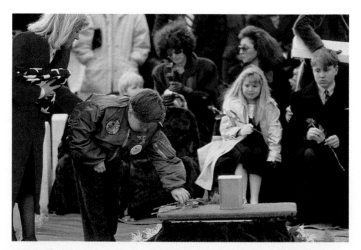

A significant loss can be particularly difficult for children.

Gender Differences in the Bereavement Experience

Although men and women suffer through similar stages of bereavement, a Harvard study pointed out interesting differences in how men and women interpret their feelings of loss immediately after the death of a spouse.

WOMEN

- Women emphasized a sense of abandonment and spoke of being alone. They felt deprived of a comforting person.

- Women tended to regard the funeral director and staff as supportive and caring people, rather than business people.
- The funeral process was important for women in reaching the realization that their spouses were gone forever.
- Widows showed more emotions to other people.
- Women most often provided help to others.

MEN

- Men reported feeling a sort of dismemberment. They felt as if both arms and legs were being cut off.
- Men expressed less gratitude toward the funeral directors and usually expressed concern over cost.

- Men felt that the funeral was just something to get through.
- Widowers showed fewer emotions to other people. Those offering help to the widower were more likely to offer practical help rather than emotional support.
- Widowers began dating and remarrying sooner than did widows. But this did not mean they had worked through their emotional attachment to their late spouse.

Source: Adapted from *Death, Society, and Human Experience* (7th ed.) by R. J. Kastenbaum (Boston: Allyn & Bacon). Copyright © 1999 by Pearson Education

going to take care of me?[11] A child's grieving period may be less stressful when adults are open and honest and include the child in the funeral process as much as possible.

Quasi-Death Experiences

Many cultures provide social and emotional support for the bereaved in the aftermath of death. Typically, however, little support is offered when people face many other significant losses in life. Losses that in many ways resemble death and that may involve a heavy burden of grief include a child running away from home, an abduction or kidnapping, a divorce, a move to a distant place, a move to a nursing home, the loss of a romance or intimate friendship, retirement, job termination, finishing a "terminal" academic degree, or ending an athletic career.

These **quasi-death experiences**[12] resemble death in that they involve separation, termination, loss, and a change in identity or self-perception. If grief results from these losses, the pattern of the grief response will probably follow the same course as responses to death. Factors that may complicate the grieving process associated with quasi-death include uncomfortable contact with the object of loss (for example, an ex-spouse) and a lack of adequate social and institutional support.

Living with Death and Loss

The reality of death and loss touches everyone. Although the accompanying grief causes painful emotions, it can also bring strength. C. M. Parkes, a British researcher in the psychiatric aspects of bereavement, observed that

the experience of grieving can strengthen and bring maturity to those who have previously been protected from misfortune. The pain of grief is just as much a part of life as the joy of love; it is, perhaps, the price we pay for love, the cost of commitment. To ignore this fact, or to pretend that it is not so [would] leave us unprepared for the losses that will inevitably occur in our lives and unprepared to help others cope with the losses in theirs.[13]

Life-and-Death Decision Making

Many complex and often expensive life-and-death decisions must be made during a highly distressing period in people's lives. These emotion-laden decisions are compounded by the stresses of dying and bereavement. We will not attempt to present definitive answers to moral and philosophical questions about death; instead, we offer these topics for your consideration. We hope that this discussion of the needs of the dying person and the bereaved will help you negotiate these difficult decisions in the future.

Grief work The process of accepting the reality of a person's death and coping with memories of the deceased.

Quasi-death experience A loss or experience that resembles death, in that it involves separation, termination, significant loss, a change of personal identity, and grief.

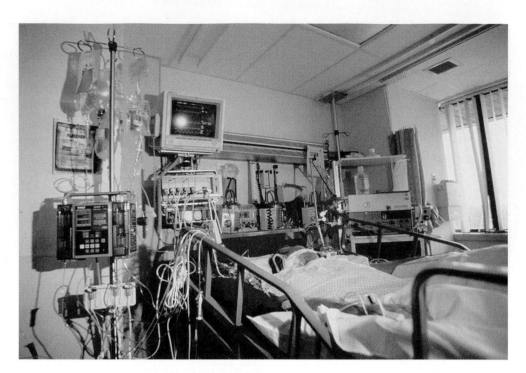

Sophisticated life-support technology allows a patient's life to be prolonged even in cases of terminal illness or mortal injury. It has also raised legal and moral questions for patients, their families, and health care professionals.

The Right to Die

Few people would object to a proposal for the right to a dignified death. Going beyond that concept, however, many people today believe that they should be allowed to die if their condition is terminal and their existence depends on mechanical life support devices or artificial feeding or hydration systems. Artificial life support techniques that may be legally refused by competent patients in some states include the following:

- Electrical or mechanical heart resuscitation.
- Mechanical respiration by machine.
- Nasogastric tube feedings.
- Intravenous nutrition.
- Gastrostomy (tube feeding directly into the stomach).
- Medications to treat life-threatening infections.

As long as a person is conscious and competent, he or she has the legal right to refuse treatment, even if this decision will hasten death. However, when a person is in a coma or otherwise incapable of speaking on his or her own behalf, medical personnel and administrative policy will dictate treatment. This issue has evolved into a battle involving personal freedom, legal rulings, health care administration policy, and physician responsibility. The living will was developed to assist in solving conflicts among these people and agencies.

Cases have been reported in which the wishes of people who had signed a living will (or advance directive) indicating their desire not to receive artificial life support were not honored by their physician or medical institution. This problem can be avoided by choosing both a physician and a hospital that will carry out the directives of the living will. Taking this precaution and discussing your personal philosophy and wishes with your family should eliminate anxiety about how you will be treated at the end of your life (see Figure 20.3).

Many legal experts suggest that you take the following steps to ensure that your wishes are carried out:

1. *Get specific.* Rather than signing an advance directive (that only speaks in generalities), fill out a directive that permits you to make specific choices about a variety of procedures, including cardiopulmonary resuscitation (CPR); dialysis; being placed on a ventilator; being given food, water, or medication through tubes; being given pain medication; and organ donation. It is also essential to attach that document to a completed copy of the standard advance directive for your state.
2. *Get an agent.* Even the most detailed directive cannot possibly anticipate every situation that may arise. You may want to also appoint a family member or friend to act as your agent, or *proxy,* by making out a form known as either a durable power of attorney for health care or a health care proxy.
3. *Discuss your wishes.* Discuss your wishes in detail with your proxy and your doctor. Your doctor or proxy may misinterpret or ignore your wishes. Going over the situations described in the form will give them a clear idea of just how much you are willing to endure to preserve your life.
4. *Deliver the directive.* Distribute several copies, not only to your doctor and your agent but also to your lawyer and to immediate family members or a close friend. Make sure *someone* knows to bring a copy to the hospital in the event you are hospitalized.[14]

Rational Suicide

We have discussed suicide in earlier chapters as a consequence of depression or other factors. The concept of **rational suicide** as an alternative to an extended dying process, however, deserves mention here. Rational suicide is a result of a reasoned, coherent process in which a person

This directive is made this _____ day of _____ (month) _____ (year). I, _____ being of sound mind, willfully and voluntarily make known my desire

    (a) ☐ **That my life shall not be artificially prolonged** and

    (b) ☐ **That my life shall be ended with the aid of a physician under circumstances set forth below, and do hereby declare:**
        (You must initial (a) or (b), or both.)

1. If at any time I should have a terminal condition or illness certified to be terminal by two physicians, and they determine that my death will occur within six months,

    (a) ☐ **I direct that life-sustaining procedures be withheld or withdrawn** and

    (b) ☐ **I direct that my physician administer aid-in-dying in a humane and dignified manner.** (You must initial (a) or (b), or both.)

    (c) ☐ **I have attached Special Instructions on a separate page to the directive.** (Initial if you have attached a separate page.)

The action taken under this paragraph shall be at the time of my own choosing if I am competent.

2. In the absence of my ability to give directions regarding the termination of my life, it is my intention that this directive shall be honored by my family, agent (described in paragraph 4), and physician(s) as the final expression of my legal right to

    (a) ☐ **Refuse medical or surgical treatment,** and

    (b) ☐ **To choose to die in a humane and dignified manner.** (You must initial (a) or (b), or both and you must initial one box below.)

        ☐ If I am unable to give directions, I *do not* want my attorney-in-fact to request aid-in-dying.

        ☐ If I am unable to give directions, I *do* want my attorney-in-fact to ask my physician for aid-in-dying.

3. I understand that a terminal condition is one in which I am not likely to live for more than six months.

4. a. I, _____
do hereby designate and appoint _____
as my attorney-in-fact (agent) to make health-care decisions for me if I am in a coma or otherwise unable to decide for myself as authorized in this document. For the purpose of this document, "health-care decision" means consent, refusal of consent, or withdrawal of consent to any care, treatment, service, or procedure to maintain, diagnose, or treat an individual's physical or mental condition, or to administer aid-in-dying.

    b. By this document I intend to create a Durable Power of Attorney for Health Care under The Oregon Death With Dignity Act and ORS Section 126.407. This power of attorney shall not be affected by my subsequent incapacity, except by revocation.

    c. Subject to any limitations in this document, I hereby grant to my agent full power and authority to make health-care decisions for me to the same extent that I could make these decisions for myself if I had the capacity to do so. In exercising this authority, my agent shall make health-care decisions that are consistent with my desires as stated in this document or otherwise made known to my agent, including, but not limited to, my desires concerning obtaining, refusing, or withdrawing life-prolonging care, treatment, services, and procedures, and administration of aid-in-dying.

5. This directive shall have no force or effect seven years from the date filled in above, unless I am competent to act on my own behalf and then it shall remain valid until my competency is restored.

6. I recognize that a physician's judgment is not always certain, and that medical science continues to make progress in extending life, but in spite of these facts, I nevertheless wish aid-in-dying rather than letting my terminal condition take its natural course.

7. My family has been informed of my request to die, their opinions have been taken into consideration, but the final decision remains mine, so long as I am competent.

8. The exact time of my death will be determined by me and my physician with my desire or my attorney-in-fact's instructions paramount.

I have given full consideration and understand the full import of this directive, and I am emotionally and mentally competent to make this directive. I accept the moral and legal responsibility for receiving aid-in-dying.

This directive will not be valid unless it is signed by two qualified witnesses who are present when you sign or acknowledge your signature. The witnesses must not be related to you by blood, marriage, or adoption; they must not be entitled to any part of your estate; and they must not include a physician or other person responsible for, or employed by anyone responsible for, your health care. If you have attached any additional pages to this form, you must date and sign each of the additional pages at the same time you date and sign this power of attorney.

Signed: _____

_____
City, County, and State of Residence

This document must be witnessed by two qualified adult witnesses. None of the following may be used as witnesses: (1) a health-care provider who is involved in any way with the treatment of the declarant, (2) an employee of a health-care provider who is involved in any way with the treatment of the declarant, (3) the operator of a community care facility where the declarant resides, (4) an employee of an operator of a community care facility who is involved in any way with the treatment of the declarant.

Figure 20.3
Directive to Physicians
Source: The Oregon Death with Dignity Act, Oregon Revised Statutes, Chapter 97, 1990.

chooses death as a preferable alternative to unbearable pain. Although exact numbers are not known, medical ethicists, experts in rational suicide, and specialists in forensic medicine (the study of legal issues in medicine) estimate that thousands of terminally ill people every year decide to kill themselves rather than endure constant pain and slow decay. To these people, the prospect of an undignified death is unacceptable. This issue has been complicated by advances in death prevention techniques that allow terminally ill patients to exist in an irreversible disease state for extended periods of time. Medical personnel, clergy, lawyers, and patients all must struggle with this ethical dilemma.

Still, questions remain. Do we have a right to die? If so, is this an unlimited right, or does it apply only to certain conditions? If terminally ill patients are allowed to commit suicide legally, what other groups will demand this option? Should the courts be involved in private decisions? Should any organization be allowed to distribute information that may encourage suicide? Should loved ones or medical caregivers be allowed to assist the person who wants to die by providing the means?

Dyathanasia is intentionally prolonging the dying process. Examples would include resuscitation of a person who is terminal or refusing to give pain control if it would shorten life. Euthanasia is often referred to as "mercy killing." The term **active euthanasia** has been given to ending the life of a person (or animal) that is suffering greatly and has no chance of recovery. An example might be a physician-prescribed lethal injection. **Passive euthanasia** refers to the intentional withholding of treatment that would prolong life. Deciding not to place a person with massive brain trauma on life support is an example of passive euthanasia.

Dr. Jack Kevorkian, a physician in Michigan, has started a one-person campaign to force the medical profession to change its position regarding physician-assisted death. Kevorkian has assisted many terminally ill patients in dying, and until recently, had escaped conviction despite being taken into court several times for his actions. Kevorkian has argued that the Hippocratic oath, an ancient ethical pledge still taken by medical students, is not binding. He believes that the present situations in our society demand a shift in the thinking and practices that medicine has had throughout most of human history. He believes that acceptance of euthanasia, specifically physician-assisted death, is one of those changes. In 1998, Kevorkian took his argument to prime time, as the CBS News program *60 Minutes* broadcast his latest case of assisting a terminally ill patient with ending his life. This time, however, the courts determined that Kevorkian's methods had gone too far, and in 1999 he was convicted of murder and sentenced to prison, where he remains.

Kevorkian's actions have focused a great deal of attention on the issue, causing many to speculate on the merits of physician-assisted suicide. A study in Michigan revealed that a greater number of physicians were in favor of legalizing assisted suicide than were against it.[15] A similar study in Oregon found that physicians have a more favorable attitude toward legalized physician-assisted suicide, are more willing to participate, and are currently participating in greater numbers than other surveyed groups in the United States.[16] In both studies, a sizable minority of physicians had a number of reservations about the practical applications of the proposed law legalizing physician-assisted suicide.

> **What do you think?**
>
> *Are there any end-of-life situations in which you would ask a physician to help you die?* ❋ *Explain your answer. Do you believe people should have the right to ask a physician to help them die?* ❋ *Why or why not?* ❋ *See the Health Ethics box for more debate on physician-assisted suicide.*

Taking Care of Business

Caring for dying people and dealing with the practical and legal questions surrounding death can be difficult and painful. The problems of the dying person and the bereaved loved ones involve a wide variety of psychological, legal, social, spiritual, economic, and interpersonal issues. We will now examine several practical problems associated with death and will present a humanitarian alternative as a possible solution.

Hospice Care: Positive Alternatives

Since the mid-1970s, **hospice** programs have grown from a mere handful to more than 2,500, available in nearly every community. Unlike even 10 years ago, families facing terminal illness are often expected to make difficult medical decisions, including where their loved ones will die. Improving the quality of care at the end of life is a top priority of the American Medical Association.

Rational suicide   The decision to kill oneself rather than endure constant pain and slow decay.

Dyathanasia   Intentionally prolonging the dying process. Examples would include resuscitation of a person who is terminal or refusing to give pain control if it would shorten life.

Active euthanasia   "Mercy killing," in which a person or organization knowingly acts to hasten the death of a terminally ill person.

Passive euthanasia   The intentional withholding of treatment that would prolong life.

Hospice   A concept of care for terminally ill patients designed to maximize quality of life.

Is Physician-Assisted Suicide Ethical?

Physician-assisted suicide (PAS) has caused a furor in the media and debate within the medical and legal professions. Consider the reasoning that follows as you develop your own position on this issue.

ARGUMENTS IN FAVOR OF PAS

Those who believe that PAS is ethically justified offer the following reasons:

1. *Respect for autonomy.* Decisions about time and circumstances of death are very personal. Competent persons should have the right to choose death.
2. *Justice.* Justice requires that we "treat like cases alike." Competent terminally ill patients are allowed to hasten death by refusing treatment. But for some patients, cutting off treatment will not suffice to hasten death; their only real option is suicide. Justice requires that we should allow assisted death for these patients.
3. *Compassion.* Suffering means more than pain; other physical and psychological burdens also accompany some forms of terminal illness. It is not always possible to relieve suffering. Thus PAS may be a compassionate response to unbearable suffering.
4. *Individual liberty versus state interest.* Though society has a strong interest in preserving life, that interest lessens when a person is terminally ill and has a strong desire to end life. A complete prohibition on assisted death excessively limits personal liberty. Therefore PAS should be allowed in certain cases.
5. *Openness of discussion.* Some would argue that assisted death already occurs, albeit in secret. For example, morphine drips ostensibly for pain relief may be a covert form of assisted death or euthanasia. The fact that PAS is illegal prevents open discussion of the issue and fosters secrecy in administration of PAS. Legalization of PAS would promote open discussion.

ARGUMENTS AGAINST PAS

Those who believe that PAS should remain illegal often present arguments like these:

1. *Sanctity of life.* This argument points out strong religious and secular traditions against taking human life. It is argued that assisted suicide is morally wrong because it contradicts these beliefs.
2. *Passive versus active distinction.* This arguments holds that there is an important difference between passively "letting die" and actively "killing." It is argued that refusing treatment or withholding treatment is equivalent to letting die (a passive measure) and therefore justifiable, whereas PAS is equivalent to killing (an active measure) and is not justifiable.
3. *Potential for abuse.* Certain groups of people, lacking access to care and support, may be pushed into assisted death. Furthermore, assisted death may become a cost-containment strategy. Burdened family members and health care providers may unscrupulously encourage the option of assisted death in certain cases. To protect against these abuses, it is argued, PAS should remain illegal.
4. *Professional integrity.* Here opponents point to the historical ethical traditions of medicine, strongly opposed to taking life. For instance, the Hippocratic oath states, "I will not administer poison to anyone where asked" and "Be of benefit, or at least do no harm." Furthermore, major professional groups (such as the American Medical Association and the American Geriatrics Society) oppose assisted death because linking PAS to the practice of medicine could harm the public's image of the profession.
5. *Fallibility of the profession.* Another concern is based on the acknowledgment that physicians will make mistakes. For instance, there may be uncertainty in diagnosis and prognosis, errors in diagnosis and treatment of depression, or inadequate treatment of pain. Thus the state has an obligation to protect lives from these inevitable mistakes.

What are your feelings about PAS? Under what circumstances might you consider it an acceptable option? Under what circumstances should it not be an option? Where should the line be drawn?

Source: Excerpted from C. H. Braddock and M. R. Tonelli, "Physician-Assisted Suicide," *Ethics in Medicine,* February 22, 1999 (see http://eduserv.hscer.washington.edu/bioethics/topics/pas.html).

The primary goals of the hospice program are to relieve the dying person's pain, offer emotional support to the dying person and loved ones, and restore a sense of control to the dying person, family, and friends. Although home care with maximum involvement by loved ones is emphasized, hospice programs are directed by cooperating physicians, coordinated by specially trained nurses, and fortified with the services of counselors, clergy, and trained volunteers. Hospital inpatient beds are available if necessary. Hospice programs usually include the following characteristics:

1. The patient and family constitute the unit of care, because the physical, psychological, social, and spiritual problems of dying confront the family as well as the patient.
2. Emphasis is placed on symptom control, primarily the alleviation of pain. Curative treatments are curtailed as requested by the patient, but sound judgment must be applied to avoid a feeling of abandonment.
3. There is overall medical direction of the program, with all health care being provided under the direction of a qualified physician.

4. Services are provided by an interdisciplinary team because no one person can provide all the needed care.
5. Coverage is provided 24 hours a day, seven days a week, with emphasis on the availability of medical and nursing skills.
6. Carefully selected and extensively trained volunteers are an integral part of the health care team, augmenting staff service but not replacing it.
7. Care of the family extends through the bereavement period.
8. Patients are accepted on the basis of their health needs, not their ability to pay.

Despite the growing number of people considering the hospice option, many people prefer to go to a hospital to die. Others choose to die at home, without the intervention of medical staff or life-prolonging equipment. Each dying person and his or her family should decide as early as possible what type of terminal care is most desirable and feasible. This will allow time for necessary emotional, physical, and financial preparations. Hospice care may also help the survivors cope better with the death experience. See the Skills for Behavior Change box for information on how to prepare yourself if you expect to be with a dying person.

Making Funeral Arrangements

Anthropological evidence indicates that all cultures throughout history have developed some sort of funeral ritual. For this reason, social scientists agree that funerals assist survivors of the deceased in coping with their loss.

In the United States, with its diversity of religious, regional, and ethnic customs, funeral patterns vary. (See the Health in a Diverse World box for information on the

---

SKILLS FOR BEHAVIOR CHANGE

Preparing to Support a Dying Person

Whether we have months to prepare for death or it comes suddenly, most people have difficulty knowing what to do. We push death from our consciousness in ways that may lead to problems as the moment of death comes for loved ones and after that moment passes. Although you can never be fully prepared for the loss of a loved one, you can learn skills that will help you through the trauma of loss. The following things to think about may help you, particularly in situations such as hospice care where you have time to prepare yourself.

1. *Follow the wishes of the patient.* Make sure that a copy of his or her advance directive is available and is accepted as the wishes of the patient. Most people, particularly in hospice, want a natural death. Think of "comfort," not "cure." Whenever possible, try to talk to the patient and allow choices to be made about the dying process. For example, if the person wants to stay in her own bed but a hospital bed would be easier for those providing care at home, talk it out with her.

2. *Help with comfort and rest.* Don't be afraid to ask for medications to help with pain, sleeping, or anxiety.

3. *Prepare a list of people to call near the time of death, including family, friends, and religious support.* Talk about who the patient wants present, if anyone. Make a list of people to notify once death occurs. Keep a list of home health nurses, hospice staff, and physicians nearby, so that they can be contacted without delays.

4. *Call for professional help if any of the following occur:*
   - Extreme pain or discomfort.
   - Difficulty breathing. Oxygen can help calm the patient and make the last hours more comfortable.
   - Trouble urinating or passing stool. Usually the urine will be dark and in small quantity. Medications can help ease discomfort.
   - Emotions getting the best of you. Thoughts of impending loss can prevent you from being supportive to the dying person.

5. *Touching is often comforting for the dying person.* Give back, hand, or foot rubs. Do not stand back and avoid contact. Help the patient adjust his or her position in bed if at all possible. Usually an extra sheet under the patient and the aid of a second person will make this easier.

6. *Moisten the eyes and lips with warm, damp cloths and apply skin lotions to ensure comfort.* Apply warm or cool compresses if the person wants them.

7. *Know what to expect.* Be ready to say goodbye. Talk to the person. In some cases soft, relaxing music may be comforting. During the last moments of life, the body begins to slow down, breathing rates slow, sometimes there are long pauses between breaths. Sometimes the person will appear to wake up. He or she may or may not be able to speak or recognize you. Usually this means patients are in or near coma state, and they may progress to longer and longer periods of sleep. The skin may be cool, especially around the feet and hands, and may become blue- or gray-tinged. In the last stages, as death nears, the person may become incontinent or lose bowel control. Finally, the chest will stop rising, the eyes may appear glassy, and there will be no more pulse.

8. *You may choose to assist with preparing the body for transport to the funeral home or other facility, or you may choose to let others take over.* Try to think about this in advance and make decisions based on your own preferences and needs.

practices of several religious traditions.) In some faiths, prior to body disposal, the deceased may be displayed to formalize last respects and increase social support of the bereaved. This part of the funeral ritual is referred to as a **wake** or **viewing.** The body of the deceased is usually embalmed prior to viewing to retard decomposition and minimize offensive odors. The funeral service may be held in a church, in a funeral chapel, or at the burial site. Some people choose to replace the funeral service with a simple memorial service held within a few days of the burial. Social interaction associated with funeral and memorial services is valuable in helping survivors cope with their losses.

Common methods of body disposal include burial in the ground, entombment above ground in a mausoleum, cremation, and anatomical donation. Expenses involved in body disposal vary according to the method chosen and the available options. It should be noted that if burial is selected, an additional charge may be assessed for a burial vault. Burial vaults—concrete or metal containers that hold the casket— are required by most cemeteries to limit settling of the gravesite as the casket disintegrates and collapses. Choosing

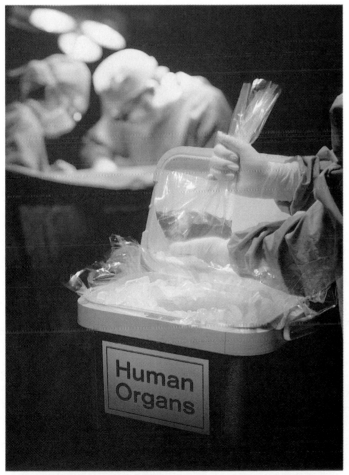

Organ donor programs provide registered donors with the satisfaction of knowing that they may save another person's life. Taking time to register with such a program also expedites the transfer of viable organs when the donor dies.

National Kidney Foundation

Please detach and give this portion
of the card to my family

This is to inform you that, should the occasion ever arise, I would like to be an organ and tissue donor. Please see that my wishes are carried out by informing the attending medical personnel that I have indicated my wishes to become a donor.
Thank you.

Signature   Date

For further information write or call:
National Kidney Foundation
30 East 33rd Street, New York, NY 10016
(800) 622-9010

- -

Uniform Donor Card

Of _____
(print or type name of donor)

In the hope that I may help others, I hereby make this anatomical gift, if medically acceptable, to take effect upon my death. The words and marks below indicate my wishes.
I give: ☐ any needed organs or parts
         ☐ only the following organs or parts

_____
(specify the organ(s), tissue(s) or part(s))

for the purposes of transplantation, therapy, medical research or education;
         ☐ my body for anatomical study if needed.
Limitations or special wishes, if any. _____

Figure 20.4
Organ Donor Card Provided by the National Kidney Foundation
Source: Reprinted with permission from "Uniform Donor Card," © National Kidney Foundation, Inc.

the actual container for the remains of the dead person is only one of many tasks that must be dealt with when a person dies. There are many other decisions concerning the funeral ritual that can be burdensome for survivors.

Pressures on Survivors

Funeral practices in the United States today are extremely varied. A great number of decisions have to be made, usually within 24 hours. These decisions relate to the method and

Wake or **viewing**   Displaying of the deceased to formalize last respects and increase social support of the bereaved.

Funeral and Mourning Customs around the World

Every culture recognizes death as a significant rite of passage. Yet the traditions associated with death vary a great deal, reflecting differing cultures and religious practices. Uncertainty or discomfort can result if you are involved in a religious mourning cermony that involves customs with which you are not familiar. For example, if you were not raised as a Catholic, you might be unsure about the significance and proper behavior at a wake. The following summaries are intended to familiarize you with some of the wonderful variety in approaches to death and grieving. We have focused on practices other than traditional Christian ones (such as Catholic, Protestant, or Baptist) in order to show the wide variety of possible practices.

Baha'i: The Baha'i faith has few teachings regarding the actual rituals of funerals. It does advise that the deceased not be embalmed, unless required by state law. Also, the deceased should be buried within one hour's travel time from the place of death, since the Baha'i faith teaches that we are all world citizens and should not be attached to a particular geographical site.

Buddhism: In several Japanese Buddhist traditions a funeral cermony resembles a Christian ceremony, with a eulogy and prayers at a funeral home. Cambodian, Thai, and Sri Lankan traditions may have up to three ceremonies. In the first, which is held two days after the death, monks hold a ceremony at the home of the bereaved. In the second, which is held two to five days after the death, monks conduct a ceremony at a funeral home, and at the third, which is held seven days after burial or cremation, monks lead a ceremony either at a temple or at the home of the bereaved. This last cermony, called a "merit transference," seeks to generate good energy for the deceased in his or her new incarnation. There is always an open casket, with the sight of the body reminding guests of the impermanence of life.

Christian Science: There are no special rituals for funerals or mourning and funeral services are optional. Since the church does not have formal clergy, if there is a service it is conducted by a church member who is an experienced Chrisitan Scientist or by a friend of the deceased. Typically the service consists of readings from the Bible and from works by the founder of Christian Science. There are usually no personal remarks or eulogy, although the family's wishes are taken into account.

Greek Orthodox Church: The Greek Orthodox funeral ceremony lasts 30 to 60 minutes and is not part of a larger service. There is usually an open casket at the ceremony. Traditionally, mourners bow in front of the casket and kiss an icon or cross placed on the chest of the deceased. Greek Orthodox traditionally say to the bereaved, "May you have an abundant life" and "May their memory be eternal." At the graveside, there is a five-minute prayer ceremony and each person present places one flower on the casket. A memorial service is held on the Sunday closest to the 40th day after the death.

Hinduism: The body remains at the home until it is taken to the place of cremation, usually 24 hours after death. It is customary to wear white at the funeral. The major officiants at the cermony are Hindu priests or senior, male members of the family. Special books containing mantras for funeral services are used, but only by the priests. At the cremation, a last food offering is symbolically made to the deceased, and then the body is cremated. An additional ceremony, performed 10 days after death for members of the Brahmin caste and 30 days after death for members of other castes, is performed at home and is intended to liberate the soul of the deceased for its ascent to heaven.

Islam: Mourners place the body of the deceased on its side and wash it with warm soap and water an odd number of times. Generally, members of the same sex as the deceased must perform the washings. The body is then dried off, perfumed, and wrapped in white cloth. Mourners face Mecca and recite prayers, and then a silent procession carries the body to its burial place. All of the mourners participate in filling the grave with soil.

Judaism: A Jewish funeral lasts between 15 and 60 minutes. It is a time of intense mourning and public grieving and is a service unto itself, not part of a larger service. Traditional Jewish law forbids cremation, but it is allowed among Reform Jews. Flowers are never appropriate for Orthodox or Conservative funerals, but are sometimes appropriate for Reform funerals. There is never an open casket and the officiants are a rabbi, who delivers a eulogy, a cantor, who sings, and family members or friends who may also deliver a eulogy or memorial. At the simplest graveside service, the rabbi recites prayers and leads the family in the mourner's *kaddish,* the prayer for the deceased. At a traditional service, once the mourners have arrived at the cemetery there is a slow procession to the grave itself with several pauses along the way. After prayers and *kaddish* have been recited, each person puts one spade of earth into the grave. The family sits in mourning for seven days after the funeral, called the *shiva* period. To symbolize the mourners' lack of interest in their comfort or how they appear to others, family members may cover mirrors in the home, wear a black ribbon that has been cut and slippers or socks rather than shoes, and, for men, refrain from shaving. A special memorial candle may be burned for seven days, and immediate family members may sit on small chairs or boxes.

Native American religions: Funeral and mourning rituals are linked to the belief that this is the beginning of a journey into the next world. Strict rules govern the behavior of the living relatives so as to ensure the deceased a good start on his or her journey. Some Potawatomi, for instance, set a place for the spirit of the deceased at a funeral feast so that the spirit can partake of the spirit food. Among the Yuchi, considered politi-

cally part of the Creek Nation of Oklahoma, personal items such as a hunting rifle, blanket, and some tobacco may be placed in an adult male's coffin, reflecting the belief that needs in the next life are not significantly different from needs in this one. While Native beliefs assert that death is not necessarily the termination of life, the bereaved still mourn the absence from this life of the one who has died. Many tribes restrict what bereaved relatives can eat or kinds of activities they can engage in. This represents a sacrifice by the living for those who have moved on.

Society of Friends (Quakers): There are two types of Quaker funerals or memorial meetings. An unpro-

grammed meeting is held in the traditional manner of Friends on the basis of silence. Worshippers sit and wait for divine guidance and inspiration. If so moved, members speak to the group. Programmed meetings are planned in advance and usually include singing, prayers, Bible reading, silent worship, and a sermon. In many cases, worship is led by a pastor. Either form of meeting usually lasts an hour.

Source: Adapted from Stuart M. Matlins and Arthur J. Magida (eds.), *How to Be a Perfect Stranger* © 2003 SkyLight Paths Publishing, P.O. Box 237, Woodstock, VT 05091. www.skylightpaths.com.

details of body disposal, the type of memorial service, display of the body, the site of burial or body disposition, the cost of funeral options, organ donation decisions, ordering floral displays, contacting friends and relatives, planning for the arrival of guests, choosing markers, gathering and submitting obituary information to newspapers, printing memorial folders, and many other details. Even though funeral directors are available to facilitate decision making, the bereaved may experience undue stress, especially in the event of a sudden death. In our society, people who make their own funeral arrangements can save their loved ones from having to deal with unnecessary problems. Even making the decision regarding the method of body disposal can greatly reduce the stress on survivors.

Wills

The issue of inheritance is controversial in some families and should be resolved before the person dies to reduce both conflict and needless expense. Unfortunately, many people are so intimidated by the thought of making a will that they never do so and die **intestate** (without a will). This is tragic, especially because the procedure for establishing a legal will is relatively simple and inexpensive. In addition, if you don't make a will before you die, the courts (as directed by state laws) will make a will for you. Legal issues, rather than your wishes, will preside.

For example, let's explore what happens if you die in Massachusetts without a will. If you are married with no children, everything goes to your spouse. If you have children, one-third of your estate goes to your spouse and two-thirds goes to the children. If you're not married, it all goes to your

parents. Think about the problems this poses for those who choose to live together or are homosexual: Without a will, their partners get *nothing*. Or think of the problems posed when stepchildren who choose not to support the surviving spouse are involved. Clearly, we all need wills, updated regularly.

In some cases, other types of wills may substitute for the traditional legal will. One of these alternatives is the **holographic will,** written in the handwriting of the **testator** (person who leaves a will) and unwitnessed. Be very cautious concerning alternatives to legally written and witnessed wills, because they are not honored in all states. For example, holographic wills are contestable in court. Think of the parents who never approved of the fact that their child lived with someone outside marriage: They could successfully challenge a holographic will in court.

Organ Donation

Another decision concerns organ donation. Organ transplant techniques have become so refined, and the demand for transplant tissues and organs has become so great, that many people are being encouraged to donate these "gifts of life." Uniform donor cards are available through the National

Intestate Not having made a will.

Holographic will A will written in the testator's own handwriting and unwitnessed.

Testator A person who leaves a will or testament at death.

Kidney Foundation, donor information is printed on the backs of drivers' licenses, and many hospitals include the opportunity for organ donor registration as a part of their admission procedures. Although some people are opposed to organ transplants and tissue donation, others experience a feeling of personal fulfillment from knowing that their organs may extend and improve someone else's life after their own deaths (see Figure 20.4).

> **What do you think?**
>
> *What can you do to ensure that your wishes will be carried out at the time of your death?*

Taking Charge **20** *20* **20**

Making Death a More Positive Journey

As you have seen in this chapter, your attitudes toward death and dying will affect not only you but also those closest to you. As you ponder the material in this chapter, think about your values and beliefs about death. What is it about the way you experience life that will have an impact on how you experience death? Is there anything in your life that you would change to prepare for your own death, or the death of people you love?

There may come a time when you need to consider how you want to live out the rest of your life and what you want others to know about your wishes. Just remember, you can make decisions that will affect the nature of your death, whatever the circumstances. Learning all that you can about issues related to the end of life may influence your own dying process and make death a much more positive event for you and for others.

Checklist for Change

Making Personal Choices

☐ What can you do to decrease your risks for dying an untimely death?

☐ Have you made a legal will? Do you update it regularly?

☐ Have you completed a directive to physicians?

☐ If you had died yesterday, would your loved ones have known what plans you had for your funeral, body disposal, and asset distribution? What steps can you take to make sure such information is known?

☐ Do you have trouble talking to people about death? If so, what steps can you take to improve your communication skills?

☐ What coping techniques will you use if someone you know dies? Do you think you would be able to help someone else who is dealing with a loss?

☐ How might you help a child understand death?

Making Community Choices

☐ What community support is available to help people cope with the death of a loved one? For example, are there widow or widower support groups?

☐ What are your state's laws regarding directives to physicians?

☐ Is physician-assisted suicide legal in your state? Are any laws pending regarding rational suicide?

Summary

* *Death* can be defined biologically in terms of brain death and/or the final cessation of vital functions. Denial of death results in limited communication about death, which can lead to further denial.

* Death is a multifaceted process and individuals may experience emotional stages of dying including denial, anger, bargaining, depression, and acceptance. Social death results when a person is no longer treated as living. Grief is the state of distress felt after loss. Men and women differ in their responses to grief. Children, too, need to be helped through the process of grieving.

* The right to die by rational suicide involves ethical, moral, and legal issues. Dyathanasia involves passive help with suicide for a terminally ill patient; euthanasia involves direct help.

* Practical and legal issues surround dying and death. Choices of care for the terminally ill include hospice care. After death, funeral arrangements must be made almost immediately, adding to pressures on survivors. Decisions should be made in advance of death through wills and organ donation cards.

Questions for Discussion and Reflection

1. Discuss why so many of us deny death. How could death become a more acceptable topic to discuss?
2. What are the stages that terminally ill patients theoretically experience? Do you agree with the five-stage theory? Explain why or why not.
3. Define *social death, near-death experiences,* and *quasi-death.*
4. Discuss coping with grief, the different grief experiences of men and women, and how to help children deal with death.
5. Identify at least one development—legal, medical, social—that has occurred in the past five years that has affected the way we view death.
6. Debate whether rational suicide should be legalized for the terminally ill. What restrictions would you include in a law?
7. Compare and contrast the hospital experience with hospice care. What must one consider before arranging for hospice care?
8. Discuss the legal matters surrounding death, including wills, physician directives, organ donations, and funeral arrangements.

Application Exercises

Reread the What Do You Think? scenarios at the beginning of the chapter and answer the following questions.

1. What can Doug do to ensure that his partner's wishes will be carried out? What legal rights does he have? What would be the "ethical" thing to do?
2. What do you think Sheila should be able to do? Present an argument as to whether or not she has the right to end her life.
3. What suggestions would you have for those closest to Sheila to help them cope with her decision and their eventual loss?

Accessing Your Health on the Internet

Visit the following Internet sites to explore further topics and issues related to personal health. To visit an organization's website, go to the Companion Website for *Access to Health, Eighth Edition* at www.aw.com/donatelle, click on the book image, and select "Accessing Your Health on the Internet" from the navigation menu on the left.

1. *Beyond Indigo.* This site addresses all aspects of grief and loss, including terminal illness, legal issues, and funeral planning.
2. *Doctor-Assisted Suicide—a Guide to Web Sites and the Literature.* A comprehensive look at the current status of doctor-assisted suicide. Sources presented are very informative and up-to-date.
3. *Funerals: A Consumer Guide.* This site guides the consumer through the thinking process of planning for a funeral, including preplanning, types of funerals, costs, choosing a casket, burial, and many other aspects of funeral preparation.
4. *GriefNet.org.* Resources to help people deal with the loss of loved ones, including memorial pages and e-mail support groups.
5. *Hospice Web.* Information and links about hospice, including frequently asked questions.
6. *Loss, Grief, and Bereavement.* This site from the National Cancer Institute covers a variety of topics related to loss, grief, and bereavement. Among the contents is a summary written by cancer experts.

Further Reading

Humphrey, D., and M. Clement. *Freedom to Die: People, Politics, and the Right-to-Die Movement.* Torrance, CA: Griffin, 2000.

Describes the history of the right-to-die movement and all sides of the debate.

Jacobs Altman, L. *Death: An Introduction to Medical–Ethical Dilemmas.* Berkeley Heights, NJ: Enslow, 2000.

A multifaceted exploration of death that gives the reader much to consider.

Mims, C. A. *When We Die: The Science, Culture, and Rituals of Death.* Torrance, CA: Griffin, 2000.

A look at how society views and portrays death in science and culture.

Muth, A. S. (ed.). *Death and Dying Sourcebook: Basic Consumer Health Information for the Layperson About End-of-Life Care and Related Ethical and Legal Issues.* Detroit, MI: Omnigraphics, 2000.

Provides up-to-date information on the issues of nursing care, living wills, pain management, and counseling.

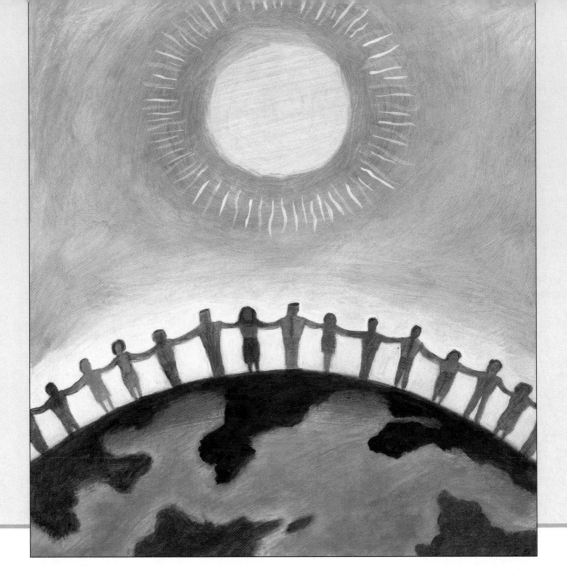

objectives

* Identify the problems and ethical issues associated with current levels of global population growth.

* Discuss major causes of air pollution, including photochemical smog and acid rain, and the global consequences of greenhouse gases and ozone depletion.

* Identify sources of water pollution and the chemical contaminants often found in water.

* Describe the physiological consequences of noise pollution.

* Distinguish between municipal solid waste and hazardous waste.

* Discuss the health concerns associated with ionizing and nonionizing radiation.

21 Environmental Health

Thinking Globally, Acting Locally

What do you think?

Since 1950, the world population has doubled, increasing the demand for water, food, firewood, and fossil fuel. Pro-growth advocates argue that these scarcities drive efforts to discover new sources of raw materials and new technologies to extract and process them, suggesting consumption is actually beneficial. However, supporters of sustainable resources maintain that resources are being depleted faster than they can be replenished: forests are shrinking, water tables are falling, soils are eroding, wetlands are disappearing, temperatures are rising, and species are disappearing.

Which view do you agree with, and why? ✳ How long might current social structures survive if population growth continues unchecked? ✳ What needs to be done to make sure the earth can support future generations?

Since 1900, the mean surface temperatures of the earth have increased by 0.6–1.2°F. Ice packs in the Arctic Ocean have decreased and sea levels have risen 4–10 inches. Greenhouse gases in the atmosphere hold on to the earth's natural outgoing energy, retaining heat necessary for life. As concentration of these gases has increased, global warming has increased, and some scientists contend that this is from heavy combustion of fossil fuels (heating; agricultural/industrial production) and predict dire health consequences from global warming. Other scientists disagree that these human activities will affect the atmosphere in catastrophic ways.

How might human health be endangered from these environmental changes? ✳ What changes can we make to prevent risks from global warming?

Human health, well-being, and the survival of all living things depend on the health and integrity of the planet on which we live. Today the natural world is under siege from the pressures of a burgeoning population that requires massive use of natural resources to survive. Consequently, many citizens are interested in the health effects of global warming and depletion of the ozone layer; increasing problems with air, water, and solid waste pollution; deforestation; endangered species; population control; and the impact of too many people on dwindling natural resources.

In response to public and political concerns, there has been a surge in federal and state regulations along with a multibillion-dollar national infrastructure—but doubt remains as to the effectiveness of that infrastructure in reducing environmental health risks.[1] In addition, during the economic downturn that began in 2001, politicians began to dismantle enironmental gains by reducing regulations, easing compliance deadlines, weakening protections for endangered species, and undermining other environmental programs labeled by some in Congress as "antibusiness." In such a period of environmental pressures, an informed citizenry with a strong commitment to be responsible for the planet and maintain it for future generations is essential to the survival of Earth and all living things. This chapter reviews some of the major global environmental issues that affect us today and will affect us in the generations to come.

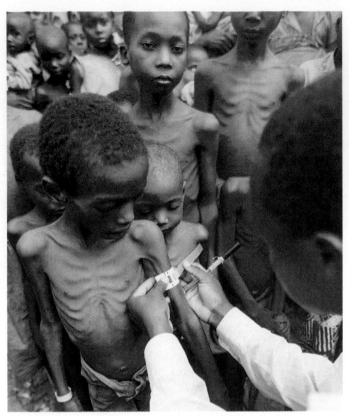

Burgeoning population puts a strain on valuable resources and leaves many parts of the world unable to meet the needs of their citizens.

Overpopulation

Anthropologist Margaret Mead wrote, "Every human society is faced with not one population problem but two: how to beget and rear enough children and how not to beget and rear too many."[2] The United Nations projects that the world population will grow from 6.3 billion in the year 2002 to 9.4 billion in 2050.[3] Though the population is expanding, the earth's resources are not. Population experts believe that many areas of the world are already struggling with "demographic fatigue" and that the most critical environmental challenge today is to slow the population growth of the world.[4] See the Health Ethics box for ethical concerns having to do with overpopulation.

The population explosion is not distributed equally. The United States and western Europe have the lowest birth rates. At the same time, these two regions produce more grain and other foodstuffs than their populations consume. Countries that can least afford a high birth rate in terms of economic, social, health, and nutritional factors are the ones with the most rapidly expanding populations. Malnutrition, high rates of infectious diseases, lack of access to health care, and a host of other problems often plague these developing countries.

The bulk of population growth in developing countries is occurring in urban areas. Third world cities' populations are doubling every 10 to 15 years, overwhelming their governments' attempts to provide clean water, sewage facilities,

adequate transportation, and other basic services. Every week, the population of the world's urban centers grows by more than 1 million.[5] In 1800, London was the only city in the world with 1 million people; today, 14 cities each have populations of over 10 million.[6]

As the global population expands, so does competition for the earth's resources. Environmental degradation caused by loss of topsoil, pesticides, toxic residues, deforestation, global warming, air pollution, acid rain, a rapidly expanding population, and increasing poverty is exerting heavy pressure on the capacity of natural resources to support human life and world health.[7]

Overpopulation threats are more evident in Latin America, Africa, and Asia. The country projected to have the largest increase in population is India, which could add another 600 million people by the year 2050 and surpass China as the most populous country in the world.[8] These projections could change, however, if governments are not able to cope with the increased resource and economic demands. For example, the AIDS epidemic has stabilized in industrial countries to an adult infection rate of under 1 percent, but countries such as Zimbabwe, Botswana, and Zambia may lose one-fifth or more of their adult population within the next decade to AIDS.[9] The loss of a significant part of the workforce would have devastating economic as well as health consequences. Diseases such as AIDS are not the only threats to countries with unstable population growth. As governments strain to support

Population Control

The world's population tops 6 billion. Ninety-seven percent of each year's population growth occurs in the poorest parts of the world. Consider the following statistics:

- An estimated 300 million women desire family planning but lack the information or the means to obtain it.
- Over 1 billion people have no access to health care.
- Roughly 1.3 billion people live in poverty.
- An estimated 840 million people are malnourished.
- Eighty-five countries lack the ability to grow or purchase enough food to feed their citizens.
- Over 1.5 billion people lack access to safe drinking water.
- Approximately 2.3 billion live without adequate sanitation.

The Population Reference Bureau projects that world population will increase to over 9 billion by 2050. The statistics listed above are sure to rise as the population increases.

According to many scientists, overpopulation has led to environmental degradation, resulting in the loss of immense tracts of forest and tons of arable topsoil.

Additionally, some scientists suggest that increased industrialization and consumption threaten the atmosphere and world climate. Many people fear that unrestricted population growth will lead to worldwide shortages of food and energy.

Already women, particularly in the developing world, suffer the ill health effects of having too many children too close together. Often these children live in poverty and are malnourished. Particularly in regions where HIV and poverty are rampant, many women neglect their own health to care for sick partners and children.

For the past half century, those concerned about overpopulation have called for population control. A number of organizations, such as the International Planned Parenthood Federation, have been advocating women's access to family planning information and contraception. Unfortunately, even if many of these women had access to family planning services, cultural mores or religious beliefs could prevent their use of these resources.

Another solution some have offered is government regulation of population growth. In the 1970s, China instituted a strictly enforced one child—one family policy that allowed each family to have only a single child. While the policy has been effective in cities, where people tend to be more educated and space is already extremely limited, it has not been successful in rural areas, where families whose survival depends on having enough labor continue to have multiple children. One unintended consequence of this policy has been female infanticide, in order for the family to make sure that its one child will be a boy.

Other recommendations are under consideration. One of these gives each woman born the right to have two babies. If the woman chooses not to exercise this right, she can sell her rights on the open market. If people want a large family, they must have enough resources to buy the baby rights and therefore, in all likelihood, the ability to support these children financially. Another option might be to pay a woman not to reproduce: Each year of her childbearing years that she does not have a child, she is rewarded financially.

Finally, some people suggest that the problem is not overpopulation but the unequal consumption of resources by a minority of the world's population. They believe that poverty results not from overpopulation but from the inequitable distribution of wealth.

Do you think overpopulation is a problem? Do you think population control is the answer? How do you think population control should be effected? Do you think inequality is a greater problem than overpopulation? If so, what do you think should be done to bring about greater equality worldwide?

growing numbers of people, they are at increased risk of developing significant problems, should any new or increased demands be placed on resources.

What can we do to alleviate these conditions? We can do our part by recognizing that the United States consumes far more energy and raw materials per person than any other nation on Earth. Many of these resources come from other countries, and our consumption is depleting the resource balances of those countries. See Table 21.1 for a comparison of U.S. oil consumption with that of selected other countries.

Perhaps the simplest course of action is to control our own reproductivity. The concept of zero population growth (ZPG) was born in the 1960s. Proponents of this idea believed that each couple should produce only two offspring. When the parents die, the two offspring are their replacements, and the population stabilizes.

The continued preference for large families in many developing nations is related to factors such as high infant mortality rates; the traditional view of children as "social security" (they work from a young age to assist families in daily survival and support parents when they grow too old to work); the low educational and economic status of women; and the traditional desire for sons that keeps parents of several daughters reproducing until they get male offspring. Education may be the single biggest contributor to zero population growth. As education levels of women increase, fertility rates drop. Moreover, some developing nations feel that overpopulation is not as great a problem as the inequitable distribution of wealth and resources, both within their countries and worldwide. For all these reasons, demographers contend that broad-based social and economic changes will be necessary before population growth can stabilize.

Table 21.1
Oil Consumption (Barrels per Day) in Selected Countries

RANK	COUNTRY	1995	2001	PERCENTAGE OF WORLD CONSUMPTION
1	United States	11,725,000	19,633,000	26.08
2	Japan	5,784,000	5,427,000	7.21
3	China	3,390,000	5,041,000	6.70
7	India	1,533,000	2,072,000	2.75
10	Canada	1,776,000	1,941,000	2.58
15	Saudi Arabia	1,123,000	1,347,000	1.79
16	Iran	1,204,000	1,131,000	1.50
19	Australia	781,000	845,000	1.1225
25	Egypt	474,000	551,000	0.73
27	South Africa	427,000	488,000	0.65
30	Argentina	415,000	404,000	0.54
	World Total	**68,175,000**	**75,291,000**	

Source: British Petroleum, "Statistical Review of World Energy June 2002," 2002, *Geohive* (see www.geohive.com/charts/en_oilcons.php).

Air Pollution

Although we often assume that the air we breathe is safe, the daily impact of a growing population makes clean air more difficult to find. Concern about air quality prompted Congress to pass the Clean Air Act in 1970 and to amend it in 1977 and again in 1990. The goal was to develop standards for six of the most widespread air pollutants that seriously affect health: sulfur dioxide, particulates, carbon monoxide, nitrogen dioxide, ozone, and lead. The Air Quality Index is the best way for the public to assess the daily quality of the air we are breathing (see the Reality Check box).

Sulfur dioxide   A yellowish brown gaseous by-product of the burning of fossil fuels.

Particulates   Nongaseous air pollutants.

Carbon monoxide   An odorless, colorless gas that originates primarily from motor vehicle emissions.

Ozone   A gas formed when nitrogen dioxide interacts with hydrogen chloride.

Nitrogen dioxide   An amber-colored gas found in smog; can cause eye and respiratory irritations.

Lead   A metal found in the exhaust of motor vehicles powered by fuel containing lead and in emissions from lead smelters and processing plants.

Sources of Air Pollution

Sulfur Dioxide   Sulfur dioxide is a yellowish brown gas that is a by-product of burning fossil fuels. Electricity-generating stations, smelters, refineries, and industrial boilers are the main sources. In humans, sulfur dioxide aggravates symptoms of heart and lung disease, obstructs breathing passages, and increases the incidence of respiratory diseases such as colds, asthma, bronchitis, and emphysema. It is toxic to plants, destroys some paint pigments, corrodes metals, impairs visibility, and is a precursor to acid rain, which we discuss later in this chapter.

Particulates   Particulates are tiny solid particles or liquid droplets that are suspended in the air. Cigarette smoke releases particulates. They are also by-products of industrial processes and the internal combustion engine. Particulates irritate the lungs and can carry heavy metals and carcinogenic agents deep into the lungs. When combined with sulfur dioxide, they exacerbate respiratory diseases. Particulates can also corrode metals and obscure visibility. Numerous scientific studies have found significant links between exposure to air particulate concentrations at or below current standards and adverse health effects, including premature death.[10]

Carbon Monoxide   Carbon monoxide is an odorless, colorless gas that originates primarily from motor vehicle emissions. Carbon monoxide interferes with the blood's ability to absorb and carry oxygen and can impair thinking, slow reflexes, and cause drowsiness, unconsciousness, and death. Many people have purchased home monitors to test for carbon monoxide.

What Is the AQI?

A ir quality affects how we live and breathe. Like the weather, it can change from day to day or even hour to hour. The U.S. Environmental Protection Agency (EPA) and other groups are working to make information about outdoor air quality as available to the public as a weather report. A key tool in this effort is the Air Quality Index, or AQI.

An index for reporting daily air quality, the AQI tells you how clean or polluted your air is and what associated health concerns you should be aware of. The AQI focuses on health effects that can happen within a few hours or days after breathing polluted air. It reflects national air quality standards for five major air pollutants regulated by the Clean Air Act: ground-level ozone, particulate matter, carbon monoxide, sulfur dioxide, and nitrogen dioxide.

HOW DOES THE AQI WORK?
Think of the AQI as a yardstick that runs from 0 to 500. The higher the AQI value, the greater the level of air pollution and associated health risks. An AQI value of 100 generally corresponds to the national air quality standard for the pollutant, which is the level the EPA has set to protect public health. AQI values below 100 are generally considered satisfactory. When AQI values rise above 100, air quality is considered to be unhealthy—at first, for certain groups of people, then for everyone.

UNDERSTANDING THE AQI
The EPA has divided the AQI scale into six categories and color codes as follows:

AQI RANGE	AIR QUALITY CONDITION/LEVEL OF HEALTH CONCERN	COLOR
0–50	Good	Green
51–100	Moderate	Yellow
101–150	Unhealthy for sensitive groups	Orange
151–200	Unhealthy	Red
201–300	Very unhealthy	Purple
301–500	Hazardous	Maroon

✔ *Good:* Air quality is satisfactory for all groups.

✔ *Moderate:* Air quality is acceptable except for a very small group of individuals. For example, people who are unusually sensitive to ozone may experience respiratory symptoms.

✔ *Unhealthy for sensitive groups:* The general public is not likely to be affected, but certain individuals may experience health effects. For example, children and adults who are active outdoors and people with respiratory disease are at greater risk from exposure to ozone, while people with heart disease are at greater risk from carbon monoxide.

✔ *Unhealthy:* At this point the general public may begin to notice symptoms.

✔ *Very unhealthy:* This may trigger a health alert, meaning everyone may experience serious health effects.

✔ *Hazardous:* The entire population is likely to be affected and a warning of emergency conditions will be triggered.

Source: United States Environmental Protection Agency, excerpt from *Air Quality Index: A Guide to Air Quality and Your Health*, 2–3, June 2002.

Ozone   Ground-level **ozone** is a form of oxygen that is produced when nitrogen dioxide reacts with hydrogen chloride. These gases release oxygen, which is altered by sunlight to produce ozone. In the lower atmosphere, ozone irritates the mucous membranes of the respiratory system, causing coughing and choking. It can impair lung functioning, reduce resistance to colds and pneumonia, and aggravate heart disease, asthma, bronchitis, and pneumonia. One of the irritants found in smog, this ozone corrodes rubber and paint and can kill vegetation. The natural ozone found in the upper atmosphere (sometimes called "good" ozone), however, serves as a protective membrane against heat and radiation from the sun. We will discuss this atmospheric ozone layer later in the chapter.

Nitrogen Dioxide   **Nitrogen dioxide** is an amber-colored gas emitted by coal-powered electrical utility boilers and motor vehicles. High concentrations of nitrogen dioxide can be fatal. Lower concentrations increase susceptibility to colds and flu, bronchitis, and pneumonia. Nitrogen dioxide is also toxic to plant life and causes a brown discoloration of the atmosphere. It is a precursor of ozone, and, along with sulfur dioxide, of acid rain.

Lead   **Lead** is a metal pollutant found in paint, batteries, drinking water, pipes, and dishes with lead-glazed bases. The elimination of lead from gasoline and auto exhaust in the 1970s was one of the great public health accomplishments of all time. Although stricter standards for all of the above prevail, almost 1 million children in the United States had elevated blood lead levels in 1997.[11] Lead impairs the circulatory, reproductive, and nervous systems. It can also affect the blood and kidneys and accumulate in bone and other tissues. Particularly detrimental to children and fetuses, lead can cause birth defects, behavioral abnormalities, and decreased learning abilities.

Hydrocarbons Although not listed as one of the six major air pollutants in the Clean Air Act, hydrocarbons encompass a wide variety of chemical pollutants in the air. Sometimes known as *volatile organic compounds (VOCs)*, **hydrocarbons** are chemical compounds containing different combinations of carbon and hydrogen. The principal source is the internal combustion engine. Most automobile engines emit hundreds of different hydrocarbon compounds. By themselves, hydrocarbons seem to cause few problems, but when they combine with sunlight and other pollutants, they form such poisons as formaldehyde, ketones, and peroxyacetylnitrate (PAN), all of which are respiratory irritants. Hydrocarbon combinations such as benzene and benzo(a)pyrene are carcinogenic. In addition, hydrocarbons play a major part in the formation of smog.

> **What do you think?**
>
> *Should automakers be responsible for developing cars with low emissions?* ✳ *As a motorist, how can you help eliminate carbon monoxide emissions?*

Photochemical Smog

Photochemical smog is a brown, hazy mix of particulates and gases that forms when oxygen-containing compounds of nitrogen and hydrocarbons react in the presence of sunlight. It is sometimes called *ozone pollution* because ozone is created when vehicle exhaust reacts with sunlight. In most cases, smog forms in areas that experience a **temperature inversion,** a weather condition in which a cool layer of air is trapped under a layer of warmer air, preventing the air from circulating. When gases such as hydrocarbons and nitrogen oxides are released into the cool air layer, they remain suspended until wind conditions move away the warmer air layer. Sunlight filtering through the air causes chemical changes in the hydrocarbons and nitrogen oxides, which results in smog. Smog is more likely to be produced in valleys blocked by hills or mountains—for example, in the Los Angeles basin, Denver, and Tokyo.

The most noticeable adverse effects of smog are difficulty in breathing, burning eyes, headaches, and nausea. Long-term exposure poses serious health risks, particularly for children, the elderly, pregnant women, and people with chronic respiratory disorders such as asthma and emphysema.

Acid Rain

Acid rain is precipitation that has fallen through acidic air pollutants, particularly those containing sulfur dioxides and nitrogen dioxides. This precipitation, in the form of rain, snow, or fog, is more acidic than unpolluted precipitation. When introduced into lakes and ponds, acid rain gradually acidifies the water. When the acid content of the water

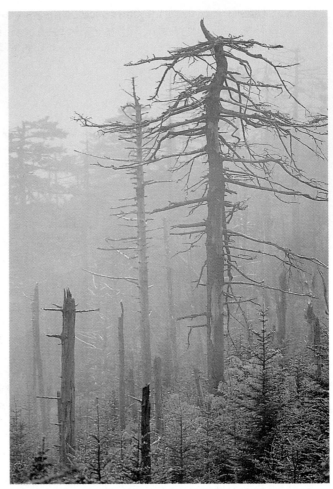

Acid rain has many harmful effects on the environment. Because its toxins seep into groundwater and enter the food chain, it also poses health hazards to humans.

reaches a certain level, plant and animal life cannot survive. Ironically, acidified lakes and ponds become a crystal-clear deep blue, giving the illusion of beauty and health.

Sources of Acid Rain More than 95 percent of acid rain originates in human actions, chiefly the burning of fossil fuels. The greatest sources of acid rain in the United States are coal-fired power plants, ore smelters, and steel mills.

When these and other industries burn fuels, the sulfur and nitrogen in the emissions combine with oxygen and sunlight in the air to become sulfur dioxide and nitrogen oxides (precursors of sulfuric acid and nitric acids, respectively). Small acid particles are then carried by the wind and combine with moisture to produce acidic rain or snow. Rain is more acidic in the summertime because of higher concentrations of sunlight. The ability of a lake to cleanse itself and neutralize its acidity depends on several factors, the most critical of which is bedrock geology.

Effects of Acid Rain In addition to damaging lakes and ponds, every year acid rain destroys millions of trees in Europe and North America. Scientists have concluded that 75 percent of Europe's forests are now experiencing damaging levels of sulfur deposition by acid rain. Forests in every country on the continent are affected.[12]

Doctors believe that acid rain aggravates and may even cause bronchitis, asthma, and other respiratory problems. People with emphysema and those with a history of heart disease may also suffer from exposure to acid rain. In addition, it may be hazardous to a pregnant woman's unborn child.

Acidic precipitation can cause metals such as aluminum, cadmium, lead, and mercury to **leach** (dissolve and filter) out of the soil. If these metals make their way into water or food supplies (particularly fish), they can cause cancer in humans who consume them. Acid rain also damages crops; laboratory experiments show that it can reduce seed yield by up to 23 percent. Actual crop losses are being reported with increasing frequency. A final consequence of acid rain is the destruction of public monuments and structures, with billions of dollars in projected building damage each year.

Indoor Air Pollution

In the last several years, a growing body of scientific evidence has indicated that the air within homes and other buildings can be even more polluted than the outdoor air in the most industrialized cities. Research also indicates that some of the most vulnerable people, particularly the young, older adults, and those who are sick, often spend over 90 percent of their time indoors.[13]

Most indoor air pollution comes from sources that release gases or particles into the air. Inadequate ventilation, particularly in heavily insulated buildings with airtight windows, may increase pollution by not allowing in outside air.

Some of the major sources of indoor air pollution and possible health effects from these pollutants are described in Table 21.2. However, the relative dose of any given chemical and the degree of toxicity of the chemical are key variables in determining risk. Some sources, such as building materials, furnishings, and household products such as air fresheners, release pollutants continuously. Others release pollutants intermittently. Health effects may develop over years of exposure or occur in response to toxic levels of pollutants. Several factors affect risk, including age, preexisting medical conditions, individual sensitivity, room temperature and humidity, and functioning of the liver, immune, and respiratory systems.[14]

Preventing indoor air pollution should focus on three main areas: source control (eliminating or reducing individual contaminants), ventilation improvements (increasing the amount of outdoor air coming indoors), and air cleaners (removing particulates from the air).[15]

Exactly how serious is the problem? Indoor air can be 10 to 40 times more hazardous than outdoor air. There are between 20 and 100 potentially dangerous chemical compounds in the average American home. Indoor air pollution comes primarily from these sources: woodstoves, furnaces, passive cigarette exposure (see Chapter 13), asbestos, formaldehyde, radon, and household chemicals. An emerging source of indoor air pollution is mold (see the New Horizons in Health box). It is not yet clear how widespread the effects of mold are.

Woodstove Smoke Woodstoves emit significant levels of particulates and carbon monoxide in addition to other pollutants, such as sulfur dioxide. If you rely on wood for heating, make sure that your stove is properly installed, vented, and maintained. Burning properly seasoned wood reduces particulates.

Furnace Emissions People who rely on oil- or gas-fired furnaces also need to make sure that these appliances are properly installed, ventilated, and maintained. Inadequate cleaning and maintenance can allow carbon monoxide to build up, which can be deadly.

Asbestos Asbestos is a mineral that was commonly used in insulating materials in buildings constructed before 1970. When bonded to other materials, asbestos is relatively harmless, but if its tiny fibers become loosened and airborne, they can embed themselves in the lungs. Their presence leads to cancer of the lungs, stomach, and chest lining, and a fatal lung disease called mesothelioma.

Formaldehyde Formaldehyde is a colorless, strong-smelling gas present in some carpets, draperies, furniture, particle board, plywood, wood paneling, countertops, and many adhesives. It is released into the air in a process called *outgassing*. Outgassing is highest in new products, but the process can continue for many years.

Exposure to formaldehyde can cause respiratory problems, dizziness, fatigue, nausea, and rashes. Long-term exposure can lead to central nervous system disorders and cancer.

Hydrocarbons Chemical compounds that contain carbon and hydrogen.

Photochemical smog The brownish yellow haze resulting from the combination of hydrocarbons and nitrogen oxides.

Temperature inversion A weather condition occurring when a layer of cool air is trapped under a layer of warmer air.

Acid rain Precipitation contaminated with acidic pollutants.

Leach To dissolve and filter through soil.

Asbestos A substance that separates into stringy fibers and lodges in the lungs, where it can cause various diseases.

Formaldehyde A colorless, strong-smelling gas released through outgassing; causes respiratory and other health problems.

Table 21.2
Health Effects of Indoor Air Pollution

TYPE OF POLLUTANT	SOURCES	HEALTH EFFECTS
Radon	Uranium in the soil or rock on which homes are built; well water can also be a source	Lung cancer from exposure in air, other health risks from swallowing in water
Environmental tobacco smoke (ETS)	Smoke that comes from burning end of cigarette, pipe, or cigar	Complex mixture of over 4,000 compounds, over 40 of which cause cancer
Biological contaminants (molds, mildew, viruses, animal dander and cat saliva, dust mites, cockroaches, and pollen)	Improper ventilation and moisture buildup, lack of cleanliness/sanitation, contaminated heating systems, household pets, rodents, insects, damp carpets, etc.	Allergic reactions, including hypersensitivity rhinitis, asthma, infectious illnesses, sneezing, watering eyes, coughing, shortness of breath, dizziness, lethargy, fever, digestive problems
Stoves, heaters, fireplaces, chimneys	Unvented kerosene heaters, woodstoves, fireplaces, gas stoves	Carbon monoxide causes headaches, dizziness, weakness, nausea, confusion and disorientation, chest pain, death. Nitrogen dioxide causes irritation of nose, eyes, respiratory distress. Particles cause lung damage and irritation.
Household chemicals (see partial list below)	Paints, varnishes; cleaning products, solvents, degreasers, and hobby products, etc.	Variable symptoms dependent on exposure level, including eye and respiratory tract problems, headaches, dizziness, visual disorders and memory impairment
Benzene	Paint, new carpet, new drapes, upholstery, fast-drying glues, caulks	Headaches, eye/skin irritation, fatigue, cancer
Formaldehyde	Tobacco smoke, plywood, cabinets, furniture, particle board, new carpet and drapes, wallpaper, ceiling tile, paneling	Headaches, eye/skin irritation, drowsiness, fatigue, respiratory problems, memory loss, depression, gynecological problems, cancer
Chloroform	Paint, new drapes, new carpet, upholstery	Headaches, asthma attacks, dizziness, eye/skin irritations
Toluene	All paper products, most finished wood products	Headaches, eye/skin irritation, sinus problems, dizziness, cancer
Hydrocarbons	Tobacco smoke, gas burners and furnaces	Headaches, fatigue, nausea, dizziness, breathing difficulty
Ammonia	Tobacco smoke, cleaning supplies, animal urine	Eye/skin irritation, headaches, nosebleeds, sinus problems
Trichlorethylene	Paints, glues, caulking, vinyl coatings, wallpaper	Headaches, eye/skin irritation, upper respiratory irritation

Source: Environmental Protection Agency, "The Inside Story: A Guide to Indoor Air Quality," EPA Document #402-K-93-007, January 2002 (see http://epa.gov/iaq/pubs/insidest.html).

Ask about the formaldehyde content of products you purchase and avoid those that contain this gas. Some houseplants, such as philodendrons and spider plants, help clean formaldehyde from the air. If you experience symptoms of formaldehyde exposure, have your home tested by a city, county, or state health agency.

Radon Radon, an odorless, colorless gas, is the natural by-product of the decay of uranium and radium in the soil. Radon penetrates homes through cracks, pipes, sump pits, and other openings in the foundation. An estimated 30,000

cancer deaths per year have been attributed to radon, making it second only to smoking as a cause of lung cancer.[16]

The EPA estimates that 1 in 15 American homes has an elevated radon level.[17] A home-testing kit from a hardware store will enable you to test your home yourself. "Alpha track" detectors are commonly used for this type of short-term testing. They must remain in your home for 2 to 90 days, depending on the device.

Household Chemicals Use cleansers and other cleaning products in a well-ventilated room, and be conservative in

Growing Concerns about Mold

WHAT IS MOLD?

Molds produce tiny spores to reproduce. Mold spores waft through the indoor and outdoor air continually. When mold spores land on a damp spot indoors, they may begin growing and digesting whatever they are growing on in order to survive. There are molds that can grow on wood, paper, carpet, and foods. When excessive moisture or water accumulates indoors, mold growth will often occur, particularly if the moisture problem remains undiscovered or unaddressed. There is no practical way to eliminate all mold and mold spores in the indoor environment; the way to control indoor mold growth is to control moisture.

Potential health effects and symptoms associated with mold exposures include allergic reactions, asthma, and other respiratory complaints.

CONTROLLING MOLD

Molds can be found almost anywhere. They can grow on virtually any substance, providing moisture is present, so the key to mold control is moisture control. It is important to dry water-damaged areas and items within 24–48 hours to prevent mold growth. If mold is a problem in your home, clean up the mold and get rid of the excess water or moisture. Fix leaky plumbing or other sources of water. Wash mold off hard surfaces with detergent and water, and dry completely. Absorbent materials (such as ceiling tiles and carpet) that become moldy may have to be replaced.

Reduce indoor humidity (to 30–60 percent) to decrease mold growth by venting bathrooms, dryers, and other moisture-generating sources to the outside; using air conditioners and dehumidifiers; increasing ventilation; and using exhaust fans whenever cooking, dishwashing, and cleaning.

Reduce the potential for condensation on cold surfaces (i.e., windows, piping, exterior walls, roof, or floors) by adding insulation.

In areas where there is a perpetual moisture problem, do not install carpeting (i.e., by drinking fountains, by sinks, or on concrete floors with leaks or frequent condensation).

Source: Environmental Protection Agency, "Mold Resources," 2002 (see http:www.epa.gov/iaq/molds/moldresources.html).

---

their use. All those caustic chemicals that zap mildew and grease cause a major risk to water and the environment. Avoid buildup. Regular cleanings will reduce the need to use potentially harmful substances. Cut down on dry cleaning, as the chemicals used by many cleaners can cause cancer. If your newly cleaned clothes smell of dry-cleaning chemicals, return them to the cleaner or hang them in the open air until the smell is gone. Avoid household air freshener products containing the carcinogenic agent *dichlorobenzene.*

Indoor air pollution is also a concern in the classroom and workplace. Studies show that one in five U.S. schools has indoor air quality problems, which affect an estimated 8.4 million students.[18] Poor air quality in classrooms may lead to drowsiness, headaches, and lack of concentration. It may also affect physical growth and development. Children with asthma are particularly at risk. Many people who work indoors complain of maladies that lessen or vanish when they leave the building. **Sick building syndrome (SBS)** is said to exist when 80 percent of a building's occupants report problems. Poor ventilation is a primary cause of sick building syndrome. Symptoms include eye irritation, sore throat, queasiness, and worsened asthma.[19]

Ozone Layer Depletion

As mentioned earlier, the *ozone* layer forms a protective layer in the earth's stratosphere—the highest level of the earth's atmosphere, located 12 to 30 miles above the earth's surface. The ozone layer in the stratosphere protects our planet and its inhabitants from ultraviolet B (UV-B) radiation, a primary cause of skin cancer. Ultraviolet B radiation may also damage DNA

and weaken immune systems in both humans and animals. Thus, the ozone layer is crucial to life on the planet's surface.

In the early 1970s, scientists began to warn of a depletion of the earth's ozone layer. Instruments developed to test atmospheric contents indicated that chemicals used on earth, **chlorofluorocarbons (CFCs),** were contributing to its rapid depletion.

At first believed to be miracle chemicals, chlorofluorocarbons were used as refrigerants (Freon), as aerosol propellants in hairsprays and deodorants, as cleaning solvents, and in medical sterilizers, rigid foam insulation, and Styrofoam. But, along with halons (found in many fire extinguishers), methyl chloroform, and carbon tetrachloride (cleaning solvents), CFCs were eventually found to be a major cause of ozone depletion. When released into the air through spraying or outgassing, CFCs migrate upward toward the ozone layer, where they decompose and release chlorine atoms. These atoms cause ozone molecules to break apart (see Figure 21.1).

Radon A naturally occurring radioactive gas resulting from the decay of certain radioactive elements.

Sick building syndrome (SBS) Problem that exists when 80 percent of a building's occupants report maladies that tend to lessen or vanish when they leave the building.

Chlorofluorocarbons (CFCs) Chemicals that contribute to the depletion of the ozone layer.

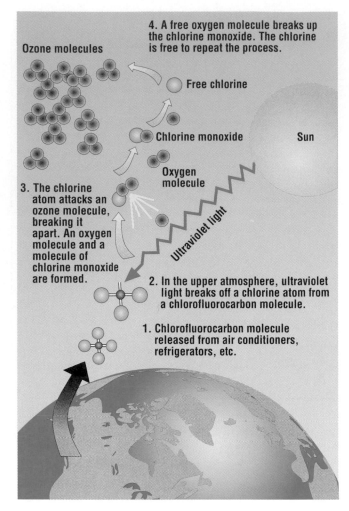

Figure 21.1
How the Ozone Layer Is Being Depleted

The labels within the figure read:

Ozone molecules

4. A free oxygen molecule breaks up the chlorine monoxide. The chlorine is free to repeat the process.

Free chlorine

Chlorine monoxide

Sun

Oxygen molecule

3. The chlorine atom attacks an ozone molecule, breaking it apart. An oxygen molecule and a molecule of chlorine monoxide are formed.

Ultraviolet light

2. In the upper atmosphere, ultraviolet light breaks off a chlorine atom from a chlorofluorocarbon molecule.

1. Chlorofluorocarbon molecule released from air conditioners, refrigerators, etc.

In the early 1970s, the U.S. government banned the use of aerosol sprays containing CFCs. The discovery of an "ozone hole" over Antarctica led to the 1987 Montreal Protocol treaty, whereby the United States and other nations agreed to reduce the use of CFCs and other ozone-depleting chemicals. The treaty was amended in 1995 to ban CFC production in developed countries. Today, over 160 countries have signed the treaty, as the international community strives to preserve the ozone layer.[20]

Global Warming

More than 100 years ago, scientists theorized that carbon dioxide emissions from fossil-fuel burning would create a buildup of *greenhouse gases* in the earth's atmosphere that could have a warming effect on the earth's surface. The

> **Greenhouse gases** Gases that contribute to global warming by trapping heat near the earth's surface.

century-old predictions now seem to be coming true, with alarming results. According to the National Academy of Sciences, the earth's surface temperature has risen 1 degree Fahrenheit in the past century, with accelerated warming in the past two decades,[21] and there is new and strong evidence that most of the warming over the last 50 years is due to human activities.[22]

With average global temperatures higher today than at any time since global temperatures were first recorded, the change in atmospheric temperature may be taking a heavy toll on human beings and crops. Climate researchers predicted in 1975 that the buildup of greenhouse gases would produce life-threatening natural phenomena, including drought in the Midwestern United States, more frequent and severe forest fires, flooding in India and Bangladesh, extended heat waves over large areas of the earth, and killer hurricanes. Recently, the planet has experienced all five of these phenomena, although whether they are connected to global warming remains a matter of debate.

Greenhouse gases include carbon dioxide, CFCs, ground-level ozone, nitrous oxide, and methane. They become part of a gaseous layer that encircles the earth, allowing solar heat to pass through and then trapping it close to the earth's surface. The most predominant is carbon dioxide, which accounts for 49 percent of all greenhouse gases. Eastern Europe and North America are responsible for approximately half of all carbon dioxide emissions. Since the late nineteenth century, carbon dioxide concentrations in the atmosphere have increased by 30 percent, with half of this increase occurring since the 1950s. Carbon emissions from the burning of fossil fuels, oil, coal, and gas continue to climb. In 2000, the United States emitted about one-fifth of total global greenhouse gases.[23]

Rapid deforestation of the tropical rain forests of Central and South America, Africa, and Southeast Asia is also contributing to the rapid rise in the presence of greenhouse gases. Trees take in carbon dioxide, transform it, store the carbon for food, and then release oxygen into the air. As we lose forests, at the rate of hundreds of acres per hour, we are losing the capacity to dissipate carbon dioxide. Forest fires in Indonesia in 1997 propelled more greenhouse gases into the atmosphere in a few months than does all of Europe's industrial activity in a year.

Reducing Air Pollution

Our national air pollution problems are rooted in our energy, transportation, and industrial practices. We must develop comprehensive national strategies to address the problem of air pollution in order to clean the air for the future. We must support policies that encourage the use of renewable resources such as solar, wind, and water power as the providers of most of the world's energy. Table 21.3 indicates global trends in sources of energy consumption.

Most experts agree that shifting away from automobiles as the primary source of transportation is the only way to reduce air pollution significantly. Many cities

Table 21.3
Global Trends in Energy Use, by Source, 1990–1997

ENERGY SOURCE	ANNUAL RATE OF GROWTH (%)
Wind power	25.7
Solar power	16.8
Geothermal power	3.0
Natural gas	21.1
Hydroelectric power	1.6
Oil	1.4
Nuclear power	0.6

Source: C. Flavin and S. Dunn, *Vital Signs Brief 98–6: Merger Signals Beginning of Geriatric Era for Oil Industry* (Washington, DC: Worldwatch Institute, 1998).

have taken steps in this direction by setting high parking fees, imposing bans on city driving, and establishing high road-usage tolls. Community governments should be encouraged to provide convenient, inexpensive, and easily accessible public transportation for citizens.

Although stricter laws on carbon emissions from cars and trucks and new cars that operate on electricity and gas are promising, we have a long way to go to reduce fossil fuel consumption. One promising initiative is "bicycle power." Bicycles are gaining popularity. Currently, China leads the world in bicycle use, followed by India. In Germany, bicycle use has increased by 50 percent, and England has a plan to quadruple bicycle use by the year 2012.[24]

Water Pollution

Seventy-five percent of the earth is covered with water in the form of oceans, seas, lakes, rivers, streams, and wetlands. Beneath the landmass are reservoirs of groundwater. We draw our drinking water from either this underground source or from surface freshwater sources. However, just 1 percent of our entire water supply is available for human use—the rest is too salty or locked away in polar ice caps.[25] Considering that this water must meet the world's agricultural, manufacturing, community, personal, and sanitation needs, it is no wonder that clean water is a precious commodity. Table 21.4 shows how much water might be saved daily through simple conservation actions.

The safety of our water supply cannot be taken for granted. Local and state governments, public water systems, and the Environmental Protection Agency (EPA) spend more than $22 billion per year to protect and maintain water quality.[26] The status of our water supply reflects the pollution level of our communities and, ultimately, of the whole earth.

Water Contamination

Many factors can contribute to water contamination. Microorganisms can flourish if water temperature and oxygen levels become hospitable to their growth, and these microbes can cause disease outbreaks. In 1993, an outbreak of cryptosporidiosis caused over 400,000 people to become sick from contaminated city water in Milwaukee, Wisconsin. Diseases such as hepatitis A, cholera, and amoebic dysentery can cause severe illness and death.

In addition to microbial contamination, water can become polluted by toxic chemicals such as pesticides, herbicides, fertilizers, and a host of other chemicals. You need only go to your local hardware store and note the aisles of chemicals that we can spray on our lawns to keep them green, to kill weeds, kill insects, and remove paint and stains to fully appreciate the magnitude of toxic load that we wash down with water every day of our lives. These substances end up in our sewers, our water supplies, and our general environment. The potential health hazards of mixing these thousands of chemicals together can barely be imagined.

Any substance that gets into the soil can potentially enter the water supply. Industrial pollutants, acid rain, and pesticides

Table 21.4
Daily per Capita Water Use (in Gallons) in Single-Family Homes

TYPE OF USE	WITHOUT	WITH WATER-CONSERVING DEVICES
Showers	12.6	10.0
Washing machines	15.1	10.6
Toilets	20.1	9.3
Dishwashers	1.0	1.0
Baths	1.2	1.2
Leaks	10.0	5.0
Faucets	11.1	10.8
Other domestic use	1.5	1.5
Total	**72.6**	**49.4**

Total savings: 23.3 gallons per day

Source: Adapted from "1999 Residential Water Use Summary," by permission. Copyright © 2002, American Water Works Association.

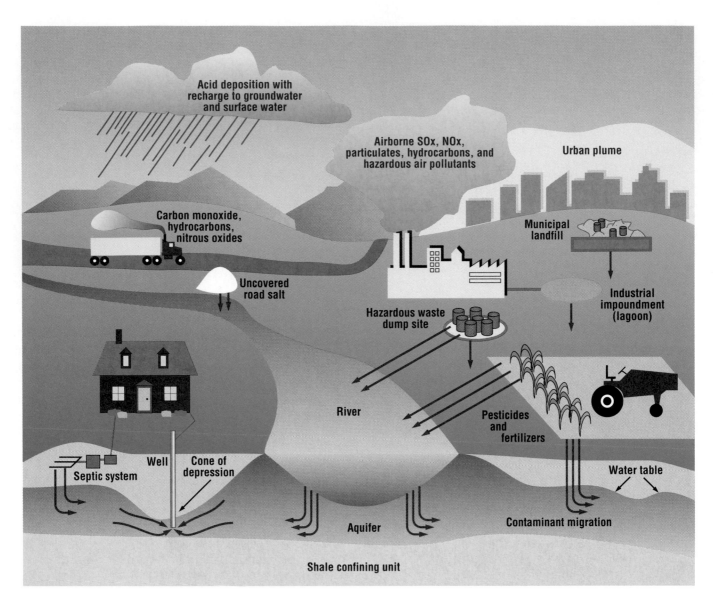

Figure 21.2
Sources of Groundwater Contamination

eventually work their way into the soil, then into groundwater. Underground storage tanks for gasoline may leak. Oil spills such as the one off the coast of Spain in November 2002 contaminate coastal waterways and spill into local rivers, along with hazardous farming and industrial wastes. Today over 1.1 billion persons (one-sixth of the world's population) do not have access to safe drinking water.[27]

Congress has coined two terms, *point source* and *nonpoint source,* to describe the two general sources of water pollution. **Point source pollutants** enter a waterway at a specific point through a pipe, ditch, culvert, or other conduit. The two major sources of this type of pollution are sewage treatment plants and industrial facilities.

Nonpoint source pollutants—commonly known as *runoff* and *sedimentation*—run off or seep into waterways from broad areas of land rather than through a discrete conduit. It is estimated that 99 percent of the sediment in our

waterways, 98 percent of the bacterial contaminants, 84 percent of the phosphorus, and 82 percent of the nitrogen come from nonpoint sources.[28] Nonpoint pollution results from a variety of human land use practices. It includes soil erosion and sedimentation, construction wastes, pesticide and fertilizer runoff, urban street runoff, wastes from engineering projects, acid mine drainage, leakage from septic tanks, and sewage sludge.[29] (See Figure 21.2.)

Septic Systems Bacteria from human waste can leach into the water supply from improperly installed septic systems. Toxic chemicals that are dumped into septic systems can also enter groundwater.

Landfills Landfills and dumps generate a liquid called **leachate,** a mixture of soluble chemicals from household garbage, office waste, biological waste, and industrial waste.

If a landfill has not been properly lined, leachate trickles through its layers of garbage and eventually into the water supply as acid and into the atmosphere as methane gas.

Gasoline and Petroleum Products   In the United States, there are more than 2 million underground storage tanks for gasoline and petroleum products, most of which are located at gasoline filling stations. One-quarter of these underground tanks are thought to be leaking.[30]

Most of these tanks were installed 25 to 30 years ago. They were made of fabricated steel that was unprotected from corrosion. Over time, pinpoint holes develop in the steel, and the petroleum products leak into the groundwater. The most common way to detect the presence of petroleum products in water is to test for benzene, a component of oil and gasoline. Benzene is highly toxic and associated with the development of cancer.

Chemical Contaminants

Organic solvents are chemicals designed to dissolve grease and oil. These extremely toxic substances, such as carbon tetrachloride, tetrachloroethylene, and trichloroethylene (TCE), are used to clean clothing, painting equipment, plastics, and metal parts. Many household products, such as stain and spot removers, degreasers, drain cleaners, septic system cleaners, and paint removers, also contain these toxic chemicals.

Organic solvents work their way into the water supply in different ways. Consumers often dump leftover products into the toilet or into street drains. Industries pour leftovers into large barrels, which are then buried. After a while, the chemicals eat their way out of the barrels and leach into groundwater.

One related group of toxic substances contains chlorinated hydrocarbons. The most notorious of these substances are the **polychlorinated biphenyls (PCBs),** their cousins the *polybromated biphenyls (PBBs),* and the *dioxins.*

PCBs   Fire resistant and stable at high temperatures, PCBs were used for many years as insulating materials in high-voltage electrical equipment such as transformers. PCBs bioaccumulate, meaning that the body does not excrete them but rather stores them in fatty tissues and the liver. PCBs are associated with birth defects, and exposure to them is known to cause cancer. The manufacture of PCBs was discontinued in the United States in 1977, but approximately 500 million pounds of them have been dumped into landfills and waterways, where they continue to pose an environmental threat.[31]

Dioxins   Dioxins are chlorinated hydrocarbons found in herbicides (chemicals that are used to kill vegetation) and produced during certain industrial processes. Dioxins have the ability to bioaccumulate and are much more toxic than PCBs.

The long-term effects of bioaccumulation of these toxic substances include possible damage to the immune system and increased risk of infections and cancer. Exposure to high concentrations of PCBs or dioxins for a short period

of time can also have severe consequences, including nausea, vomiting, diarrhea, painful rashes and sores, and chloracne, an ailment in which the skin develops hard, black, painful pimples that may never go away. See the Men's Health/Women's Health Box for other risks that toxics exposures may pose for women.

Pesticides   Pesticides are chemicals that are designed to kill insects, rodents, plants, and fungi. Americans use more than 1.2 billion pounds of pesticides each year, but only 10 percent actually reach the targeted organisms. The remaining 1.1 billion pounds of pesticides settle on the land and in our water. Pesticide residues also cling to many fresh fruits and vegetables and are ingested when people eat these items.

Most pesticides remain in the environment and accumulate in the body. A recent study found a correlation between breast cancer and dieldrin, a popular pesticide used until the 1970s.[32] Women who had the highest traces of dieldrin in their blood were twice as likely as women with the lowest levels to develop breast cancer. Other potential hazards associated with exposure to pesticides include birth defects, liver and kidney damage, and nervous system disorders.

Lead   The Environmental Protection Agency has issued new standards to reduce dramatically the levels of lead in U.S. drinking water. These standards are already in place in many municipalities and will eventually reduce lead exposure for approximately 130 million people. The new rules stipulate that tap water lead values must not exceed 15 parts per billion (the previous standard allowed an average lead level of 50 parts per billion). When water suppliers identify problem areas, they will have to lower the water's acidity with chemical treatment because acidity increases water's ability to leach lead from the pipes through which it passes, or they will have to replace old lead plumbing in the service lines.

If lead does exist in your home's water, you can reduce your risk by running tap water for several minutes before taking a drink or cooking with it. This flushes out water that

---

Point source pollutants   Pollutants that enter waterways at a specific point.

Nonpoint source pollutants   Pollutants that run off or seep into waterways from broad areas of land.

Leachate   A liquid consisting of soluble chemicals that come from garbage and industrial waste that seeps into the water supply from landfills and dumps.

Polychlorinated biphenyls (PCBs)   Toxic chemicals that were once used as insulating materials in high-voltage electrical equipment.

Dioxins   Highly toxic chlorinated hydrocarbons contained in herbicides and produced during certain industrial processes.

Pesticides   Chemicals that kill pests.

Women's Health and the Environment

In addition to the common environmental health threats faced by both women and men, as we have seen in earlier chapters, women encounter particular diseases that are specific to their sex. The following conditions are currently being studied to determine specific environmental influences.

BREAST CANCER

Scientists are studying possible links between environmental estrogens and breast cancer. Environmental estrogens are synthetic and natural compounds scientists believe may mimic the female hormone estrogen and either act like estrogens or block the body's natural hormone. Environmental estrogens are found in pesticides, PCBs, and even natural plant products in our diet.

ENDOMETRIOSIS

Endometriosis is a condition in which the tissue that lines the uterus and is shed during menstruation grows outside the uterus, often creating painful implants on the ovaries, fallopian tubes, and ligaments that support the uterus. Again, environmental estrogens are suspect.

OSTEOPOROSIS

Osteoporosis, a debilitating bone fragility, commonly occurs in postmenopausal women. Scientists think that cadmium, lead, and possibly other heavy metals in the environment may contribute to the development of this disease.

AUTOIMMUNE DISEASES

Women are more susceptible to autoimmune diseases such as multiple sclerosis, rheumatoid arthritis, scleroderma (a connective tissue disease), and systemic lupus erythematosus. Scientists have linked autoimmune diseases to chemicals such as pharmaceuticals, solvents, and food additives.

Source: National Institute of Environmental Health Sciences, National Institutes of Health, "Women's Health and the Environment," NIEHS Fact Sheet #10, 1997.

---

has been standing overnight in lead-contaminated lines. Although leaded paints and ceramic glazes used to pose health risks, particularly for small children who put painted toys in their mouths, the use of lead in such products has been effectively reduced in recent years.

What do you think?

Who should bear the financial responsibility for cleaning up hazardous waste leaks? ✷ What can you do to avoid contributing to water contamination?

Noise Pollution

Loud noise has become commonplace. We are often painfully aware of construction crews in our streets, jet airplanes roaring overhead, stereos blaring next door, and trucks rumbling down nearby freeways.

Our bodies show definite physiological responses to noise, and it can become a source of physical or mental distress. Short-term exposure to loud noise reduces productivity, concentration levels, and attention spans and may affect mental and emotional health. Symptoms of noise-related distress include disturbed sleep patterns, headaches, and tension. Physically, our bodies respond to noise in a variety of ways. Blood pressure increases, blood vessels in the brain dilate, and vessels in other parts of the body constrict. The pupils of the eye dilate. Cholesterol levels in the blood rise, and some endocrine glands secrete additional stimulating hormones, such as adrenaline, into the bloodstream.

Sounds are measured in decibels. Table 21.5 shows the decibel levels for various sounds. Hearing can be damaged by varying lengths of exposure to sound. If the duration of allowable daily exposure to different decibel levels is exceeded, hearing loss will result.

Unfortunately, despite increasing awareness that noise pollution is more than just a nuisance, noise control programs at federal, state, and local levels have received low budgetary priority. To protect your hearing, you must take it upon yourself to avoid exposure to excessive noise. Playing stereos in your car and home at reasonable levels, wearing ear plugs when you use power equipment, and establishing barriers (closed windows, etc.) between you and noise will help keep your hearing intact.

What do you think?

What do you currently do that places your hearing at risk? ✷ What changes can you make in your lifestyle to protect your hearing?

Land Pollution

Solid Waste

Each day, every person in the United States generates about 4 pounds of **municipal solid waste**—containers and packaging, discarded food, yard debris, and refuse from residential, commercial, institutional, and industrial sources.

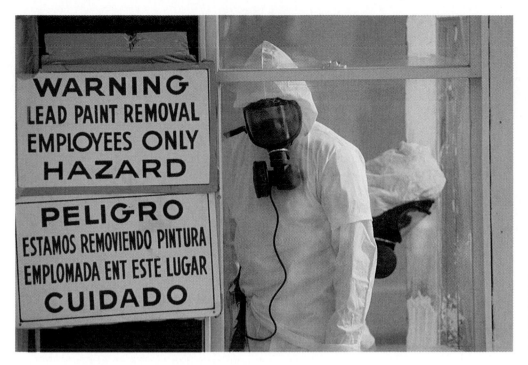

Although an expensive and cumbersome project, deleading a house is now one of the most important considerations of prospective homeowners, especially those with children.

Approximately 73 percent of this waste is buried in landfills. Cities throughout the country are in danger of exhausting their landfill space.

As communities run out of landfill space, it is becoming more common to haul garbage out to sea to dump it or ship it to landfills in developing countries. Figure 21.3 shows the composition of our trash and what happens to our garbage after disposal. Although experts believe that up to 90 percent of our trash is recyclable, only 26 percent of it is currently recycled. In today's throwaway society, we need to become aware of the amount of waste we generate every day and to look for ways to recycle, reuse, and—most desirable of all—reduce the products we use.

Hazardous Waste

The community of Love Canal, New York, has come to symbolize **hazardous waste** dump sites. The Hooker Chemical Company used Love Canal as a chemical dump site for nearly 30 years, starting in the 1920s. Then the area was filled in by land developers and built up with homes and schools.

In 1976, homeowners began noticing strange seepage in their basements and strong chemical odors. Babies were born with abnormal hearts and kidneys, two sets of teeth, mental handicaps, epilepsy, liver disease, and abnormal rectal bleeding. The rate of cancer and miscarriages was far above normal.

The New York State Department of Health investigated the Love Canal area and found high concentrations of PCBs in the storm sewers near the old canal, but it took the

---

Table 21.5
Noise Levels of Various Activities (in Decibels)

Decibels (db) measure the volume of sounds. Here are the decibel levels of some common sounds.

TYPE OF SOUND	NOISE LEVEL (DB)
Carrier deck jet operation	150
Jet takeoff from 200 feet	140
Rock concert	120 (painful)
Auto horn (3 feet)	110 (extremely loud)
Motorcycle	100
Garbage truck	100
Pneumatic drill	90
Lawnmower	90
Heavy traffic	80
Alarm clock	80
Shouting, arguing	80 (very loud)
Vacuum cleaner	75 (loud)
Freight train from 50 feet	70
Freeway traffic	65
Normal conversation	60
Light auto traffic	50 (moderate)
Library	40
Soft whisper	30 (faint)

Municipal solid waste   Solid wastes such as durable goods, nondurable goods, containers and packaging, food wastes, yard wastes, and miscellaneous wastes from residential, commercial, institutional, and industrial sources.

Hazardous waste   Solid waste that, due to its toxic properties, poses a hazard to humans or to the environment.

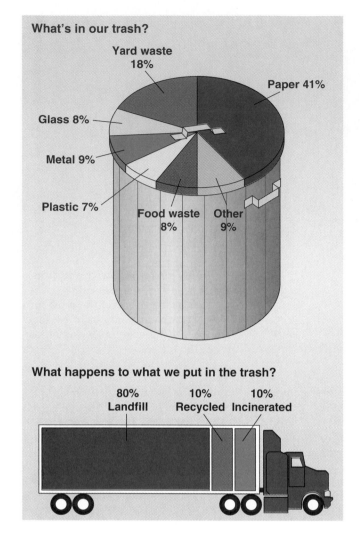

What's in our trash?

Yard waste 18%

Paper 41%

Glass 8%

Metal 9%

Plastic 7%

Food waste 8%

Other 9%

What happens to what we put in the trash?

80% Landfill

10% Recycled

10% Incinerated

Figure 21.3
The Composition and Disposal of Trash

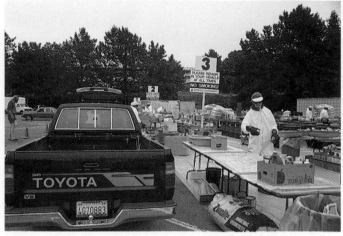

Many communities now provide special programs where their residents can drop off any kind of hazardous waste for safe disposal.

department another two years to order the evacuation of Love Canal homes. Over 900 families were evacuated, and the state purchased their homes. Finally, in 1978, the expensive process of cleaning up the waste dump began. Many lawsuits for damages are still being litigated.

In 1980, the Comprehensive Environmental Response Compensation and Liability Act **(Superfund)** was enacted to provide funds for cleaning up chemical dump sites that endanger public health and land. This fund is financed through taxes on the chemical and petroleum industries (87 percent) and through general federal tax revenues (13 percent). Cleanup cost estimates from the year 1990 through 2020 range from $106 billion to as high as $500 billion.[33]

Superfund Fund established under the Comprehensive Environmental Response Compensation and Liability Act to be used for cleaning up toxic waste dumps.

To date, 32,500 potentially hazardous waste sites have been identified across the nation. After investigation, 17,800 of these sites were determined to require no further action. But about 1,300 sites are listed on the National Priorities List (NPL), and 46 percent of the sites assessed from 1992 through 1996 are a hazard to human health.[34] The large number of hazardous waste dump sites in the United States indicates the severity of our toxic chemical problem. American manufacturers generate more than 1 ton of chemical waste per person per year (approximately 275 million tons). The *Agency for Toxic Substances and Disease Registry (ATSDR)* and the *EPA* evaluate and rank the chemicals that are considered hazardous substances (see Table 21.6).

The EPA and the states have undertaken a "cradle-to-grave" program to manage hazardous wastes by monitoring their generation, transportation, storage, treatment, and final disposal.[35] To ensure that hazardous wastes being generated

---

Table 21.6
Top 20 Hazardous Substances: ATSDR/EPA Priority List for 2001

1.	Arsenic	11.	Chloroform
2.	Lead	12.	DDT, P′P′-
3.	Mercury	13.	Aroclor 1254
4.	Vinyl chloride	14.	Aroclor 1260
5.	Polychlorinated biphenyls (PCBs)	15.	Trichlorethylene
		16.	Dibenz[a, h]anthracene
6.	Benzene	17.	Dieldrin
7.	Cadmium	18.	Chromium, Hexavalent
8.	Benzo(a)pyrene	19.	Chlordane
9.	Polycyclic aromatic hydrocarbons	20.	Hexachlorobutadiene
10.	Benzo(b)fluoranthene		

Source: Agency for Toxic Substances and Disease Registry (ATSDR), 2001 (see http://www.atsdr.cdc.gov/cxcx3.html).

Environmental Racism

Environmental racism has meant, among other things, that toxic waste dumps, landfills, and industrial plants are much more likely to be placed in communities of color and in the developing world than in predominantly white communities. The adverse health effects of environmental racism have been devastating for people of color in the United States and throughout the world.

A clear example comes from the Amazon rain forest of Ecuador. Over a 21-year period, an American oil company systematically dumped more than 16 million gallons of oil and toxic wastewater into the Ecuadorian Amazon. Three indigenous groups lived in the area where the oil company operated—the Cofan, the Secoya, and the Siona. The Cofan, who numbered approximately 15,000 when the oil company built its first well in 1971, now number only a few hundred. The Secoya and Siona populations have also declined. Each of these three groups was a fishing culture when the oil company first came to the Amazon. Now, because of oil contamination, they can no longer fish in the rivers and so face malnourishment. Often young people migrate to the cities and take low-wage jobs. The result of the contamination of the environment has been the practical decimation of these three cultures.

In the mid-1990s, the remaining indigenous people filed suit against the oil company, claiming that it had violated their right to a healthy environment. They alleged that the company's decision to dump millions of gallons of toxins in the rain forest led to the cultural genocide of the three tribes, amounting to racial and ethnic discrimination. One of the tribes' attorneys commented, "The fact is when [the oil company] drills for oil where white people live, they do it safely and according to industry standards. When they drilled in the headwaters of the Amazon River, however, they blatantly ignored these standards while knowingly wreaking havoc on the local people, almost all of whom are people of color." As late as September 1999, the oil company was continuing to fight the lawsuit and refusing to clean up the Amazon. Indigenous leaders launched a national media campaign in the United States, charging the oil company with racism. The company denied that race played any role in its actions.

Scientific literature clearly demonstrates that crude oil and toxic wastewater produced by oil drilling are highly carcinogenic. A public health study of San Carlos, an Ecuadorian town containing more than 30 oil wells, found cancer rates 30 times greater than normal, despite the fact that local inhabitants do not smoke, eat a healthy diet, and are not exposed to urban contamination. Additionally, no other industries in the area release cancer-causing toxins. The water in San Carlos had nearly 150 times the amount of hydrocarbons considered safe by internationally recognized limits.

Examples of environmental racism can also be found throughout the United States:

- In Los Angeles, recycling plants were located in low-income, primarily Latino neighborhoods. Local residents consistently complained of dustlike glass particles in the air.
- In Augusta, Georgia, a wood preservant factory leaked creosote into the ground, and a scrap metal company leaked arsenic. This ethnic minority community now evidences high rates of cancer and skin disease. The plants are also located near an elementary school, and students there experience high rates of learning disabilities, allergies, and asthma.
- In the predominantly African American area of Chester, Pennsylvania, four hazardous and municipal waste facilities are located. That area has the highest percentage of low-weight births in the state as well as mortality and lung cancer rates 60 percent higher than in the rest of the county.

Many health, civil rights, and environmental activists have become proponents of environmental justice. They argue that people of color have the right to be protected from hazardous substances and that public policy be developed based on mutual respect and justice for all people.

today do not become complex and expensive cleanup problems tomorrow, the following steps are being taken:

- Many wastes are now banned from land disposal or are being treated to reduce their toxicity before they become part of land disposal sites.
- The EPA has developed protective requirements for land disposal facilities, such as double liners, detection systems for substances that may leach into groundwater, and groundwater monitoring systems.
- Hazardous waste handlers must now clean up contamination resulting from past waste management practices as well as from current activities.
- The EPA is exploring economic incentives to encourage ingenuity in waste minimization practices and recycling.[36]

See the Health in a Diverse World box for a description of the devastating effects of hazardous waste, oil contamination, and other environmental problems on minority communities.

What do you think?

*What items do you currently recycle? * What are some of the reasons you do not recycle? * What might encourage you to recycle more than you do? * What concerns would you have about living near a landfill or hazardous waste disposal site?*

Radiation

A substance is said to be radioactive when it emits high-energy particles from the nuclei of its atoms. There are three types of radiation: alpha particles, beta particles, and gamma rays. *Alpha* particles are relatively massive and are not capable of penetrating human skin. They pose health hazards only when inhaled or ingested. *Beta* particles can penetrate the skin slightly and are harmful if ingested or inhaled. *Gamma* rays are the most dangerous because they can pass straight through the skin, causing serious damage to organs and other vital structures.

Ionizing Radiation

Exposure to ionizing radiation is an inescapable part of life on this planet. **Ionizing radiation** is caused by the release of particles and electromagnetic rays from atomic nuclei during the normal process of disintegration. Some naturally occurring elements, such as uranium, emit radiation. Radiation can wreak havoc on human cells, leading to mutations, cancer, miscarriages, and other problems.

Reactions to radiation differ from person to person. Exposure is measured in **radiation absorbed doses, or rads** (also called *roentgens*). Recommended maximum "safe" dosages range from 0.5 rads to 5 rads per year. Approximately 50 percent of the radiation to which we are exposed comes from natural sources, such as building materials. Another 45 percent comes from medical and dental x-rays. The remaining 5 percent comes from computer display screens, microwave ovens, television sets, luminous watch dials, and radar screens and waves. Most of us are exposed to far less radiation than the "safe" maximum dosage per year.

Radiation can cause damage at dosages as low as 100 to 200 rads. At this level, signs of radiation sickness include nausea, diarrhea, fatigue, anemia, sore throat, and hair loss, but death is unlikely. At 350 to 500 rads, these symptoms become more severe, and death may result because the radiation hinders bone marrow production of the white blood cells we need to protect us from disease. Dosages above 600 to 700 rads are invariably fatal. The effects of long-term exposure to relatively low levels of radiation are unknown. Some scientists believe that such exposure can cause lung cancer, leukemia, skin cancer, bone cancer, and skeletal deformities.

Ionizing radiation   Radiation produced by photons having high enough energy to ionize atoms

Radiation absorbed doses (rads)   Units that measure exposure to radioactivity.

Meltdown   An accident that results when the temperature in the core of a nuclear reactor increases enough to melt the nuclear fuel and the containment vessel housing it.

Researchers are now investigating links between the radio frequency waves generated by cell phones and cancer, but results are inconclusive (see the New Horizons in Health box).

EMFs: Emerging Risks?

If you believe what you hear on TV or read in the papers, electric and magnetic fields (EMFs) generated by electric power delivery systems are responsible for risks for cancer (particularly among children), reproductive dysfunction, birth defects, neurological disorders, Alzheimer's disease, and other ailments. But does research support these claims about EMFs? Though many believe that the threat is legitimate, others point to major discrepancies and inconsistencies in the research. In spite of many questions, fears have increased, and there is probably more potential for exploitation of consumers than real hazard to health from this nonionizing form of exposure.

A six-year study by the National Institute of Environmental Health Sciences (NIEHS) found that the evidence for a link between cancer and EMFs is "weak," although the director of NIEHS warned that efforts to reduce exposure should continue. The study did find a slight increase in risk for childhood leukemia, as well as chronic lymphocytic leukemia in occupationally exposed adults such as utility workers, machinists, and welders. However, NIEHS suggests that the lack of consistent, positive findings weakens the contention that this association is actually due to EMFs.[37]

Nuclear Power Plants

Nuclear power plants account for less than 1 percent of the total radiation to which we are exposed. Other producers of radioactive waste include medical facilities that use radioactive materials as treatment and diagnostic tools and nuclear weapons production facilities.

Proponents of nuclear energy believe that it is a safe and efficient way to generate electricity. Initial costs of building nuclear power plants are high, but actual power generation is relatively inexpensive. A 1,000-megawatt reactor produces enough energy for 650,000 homes and saves 420 million gallons of fossil fuels each year. In some areas where nuclear power plants were decommissioned, electricity bills tripled when power companies turned to hydroelectric or fossil fuel sources to generate electricity.

Nuclear reactors also discharge fewer carbon oxides into the air than fossil fuel–powered generators. Advocates believe that conversion to nuclear power could help slow the global warming trend. Over the past 15 years, carbon emissions were reduced by 298 million tons, or 5 percent.

All these advantages of nuclear energy must be weighed against the disadvantages. First, disposal of nuclear wastes is extremely problematic for the entire world. Additionally, a reactor core meltdown could pose serious threats to a plant's immediate environment and to the world in general.

A **meltdown** occurs when the temperature in the core of a nuclear reactor increases enough to melt both the

Wireless Worries: Cell Phones and Risks to Health

In less than a decade, cell phones have become a household staple, with the number of subscribers skyrocketing from a mere 16 million in 1994 to over 110 million in 2001, a number that continues to increase by a rate of 1 million per month.

Although the sight of people chatting on cell phones is commonplace, such use continues to spur controversy, particularly when issues of potential health risks are discussed. While the cell phone industry has assured consumers for years that phones are completely safe, a former industry research director, Dr. George Carlo, stated in 2002 that such assurances of safety may not be reliable. He argues that past studies have not provided conclusive evidence of safety and that we do not know what the effects of current cell phone usage may be on future generations. He observed, "This is the first generation that has put relatively high-powered transmitters against the head, hour after hour, day after day." Depending on how close the cell phone antenna is to the head, as much as 60 percent of microwave radiation may be absorbed by and actually penetrate the area around the head, some reaching an inch to an inch and a half into the brain.

Are increases in the incidence and prevalence of brain tumors and other neurological conditions in the last decade related to cell phone use? At high power levels, radio frequency energy, which is the energy used in cell phones, can rapidly heat biological tissue and cause damage, such as burns. However, it is important to note that cell phones operate at power levels well below the level at which such heating effects occur. Many countries, including the United States and most of Europe, use standards set by the FCC for radio frequency energy based on research by several scientific groups. These groups identified a whole-body *specific absorption rate (SAR)* value for exposure to radio frequency energy. Four watts per kilogram was identified as a threshold level of exposure at which harmful biological effects may occur. Every phone distributed has a specific SAR level associated with it. The FCC requires wireless phones to comply with a safety limit of 1.6 watts per kilogram. To find out what the SAR for your phone is, see this website: http://www.fda.gov/cellphones/qa.html.

Should you be foregoing those long hours of chatting with friends and loved ones? Should you wear an ear bud or get a phone jack for your car to keep that phone at a distance from your head? The consensus of the Food and Drug Administration (FDA), the World Health Organization, and other major health agencies is that the research to date has not yet shown radio frequency energy emitted from cell phones to be harmful. However, they all point to the need for more research and caution that because cell phones have only been widely used for less than a decade, and because no long-term studies have been done, there is not yet enough information available to say that they pose no risk. Three recently published, large, case control studies and one large cohort study have compared cell phone use among brain cancer patients and individuals free of brain cancer. Some key findings from these studies are the following:

- Brain cancer patients did not report more cellular phone use overall than controls. In fact, most of the studies showed a tendency toward lower risk of brain cancer among cell phone users, for unclear reasons.
- None of the studies showed a clear link between the side of the head on which the cancer occurred and the side on which the phone was used.
- There was no correlation between brain tumor risk and dose of exposure, as assessed by duration of use, date since first subscription, age at first subscription, or type of cellular phone used.

Although these studies are inconclusive, preliminary results from smaller studies have continued to raise questions. The biggest risk from using cell phones today appears to be in using them during driving and a corresponding risk from crashes. However, if you would rather err on the side of caution, a few simple hints to reduce your risk may be in order:

- Use lighter- or dash-mounted phones or headphones/ear buds when driving. This not only helps keep your hands free and avoids crashes, but, if subsequent studies indicate the potential for health risks, you will have kept your brain away from the highest levels of radio frequency energy. Exposure levels drop dramatically with distance.
- Limit cell phone usage. Use land-based phones whenever possible.
- Check the SAR level of your phone. Purchase one with a lower level if yours is near the FCC limit.
- Digital phones have lower RFs than analog phones. An upgrade might be in order.

Sources: U.S. General Accounting Office (GAO), "Research and Regulatory Efforts on Mobile Cell Phone Health Issues" (GAO-01-545), Washington, DC. USGAO, 2001; H. Frumkin and M. Thun, "Environmental Carcinogens—Cellular Phones and Risk of Brain Tumors," *California Cancer Journal for Clinicians* 51 (2001): 137–141 (see http://www.cancer.org/eprise/main/docroot/PUB/content/PUB_3_8X_Environmtnal_Carcino); Brian Ross, "Wireless Worries?" ABC News 20/20, December 8, 2002 (see http://abcnews.go.com/onair/2020/2020_991020cellphones.html); Food and Drug Administration, FCC report, "Questions and Answers about Wireless Telephones," updated April 3, 2002 (see http://www.fda.gov/cellphones/qa.html).

Speaking Out on the Environment

Here are eight ways to get involved in the crusade against environmental pollution:

- Monitor legislation. All of the key environmental organizations keep tabs on state and national laws being considered in order to offer testimony and to generate letter-writing campaigns on behalf of (or against) proposed laws.
- Write letters or send e-mails. These communications may not seem like a potent weapon, but letters to state and federal legislators on pending bills do influence their opinions. When writing to any public official, keep your letter simple. Focus on one subject and identify a particular piece of legislation, request a specific action, and state your reasons for taking your position. If you live or work in the legislator's district, make sure to say so. Keep the letter to one or two paragraphs, and never write more than one page. Send your letters to:

Hon. _____
House Office Building
Washington, DC 20515

Senator _____
Senate Office Building
Washington, DC 20515

Find your senators' e-mail addresses online at www.senate.gov and your representative's address at www.house.gov.

- Fill out customer comment cards and phone toll-free numbers on packages. Let companies know your concerns.
- Educate others. You can do this in a variety of ways, from talking to your friends, coworkers, and neighbors to organizing an educational activity.
- Campaign for environmental candidates. Don't just be concerned about someone claiming to be an "environmental president." Look at the environmental positions of candidates at all levels of government.
- Launch a campaign at school or work. At Rutgers University, for example, members of the law association decided to target the use of plastic foam in the cafeterias. The students spoke with the director of food services, who readily agreed to stop using foam cups and foam food containers. Sometimes all you have to do is ask.

- Invite speakers to your organization. Most environmental organizations offer speakers on a wide range of topics who will speak at no charge to your civic, school, religious, or social organization. For maximum impact, consider scheduling a debate or panel discussion among representatives of environmental groups, government agencies, and industry.
- Get involved with government. Most communities offer a variety of boards, commissions, and committees that deal with environmental issues: planning commissions, zoning and land-use commissions, parks commissions, transit boards, and so on. Each can play a role in setting policies that affect the quality of the environment in your area.

Source: Except for the first paragraph, from *The Green Consumer Supermarket Guide*, 260–264, by J. Makower, J. Elkington, and J. Hailes. Copyright © 1991 by John Elkington, Julia Hailes, and Viking Penguin. Used by permission of Viking Penguin, a division of Penguin Putnam Inc. and Victor Gollancz Ltd.

---

nuclear fuel and the containment vessel that holds it. Most modern facilities seal their reactors and containment vessels in concrete buildings having pools of cold water on the bottom. If a meltdown occurs, the building and the pool are supposed to prevent the escape of radioactivity.

Two serious nuclear accidents within seven years of each other caused a steep decline in public support for nuclear energy. The first occurred in 1979 at Three Mile Island near Harrisburg, Pennsylvania, when a mechanical failure caused a partial meltdown of one reactor core and small amounts of radioactive steam were released into the atmosphere. No loss of human life was reported, although residents in the area were evacuated. Miscarriages, birth defects, and cancer rates in the area are reported to have increased, but no public health statistics have been released.

Human error and mechanical failure were the reported causes of the 1986 reactor core fire and explosion at the Chernobyl nuclear power plant in the Soviet Union. In just 4.5 seconds, the temperature in the reactor rose to 120 times normal, causing the explosion. Eighteen people were killed immediately, 30 workers died later from radiation sickness, and 200 other workers were hospitalized for severe radiation sickness. Soviet officials evacuated towns and villages near the plant. Some medical workers estimate that the eventual death toll from radiation-induced cancers related to the Chernobyl incident could top 100,000.

Radioactive fallout from the Chernobyl disaster spread over most of the Northern Hemisphere. Milk, meat, and vegetables in Scandinavian countries were contaminated with radioactive iodine and cesium and were declared unfit for human consumption. Thousands of reindeer in Lapland were contaminated and had to be destroyed. In Great Britain, thousands of sheep had to be destroyed, and three years later sheep in the northern regions of the country were still found to be contaminated. Direct costs of the disaster totaled more than $13 billion, including lost agricultural output and the cost of replacing the power plant. Nuclear accidents continue to pose risks to human health, even in well-controlled settings.

What do you think?

How much exposure do you have to ionizing and nonionizing radiation in a year? ✳ What measures could you take to reduce your exposure? ✳ Do you feel the advantages outweigh the disadvantages of nuclear power? ✳ Explain why or why not.

Taking Charge **21** 21 **21**

Managing Environmental Pollution

Caring for the environment is everyone's responsibility. See the Skills for Behavior Change box for ideas on what you can do to protect the environment. Personally, you can recycle, conserve energy, drive less, and pay attention to the products you buy and the practices these products support. As a consumer, you can make your opinions known by contacting corporations whose practices are unfriendly to the environment, and you can refuse to use their products. As a citizen, you can influence the government by voting and by contacting government officials and agencies to express your opinions about environmental issues.

Checklist for Change

Making Personal Choices

- ☐ Do you recycle newspaper, tin cans, glass, paper, plastic, and cardboard?
- ☐ Do you take short showers?

- ☐ Do you heat only rooms that are being used?
- ☐ Do you turn off lights when you leave a room?
- ☐ Do you use cold water and run your washing machine fully loaded?
- ☐ Do you dry clothes on a line when possible?
- ☐ Do you carpool or take public transportation whenever possible?
- ☐ Do you drive a car that gets good gas mileage?
- ☐ Do you purchase only the things you need?
- ☐ Do you recycle used oil?
- ☐ Do you use low-phosphorus fertilizers?
- ☐ Do you compost leaves, clippings, and kitchen scraps?
- ☐ Do you dispose of household chemicals safely?
- ☐ Do you buy products in recyclable packaging?
- ☐ Do you reuse containers rather than buy new ones?

- ☐ Do you refuse to use products that contribute to deforestation, wetland extinction, and water or air pollution?

Making Community Choices

- ☐ Do you write or call politicians to advocate for environmental legislation?
- ☐ Do you protest the location of hazardous waste sites and toxic chemical use in communities of color?
- ☐ Do you support candidates who have strong environmental records?
- ☐ Do you contact manufacturers to discourage overpackaging, nonrecyclable packaging, and environmentally harmful products?
- ☐ Do you encourage your school to recycle?

Summary

* Population growth is the single largest factor affecting the demands made on the environment. Demand for more food, products, and energy—as well as places to dispose of waste, particularly in the industrialized world—places great strains on the earth's resources.
* The primary constituents of air pollution are sulfur dioxide, particulate matter, carbon monoxide, nitrogen dioxide, ozone, lead, and hydrocarbons. Air pollution takes the forms of photochemical smog and acid rain, among others. Indoor air pollution is caused primarily by woodstove smoke, furnace emissions, asbestos, passive smoke, formaldehyde, radon, and household chemicals. Pollution is depleting the earth's protective ozone layer, contributing to global warming.
* Water pollution can be caused by either point (direct entry through a pipeline, ditch, etc.) or nonpoint (runoff or seepage from a broad area of land) sources. Chemicals that are major contributors to water pollution include dioxins, pesticides, and lead.
* Noise pollution affects our hearing and produces other symptoms such as reduced productivity, reduced concentration, headaches, and tension.
* Solid waste pollution includes household trash, plastics, glass, metal products, and paper; limited landfill space creates problems. Hazardous waste is toxic; its improper disposal creates health hazards for those in surrounding communities.
* Ionizing radiation results from the natural erosion of atomic nuclei. Nonionizing radiation is caused by the electric and magnetic fields around power lines and household appliances, among other sources. The disposal and storage of radioactive wastes from nuclear power plants and weapons production pose serious potential problems for public health.

Questions for Discussion and Reflection

1. How are the rapidly increasing global population and consumption of resources related? Is population control the best solution? Why or why not?
2. What are the primary sources of air pollution? What can be done to reduce air pollution?
3. What causes poor indoor air quality? How does indoor air pollution affect schoolchildren?
4. What are the causes and consequences of global warming?
5. What are point and nonpoint sources of water pollution? What can be done to reduce or prevent water pollution?
6. What are the physiological consequences of noise pollution? What can you do to lessen your exposure to noise pollution?
7. Why do you think so little recycling occurs in the United States?
8. Would you feel comfortable living near a nuclear power plant? Do you think nuclear power is an important source of energy in the future? Why or why not?

Application Exercises

Reread the What Do You Think? scenarios at the beginning of the chapter and answer the following questions.

1. What are the arguments in favor of and against population growth?
2. According to the sustainable resources proponents, what signs show that renewable resources are being depleted?
3. A larger population creates greater demand for resources and in turn generates greater amounts of waste. What steps could be taken worldwide to prevent population growth from depleting resources and polluting the environment? Describe components of a U.S. program to decrease consumption and pollution.
4. Do you agree with the scientists who believe that the increase in greenhouse gases is a result of human activities, or do you agree with those scientists who feel there is little evidence to suggest that humans have created this threat to the environment? Support your answer with examples.
5. Who do you think is responsible for the environment? Is there anything that you, as an individual, can do to slow the negative effects of greenhouse gases?

Accessing Your Health on the Internet

Visit the following Internet sites to explore further topics and issues related to personal health. To visit an organization's website, go to the Companion Website for *Access to Health, Eighth Edition* at www.aw.com/donatelle, click on the book image, and select "Accessing Your Health on the Internet" from the navigation menu on the left.

1. ***American Cancer Society Environmental Cancer Risks.*** Provides a searchable database of information about specific cancers and environmental risks, as well as a risk assessment and information about carcinogens.

2. ***Data Online for Population, Health, and Nutrition (DOLPHN) Database.*** DOLPHN provides demographic and health trend data relevant to the U.S. Agency for International Development. Subjects include child survival, family planning, access to clean water, and many other subjects.

3. ***GeoHive.*** A resource for general statistics on human population and health-related factors.

4. ***National Center for Environmental Health.*** A section of the Centers for Disease Control and Prevention, with information on a wide variety of environmental health issues, including a series of helpful fact sheets.

5. ***National Environmental Health Association.*** This organization provides educational resources and opportunities for environmental health professionals. The NEHA website lists conferences, training, and publications and offers informational position papers.

Further Reading

Cayne, B., and J. Tesar. *Food and Water: Threats, Shortages, and Solutions.* New York: Facts on File, 2002.

A basic introduction that discusses the vital importance of having an adequate supply of food and water and the need for alternative water storage and agricultural strategies.

Godish, T. *Indoor Environmental Quality.* Boca Raton, FL: Lewis Publishers, 2000.

Explores the scope of the indoor environment, both in the home and workplace, and major indoor contaminants.

Hofrichter, R., ed. *Reclaiming the Environmental Debate: The Politics of Health in a Toxic Culture.* Boston: MIT Press, 2000.

Examines the links between the threat of hazardous substances to public health and the social arrangements that encourage and excuse the deterioration of human health and the environment.

Nadakavukaren, N. *Our Global Environment: A Health Pespective.* Prospect Heights, II.: Waveland, 2000.

A survey of major global environmental issues and their ecological impact on personal and community health.

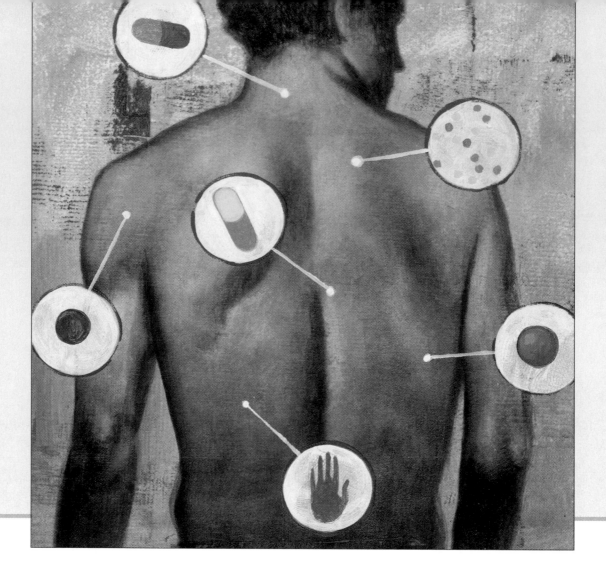

objectives

22

Consumerism

Selecting Health Care Products and Services

What do you think?

Beth has been fighting a sore throat and elevated temperature for several days and is worried she may be getting strep throat. It's the end of the term, she's short on time and money, and she just needs to make it through her last final. A friend offers Beth some leftover antibiotics she had received from the Student Health Center last month.

What risks are associated with taking someone else's prescription drug? ✷ What part of the directions for taking the antibiotic did Beth's friend ignore? ✷ What are the dangers of taking only a part of the dose of an antibiotic that have been prescribed?

Ira and Sarah Lamm belong to a privately managed health care plan. Other than covering their own care, this plan pays an independent pediatrician in the community a set monthly fee to provide care for the Lamms' two young children. Recently, their seven-year-old son, Randy, was diagnosed with leukemia. The family pediatrician informed the parents that she could no longer provide the advanced level of treatment that Randy now needs and would be transferring his care to someone who specializes in treating childhood cancers. The only pediatric oncologist covered by the plan is in a town 50 miles away, and this doctor has been designated as Randy's primary health care provider.

Why might such a change upset the Lamms? ✷ Some people feel that managed care has depersonalized health care and that there are built-in incentives for health care providers to care for patients only when they are essentially well. Do you agree with this viewpoint? ✷ How does the Lamms' current plan limit options for Randy's care? ✷ What are the benefits of such a plan?

There are many reasons to be an informed health care consumer. Most important, you have only one body and if you don't treat it with care, you will pay a major price in terms of financial costs and health consequences. Doing everything you can to prevent illness, stay healthy, and recover rapidly when you do get sick will enhance every other part of your life.

Another reason to be an active health consumer is that as a citizen or resident of the United States, you have no constitutional right to health care. Our society generally treats health care as a private-consumption good or service to be bought and sold rather than as a social good to which everyone is entitled. Therefore, to obtain high-quality health care at an affordable cost, you need to be both informed and assertive. But, as you may already know, medical and health care services are much harder to evaluate for need, availability, cost, and quality than are, say, articles of clothing or vegetables. In addition, you may seek health care services in circumstances of physical or emotional distress when your decision-making powers are compromised and you may find yourself very vulnerable.

This chapter will help you make better decisions about your health and health care. Our health care system is a maze of health care providers, payers (insurance, government, and individuals), and products, and many of us find it hard to thread our way through it. Health care is the fifth-largest industry in our country, accounting for over 10 percent of our workforce, and many different companies aggressively market health products and services to the public. Increasingly, health care organizations are "for-profit" businesses, sold and traded on the stock market, and making a profit is the goal. Medical professionals and consumers report that they feel overwhelmed, confused, and frustrated by the multitude of choices, seemingly divergent interests, and lack of coordination in our system.

Responsible Consumerism: Choices and Challenges

Perhaps the single greatest difficulty that we face as health consumers is the sheer magnitude of choices available to us. If you try to select a general practitioner from the telephone book when you are sick, you have to thumb through dozens of pages of specialists. When you want to purchase cough syrup, you are confronted with hundreds of options, each

---

Spontaneous remission The disappearance of symptoms without any apparent cause or treatment.

Placebo effect An apparent cure or improved state of health brought about by a substance or product that has no medicinal value.

---

claiming to do more for you than the brand next to it. Even trained pharmacists find it impossible to keep up with the explosion of new drugs and health-related products.

Because there are so many profit-seekers competing for a share of the lucrative health market and because misinformation is so common, wise health consumers use every means at their disposal to ensure that they are acting responsibly and economically.

Attracting Consumers' Dollars

Today's marketing specialists can identify a target audience for a given product and carefully go after it with an arsenal of gimmicks, subtle persuaders, and sophisticated strategies. Different techniques are used to attract new customers, maintain existing customers, and encourage former consumers to come back. Many advertisements present a product as a status symbol or play on inner fears and insecurities, causing you to wonder whether your deodorant is working, your breath is bad, or your skin is greasy.

Whatever your desires, countless products and services are available to meet them. Although some marketing tactics are obvious, others are subtle and difficult to discern. Perfume advertisements that depict passionate embraces and automobile ads that feature expensive sports cars with beautiful young men and women are common. The implied message is that if you purchase a given perfume, your love life will improve, and if you buy that flashy car, attractive people will flock to you.

Many other marketing strategies revolve around "trendy" news items. A good example of this is the current fascination with the use of herbs to treat the common cold and wearable magnets to treat arthritis and painful joints.

Putting *Cure* into Better Perspective

People often fall victim to false health claims because they mistakenly believe that a product or provider has helped them. Frequently this belief arises from two conditions: spontaneous remission and the placebo effect.

Spontaneous Remission It is commonly said that if you treat a cold, it will disappear in a week, but if you leave it alone, it will last seven days. A **spontaneous remission** from an ailment refers to the disappearance of symptoms without any apparent cause or treatment. Many illnesses, like the common cold and even back strain, are self-limiting and will improve in time, with or without treatment. Other illnesses, such as multiple sclerosis and some cancers, are characterized by alternating periods of severe symptoms and sudden remissions. People experiencing spontaneous remissions can easily attribute their "cure" to a treatment that in fact had no real effect.

Placebo Effect The **placebo effect** is an apparent cure or improved state of health brought about by a substance, product, or procedure that has no generally recognized therapeutic value. It is not uncommon for patients to report

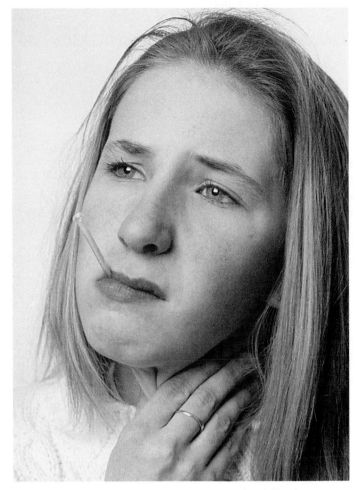

Deciding when to contact a physician can be difficult. Most people first try to diagnose and treat their conditions themselves.

improvements based on what they expect, desire, or were told would happen after taking simple sugar pills that they believed were powerful drugs. About 10 percent of the population is believed to be exceptionally susceptible to the power of suggestion and may be easy targets for such aggressive marketing. Although the placebo effect is generally harmless, it does account for the expenditure of millions of dollars on health products and services every year. Megadoses of vitamin C have never been proven to treat cancer. Mud baths do not smooth wrinkled skin, nor do electric shocks reduce muscle pain. People who mistakenly use placebos when medical treatment is urgently needed increase their risk for health problems. Those who use low-cost, no-risk placebos and find relief, even for just a short time, should not be criticized.

Taking Responsibility for Your Health Care

As the health care industry has become more sophisticated about seeking your business, so must you become more sophisticated about purchasing its products and services. Learn how, when, and where to enter the massive technological maze that is our health care system without incurring unnecessary risk and expense. Acting responsibly in times of illness can be difficult, but the person best able to act on your behalf is you.

If you are not feeling well, you must first decide whether you really need to seek outside medical advice. Not that long ago, as many as 70 percent of all trips to the doctor and nearly half of all hospital stays were believed to be unnecessary and potentially harmful.[1] These figures have been reduced considerably, however, with the advent of managed care, which carries with it a degree of out-of-pocket shared costs. Theoretically, patients who have to pay for a portion of their care will not seek care that is not needed. Managed care involves a number of measures designed to keep people out of the hospitals and emergency rooms.[2] Although there are no exact figures, respected sources indicate that the number of emergency room visits has decreased dramatically and that the cost of emergency room care for nonemergencies has declined as well.[3]

Yet critics of managed care point to cost savings as a part of the problem with quality and access. Not seeking treatment, whether due to high costs or limited coverage, or trying to medicate yourself when more rigorous methods of treatment are needed, is dangerous. Being knowledgeable about the benefits and limits of self-care is critical for responsible consumerism.

Self-Help or Self-Care

A recent concept in health consumerism proposes that the patient is the primary health care provider or first line of defense in health. We can practice behaviors that promote health, prevent disease, and minimize reliance on the formal medical system. We can also interpret basic changes in our own physical and emotional health and treat minor afflictions without seeking professional help. Self-care consists of knowing your body, paying attention to its signals, and taking appropriate action to improve your health and stop the progression of illness or injury. See the New Horizons in Health box for suggestions about seeking advice online. Common forms of self-care include the following:

- Diagnosing symptoms or conditions that occur frequently but may not need physician visits (e.g., the common cold, minor abrasions).
- Performing breast and testicular self-examinations (monthly).
- Learning first aid for common, uncomplicated injuries and conditions.
- Checking blood pressure, pulse, and temperature.
- Using home pregnancy and ovulation kits and HIV test kits.
- Monitoring cervical mucus for natural family planning.
- Doing periodic checks for blood cholesterol.
- Using home stool test kits for blood and early colon cancer detection.
- Using self-help books, tapes, software, websites, and videos.

Doc.com Surfer Beware!

Mary, an avid fitness proponent with no formal academic training in health, took her first webpage-building class in August. Today, because of her interest and enthusiasm for health topics, she has a comprehensive medical advice website on which she talks with great authority about a variety of interesting health topics. It includes self-assessment exercises and numerous links to other health sites. But does her glitzy, interactive page provide accurate, well-researched advice? Or is she just picking up bits and pieces of information from the same, often questionable sites to which we all have access? Mary is just as vulnerable to bad information as the rest of us. She may not even realize when her information is based on weak science. So, while her intentions are good, Mary's website has the potential to harm others seriously.

Although Mary is a fictional character, invented to make a point, such a scenario is more than possible. A great many "Marys" abound on the Internet today, because anyone capable of creating a webpage has the tools to put up anything he or she wants. Sometimes what is put online for the world lacks the backing of reputable scientists, medical and health care groups, and educational counsel. It can be misleading and possibly even harmful. This is certainly the case with the surge of sites devoted to health and medical information. The World Wide Web is filled with self-appointed health experts, with legitimate professional health agencies, and, more recently, with what have come to be known as doc.coms—websites that provide everything from online diagnoses, chatroom support groups, and detailed information on conditions and procedures to opportunities to observe surgical procedures. Today, millions of people throughout the world are turning to these sources for help and self-diagnosis of symptoms. While this could encourage people to be more proactive in their own care, the potential for harm should make us proceed with caution.

In an article for *The Wall Street Journal* in 1999, columnist Marilyn Chase reported her experiences seeking information on the Internet about headaches. Her search focused on finding chatrooms and doctors online offering information. Her conclusion? "In short, browsers in the e-marketplace of medical information will find that the quality is very diverse. Some sites offer depth of data, with credentials to back them up. Others display nice site design or easy access but have thin content. Randomly [hopping] from link to link can leave you with a handful of commercial pitches or fringe benefits."

How can you make sure you get the best information possible? Follow these strategies:

- Don't forget the wealth of information at your school's library. Ask the reference librarian at your school to recommend health-related information data banks that the school subscribes to. Institutions of higher education generally subscribe to peer-reviewed journals, which are written by professionals and reviewed by the writers' peers. In addition, universities often subscribe to services that compile journal articles from the social and health sciences and meet the criteria for peer review. Many of these publications are online. Those that are not will probably be on your library's shelves.
- Seek information from several different types of sources. Check author credentials and cross-check information from different sources to find areas of consensus. Taking information from only one source and assuming it to be true is a bad idea.
- Reputable information in the health area often includes complete references. Find out if the site is professionally managed, peer-reviewed, and updated regularly.
- Professional and nationally recognized organizations, including government agencies, are good places to start. Although still possessing inaccuracies, many of these sites include the latest data-based statistics from randomized clinical trials.
- Remember that just because a site is "linked" to a government source doesn't mean that the government source is aware of the site or endorses it.
- Look at the credentials of the authors of any papers posted online. With what organizations, if any, are they affiliated?
- Avoid online health professionals who diagnose or make blanket statements about your health without requiring a formal examination or referring you to others.
- Look at the advertisements on the page. If they are part of the text or if they appear to promise quick cures or easy solutions, beware.
- Note the date of the article and all references. Citations that are more than a couple of years old are too old.
- If the site is from a reputable institution of higher education, determine whether it is managed by faculty, students, or laboratories on campus.
- Look to see if the site provides both sides of controversial issues, including references. Reputable sites want you to consider your options, not force you to buy their product or endorse their view.
- Be cautious when purchasing health products and services over the Internet. Check out your options and consider the costs and benefits.
- For personal health issues, weigh all the information you gather from the Internet with what you learn from your health care provider. Your health care providers are still some of the best resources at your disposal.

- Benefiting from relaxation techniques, including meditation, nutrition, rest, and exercise.

When to Seek Help

Effective self-care also means understanding when to seek professional medical attention rather than treating a condition yourself. Deciding which conditions warrant professional advice is not always easy. Generally, you should consult a physician if you experience any of the following:

- A serious accident or injury.
- Sudden or severe chest pains causing breathing difficulties.
- Trauma to the head or spine accompanied by persistent headache, blurred vision, loss of consciousness, vomiting, convulsions, or paralysis.
- Sudden high fever or recurring high temperature (over 102°F for adults and 103°F for children) and/or sweats.
- Tingling sensation in the arm accompanied by slurred speech or impaired thought processes.
- Adverse reactions to a drug or insect bite (shortness of breath, severe swelling, dizziness).
- Unexplained bleeding or loss of bodily fluid from any body opening.
- Unexplained sudden weight loss.
- Persistent or recurrent diarrhea or vomiting.
- Blue-colored lips, eyelids, or nail beds.
- Any lump, swelling, thickness, or sore that does not subside or that grows for over a month.
- Any marked change or pain in bowel or bladder habits.
- Yellowing of the skin or the whites of the eyes.
- Any symptom that is unusual and recurs over time.
- Pregnancy.

With the vast array of home diagnostic devices currently available, it appears to be relatively easy for most people to take care of themselves. But some caution is in order here: Although many of these devices are valuable for making an initial diagnosis, home health tests cannot substitute for regular, complete examinations by a trained practitioner. The Skills for Behavior Change box offers valuable information about taking an active role in your own health care.

Assessing Health Professionals

Suppose you decide that you do need medical help. You must then identify what type of help you need and where to obtain it. Initially, selecting a professional may seem a simple matter, yet many people have no idea how to assess the qualifications of a health care provider.

Knowledge of both traditional medical specialties and alternative, or complementary, medical treatment is critical to making an intelligent selection. You also need to be aware of your own criteria for evaluating a health professional. Several studies have pointed to bedside manner and positive interactions with doctors as key to patient satisfaction. In a survey of HMO members, it was shown that even in a setting of limited physician choice, the opportunity to select one's

personal physician had a positive influence on patient satisfaction with that physician.[4] When selecting from a network of providers, make sure you fully understand your coverage options. Carefully consider the following factors about all prospective health care providers:

- What professional educational training have they had? What license or board certification do they hold? Note that there is a difference between "board eligible" and "board certified." *Board certified* indicates that they have passed the national board examination for their specialty (e.g., pediatrics) and have been certified as competent in that specialty. In contrast, *board eligible* merely means that they are eligible to take the specialty board's exam or even that they may have failed the exam.
- Are they affiliated with an accredited medical facility or institution? The Joint Commission on the Accreditation of Healthcare Organizations (JCAHO) requires these institutions to verify all education, licensing, and training claims of their affiliated practitioners. What other doctors are in their group, and who will assist in my treatment?
- Are they open to complementary or alternative strategies? Would they refer me for different treatment modalities, when appropriate?
- Do they indicate clearly how long a given treatment may last, what side effects I might expect, and what things I should be on the alert for?
- Do their diagnoses, treatments, and general statements appear to be consistent with established scientific theory and practice?
- Who will be responsible for my care when the doctor is on vacation or off call?
- Do they listen to me, respect me as an individual, and give me time to ask questions? Do they return my calls, and are they available to answer questions?
- How often has the doctor performed this test, surgery, or procedure and with what proportion of successful outcome?

When a doctor orders a test, treatment, or medication, you might ask questions like these:

- What are the side effects, and can these side effects be treated or reduced?
- Does this procedure require an overnight stay at a hospital or can it be performed in a doctor's office?
- Why has this test been ordered? What is the doctor trying to find or exclude?

Asking the right questions at the right time may save you personal suffering and expense. Many patients find that writing their questions down before an appointment helps them get answers to all their questions. You should not accept a defensive or hostile response; asking questions is your right as a patient.

A 2002 survey found that nearly two-thirds of Americans are confident that the medical information given to them by their doctor is accurate, while the remaining third opt for a second opinion on important issues or do independent research.[5]

Being Proactive in Your Own Health Care

Throughout this book, we have emphasized the importance of healthy preventive behaviors. Sometimes, however, regardless of the steps you take to care for yourself, you still get sick. At such times, it is important that you continue to be actively involved in your care. The more you know about your own body and the factors that can affect your health, the better you will be at communicating with your doctor. It also helps you make informed decisions and recognize when a certain treatment may not be right for you. The following points can help:

- Know your own and your family's medical history.
- Be knowledgeable about your condition—causes, physiological effects, possible treatments, prognosis. Don't rely on the doctor for this information. Do some research.
- Bring a friend or relative along for medical visits to help you review what the doctor says. Or take notes if you go alone.
- Ask the practitioner to explain the problem and possible treatments, tests, and drugs in a clear and understandable way. If you don't understand something, ask for clarification.
- If the doctor prescribes any medications, ask whether you can take generic equivalents that cost less.

- Ask for a written summary of the results of your visit and any lab tests.
- If you have any doubt about the doctor's recommended treatment, seek a second opinion.
- If you will need to take a prescription medication for an extended time, ask for the maximum number of doses allowed by your plan if you have a small pharmacy copayment.

After seeing a health care professional, consider these ideas:

- Write down an accurate account of what happened and what was said. Be sure to include the names of the doctor and all other people involved in your care, the date, and the place.
- Shop around drugstores for the best prices in the same way that you would when shopping for clothes.
- When filling prescriptions, ask to see the pharmacist's package inserts that list medical considerations concerning the medicines. Request detailed information about potential drug and food interactions.
- Write clear instructions on the label to avoid risk to others who may take the drug in error.

Just like you, doctors are human. Their decisions are based on the best information they have available to them and may be influenced by a number of factors—workload, limited information, personal views. Therefore, in addition to following the practical steps listed above, being proactively involved in your health care also means that you should be aware of

your rights as a patient. Your rights include the following:

1. The right of informed consent means that before receiving any care, you should be fully informed of what is being planned, the risks and potential benefits, and possible alternative forms of treatment, including the option of no treatment. Your consent must be voluntary and without any form of coercion. It is critical that you read any consent forms carefully and amend them as necessary before signing.
2. You are entitled to know whether the treatment you are receiving is standard or experimental. In experimental conditions, you have the legal and ethical right to know if the study is one in which some people receive treatment while others do not in order to compare the results and if any drug is being used in the research project for a purpose not approved by the Food and Drug Administration (FDA).
3. You have the right to privacy, which includes the source of payment for treatment and care. It also includes protecting your right to make personal decisions concerning all reproductive matters.
4. You have the right to receive care. You also have the legal right to refuse treatment at any time and to cease treatment at any time.
5. You are entitled to access all your medical records and to have those records remain confidential.
6. You have the right to seek the opinions of other health care professionals regarding your condition.

Choices in Health Products: Prescription and Over-the-Counter Drugs

Recall from Chapter 14 that prescription drugs can be obtained only with a written prescription from a physician, while over-the-counter (OTC) drugs can be purchased without a prescription. Just as making wise decisions about providers is an important aspect of responsible health care, so is making wise decisions about these medications. A number of

factors must be taken into account, and it is important to understand the benefits, risks, and possible interactions related to a given drug.

Prescription Drugs

Even though prescription drugs are administered under medical supervision, the wise consumer still takes precautions. Hazards and complications arising from the use of prescription drugs are common. Responsible decision making requires the consumer to acquire basic drug knowledge.

Preserving the Usefulness of Antibiotics

In the 1300s, the scourge known as bubonic plague killed up to one-third of Europe's population. In modern times, we've been told that such a plague isn't possible. It would be controlled handily with the help of antibiotic drugs such as streptomycin, gentamicin, and chloramphenicol, drugs once thought to be invincible—that is, until 1995, when a 16-year-old boy from Madagascar, infected with bubonic plague, failed to respond to the usual antibiotic treatments. This was the first documented case of an antibiotic-resistant plague, which did eventually succumb to another antibiotic.

To some, this development was not all that surprising. Throughout the world, many other infectious bacteria, including those that cause pneumonia, ear infections, acne, gonorrhea, urinary tract infections, meningitis, and tuberculosis, can now outwit commonly used antibiotics and their synthetic counterparts, antimicrobials. Every time a patient takes penicillin or another antibiotic for a bacterial infection, the drug kills most of the bacteria. But a few tenacious germs may survive by mutating or acquiring resistance genes from other bacteria. These surviving genes can multiply quickly, creating drug-resistant strains. The presence of these strains may mean the patient's next infection may not respond to the first-choice antibiotic therapy. Also, the resistant bacteria may be transmitted to other people in the community.

According to the Centers for Disease Control, each year nearly 2 million people in the United States acquire an infection while in the hospital, resulting in 90,000 deaths. More than 70 percent of the bacteria that cause these infections are resistant to at least one of the antibiotics commonly used to treat them. Although resistant bacteria have been around a long time, the number of bacteria resistant to many different antibiotics has increased tenfold or more in the past 10 years.

What is causing the increase in drug-resistant strains? Two factors: One has to do with the medical community, the other with patients. Experts say that doctors are sometimes too quick to prescribe antibiotics for all sorts of symptoms, despite the fact that antibiotics work only against bacteria, not viruses or the common cold. It is estimated that more than 50 to 150 million antibiotic prescriptions written for patients each year outside of hospitals are unnecessary. As for patients, even when they need the antibiotics that are prescribed, they don't always follow instructions properly. To be completely effective, antibiotics should be taken for a specific number of days. Many people, however, often stop taking the drug after symptoms have cleared or they start feeling better. Unfortunately, some of the bacteria may still be present in their systems, free to attack again and able to mutate.

Organisms that have already developed defenses against antibiotic attack include the following:

✔ *Staphylococcus aureus.* One of the primary causes of infections in patients in U.S. hospitals; can infect burns, skin, and surgical wounds.
✔ *Enterococcus.* Can cause everything from urinary tract infections to heart valve infections.
✔ *Streptococcus pneumoniae.* Up to 30 percent of the strains of this bacterium, which can cause pneumonia, meningitis, and ear infections, are at least partially resistant to antibiotics in the penicillin family.

Other bacteria that have grown resistant to once-reliable antibiotics are *Neisseria gonorrhoeae,* which causes the sexually transmitted infection gonorrhea; *Salmonella; Escherichia coli (E. coli),* the culprit behind food poisoning; and *Mycobacterium tuberculosis,* which causes tuberculosis.

What can you do to help curb the problem of antibiotic-resistant bacteria?

✔ Don't demand an antibiotic when your health care provider determines that one is not appropriate. Remember, antibiotics won't help a cold or flu.
✔ Finish each prescription. Even when the symptoms of an illness have disappeared, some bacteria may still survive and reproduce if you don't complete the course of treatment.
✔ Don't take leftover antibiotics or antibiotics prescribed for someone else.

Sources: FDA Consumer Magazine (July–August 2002); downloaded December 6, 2002; *FDA Consumer Magazine* (November–December 1998); downloaded October 22, 1998.

Types of Prescription Drugs Prescription drugs can be divided into dozens of categories. Some of the most common are discussed here. Others are explored in the chapters on birth control, infectious and sexually transmitted diseases, cancer, and cardiovascular disease.

Antibiotics are drugs used to fight bacterial infection. Bacterial infections continue to be the most common serious diseases in the United States and throughout the world. The vast majority of these can be cured with antibiotic treatment. There are currently close to 100 different antibiotic drugs used to kill or stop bacterial growth. They may be dispensed by intramuscular injection or in tablet or capsule form.

Some, called broad-spectrum antibiotics, are designed to control disease caused by a number of bacterial species. These medications may also kill off helpful bacteria in the body, thus triggering secondary infections. For example, some vaginal infections are related to long-term use of antibiotics. See the Reality Check box for other issues concerning antibiotic use and overuse.

Antibiotics Prescription drugs designed to fight bacterial infection.

Sedatives are central nervous system depressants that induce sleep and relieve anxiety. Because of the high incidence of anxiety and sleep disorders in the United States, drugs that encourage relaxation and drowsiness are frequently prescribed. The potential for addiction is high. Detoxification can be life-threatening and must be medically supervised. Because doctors do not prescribe sedatives as frequently as they did in past decades, users often purchase them illegally.

Tranquilizers, another form of central nervous system depressant, are classified as major and minor tranquilizers. The most powerful tranquilizers are used to treat major psychiatric illnesses. When used appropriately, these strong sedatives can reduce violent aggressiveness and self-destructive impulses.

The so-called minor tranquilizers gained much notoriety in the 1970s when consumer groups discovered that these drugs—known by their trade names Valium, Librium, and Miltown—were the most commonly prescribed medications in the United States. They were often prescribed for women who suffered from anxiety. These drugs have a high potential for addiction, and many people became physically and psychologically dependent on them. When the media reported on the widespread and casual prescribing of these drugs, physicians were forced to reevaluate the practice. Today a doctor is more likely to suggest psychotherapy or counseling for patients suffering from anxiety.

Antidepressants are medications typically used to treat major depression, although occasionally they are used to treat other forms of depression that may be resistant to conventional therapy. There are several groups of antidepressant medications approved for use in the United States (see Table 22.1). The first to be used to treat depression were monoamine oxidase (MAO) inhibitors, which were discovered in the

Table 22.1 Antidepressants	
TYPE/GENERIC NAME	**TRADE NAME**
MAO INHIBITORS	
Phenelzine	Nardil
Tranylcypromine	Parnate
TRICYCLIC MEDICATIONS	
Amitriptyline	Elavil, Endep, Tryptanol
Amoxapine	Asendin
Clomipramine	Anafranil
Desipramine	Norpramin, Pertofran
Doxepin	Adapin, Sinequan
Imipramine	Janimine, Tofranil
Maprotiline	Ludiomil
Nortriptyline	Aventyl, Pamelor
Protriptyline	Concordin, Triptil, Vivactil
Trazodone	Desyrel, Molipaxin
Trimipramine	Surmontil
SSRIs	
Fluoxetine	Prozac
Fluvoxamine	Luvox
Paroxetine	Paxil
Sertraline	Lustral, Zoloft
Citalopram	Cipramil
OTHER ANTIDEPRESSANTS	
Bupropion	Wellbutrin
Nefazodone	Serzone
Venlafaxine	Effexor

1960s. The most commonly used antidepressants are the tricyclic medications, but perhaps the best known are the SSRIs, or selective serotonin reuptake inhibitors, which include the drugs Prozac and Zoloft. Although, as a group, tricyclic medications are most commonly prescribed, Prozac is the most frequently prescribed antidepressant and in 1999 was the eighth most frequently prescribed drug in the United States.

Amphetamines are stimulants that are prescribed less commonly now than in the past. Like many psychoactive drugs, they are purchased both legally and illegally. Amphetamines suppress appetite and elevate respiration, blood pressure, and pulse rate. Ritalin and Cylert are prescription amphetamines that are used to treat attention-deficit/hyperactivity disorder in children, and Pondimin is used to treat obesity.

Tolerance to these powerful stimulants develops rapidly, and the user trying to cut down or quit may experience unpleasant **rebound effects.** These severe withdrawal symptoms, peculiar to stimulants, include depression, irritability, violent behavior, headaches, nausea, and deep fatigue.

Generic Drugs Generic drugs, medications sold under a chemical name rather than under a brand name, have gained popularity in recent years. They contain the same active ingredients as brand-name drugs but are less expensive.

Sedatives Central nervous system depressants that induce sleep and relieve anxiety.

Tranquilizers Central nervous system depressants that relax the body and calm anxiety.

Antidepressants Prescription drugs used to treat clinically diagnosed depression.

Amphetamines Prescription stimulants not commonly used today because of the dangers associated with them.

Rebound effects Severe withdrawal effects experienced by users of stimulants, including depression, nausea, and violent behavior.

Generic drugs Drugs marketed by chemical name rather than brand name.

Analgesics Pain relievers.

Prostaglandin inhibitors Drugs that inhibit the production and release of prostaglandins associated with arthritis or menstrual pain.

Generic drugs can help reduce health care costs because their price is often less than half that of brand-name medications. If your doctor prescribes a drug, always ask if a generic equivalent exists and if it would be safe and effective for you to try.

Be aware, though, that there is some controversy about the effectiveness of generic drugs because substitutions are often made in minor ingredients that can affect the way the drug is absorbed, causing discomfort or even an allergic reaction in some users. Always note any reactions you have to medications and tell your doctor. Also, not all drugs are available as generics.

Over-the-Counter (OTC) Drugs

Over-the-counter (OTC) drugs are nonprescription substances we use in the course of self-diagnosis and self-medication. More than one-third of the time people treat their routine health problems with OTC medications. Self-care for many of us results from an eagerness to save money and time on an office visit to the physician. We therefore diagnose our own illnesses and go to the nearest discount pharmacy to stock up on the latest and best-advertised cure for what we think ails us.

In fact, American consumers spend billions of dollars yearly on OTC preparations for relief of everything from runny noses to ingrown toenails. There are 40,000 OTC drugs and more than 300,000 brand names for those drugs. Most of these products are manufactured from a basic group of 1,000 chemicals. The many different OTC drugs available to us are produced by combining as few as 2 and as many as 10 substances.

How Prescription Drugs Become OTC Drugs
The Food and Drug Administration (FDA) regularly reviews prescription drugs to evaluate how suitable they would be as OTC products. (See the Health Ethics box.) Typically, these are drugs that treat conditions that consumers can diagnose readily and manage themselves and include clear, understandable directions. For a drug to be switched from prescription to OTC status, it must meet the following criteria:

1. The drug has been marketed as a prescription medication for at least three years.
2. The use of the drug has been relatively high during the time it was available as a prescription drug.
3. Adverse drug reactions are not alarming, potential adverse effects are printed on the drug label and the frequency of side effects has not increased during the time it was available to the public.

Since this policy has been in effect, the FDA has switched hundreds of drugs from prescription to OTC status. Some examples are ibuprofen (Advil, Nuprin), the analgesic/anti-inflammatory medicine naproxen sodium (Aleve), the antihistamine Benadryl, the vaginal antifungal Gyne-Lotrimin, the bronchodilator Bronkaid Mist, the hydrocortisone, Cortaid, and Claritin, for allergy relief. Many more prescription drugs are currently being considered for OTC status.

Types of OTC Drugs
The FDA has categorized 26 types of OTC preparations. Those most commonly used are analgesics, cold/cough/allergy and asthma relievers, stimulants, sleeping aids and relaxants, and dieting aids.

Analgesics
We spend more than $2 billion annually on **analgesics** (pain relievers), the largest sales category of OTC drugs in the United States. Although these pain relievers come in several forms, aspirin, acetaminophen (Tylenol, Pamprin, Panadol), and ibuprofen-like drugs such as naproxen (Aleve) and ketoprofen (Orudis) are the most common.

Most pain relievers work at receptor sites by interrupting pain signals. Some are categorized as NSAIDs (nonsteroidal anti-inflammatory drugs), also called **prostaglandin inhibitors.** Prostaglandins are chemicals that resemble hormones and are released by the body in response to pain. (Scientists believe that the additional pain caused by the release of prostaglandins signals the body to begin the healing process.) Prostaglandin inhibitors restrain the release of prostaglandins, thereby reducing the pain. Common NSAIDs include ibuprofen (Motrin), naproxen sodium (Anaprox), and aspirin.

In addition to relieving pain, aspirin lowers fever by increasing the flow of blood to the skin surface, which causes sweating, thereby cooling the body. Aspirin has also long been used to reduce the inflammation and swelling associated with arthritis. Recently it has been discovered that aspirin's anticoagulant (interference with blood clotting) effects make it useful for reducing the risk of heart attack and stroke.

Although aspirin has been popular for nearly a century, it is not as harmless as many people think. Possible side effects—for it and many other NSAIDS—include allergic reactions, ringing in the ears, stomach bleeding, and ulcers. Combining aspirin with alcohol can compound aspirin's gastric irritant properties. As with all drugs, read the labels. Some analgesic labels caution against driving or operating heavy machinery when using the drug, and most warn that analgesics should not be taken with alcohol.

In addition, research has linked aspirin to a potentially fatal condition called Reye's syndrome. Children, teenagers, and young adults (up to age 25) who are treated with aspirin while recovering from the flu or chicken pox are at risk for developing the syndrome. Aspirin substitutes are recommended for people in these age groups.

Acetaminophen is an aspirin substitute found in Tylenol and related medications. Like aspirin, acetaminophen is an effective analgesic and antipyretic (fever-reducing drug). It does not, however, relieve inflamed or swollen joints. The side effects associated with acetaminophen are generally minimal, though overdose can cause liver damage.

Several analgesics are available as prescription or OTC drugs. Generally, the OTC drugs (for example, Nuprin, Advil, and Aleve) are milder versions of the prescription varieties. Aleve's main distinction is its lasting effect: While other analgesics must be taken every 4 to 6 hours, once every 8 to 12 hours is sufficient for Aleve.

FDA: Rejecting Advice and Risking Lives

Hundreds of new drugs have been approved for OTC status since 1993, when the Food and Drug Administration changed its policies to speed the approval process. The changes came in response to activists seeking fast approval of experimental drugs that offered at least a ray of hope to AIDS patients who otherwise faced certain death.

Of the hundreds of drugs approved since 1993, seven have been withdrawn after reports of deaths and severe side effects. Examples of drugs that have been placed on the pharmacy shelves as a result of the FDA's more lenient approach, but have yielded fatal results, include Redux and Lotronex. Redux, the diet pill approved in 1996 despite an advisory committee's vote against it, was taken off the shelves in 1997 after some patients taking it developed heart-valve damage. Lotronex, a drug for treating irritable bowel syndrome, was approved despite warnings. It has now been linked to five deaths, the removal of one patient's colon, and other bowel surgeries. Lotronex was pulled from the market after only 10 months.

Reports of adverse drug reactions made to the Food and Drug Administration are considered by public health officials to be the most reliable early warning that a product may be dangerous. The reports are filed to the FDA by health professionals, consumers, and drug manufacturers. More than 250,000 side effects linked to prescription drugs, including injuries and deaths, are reported each year. Since these "adverse-event" reports are voluntary, experts, including Dr. Brian L. Strom, chair of epidemiology at the University of Pennsylvania, believe they represent only 1 percent to 10 percent of all such events. "There is no incentive at all for a physician to report [an adverse drug reaction]," said Strom, who has documented the process. "The underreporting is vast."

Even when deaths are reported, companies consistently dispute that their product is responsible by pointing to other factors, such as another medicine or pre-existing disease. To be sure, a chain of events does affect safe use of a prescription drug. A lapse at any link could prove fatal. The chain includes these steps:

- The companies' conduct of clinical studies.
- The FDA's regulatory actions.
- The doctor's decision to prescribe.
- The pharmacist's filling of a handwritten prescription.
- The patient's ability to take the drug as directed.

When serious side effects emerge, FDA officials have championed using package labeling to warn of potential risks as a way to, in their words, "manage" risks. Yet the agency typically has no way to know if the labels—dense, lengthy, and in tiny print—are read or followed by doctors and their patients. The FDA often addresses unresolved safety questions by asking companies to conduct studies after the product is approved. However, this research frequently has not been performed.

To address this lack of follow-through, the inspector general of the Department of Health and Human Services issued a statement in 1996, stating that "the FDA can move to withdraw drugs from the market if the post-marketing studies are not completed with due diligence." However, since then the FDA has not withdrawn any drug because of a company's failure to complete a postapproval safety study.

What standards should the FDA use in deciding whether a drug can be sold over the counter? Are its current standards too strict or too lenient? Explain your answer. What assumptions has the FDA made about the way consumers use drug labels?

Source: Adaptation of "How a New Policy Led to Seven Deadly Drugs" by David Willman, *Los Angeles Times,* December 20, 2000. Reprinted by permission of Tribune Media Services International.

Cold, Cough, Allergy, and Asthma Relievers The operative word in this category is *reliever.* Most of these medications are designed to alleviate the discomforting symptoms associated with maladies of the upper respiratory tract. Unfortunately, no drugs exist to cure the actual diseases. The drugs available provide only temporary relief until the sufferer's immune system prevails over the disease. Aspirin or acetaminophen is used in some cold preparations, as are several other ingredients. Both aspirin and acetaminophen are on the government's lists of medications that are Generally Recognized as Safe (**GRAS**) and Generally Recognized as Effective (**GRAE**).

Basic types of OTC cold, cough, and allergy relievers include the following:

- *Expectorants.* These drugs are formulated to loosen phlegm, allowing the user to cough it up and clear congested respiratory passages. GRAS and GRAE reviewers question the effectiveness of many expectorants. In addition, when combined with other medications particularly among frail or very ill individuals, safety issues may arise.
- *Antitussives.* These OTC drugs calm or curtail the cough reflex. They are most effective when the cough is "dry," or does not produce phlegm. Oral codeine, dextromethorphan, and diphenhydramine are the most common antitussives that are on both the GRAE and GRAS lists.
- *Antihistamines.* These central nervous system depressants dry runny noses, clear postnasal drip, clear sinus congestion, and reduce tears.

- *Decongestants.* These remedies reduce nasal stuffiness due to colds.
- *Anticholinergics.* These substances are often added to cold preparations to reduce nasal secretions and tears. None of the preparations tested was found to be GRAE/GRAS. Some cold compounds contain alcohol in concentrations that may exceed 40 percent as well as making users extremely drowsy.

Stimulants Nonprescription stimulants are sometimes used by college students who have neglected assignments and other obligations until the last minute. The active ingredient in OTC stimulants is caffeine, which heightens wakefulness, increases alertness, and relieves fatigue. None of the OTC stimulants has been judged GRAS or GRAE.

Sleeping Aids Nearly 50 percent of the U.S. population experiences insomnia at least five nights each month. About 1 percent of the adult population routinely treat their insomnia with OTC sleep aids (such as Nytol, Sleep-Eze, and Sominex) that are advertised as providing a "safe and restful" sleep.[6] These drugs are often used to induce the drowsy feelings that precede sleep. The principal ingredient in OTC sleeping aids is an antihistamine called pyrilamine maleate. Chronic reliance on sleeping aids may lead to addiction; people accustomed to using these products may eventually find it impossible to sleep without them.

Dieting Aids In the United States, there is a $200 million market for dieting aids. Some of these drugs (e.g., Acutrim, Dexatrim) are advertised as "appetite suppressants." The FDA has pulled several appetite suppressants off the market because their active ingredient was phenylpropanolamine (PPA), which is a **sympathomimetic** (affecting the sympathetic nervous system). This causes reactions similar to those experienced when angry or excited, such as dry mouth and lack of appetite. PPA has been linked to increased risk of stroke.[7]

Estimates show that, when taken as recommended, even the best OTC dieting aids significantly reduce appetite in less than 30 percent of users, and tolerance occurs in only one to three days of use. Manufacturers of appetite suppressants often include a written 1,200-calorie diet to complement their drug. However, most people who limit themselves to 1,200 calories per day will lose weight—without any help from appetite suppressants. Clearly, these products have no value in treating obesity.

Some people rely on **laxatives** and **diuretics** ("water pills") to lose weight. Frequent use of laxatives disrupts the body's natural elimination patterns and may cause constipation or even obstipation (inability to have a bowel movement). The use of laxatives to produce weight loss has generally unspectacular results and can rob the body of needed fluids, salts, and minerals.

Taking diuretics to lose weight is also dangerous. Not only will the user gain the weight back upon drinking fluids, but diuretic use may contribute to dangerous chemical imbalances. The potassium and sodium eliminated by diuretics play important roles in maintaining electrolyte balance. Depletion of these vital minerals may cause weakness, dizziness, fatigue, and sometimes death. (See Table 22.2 on page 612 for side effects of other OTC drugs.)

Rules for Proper OTC Drug Use Despite a common belief that OTC products are safe and effective, indiscriminate use and abuse can occur with these drugs as with all others. For example, people who frequently drop medication into their eyes to "get the red out" or pop antacids after every meal are likely to be addicted. Many people also experience adverse side effects because they ignore warning labels or simply do not read them. The FDA has developed a standard label that appears on most OTC products (see Figure 22.1 on page 613). It provides directions for use, warnings, and other useful information. (Diet supplements, which are regulated as food products, have their own type of label that includes a Supplements Facts panel.)

OTC medications are far more powerful than ever before, and the science behind them is stronger as well. Most of us are self-medicators at one time or another. We find it easier to function, for example, if the headache and stuffiness of the common cold do not interfere with our studies or work. Most of us can use OTC products safely with adequate precautions, but for some people, OTCs can be as toxic as the most dangerous chemicals. Therefore, when you use any type of medication, do your homework. Observe the following rules when taking nonprescription drugs:

1. Always know what you are taking. Identify the active ingredients in the product.
2. Know the effects. Be sure you know both the desired and potentially undesired effects of each active ingredient.
3. Read the warnings and cautions.
4. Don't use anything for more than one or two weeks. If your symptoms persist, consult a doctor.
5. Be particularly cautious if you are also taking prescription drugs.
6. If you have questions, ask your pharmacist.
7. *If you don't need it, don't take it!*

GRAS list A list of drugs generally recognized as safe, which seldom cause side effects when used properly.

GRAE list A list of drugs generally recognized as effective, which work for their intended purpose when used properly.

Sympathomimetics Drugs found in appetite suppressants that affect the sympathetic nervous system.

Laxatives Medications used to soften stool and relieve constipation.

Diuretics Drugs that increase the excretion of urine from the body.

Table 22.2
Some Side Effects of OTC Drugs

DRUG	POSSIBLE HAZARDS
Acetaminophen	• Bloody urine, painful urination, skin rash, bleeding and bruising, yellowing of the eyes or skin (even for normal doses) • Difficulty in diagnosing overdose because reaction may be delayed up to a week • Severe liver damage and death (for dose of about 50 tablets) • Liver damage from chronic low-level use
Antacids	• Reduced mineral absorption from food • Possible concealment of ulcer • Reduction of effectiveness for anticlotting medications • Prevention of certain antibiotics' functioning (for antacids that contain aluminum) • Worsening of high blood pressure (for antacids that contain sodium) • Aggravation of kidney problems
Aspirin	• Stomach upset and vomiting, stomach bleeding, worsening of ulcers • Enhancement of the action of anticlotting medications • Potentiation of hearing damage from loud noise • Severe allergic reaction • Association with Reye's syndrome in children and teenagers • Prolonged bleeding time (when combined with alcohol)
Cold medications	• Loss of consciousness (if taken with prescription tranquilizers)
Diet pills, caffeine, decongestants	• Organ damage or death from cerebral hemorrhage
Ibuprofen	• Allergic reaction in some people with aspirin allergy • Fluid retention or edema • Liver damage similar to that from acetaminophen • Enhancement of action of anticlotting medications • Digestive disturbances (half as often as with aspirin)
Laxatives	• Reduced absorption of minerals from food • Creation of dependency
Naproxen sodium	• Potential digestive tract bleeding • Possible stomach cramps • May cause ulcers
Toothache medications	• Destruction of the still-healthy part of a damaged tooth (for medications that contain clove oil)

Drug Interactions Sharing medications, using outdated prescriptions, taking higher doses than recommended, or using medications as a substitute for dealing with personal problems may result in serious health consequences. But so may **polydrug use:** taking several medications or illegal drugs simultaneously may result in very dangerous problems associated with drug interactions. The most hazardous interactions are synergism, antagonism, inhibition, and intolerance. Hazardous interactions may also occur between drugs and foods and nutrients (see Table 22.3 on page 614 for common drug-nutrient interactions).

Synergism, also known as potentiation, is an interaction of two or more drugs in which the effects of the individual drugs are multiplied beyond what would normally be expected if they were taken alone. Synergism can be expressed mathematically as 2 + 2 = 10.

A synergistic interaction is most likely to occur when *central nervous system depressants* are combined. Included in this category are alcohol, opiates (morphine, heroin), antihistamines (cold remedies), sedative hypnotics (Quaaludes), minor tranquilizers (Valium, Librium, and Xanax), and barbiturates. The worst possible combination is alcohol and barbiturates (sleeping preparations such as Seconal and phenobarbital) because combining these depressants slows down the brain centers that normally control vital functions. Respiration, heart rate, and blood pressure can drop to the point of inducing coma and even death.

Prescription and OTC drugs carry labels warning the user not to combine the drug with certain other drugs or with alcohol. Because the dangers associated with synergism are so great, you should always verify any possible drug interactions before using a prescribed or OTC drug.

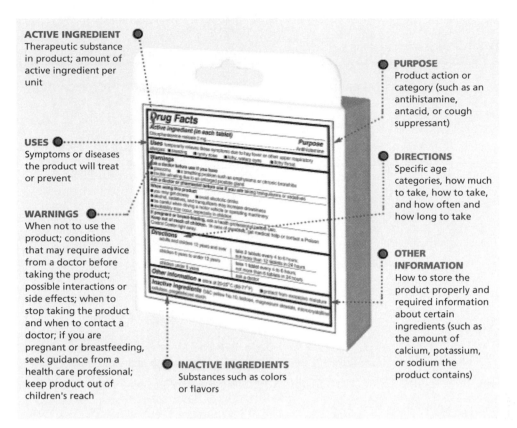

ACTIVE INGREDIENT Therapeutic substance in product; amount of active ingredient per unit

USES Symptoms or diseases the product will treat or prevent

WARNINGS When not to use the product; conditions that may require advice from a doctor before taking the product; possible interactions or side effects; when to stop taking the product and when to contact a doctor; if you are pregnant or breastfeeding, seek guidance from a health care professional; keep product out of children's reach

INACTIVE INGREDIENTS Substances such as colors or flavors

PURPOSE Product action or category (such as an antihistamine, antacid, or cough suppressant)

DIRECTIONS Specific age categories, how much to take, how to take, and how often and how long to take

OTHER INFORMATION How to store the product properly and required information about certain ingredients (such as the amount of calcium, potassium, or sodium the product contains)

Figure 22.1
The New Over-the-Counter Medicine Label
Source: Consumer Healthcare Products Association, "The New Over-the-Counter Medicine Label," 2002. Reprinted by permission.

Pharmacists, physicians, drug information centers, or community drug education centers can answer your questions. Even if one of the drugs in question is an illegal substance, you should still attempt to determine the dangers involved in combining it with other drugs. Health care professionals are legally bound to maintain confidentiality even when they know that a client is using illegal substances.

Antagonism, although not usually as serious as synergism, can produce unwanted and unpleasant effects. In an antagonistic reaction, drugs work at the same receptor site so that one drug blocks the action of the other. The "blocking" drug occupies the receptor site and prevents the other drug from attaching, thus altering its absorption and action.

With **inhibition,** the effects of one drug are eliminated or reduced by the presence of another drug at the receptor site. One common inhibitory reaction occurs between antacid tablets and aspirin. The antacid inhibits the absorption of aspirin, making it less effective as a pain reliever. Other inhibitory reactions occur between alcohol and contraceptive pills and between antibiotics and contraceptive pills. Both alcohol and antibiotics may make birth control pills less effective.

Intolerance occurs when drugs combine in the body to produce extremely uncomfortable reactions. The drug Antabuse, used to help alcoholics give up alcohol, works by producing this type of interaction. It binds liver enzymes (the chemicals the liver produces to break down alcohol), making it impossible for the body to metabolize alcohol. As a result, an Antabuse user who drinks alcohol experiences nausea, vomiting, and, occasionally, fever.

Polydrug use The use of multiple medications or illicit drugs simultaneously.

Synergism An interaction of two or more drugs that produces more profound effects than would be expected if the drugs were taken separately.

Antagonism A type of interaction in which two or more drugs work at the same receptor site.

Inhibition A type of interaction in which the effects of one drug are eliminated or reduced by the presence of another drug at the receptor site.

Intolerance A type of interaction in which two or more drugs produce extremely uncomfortable symptoms.

Table 22.3
Foods and Drugs That Don't Mix

DRUGS	COMMON BRANDS	EFFECTS AND PRECAUTIONS
ALLERGY AND COLD MEDICATIONS		
Antihistamines	Hismanal, Seldand, Tavist, Dimetane	Large quantities of grapefruit juice may decrease absorption of the drug. Antihistamines should be taken on an empty stomach to increase their effectiveness. Avoid alcohol; some antihistamines may increase drowsiness and slow mental function and motor performance when taken with alcohol.
ANTIBIOTICS		
Erythromycin	ERYC, Erythrocot, Erythrocin	Best taken with water. Fruit juice, vegetable juice, and soda may interfere with drug absorption.
Sulfonamides	Gantanal, Gantrisin, Renoquid	Long-term therapy may cause a deficiency in folic acid; talk with your doctor about adding a multivitamin or folate-rich foods to your diet.
Tetracycline	Declomycin, Terramycin, Tetracyn	Dairy products and other foods rich in calcium may interfere with drug absorption.
ANALGESICS		
Acetaminophen	Tylenol, Tempra	Avoid or limit the use of alcohol because chronic alcohol use can increase the risk of liver damage or stomach bleeding.
NONSTEROIDAL ANTI-INFLAMMATORY DRUGS (NSAIDs)		
Aspirin, ibuprofen, naproxen, ketoprofen	Bayer, Motrin, Advil, Aleve, Orudis	Because these medications can irritate the stomach, it is best to take them with food or milk. Avoid or limit the use of alcohol; chronic alcohol use can increase the risk of liver damage or stomach bleeding.
ANTIDEPRESSANTS		
Paroxetine, sertaline, fluoxetine	Paxil, Zoloft, Prozac	Individuals taking these drugs should avoid the use of alcohol.
MONOAMINE OXIDASE (MAO) INHIBITORS		
Phenelzine, tranylcypromine	Nardil, Parnate	Foods high in tyramine should be avoided. Check with physician for complete list; examples include Parmesan cheese, cured meats, avocados, caffeine-containing products, alcoholic beverages, and nonalcoholic beer and wine.
HORMONE PREPARATIONS		
Oral contraceptives	Demulen, Loestrin, Triphasil	Salty foods increase fluid retention. Increase intake of foods high in calcium, vitamin K, potassium, and protein to avoid deficiencies.
Steroids	Cortef, Deltasone, Prednisone, Sterapred	Salty foods increase fluid retention. Increase intake of foods high in calcium, vitamin K, potassium, and protein to avoid deficiencies.
Thyroid drugs	Propylthiouracil, Tapazole	Avoid taking with iodine-rich foods, which can reduce the drug's efficacy.
LAXATIVES		
Mineral Oil	Lansoyl, Liqui-Doss, Magnolax	Frequent use can lead to deficiency in vitamins A, D, E, and K.

Source: Food and Drug Administration, "Food and Drug Interactions," National Consumers League, 2000.

Cross-tolerance occurs when a person develops a physiological tolerance to one drug and shows a similar tolerance to selected other drugs as a result. Taking one drug may actually increase the body's tolerance to another drug. For example, cross-tolerance can develop between alcohol and barbiturates, two depressant drugs.

> **What do you think?**
>
> *What are some situations in which students misuse drugs?* ✳ *Other than alcohol, which drugs (prescription or OTC) do students tend to abuse while they are at college?*

Table 22.4
Allopathic/Traditional Medical Professionals

Allergist	A specialist who diagnoses and treats allergies
Anesthesiologist	A specialist who administers drugs during surgical procedures to reduce pain or induce unconsciousness
Cardiologist	A specialist in the diagnosis and treatment of heart and blood vessel disorders
Dematologist	A specialist in the diagnosis and treatment of skin disorders
Dietitian	A specialist in the field of diet and human nutrition
Endocrinologist	A specialist in the diagnosis and treatment of glandular disorders
Family practitioner	A physician who offers routine medical service for a variety of ailments
Gastroenterologist	A specialist who diagnoses and treats disorders of the stomach and intestinal tract
Geneticist	A specialist who diagnoses and treats genetic diseases
Health educator	A specialist in the field of health education and health promotion who holds a degree in a health-related area (look for Comprehensive Health Education Specialist [CHES] certification)
Hematologist	A specialist who diagnoses and treats blood-related disorders
Neurologist	A specialist who diagnoses and treats diseases of the brain, nervous system, and spinal cord
Nurse practitioner	Nurse specialist with additional training in a specific area, such as OB/GYN
Obstetrician/gynecologist (OB/GYN)	A specialist who diagnoses and treats problems of the female reproductive system
Oncologist	A specialist who diagnoses and treats cancerous growths and tumors
Ophthalmologist	A specialist who diagnoses, treats, and provides general care of eye disorders
Orthopedist/orthopedic surgeon	A specialist who diagnoses, treats, or provides surgical care for bone and joint injuries and problems
Otolaryngologist	A specialist who specializes in ear, nose, and throat disorders
Pediatrician	A physician who treats childhood diseases
Physical therapist	A specialist who rehabilitates people after impairment due to injury or disease
Physician assistant	Health care professional trained to assist physicians
Plastic surgeon	A specialist who provides corrective surgery for irregularities of body or facial contours
Podiatrist	A specialist who diagnoses and treats disorders of the feet
Psychiatrist	A physician who diagnoses and treats mental and emotional disorders
Pulmonary specialist	A specialist who diagnoses and treats disorders of the respiratory system
Radiologist	A specialist in the diagnosis of disease by using x-rays and other imaging techniques
Rheumatologist	A specialist who diagnoses and treats medical conditions of joints and surrounding tissues
Urologist	A specialist who diagnoses and treats disorders of the urinary tract

Gender and Medications

Women menstruate, can become pregnant, and go through menopause. These normal conditions all affect how women's bodies react to medication. On average, women take more prescription and nonprescription medications than do men. For these reasons, women should be especially concerned about which medications they take and about how and when they take them.

Many women use oral contraceptives, commonly known as "the pill." Failure to take the pill each day can result in pregnancy, yet 25 percent of women on the pill miss or skip days. Women may also become pregnant accidentally because some medicines—such as penicillin, some sleeping pills, tuberculosis medicines, and anxiety medicines—can keep oral contraceptives from working. When a woman is prescribed a new medication, she should inform her health care provider that she is on the pill.

If a woman is taking medication while pregnant or breastfeeding, she should make sure to inform her physician. Medications taken during these times may be passed to her fetus or child. The physician may be able to prescribe a different drug or a different way to take the medication that will not affect the fetus or baby.

Choices in Medical Care

How can you choose the best health care provider for your needs? Familiarize yourself with the various health professions and subspecialties (see the list in Table 22.4). These professionals all subscribe to allopathic medical procedures. Most people believe that **allopathic medicine,** or traditional

---

Cross-tolerance The development of a tolerance to one drug that reduces the effects of another, similar drug.

Allopathic medicine Traditional, Western medical practice; in theory, based on scientifically validated methods and procedures.

Western medical practice, is based on scientifically validated methods, but you should consider the fact that only about 20 percent of all allopathic treatments have been proved clinically efficacious in scientific trials. Medical practitioners who adhere to allopathic principles are bound by a professional code of ethics.

Traditional Western (Allopathic) Medicine

Selecting a **primary care practitioner**—a medical practitioner whom you can go to for routine ailments, preventive care, general medical advice, and appropriate referrals— is not an easy task. The primary care practitioner for most people is a family practitioner, an internist, a pediatrician, or an obstetrician/gynecologist. Many people routinely see nurse practitioners or physician assistants who work for an individual doctor or a medical group, and others use nontraditional providers as their primary source of care.

Active participation in your own treatment is the only sensible course in a health care environment that encourages "defensive medicine." That is, physicians will frequently order tests to rule out rare or unlikely diagnoses simply because they are worried about possible malpractice suits. Researchers have documented that this practice often leads to unnecessary tests and overtreatment. By some estimates, between 20 and 70 percent of what is done in medicine either does not improve health outcomes or creates iatrogenic disease (illness caused by the medical process itself). *Informed consent* refers to your right to have explained to you—in nontechnical language you can understand—all possible side effects, benefits, and consequences of a procedure as well as available alternatives to it. It also means that you have the right to refuse a treatment and to seek a second or even third opinion from unbiased, noninvolved providers.[8]

> **What do you think?**
>
> *Have you ever opted for a treatment other than what was recommended by your allopathic medical provider? ✳ What was the response? ✳ Did your health insurer cooperate fully and pay the bill?*

Other Forms of Allopathic Specialties

Although Table 22.4 provides an overview of common sources of health care, it is by no means all-inclusive. Other specialists include **osteopaths,** general practitioners who receive training similar to a medical doctor's but who put special emphasis on the skeletal and muscular systems. Their treatments may involve manipulation of the muscles and joints. Osteopaths receive the degree of doctor of osteopathy (D.O.) rather than doctor of medicine (M.D.).

Much confusion exists about the roles of optometrists and ophthalmologists. An **ophthalmologist** holds a medical degree and can perform surgery and prescribe medications. An **optometrist** typically evaluates visual problems and fits glasses but is not a trained physician. If you have an eye infection, glaucoma, or other eye condition needing diagnosis and treatment, you need to see an ophthalmologist.

Dentists are specialists who diagnose and treat diseases of the teeth, gums, and oral cavity. They attend dental school for four years and receive the title of doctor of dental surgery (D.D.S.) or doctor of medical dentistry (D.M.D.). They must also pass both state and national board examinations before receiving their licenses to practice. The field of dentistry includes many specialties. For example, **orthodontists** are specialists in the alignment of teeth. **Oral surgeons** perform surgical procedures to correct problems of the mouth, face, and jaw.

Nurses are highly trained and strictly regulated health practitioners who provide a wide range of services for patients and their families, including patient education, counseling, provision of community health and disease prevention information, and administration of medications.

Primary care practitioner A medical practitioner who treats routine ailments, advises on preventive care, gives general medical advice, and makes appropriate referrals when necessary.

Osteopath General practitioner who receives training similar to a medical doctor's but with an emphasis on the skeletal and muscular systems, often using spinal manipulation as part of treatment.

Ophthalmologist Physician who specializes in the medical and surgical care of the eyes, including prescriptions for glasses.

Optometrist Eye specialist whose practice is limited to prescribing and fitting lenses.

Dentist Specialist who diagnoses and treats diseases of the teeth, gums, and oral cavity.

Orthodontist Dentist who specializes in the alignment of teeth.

Oral surgeon Dentist who performs surgical procedures to correct problems of the mouth, jaw, and face.

Nurse Health practitioner who provides many services for patients and who may work in a variety of settings.

Physician assistant A midlevel practitioner trained to handle most standard cases of care.

Group practice A group of physicians who combine resources, sharing offices, equipment, and staff costs, to render care to patients.

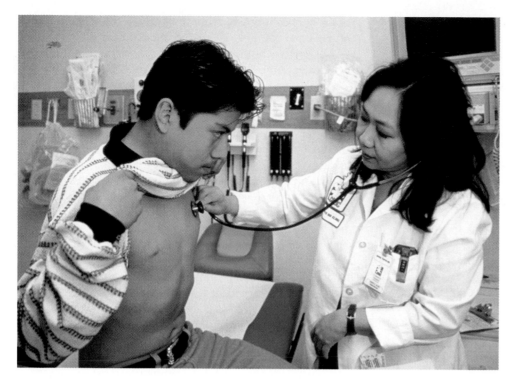

People who largely rely on student health centers, clinics, and hospital emergency rooms for treatment miss out on the benefits of continuity of care offered by a primary care physician.

Nurses may today choose from several training options. There are over 2.4 million licensed registered nurses (R.N.s) in the United States who have completed either a four-year program leading to a bachelor of science in nursing (B.S.N.) degree or a two-year associate degree program. More than half a million lower-level licensed practical or vocational nurses (L.P.N.s or L.V.N.s) have completed a one- to two-year training program, which may be community college–based or hospital-based.

Nurse practitioners (N.P.s) are professional nurses having advanced training obtained through either a master's degree program or a specialized nurse practitioner program. Nurse practitioners have the training and authority to conduct diagnostic tests and prescribe medications (in some states). They work in a variety of settings, particularly in HMOs, clinics, and student health centers. Nurses may also earn the clinical doctor of nursing degree (N.D.) or doctor of nursing science (D.N.S. and D.N.Sc.), or a research-based Ph.D. in nursing.

More than 30,000 **physician assistants** (P.A.s) currently practice in the United States. Most of these are in office-based practices, including school health centers, but approximately 40 percent practice in areas where physicians are in short supply. Studies have shown that this relatively new class of midlevel practitioners may competently care for the majority of patients seeking primary care. All physician assistants must work under the supervision of a licensed physician, but most states do allow physician assistants to prescribe drugs.[9]

Health Care Organizations, Programs, and Facilities

Today, managed care is the dominant health payer system in the United States. Because of this, many people are restricted in their choice of a health care provider. Selective contracting between insurers or employers and health providers has limited the freedom of choice that some Americans previously enjoyed under a fee-for-service system. Two critical decisions to make are (1) choosing an insurance carrier or type of plan, and then (2) choosing from among the health care providers who participate in that plan. This section lists the most common choices.

Types of Medical Practices

In the highly competitive market for patients, many health care providers have found it essential to combine resources into a **group practice,** which can be single-specialty or multi-specialty. Physicians share offices, equipment, utility bills, and staff costs. Besides sharing costs, they may also share profits. Proponents of group practice maintain that it provides better coordination of care, reduces unnecessary duplication of equipment, and improves the quality of health care through peer review. Critics argue that group practice may limit competition and patients' access to services.

Solo practitioners are medical providers who practice independently of other practitioners. It is hard for solo practitioners to survive in today's high-cost, high-technology health care market. Additionally, they often have little time away from their offices and have to trade on-call hours with other doctors. For these reasons, there are far fewer solo practices today than in the past. Most solo practitioners are doctors who established their practices years ago, have a specialty that's in high demand, or work in a rural or underserved area.

Integrated Health Care Organizations

Both hospitals and clinics provide a range of health care services, including emergency treatment, diagnostic tests, and inpatient and outpatient (ambulatory) care. Your selection of a hospital or clinic will depend on your particular needs, income, and insurance coverage, plus the availability of services in your community. As the number of hospitals has decreased in recent years due to an oversupply of hospital beds, a decreasing need for inpatient care, and an increase in competition, the number of hospital-based outpatient clinics has grown. These integrated health care organizations range from groups of loosely affiliated health service organizations and hospitals to HMOs that control their own very tightly joined hospitals, clinics, pharmacies, and even home health agencies.

There are several ways to classify hospitals: by profit status (nonprofit or for-profit), by ownership (private, city, county, state, federal), by specialty (children's, maternity, chronic care, psychiatric, general acute), by teaching status (teaching-affiliated or not), by size, and by whether they are part of a chain of hospitals.

Nonprofit (voluntary) hospitals have traditionally been run by religious or other humanitarian groups. Earnings have generally been reinvested in the hospital to improve health care. These hospitals have often cared for patients whether they could pay or not.

The number of **for-profit (proprietary) hospitals** has multiplied over the past two decades. Today they constitute over 20 percent of nongovernmental acute-care hospitals.

For-profit hospitals, which do not receive tax breaks, are not compelled to operate as a charity and typically provide fewer free services to the community than do nonprofit hospitals. Historically, some for-profit hospitals have quickly transferred indigent (poor) or uninsured patients to public hospitals (those that are not heavily supported by taxes) or to nonprofit hospitals.[10] This practice, known as *patient dumping,* was prohibited by federal law in 1986. Today, all hospital emergency rooms are required to perform a screening medical exam on all patients, regardless of their ability to pay. Patients must be determined to be "medically stable" before they can be transferred to another facility or discharged from the emergency room.

More treatments or services, including surgery, are delivered on an **outpatient (ambulatory) care** basis (care that does not involve an overnight stay) by hospitals, traditional clinics, student health clinics, and nontraditional clinical centers. One type of ambulatory facility that is becoming common is the *surgicenter*—a place where minor, low-risk procedures such as vasectomies, tubal ligations, tissue biopsies, cosmetic surgery, abortions, and minor eye operations are performed. In 1982, nearly 85 percent of all surgeries in the United States involved an overnight hospital stay; by 2000, less than 30 percent of surgeries did so.

To reduce the distance patients have to travel, many hospitals locate satellite clinics in cities' outlying areas, sometimes in shopping centers. A few hospitals have designated their satellites as freestanding emergency centers, or surgicenters, that function like hospital emergency rooms for uncomplicated immediate-care cases but have lower operating costs. Some consumers refer to these as "doc-in-the-box" centers.

Many hospitals and group practices have freestanding imaging and diagnostic laboratory centers affiliated with them through either direct ownership or other profit-sharing arrangements. Significant debate surrounds this practice because research has found that when doctors own the diagnostic and laboratory services to which they refer patients, they tend to order an excessive number of tests. Today, these practices are prohibited by antikickback legislation.

Most health clinics were once located within hospitals. Today they are more likely to be independent facilities run by medical practitioners. Other health clinics are run by county health departments; these offer low-cost diagnosis and treatment for financially needy patients. Additionally, some 1,500 college campuses have student health centers that, along with county, city, or community clinics, supply low-cost family planning, tests and services related to sexually transmitted infection, gynecological services, and vaccination services.

Consumers who consider using a hospital or clinic should scrutinize the facility's accreditation. Accredited hospitals have met rigorous standards set by the Joint Commission on the Accreditation of Healthcare Organizations (JCAHO). If you choose an institution having this accreditation, you have a high likelihood of obtaining quality care.

Solo practitioner   Physician who renders care to patients independently of other practitioners.

Nonprofit (voluntary) hospitals   Hospitals run by religious or other humanitarian groups that reinvest their earnings in the hospital to improve health care.

For-profit (proprietary) hospitals   Hospitals that provide a return on earnings to the investors who own them.

Outpatient (ambulatory) care   Treatment that does not involve an overnight stay in a hospital.

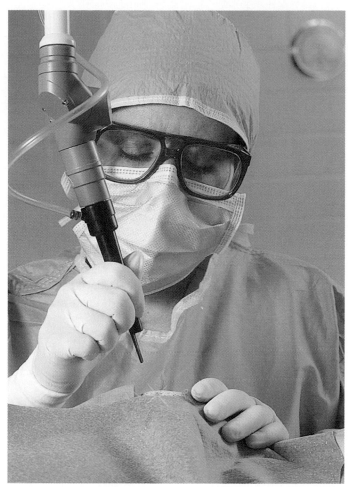

Modern technology has vastly improved treatment for many illnesses, but it has also played a major role in the escalating costs of medical care.

With the growth of managed care organizations, concerns have arisen about the quality of care offered under this type of payment system. These concerns compelled consumer groups and public health organizations to require managed care insurers to compile quality care "report cards," known as HEDIS (Health Employer Data Information Set) Reports, so that health outcomes could be compared across different plans. The quality measures include preventive services (childhood immunizations, Pap smears, mammograms), disease indicators (eye exams and glucose control tests for diabetics), and screening exams (routine physical exams, including gynecological exams). These reports are available from most managed care health plans on request. Still, such information is difficult for the consumer to evaluate due to inconsistent data collection and reporting techniques. This problem has given rise to skepticism and controversy over the validity of these reports.

Consumers can obtain additional information regarding prior provider malpractice insurance or sanctions from state licensure boards and the National Practitioner Data Bank. It is the responsibility of every health care consumer to report concerns about their health care providers to local or state medical societies or licensing agencies for investigation. If you have any concerns about billing-related fraud or abuse, report them directly to the Health Care Finance Administration (HCFA).

> ### What do you think?
>
> *If you had access to a HEDIS health care report card for the hospitals in your area, would you try to switch your upcoming surgery to the hospital having the lowest complication and mortality rate? ✳ Have you ever checked on a doctor's or health care facility's credentials, or do you take it for granted that they are licensed, certified, or accredited?*

Issues Facing Today's Health Care System

Many Americans believe that our health care system needs fundamental reform. What are the problems that have brought us to this point? Cost, access, malpractice, restriction of provider and treatment modality choice, unnecessary procedures, complicated and cumbersome insurance rules, and dramatic ranges in quality are among the issues of concern. One of the most frequently voiced criticisms concerns lack of access to adequate health insurance, as many Americans have had increasing difficulty obtaining comprehensive coverage from their employers. Until recently, insurance benefits were often lost when employees changed jobs, causing many to remain in undesirable positions in order to avoid losing health benefits. This phenomenon, known as *job lock,* led the federal government to pass legislation mandating the "portability" of health insurance benefits from one job to the next, thereby guaranteeing coverage during the transition.

Over 90 million people in the United States suffer from chronic health conditions that should be at least monitored by medical practitioners.[11] Their access to care is largely determined by whether they have health insurance. Catastrophic or chronic illness among only 10 percent of the population accounts for 75 percent of all health expenditures.[12] Since we cannot perfectly predict who will fall into that 10 percent, every American is potentially vulnerable to the high cost and devastating effects of such illnesses.

Cost

Both per capita and as a percent of gross domestic product (GDP), we spend more on health care than any other nation, yet, unlike the rest of the industrialized world, we do not provide access for our entire population. In 2000, we spent over

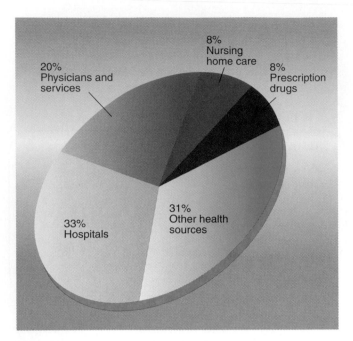

Figure 22.2

How Health Care Dollars Are Spent in the United States—1998

Source: Health Care Financing Administration, Office of the Actuary, data from the National Health Statistics Group, as printed in K. Levit et al., "Health Spending in 1998: Signals of Change," (2000) *Health Affairs* 19(1): 124–132.

$1.3 trillion on health care, up nearly 7 percent since 1997.[13] This translates into nearly 13 percent of our GDP, up from 5 percent of the GDP in 1960.

Why do health care costs continue to spiral upward? There are a variety of theories, including excess administrative costs, duplication of services, an aging population, demand for new diagnostic and treatment technologies, an emphasis on crisis-oriented care instead of preventive care, inappropriate utilization of services by consumers, and related factors.

Our system has more than 2,000 health insurance companies, each with different coverage structures and administrative requirements. This lack of uniformity prevents our system from achieving the *economies of scale* (bulk purchasing at a reduced cost) and administrative efficiency realized in countries where there is a single-payer delivery system. According to the Health Insurance Association of America (HIAA), commercial insurance companies commonly experience administrative costs greater than 10 percent of the total health care insurance premium, whereas the administrative cost of the government's Medicare program is less than 4 percent. Administrative expenses in the private sector contribute to the high cost of health care and force companies to require employees to share more of the costs, cut back on benefits, and drop some benefits altogether. These costs are largely passed on to consumers in the form of higher prices for goods and services. See Figure 22.2 for a breakdown of how health care dollars are spent.

The declining availability of health insurance coverage means more Americans are uninsured or underinsured. These people are unable to access preventive care and seek care only in the event of an emergency or crisis. Since emergency care is extraordinarily expensive, they often are unable to pay, and the cost is absorbed by those who *can* pay—the insured or taxpayers. This process is known as *cost shifting*.

Access

Access to health care is determined by numerous factors, including the supply of providers and facilities, proximity to care, ability to maneuver in the system, health status, and insurance coverage. Although there are approximately 700,000 physicians in the United States, many Americans do not have adequate access to health services because of insurance barriers or maldistribution of providers. There is an oversupply of higher-paid specialists and a shortage of lower-paid primary care physicians (family practitioners, pediatricians, internists, OB/GYNs, geriatricians). Inner cities and some rural areas face constant shortages of physicians.

Managed-care health plans determine access on the basis of the participating providers, health plan benefits, and administrative rules. Often this means that consumers do not have the freedom to choose specialists, facilities, or treatment options beyond those contracted with the health plan and recommended by their primary care provider (also known as *gatekeeper*). In the United States, consumer demand has led to an expansion of benefits to include nonallopathic therapies such as chiropractic and acupuncture (see Chapter 23). However, many nonallopathic treatments remain unavailable, even to a limited degree, through available health plans.

Quality and Malpractice

The U.S. health care system employs several mechanisms for ensuring quality services: education, licensure, certification/registration, accreditation, peer review; and, as a last resort, the legal system of malpractice litigation. Some of these mechanisms are mandatory before a professional or organization may provide care, whereas others are purely voluntary. (Be aware that licensure, although state mandated for some practitioners and facilities, is only a minimum guarantee of quality.) Insurance companies and government payers may also require a higher level of quality by linking payment to whether a practitioner is board certified or a facility is accredited by the appropriate agency. In addition, most insurance plans now require prior authorization and/or second opinions not only to reduce costs but also to improve quality of care.

Consumer, provider, and advocacy groups focus on the great variation in quality as a main problem in our health care system. A newer form of quality measurement uses "outcome" as the primary indicator for measuring health care quality at the individual level. With outcome measurements, we don't look just at what is done to the patient but

"Actionable" Medical Malpractice: What Is It, and When Should You Consider It?

Actionable medical malpractice or medical negligence occurs when a physician fails to properly treat a medical condition and the negligent act or omission causes a new or aggravated injury to the patient. Obviously, the physician cannot be held responsible for the original underlying health problem. The negligence in medical malpractice cases can occur in a variety of situations including, but not limited to, the following:

✔ Delay or failure in diagnosing a disease.
✔ Surgical or anesthesia-related mishap during an operative procedure.
✔ Failure to gain the informed consent of the patient for an operation or surgical procedure.
✔ Failure to properly treat the disease process after making the correct diagnosis.
✔ Misuse of prescription drugs or a medical device or implant.

Typically, patients must secure an attorney who is well versed in medical law and who can quickly determine whether there is an actionable case. Usually, a medical expert who is qualified to give a medical opinion and board certified in the relevant field of medicine is also necessary. The attorney agrees up front to advance costs and to be repaid in the event the case is won, with a percentage of the gross recovery as the established fee for service. Medical malpractice lawsuits are costly and complex and may take years to win. Careful record keeping of procedures and actions is an important part of the entire case. Having a health advocate who has witnessed the events is another key element in determining the success or failure of a case.

Source: "Actionable Medical Malpractice Civil Rights and the Law," January 2002 (see http://www.civilrights.com/medical.html).

---

at what subsequently happens to the patient's health status. Thus, mortality rates and complication rates (such as infections) become very important statistics in assessing individual practitioners and facilities. The Reality Check box discusses what "actionable" malpractice really is.

What do you think?

Do you believe prospective patients should have access to information about practitioners' and facilities' malpractice records? ✳ *How about their success and failure rates or outcomes of various procedures?*

Third-Party Payers

The fundamental principle of insurance underwriting is that the cost of health care can be predicted for large populations. This is how health care premiums (payments) are determined. Policyholders pay premiums into a pool, which fills as reserves until needed. When you are sick or injured, the insurance company pays out of the pool, regardless of your total amount of contribution. Depending on circumstances, you may never pay for what your medical care costs or you may pay much more for insurance than your medical bills ever total. The idea is that you pay in affordable premiums so that you never have to face catastrophic bills. In today's profit-oriented system, insurers prefer to have healthy people in their plans who pour money into risk pools without taking money out.

Unfortunately, not everyone has health insurance. Almost 40 million Americans are uninsured at any given point in time—that is, they have no private health insurance and are not eligible for Medicare, Medicaid, or other health programs. The number of uninsured has been growing since the late 1970s. Lack of health insurance has been associated with delayed health care and increased mortality. *Underinsurance* (i.e., the inability to pay out-of-pocket expenses despite having insurance) also may result in adverse health consequences. Findings from the CDC's latest Behavior Risk Factor Surveillance System (BRFSS) indicate that a large proportion of all adults are either uninsured or underinsured. People lacking any type of health insurance make up just over 15 percent of the nonelderly population. Another 20 million to 40 million Americans are estimated to be *underinsured* (at risk for spending more than 10 percent of their income on medical care because their insurance is inadequate).[14]

Contrary to the common belief that the uninsured are unemployed, 75 percent of them are either workers or the dependents of workers. One-quarter of all the uninsured are children under age 16. College students are one of the largest groups of the uninsured not in the labor force. This presents a difficult dilemma for both universities and students when they must seek care because most university insurance plans are designed as short-term, noncatastrophic plans having low upper limits of benefits. As a full-time student, you should consider purchasing a higher level catastrophic plan to protect yourself in the event of a rare, but very costly, illness or accident.

For the uninsured and many of the underinsured, health care may not be available through any source because of their inability to pay. Many either will not or cannot seek care from charitable providers, so they fail to receive the medical care they need. People without health care coverage are less likely than other Americans to have their children immunized, seek early prenatal care, obtain annual blood pressure checks, and seek attention for serious symptoms of illness. Many experts believe that this ultimately leads to higher system costs because their conditions deteriorate to a more debilitating and costly stage before they are forced to seek help.

Private Health Insurance

Our current health system began in the past century and its growth accelerated in the post–World War II era to its current massive, complex web. Hospitals became the engines of medicine in the mid-twentieth century. Doctors became the drivers or conductors of this rapidly moving system. The system was fueled by a variety of funding sources but, chiefly, first by the growth of tax-exempt, nonprofit private insurance companies established in the 1940s and later by the growth of for-profit insurance companies.

Health insurance originally consisted solely of coverage for hospital costs (it was called *major medical*), but gradually coverage was extended to routine physicians' treatment and to other areas such as dental services and pharmaceuticals. Payment mechanisms used until recently laid the groundwork for today's ever-rising health care costs. Hospitals were reimbursed on a cost-plus basis after services were rendered. That is, they billed for the costs of providing care plus an amount for profit. This system provided no incentive to contain costs, limit the number of procedures, or curtail capital investment in redundant equipment and facilities. Physicians were reimbursed on a fee-for-service (indemnity) basis determined by "usual, customary, and reasonable" fees. These were arrived at by comparing what a doctor charged for a service with what that same doctor charged last year for the service and with what other doctors in the area were charging. This system encouraged physicians to charge high fees, raise them often, and perform as many procedures as possible. At the same time, because most insurance did not cover routine or preventive services, consumers were encouraged to use hospitals whenever possible (the coverage was better) and to wait until illness developed to seek help instead of seeking preventive care. Consumers were also free to choose any provider or service they wished, including even inappropriate—and often very expensive—levels of care.

Private insurance companies have increasingly employed several mechanisms to limit potential losses and control consumers' use of insurance. These mechanisms include cost sharing (in the form of deductibles, copayments, and coinsurance), exclusions, "preexisting condition" clauses, waiting periods, and upper limits on payments. *Deductibles* are front-end payments (commonly $250 to $1,000) that you must make to your provider before your insurance com-

pany will start paying for any services you use. *Copayments* are set amounts that you pay per service received regardless of the cost of the services (e.g., $10 per doctor visit or per prescription). *Coinsurance* is the percentage of the bill that you must pay throughout the course of treatment (e.g., 20 percent of whatever the total is). *Preexisting condition clauses* limit the insurance company's liability for medical conditions that a consumer had before obtaining insurance coverage (i.e., if a woman takes out coverage while she is pregnant, the insurance company may cover pregnancy complications and infant care but not charges related to "normal pregnancy"). Because many insurance companies use a combination of these mechanisms, keeping track of the costs you are responsible for can become very difficult.

Group plans of large employers (government agencies, school districts, or corporations, for example) generally do not have preexisting condition clauses in their plans. But smaller group plans (a group may be as small as two) often do. Some plans never cover services for preexisting conditions, while others specify a waiting period (such as six months) before they will provide coverage. All insurers set some limits on the types of services they will cover (e.g., most exclude cosmetic surgery, private rooms, and experimental procedures). Some insurance plans may also include an upper or lifetime limit, after which coverage will end. Although $250,000 may seem like an enormous sum, medical bills for a sick child or chronic disease can easily run this high within a few years.

Medicare and Medicaid (Social Insurance versus Welfare)

After years of debate about whether we should have a national health program like those of most industrialized countries, the U.S. government directed the system toward a mixed private and public approach in the 1960s. Most Americans obtained their health insurance through their employers. But this left out two groups—the nonworking poor and the aged. In 1965, amendments to the 1935 Social Security Act established Medicare and Medicaid. Although enacted simultaneously, these programs were vastly different.

Medicare, basically a federal social insurance covering 99 percent of the elderly over 65 years of age, all totally and permanently disabled people (after a waiting period), and all people with end-stage kidney failure, is a universal program that covers a broad range of services except long-term care and pharmaceuticals. It currently covers 36 million people. Medicare is widely accepted by physicians and hospitals and has relatively low administrative costs.

On the other hand, **Medicaid,** covering approximately 35 million people, is a federal-state matching funds welfare program for the categorically eligible poor (blind, disabled, aged, or those receiving Aid to Families with Dependent Children). Because each state determines income eligibility levels and payments to providers, there are vast differences in the way Medicaid operates from state to state.

To control hospital costs, in 1983 the federal government set up a prospective payment system based on **diagnosis related groups (DRGs)** for Medicare. Using a complicated formula, nearly 500 groupings of diagnoses were created to establish how much a hospital would be reimbursed for a particular patient. If a hospital can treat the patient for less than that amount, it can keep the difference. However, if a patient's care costs more than the set amount, the hospital must absorb the difference (with a few exceptions that must be reviewed by a panel). This system gives hospitals the incentive to discharge patients quickly after doing as little as possible for them, provide more ambulatory care, and admit only patients with favorable (profitable) DRGs. Many private health insurance companies have followed the federal government in adopting this type of reimbursement. In 1998, the federal HCFA expanded the prospective payment system to include payments for outpatient surgery and skilled nursing care.

In its continued efforts to control rising costs, HCFA has encouraged the growth of prepaid HMO senior plans for Medicare-eligible persons. Under this system, commercial managed care insurance plans receive a fixed per-capita premium from HCFA and then offer more preventive services with lower out-of-pocket copayments. These managed care plans encourage providers and patients to utilize health care resources under administrative rules similar to commercial HMO plans. Similarly, states have encouraged the growth of managed Medicaid programs.

Managed Care

Managed care describes a health care delivery system with the following elements:

1. A budget based on an estimate of the annual cost of delivering health care for a given population.
2. A network of physicians, hospitals, and other providers and facilities linked contractually to deliver comprehensive health benefits within that predetermined budget, sharing economic risk for any budget deficit or surplus.
3. An established set of administrative rules requiring patients to follow the advice of the participating health care providers in order to have their health care paid for under the terms of the health plan.

Many such plans pay their contracted health care providers through **capitation,** that is, prepayment of a fixed monthly amount for each patient without regard for the type or number of health services provided. Some plans pay health care providers salaries and some are still fee-for-service plans. As with other insurance plans, enrollees are members of a risk pool, and it is expected that some persons will use no services, some will use a modest amount of services, and others will have high-cost utilization over a given year. Doctors have the incentive to keep their patient pool healthy and avoid catastrophic ailments that are preventable; usually such incentives come back in terms of increased salaries, bonuses, and other benefits. As such, prevention and health education

to reduce risk and intervene early to avoid major problems should be capstone components of such plans.

Managed care plans have grown steadily over the past decade with a proportionate decline of enrollment in traditional indemnity insurance plans. The reason for this shift is that indemnity insurance, which pays providers and hospitals on a fee-for-service basis with no built-in incentives to control costs, has become unaffordable or unavailable for most Americans.

Today, managed care plans are sweeping the nation, with over 60 million Americans enrolled in one type, the health maintenance organization, and another 90 million in other forms of managed care. Four million beneficiaries are in Medicare HMOs, with enrollment growing by about 80,000 people a month.[15] Types of managed care plans include HMOs, point of service (POS), and preferred provider organizations (PPOs).

Health Maintenance Organizations (HMOs) HMOs provide a wide range of covered health benefits (such as checkups, surgery, doctor visits, lab tests) for a fixed amount prepaid by you, the employer, Medicaid, or Medicare.[16] Usually, HMO premiums are the least expensive, but HMOs are the most restrictive type of managed care (little or no choice in doctors and/or certain services). These premiums are 8 to 10 percent lower than for traditional plans, there are low or no deductibles or coinsurance payments, and copayments are $10 to $20 per office visit. HMOs contract with providers to supply health services for enrollees through various systems,[17] such as these:

- *The staff model.* You receive care from salaried staff doctors at the HMO's facility.
- *The group network model.* The HMO contracts with one or several groups of doctors, who provide care for a fixed amount per plan member. Groups often practice in one facility.
- *The independent practice association (IPA).* Doctors in private practice form an association that contracts with HMOs. The physicians generally work in their own offices.

Medicare   Federal health insurance program for the elderly and the permanently disabled.

Medicaid   Federal-state health insurance program for the poor.

Diagnosis related groups (DRGs)   Diagnostic categories established by the federal government to determine in advance how much hospitals will be reimbursed for the care of a particular Medicare patient.

Managed care   Cost-control procedures used by health insurers to coordinate treatment.

Capitation   Prepayment of a fixed monthly amount for each patient without regard to the type or number of services provided.

The downside of these plans is the typical requirement to use the plan's doctors and hospitals and to get approval from a "gatekeeper" or primary care physician for treatment and referrals. Although more and more people are opting for HMOs, some people continue to be skeptical. Concerns leveled against HMOs include such issues as the following:

- Do high-paid administrators and stockholders ration care, providing only for the upper end of the paying and health continuums?
- Does the huge administrative structure imposed by the HMO make it virtually impossible for patients to sue in the event of clear violations?
- Are patients denied costly diagnostic tests because such tests cut into bottom-line profits? Are some tests given too late because of concerns over costs?
- Do HMOs really focus on prevention or intervention? Evidence exists that the fee structure of many HMOs actually discourages basic preventive services, such as immunizations.
- Are doctors allowed to treat patients using their best judgment and skills, or do policies and profit-motivated concerns interfere with the doctors' roles as advocates for their patients?
- Are the obstacles imposed by HMOs too daunting for patients in need of urgent care?
- Do HMO cost-saving policies force patients out of hospitals and treatment centers too early?

Point of Service (POS)   This option often provides a more acceptable form of managed care for those used to the traditional indemnity plan of insurance, which probably explains why it is among the fastest growing of the managed care plans. Under POS, patients can go to providers outside of their HMO for care but must pay for the extra cost. Usually this is a reasonable alternative for middle-class or wealthy Americans who are willing to pay the extra cost for choices in care.[18]

Preferred Provider Organization (PPO)   PPOs are networks of independent doctors and hospitals that contract to provide care at discounted rates. Although they offer greater choices in doctors than HMOs do, they are less likely to coordinate a patient's care. In addition, while members have a choice of seeing doctors who are not on the preferred list, this choice may come at considerable cost (such as having to pay 30 percent of the charges out of pocket, rather than 10 to 20 percent for PPO doctors and services).[19]

What do you think?

Why is it important that private insurance cover preventive or lower-level care as well as hospitalization and high-technology interventions? ✷ *What kinds of incentives would cause you to seek help early rather than to delay care?*

What Are Your Options?

The United States and South Africa are currently the only industrialized nations that do not have a national health program that guarantees all citizens access to at least a basic set of health benefits. The United States has seen four major political movements supporting national health insurance during the twentieth century, but none has succeeded. Whether universal coverage will—or should—be achieved and through what mechanism are hotly debated topics. Many analysts believe that health-care reformers have failed due to a combination of circumstances and influences: lobbying efforts by the insurance industry and the medical community, proposed plans that were too complicated, and interest groups who felt that the plans either went "too far" or "not far enough." But some people also believe that our current system serves people well.

One critical point must be made, though: We are paying for the most expensive system in the world without obtaining full coverage. We pay for people who don't have insurance through cost shifting that increases premiums and taxes, and we spend more than necessary because prevention and early treatment are not emphasized. We also pay for much duplication of services and technologies, for practitioners who practice defensive medicine and who refer patients to their own diagnostic labs for profit reasons, and for the vast bureaucracy made inevitable by over 2,000 private health insurance companies.

The managed competition model proposed by the Clinton administration called for employers and major insurance companies to play a central role. This appealed to those who don't wish to change the structure of the system radically or place a great deal of power in the hands of one institution but do want to do more than merely provide incentives through the tax system. It did not appeal to those who believe that a system based on competition actually fuels costs and increases the emphasis on high technology while leaving the sickest and poorest at a severe disadvantage.

Another proposal involves the federalization and incremental expansion of Medicaid. The idea is to eliminate state disparities and improve coverage gradually through progressive general tax financing. First would come federalization of Medicaid eligibility, benefits, and reimbursement to improve access for those determined eligible. Next would come a step-by-step expansion raising the age limits for children, then covering all pregnant women, then allowing "intact" poor families to obtain coverage, then increasing the income limit to incorporate the uninsured near-poor, and finally allowing the middle class to buy into the program. This type of plan could work well if reimbursements were set high enough to encourage provider participation. But it would take a long time to provide universal coverage, and it is not a likely option at this time.

Either approach could evolve into a single-payer, tax-financed scheme that severs insurance ties from employment. Similar to the Canadian model, it would cover everyone—regardless of income or other factors such as health status. It would offer many different ways to tailor a plan to the needs of U.S. citizens. A single federal plan or a privately administered plan paid for by general tax funds or earmarked taxes could be created. Thus, all (or most) private insurers would be eliminated or would see their role limited to that of fiscal administrators. Benefits would be comprehensive and provide incentives for cost-effective care. In addition, benefits would be "portable": They would remain in effect when individuals changed jobs or moved to a different area of the country. Freedom of choice in terms of providers might actually improve in a single-payer system, given how restrictive our current private health insurance system has become. Such a plan would allow far greater control over resource and personnel planning and improve access to preventive services, and it could eliminate duplicate services and technology. Researchers have estimated that adopting a single-payer system would save upward of $130 billion annually in administrative costs—enough to provide coverage to all uninsured Americans.[20] Claims that the Canadian system has long waiting lists have either proved entirely untrue or exaggerated: Modest waits do not appear to result in any reduction of health status.

Given the delay in realizing national health care reform, several states have sought ways to contain costs and improve access for their populations. Currently, Congress is grappling with several strategies for bolstering Social Security and Medicare.

What do you think?

Do you believe that the time is right for another national discussion on health care reform? ✷ *Do you think we are moving to a more profit-oriented health care system or a single-payer system?* ✷ *Which would you prefer?* ✷ *Is health care a right or a privilege?*

Taking Charge **22** 22 **22**

Managing Your Health Care Needs

Throughout this text, we have emphasized behaviors important to staying healthy. How can you promote your health when seeking medical attention? Many people wait until a problem arises to seek medical care, and they either take the first available physician or go to the nearest facility. This is not always the best choice. When you have a medical problem (even a minor one), you need to decide how best to treat it. Do your research. Be aware of your options. Then you will be able to make informed decisions that will lead to better health care.

Some health care decisions are dictated by physicians, insurance companies, and government agencies, but many decisions still rest with you. Are you a good health consumer? Start by learning about your own insurance protection. What coverage do you currently have? If you don't have coverage, how would you pay for a medical emergency? What coverage is available to you as a student? Learn how your insurance plan works and what it does and does not cover. Can you choose your physicians and hospitals? Remember that you have rights as a patient and a consumer. Don't be afraid to ask questions. Consider the following issues.

Checklist for Change

Making Personal Choices

☐ Do you feel comfortable discussing your problems with your health care provider?

☐ Are you confident that your doctor knows what he or she is talking about?

☐ Is the doctor willing to talk about issues such as credentials, hospital affiliations, qualifications of referrals for special problems, and fees?

☐ Are you able to understand answers to your questions? Does the doctor seem interested in whether you understand? Is he or she willing to answer questions?

☐ Does the physician tell you why one test is being given rather than another? About risks of the test? About preparation for the tests? About what to expect concerning certain results?

☐ Is the physician willing to refer you to a nongroup specialist in a location of your choice?

☐ Does the doctor support your obtaining a second opinion or seem irritated by such a request?

☐ Suppose you became seriously ill and had to see a lot of this doctor. Would you feel comfortable, or would you rather see someone else?

☐ When you start taking a medication, do you find out about its active ingredients? Its potential side effects? What to do if you experience side effects? What foods or beverages you should avoid while taking the medication? Adverse consequences of long-term use?

Making Community Choices

☐ How long has your doctor been in your community?

☐ How many hospitals are within a 30-minute drive of your home? Are any of them teaching hospitals?

☐ What percentage of people in your community lack health insurance?

☐ What services are available in your community to help people

who are underinsured or uninsured?

☐ What are the policies of local hospitals concerning uninsured individuals who need care?

☐ Have you written to your congressional leaders concerning your views about health care legislation?

Summary

✳ Advertisers of health care products and services use sophisticated tactics to attract attention and get business. Advertising claims sometimes appear to be supported by spontaneous remission (symptoms disappearing without any apparent cause) or the placebo effect (symptoms disappearing because people think they should), rather than the efficacy of the product or service.

✳ Self-care and individual responsibility are key factors in reducing rising health care costs and improving health status. Advance planning can help a person navigate health care treatment in unfamiliar situations or emergencies. Assess health professionals by considering their qualifications, their record of treating problems like yours, and their ability to work with you.

✳ In theory, allopathic ("traditional") medicine is based on scientifically validated methods and procedures. Medical doctors, specialists of various kinds, nurses, physician assistants, and other health professionals practice allopathic medicine.

✳ Prescription drugs are administered under medical supervision. Categories include antibiotics, sedatives, tranquilizers, antidepressants, and amphetamines. Generic drugs can often be substituted for more expensive brand-name

drugs. Over-the-counter drug categories include analgesics; cold, cough, allergy, and asthma relievers; stimulants; sleeping aids and relaxants; and dieting aids. Exercise personal responsibility by reading directions for OTC drugs and asking your pharmacist or doctor if any special precautions are advised when taking these substances.

✳ Health care providers may provide services as solo practitioners or in group practices (in which overhead cost is shared). Hospitals and clinics are classified by profit status, ownership, specialty, and teaching status.

✳ Concerns about the U.S. health care system include cost, access, choice of treatment modality, quality and malpractice, and fraud and abuse.

✳ Health insurance is based on the concept of spreading risk. Insurance is provided by private insurance companies (who charge premiums) and the government Medicare and Medicaid programs (funded by taxes). Managed care (in the form of HMOs, PPOs, etc.) attempts to keep costs lower by streamlining administrative procedures and stressing preventive care (among other initiatives).

Questions for Discussion and Reflection

1. What claims do marketers use to get people to try health-related products? Why are consumers susceptible to such ploys? What could be done to increase the accuracy of messages related to health care?

2. List several conditions (resulting from illness or accident) for which you don't need to seek medical help. When would you consider each condition to be bad enough to require medical attention? How would you decide to whom and where to go for treatment?

3. Explain the terms *synergism, antagonism,* and *inhibition.*

4. What are the advantages and disadvantages associated with generic drug use?

5. What are the pros and cons of group practices? Of non-profit and for-profit hospitals? If you had health insurance, where do you believe you would get the best care? On what do you base your answer?

6. What are the inherent benefits and risks of managed care organizations?

7. Discuss the problems of the U.S. health care system. If you were president, what would you propose as a solution? Which groups might oppose your plan? Which groups might support it?

8. Explain the differences between traditional indemnity insurance and managed health care. Which would you feel more comfortable with? Should insurance companies dictate rates for various medical tests and procedures in an attempt to keep prices down?

Application Exercises

Reread the What Do You Think? scenarios at the beginning of the chapter and answer the following questions.

1. If you were faced with a situation like the Lamms', would you have any other option but to switch to another pediatrician? What type of health policy or law would be necessary to avoid this situation in the future?
2. When is it appropriate to diagnose and medicate oneself? What would you recommend to Beth if she came to you to discuss her symptoms?

3. What risk does Beth run in using someone else's prescription medication? Is it ever safe to share a prescription? Is it legal?
4. If Beth is using an oral contraceptive, what impact may antibiotic use have on the efficacy of the pill? What precautions should she take?

Accessing Your Health on the Internet

Visit the following Internet sites to explore further topics and issues related to personal health. To visit an organization's website, go to the Companion Website for *Access to Health, Eighth Edition* at www.aw.com/donatelle, click on the book image, and select "Accessing Your Health on the Internet" from the navigation menu on the left.

1. *Agency for Health Care Research and Quality.* A gateway to consumer health information, providing links to sites that can address health care concerns and provide information on questions to ask, what to look for, and what you should know when making critical decisions about personal care.

2. *Food and Drug Administration.* News on the latest government-approved generic drugs and investigations.
3. *Health Touch.* Search for prescription and over-the-counter drug uses and side effects, plus other health-related resources.
4. *National Committee for Quality Assurance.* The NCQA assesses and reports on the quality of managed care plans, including health maintenance organizations.

Further Reading

Anders, G. *Health Against Wealth: HMOs and the Breakdown of Medical Trust.* Boston: Houghton Mifflin, 1997.

A series of cases that outline some of the severe problems of managed care.

Greenburg, S. *2002 Physician's Desk Reference for Nonprescription Drugs,* 21th ed. Oradell, NJ: Medical Economics Data, 2002.

Outlines proper uses, possible dangers, and effective ingredients of nonprescription medications.

Griffith, W. H. *A Complete Guide to Prescription and Nonprescription Drugs, 2001.* Berkeley Publishing Group, San Francisco, CA, 2001.

This essential guide answers every conceivable question about prescription and nonprescription drugs and contains information about dosages, side effects, precautions, interactions, and more. More than 5,000 brand-name and 700 generic drugs are profiled in an easy-to-use format.

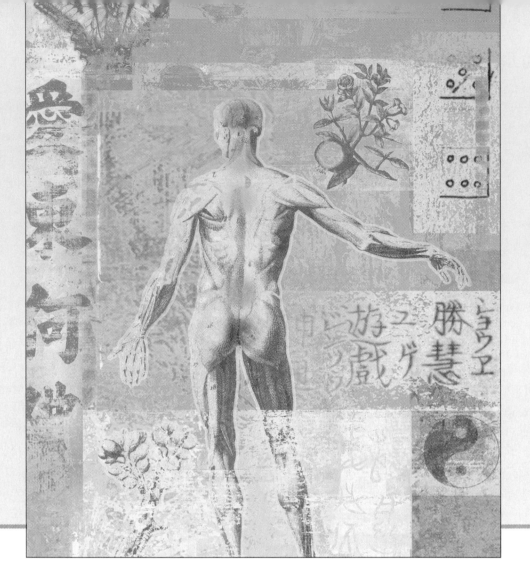

Objectives

* Describe complementary and alternative medicine (CAM) and identify its typical domains. Explain why it is growing in popularity in the United States and throughout the world and who is most likely to use it.

* Describe the major types of complementary and alternative medicine providers, and list some of the common treatments that they offer.

* Discuss the various types of complementary and alternative medicines being used in America today, their patterns of use, and their potential benefits and risks.

* Describe why you must be cautious as you evaluate testimonials and claims related to complementary and alternative products and services, and what you can do to ensure that you are getting reliable, accurate information and sound treatment.

* Discuss the challenges and opportunities related to complementary and alternative medicine in ensuring our health and wellness.

23 Complementary and Alternative Medicine

New Choices and Responsibilities for Healthwise Consumers

What do you think?

For over a year, Mia has been suffering from chronic knee pain. When an MRI reveals no structural damage to the knee, her doctor recommends limited activity, rest, over-the-counter pain and anti-inflammatory medications, and four weeks of physical therapy. After four weeks, Mia is still in pain. Looking for another strategy, she visits a chiropractor, who tells her that she needs joint manipulation, acupuncture, and pain medication. Her best friend tells her to take chondroitin and glucosamine to rebuild cartilage. A quick check of the Web yields numerous herbal medications and exercises to help her knee. Mia's mother suggests that Mia should be eating functional foods to rebuild tissue. Mia doesn't know *what* to do.

What are Mia's options? ✻ *What are the potential risks and benefits of each option?* ✻ *Where can Mia get the most reliable information?* ✻ *How would you recommend that she proceed?*

Jared goes to his hometown doctor, who has a small practice in the rural community where Jared was raised. As he is sitting in the waiting room, Jared notes that one entire wall is used to display nutritional supplements, herbal medications, and various health foods. The products are very expensive, and when Jared asks about them, the doctor hands him pamphlets from the company that supplies these products.

Do you think it is appropriate for a licensed health care provider to make a profit by selling nonallopathic products and services at the office? ✻ *Would you assume that a health professional has in-depth knowledge of such products?* ✻ *What obligations do health providers have to inform the public about risks and dangers associated with alternative therapies and products?*

Consumers today face an amazing array of choices when they consider taking action to improve their health or seek care for a health problem. In increasing numbers they are looking beyond conventional medicine for at least some of their health care. One of the newest movements toward self-care and health promotion focuses on *complementary and alternative medicine (CAM)*. Whether taking herbs to lift their mood or reduce pain, engaging in yoga or Pilates to reduce stress and increase strength, receiving acupuncture for low back pain, or following naturopathic tenets for cancer treatment, over half of all Americans will go outside the traditional health care system in 2003 to prevent disease, enhance health, or treat symptoms.

After dismissing CAM therapies as quackery for the better part of a century, the medical establishment now finds itself racing to evaluate them. Many of the country's leading hospitals and research institutions are studying the effects of herbs, acupuncture, tai chi, and biofeedback as rigorously as they would a new antibiotic.[1] The short-term goal of this investigation is to identify the CAM practices with the greatest benefits and the fewest hazards and to make these part of clinical practice; the long-term goal is to spawn a new kind of medicine—an *integrative* medicine that employs the rigor of modern science without being constrained by it.[2] If these CAM remedies prove effective, a merger of traditional medicine and CAM will change the face of modern medicine in ways that few would have imagined only a decade ago.

Until reports from clinical trials are in, consumers must remember that few CAM therapies have been thoroughly evaluated in controlled studies, so their effectiveness is still widely debated. While there has been much progress in research and testing since the National Institutes of Health opened a full-strength federal agency—the National Center for Complementary and Alternative Medicine (NCCAM)—in 1998, the science of CAM is still in its infancy.

The challenge for consumers is to keep informed of current research, to know how and where to find information about the effectiveness and risks of particular therapies, and to examine any therapy (traditional or alternative) thoroughly. Although the excitement and enthusiasm for CAM are unmistakable, wise consumers will apply the same caution to CAM therapies they would employ in any health decision making, and stay informed. Many consu-mers will use the Internet to research CAM therapies, so the NCCAM has developed guidelines for evaluating health-related websites (see the Reality Check box).

How does the average consumer know what to believe? How do we separate genuinely helpful CAM therapies from those that might be risky? This chapter attempts to present a research-based and unbiased perspective on the modern CAM movement. As you read, look for answers to your own questions, and think about how this information feeds into your interests and lifestyle.

CAM: What Is It and Who Uses It?

If you think that alternative medicine is just a fad, you are in for a surprise. Today, Americans and people from most other cultures of the world are much more likely to try therapies once considered exotic and strange. This is particularly true as America becomes a composite of people from different regions and cultures of the world. Many of these cultures are contributing their unique beliefs about remedies to restore health and treat afflictions. Referred to as **complementary and alternative medicine (CAM),** these therapies are generically defined as "neither being taught widely in U.S. medical schools nor generally available in U.S. hospitals during the previous year."[3] Although often used interchangeably, the terms *complementary* and *alternative* have actually been defined as being slightly different as the field has evolved. **Complementary medicine** is used with conventional medicine, as part of the modern integrative medicine approach. An aromatherapist might work with an oncologist to reduce a patient's nausea during chemotherapy, for example. **Alternative medicine** is used in place of conventional medicine. An example of this would be using a special diet or an herbal remedy to treat cancer instead of using radiation, surgery, or other traditional treatments.[4]

Complementary and alternative therapies vary widely in terms of nature of treatment, extent of therapy, and types of problems for which they offer help. Typically, CAM therapies are compared with the more traditional, allopathic treatments offered by individuals who graduate from U.S.–sanctioned schools of medicine or are licensed medical practitioners recognized by the American Medical Association and its governing board.[5]

The list of practices that are considered CAM changes continually as CAM therapies are proven safe and effective and become accepted as "mainstream."[6] CAM therapies, in general, serve as alternatives to an allopathic system that some people regard as too invasive, too high tech, and too toxic in terms of laboratory-produced medications. CAM users are often people who are seeking what they perceive to be a more natural, gentle approach to healing. Other CAM patients distrust the traditional medical approach and believe that they will have more personal control of their health care decisions with CAM. People choose alternative therapies for a variety of practical and deeply personal reasons (see Table 23.1 and the Reality Check box). Others continue to consult traditional medical providers, believing that there is safety in

---

Complementary and alternative medicine (CAM) Forms of treatment distinct from traditional allopathic medicine that until recently were neither taught widely in U.S. medical schools nor generally available in U.S. hospitals.

Complementary medicine Treatment used in conjunction with conventional medicine.

Alternative medicine Treatment used in place of conventional medicine.

Evaluating Medical Resources on the Web

The National Center for Complementary and Alternative Medicine recommends that you ask these 10 questions about any health-related site you visit online.

1. *Who runs this site?* Any good health-related website should make it easy for you to learn who is responsible for the site and its information, with the name of the site's sponsor and a link to its homepage on every major page of the site.

2. *Who pays for the site?* It costs money to run a website. The source of a website's funding should be clearly stated or readily apparent. For example, Web addresses ending in ".gov" denote a federal government–sponsored site. You should know how the site pays for its existence. Does it sell advertising? Is it sponsored by a drug company? The source of funding can affect what content is presented, how the content is presented, and what the site owners want to accomplish on the site.

3. *What is the purpose of the site?* This question is related to who runs and pays for the site. An "About This Site" link appears on many sites; if it's there, use it. The purpose of the site should be clearly stated and should help you evaluate the trustworthiness of the information.

4. *Where does the information come from?* Many health/medical sites post information collected from other websites or sources. If the person or organization in charge of the site did not create the information, the original source should be clearly labeled.

5. *What is the basis of the information?* In addition to identifying who wrote the material you are reading, the site should describe the evidence that the material is based on. Medical facts and figures should have references (such as to articles in medical journals). Also, opinions or advice should be clearly set apart from information that is "evidence-based" (that is, based on research results).

6. *How is the information selected?* Is there an editorial board? Do people with excellent professional and scientific qualifications review the material before it is posted?

7. *How current is the information?* Websites should be reviewed and updated on a regular basis. It is particularly important that medical information be current. The most recent update or review date should be clearly posted. Even if the information has not changed, you want to know whether the site owners have reviewed it recently to ensure that it is still valid.

8. *How does the site choose links to other sites?* Websites usually have a policy about how they establish links to other sites. Some medical sites take a conservative approach and don't link to any other sites. Some link to any site that asks, or pays, for a link. Others link only to sites that have met certain criteria.

9. *What information about you does the site collect, and why?* Websites routinely track the paths visitors take through their sites to determine what pages are being used. However, many health websites ask for you to "subscribe" or "become a member." In some cases, this may be so that they can collect a user fee or select information for you that is relevant to your concerns. In all cases, this will give the site personal information about you.

Any credible health site asking for this kind of information should tell you exactly what will and will not be done with it. Many commercial sites sell "aggregate" (collected) data about their users to other companies—information such as what percentage of their users are women with breast cancer, for example. In some cases they may collect and reuse information that is "personally identifiable," such as your ZIP code, gender, and birth date. Be certain that you read and understand any privacy policy or similar language on the site, and don't sign up for anything that you are not sure you fully understand.

10. *How does the site manage interactions with visitors?* There should always be a way for you to contact the site owner if you run across problems or have questions or feedback. If the site hosts chatrooms or other online discussion areas, it should tell visitors what the terms of using this service are. Is it moderated? If so, by whom, and why? It is always a good idea to spend time reading the discussion without joining in, so that you feel comfortable with the environment before becoming a participant.

Source: National Center for Complementary and Alternative Medicine, "Ten Things to Know about Evaluating Medical Resources on the Web," 2002 (see http://nccam.nih.gov/health/webresources).

---

government-controlled licensing, regulation of procedures, and drug testing and approval.

A Historical Perspective

America's zeal for the healing power of herbs and plant medicines marks a return to a simpler life. In fact, it takes us back thousands of years. Poppy extract was used to quiet crying children in the time of the pharaohs, eons before the medical use of opiates. Ephedra, the main ingredient of some over-the-counter asthma treatments, has relieved breathing problems in China for 5,000 years. Although the United States has been somewhat slow in accepting plant remedies as standard treatment, it should be noted that an

Table 23.1
Trends in the Use of Alternative Therapies

AILMENT	PERCENTAGE OF CAM USE AMONG STUDY PARTICIPANTS
Chronic pain	37%
Anxiety, chronic fatigue, other conditions	31%
Sprains and strains	26%
Addiction problems	25%
Arthritis	25%
Headaches	24%
Depression, digestive problems, diabetes	20%+

OTHER CONDITIONS TREATED WITH ALTERNATIVE THERAPIES

- An *unrelenting* chronic problem, for which any chance of complete cure or remediation of symptoms is limited
- A large measure of *discomfort* or pain that causes the patient to focus on the disease, rather than on health
- Situations in which traditional medications have been used, but must be discontinued because they *carry substantial side effects or contraindications* if used for long periods of time
- Symptoms that affect activities or tasks of daily living
- A need to consult a health care specialist for a particular health problem

Source: Adapted from "Why Patients Use Alternative Medicine: Results of a National Study" by J. Astin, *Journal of the American Medical Association,* 279, 1998, pp. 1548–1552. Reprinted by permission of the American Medical Association.

estimated 25 percent of all modern pharmaceutical drugs are derived from herbs, including aspirin (white willow bark), the heart medication digitalis (foxglove), and the cancer treatment Taxol (Pacific yew tree).

Although plant-based medicines were used widely in the United States until World War II, a new generation of pharmaceuticals that were FDA tested and safe took over in the later years of the twentieth century. Nontraditional treatments fell out of favor among all but a few segments of the U.S. population and became symbols of the undeveloped and impoverished parts of the world. After decades of languishing, however, and with a growing dissatisfaction of the populace with the technowizardry of late twentieth- and early twenty-first-century U.S. medicine, many nontraditional treatments reemerged in treatment arsenals.

To better understand why Americans behave as they do when confronted with an illness or disorder, it is necessary to understand fears, concerns, and sources of hope for a positive outcome. Many of us have a powerful distrust of traditional medical practice. Through either direct experience or media portrayals of problems with today's health care sys-

tem, many people believe that when sick, the worst place to be is in a hospital or health care setting.

The shift to alternatives is not surprising, considering what has happened in other regions of the world. Reports of miracle cures from ancient remedies, more gentle and holistic means of treatment, and positive outcomes from alternative treatments have led many to seek answers from other cultures. In fact, a number of our recent pharmacological advances have their roots in the herbal remedies used in cultures throughout the world. Eastern medicine, in particular, has been very influential in today's alternative therapies. Chinese medicine and some of the world's ancient healing practices, such as Ayurvedic medicine, provide reasonable alternatives to traditional treatment.

CAM in the United States Today

In 1993, a landmark study showed that one in three Americans sought some form of alternative care.[7] A follow-up study five years later found that these numbers had jumped to 47 percent, reflecting an unprecedented explosion in use. In fact, in 2001, people were more likely to seek out and use some form of alternative care than they were to seek out and use a form of what we've long regarded as traditional medicine, making over 600 million visits to CAM providers.[8] By 2002, total out-of-pocket expenditures for alternative care were conservatively estimated at $307 billion, which is comparable to out-of-pocket expenditures for all U.S. physician services. Additionally, an estimated 15 million Americans took prescription medications concurrently with herbal remedies or high-dose vitamins and supplements, which are not considered in these estimates.[9]

Although it is widely assumed that increasing numbers of us are choosing alternative care, we have known little about the nature and extent of CAM use until fairly recently. According to the studies cited above, the most frequently used alternatives to conventional medicine are the following:

- Relaxation techniques (16.9 percent of respondents).
- Chiropractic (31 percent).
- Massage (18 percent).
- Self-help (13 percent).
- Energy healing (6 percent).
- Other therapies (16 percent).

Major Domains of CAM

Today, the United States government not only has sanctioned the concept of CAM in prevention and treatment, but also has moved aggressively to create the Center for Complementary and Alternative Medicine (NCCAM) within the National Institutes of Health. This center serves as a clearinghouse for CAM information and a focal point for research initiatives, policy development, and general recommendations for CAM use. NCCAM broadly groups CAM practices into five major domains: (1) alternative medical systems, (2) manipulative and body-based methods, (3) energy therapies, (4) mind-body

Who Seeks Alternative Medical Treatment?

Those who choose complementary and alternative medicine tend not to make this decision on a whim. In fact, in many cases, they are more educated than those who rely solely on traditional health care. They are also more likely to be middle-aged and have a middle-class socioeconomic status. A randomized study of several thousand patients seeking care for low back pain through traditional, allopathic providers versus chiropractic providers found that those opting for chiropractic health were more likely to question their providers about the nature and extent of recommended treatments. Generally, people who seek alternative care do so for one of three reasons:

1. *Dissatisfaction.* Patients are unhappy with ineffective treatment or treatment that has resulted in adverse effects, they find traditional allopathic medicine too impersonal and technologically

oriented, and some find it too costly. Also, it appears that managed care may have pushed some people out of the allopathic system. Many began to distrust it after they or family members experienced problems with the system.
2. *Need for personal control.* They view CAM therapies as less authoritarian and more empowering.
3. *Philosophical congruence.* For some, CAM is just a better fit. Referred to as *cultural creatives,* these CAM users tend to be committed to the environment; to feminism; to involvement with esoteric forms of spirituality and personal growth psychology, including self-actualization and self-expression; and to exploring anything foreign and exotic. They also identify with cultural change and innovation and are among those most likely to adopt one of the more alternative treatments.

Other findings include the following:

✔ CAM users didn't have a particularly negative attitude toward traditional medicine.
✔ Racial or ethnic status didn't predict CAM usage.

✔ Men and women were equally likely to use CAM.
✔ Those with poorer health status were more likely to use CAM.
✔ Some conditions, particularly low back pain and other chronic pain conditions, predict higher CAM usage.
✔ Those who had gone through a transformational experience that had changed their worldview were more likely to use CAM, as are cultural creatives.

Sources: J. Astin, "Why Patients Use Alternative Medicine: Results of a National Study," *Journal of the American Medical Association* 279 (1998): 1548–1552; D. Eisenberg et al., "Trends in Alternative Medicine Use in the United States, 1990–1997: Results of a Follow-up National Study," *Journal of the American Medical Association* 280 (1998): 1569–1579; R. Donatelle, J. Nyiendo, and M. Haas, "Health Care Decision-Making among Those Seeking Care for Low Back Pain from Traditional Medical and Chiropractic Physicians," paper presented at the American Public Health Association's annual meeting, 1998; R. H. Ray, "The Emerging Culture," *American Demographics* (Intertec Publishing, 1997) (see http://www.demographics.com).

interventions, and (5) biologically based treatments. Many of these alternatives are discussed in other parts of this book. In this chapter, we focus on alternatives that have become increasingly popular in recent years or that might be of particular interest to young adults.

Alternative Medical Systems

Alternative medical systems involve complete systems of theory and practice that have evolved independently of, and often prior to, the conventional biomedical approach that we tend to consider "traditional." In the United States, the term *traditional* or *allopathic* has historically referred to a system that is directed by the American Medical Association guidelines for licensing and that most insurance plans cover as fairly standard and acceptable procedure. In contrast, *nonallopathic* medicine has been dubbed "alternative." This situation is changing. In the past decade, some specialists in nonallopathic medicine have been accepted by professional groups, and their inclusion in mainstream medicine

is growing daily. Many traditional medical schools are now offering coursework in CAM, and many traditional doctors refer patients to alternative providers, who are in turn reimbursed by the patients' health insurance plans. Modalities that have received the greatest degree of acceptance include chiropractic medicine, acupuncture, herbal and homeopathic medicine, and naturopathy. However, it is important to realize that there are many "other" traditional systems of medicine that have been practiced by various cultures throughout the world. Many come from venerable Asian approaches.

Traditional Oriental Medicine and Ayurveda

Two major systems that are at the root of much of our CAM thinking today are traditional Oriental medicine and Ayurveda, which is India's traditional system of medicine. **Traditional Oriental medicine (TOM)** emphasizes the proper balance or disturbances of *qi* (pronounced "chi"), or vital energy in health and disease, respectively. In TOM, diagnosis is based on history, on observation of the body (especially the

Tibetan Medicine Strikes a Balance

As society becomes faster paced, more technological, and ever more competitive, we are bombarded by daily stressors. We are advised to "stop and smell the roses," but who has time?

According to Tibetan medicine, our health depends on finding balance in our lives—specifically, a balance among our three bodily "humors." These refer to the water humor (bad-kan), responsible for support and cohesion; the fire humor (mkhris-pa), responsible for heat and digestion; and the wind humor (rlung), responsible for breath and mobility. When these humors fall out of balance, disease results.

Tibetan physicians look to behavior as a catalyst for health or disease. Their belief that the mind and body are one makes it mandatory for behavior to encourage equilibrium. For example, doctors prescribe changes in lifestyle and diet to effect change in the body. Behaviors considered unhealthy may be evil deeds in present or past lives, sexual indiscretions, or unhealthy diets. In fact, a Tibetan painting that illustrates the general rules of healthy conduct specifies: "Do not take what is not yours," "Do not lie," "Do not gossip," and "Do not be covetous."

The information gathering that takes place when a Tibetan physician diagnoses an illness differs from that of an American doctor. Diagnosis relies on careful observation and conversation. Tibetan physicians use their senses of smell, touch, sight, and hearing to draw conclusions.

Tibetan physicians begin their training at about 13 years of age and continue for the next 11 years, following a strict daily regimen that starts at 4 a.m. and ends at 10 p.m. Special training is provided in subjects such as pulse diagnosis and herb identification, as herbs are key in Tibetan medicines. Four-year internships are then required before one becomes a full-fledged physician.

In the United States there is an increased interest in Tibetan medicine, just as there is in all forms of alternative medical care. Our newspapers, magazines, medical journals, and even yearly visits to doctors point to the importance of finding a balance. More than ever, the American medical community is urging the general public to eat a balanced diet, exercise, and avoid harmful habits such as smoking, irresponsible drinking, and substance abuse. We are encouraged to use our senses, and our common sense, to stay healthy. Although some view Tibetan medical practice as extreme, the message of balance as the central theme of care appeals to many. Above all else, the arrival of Tibetan medicine in the United States indicates the growth of alternative care and the blending of cultures within this country.

Source: S. Okie, The Washington Post, Health Section, October 27, 1998. © 1998 The Washington Post. Reprinted with permission.

tongue), on palpation, and on pulse diagnosis, an elaborate procedure requiring considerable skill and experience by the practitioner. Techniques such as acupuncture, herbal medicine, Oriental massage, and *qi gong* (a form of energy therapy described in more detail later in this chapter) are among the TOM approaches to health and healing. See the Health in a Diverse World box about the Tibetan perspective on medicine.

Ayurveda (or **Ayurvedic medicine**) relates to the "science of life," which places equal emphasis on body, mind, and spirit and strives to restore the innate harmony of the individual. Ayurvedic practitioners diagnose mainly by observation and touch and assign patients to one of three major body types and a variety of subtypes. Once classified, patients are treated mostly through dietary modifications and herbal remedies that have been drawn from the vast botanical wealth of the Indian subcontinent. Treatments may also include animal and mineral ingredients, even powdered gemstones. Massage, steam baths, exposure to sunlight, and controlled breathing are among the more common Ayurvedic treatments.[10]

Homeopathy and Naturopathy

Other alternative systems of medicine include **homeopathy** and **naturopathy**. *Homeopathic medicine* is an unconventional Western system based on the principle that "like cures like." In other words, the same substance that in large doses produces the symptoms of an illness will in very small doses cure the illness.[11] Essentially, homeopathic physicians use herbal medicine, minerals, and chemicals in extremely diluted forms as natural agents to kill or ward off illnesses that are caused by more potent forms or doses of those agents.

Traditional Oriental medicine (TOM) Comprehensive system of diagnosis and treatment in which dietary change, touch, massage, medicinal teas, and other herbal medicines are used extensively.

Qi Element of traditional Oriental medicine that refers to the vital energy force that courses through the body. When qi is in balance, health is restored.

Ayurveda (Ayurvedic medicine) A method of treatment derived largely from ancient India, in which practitioners diagnose by observation and touch and then assign a largely dietary treatment laced with herbal medicines.

Homeopathy Unconventional Western system of medicine based on the principle that "like cures like."

Naturopathy System of medicine that attempts to restore natural processes of the body and promote healing through natural means.

Table 23.2
Popular Complementary Treatments

Energy healing	Different therapies are based on the philosophy that humans produce waves of energy that are disrupted during illness.
Food therapy	Treatment is based on the belief that many disorders are based on allergies and toxic synergism among food combinations. Naturopaths test for and treat food allergies and assign special diets designed to produce nutritional balance.
Hypnosis	The treatment of disease by suggestion while the patient is in a hypnotic trance.
Relaxation techniques	The goal is to remove stress and promote healing. Techniques include yoga, meditation, breathing and posture exercises, and visualization.
Megavitamins	Treatment with megavitamins promotes the consumption of large doses of common essential vitamins and minerals to prevent disease and heal illness.
Massage	Massage involves rubbing, stroking, kneading, or lightly pounding the body with the hands or other instruments.
Aromatherapy	Aromatherapists use scented materials to evoke sensations through the smell centers of the body. Treatment focuses on odors regarded as pleasurable.

Naturopathic medicine views disease as a manifestation of an alteration in the processes by which the body naturally heals itself. Disease results from the body's effort to ward off impurities and harmful substances from the environment. Naturopathic physicians emphasize restoring health rather than curing disease. They employ an array of healing practices, including diet and clinical nutrition; homeopathy; acupuncture; herbal medicine; hydrotherapy (the use of water in a range of temperatures and methods of application); spinal and soft-tissue manipulation; physical therapies involving electric currents, ultrasound, and light therapy; therapeutic counseling; and pharmacology. Three major naturopathic schools in the United States and Canada provide thorough training, conferring the *naturopathic doctor (N.D.)* degree on students who have completed a four-year graduate program that emphasizes humanistically oriented family medicine.

While these medical philosophies and patterns of treatment have exerted great influence on populations worldwide, other, more regionally limited, medical traditions are also noteworthy. Native American, aboriginal, African, Middle Eastern, Tibetan, and South American cultures also have their own unique alternative systems. International surveys of CAM outside the United States suggest that alternative therapies are popular throughout most of the world. Public opinion polls and consumer surveys in Europe and the United Kingdom suggest high CAM use in Italy, France, Denmark, Finland, and Australia, in addition to most Asian cultures.[12]

As the number of alternative therapists grows and systems become intertwined, so do the number of health care options available to consumers (see Table 23.2 for some examples). Before considering the practices of any medical systems, wise consumers will consult the most reliable resources to thoroughly evaluate risks, the scientific basis of claimed benefits, and any contraindications to using the CAM product or service. Avoid practitioners who promote their treatments as a cure-all for every health problem or who seem to promise remedies that have thus far defied the best scientific efforts of mainstream medicine. Asking questions, seeking reputable resources for information, and other strategies used by wise consumers of traditional medical care in the United States (see Chapter 22) should also be applied to CAM.

Manipulative and Body-Based Methods

Another category of CAM includes methods that are based on manipulation and/or movement of the body. For example, chiropractors focus on the relationship between the body's structures (primarily the spine) and functions and on how that relationship affects the preservation and restoration of health. Chiropractors employ manipulation as a key therapy.

Chiropractic Medicine

Chiropractic medicine has been practiced for over 100 years. Allopathic medicine and chiropractic medicine were in direct competition over a century ago.[13] But today, many managed care organizations work closely with chiropractors. Many insurance companies will now pay for chiropractic treatment if a medical doctor recommends it. More than 20 million Americans now visit chiropractors each year.

Chiropractic medicine is based on the idea that a life-giving energy flows through the spine via the nervous system. If the spine is subluxated (partly misaligned or dislocated), that force is disrupted. Chiropractors use a variety of techniques to manipulate the spine back into proper alignment so the life-giving energy can flow unimpeded through the nervous system. It has been established that their treatment can be effective for back pain, neck pain, and headaches.

The average chiropractic training program requires four years of intensive courses in biochemistry, anatomy, physiology, diagnostics, pathology, nutrition, and so forth, combined

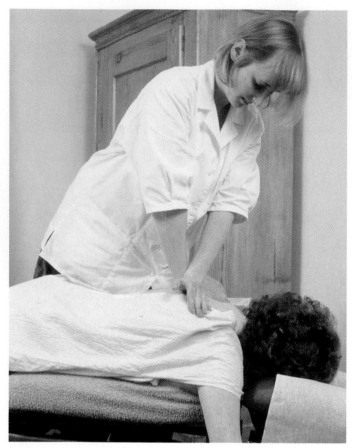

A chiropractor treats a patient using a variety of techniques to manipulate the spine into proper alignment.

with hands-on clinical training. Moreover, many chiropractors continue their training to obtain specialization certification, for instance, in women's health, gerontology, or pediatrics. Like allopathic physicians, chiropractors are licensed and regulated by the states in which they practice. You should investigate and question a chiropractor as carefully as you would a licensed medical doctor. As with many health professionals, you may note vast differences in technique among specialists. It is recommended that you choose a chiropractor who follows standard chiropractic regimens for treating musculoskeletal conditions and avoid those who promote adjustment as a cure-all for all disorders or whose treatments are not based on manipulation of the spine.

Other Manipulation Therapies

There are other specialties that involve manipulation of the body. *D.O.s,* or *doctors of osteopathy,* place particular emphasis on the musculoskeletal system. Osteopathic practitioners believe that all of the body's systems work together and that disturbances in one system may have an impact upon function elsewhere in the body.[14] As such, they specialize in body manipulation yet also have a more traditional form of medical school training.

Energy Therapies

Energy therapies focus either on energy fields originating with the body (biofields) or on fields from other sources (electromagnetic fields). Biofield therapies are intended to affect energy fields (whose existence is not experimentally proven) that surround and penetrate the human body. Some forms of energy therapy manipulate biofields by applying pressure and/or manipulating the body by placing the hands in, or through, these fields.[15]

Popular examples of biofield therapy include *qi gong, reiki,* and *therapeutic touch. Qi gong,* a component of traditional Chinese medicine, combines movement, meditation, and regulation of breathing to enhance the flow of vital energy (qi), improve blood circulation, and enhance immune function.[16] *Reiki,* whose name derives from the Japanese word representing "universal life energy," is based on the belief that by channeling spiritual energy through the practitioner the spirit is healed, and it in turn heals the physical body.[17] *Therapeutic touch* derives from the ancient technique of "laying on" of hands and is based on the premise that the healing force of the therapist effects the patient's recovery and that healing is promoted when the body's energies are in balance. By passing the hands over the body, the healers identify body imbalances.[18]

Bioelectromagnetic-based therapies involve the unconventional use of electromagnetic fields, such as pulsed fields, magnetic fields, or alternating current or direct current fields, to treat asthma, cancer, pain, migraines, and other conditions. The energy field techniques mentioned above have little scientific documentation to support their claims at this point. However, two derivatives of energy therapy have gained much wider acceptance in recent years: acupuncture and acupressure.

Acupuncture

Chinese medical treatments are growing in popularity and offer an important complement to Western biomedical care. Acupuncture, one of the more popular forms of Chinese medicine among Americans, is sought for a wide variety of health conditions, including musculoskeletal dysfunction, mood enhancement, and wellness promotion. Following acupuncture, most respondents report high satisfaction with the treatment, improved quality of life, improvement in or cure of the condition, and reduced reliance on prescription drugs and surgery.[19]

Acupuncturists in the United States are state-licensed, and each state has specific requirements regarding training programs. Most acupuncturists have either completed a two-to three-year postgraduate program to obtain a master of traditional Oriental medicine (M.T.O.M.) degree or attended a shorter certification program here or in Asia. They may be licensed in multiple areas—for example, the M.T.O.M. is also trained in the use of herbs and moxabustion (the application of a heated herbal moxa stick). Some licensed M.D.s and

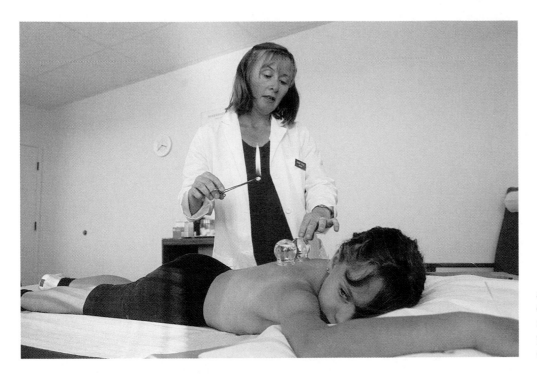

A popular form of Chinese medicine, moxabustion (use of a moxa stick) warms certain acupuncture points to treat a variety of conditions.

chiropractors have trained in acupuncture and obtained certification to use this treatment.

Acupressure

Acupressure is similar to acupuncture, but does not use needles. Instead, the practitioner applies pressure to points critical to balancing yin and yang. Practitioners must have the same basic understanding of energy pathways as do acupuncturists. Acupressure should not be applied by an untrained person to pregnant women or to anyone with a chronic health condition.

> **What do you think?**
>
> *Why do you think more and more people are opting for complementary and alternative treatments? ✻ What are the potential benefits of these treatments? ✻ What are the potential risks? ✻ What types of controls are reasonable to regulate the quality and consistency of foreign trained health care providers?*

Mind-Body Interventions

Mind-body interventions employ a variety of techniques to facilitate the mind's capacity to affect bodily functions and symptoms. Many therapies might fall under this category but some areas, such as biofeedback, patient education, and cognitive-behavioral techniques, have been so well investigated that they are no longer considered alternative therapies. However, meditation, yoga, tai chi, certain uses of hypnosis, dance, music and art therapy, prayer and mental healing, and others are still categorized as complementary and alternative.

Body Work

Body work actually consists of several different forms of exercise. *Feldenkrais* work is a system of the movements, floor exercises, and body work designed to retrain the central nervous system to help it find new pathways around areas of blockage or damage. It is gentle and effective in rehabilitating trauma victims. *Rolfing* is a more invasive form of body work, aimed at restructuring the musculoskeletal system by working on patterns of tension held in deep tissue. The therapist applies firm pressure to different areas of the body, and this pressure may be painful. Rolfing can release repressed emotions as well as dissipate muscle tension. *Shiatsu* is a traditional healing art from Japan that makes use of firm finger pressure applied to specified points on the body and is intended to increase the circulation of vital energy. The client lies on the floor, with the therapist seated alongside. *Trager work,* one of the least invasive forms of body work, employs gentle rocking and bouncing motions to induce states of deep, pleasant relaxation.[20]

> **What do you think?**
>
> *Have you ever tried any of these CAM therapies? ✻ Which of them are offered on your campus or in your community? ✻ What role do CAM exercises have in your personal quest for physical fitness? ✻ Spiritual fitness?*

Biologically Based Therapies

Biologically based therapy is perhaps one of the most controversial domains of CAM practice, largely because of the sheer numbers of options that are available and the myriad claims that are made about the magic effects of these products and services. To date, many of these claims have not been thoroughly investigated, and regulation of this aspect of CAM has been relatively slow in coming.

Biologically based therapies include natural and biologically based practices, interventions, and products, many of which overlap with conventional medicine's use of dietary supplements. Included are *herbal, special dietary, orthomolecular,* and *individual* biological therapies.

Practitioners who base their therapies primarily on the medicinal qualities of plants and herbs are referred to as *herbalists.*

Herbal remedies are not to be taken lightly. Just because something is natural does not necessarily mean that it is safe. For example, a recent FDA Consumer Advisory warned that kava products may be associated with severe liver damage.[21] Other reports remind consumers that even rigorously tested products may carry risks. Many plants are poisonous, and some can be toxic if ingested in high doses. Others may be dangerous when combined with prescription or over-the-counter drugs, or they could disrupt the normal action of the drugs. Properly trained herbalists and homeopaths have received graduate-level training in special programs such as herbal nutrition or traditional Oriental medicine. These practitioners have been trained in diagnosis; in mixing herbs, titrations, and dosages; and in the follow-up care of patients.

Checking on the education and training of anyone who recommends or sells herbal medications is a part of intelligent consumerism as well as just plain good sense. Also, it is important to look at the research surrounding individual substances and remedies. The NCCAM website is a good place to start, since it includes summaries of recent research.

Herbal Remedies

Largely derived from Ayurvedic or traditional Chinese medicine, herbal medications are widely available in the United States. Fueled by mass advertising and promoted as part of multiple vitamin and mineral regimens by major drug manufacturers, herbal supplements represent the hottest trend in the health market.

Herbal remedies come in several different forms. **Tinctures** (extracts of fresh or dried plants) usually contain a high

---

Biologically based therapies Combination of natural and biologically based therapies and products used to restore health.

Tinctures Herbal extracts usually combined with grain alcohol to prevent spoilage.

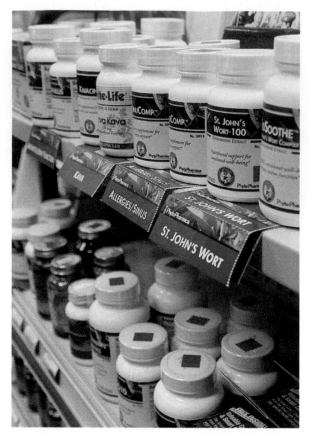

Buying herbal supplements can be confusing, since so many brands exist and their manufacture is not strictly regulated for potency or quality.

percentage of grain alcohol to prevent spoilage and are among the best herbal options. Freeze-dried extracts are very stable and offer good value for your money. Standardized extracts are also among the more reliable forms of herbal preparations.

In general, herbal medicines tend to be milder than chemical drugs and produce their effects more slowly; they also are much less likely to cause toxicity because they are diluted forms of drugs rather than concentrated forms.[22] But diluted or not, herbals are still drugs. They should not be taken casually, any more than you would take over-the-counter or prescription drugs without really needing them or knowing their side effects. No matter how natural they are, they still contain many of the same chemicals as synthetic prescription drugs. Too much of an herb can cause problems, particularly one from nonstandardized extracts. Some herbs and specific dietary supplements can pose risks to consumers by interacting with prescription drugs or causing unusual side effects. (See the New Horizons in Health box.)

The following discussion gives an overview of some of the most common herbal supplements on the market.

Ginkgo Biloba Ginkgo biloba is an extract from the leaves of a deciduous tree that lives up to 1,000 years, making it one of the world's oldest living tree species, one that can be traced back more than 200 million years. The ginkgo was almost

Mixing Foods, Supplements, and Medicines

You probably know that you shouldn't take medications in certain combinations or with alcohol. But did you know that certain foods can cause serious reactions when combined with medications? According to a National Consumer Alert from the Food and Drug Administration, here are some combinations to avoid:

- Never drink grapefruit juice less than two hours before or five hours after taking heart drugs called calcium channel blockers, such as Procardia. This combination can kill.

- Grapefruit juice taken with cyclosporin, which fights organ rejection in transplant recipients, can cause confusion and trembling.
- Combining grapefruit juice with antihistamines, either prescription versions such as Allegra or over-the-counter types such as Claritin or Benadryl, can cause serious heart problems.
- High doses of vitamin E thin the blood. If taken by heart patients along with the popular blood thinner Coumadin, the risk of serious bleeding increases.
- Foods high in vitamin K, such as broccoli, spinach, and turnip greens, can reduce the effectiveness of Coumadin.
- Antidepressants called MAO inhibitors can cause a potentially fatal blood pressure rise when taken with foods high in the chemical tyramine, such as cheese and sausage.
- Drinking coffee or colas with certain antibiotics, such as Cipro, or the ulcer drugs Tagamet, Zantac, and Pepcid, can increase caffeine levels, causing jitters and stomach irritation.
- Consuming bananas or potassium supplements along with heart drugs called ACE inhibitors, such as Capoten and Vasotec, can cause harmful potassium buildup if not monitored carefully.

Source: Food and Drug Interactions, Food and Drug Administration, 1998. For a free copy, call 1-800-639-8140 or visit the Internet site www.nclnet.org.

destroyed during the last ice age in all regions of the world except China, where it is considered a sacred tree with medicinal properties.[23] Today, ginkgo leaf extracts are among the leading prescription medicines in Germany and France, where they account for nearly 2 percent of total prescription sales.[24]

Purported benefits are many, and ginkgo biloba is used to treat depression; impotence; premenstrual syndrome; diseases of the eye, such as retinopathy and macular degeneration; and general vascular disease. In particular, it has been shown to improve short-term memory and concentration for individuals with impaired blood flow to the brain due to narrowing of vessels or clogging of key arteries. A Harvard-based study of 202 men and women with mild to moderately severe dementia caused by stroke or Alzheimer's disease was among the first to promote ginkgo in the United States. After one year, the group receiving ginkgo experienced significant improvement in cognitive performance (memory, learning, reading) and social functioning (carrying on conversations, recognizing familiar faces) compared to those in the placebo (non-ginkgo) group.[25] Much of this improvement was believed to be due to the antioxidant properties of the herb, as well as to the blood-thinning properties that seem to improve blood and oxygen flow to clogged blood vessels. Whether this herb will improve memory in people with normal blood flow remains largely unexplored. Claims that ginkgo will improve short-and long-term memory in the typical person are not scientifically based.

Most nutritional experts and physicians recommend that people who are considering using ginkgo take a 40-milligram tablet three times a day for a month or so to determine whether there is any improvement. If there is none, continuing to take this supplement is largely unwarranted.

Also, remember that disturbing memory loss or difficulty thinking, regardless of age, should be checked by a doctor to determine underlying causes.

Because the main action of ginkgo appears to be as a blood thinner, it should not be taken with other blood-thinning agents, such as aspirin, vitamin E, garlic, ginger, the prescription drug warfarin (trade name: Coumadin), or any other medications that list thinning of the blood as a potential side effect.[26] Doing so could increase the risk of hemorrhage.

St. John's Wort   The bright yellow, star-shaped flowers of St. John's wort (SJW) have a rich and varied history in Europe, Asia, and Africa. The name for this herb dates back to early Christian times and relates to the red oil that glands in the flowers secrete when they are pinched or cut. Christians believed that the flowers secreted this blood-red oil on August 29, the anniversary of the beheading of St. John the Baptist, and that they bloomed on June 24, St. John's birthday. The term *wort* is Old English for "plant." In addition, John the Baptist represents light, and the flowers themselves seemed to represent the bright yellow light of the sun.[27] Colonists who came to the United States brought SJW with them, only to find that Native Americans were already using it for everything from snake bite to general health enhancement. In the United States, SJW grows in abundance in northern California and southern Oregon and is also referred to as *klammath weed*.[28]

Today, SJW enjoys global popularity. It is the favored therapy for depression in a number of countries, including Germany, actually surpassing most standard antidepressants as the first mode of treatment for clinical depression. German researchers report that it is decidedly better than placebos in medical trials and at least as good as some prescription antidepressants for treatment of mild depression. It is also cheaper and appears to cause fewer side effects than drugs such as Prozac, Paxil, and Zoloft.[29] SJW is believed to have the following effects:

- Acts as a positive mood enhancer by helping maintain serotonin levels, and as natural neurotransmitters that help brain function and calm the body.[30]
- Helps as a sleep enhancer for those having difficulty sleeping.[31]
- Supports immune function by suppressing the release of interleukin-6, a protein that controls certain aspects of the immune response.[32]

A review of 23 well-designed clinical trials published in *The British Medical Journal* concluded that extracts of SJW "are more effective than placebo for the treatment of mild to moderately severe depressive disorders." This review also found evidence from eight other studies that SJW may work as well as some other drugs in countering mild depression. The research team called for more rigorously controlled, larger sample–sized studies comparing this herb with prescription doses of Prozac and other drugs.[33] The results of one such study, a randomized, double-blind trial conducted at multiple sites and reported in the *Journal of the American Medical Association,* found that SJW was no more effective for treating major depression of moderate severity than a placebo.[34] As this study refutes the results of several less rigorously controlled trials, reports on it were front-page news. As other well-designed studies are published, consumers will have more information on which to base their decision.

Like other plants, SJW contains a number of different chemicals, many of which are not clearly understood. Why it seems to lift depression and possess antiviral properties remains largely unknown. Although there may be more to SJW than the myths and simplistic explanations that many health food stores tend to give their customers, researchers are beginning to view SJW in a less favorable light.

The herb does have several side effects. Most are more bothersome than severe and range from slight gastrointestinal upset to fatigue, dry mouth, dizziness, skin rashes, and itching. Some people have noted sensitivity to sunlight. Most of these side effects are minor, however, when compared with those of major antidepressant medicines.

Due to conflicting news about SJW, consumers should proceed with caution. Since the herb is sold in the United States as a dietary supplement, not a drug, it is not regulated by the FDA and rigorous testing has not been done. Anyone suffering from clinical depression should be under a physician's and psychologist's care.

In addition, SJW should never be taken in combination with prescription antidepressants. When combined with other serotonin-enhancing drugs, such as Prozac, SJW may result in serotonin overload, leading to tremors, agitation, or convulsions. SJW also should not be used by pregnant women or women who are nursing, by young children, or by the frail elderly, because the safety margins have not been established.

Echinacea Echinacea, or the *purple coneflower,* is found primarily in the Midwest and the prairie regions of the United States. Two of the nine species of echinacea in the United States are now on the federal endangered species list, a cause of growing concern for many environmentalists as the herb's popularity has grown. Believed to be used extensively by Native Americans for centuries, echinacea eventually gained widespread acceptance in the United States before being shipped to Europe, where its use grew gradually over the eighteenth and nineteenth centuries.

Today, echinacea is the best-selling herb in health and natural food stores in the United States and is widely used throughout most of the world. It is said to stimulate the immune system and increase the effectiveness of the white blood cells that attack bacteria and viruses. Many people believe it to be helpful in preventing and treating the symptoms of a cold or flu. However, echinacea remains controversial. While many studies in Europe have provided preliminary evidence of its effectiveness, recent controlled trials in the United States indicate that echinacea is no more effective than a placebo in preventing a cold. [35]

As with many herbal treatments, little research has been conducted on the benefits and risks of echinacea. Because it can affect the immune system, people with auto-immune diseases such as arthritis should not take it. Other people who should avoid echinacea include pregnant women, people with diabetes or multiple sclerosis, and anyone allergic to the daisy family of plants. See Table 23.3 for other herbal remedies that are popular for treating common health conditions.

Green Tea Several studies have shown promising links between green and white tea consumption and cancer prevention, although investigation continues. Now, new research from Japan suggests that drinking one or two cups of green tea per day may keep the heart attack doctors away.[36] Findings suggested that those who drank the tea had lower rates of heart attack, indicating a possible protective effect. Some scientists suspect that green tea may boost heart health because it contains high levels of flavonoids. These plant compounds, which are found in a variety of fruits and vegetables as well as in tea and red wine, are thought to boost health in part by combating oxidation, a process in which cell-damaging free radicals (see Chapter 8) accumulate. Oxidative damage can be caused by outside factors, such as cigarette smoking, or by factors on the cellular level. Oxidation is suspected of increasing the risk of heart disease, stroke, and several other diseases. Although promising, more research on the role of green tea in CVD risk must be conducted to determine whether the effect is due to the tea itself or some other characteristic that tea drinkers have in common.

Special Supplements

Dietary supplements are defined as "products (other than tobacco) that are intended to supplement or add to the diet and contain one or more of the following ingredients: vitamins,

Table 23.3
Herbal Remedies for Common Conditions

CONDITION	HERBAL PRODUCT	DOSE	SIDE EFFECTS
Constipation	Aloe	20–30 mg hydroxyanthracene derivatives/day	Electrolyte and fluid imbalance
	Buckthorn	20–30 mg glycofrangulin per day	
	Cascara	20–30 mg cascaroside/day	
	Flaxseed	1 tbs. whole flaxseed with 8 oz. water 2–3 times/day	None if taken as directed
	Manna	20–30 gm/day	Nausea, flatulence
	Psyllium	12–40 gm (seed) or 4–20 gm (husk) daily with 8 oz. water for every 5 gm drug	Allergic reaction (rare)
	Senna leaf	20–30 mg sennoside per day	Electrolyte and fluid imbalance; can produce rebound constipation if used longer than 1–2 weeks
Dysmenorrhea (menstrual cramps)	Black cohosh Potentilla	40–60% extract with alcohol 4–6 gm powdered herb	Occasionally, gastric discomfort Aggravates any gastric discomforts
Leg cramps and swelling	Butcher's broom Horse chestnut Sweet clover	7–11 mg ruscogenin in extract 250–312.5 mg extract 2 times/day 3–30 mg coumarin/day	Gastric disturbance, nausea in rare cases Itching, nausea in rare cases May cause headache
Memory loss	Ginkgo biloba	60–80 mg extract 2–3 times/day	Rarely, headache, stomach upsets
Menopausal symptoms	Black cohosh Chaste tree fruit	40–60% extract with alcohol 30–40 mg in aqueous-alcohol extracts	Occasionally, gastric discomfort May cause itching, rash
Premenstrual syndrome	Black cohosh Chaste tree fruit Yarrow	40–60% extract with alcohol 30–40 mg in aqueous-alcohol extracts 4.5 gm powder for infusion	Occasionally, gastric discomfort May cause itching, rash None known
Sleep disturbances	Hops flower Valerian root	0.5 gm powder for infusion 2–3 gm powder for infusion	None known None known

Source: From "New Guides to Herbal Remedies: Examples of Herbs Approved by German Commission E," *Harvard Women's Health Watch,* February 1999, © 1999, President and Fellows of Harvard College. Reprinted by permission.

minerals, amino acids, herbs, or other substance that increases total dietary intake, and that is intended for ingestion in the form of a capsule, powder, soft gel, or gelcap, and is not represented as a conventional food or as a sole item" (Dietary Supplement Health and Education Act). Typically, these supplements are taken to enhance health, prevent disease, or enhance mood. In recent years, we've heard increasing reports on the health benefits of a number of vitamins and minerals.

When taken to increase work output or the potential for it, dietary supplements are labeled as **ergogenic aids.** Examples include bee pollen, caffeine, glycine, carnitine, lecithin, brewer's yeast, and gelatin. In recent years, a new generation of performance-enhancing ergogenic aids has hit the market. Many of these claim to increase muscular strength and performance, boost energy, and enhance resistance to disease.

Muscle Enhancers In 1998, Mark McGwire made headline news for his home run records. At the same time, he also made news for his admission that he was a regular user of the diet supplement androstenedione, a substance found naturally in meat and some plants and which is also produced in the human body by the adrenal glands and gonads. The synthetic version, sold in concentrated form, is known in locker room talk as "andro," a precursor to the human hormone testosterone (see Chapter 14 for more on andro). In other words, the body converts andro directly into testosterone, which enables an athlete to train harder and recover more quickly. Ironically, although the NCAA, the NFL, and the International Olympic Committee have banned andro, it is readily available over the counter.

The McGwire controversy has encouraged new research into the compound. Early results indicate that andro has a chemical structure that is very similar to anabolic

Ergogenic aids Special dietary supplements taken to increase strength, energy, and the ability to work.

steroids, which may result in long-term risks similar to those of the illegal androgens.[37]

Creatine is a naturally occurring compound found primarily in skeletal muscle that helps to optimize the muscles' energy levels. In recent years, the use of creatine supplements has increased dramatically because of claims that it increases muscle energy and allows a person to work harder with less muscle fatigue and build muscle mass with less effort. Reports of creatine's benefits, however, appear exaggerated. Over one-third of those taking creatine are unable to absorb it in the muscles and thus achieve no benefit. Side effects include muscle cramping, muscle strains, and possible liver and kidney damage.[38]

Ginseng Grown commercially throughout many regions of North America, ginseng is much prized for its reported sexual restorative value. It is believed that ginseng affects the pituitary gland, increasing resistance to stress, affecting metabolism, aiding skin and muscle tone, and providing the hormonal balance necessary for a healthy sex life. Other purported benefits include improved endurance, muscle strength, recovery from exercise, oxygen metabolism during exercise, auditory and visual reaction time, and mental concentration.[39] Studies of the effectiveness of ginseng, however, have raised questions about it: primarily, what are appropriate dosages, and how long should it be taken to realize benefits? Because the potency of plants varies considerably, dosage is difficult to control and side effects are fairly common. Noteworthy side effects of high doses include nervousness, insomnia, high blood pressure, headaches, skin eruptions, chest pain, depression, and abnormal vaginal bleeding.[40]

Glucosamine Glucosamine is a substance produced by the body that plays a key role in the growth and development of cartilage. When present in sufficient amounts, it stimulates the manufacture of substances necessary for proper joint function and joint repair. It is manufactured commercially and sold under a variety of different names, usually glucosamine sulfate. Glucosamine has been shown to be effective for treating osteoarthritis and related degenerative joint diseases and appears to relieve swelling and decrease pain. Unlike many other herbal supplements, glucosamine sulfate has an excellent safety record with few noteworthy side effects.[41]

Chromium Picolinate A few years ago, chromium picolinate was believed to be the new miracle for anyone interested in weight loss. Since then, at least two major studies at the U.S. Department of Agriculture Human Nutrition Research Center have shown no benefit.[42]

SAMe SAMe (pronounced "Sammy") is the nickname for S-adenosyl-L-methionine, a compound produced biochemically in all humans to help perform some 40 functions in the body, ranging from bone preservation (hence its purported osteoarthritis benefits) to DNA replication.

SAMe has been reported to have a significant effect on mild-to-moderate depression without many of the typical side effects of prescription medications, such as sexual dysfunction, weight gain, and sleep disturbance. Scientists speculate that SAMe somehow affects brain levels of the neurotransmitters noradrenaline, serotonin, and, possibly, dopamine, all of which are related to the human stress response and the origins of depression in the body.[43]

While there has been much ado about the wonders of this natural antidepressant, much of the hype has not been substantiated in large, randomized clinical trials, the type of research necessary to validate drug claims. Also, the research has been of short duration, meaning that little is known of any long-term side effects such as toxicity to the liver or carcinogenic properties. In addition, questions exist over how much SAMe a person should take and in what form it should be administered.

Anyone interested in SAMe should consider these factors:[44]

- While one large, randomized trial showed modest pain relief in osteoarthritis patients using SAMe, results were not significantly better than results obtained using standard treatments.
- Many question the high cost of SAMe (between $15 and $35 or higher for 20 pills).
- Clinical depression requires more than self-treatment. Any depressed person should consult a physician to explore all options, including counseling as well as pharmaceutical and natural remedies.
- People with a family history of cardiovascular disease should not take SAMe, due to preliminary indications that it may trigger heart problems.
- Side effects such as restlessness, anxiety, insomnia, and mania occasionally occur with use and are more common in people with bipolar disorder.

Under no circumstances should SAMe be taken by anyone on prescription antidepressants, and the time lag between taking the prescription and beginning SAMe, and vice versa, should be carefully considered.[45]

Antioxidants Although covered in depth in the chapter on nutrition, it should be noted that antioxidants are among the most sought-after supplements on the market. Primary antioxidants include beta-carotene, selenium, vitamin C, and vitamin E.

Foods as Healing Agents

It has been widely documented that many Americans rely on *functional foods*—foods or supplements designed to improve some aspect of physical or mental functioning. Sometimes referred to as **nutraceuticals,** for their combined nutritional and pharmaceutical benefit, several are believed to actually work in much the same way as pharmaceutical drugs in making a person well or bolstering the immune system.

Foods contain many "nonnutrient" active ingredients that can affect us in different ways. For example, chili peppers contain ingredients that make your eyes water and clear your sinuses. Many of these active ingredients, or consti-tuents, can promote good health. A number of foods, such as sweet potatoes, tangerines, and red peppers, are recog-nized as excellent sources of antioxidants. Onion and garlic contain allium compounds that reduce blood clotting. Other foods have natural anti-inflammatory properties or aid digestion. Some are known by the term *prebiotics,* foods that promote good bacteria in the body that may help fight off infection.[46]

Some of the most common healthful foods and their purported benefits include the following:

* *Plant stanol.* Can lower "bad" LDL cholesterol.
* *Oat fiber.* Can lower "bad" LDL cholesterol; serves as a natural soother of nerves; stabilizes blood sugar levels.
* *Sunflower.* Can lower risk of heart disease; may prevent angina.
* *Soy protein.* May lower heart disease risk; provides protective phytoestrogen effect; may reduce risk from certain cancers.
* *Red meats and dark green, leafy vegetables.* Contain B vita-mins (B_6, B_{12}, folate), which can lower levels of homocys-teine, an amino acid associated with heart disease.
* *Garlic.* Lowers cholesterol and reduces clotting tendency of blood; lowers blood pressure; may serve as form of antibiotic.
* *Green tea.* Lowers cholesterol; may have a role in fighting certain cancers (see earlier section).
* *Ginger.* Fights motion sickness, stomach pain and upset; discourages blood clots; may relieve rheumatism.
* *Yogurt.* Untreated, nonpasteurized yogurt contains active, friendly bacteria that can fight off infections.

Table 23.4 on page 644 lists other foods and supple-ments with their risks and benefits.

Many people purchase foods labeled *organic* because they expect these products to contain only health-promoting substances. See Chapter 8 for a complete discussion of what it means for a food to be labeled organic.

> ### What do you think?
>
> *Why do you think the government has not acted more aggressively to regulate or control herbal and other dietary supplements?* ✳ *Why are many CAM treatments not covered under typical insurance plans?*

Protecting Consumers and Regulating Claims

While many CAM products appear promising, be aware that most of them are not regulated in the United States as strictly as are foods and drugs. This is in sharp contrast to nations such as Germany, where the government holds com-panies to strict standards for ingredients and manufacturing.

In the United States, nutritional supplements, genetically en-gineered foods, and organic foods have had a long history of unregulated growth, including an abundance of claims and testimonials about their health-enhancing attributes. With few regulatory controls in place, many get-rich-quick charla-tans have jumped into the health food and CAM market. As their profits soar, more and more companies eagerly join them. Unfortunately, this trend means that issues related to consumer safety and protection from fraudulent claims will also grow more urgent and continue to raise serious ques-tions about our current regulatory system.

Strategies to Protect Consumers' Health

The burgeoning popularity of nutraceuticals and functional foods concerns many scientists. According to National Institutes of Health (NIH) nutritional biochemist Dr. Terry Krakower,

> NIH does have some concerns about them and we are look-ing into them, especially the potential for interaction with other medications. We advise anyone who uses them to talk to their physician. [Functional foods] are so new we don't know yet if they are good, bad, or indifferent. [Much] of the herb content in these food products is so small that it's proba-bly ineffective, and if it were included in large amounts, it could be harmful. Anyone taking these supplements, whether in pill form or in foods, should do their homework and thor-oughly research them rather than rely on health claims made by manufacturers.[47]

By legal definition, herbal supplements and functional foods are neither prescription drugs nor over-the-counter medications. Instead, classified as food supplements, they can be sold without FDA approval. Since they are not regu-lated by the FDA, these products are not subject to the strict guidelines that govern the research and development of medications. Many are not labeled with the precise amount of chemicals in the product, and the labels provide little guidance on how they should be used. They are not supposed to be accompanied by claims of therapeutic bene-fit, but they often are. Since they are available without a prescription, this poses risks for unsuspecting consumers, raising issues of consumer safety to new levels.

Creatine A naturally occurring compound found primarily in skeletal muscle that helps optimize the muscles' energy levels.

Nutraceuticals Term often used interchangeably with *functional foods;* refers to the combined nutritional and pharmaceutical benefit derived through use of foods or food supplements.

Table 23.4
Common Herbal, Vitamin, and Mineral Supplements: Benefits versus Risks

SUPPLEMENT	USE	CLAIMS OF BENEFITS	RISKS
Ephedra (*ma huang, epitonin,* and *sida cordifolia*)	Serves as a stimulant and bronchodilator	Natural source of ephedrine for use as bronchodilator in asthmatic attack	Numerous reports of side effects including heart palpitations and psychosis, heart attacks and strokes; banned in several states; TOXIC
Chaparral	Sold as teas and pills	Fights cancer and purifies blood	Linked to serious liver damage
Comfrey	Originated as a poultice to reduce swelling, but later used internally	Wound healing, infection control	Contains alkaloids toxic to the liver, and animal studies suggest it is carcinogenic
Melatonin	"Clock hormone"	Role in regulating circadian rhythms and sleep patterns	Anti-aging claims unfounded
DHEA	Hormone that turns into estrogen and testosterone in the body	Fights aging, boosts immunity, strengthens bones, and improves brain functioning	No anti-aging benefits proven; could increase cancer risk and lead to liver damage, even when taken briefly
Dieter's teas	Herbal blends containing senna, aloe, rhubarb root, buckthorn, cascara, and castor oil	Act as laxatives	Can disrupt potassium levels and cause heart arrhythmias; linked to diarrhea, vomiting, chronic constipation, fainting, and death
Pennyroyal (member of the mint family)		Soothing effect in teas	Pregnancy-related complications, heart arrhythmias, death
Sassafras	Once a flavoring in root beer, used in tonics and teas	No real claims	Shown to cause liver cancer in animals
Flaxseeds	Produce linseed oil	Omega-3 fatty acid benefits	Delay absorption of medicine
Kava kava			Increases the effects of alcohol and other drugs
High-dose vitamin E	Antioxidants	Reduces risk of heart disease; better survivability after heart attack	Causes bleeding when taking blood thinners
Vitamin C	Antioxidant, manufactures collagen, wound repair, nerve transmission	Improves blood vessel relaxation in people with CVD, diabetes, hypertension, and other problems; can relieve pain of angina pectoris	
L-Carnitine	Amino acid	Improves metabolism in heart muscle, purported to increase fat-burning enzymes	Heart palpitations, arrhythmias, sudden death; claims largely unsubstantiated
Licorice root		None proven	Speeds potassium loss
Niacin (vitamin B_3)	Reduces serum lipids, vasodilation, and increases blood flow		Skin flushing, gastrointestinal distress, stomach pain, nausea and vomiting
Chondroitin (shark cartilage or sea cucumber)		Improves osteoporosis and arthritis by improving cartilage function	Fewer benefits than glucosamine; benefits still unproven

Even when products are dispensed by CAM practitioners, the situation can be risky. Some homeopaths and herbalists who mix their own tonics may not use standardized measures. Unfortunately, some unskilled and untrained people, who do not fully understand the potential chemical interactions of their preparations, are treating patients.

Consumer groups, members of the scientific community, and government officials are calling for action. Pressure is mounting to establish consistent standards for herbal supplements and functional foods similar to those used in Germany and other countries. Many scientists advocate a more stringent FDA approval process for virtually all supplements sold in the United States.

The German Commission E

The German Commission E is among the most noteworthy of the international groups attempting to regulate the sale of alternative medicines and supplements. Consisting of an expert panel established in 1970, its mission was to conduct a formal evaluation of the hundreds of herbal remedies that have been part of traditional German medicine for centuries. Commission members carefully analyzed data from clinical trials, observational studies, biological experiments, and chemical analyses, and between 1983 and 1996, evaluated 383 herbal remedies, approving almost two-thirds of them for use, but discounting nearly another third, some of which continue to be sold in America.[48]

Essentially, the German Commission E analyzed a growing list of **phytomedicines,** another name for medicinal herbs, many of which are sold over the counter in Europe. Typically, phytomedicines are integrated into conventional medical practice and are prepared in several different ways, usually as tablets or powders.[49] Many are sold in much the same way as over-the-counter remedies in the United States.

Looking to Science for More Answers

Even as CAM treatments gain credibility, this credibility must be tempered with good science. Although slow in coming, legislators have pushed for better science, increased funding, and an agency designed to garner information useful to consumers.

In 1993 Congress established the Office of Alternative Medicine (OAM) at the NIH. Now much larger and renamed the National Center for Complementary and Alternative Medicine (NCCAM) and with a budget of nearly $70 million, it can fund its own projects and has established research centers at universities and other institutions throughout the United States, where many clinical trials are being conducted[50] (see Table 23.5). In addition, numerous other studies into alternative treatments for ailments from arthritis to depression to high blood cholesterol are taking place across the United States. One of the most promising aspects of this research is the enthusiastic support of professionals who have the training and laboratory expertise to evaluate the efficacy of current market-driven claims.

Healthy Living in the New Millennium

Clearly, CAM is here to stay. It appears to serve a very real need for consumers. While consumers are making the adjustment to CAM in record numbers, members of the health care delivery system seem slow to act. Although progress has been noted, there is still a long way to go before CAM becomes fully accepted in mainstream medical practice.

Enlisting Support from Insurers and Providers

More and more insurers are hiring alternative practitioners as staff or covering alternative care as a routine benefit, at least to some degree. This is especially true as criticisms of managed care increase and government agencies get involved.

In 1999, over 60 health maintenance groups throughout the United States covered some form of alternative care, nearly three times the number in 1994. The changing nature of HMOs and health care insurers makes it impossible to determine exactly how many insurance companies currently cover CAM therapies today. What is known is that the numbers are increasing despite a reimbursement system that is biased in favor of traditional treatments. While the nation's insurers spend over $30 billion a year on bypass and angioplasty for CVD, only 40 companies cover the lifestyle-based program developed by Dr. Dean Ornish. This despite repeated compelling research that demonstrates that the program is safe, effective, and much cheaper than surgery.[51] In some cases, consumers are offered an optional "extra-cost" rider on their insurance policy, through which they may choose to consult alternative practitioners for a higher premium and co-pay agreement. For many consumers, just knowing they have a choice seems to be worth the extra cost.

Support from professional organizations, such as the American Medical Association (AMA), is also increasing, as more physician training programs require or offer electives in alternative treatment modalities. In many cases, medical schools are educating a new generation of medical doctors to be better prepared to advise patients about the pros and cons of alternative treatments and how to follow integrative practices. Studies comparing the efficacy of alternative strategies compared to that of traditional treatments are becoming more comprehensive. Although alternative medicine is becoming increasingly integrated into today's health care programs and plans, there is still a long way to go. As we learn more, we will be better able to apply both traditional and alternative care.

> **Phytomedicines** Another name for medicinal herbs, many of which are sold over the counter in Europe.

Table 23.5
NCCAM-Funded Centers of Research on Complementary and Alternative Medicine

NAME/WEBSITE OF CENTER	INSTITUTION	RESEARCH SPECIALTY
Center for Addiction and Alternative Medicine Research www.mmrf.web.org/research/addiction&alt_med/index.html	Minneapolis Medical Research Foundation	Addictions
Center for CAM Research in Aging and Women's Health cpmcnet.Columbia.edu/dept/Rosenthal	Columbia University	Aging and women's health
Center for Alternative Medicine Research on Arthritis www.compmed.ummc.umaryland.edu	University of Maryland	Arthritis
Center for Frontier Medicine in Biofield Science	University of Arizona	Energy fields
Botanical Center for Age-Related Diseases	Purdue University West Lafayette	Plant-based treatments for CVD, cancer, osteoporosis, cognitive decline
Botanical Dietary Supplements for Women's Health	University of Illinois at Chicago	Herbal supplements and women's health
Center for Dietary Supplements Research: Botanicals	University of California at Los Angeles	Botanicals and cholesterol
Center for Phytomedicine Research	University of Arizona	Botanicals and inflammatory conditions
The Center for Cancer Complementary Medicine www.hopkins-cam.org	Johns Hopkins University	Cancer
Specialized Center of Research in Hyperbaric Oxygen Therapy	University of Pennsylvania	Cancer
CAM Research Center for Cardiovascular Diseases www.med.umich.edu/camrc/index.html	University of Michigan	Cardiovascular disease
Center for Natural Medicine and Prevention www.mum.edu/CNMP	Maharishi University of Management	CVD in older African Americans
Consortial Center for Chiropractic Research www.palmer.edu	Palmer College	Chiropractic
Oregon Center for CAM Research in Craniofacial Disorders	Kaiser Foundation Hospitals	Craniofacial disorders
Oregon Center for CAM Research in Neurological Disorders	Oregon Health Sciences University	Neurological disorders
Center for CAM Research in Neurodegenerative Diseases www.emory.edu/WHSC/MED/NEUROLOGY/CAM/index.html	Emory University	Neurodegenerative diseases
Pediatric Center for Complementary and Alternative Medicine	University of Arizona	Pediatrics
Exploratory Program Grant for Frontier Medicine	University of Connecticut	Touch

Source: National Center for Complementary and Alternative Medicine, "NCCAM's Research Centers Program," 2002 (see http://nccam.nci.nih.gov/training/centers).

What do you think?

*What can you do as a consumer to obtain the greatest benefit from CAM? * How can you protect yourself from possible negative risks?*

Self-Care: Protecting Yourself

Like no other time in human history, we are faced with an astounding array of possible health choices. Be aware that, with a few notable exceptions, much of what we read on the Internet about functional foods, herbal medicines, and CAM is unreliable at best—and strewn with potentially harmful and downright false information at worst. See the Skills for Behavior Change box for strategies on choosing a CAM therapy.

When considering alternative treatments, do your homework and protect yourself by remembering the following points:

• Consult only reliable sources—texts, journals, periodicals, and government resources. Start with the websites listed at the end of this and every chapter.
• Remember that *natural* and *safe* are not necessarily synonyms. Many people have become seriously ill from seemingly harmless products. For example, some have suffered

Selecting a CAM Provider

Selecting a CAM practitioner or any health care provider can be difficult. Although these recommendations apply to CAM, you should also consider them when selecting any health care product or service. Before starting a CAM therapy or choosing a practitioner, talk with your primary health care provider(s) and anyone else who is knowledgeable about CAM. If they dismiss the therapy, listen and ask them what they base their opinion on. Check their explanations with other sources to see if their insights are confirmed.

FINDING A CAM PRACTITIONER

- Ask your doctor or other health professional to recommend or refer you to a CAM therapist.
- Ask someone you trust who has used CAM practices if they have any recommendations based on experience.
- Contact a nearby hospital or medical school and ask if they maintain a list of area CAM practitioners and could recommend some to you. Some may actually have CAM providers on staff or as part of their group.
- If your therapy will be covered by insurance, ask your carrier for a list of CAM providers covered by your insurance.
- Contact a professional organization for the type of practitioner you are seeking. Often they have standards of practice

and websites or publications that list recommended providers. These resources will also answer common questions that you might have. If there is a regulatory or licensing board for this specialty, check to see that your practitioner has the proper credentials.

INTERVIEWING A CAM PRACTITIONER

- Make a list of your options and gather information about each before making your first visit. Ask basic questions about the credentials and experience of the provider. Where did he or she obtain his or her training? What supporting degrees does he or she have? What licenses or certifications? How much will the treatment cost?
- Make a list of questions to ask at your first visit. You may want to bring a friend or family member who can help you ask questions and note answers.
- Bring medical information with you, including any tests you've had, information about your health history, surgical history, allergies, and any medications (including prescription, over-the-counter, and herbal or other supplements).
- Ask if there are diseases/health conditions in which the practitioner specializes and how frequently he or she treats patients with conditions like yours.
- Ask if the practitioner believes the therapy can effectively address your complaint and if there is any scientific research supporting the treatment's use for your condition.

- Is the provider supportive of conventional as well as CAM treatments? Does he or she have a good referral relationship with conventional practitioners?
- Were questions answered to your satisfaction? Did the therapist seem interested in you as a person?
- How many patients per day does the provider see and how much time is spent with each one?
- Ask about charges and payment options. What percentage of the payment might you have to pay out of pocket?

After the visit, assess the interaction and how you felt about the practitioner, your comfort level, how your questions were answered, and any other issues.

UNDERSTANDING THE RECOMMENDED TREATMENT

- What benefits can I expect from this therapy?
- What are the risks associated with this therapy?
- Do the benefits outweigh the risks?
- Will I need to buy any special equipment or take any special supplements?
- Will this therapy interfere with any conventional medicine treatments?
- Are there any side effects?
- If there are problems, where would you be referred for further treatment?
- What is the history of success in treating this type of condition for someone of your age, health status, and other characteristics?

---

serious liver damage from sipping teas brewed with comfrey, an herb used in poultices and ointments to treat sprains and bruises and that should not be taken internally. Pregnant women face special risks from herbs such as echinacea, senna, comfrey, and licorice.

- Realize that no one is closely monitoring the purity of herbal supplements. The FDA has verified industry reports that certain shipments of ginseng were contaminated with high levels of fungicides. Other problems with imported herbs have been noted.
- Recognize that dosage levels in many herbal products are not regulated. German manufacturers produce identical

batches of herbal remedies as required by law. Look for reputable manufacturers.

- Tell your doctor if you are taking herbal medications. Several may interact with prescription (and over-the-counter) medications.
- Remember that no herbal medicine is likely to work miracles. Monitor your health, and seek help if you notice any unusual side effects from herbal products.
- Always look for the word *standardized* on any herbal product you buy. This indicates that manufacturing is monitored to ensure that the dosage and content are the same in every pill or tablet.

News from the World of CAM Research

Research is being conducted on complementary and alternative therapies in all areas of health, with investigations into treatments for some conditions making headlines. A recent special report in *Newsweek* magazine showed the widespread interest in complementary and alternative medicine. Experts from Harvard Medical School shared their insights about selected treatments for certain conditions:

Cancer: Although CAM therapies for cancer abound on the Internet and among the public at large, choosing a CAM therapy over a conventional therapy is risky business. However, promising new research focusing on diet, mind-body techniques, and even things like shark-cartilage supplements may provide evidence that CAM coupled with traditional medicine may make treatment more bearable, as well as improve survival. Some interesting points include the following:

- "Natural" doesn't always mean "safe." High doses of vitamin E and the herbal remedy of ginkgo biloba have anticoagulant effects that could cause excessive bleeding during surgery, particularly in those already taking aspirin. Soy contains plant estrogens that have not been ruled out in causing breast or endometrial cancer.
- Some supplements, such as St. John's wort, seem to counteract the effects of conventional cancer treatment drugs.
- Antioxidants may help limit adverse effects of radiation and chemotherapy; however, recent studies suggest they may also sometimes make these treatments less effective.
- Mind-body therapies, acupuncture, massage, and other remedies may help comfort patients, relieve physical symptoms such as pain and insomnia, alleviate nausea, and improve recovery from treatment.
- Complementary therapies can make cancer treatments more bearable and improve quality of life.
- Risks and benefits of any CAM therapy should be discussed with an oncologist.

Cardiovascular disease: Diet and exercise provide nearly undisputable benefits for reducing CVD risks. Diets low in saturated fats and trans fats—and high in fruits, vegetables, fish, and whole grains—can reduce your risk of a heart attack or stroke by anywhere from 20 to 80 percent, depending on other factors. Moderate exercise can reduce your risk by 30 to 40 percent. Research on other natural supplements is promising, although not conclusive at this time. Findings of other benefits and risks include the following:

- The Harvard Nurses' Health Study and Health Professionals' Follow-Up Study found reduced rates of CVD in people whose diets are rich in antioxidants such as vitamin E, vitamin A, and beta-carotene. However, other studies have refuted these results.
- A large study of chelation therapy (a technique used to clear toxic metals from the bloodstream) may provide results within the next five years. Until this time, the jury is out on this one.
- Supplements to watch out for include ginkgo biloba (can cause excessive bleeding) and ephedra (ma huang), which has been banned in several states and can have serious side effects, including high blood pressure and irregular heartbeat.

Arthritis: Current treatment for the 20-million-plus sufferers of arthritis has been primarily exercise and acetaminophen (Tylenol) plus NSAIDs (nonsteroidal anti-inflammatory drugs) such as aspirin, ibuprofen (Advil), naproxen (Aleve), or celecoxib (Celebrex) and rofecoxib (Vioxx). Many of these, particularly Celebrex and Vioxx, have side effects that cause people to seek alternatives. Summary points about the most commonly used alternatives include the following:

- *Glucosamine.* Although critics abound, many believe that glucosamine may help those suffering from arthritis pain while reducing the gastrointestinal irritation of NSAIDs. However, newer research also indicates that it can interfere with insulin, causing increases in blood sugar.
- *Chondroitin.* Often used with glucosamine, chondroitin may also elevate blood sugar levels and lead to excessive bleeding, particularly among those already on blood thinners and with other risks.
- *Herbs and supplements.* Although many are touted as arthritis treatments, scientific evidence of pain and symptom relief is lacking for many of these.

Memory loss: While Americans have been buying ginkgo biloba in search of supposed memory-aiding benefits, a study in the August 2002 edition of the *Journal of the American Medical Association* suggests that the herb does not help healthy people. Another study has shown that it may slow the rate of decline among Alzheimer's patients. A six-year trial started in 1999 and due to be completed in 2005 may shed more light on this. Most research supports the idea that mental activities, such as playing brain teasers and working on puzzles, are the best remedy for slowed memory.

Sources: Adapted from Wendy Weiger and David Eisenberg, "Health for Life: The New Science of Alternative Medicine: Cancer: Easing the Treatment," *Newsweek,* December 2, 2002, p. 49; William Haskell and David Eisenberg, "Health for Life: The New Science of Alternative Medicine: Cardiac Disease: Ways to Heal Your Heart," *Newsweek,* December 2, 2002, p. 52.

As we enter a new era of medicine, more than ever, you are being called upon to take responsibility for what goes into your body. This means you must educate yourself. CAM can offer new avenues toward better health, but it is up to you to make sure that you are on the right path. See Figure 23.1 for a recommended method of evaluating basic CAM alternatives.

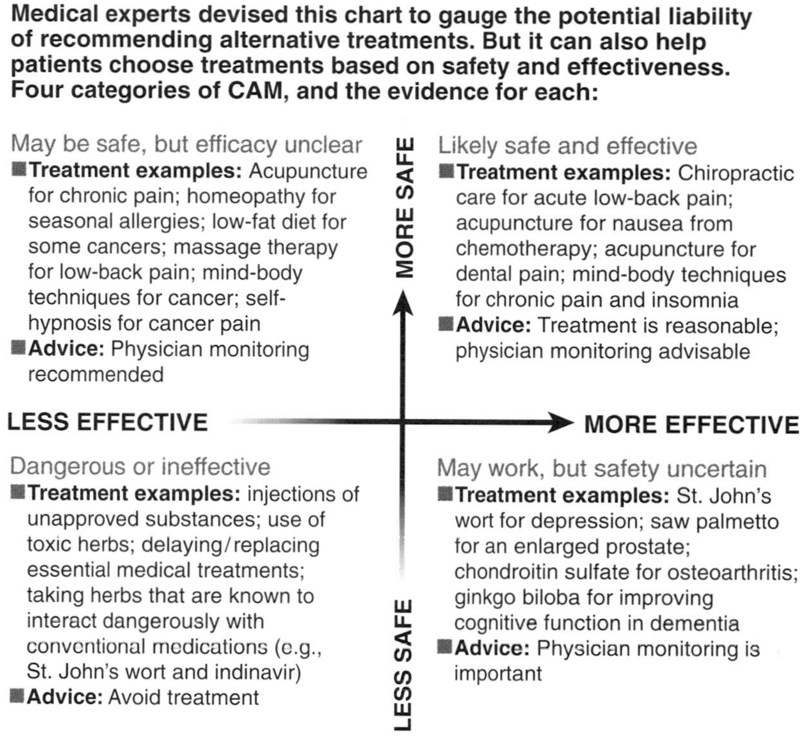

Medical experts devised this chart to gauge the potential liability of recommending alternative treatments. But it can also help patients choose treatments based on safety and effectiveness. Four categories of CAM, and the evidence for each:

May be safe, but efficacy unclear
- **Treatment examples:** Acupuncture for chronic pain; homeopathy for seasonal allergies; low-fat diet for some cancers; massage therapy for low-back pain; mind-body techniques for cancer; self-hypnosis for cancer pain
- **Advice:** Physician monitoring recommended

Likely safe and effective
- **Treatment examples:** Chiropractic care for acute low-back pain; acupuncture for nausea from chemotherapy; acupuncture for dental pain; mind-body techniques for chronic pain and insomnia
- **Advice:** Treatment is reasonable; physician monitoring advisable

MORE SAFE

LESS EFFECTIVE ⟶ MORE EFFECTIVE

Dangerous or ineffective
- **Treatment examples:** injections of unapproved substances; use of toxic herbs; delaying/replacing essential medical treatments; taking herbs that are known to interact dangerously with conventional medications (e.g., St. John's wort and indinavir)
- **Advice:** Avoid treatment

May work, but safety uncertain
- **Treatment examples:** St. John's wort for depression; saw palmetto for an enlarged prostate; chondroitin sulfate for osteoarthritis; ginkgo biloba for improving cognitive function in dementia
- **Advice:** Physician monitoring is important

LESS SAFE

Figure 23.1

Assessing Risks and Benefits of CAM Treatments

Source: Adapted from an article by Michael J. Cohn, J.D., and David M. Eisenberg, M.D., *The Annals of Internal Medicine,* vol. 136, no. 8. Published in "Health for Life: The New Science of Alternative Medicine," *Newsweek,* December 2, 2002.

Taking Charge

23 23 **23**

Making Healthful Decisions about CAM

Based on the information in this chapter, you can see that you should not use CAM products and services lightly, just as you should not take decision making about the traditional allopathic health care system lightly. Though the U.S. government has stepped up research and testing, we have addressed only the tip of the iceberg regarding information about the benefits and risks from CAM.

You need to constantly remain aware of the risks facing you in all of your decisions about health. As long as you are armed with the best sources of information, reading widely from reputable sources, and questioning the basis of claims and testimonials, you are taking critical steps in reducing risks. Consider the following as you make decisions about any health care product or service.

Checklist for Change

Making Personal Choices

☐ Find the most reputable sources for CAM-related information. Determine whether the information is current and whether it represents a single finding or one that is consistent with other research. Also, check the qualifications of the people who wrote the materials. Pay more heed to professionals with recognized credentials in specific areas such as an M.D. or Ph.D. in a particular specialty. Find out whether such authors are conducting active research using randomized, controlled trials.

☐ Focus on websites sponsored by professional organizations such as the American Dietetic Association, the Centers for Disease Control and Prevention, the American Public Health Association, and the American Medical Association.

☐ Consider your current health status, the areas you would like to improve, and the wide array of options that may help. Ask questions of other people who have experienced similar conditions or situations. What worked for them? Consult people whose judgment and knowledge you trust. Then itemize your options, and choose those that appear to offer the most benefit and the least risk.

☐ When shopping at health food stores or fitness centers that sell supplements and other purported health products, request the qualifications of those who are selling the products. Have they graduated with degrees in health education, nutrition, pharmacology, exercise physiology, or other reputable fields? Or have they simply attended a 1–2 week training program provided by their employer? Do they offer you choices and talk about risks and concerns, or are they primarily in SELL mode?

☐ Does your student health center have anyone available to answer your questions? Is there a certified health educator on staff? A dietitian? Does your doctor have time to answer some of your questions? Prepare a list, and ask for advice from experts on your own campus. Also, ask where you can go for reputable, easy-to-understand information about a given topic.

☐ Consider a balance in all things. Just because CAM modalities are available, it doesn't mean that you should toss out all the options in the traditional health care system. Optimize your health by utilizing the most effective modalities from both systems of treatment.

Making Community Choices

☐ Assess CAM providers in your community. Support those that are reputable and offer products and services including appropriate scientific information for consumers. Report those who offer questionable products and services.

☐ Write to congressional leaders in support of insurance provisions that allow consumers to choose CAM therapies that have been shown through scientific evidence to be safe and effective.

☐ Review policies about CAM products and services on your campus. What is offered? Who is using the services? How aware are other students of these services?

☐ Act responsibly, and stay informed about CAM and traditional medicine practices. Whenever someone is treated unfairly or inappropriately, make your concerns known. Be an advocate for good information and ethical treatment of all health problems.

Summary

✳ People throughout the world are choosing complementary and alternative medicine options, and these numbers are growing exponentially. Compared to other countries, the United States has been relatively slow to turn to alternative treatment and medicine.

✳ The National Center for Complementary and Alternative Medicine groups CAM practices into five major domains: (1) alternative medical systems (such as traditional Oriental medicine [TOM], Ayurveda, homeopathy, and naturopathy); (2) manipulative and body-based methods (such as chiropractic medicine and osteopathy); (3) energy therapies (including qi gong, reiki, therapeutic touch, and electromagnetic fields); (4) mind-body interventions (for example, body work, meditation, yoga, and tai chi); and (5) biologically based treatments (such as herbal, special dietary, orthomolecular, and individual biological therapies). Acupuncture and acupressure, two derivatives of energy therapy, are among the more popular forms of Oriental medicine in the United States.

✳ Herbal remedies, largely derived from traditional Chinese medicine, include ginkgo biloba, St. John's wort, echinacea, and green tea. Other herbal remedies have also received widespread attention as potential miracle drugs without having harmful side effects. Special supplements include muscle enhancers, ginseng, glucosamine, chromium picolinate, SAMe, and antioxidants. A number of functional foods may also serve as healing agents.

✳ Though many positive effects are associated with CAM, there are also many risks. The drive for profits and the lack of strict government regulation make the CAM market a free-for-all. As a consumer, you must be aware of the risks and check reputable sources to ensure that you are not being lured by false claims and promises.

✳ Health in the new millennium will provide an interesting assortment of choices for health care consumers. By enlisting the support of health professionals and health care services and by making informed decisions, you will reap positive rewards in your quest for health enhancement in the days ahead.

Questions for Discussion and Reflection

1. What are some of the potential benefits and risks of CAM? Why do you think these practices and products are growing in popularity so rapidly?
2. What are the major domains of CAM treatments? Have you tried any of them? Would you feel comfortable trying any new ones? Why or why not?
3. What are the major herbal remedies? Special supplements? What are some of the risks and benefits associated with each?
4. What can you do to ensure that you are receiving accurate information regarding CAM treatments or medicines? What is the name of the federal agency that oversees CAM in the United States?
5. What is being done in the United States to ensure continued growth of CAM?

Application Exercises

Reread the What Do You Think? scenarios at the beginning of the chapter and answer the following questions.

1. Why are there so many conflicting sources of information in today's health care system about even a seemingly simple problem? What could we do to streamline or synthesize sources and give consumers access to the best information available? Would you favor a government watchdog agency to monitor such a source of information? Why or why not? In the absence of such a resource, what actions can consumers like Mia take to protect themselves from misleading information about important health concerns?

2. Who should be allowed to sell CAM products and services? Should everyone who is looking to make money be allowed to set up websites and post claims that their products improve health? If not, what would you propose instead? Are all M.D.s qualified to give advice with regard to CAM? Who is qualified to offer information about specific CAM products and services? Should doctors prescribe supplements and other products from which the doctors gain profit, or should only licensed, trained providers who aren't motivated by profit be allowed to dispense such products and services? Explain your answer.

Accessing Your Health on the Internet

Visit the following Internet sites to explore further topics and issues related to personal health. To visit an organization's website, go to the Companion Website for *Access to Health, Eighth Edition,* at www.aw.com/donatelle, click on the book image, and select "Accessing Your Health on the Internet" from the navigation menu on the left.

1. *Acupuncture.com.* Provides resources for consumers regarding traditional Asian therapies, geared to students and practitioners.

2. *Alternative Medicine Links.* Provides links to a number of the best alternative, complementary, and preventive health news pages.
3. *National Center for Complementary and Alternative Medicine.* A division of the National Institutes of Health dedicated to providing the latest information on complementary and alternative practices.
4. *National Institutes of Health, Office of Dietary Supplements.* An excellent resource for information on dietary supplements.

Further Reading

Blumenthal, M., ed. *Complete German Commission E Monographs: Therapeutic Guide to Herbal Medicines.* Mark Blumenthal (Editor), Austin, TX: The American Botanical Council, 1998.

Overview of German E commission findings and relevant information about supplement research for consumers. Provides an interesting perspective on international herbal research, policies, recommendations, and future directions.

Cassileth, B. R. *The Alternative Medicine Handbook: The Complete Reference Guide to Alternative and Complementary Therapies.* New York: W. W. Norton & Co., 1998.

A complete reference for patients and physicians alike on possible alternative treatments.

Pelletier, Ken. *The Best Alternative Medicine: What Works? What Does Not.* New York: Simon & Schuster, 2000.

Excellent overview of commonly used CAM techniques with scientific information for consumers.

Turchaninov, R., and C. A. Cox. *Medical Massage.* Scottsdale, AZ: Stress Less Publishing and Phoenix: Aesculapius Books, 1998.

An in-depth review of therapeutic practices from around the world.

Appendix A

Injury Prevention and Emergency Care

Injury Prevention

Unintentional injuries are one of the major public health problems facing the United States today. On an average day, more than a million people will suffer a nonfatal injury; almost 100,000 people die each year as a result of unintentional injuries. Unintentional injuries are the leading cause of death for Americans under the age of 44. In the United States, unintentional injuries are the fifth leading cause of death, after heart disease, cancer, stroke, and lung disease.

Vehicle Safety

The risk of dying in an auto crash is related to age. Young drivers (ages 16–24) have the highest death rate, owing to their inexperience and immaturity. In 2001, 42,900 Americans died in automobile crashes. Each year another 1.6 million are disabled, 140,000 permanently. Most of these car crashes were avoidable. The best line of prevention against car crashes is to practice risk management driving and accident-avoidance techniques and to be aware of safety technology when purchasing a car.

Risk Management Driving Practicing risk management driving techniques helps reduce chances of being involved in a collision. Techniques include the following:

- *Surround your car with a bubble space.* The rear bumper of the car ahead of you should be three seconds away. To measure your safety bubble, choose a roadside landmark such as a signpost or light pole as a reference point. When the car in front of you passes this point, count "one-one-thousand, two-one-thousand." Make sure you are not passing the reference point before you've finished saying "three-one-thousand."
- *Scan the road ahead of you and to both sides.*
- *Drive with your low-beam headlights on.* Being seen is an important safety factor. Driving with your low-beam headlights on, *day or night,* makes you more visible to other drivers.

In addition, remember these points:

- Anticipate other drivers' actions.
- Drive refreshed.
- Drive sober.
- Obey all traffic laws.
- Use safety belts.

Accident-Avoidance Techniques Sometimes when driving, you need to react instantly to a situation. To avoid a more severe accident, you may need to steer into another, less severe collision. The point of accident evasion is to save lives. Here are AAA's rules for avoidance:

1. Generally, veer to the right.
2. Steer, don't skid, off the road.
3. If you have to hit a vehicle, hit one moving in the same direction as your own.
4. If you have to hit a stationary object, try to hit a soft one (bushes, small trees, etc.) rather than a hard one (boulders, brick walls, giant oaks).
5. If you have to hit a hard object, hit it with a glancing blow.
6. Avoid hitting pedestrians, motorcyclists, and bicyclists at all costs.

Safety Technology The last line of defense against a collision is the car itself. How a car is equipped can mean the difference between life and death. When purchasing a car, the Insurance Institute for Highway Safety recommends that you look for the following features:

- Does the car have airbags? Remember, airbags do not eliminate the need for everyone to wear safety belts. Airbags inflate only in the case of frontal crashes.
- Does the car have antilock brakes? Antilock brakes help pump the brakes and prevent them from locking up and, hence, prevent the car from skidding.
- Does the car have impact-absorbing crumple zones?
- Are there strengthened passenger compartment side walls?
- Is there a strong roof support? (The center door post on four-door models gives you an extra roof pillar.)

In Case of Mechanical Breakdown

- Try to get off the road as far as possible.
- Turn on your car's emergency flashers and raise the hood. Set out flares or reflective triangles.
- Stay in the car until a law enforcement officer arrives. If others stop to help, ask them to contact the police, sheriff's office, or the state patrol.
- If you must leave your car, leave a note with the car explaining the problem (as best you can), the time and date, your name, the direction in which you are walking, and what you are wearing. This information will help anyone who needs to look for you.
- Remove all valuables from the car if you must leave it.

Safe Refueling

Gasoline is a flammable substance. Follow these guidelines from the Petroleum Equipment Institute any time you are filling up a car, truck, or motorcycle:

- Turn off the engine while refueling.
- Do not reenter your vehicle during refueling. In the unlikely event of a static-caused fire, leave the nozzle in the tank and back away from the vehicle. Notify the attendant immediately.
- Avoid prolonged breathing of gasoline vapors. Keep gasoline away from your eyes and skin; it can cause irritation. Never use it to wash your hands or as a cleaning solvent.
- If you are dispensing gasoline into a container or storing it, be sure the container is approved for such a use.
- Never siphon gasoline by mouth; it can be harmful or fatal if swallowed.

Pedestrian Safety

Each year approximately 13 percent of all motor vehicle deaths involve pedestrians, and another 82,000 pedestrians are injured each year. The highest death rates involving pedestrians occur among the very young and elderly populations. Pedestrian injuries occur most frequently after dark, in urban settings, and primarily in intersections where pedestrians may walk or dart into traffic. It is not uncommon for alcohol to play a role in the death or injury of a pedestrian. How can you protect yourself from being injured or becoming a fatality? AAA has the following suggestions for joggers and walkers:

- Carry or wear reflective material at night to help drivers see you.
- Cross only at crosswalks. Keep to the right in crosswalks.
- Before crossing, look both ways. Be sure the way is clear before you cross.
- Cross only on the proper signal.
- Watch for turning cars.
- Never go into the roadway from between parked cars.
- Where there is no sidewalk and it is necessary to walk in a roadway, walk on the left side, facing traffic.

- Don't wear headphones for a radio or CD player. These may interfere with your ability to hear sounds of motor vehicles.

Cycling Safety

Currently over 63 million Americans of all ages ride bicycles for transportation, recreation, and fitness. The Consumer Product Safety Commission reports about 800 deaths per year from cycling accidents. The biggest risk factors are failure to wear a helmet, being male, and riding after dark. Children age 10 to 14 also are at higher risk for injury. Approximately 87 percent of fatal collisions were due to cyclists' errors, usually failure to yield at intersections. Alcohol also plays a significant role in bicycle deaths and injuries. The following are suggestions cyclists should consider to reduce risk of injury or death.

- Wear a helmet. It should be ANSI or Snell approved. This can reduce head injuries by 85 percent.
- Don't drink and ride.
- Respect traffic.
- Wear light reflective clothing that is easily seen at night and during the day.
- Avoid riding after dark.
- Ride with the flow of traffic.
- Know and use proper hand signals.
- Keep your bicycle in good working condition.
- Use bike paths whenever possible.
- Stop at stop signs and traffic lights.

Water Safety

Drowning is the third most common cause of accidental death in the United States, according to the National Safety Council. About 85 percent of drowning victims are teenage males. Many drowned swimmers are strong swimmers. Alcohol plays a significant role in many drowning cases. Most drownings occur in unorganized or unsupervised facilities, such as ponds or pools with no lifeguards present. Swimmers should take the following precautions:

- Don't drink alcohol before or while swimming.
- Don't enter the water unless you can swim at least 50 feet unassisted.
- Know your limitations; get out of the water as soon as you start to feel even slightly fatigued.
- Never swim alone, even if you are a skilled swimmer. You never know what might happen.
- Never leave a child unattended, even in extremely shallow water or wading pools.
- Before entering the water, check the depth. Most neck and back injuries result from diving into water that is too shallow.
- Never swim in muddy or dirty water that obstructs your view of the bottom.
- Never swim in a river with currents too swift for easy, relaxed swimming.

Emergency Care

In certain situations, it may be necessary to administer first aid. Ideally, first-aid procedures should be performed by someone who has received formal training from the American Red Cross or some other reputable institution. If you do not have such training, contact a physician or call your local emergency medical service (EMS) by dialing 911 or your local emergency number. In life-threatening situations, however, you may not have time to call for outside assistance.

In cases of serious injury or sudden illness, you may need to begin first aid immediately and continue until help arrives. The remainder of this appendix contains basic information and general steps to follow for various emergency situations. Simply reading these directions, however, may not prepare you fully to handle these situations. For this reason, you may want to enroll in a first-aid course.

Calling for Emergency Assistance

When calling for emergency assistance, be prepared to give exact details. Be clear and thorough, and do not panic. Never hang up until the dispatcher has all the information needed. Be ready to answer the following questions:

1. Where are you and the victim located? This is the most important information the EMS will need.
2. What is your phone number and name?
3. What has happened? Was there an accident, or is the victim ill?
4. How many people need help?
5. What is the nature of the emergency? What is the victim's apparent condition?
6. Are there any life-threatening situations that the EMS should know about (for example, fires, explosions, or fallen electrical lines)?
7. Is the victim wearing a medic-alert tag (a tag indicating a specific medical problem such as diabetes)?

Are You Liable?

According to the laws in most states, you are not required to administer first aid unless you have a special obligation to the victim. For example, parents must provide first aid for their children, and a lifeguard must provide aid to a swimmer.

Before administering first aid, you should obtain the victim's consent. If the victim refuses aid, you must respect that person's rights. However, you should make every reasonable effort to persuade the victim to accept your help. In emergency situations, consent is *implied* if the victim is unconscious.

Once you begin to administer first aid, you are required by law to continue. You must remain with the victim until someone of equal or greater competence takes over.

Can you be held liable if you fail to provide adequate care or if the victim is further injured? To help protect people who render first aid, most states have "Good Samaritan"

laws. These laws grant immunity (protection from civil liability) if you act in good faith to provide care to the best of your ability, according to your level of training. Because these laws vary from state to state, you should become familiar with the Good Samaritan laws in your state.

When Someone Stops Breathing

If someone has stopped breathing, you should perform mouth-to-mouth resuscitation. This involves the following steps:

1. Check for responsiveness by gently tapping or shaking the victim. Ask loudly, "Are you OK?"
2. Call the local EMS for help (usually 911).
3. Gently roll the victim onto his or her back.
4. Open the airway by tilting the victim's head back, placing your hand nearest the victim's head on the victim's forehead, and applying backward pressure to tilt the head back and lift the chin.
5. Check for breathing (3 to 5 seconds): look, listen, and feel for breathing.
6. Give 2 slow breaths.

- Keep the victim's head tilted back.
- Pinch the victim's nose shut.
- Seal your lips tightly around the victim's mouth.
- Give 2 slow breaths, each lasting 1½ to 2 seconds.

7. Check for pulse at side of neck; feel for pulse for 5 to 10 seconds.
8. Begin rescue breathing.

- Keep the victim's head tilted back.
- Pinch the victim's nose shut.
- Give one breath every 5 to 6 seconds.
- Look, listen, and feel for breathing between breaths.

9. Recheck pulse every minute.

- Keep the victim's head tilted back.
- Feel for pulse for 5 to 10 seconds.
- If the victim has a pulse but is not breathing, continue rescue breathing. If there is no pulse, begin CPR.

There are some variations when performing this procedure on infants and children. For children ages one to eight, at step 8, give one slow breath every 4 seconds. For infants, you should not pinch the nose. Instead, seal your lips tightly around the infant's nose and mouth. Also, at step 8, you should give one slow breath every 3 seconds.

In cases in which the victim has no pulse, cardiopulmonary resuscitation (CPR) should be performed. This technique involves a combination of artificial respiration and chest compressions. You should not perform CPR unless you have received training in it. You cannot learn CPR simply by reading directions, and without training, you could cause further injury to the victim. The American Red Cross offers courses in mouth-to-mouth resuscitation and CPR as well as general first aid. If you have taken a CPR course in the past, you should be aware that certain changes have been made in the procedure. You should, therefore, consider taking a refresher course.

When Someone Is Choking

Choking occurs when an object obstructs the trachea (windpipe), thus preventing normal breathing. Failure to expel the object and restore breathing can lead to death within 6 minutes. The universal signal of distress related to choking is the clasping of the throat with one or both hands. Other signs of choking include not being able to talk and/or noisy and difficult breathing. If a victim can cough or speak, do not interfere. The most effective method for assisting choking victims is the Heimlich maneuver, which involves the application of pressure to the victim's abdominal area to expel the foreign object.

The Heimlich maneuver involves the following steps:

If the Victim Is Standing or Seated

1. Recognize that the victim is choking.
2. Wrap your arms around the victim's waist, making a fist with one hand.
3. Place the thumb side of the fist on the middle of the victim's abdomen, just above the navel and well below the tip of the sternum.
4. Cover your fist with your other hand.
5. Press fist into victim's abdomen, with up to five quick upward thrusts.
6. After every five abdominal thrusts, check the victim and your technique.
7. If the victim becomes unconscious, gently lower him or her to the ground.
8. Try to clear the airway by using your finger to sweep the object from the victim's mouth or throat.
9. Give two rescue breaths. If the passage is still blocked and air will not go in, proceed with the Heimlich maneuver.

If the Victim Is Lying Down

1. Facing the person, kneel with your legs astride the victim's hips. Place the heel of one hand against the abdomen, slightly above the navel and well below the tip of the sternum. Put the other hand on top of the first hand.
2. Press inward and upward using both hands with up to five quick abdominal thrusts.
3. Repeat the following steps in this sequence until the airway becomes clear or the EMS arrives:
   a. Finger sweep.
   b. Give two rescue breaths.
   c. Do up to five abdominal thrusts.

Alcohol Poisoning

Alcohol overdose is considered a medical emergency when one or both of the following occur: an irregular heartbeat or coma. The two immediate causes of death in such cases are cardiac arrhythmia and respiratory depression. If a person is seriously uncoordinated and has possibly also taken a depressant, the risk of respiratory failure is serious enough that a physician should be contacted. When dealing with someone who is drunk, remember these points:

1. Stay calm. Assess the situation.
2. Keep the person still and comfortable.
3. Stay with the person if she or he is vomiting. When lying him or her down, turn the head to the side to prevent it from falling back. This helps to keep the person from choking on vomit.
4. Monitor the person's breathing.
5. Keep your distance. Before approaching or touching the person, explain what you intend to do.
6. Speak in a clear, firm, reassuring manner.

When Someone Is Bleeding

External Bleeding   Control of external bleeding is an important part of emergency care. Survival is threatened by the loss of one quart of blood or more. There are three major procedures for the control of external bleeding.

1. *Direct pressure.* The best method is to apply firm pressure by covering the wound with a sterile dressing, bandage, or clean cloth. Wearing disposable latex gloves or an equally protective barrier, apply pressure for 5 to 10 minutes to stop bleeding.
2. *Elevation.* Elevate the wounded section of the body to slow bleeding. For example, a wounded arm or leg should be raised above the level of the victim's heart.
3. *Pressure points.* Pressure points are sites where an artery that is close to the body's surface lies directly over a bone. Pressing the artery against the bone can limit the flow of blood to the injury. This technique should be used only as a last resort when direct pressure and elevation have failed to stop bleeding.

Knowing where to apply pressure to stop bleeding is critical (see Figure A.1). For serious wounds, seek medical attention immediately.

Internal Bleeding   Although internal bleeding may not be immediately obvious, you should be aware of the following signs and symptoms:

- Symptoms of shock (discussed later in this appendix).
- Coughing up or vomiting blood.
- Bruises or contusions of the skin.
- Bruises on chest or fractured ribs.
- Black, tarlike stools.
- Abdominal discomfort or pain (rigidity or spasms).

In some cases, a person who has suffered an injury (such as a blow to the head, chest, or abdomen) that does not cause external bleeding may experience internal bleeding. If you suspect that someone is suffering from internal bleeding, follow these steps:

1. Have the person lie on a flat surface with knees bent.

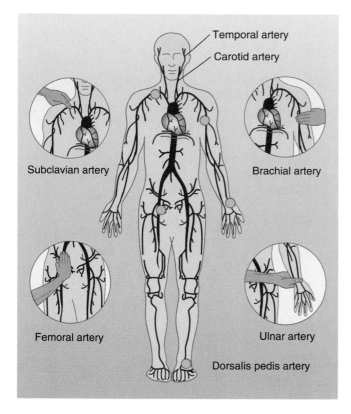

Figure A.1
Pressure Points
Pressure can be applied to these points to stop bleeding. However, unless absolutely necessary, avoid applying pressure to the carotid arteries, which supply blood to the brain. Also, never apply pressure to both carotid arteries at the same time.

2. Treat for shock. Keep the victim warm. Cover the person with a blanket, if possible.
3. Expect vomiting. If vomiting occurs, keep the victim on his or her side for drainage, to prevent inhalation of vomit, and to prevent expulsion of vomit from the stomach.
4. Do *not* give the victim any medications of fluids.
5. Send someone to call for emergency medical help immediately.

Nosebleeds To control a nosebleed, follow these steps:

1. Have the victim sit down and lean slightly forward to prevent blood from running into the throat. If you do not suspect a fracture, pinch the person's nose firmly closed using the thumb and forefinger. Keep the nose pinched for at least 5 minutes.
2. While the nose is pinched, apply a cold compress to the surrounding area.
3. If pinching does not work, gently pack the nostril with gauze or a clean strip of cloth. Do not use absorbent cotton, which will stick. Be sure that the ends of the gauze or

cloth hang out so that it can be easily removed later. Once the nose is packed with gauze, pinch it closed again for another 5 minutes.
4. If the bleeding persists, seek medical attention.

Treatment for Burns

Minor Burns For minor burns caused by fire or scalding water, apply running cold water or cold compresses for 20 to 30 minutes. Never put butter, grease, salt water, aloe vera, or topical burn ointments or sprays on burned skin. If the burned area is dirty, gently wash it with soap and water and blot it dry with a sterile dressing.

Major Burns For major burn injuries, call for help immediately. Wrap the victim in a dry sheet. Do not clean the burns or try to remove any clothing attached to burned skin. Remove jewelry near the burned skin immediately, if possible. Keep the victim lying down and calm.

Chemical Burns Remove clothing surrounding the burn. Wash skin that has been burned by chemicals by flushing with water for at least 20 minutes. Seek medical assistance as soon as possible.

Shock

Shock is a condition in which the cardiovascular system fails to provide sufficient blood circulation to all parts of the body. Victims of shock display the following symptoms:

- Dilated pupils.
- Cool, moist skin.
- Weak, rapid pulse.
- Vomiting.
- Delayed or unrelated responses to questions.

All injuries result in some degree of shock. Therefore, treatment for shock should be given after every major injury. The following are basic steps for treating shock:

1. Have the victim lie flat with his or her feet elevated approximately 8 to 12 inches. (In the case of chest injuries, difficulty breathing, or severe pain, the victim's head should be slightly elevated if there is no sign of spinal injury.)
2. Keep the victim warm. If possible, wrap him or her in blankets or other material. Keep the victim calm and reassured.
3. Seek medical help.

Electrical Shock

Do not touch a victim of electrical shock until the power source has been turned off. Approach the scene carefully, avoiding any live wires or electrical power lines. Pay attention to the following:

1. If the victim is holding onto the live electrical wire, do not remove it unless the power has been shut off at the plug, circuit breaker, or fuse box.

2. Check the victim's breathing and pulse. Electrical current can paralyze the nerves and muscles that control breathing and heartbeat. If necessary, give mouth-to-mouth resuscitation. If there is no pulse, CPR might be necessary. (Remember that only trained people should perform CPR.)
3. Keep the victim warm and treat for shock. Once the person is breathing and stable, seek medical help or send someone else for help.

Poisoning

Of the 1 million cases of poisoning reported in the United States each year, about 75 percent occur in children under age five, and the majority are caused by household products. Most cases of poisoning involving adults are attempted suicides or attempted murders.

You should keep emergency telephone numbers for the poison control center and the local EMS close at hand. Many people keep these numbers on labels on their telephones. Check the front of your telephone book for these numbers. The National Safety Council recommends that you be prepared to give the following information when calling for help:

- What was ingested? Have the container of the product and the remaining contents ready so you can describe it. You should also bring the container to the emergency room with you.
- When was the substance taken?
- How much was taken?
- Has vomiting occurred? If the person has vomited, save a sample to take to the hospital.
- Are there any other symptoms?
- How long will it take to get to the nearest emergency room?

When caring for a person who has ingested a poison, keep these basic principles in mind:

1. Maintain an open airway. Make sure the person is breathing.
2. Call the local poison control center. Follow their advice for neutralizing the poison.
3. If the poison control center or another medical authority advises you to induce vomiting, then do so.
4. If a corrosive or caustic (i.e., acid or alkali) substance was swallowed, immediately dilute it by having the victim drink at least one or two 8-ounce glasses of cold water or milk.
5. Place the victim on his or her left side. This position will delay advancement of the poison into the small intestine, where absorption into the victim's circulatory system is faster.

Injuries of Joints, Muscles, and Bones

Sprains   Sprains result when ligaments and other tissues around a joint are stretched or torn. The following steps should be taken to treat sprains:

1. Elevate the injured joint to a comfortable position.

2. Apply an ice pack or cold compress to reduce pain and swelling.
3. Wrap the joint firmly with a (roller) bandage.
4. Check the fingers or toes periodically to ensure that blood circulation has not been obstructed. If the bandage is too tight, loosen it.
5. Keep the injured area elevated, and continue ice treatment for 24 hours.
6. Apply heat to the injury after 48 hours if there is no further swelling.
7. If pain and swelling continue or if a fracture is suspected, seek medical attention.

Fractures   Any deformity of an injured body part usually indicates a fracture. A fracture is any break in a bone, including chips, cracks, splinters, and complete breaks. Minor fractures (such as hairline cracks) might be difficult to detect and might be confused with sprains. If there is doubt, treat the injury as a fracture until x-rays have been taken.

Do not move the victim if a fracture of the neck or back is suspected because this could result in a spinal cord injury. If the victim must be moved, splints should be applied to immobilize the fracture, to prevent further damage, and to decrease pain. Following are some basic steps for treating fractures and applying splints to broken limbs:

1. If the person is bleeding, apply direct pressure above the site of the wound.
2. If a broken bone is exposed, do not try to move it back into the wound. This can cause contamination and further injury.
3. Do not try to straighten out a broken limb. Splint the limb as it lies.
4. The following materials are needed for splinting:

- *Splint:* wooden board, pillow, or rolled up magazines and newspapers.
- *Padding:* towels, blankets, socks, or cloth.
- *Ties:* cloth, rope, or tape.

5. Place splints and padding above and below the joint. Never put padding directly over the break. Padding should protect bony areas and the soft tissue of the limb.
6. Tie splints and padding into place.
7. Check the tightness of the splints periodically. Pay attention to the skin color, temperature, and pulse below the fracture to make sure the blood flow is adequate.
8. Elevate the fracture and apply ice packs to prevent swelling and reduce pain.

Head Injuries

A head injury can result from an auto accident, a fall, an assault, or a blow from a blunt object. All head injuries can potentially lead to brain damage, which may resulting a cessation of breathing and pulse.

For Minor Head Injuries
1. For a minor bump on the head resulting in a bruise without bleeding, apply ice to decrease the swelling.

2. If there is bleeding, apply even, moderate pressure. Because there is always the danger that the skull may be fractured, excessive pressure should not be used.
3. Observe the victim for a change in consciousness. Observe the size of pupils and note signs of inability to think clearly. Check for any signs of numbness or paralysis. Allow the victim to sleep, but wake him or her periodically to check for awareness.

For Severe Head Injuries

1. If the victim is unconscious, check the airway for breathing. If necessary, perform mouth-to-mouth resuscitation.
2. If the victim is breathing, check the pulse. If it is less than 55 or more than 125 beats per minute, the victim may be in danger.
3. Check for bleeding. If fluid is flowing from the ears or nose, do not stop it.
4. Do not remove any objects embedded in the victim's skull.
5. Cover the victim with blankets to maintain body temperature, but guard against overheating.
6. Seek medical help as soon as possible.

Temperature-Related Emergencies

Frostbite Frostbite is damage to body tissues caused by intense cold. Frostbite generally occurs at temperatures below 32°F. The body parts most likely to suffer frostbite are the toes, ears, fingers, nose, and cheeks. When skin is exposed to the cold, ice crystals form beneath the skin. Avoid rubbing frostbitten tissue, because the ice crystals can scrape and break blood vessels.

To treat frostbite, follow these steps:

1. Bring the victim to a health facility as soon as possible.
2. Cover and protect the frostbitten area. If possible, apply a steady source of external warmth, such as a warm compress. The victim should avoid walking if the feet are frostbitten.
3. If the victim cannot be transported, you must rewarm the body part by immersing it in warm water (100°F to 105°F). Continue to rewarm until the frostbitten area is warm to the touch when removed from the bath. Do not allow the body part to touch the sides or bottom of the water container. After rewarming, dry gently and wrap the body part in bandages to protect from refreezing.

Hypothermia Hypothermia is a condition of generalized cooling of the body, resulting from exposure to cold temperatures or immersion in cold water. It can occur at any temperature below 65°F and can be made more severe by wind chill and moisture. The following are key symptoms of hypothermia:

- Shivering.
- Vague, slow, slurred speech.
- Poor judgment.
- A cool abdomen.
- Lethargy, or extreme exhaustion.
- Slowed breathing and heartbeat.
- Numbness and loss of feeling in extremities.

After contacting the EMS, you should take the following steps to provide first aid to a victim of hypothermia:

1. Get the victim out of the cold.
2. Keep the victim in a flat position. Do not raise the legs.
3. Squeeze as much water from wet clothing, and layer dry clothing over wet clothing. Removal of clothing may jostle victim and lead to other problems.
4. Give the victim warm drinks only if he or she is able to swallow. Do not give the victim alcohol or caffeinated beverages, and do not allow the victim to smoke.
5. Do not allow the victim to exercise.

Heatstroke Heatstroke, the most serious heat-related disorder, results from the failure of the brain's heat-regulating mechanism (the hypothalamus) to cool the body. The following are signs and symptoms of heatstroke:

- Rapid pulse.
- Hot, dry, flushed skin (absence of sweating).
- Disorientation leading to unconsciousness.
- High body temperature.

As soon as these symptoms are noticed, the body temperature should be reduced as quickly as possible. The victim should be immersed in a cool bath, lake, or stream. If there is no water nearby, a fan should be used to help lower the victim's body temperature.

Heat Exhaustion Heat exhaustion results from excessive loss of salt and water. The onset is gradual, with the following symptoms:

- Fatigue and weakness.
- Anxiety.
- Nausea.
- Profuse sweating.
- Clammy skin.
- Normal body temperature.

To treat heat exhaustion, move the victim to a cool place. Have the victim lie down flat, with feet elevated 8 to 12 inches. Replace lost fluids slowly and steadily. Sponge or fan victim.

Heat Cramps Heat cramps result from excessive sweating, resulting in an excessive loss of salt and water. Although heat cramps are the least serious heat-related emergency, they are the most painful. The symptoms include muscle cramps, usually starting in the arms and legs. To relieve symptoms, the victim should drink electrolyte-rich beverages or a light saltwater solution or eat salty foods.

First-Aid Supplies

Every home, car, or boat should be supplied with a basic first-aid kit. In order to respond effectively to emergences, you must have the basic equipment. This kit should be stored in a convenient place, but it should be kept out of the reach of children. Following is a list of supplies that should be included:

- Bandages, including triangular bandages (36 inches by 36 inches), butterfly bandages, a roller bandage, rolled white gauze bandages (2- and 3-inch widths), adhesive bandages.
- Sterile gauze pads and absorbent pads.
- Adhesive tape (2- and 3-inch widths).
- Cotton-tip applicators.
- Scissors.
- Thermometer.
- Antibiotic ointment.
- Syrup of ipecac (to induce vomiting).
- Aspirin.
- Calamine lotion.
- Antiseptic cream or petroleum jelly.
- Safety pins.
- Tweezers.
- Flashlight.
- Paper cups.
- Blanket.

You cannot be prepared for every medical emergency. Yet these essential tools and a knowledge of basic first aid will help you cope with many emergency situations.

Appendix B

Nutritive Value
of Selected Foods

DESCRIPTION OF FOOD	SERVING SIZE	WT (G)	CAL (KCAL)	PROT (G)	FAT (G)	SAT FAT (G)	CHOL (MG)	CARBO (G)	CALC (MG)	SOD (MG)
BEVERAGES										
Beer, light	12 fl oz	355	95	1	0	0	0	5	14	11
Beer, regular	12 fl oz	360	150	1	0	0	0	13	14	18
Club soda	12 fl oz	355	0	0	0	0	0	0	18	78
Coffee, brewed	6 fl oz	180	0	0	0	0	0	0	4	2
Cola, diet	12 fl oz	355	0	0	0	0	0	0	14	32
Cola, regular	12 fl oz	369	160	0	0	0	0	41	11	18
Fruit punch drink, canned	6 fl oz	190	85	0	0	0	0	22	15	15
Gin, rum, vodka, whiskey, 80 proof	1.5 fl oz	42	95	0	0	0	0	0	0	0
Ginger ale	12 fl oz	366	125	0	0	0	0	32	11	29
Grape soda	12 fl oz	372	100	0	0	0	0	46	15	48
Lemon-lime soda	12 fl oz	372	155	0	0	0	0	39	7	33
Orange soda	12 fl oz	372	180	0	0	0	0	46	15	52
Pineapple-grapefruit juice drink	6 fl oz	187	90	0	0	0	0	23	13	24
Root beer	12 fl oz	370	165	0	0	0	0	42	15	48
Tea, brewed	8 fl oz	240	0	0	0	0	0	0	0	1
Wine, dessert	3.5 fl oz	103	140	0	0	0	0	8	8	9
Wine, table, red	3.5 fl oz	102	75	0	0	0	0	3	8	5
Wine, table, white	3.5 fl oz	102	80	0	0	0	0	3	9	5
BREADS										
Bagels, egg	1 bagel	68	200	7	2	0.3	44	38	29	245
Bagels, plain	1 bagel	68	200	7	2	0.3	0	38	29	245
Baking powder biscuits, from mix	1 biscuit	28	95	2	3	0.8	0	14	58	262
Bread crumbs, dry, grated	1 cup	100	390	13	5	1.5	5	73	122	736
Bread stuffing, from mix, moist	1 cup	203	420	9	26	5.3	67	40	81	1,023
French bread	1 slice	35	100	3	1	0.3	0	18	39	203
Italian bread	1 slice	30	85	3	0	0	0	17	5	176
Mixed-grain bread	1 slice	25	65	2	1	0.2	0	12	27	106
Oatmeal bread	1 slice	25	65	2	1	0.2	0	12	15	124
Pita bread	1 pita	60	165	6	1	0.1	0	33	49	339
Pumpernickel bread	1 slice	32	80	3	1	0.2	0	16	23	177
Raisin bread	1 slice	25	65	2	1	0.2	0	13	25	92
Rolls, dinner, commercial	1 roll	28	85	2	2	0.5	0	14	33	155
Rolls, frankfurter or hamburger	1 roll	40	115	3	2	0.5	0	20	54	241
Rolls, hoagie or submarine	1 roll	135	400	11	8	1.8	0	72	100	683
Rye bread, light	1 slice	25	65	2	1	0.2	0	12	20	175

DESCRIPTION OF FOOD	SERVING SIZE	WT (G)	CAL (KCAL)	PROT (G)	FAT (G)	SAT FAT (G)	CHOL (MG)	CARBO (G)	CALC (MG)	SOD (MG)
Wheat bread	1 slice	25	65	2	1	0.2	0	12	32	138
Whole-wheat bread	1 slice	28	70	3	1	0.4	0	13	20	180
CEREALS										
All-bran cereal	1 oz	28.35	70	4	1	0.1	0	1	23	320
Cap'n Crunch cereal	1 oz	28.35	120	1	3	1.7	0	23	5	213
Cheerios cereal	1 oz	28.35	110	4	2	0.3	0	20	48	307
Corn flakes, Kellogg's	1 oz	28.35	110	2	0	0	0	24	1	351
Cream of wheat, cooked	1 pkt	142	100	3	0	0	0	21	20	241
Froot Loops cereal	1 oz	28.35	110	2	1	0.2	0	25	3	145
Golden Grahams cereal	1 oz	28.35	110	2	1	0.7	0	24	17	346
Grape-Nuts cereal	1 oz	28.35	100	3	0	0	0	23	11	197
Honey-Nut Cheerios cereal	1 oz	28.35	105	3	1	0.1	0	23	20	257
Lucky Charms cereal	1 oz	28.35	110	3	1	0.2	0	23	32	201
Nature Valley Granola cereal	1 oz	28.35	125	3	5	3.3	0	19	18	58
Oatmeal, cooked, instant, flavored, fortified	1 pkt	164	160	5	2	0.3	0	31	168	254
Oatmeal, cooked, regular, quick, instant, w/salt	1 cup	234	145	6	2	0.4	0	25	19	374
100% Natural cereal	1 oz	28.35	135	3	6	4.1	0	18	49	12
Product 19 cereal	1 oz	28.35	110	3	0	0	0	24	3	325
Raisin Bran, Kellogg's	1 oz	28.35	90	3	1	0.1	0	21	10	207
Raisin Bran, Post	1 oz	28.35	85	3	1	0.1	0	21	13	185
Rice Krispies cereal	1 oz	28.35	110	2	0	0	0	25	4	340
Shredded Wheat cereal	1 oz	28.35	100	3	1	0.1	0	23	11	3
Special K cereal	1 oz	28.35	110	6	0	0	0	21	8	265
Sugar Frosted Flakes, Kellogg's	1 oz	28.35	110	1	0	0	0	26	1	230
Sugar Smacks cereal	1 oz	28.35	105	2	1	0.1	0	25	3	75
Super Sugar Crisp cereal	1 oz	28.35	105	2	0	0	0	26	6	25
Total cereal	1 oz	28.35	100	3	1	0.1	0	22	48	352
Wheaties cereal	1 oz	28.35	100	3	0	0.1	0	23	43	354
DAIRY PRODUCTS										
Cheddar cheese	1 oz	28.35	115	7	9	6	30	0	204	176
Chocolate milk, regular	1 cup	250	210	8	8	5.3	31	26	280	149
Cottage cheese, creamed, large curd	1 cup	225	235	28	10	6.4	34	6	135	911
Cream cheese	1 oz	28.35	100	2	10	6.2	31	1	23	84
Half and half, cream	1 Tbsp	15	20	0	2	1.1	6	1	16	6
Milk, low fat, 2%	1 cup	244	120	8	5	2.9	18	12	297	122
Milk, skim	1 cup	245	85	8	0	0.3	4	12	302	126
Milk, whole, 3.3% fat	1 cup	244	150	8	8	5.1	33	11	291	120
Pasteurized processed cheese food, American	1 oz	28.35	95	6	7	4.4	18	2	163	337
Ricotta cheese, whole milk	1 cup	246	430	28	32	20.4	124	7	509	207
Shakes, thick, chocolate	10 oz	283	335	9	8	4.8	30	60	374	314
Shakes, thick, vanilla	10 oz	283	315	11	9	5.3	33	50	413	270
Sherbet, 2% fat	1 cup	193	270	2	4	2.4	14	59	103	88
Sour cream	1 Tbsp	12	25	0	3	1.6	5	1	14	6
Swiss cheese	1 oz	28.35	105	8	8	5	26	1	272	74
Whipped topping, pressurized	1 Tbsp	3	10	0	1	0.4	2	0	3	4
Yogurt, w/low-fat milk, fruit flavored	8 oz	227	230	10	2	1.6	10	43	345	133
Yogurt, w/low-fat milk, plain	8 oz	227	145	12	4	2.3	14	16	415	159

DESCRIPTION OF FOOD	SERVING SIZE	WT (G)	CAL (KCAL)	PROT (G)	FAT (G)	SAT FAT (G)	CHOL (MG)	CARBO (G)	CALC (MG)	SOD (MG)
DESSERTS, CRACKERS, AND SNACKS										
Angel food cake, from mix	1 piece	53	125	3	0	0	0	29	44	269
Apple pie	1 piece	158	405	3	18	4.6	0	60	13	476
Blueberry muffins, from commercial mix	1 muffin	45	140	3	5	1.4	45	22	15	225
Blueberry pie	1 piece	158	380	4	17	4.3	0	55	17	423
Bran muffins, from commercial mix	1 muffin	45	140	3	4	1.3	28	24	27	385
Brownies w/nuts, frosting, commercial	1 brownie	25	100	1	4	1.6	14	16	13	59
Carrot cake, cream cheese frosting	1 piece	96	385	4	21	4.1	74	48	44	279
Cheesecake	1 piece	92	280	5	18	9.9	170	26	52	204
Cheese crackers, plain	10 crackers	10	50	1	3	0.9	6	6	11	112
Cheese crackers, sandwich, peanut	1 sandwich	8	40	1	2	0.4	1	5	7	90
Cherry pie	1 piece	158	410	4	18	4.7	0	61	22	480
Chocolate chip cookies, commercial	4 cookies	42	180	2	9	2.9	5	28	13	140
Coffee cake, crumb, from mix	1 piece	72	230	5	7	2	47	38	44	310
Corn chips	1 oz	28.35	155	2	9	1.4	0	16	35	233
Corn muffins, from commercial mix	1 muffin	45	145	3	6	1.7	42	22	30	291
Croissants	1 croissant	57	235	5	12	3.5	13	27	20	452
Custard pie	1 piece	152	330	9	17	5.6	169	36	146	436
Danish pastry, fruit	1 pastry	65	235	4	13	3.9	56	28	17	233
Devil's food cake, chocolate frosting, from mix	1 piece	69	235	3	8	3.5	37	40	41	181
Doughnuts, cake type, plain	1 donut	50	210	3	12	2.8	20	24	22	192
English muffins, plain	1 muffin	57	140	5	1	0.3	0	27	96	378
French toast, home recipe	1 slice	65	155	6	7	1.6	112	17	72	257
Gingerbread cake, from mix	1 piece	63	175	2	4	1.1	1	32	57	192
Graham crackers, plain	2 crackers	14	60	1	1	0.4	0	11	6	86
Lemon meringue pie	1 piece	140	355	5	14	4.3	143	53	20	395
Oatmeal cookies w/raisins	4 cookies	52	245	3	10	2.5	2	36	18	148
Peanut butter cookies, home recipe	4 cookies	48	245	4	14	4	22	28	21	142
Popcorn, air-popped, unsalted	1 cup	8	30	1	0	0	0	6	1	0
Popcorn, popped, vegetable oil, salted	1 cup	11	55	1	3	0.5	0	6	3	86
Pound cake, from home recipe	1 slice	30	120	2	5	1.2	32	15	20	96
Pretzels, stick	10 pretzels	3	10	0	0	0	0	2	1	48
Pumpkin pie	1 piece	152	320	6	17	6.4	109	37	78	325
Rye wafers, whole-grain	2 wafers	14	55	1	1	0.3	0	10	7	115
Saltines	4 crackers	12	50	1	1	0.5	4	9	3	165
Sandwich-type cookies	4 cookies	40	195	2	8	2	0	29	12	189
Sugar cookies	4 cookies	48	235	2	12	2.3	29	31	50	261
Toaster pastries	1 pastry	54	210	2	6	1.7	0	38	104	248
Wheat, thin crackers	4 crackers	8	35	1	1	0.5	0	5	3	69
EGGS										
Eggs, cooked, fried	1 egg	46	90	6	7	1.9	211	1	25	162
Eggs, cooked, hard-cooked	1 egg	50	75	6	5	1.6	213	1	25	62
Eggs, cooked, scrambled/omelet	1 egg	61	100	7	7	2.2	215	1	44	171
Eggs, raw, whole	1 egg	50	75	6	5	1.6	213	1	25	63
FATS, OILS, AND DRESSINGS										
Butter, salted	1 Tbsp	14	100	0	11	7.1	31	0	3	116
Corn oil	1 Tbsp	14	125	0	14	1.8	0	0	0	0
Fats, cooking/vegetable shortening	1 Tbsp	13	115	0	13	3.3	0	0	0	0

DESCRIPTION OF FOOD	SERVING SIZE	WT (G)	CAL (KCAL)	PROT (G)	FAT (G)	SAT FAT (G)	CHOL (MG)	CARBO (G)	CALC (MG)	SOD (MG)
French salad dressing, regular	1 Tbsp	16	85	0	9	1.4	0	1	2	188
Italian salad dressing, regular	1 Tbsp	15	80	0	9	1.3	0	1	1	162
Margarine, imitation, 40% fat	1Tbsp	14	50	0	5	1.1	0	0	2	134
Margarine, regular, soft, 80% fat	1 Tbsp	14	100	0	11	1.9	0	0	4	151
Mayonnaise, imitation	1 Tbsp	15	35	0	3	0.5	4	2	0	75
Mayonnaise, regular	1 Tbsp	14	100	0	11	1.7	8	0	3	80
Mayonnaise-type salad dressing	1 Tbsp	15	60	0	5	0.7	4	4	2	107
Olive oil	1 Tbsp	14	125	0	14	1.9	0	0	0	0
Safflower oil	1 Tbsp	14	125	0	14	1.3	0	0	0	0
Tartar sauce	1 Tbsp	14	75	0	8	1.2	4	1	3	182
Vinegar and oil salad dressing	1 Tbsp	16	70	0	8	1.5	0	0	0	0
FISH AND SHELLFISH										
Fish sticks, frozen, reheated	1 stick	28	70	6	3	0.8	26	4	11	53
Flounder or sole, baked, butter	3 oz	85	120	16	6	3.2	68	0	13	145
Oysters, breaded, fried	1 oyster	45	90	5	5	1.4	35	5	49	70
Salmon, baked, red	3 oz	85	140	21	5	1.2	60	0	26	55
Salmon, smoked	3 oz	85	150	18	8	2.6	51	0	12	1,700
Sardines, canned, oil, drained	3 oz	85	175	20	9	2.1	85	0	371	425
Scallops, breaded, frozen, reheated	6 scallops	90	195	15	10	2.5	70	10	39	298
Shrimp, canned, drained	3 oz	85	100	21	1	0.2	128	1	98	1,955
Trout, broiled, w/butter, lemon juice	3 oz	85	175	21	9	4.1	71	0	26	122
Tuna, canned, drained, oil, chunk, light	3 oz	85	165	24	7	1.4	55	0	7	303
Tuna, canned, water, white	3 oz	85	135	30	1	0.3	48	0	17	468
FRUITS AND FRUIT JUICES										
Apple juice, canned	1 cup	248	115	0	0	0	0	29	17	7
Apples, dried, sulfured	10 rings	64	155	1	0	0	0	42	9	56
Apples, raw, unpeeled, 3 per lb	1 apple	138	80	0	0	0.1	0	21	10	0
Applesauce, canned, sweetened	1 cup	255	195	0	0	0.1	0	51	10	8
Apricots, dried, uncooked	1 cup	130	310	5	1	0	0	80	59	13
Apricots, raw	3 apricots	106	50	1	0	0	0	12	15	1
Avocados	1 avocado	304	340	5	27	5.3	0	27	33	15
Bananas	1 banana	114	105	1	1	0.2	0	27	7	1
Blackberries, raw	1 cup	144	75	1	1	0.2	0	18	46	0
Blueberries, raw	1 cup	145	80	1	1	0	0	20	9	9
Cantaloupe, raw	1/2 melon	267	95	2	1	0.1	0	22	29	24
Cherries, sweet, raw	10 cherries	68	50	1	1	0.1	0	11	10	0
Cranberry juice cocktail w/vitamin C	1 cup	253	145	0	0	0	0	38	8	10
Cranberry sauce, canned, sweetened	1 cup	277	420	1	0	0	0	108	11	80
Fruit cocktail, canned, juice pack	1 cup	248	115	1	0	0	0	29	20	10
Grapefruit juice, canned, sweetened	1 cup	250	115	1	0	0	0	28	20	5
Grapefruit, raw, white	½ fruit	120	40	1	0	0	0	10	14	0
Grape juice, frozen, diluted, sweetened, w/vitamin C	1 cup	250	125	0	0	0.1	0	32	10	5
Grapes, raw	10 grapes	50	35	0	0	0.1	0	9	6	1
Honeydew melon, raw	¹⁄₁₀ melon	129	45	1	0	0	0	12	8	13
Kiwifruit, raw	1 kiwi	76	45	1	0	0	0	11	20	4
Lemons, raw	1 lemon	58	15	1	0	0	0	5	15	1
Mangos, raw	1 mango	207	135	1	1	0.1	0	35	21	4
Nectarines, raw	1 nectarine	136	65	1	1	0.1	0	16	7	0
Orange juice, concentrate, diluted	1 cup	249	110	2	0	0	0	27	22	2

DESCRIPTION OF FOOD	SERVING SIZE	WT (G)	CAL (KCAL)	PROT (G)	FAT (G)	SAT FAT (G)	CHOL (MG)	CARBO (G)	CALC (MG)	SOD (MG)
Oranges, raw	1 orange	131	60	1	0	0	0	15	52	0
Papayas, raw	1 cup	140	65	1	0	0.1	0	17	35	9
Peaches, canned, heavy syrup	1 cup	256	190	1	0	0	0	51	8	15
Peaches, canned, juice pack	1 cup	248	110	2	0	0	0	29	15	10
Peaches, raw	1 peach	87	35	1	0	0	0	10	4	0
Pears, raw, Bartlett	1 pear	166	100	1	1	0	0	25	18	0
Pineapple, canned, heavy syrup	1 cup	255	200	1	0	0	0	52	36	3
Pineapple, raw, diced	1 cup	155	75	1	1	0	0	19	11	2
Plums, raw, 1½-in diam	1 plum	28	15	0	0	0	0	4	1	0
Prunes, dried	5 large	49	115	1	0	0	0	31	25	2
Raisins	1 cup	145	435	5	1	0.2	0	115	71	17
Raspberries, frozen, sweetened	1 cup	250	255	2	0	0	0	65	38	3
Raspberries, raw	1 cup	123	60	1	1	0	0	14	27	0
Strawberries, frozen, sweetened	1 cup	255	245	1	0	0	0	66	28	8
Strawberries, raw	1 cup	149	45	1	1	0	0	10	21	1
Tangerines, raw	1 tangerine	84	35	1	0	0	0	9	12	1
Watermelon, raw	1 piece	482	155	3	2	0.3	0	35	39	10
GRAINS										
Bulgur, uncooked	1 cup	170	600	19	3	1.2	0	129	49	7
Macaroni, cooked, firm	1 cup	130	190	7	1	0.1	0	39	14	1
Noodles, chow mein, canned	1 cup	45	220	6	11	2.1	5	26	14	450
Noodles, egg, cooked	1 cup	160	200	7	2	0.5	50	37	16	3
Rice, brown, cooked	1 cup	195	230	5	1	0.3	0	50	23	0
Rice, white, cooked	1 cup	205	225	4	0	0.1	0	50	21	0
Rice, white, instant, cooked	1 cup	165	180	4	0	0.1	0	40	5	0
Spaghetti, cooked, firm	1 cup	130	190	7	1	0.1	0	39	14	1
Tortilla, corn	1 tortilla	30	65	2	1	0.1	0	13	42	1
Waffles, from mix	1 waffle	75	205	7	8	2.7	59	27	179	515
LEGUMES, NUTS, AND SEEDS										
Almonds, whole	1 oz	28.35	165	6	15	1.4	0	6	75	3
Beans, dry, canned, w/pork and tomato sauce	1 cup	255	310	16	7	2.4	10	48	138	1,181
Black beans, dry, cooked, drained	1 cup	171	225	15	1	0.1	0	41	47	1
Black-eyed peas, dry, cooked	1 cup	250	190	13	1	0.2	0	35	43	20
Brazil nuts	1 oz	28.35	185	4	19	4.6	0	4	50	1
Cashew nuts, dry-roasted, salted	1 oz	28.35	165	4	13	2.6	0	9	13	181
Cashew nuts, oil-roasted, salted	1 cup	130	750	21	63	12.4	0	37	53	814
Chickpeas, cooked, drained	1 cup	163	270	15	4	0.4	0	45	80	11
Coconut, dried, sweetened, shredded	1 cup	93	470	3	33	29.3	0	44	14	244
Filberts (hazelnuts), chopped	1 cup	115	725	15	72	5.3	0	18	216	3
Lentils, dry, cooked	1 cup	200	215	16	1	0.1	0	38	50	26
Lima beans, dry, cooked, drained	1 cup	190	260	16	1	0.2	0	49	55	4
Macadamia nuts, oil roasted, salted	1 cup	134	960	10	103	15.4	0	17	60	348
Mixed nuts w/peanuts, dry, salted	1 oz	28.35	170	5	15	2	0	7	20	190
Peanut butter	1 Tbsp	16	95	5	8	1.4	0	3	5	75
Peanuts, oil roasted, salted	1 cup	145	840	39	71	9.9	0	27	125	626
Peas, split, dry, cooked	1 cup	200	230	16	1	0.1	0	42	22	26
Pine nuts	1 oz	28.35	160	3	17	2.7	0	5	2	20
Pinto beans, dry, cooked, drained	1 cup	180	265	15	1	0.1	0	49	86	3
Pumpkin and squash kernels	1 oz	28.35	155	7	13	2.5	0	5	12	5
Red kidney beans, dry, canned	1 cup	255	230	15	1	0.1	0	42	74	968
Walnuts, black, chopped	1 cup	125	760	30	71	4.5	0	15	73	1

DESCRIPTION OF FOOD	SERVING SIZE	WT (G)	CAL (KCAL)	PROT (G)	FAT (G)	SAT FAT (G)	CHOL (MG)	CARBO (G)	CALC (MG)	SOD (MG)
MEATS AND MEAT PRODUCTS										
Beef, canned, corned	3 oz	85	185	22	10	4.2	80	0	17	802
Beef roast, eye round, lean	2.6 oz	75	135	22	5	1.9	52	0	3	46
Beef roast, rib, lean	2.2 oz	61	150	17	9	3.6	49	0	5	45
Beef steak, sirloin, broiled, lean	2.5 oz	72	150	22	6	2.6	64	0	8	48
Bologna	2 slices	57	180	7	16	6.1	31	2	7	581
Brown and serve sausage, browned	1 link	13	50	2	5	1.7	9	0	1	105
Frankfurter (hot dog), cooked	1 frank	45	145	5	13	4.8	23	1	5	504
Ground beef, broiled, lean	3 oz	85	230	21	16	6.2	74	0	9	65
Ground beef, broiled, regular	3 oz	85	245	20	18	6.9	76	0	9	70
Lamb chops, loin, broiled, lean	2.3 oz	64	140	19	6	2.6	60	0	12	54
Pork chop, loin, pan fried, lean	2.4 oz	67	180	19	11	3.7	72	0	3	57
Pork, cured, bacon, Canadian, cooked	2 slices	46	85	11	4	1.3	27	1	5	711
Pork, cured, bacon, regular, cooked	3 slices	19	110	6	9	3.3	16	0	2	303
Pork, cured, ham, roasted, lean	2.4 oz	68	105	17	4	1.3	37	0	5	902
Pork, luncheon meat, cooked ham, regular	2 slices	57	105	10	6	1.9	32	2	4	751
Salami, cooked type	2 slices	57	145	8	11	4.6	37	1	7	607
Sandwich spread, pork, beef	1 Tbsp	15	35	1	3	0.9	6	2	2	152
Veal cutlet, med. fat, braised, broiled	3 oz	85	185	23	9	4.1	86	0	9	56
MIXED DISHES										
Beef and vegetable stew, home recipe	1 cup	245	220	16	11	4.4	71	15	29	292
Beef potpie, home recipe	1 piece	210	515	21	30	7.9	42	39	29	596
Cheeseburger, 4-oz patty	1 sandwich	194	525	30	31	15.1	104	40	236	1,224
Cheeseburger, regular	1 sandwich	112	300	15	15	7.3	44	28	135	672
Chicken à la king, home recipe	1 cup	245	470	27	34	12.9	221	12	127	760
Chicken and noodles, home recipe	1 cup	240	365	22	18	5.1	103	26	26	600
Chicken chow mein, canned	1 cup	250	95	7	0	0.1	8	18	45	725
Chili con carne w/beans, canned	1 cup	255	340	19	16	5.8	28	31	82	1,354
Chop suey w/beef and pork, home recipe	1 cup	250	300	26	17	4.3	68	13	60	1,053
English muffin, egg, cheese, bacon	1 sandwich	138	360	18	18	8	213	31	197	832
Fish sandwich, reg, w/cheese	1 sandwich	140	420	16	23	6.3	56	39	132	667
Hamburger, regular	1 sandwich	98	245	12	11	4.4	32	28	56	463
Macaroni and cheese, home recipe	1 cup	200	430	17	22	9.8	44	40	362	1,086
Pizza, cheese	1 slice	120	290	15	9	4.1	56	39	220	699
Quiche lorraine	1 slice	176	600	13	48	23.2	285	29	211	653
Roast beef sandwich	1 sandwich	150	345	22	13	3.5	55	34	60	757
Spaghetti, meatballs, tomato sauce	1 cup	248	330	19	12	3.9	89	39	124	1,009
Spaghetti, tomato sauce, cheese	1 cup	250	260	9	9	3	8	37	80	955
POULTRY AND POULTRY PRODUCTS										
Chicken frankfurter	1 frank	45	115	6	9	2.5	45	3	43	616
Chicken, fried, batter, breast	4.9 oz	140	365	35	18	4.9	119	13	28	385
Chicken, fried, batter, drumstick	2.5 oz	72	195	16	11	3	62	6	12	194
Chicken, roasted, breast	3.0 oz	86	140	27	3	0.9	73	0	13	64
Turkey, roasted, dark meat	4 pieces	85	160	24	6	2.1	72	0	27	67
Turkey, roasted, light meat	2 pieces	85	135	25	3	0.9	59	0	16	54
SAUCES AND GRAVIES										
Barbecue sauce	1 Tbsp	16	10	0	0	0	0	02	3	130
Beef gravy, canned	1 cup	233	125	9	5	2.7	7	11	14	1,305
Brown gravy from dry mix	1 cup	261	80	3	2	0.9	2	14	66	1,147

DESCRIPTION OF FOOD	SERVING SIZE	WT (G)	CAL (KCAL)	PROT (G)	FAT (G)	SAT FAT (G)	CHOL (MG)	CARBO (G)	CALC (MG)	SOD (MG)
Cheese sauce w/milk, from mix	1 cup	279	305	16	17	9.3	53	23	569	1,565
Chicken gravy, canned	1 cup	238	190	5	14	3.4	5	13	48	1,373
Soy sauce	1 Tbsp	18	10	2	0	0	0	2	3	1,029
SOUPS										
Bean with bacon soup, canned	1 cup	253	170	8	6	1.5	3	23	81	951
Beef broth, bouillon, consommé, canned	1 cup	240	15	3a	1	0.3	0	0	14	782
Beef noodle soup, canned	1 cup	244	85	5	3	1.1	5	9	15	952
Bouillon, dehydrated, unprepared	1 packet	6	15	1	1	0.3	1	1	4	1,019
Chicken noodle soup, canned	1 cup	241	75	4	2	0.7	7	9	17	1,106
Chicken noodle soup, dehydrated, prepared	1 packet	188	40	2	1	0.2	2	6	24	957
Chicken rice soup, canned	1 cup	241	60	4	2	0.5	7	7	17	815
Clam chowder, Manhattan, canned	1 cup	244	80	4	2	0.4	2	12	34	1,808
Clam chowder, New England, w/milk	1 cup	248	165	9	7	3	22	17	186	992
Cream of chicken soup w/milk, canned	1 cup	248	190	7	11	4.6	27	15	181	1,047
Cream of mushroom soup w/milk canned	1 cup	248	205	6	14	5.1	20	15	179	1,076
Minestrone soup, canned	1 cup	241	80	4	3	0.6	2	11	34	911
Onion soup, dehydrated, prepared	1 packet	184	20	1	0	0.1	0	4	9	635
Pea, green, soup, canned	1 cup	250	165	9	3	1.4	0	27	28	988
Tomato soup w/milk, canned	1 cup	248	160	6	6	2.9	17	22	159	932
Tomato soup w/water, canned	1 cup	244	85	2	2	0.4	0	17	12	871
Tomato vegetable soup, dehydrated, prepared	1 packet	189	40	1	1	0.3	0	8	6	856
Vegetable beef soup, canned	1 cup	244	80	6	2	0.9	5	10	17	956
Vegetarian soup, canned	1 cup	241	70	2	2	0.3	0	12	22	822
SUGAR AND SWEETS										
Caramels, plain or chocolate	1 oz	28.35	115	1	3	2.2	1	22	42	64
Custard, baked	1 cup	265	305	14	15	6.8	278	29	297	209
Fudge, chocolate, plain	1 oz	28.35	115	1	3	2.1	1	21	22	54
Gelatin desert, prepared	½ cup	120	70	2	0	0	0	17	2	55
Gumdrops	1 oz	28.35	100	0	0	0	0	25	2	10
Hard candy	1 oz	28.35	110	0	0	0	0	28	0	7
Honey	1 Tbsp	21	65	0	0	0	0	17	1	1
Jams and preserves	1 Tbsp	20	55	0	0	0	0	14	4	2
Jellies	1 Tbsp	18	50	0	0	0	0	13	2	5
Jelly beans	1 oz	28.35	105	0	0	0	0	26	1	7
Marshmallows	1 oz	28.35	90	1	0	0	0	23	1	25
Milk chocolate candy, plain	1 oz	28.35	145	2	9	5.4	6	16	50	23
Milk chocolate candy, w/almonds	1 oz	28.35	150	3	10	4.8	5	15	65	23
Milk chocolate candy, w/peanuts	1 oz	28.35	155	4	11	4.2	5	13	49	19
Molasses, cane, blackstrap	2 Tbsp	40	85	0	0	0	0	22	274	38
Pudding, chocolate, cooked from mix	½ cup	130	150	4	4	2.4	15	25	146	167
Pudding, chocolate, instant, from mix	½ cup	130	155	4	4	2.3	14	27	130	440
Pudding, vanilla, cooked, from mix	½ cup	130	145	4	4	2.3	15	25	132	178
Pudding, vanilla, instant, from mix	½ cup	130	150	4	4	2.2	15	27	129	375
Semisweet chocolate	1 cup	170	860	7	61	36.2	0	97	51	24
Sugar, brown, packed	1 cup	220	820	0	0	0	0	212	187	97
Sugar, white, granulated	1 Tbsp	12	45	0	0	0	0	12	0	0
Table syrup (corn and maple)	2 Tbsp	42	122	0	0	0	0	32	1	19

DESCRIPTION OF FOOD	SERVING SIZE	WT (G)	CAL (KCAL)	PROT (G)	FAT (G)	SAT FAT (G)	CHOL (MG)	CARBO (G)	CALC (MG)	SOD (MG)
VEGETABLES AND VEGETABLE PRODUCTS										
Beets, cooked, drained, diced	1 cup	170	55	2	0	0	0	11	19	83
Broccoli, raw	1 spear	151	40	4	1	0.1	0	8	72	41
Cabbage, common, raw	1 cup	70	15	1	0	0	0	4	33	13
Carrots, raw, whole	1 carrot	72	30	1	0	0	0	7	19	25
Cauliflower, raw	1 cup	100	25	2	0	0	0	5	29	15
Corn, cooked from frozen, yellow	1 ear	63	60	2	0	0.1	0	14	2	3
Cucumber, w/peel	6 slices	28	5	0	0	0	0	1	4	1
Eggplant, cooked, steamed	1 cup	96	25	1	0	0	0	6	6	3
Endive, curly, raw	1 cup	50	10	1	0	0	0	2	26	11
Lettuce, crisphead, raw, head	1 head	539	70	5	1	0.1	0	11	102	49
Lettuce, looseleaf	1 cup	56	10	1	0	0	0	2	38	5
Mushrooms, raw	1 cup	70	20	1	0	0	0	3	4	3
Onions, raw, sliced	1 cup	115	40	1	0	0.1	0	8	29	2
Peas, edible pod, cooked, drained	1 cup	160	65	5	0	0.1	0	11	67	6
Peas, green, frozen, cooked, drained	1 cup	160	125	8	0	0.1	0	23	38	139
Peppers, sweet, raw	1 pepper	74	20	1	0	0	0	4	4	2
Potato chips	10 chips	20	105	1	7	1.8	0	10	5	94
Potatoes, au gratin, from mix	1 cup	245	230	6	10	6.3	12	31	203	1,076
Potatoes, baked with skin	1 potato	202	220	5	0	0.1	0	51	20	16
Potatoes, boiled, peeled after	1 potato	136	120	3	0	0	0	27	7	5
Potatoes, french-fried, frozen, fried	10 strips	50	160	2	8	2.5	0	20	10	108
Potatoes, french-fried, frozen, oven	10 strips	50	110	2	4	2.1	0	17	5	16
Potatoes, mashed, from dehydrated	1 cup	210	235	4	12	7.2	29	32	103	697
Potatoes, mashed, recipe, milk and margarine	1 cup	210	225	4	9	2.2	4	35	55	620
Potato salad made w/mayonnaise	1 cup	250	360	7	21	3.6	170	28	48	1,323
Radishes, raw	4 radishes	18	5	0	0	0	0	1	4	4
Sauerkraut, canned	1 cup	236	45	2	0	0.1	0	10	71	1,560
Snap bean, frozen, cooked, drained, green	1 cup	135	35	2	0	0	0	8	61	18
Snap bean, raw, cooked, drained, green	1 cup	125	45	2	0	0.1	0	10	58	4
Spinach, raw	1 cup	55	10	2	0	0	0	2	54	43
Squash, summer, cooked, drained	1 cup	180	35	2	1	0.1	0	8	49	2
Squash, winter, baked	1 cup	205	80	2	1	0.3	0	18	29	2
Sweet potatoes, baked, peeled	1 potato	114	115	2	0	0	0	28	32	11
Tomato juice, canned with salt	1 cup	244	40	2	0	0	0	10	22	881
Tomato paste, canned with salt	1 cup	262	220	10	2	0.3	0	49	92	2,070
Tomato purée, canned with salt	1 cup	250	105	4	0	0	0	25	38	998
Tomato sauce, canned with salt	1 cup	245	75	3	0	0.1	0	18	34	1,482
Tomatoes, canned w/salt	1 cup	240	50	2	1	0.1	0	10	62	391
Tomatoes, raw	1 tomato	123	25	1	0	0	0	5	9	10
Vegetable juice cocktail, canned	1 cup	242	45	2	0	0	0	11	27	883
Vegetables, mixed, cooked from frozen	1 cup	182	105	5	0	0.1	0	24	46	64
MISCELLANEOUS										
Catsup	1 Tbsp	15	15	0	0	0	0	4	3	156
Gelatin, dry	1 envelope	7	25	6	0	0	0	0	1	6
Mustard, prepared, yellow	1 tsp	5	5	0	0	0	0	0	4	63
Olives, canned, green	4 medium	13	15	0	2	0.2	0	0	8	312
Olives, canned, ripe	3 small	9	15	0	2	0.3	0	0	10	68
Pickles, cucumber, dill	1 pickle	65	5	0	0	0	0	1	17	928
Pickles, cucumber, fresh pack	2 slices	15	10	0	0	0	0	3	5	101
Relish, sweet	1 Tbsp	15	20	0	0	0	0	5	3	107
Salt	1 tsp	5.5	0	0	0	0	0	0	14	2,132

Source: Summarized from U.S. Department of Agriculture, Agricultural Research Department, 1997. USDA Nutrient Database for Standard Reference, Release 11-1. Nutrient Data Laboratory Home Page (see http://www.nal.usda.gov/fnic/foodcomp).

Glossary

Abortion   The medical means of terminating a pregnancy.

Abstinence   Refraining from an addictive behavior.

Accessory glands   The seminal vesicles, prostate gland, and Cowper's glands.

Accountability   Accepting responsibility for personal decisions, choices, and actions.

Acid rain   Precipitation contaminated with acidic pollutants.

Acquired immune deficiency syndrome (AIDS)   Extremely virulent sexually transmitted disease that renders the immune system inoperative.

Acquired immunity   Immunity developed during life in response to disease, vaccination, or exposure.

Active euthanasia   "Mercy killing" in which a person or organization knowingly acts to hasten the death of a terminally ill person.

Activities of daily living (ADLs)   Tasks of everyday living, such as bathing and walking up the stairs.

Acute bronchitis   A form of bronchitis most often caused by viruses.

Adaptive response   Form of adjustment in which the body attempts to restore homeostasis.

Adaptive thermogenesis   Theoretical mechanism by which the brain regulates metabolic activity according to caloric intake.

Addiction   Continued involvement with a substance or activity despite ongoing negative consequences.

Addictive exercisers   People who exercise compulsively to try to meet needs of nurturance, intimacy, self-esteem, and self-competency.

Adequate intakes (AIs)   Best estimates of nutritional needs.

Adjustment   The attempt to cope with a given situation.

Adrenocorticotrophic hormone (ACTH)   A pituitary hormone that stimulates the adrenal glands to secrete cortisol.

Aerobic capacity   The current functional status of a person's cardiovascular system; measured as $VO_{2\,max}$.

Aerobic exercise   Any type of exercise, typically performed at moderate levels of intensity for extended periods of time (20 to 30 minutes or longer), that increases heart rate.

Afterbirth   The expelled placenta.

Ageism   Discrimination based on age.

Aggravated rape   Rape that involves multiple attackers, strangers, weapons, or a physical beating.

Aggressive communicators   People who use hostile, loud, and blaming communication styles.

Aging   The patterns of life changes that occur in members of all species as they grow older.

Alcohol abuse (alcoholism)   Use of alcohol that interferes with work, school, or personal relationships or that entails violations of the law.

Alcoholic hepatitis   Condition resulting from prolonged use of alcohol in which the liver is inflamed. It can result in death.

Alcoholics Anonymous (AA)   An organization whose goal is to help alcoholics stop drinking; includes auxiliary branches such as Al-Anon and Alateen.

Allergy   Hypersensitive reaction to a specific antigen or allergen in the environment in which the body produces excessive antibodies to that antigen or allergen.

Allopathic medicine   Traditional, Western medical practice; in theory, based on scientifically validated methods and procedures.

Alternative insemination   Fertilization accomplished by depositing a partner's or a donor's semen into a woman's vagina via a thin tube; almost always done in a doctor's office.

Alternative medicine   Treatment used in place of conventional medicine.

Alveoli   Tiny air sacs of the lungs.

Alzheimer's disease   A chronic condition involving changes in nerve fibers of the brain that results in mental deterioration.

Amino acids   The building blocks of protein.

Amniocentesis   A medical test in which a small amount of fluid is drawn from the amniotic sac to test for Down syndrome and genetic diseases.

Amniotic sac   The protective pouch surrounding the baby.

Amphetamines   Prescription stimulants not commonly used today because of the dangers associated with them.

Amyl nitrite   A drug that dilates blood vessels and is properly used to relieve chest pain.

Anabolic steroids   Artificial forms of the hormone testosterone that promote muscle growth and strength.

Anal intercourse   The insertion of the penis into the anus.

Analgesics   Pain relievers.

Androgyny   Combination of traditional masculine and feminine traits in a single person.

Anemia   Iron deficiency disease that results from the body's inability to produce hemoglobin.

Aneurysm   A weakened blood vessel that may bulge under pressure and, in severe cases, burst.

Angina pectoris   Chest pain occurring as a result of reduced oxygen flow to the heart.

Angiography   A technique for examining blockages in heart arteries. A catheter is inserted into the arteries, a dye is injected, and an x-ray is taken to find the blocked areas. Also called *cardiac catheterization*.

Angioplasty   A technique in which a catheter with a balloon at the tip is inserted into a clogged artery; the balloon is inflated to flatten fatty deposits against artery walls, allowing blood to flow more freely.

Anorexia nervosa   Eating disorder characterized by excessive preoccupation with food, self-starvation, and/or extreme exercising to achieve weight losses.

Antagonism   A type of interaction in which two or more drugs work at the same receptor site.

Antibiotics   Prescription drugs designed to fight bacterial infection.

Antibodies   Substances produced by the body that are individually matched to specific antigens.

Antidepressants   Prescription drugs used to treat clinically diagnosed depression.

Antigen   Substance capable of triggering an immune response.

Antioxidants   Substances believed to protect active people from oxidative stress and resultant tissue damage at the cellular level.

Anxiety disorders   Disorders characterized by persistent feelings of threat and anxiousness in coping with everyday problems.

Appetite   A learned desire to eat that is tied to an emotional or psychological craving for food; often unrelated to nutritional or physiological need.

Arrhythmia   An irregularity in heartbeat.

Arteries   Vessels that carry blood away from the heart to other regions of the body.

Arterioles   Branches of the arteries.

Arteriosclerosis   Condition characterized by deposits of fatty substances, cholesterol, cellular waste products, calcium, and fibrin in the inner lining of an artery.

Arthritis   Painful inflammatory disease of the joints.

Asbestos   A substance that separates into stringy fibers and lodges in the lungs, where it can cause various diseases.

Assertive communicators   People who use direct, honest communication that maintains and defends their rights in a positive manner.

Asthma   A chronic respiratory disease characterized by attacks of wheezing, shortness of breath, and coughing spasms.

Asymptomatic   Without symptoms, or symptom-free.

Atherosclerosis   A general term for thickening and hardening of the arteries.

Atria   The two upper chambers of the heart, which receive blood.

Attitude   Relatively stable set of beliefs, feelings, and behavioral tendencies in relation to something or someone.

Autoerotic behaviors   Sexual self-stimulation.

Autoinoculation   Transmission of a pathogen from one part of the body to another.

Autonomic nervous system (ANS)   The portion of the central nervous system that regulates bodily functions that a person does not normally consciously control.

Autonomy   The ability to care for oneself emotionally, socially, and physically.

Ayurveda (Ayurvedic medicine)   A method of treatment derived largely from ancient India, in which practitioners diagnose by observation and touch and then assign a largely dietary treatment laced with herbal medicines.

Background distressors   Environmental stressors of which people are often unaware.

Bacteria   Single-celled organisms that may cause disease.

Barrier methods   Contraceptive methods that block the meeting of egg and sperm by means of a physical barrier (e.g., condom, diaphragm, or cervical cap), a chemical barrier (e.g., spermicide), or both.

Basal metabolic rate (BMR)   The energy expenditure of the body under resting conditions at normal room temperature.

Belief   Appraisal of the relationship between some object, action, or idea and some attribute of that object, action, or idea.

Benign   Harmless; refers to a noncancerous tumor.

Bereavement   The loss or deprivation experienced by a survivor when a loved one dies.

Bidis   Hand-rolled flavored cigarettes.

Binge drinking   Drinking for the express purpose of becoming intoxicated; five drinks in a single sitting for men and four drinks in a sitting for women.

Binge eating disorder (BED)   Eating disorder characterized by recurrent binge eating, without excessive measures to prevent weight gain.

Bioelectrical impedance analysis (BIA)   A technique of body fat assessment in which electrical currents are passed through fat and lean tissue.

Biofeedback   A technique involving machine self-monitoring of physical responses to stress.

Biologically based therapies   Combination of natural and biologically based therapies and products used to restore health.

Biopsy   Microscopic examination of tissue to determine if a cancer is present.

Biopsychosocial model of addiction   Theory of the relationship between an addict's biological (genetic) nature and psychological and environmental influences.

Bisexual   Experiencing attraction to and preference for sexual activity with people of both sexes.

Black tar heroin   A dark brown, sticky form of heroin.

Blood alcohol concentration (BAC)   The ratio of alcohol to total blood volume; the factor used to measure the physiological and behavioral effects of alcohol.

Body mass index (BMI)   A technique of weight assessment based on the relationship of weight to height.

Body temperature method   A birth control method in which a woman monitors her body temperature for the rise that signals ovulation in order to abstain from intercourse around this time.

Botulism   A resistant food-borne organism that is extremely virulent.

Brain death   The irreversible cessation of all functions of the entire brain stem.

Bronchitis   An inflammation of the lining of the bronchial tubes.

Brown fat cells   Specialized type of fat cell that affects the ability to regulate fat metabolism.

Bulimia nervosa   Eating disorder characterized by binge eating followed by inappropriate measures to prevent weight gain.

Burnout   Physical and mental exhaustion caused by excessive stress.

Caffeine   A stimulant found in coffee, tea, chocolate, and some soft drinks.

Caffeinism   Caffeine intoxication brought on by excessive caffeine use; symptoms include chronic insomnia, irritability, anxiety, muscle twitches, and headaches.

Calendar method   A birth control method in which a woman's menstrual cycle is mapped on a calendar to determine presumed fertile times in order to abstain from penis-vagina contact during those times.

Calorie   A unit of measure that indicates the amount of energy obtained from a particular food.

Cancer   A large group of diseases characterized by the uncontrolled growth and spread of abnormal cells.

Candidiasis   Yeastlike fungal disease often transmitted sexually.

Capillaries   Minute blood vessels that branch out from the arterioles; their thin walls allow for the exchange of oxygen, carbon dioxide, nutrients, and waste products among body cells.

Capitation   Prepayment of a fixed monthly amount per patient without regard to the type or number of services provided.

Carbohydrates   Basic nutrients that supply the body with the energy needed to sustain normal activity.

Carbon monoxide   An odorless, colorless gas that originates primarily from motor vehicle emissions. Also found in cigarette smoke and binds at oxygen receptor sites in the blood.

Carcinogens   Cancer-causing agents.

Cardiorespiratory fitness   The ability of the heart, lungs, and blood vessels to supply oxygen to skeletal muscles during sustained physical activity.

Cardiovascular disease (CVD)   Disease of the heart and blood vessels.

Cardiovascular system   A complex system consisting of the heart and blood vessels that transports nutrients, oxygen, hormones, and enzymes throughout the body and regulates temperature, the water levels of cells, and the acidity levels of body components.

Carotenoids   Fat-soluble compounds with antioxidant properties.

Carpal tunnel syndrome   A common occupational injury in which the median nerve in the wrist becomes irritated, causing numbness, tingling, and pain in the fingers and hands.

Cataracts   Clouding of the lens that interrupts the focusing of light on the retina, resulting in blurred vision or eventual blindness.

Celibacy   State of not being involved in a sexual relationship.

Cellulose   Fiber; a major form of complex carbohydrates.

Cerebrospinal fluid   Fluid within and surrounding the brain and spinal cord tissues.

Certified Health Education Specialists (CHESs)   Academically trained health educators who have passed a national competency examination for prevention and intervention programming.

Cervical cap   A small cup made of latex that is designed to fit snugly over the entire cervix.

Cervical mucous method   A birth control method that relies upon observation of changes in cervical mucous to determine when the woman is fertile so the couple can abstain from intercourse during those times.

Cervix   Lower end of the uterus that opens into the vagina.

Cesarean section (C-section)   A surgical procedure in which a baby is removed through an incision made in the mother's abdominal and uterine walls.

Chancre   Sore often found at the site of syphilis infection.

Chemotherapy   The use of drugs to kill cancerous cells.

Chewing tobacco   A stringy type of tobacco that is placed in the mouth and then sucked or chewed.

Child abuse   The systematic harming of a child by a caregiver, typically a parent.

Chlamydia   Bacterially caused STI of the urogenital tract.

Chlorofluorocarbons (CFCs)   Chemicals that contribute to the depletion of the ozone layer.

Cholesterol   A form of fat circulating in the blood that can accumulate on the inner walls of arteries.

Chronic bronchitis   A serious respiratory disorder in which the bronchial tubes become so inflamed and swollen that respiratory function is impaired.

Chronic mood disorder   Experience of persistent sadness, despair, and hopelessness.

Chronic obstructive pulmonary diseases (COPDs)   A collection of chronic lung diseases including asthma, emphysema, and chronic bronchitis.

Cirrhosis   The last stage of liver disease associated with chronic heavy use of alcohol, during which liver cells die and damage becomes permanent.

Clitoris   A pea-sized nodule of tissue located at the top of the labia minora.

Cocaine   A powerful stimulant drug made from the leaves of the South American coca shrub.

Codeine   A drug derived from morphine; used in cough syrups and certain painkillers.

Codependence   A self-defeating relationship pattern in which a person is "addicted to the addict."

Cognitive stress system   The psychological system that governs emotional responses to stress.

Cohabitation   Living together without being married.

Collateral circulation   Adaptation of the heart to partial damage accomplished by rerouting needed blood through unused or underused blood vessels while the damaged heart muscle heals.

Commercial preparations   Commonly used chemical substances including cosmetics, household cleaning products, and industrial by-products.

Common-law marriage   Cohabitation lasting a designated period of time (usually seven years) that is considered legally binding in some states.

Communication   The transmission of information and meaning from one individual to another.

Comorbidity   The presence of a number of diseases at the same time.

Complementary and alternative medicine (CAM)   Forms of treatment distinct from traditional allopathic medicine that until recently were neither taught widely in U.S. medical schools nor generally available in U.S. hospitals.

Complementary medicine   Treatment used in conjunction with conventional medicine.

Complete (high-quality) proteins   Proteins that contain all of the nine essential amino acids.

Complex carbohydrates   A major type of carbohydrate, which provides sustained energy.

Compulsion   Obsessive preoccupation with a behavior and an overwhelming need to perform it.

Compulsive gambler   A person addicted to gambling.

Computerized axial tomography scan (CAT scan)   Diagnostic tool in which a machine uses radiation to view internal organs not normally visible on x-rays.

Concentric muscle action   Force produced while the muscle is shortening.

Conception   The fertilization of an ovum by a sperm.

Condom   A single-use sheath of thin latex or other material designed to fit over an erect penis and to catch semen upon ejaculation.

Conflict   An emotional state that arises when the behavior of one person interferes with the behavior of another.

Conflict resolution   A concerted effort by all parties to resolve points in contention in a constructive manner.

Congeners   Forms of alcohol that are metabolized more slowly than ethanol and produce toxic by-products.

Congenital heart disease   Heart disease that is present at birth.

Congestive heart failure (CHF)   An abnormal cardiovascular condition that reflects impaired cardiac pumping and blood flow; pooling blood leads to congestion in body tissues.

Conjunctivitis   Serious inflammation of the eye caused by any number of pathogens or irritants; can be caused by STDs such as chlamydia.

Contraception   Methods of preventing conception.

Coronary bypass surgery   A surgical technique whereby a blood vessel is implanted to bypass a clogged coronary artery.

Coronary thrombosis   A blood clot occurring in the coronary artery.

Cortisol   Hormone released by the adrenal glands that makes stored nutrients more readily available to meet energy demands.

Counselor   A person having a variety of academic and experiential training who deals with the treatment of emotional problems.

Cowper's glands   Glands that secrete a fluid that lubricates the urethra and neutralizes any acid remaining in the urethra after urination.

Crack   A distillate of powdered cocaine that comes in small, hard "chips" or "rocks."

Creatine   A naturally occurring compound found primarily in skeletal muscle that helps optimize the muscles' energy levels.

Cross-tolerance   The development of a tolerance to one drug that reduces the effects of another, similar drug.

Cunnilingus   Oral stimulation of a female's genitals.

Daily Reference Values (DRVs)   Recommended amounts for micronutrients such as total fat, saturated fat, and cholesterol.

Daily Values (DVs)   The RDIs and DRVs together make up the Daily Values, seen on food and supplement labels.

Death   The permanent ending of all vital functions.

Dehydration   Abnormal depletion of body fluids; a result of lack of water or acute loss of fluids from sweating, blood loss, excessive vomiting and/or diarrhea, etc.

Delirium tremens (DTs)   A state of confusion brought on by withdrawal from alcohol. Symptoms include hallucinations, anxiety, and trembling.

Dementias   Progressive brain impairments that interfere with memory and normal intellectual functioning.

Dengue   A disease transmitted by mosquitoes, which causes flulike symptoms.

Dengue hemorrhagic fever   A more serious form of dengue.

Denial   Inability to perceive or accurately interpret the effects of an addictive behavior.

Dentist   Specialist who diagnoses and treats diseases of the teeth, gums, and oral cavity.

Depo-Provera   An injectable method of birth control that lasts for three months.

Designer drug   A synthetic analog (a drug that produces similar effects) of an existing illicit drug.

Detoxification   The early abstinence period during which an addict adjusts physically and cognitively to being free from the influences of the addiction.

Diabetes mellitus   A disease in which the pancreas fails to produce enough insulin or the body fails to use insulin effectively.

Diagnosis related groups (DRGs)   Diagnostic categories established by the federal government to determine in advance how much hospitals will be reimbursed for the care of a particular Medicare patient.

Diaphragm   A latex, saucer-shaped device designed to cover the cervix and block access to the uterus; should always be used with spermicide.

Diastolic blood pressure   The lower number in the fraction that measures blood pressure, indicating pressure on the walls of the arteries during the relaxation phase of heart activity; abnormal if consistently 95 mm Hg or above.

Dietary Reference Intake (DRI)   A new, combined listing of over 26 essential vitamins and minerals developed by Canadian and U.S. researchers.

Digestive process   The process by which foods are broken down and either absorbed or excreted by the body.

Dilation and curettage (D&C)   An abortion technique in which the cervix is dilated with laminaria for one to two days, after which the uterine walls are scraped clean.

Dilation and evacuation (D&E)   An abortion technique that combines vacuum aspiration with dilation and curettage; fetal tissue is both sucked and scraped out of the uterus.

Dioxins   Highly toxic chlorinated hydrocarbons contained in herbicides and produced during certain industrial processes.

Dipping   Placing a small amount of chewing tobacco between the front lip and teeth for rapid nicotine absorption.

Disaccharide   A combination of two monosaccharides.

Discrimination   Actions that deny equal treatment or opportunities to a group, often based on bias and prejudice.

Disease prevention   Actions or behaviors designed to keep people from getting sick.

Disenfranchised grief   Grief concerning a loss that cannot be openly acknowledged, publicly mourned, or socially supported.

Distillation   The process whereby mash is subjected to high temperatures to release alcohol vapors, which are then condensed and mixed with water to make the final product.

Distress   Stress that can have a negative effect on health.

Diuretics   Drugs that increase the excretion of urine from the body.

Diverticulosis   A condition in which bulges form in the walls of the intestine; results in irritation and infection of the intestine.

Documenting   Giving specific examples of issues being discussed.

Domestic violence   The use of force to control and maintain power over another person in the home environment, including both actual harm and the threat of harm.

Down syndrome   A condition characterized by mental retardation and a variety of physical abnormalities.

Downshifting   Conscious attempt to simplify life in an effort to reduce the stresses and strains of modern living.

Drug abuse   The excessive use of a drug.

Drug misuse   The use of a drug for a purpose for which it was not intended.

Dyathanasia   The passive form of "mercy killing," in which life-prolonging treatments or interventions are not offered or are withheld, thereby allowing a terminally ill person to die naturally.

Dying   The process of decline in body functions, resulting in the death of an organism.

Dysfunctional families   Families in which there is violence; physical, emotional, or sexual abuse; parental discord; or other negative family interactions. Interactions between family members tend to inhibit psychological growth rather than serving to enhance it.

Dysmenorrhea   Condition that causes pain or discomfort in the lower abdomen just before or after menstruation.

Dyspareunia   Pain experienced by women during intercourse.

Dyspnea   Chronic breathlessness.

Eccentric muscle action   Force produced while the muscle is lengthening.

Eclampsia   Untreated preeclamsia can develop into this potentially fatal complication that involves maternal strokes and seizures.

Ecological or Public Health Model   A model in which diseases and other negative health events are viewed as a result of an individual's interaction with his/her social and physical environment.

Ecstasy   A "club drug" that creates feelings of openness and warmth but also raises heart rate and blood pressure.

Ectopic pregnancy   Implantation of a fertilized egg outside the uterus, usually in a fallopian tube; a medical emergency that can end in death from hemorrhage for the mother.

Editing   The process of censoring comments that would be intentionally hurtful or irrelevant to the conversation.

Ejaculation   The propulsion of semen from the penis.

Electrocardiogram (ECG)   A record of the electrical activity of the heart measured during a stress test.

ELISA   Blood test that detects presence of antibodies to HIV virus.

Embolus   Blood clot that is forced through the circulatory system.

Embryo   The fertilized egg from conception until the end of two months' development.

Embryo adoption programs   A procedure whereby an infertile couple is able to purchase frozen embryos donated by another couple.

Embryo freezing   The freezing of an embryo for later implantation.

Embryo transfer   Artificial insemination of a donor with male partner's sperm; after a time, the embryo is transferred from the donor to the female partner's body.

Emergency contraceptive pills (ECPs)   Drugs taken within three days after intercourse to prevent fertilization or implantation.

Emergency minipills   Contraceptive pills containing only progestin that can be taken up to three days after unprotected intercourse.

Emotional health   The "feeling" part of psychosocial health. Includes your emotional reactions to life.

Emotions   Intensified feelings or complex patterns of feelings we constantly experience.

Emphysema   A chronic lung disease in which the tiny air sacs in the lungs are destroyed, making breathing difficult.

Enablers   People who knowingly or unknowingly protect addicts from the natural consequences of their behavior.

Endemic   Describing a disease that is always present to some degree.

Endometriosis A disorder in which uterine lining tissue establishes itself outside the uterus leading to feelings of bloating, discomfort, and other side effects; the leading cause of infertility in the United States.

Endometrium Soft, spongy matter that makes up the uterine lining.

Endorphins Opiate-like hormones that are manufactured in the human body and contribute to natural feelings of well-being.

Environmental tobacco smoke (ETS) Smoke from tobacco products, including sidestream and mainstream smoke.

Enzymes Organic substances that cause bodily changes and destruction of microorganisms.

Epidemic Disease outbreak that affects many people in a community or region at the same time.

Epidermis The outermost layer of the skin.

Epididymis A comma-shaped structure atop the testis where sperm mature.

Epilepsy A neurological disorder caused by abnormal electrical brain activity; can be accompanied by altered consciousness or convulsions.

Epinephrine Also called adrenaline, a hormone that stimulates body systems in response to stress.

Episiotomy A straight incision in the mother's perineum.

Erectile dysfunction (impotence) Difficulty in achieving or maintaining a penile erection sufficient for intercourse.

Ergogenic aids Special dietary supplements taken to increase strength, energy, and the ability to work.

Ergogenic drug Substance that enhances athletic performance.

Erogenous zones Areas of the body of both males and females that, when touched, lead to sexual arousal.

Esophagus Tube that transports food from the mouth to the stomach.

Essential amino acids Nine of the basic nitrogen-containing building blocks of protein that must be obtained from foods to ensure health.

Essential hypertension Hypertension that cannot be attributed to any cause.

Estrogen replacement therapy (ERT) Use of synthetic or animal estrogens to compensate for decreases in estrogens in a woman's body.

Estrogens Hormones that control the menstrual cycle.

Ethnoviolence Violence directed randomly at persons affiliated with a particular group.

Ethyl alcohol (ethanol) An addictive drug produced by fermentation and found in many beverages.

Eustress Stress that presents opportunities for personal growth.

Exercise metabolic rate (EMR) The energy expenditure that occurs during exercise.

Exercise training The systematic performance of exercise at a specified frequency, intensity, and duration to achieve a desired level of physical fitness.

External female genitals The mons pubis, labia majora and minora, clitoris, urethral and vaginal openings, and the vestibule of the vagina and its glands.

External male genitals The penis and scrotum.

Faith Belief that helps each person realize a unique purpose in life.

Fallopian tubes Tubes that extend from the ovaries to the uterus.

Family of origin People present in the household during a child's first years of life-usually parents and siblings.

Fats Basic nutrients composed of carbon and hydrogen atoms; needed for the proper functioning of cells, insulation of body organs against shock, maintenance of body temperature, and healthy skin and hair.

Fellatio Oral stimulation of a male's genitals.

Female condom A single-use polyurethane sheath for internal use by women.

Female orgasmic disorder The inability to achieve orgasm.

Fermentation The process whereby yeast organisms break down plant sugars to yield ethanol.

Fertility A person's ability to reproduce.

Fertility awareness methods (FAMs) Several types of birth control that require alteration of sexual behavior rather than chemical or physical intervention in the reproductive process.

Fertility drugs Hormones that stimulate ovulation in women who are not ovulating; often responsible for multiple births.

Fetal alcohol effects (FAE) A syndrome describing children with a history of prenatal alcohol exposure but without all the physical or behavioral symptoms of FAS. Among its symptoms are low birth weight, irritability, and possible permanent mental impairment.

Fetal alcohol syndrome (FAS) A disorder that may affect the fetus when the mother consumes alcohol during pregnancy. Among its effects are mental retardation, small head, tremors, and abnormalities of the face, limbs, heart, and brain.

Fetus The name given the developing baby from the third month of pregnancy until birth.

Fiber The indigestible portion of plant foods that helps move foods through the digestive system and softens stools by absorbing water.

Fibrillation A sporadic, quivering pattern of heartbeat resulting in extreme inefficiency in moving blood through the cardiovascular system.

Fibrocystic breast condition A common, noncancerous condition in which a woman's breasts contain fibrous or fluid-filled cysts.

Fibromyalgia A chronic, rheumatoid-like disorder that can be highly painful and difficult to diagnose.

Fight-or-flight response Physiological arousal response in which the body prepares to combat a real or perceived threat.

Flexibility The measure of the range of motion, or the amount of movement possible, at a particular joint.

Folate A type of vitamin B that is believed to decrease levels of homocysteine, an amino acid that has been linked to vascular diseases.

Follicle-stimulating hormone (FSH) Hormone that signals the ovaries to prepare to release eggs and to begin producing estrogens.

Food allergies Overreaction by the body to normally harmless proteins, which are perceived as allergens. In response, the body produces antibodies, triggering allergic symptoms.

Food intolerance Adverse effects resulting when people who lack the digestive chemicals needed to break down certain substances eat those substances.

Food irradiation Treating foods with gamma radiation from radioactive cobalt, cesium, or some other source of x-rays to kill microorganisms.

Formaldehyde A colorless, strong-smelling gas released through outgassing; causes respiratory and other health problems.

For-profit (proprietary) hospitals Hospitals that provide a return on earnings to the investors who own them.

Fourth trimester The first six weeks of an infant's life outside the womb.

Freebase The most powerful distillate of cocaine.

Functional foods Foods believed to be beneficial and/or to prevent disease.

Fungi A group of plants that lack chlorophyll and do not produce flowers or seeds; several microscopic varieties are pathogenic.

Gamete intrafallopian transfer (GIFT) Procedure in which an egg harvested from the female partner's ovary is placed with the male partner's sperm in her fallopian tube, where it is fertilized and then migrates to the uterus for implantation.

Gamma-hydroxybutrane (GHB) A "date rape drug" sometimes used in combination with alcohol to facilitate rape by making a woman unaware of what is happening to her.

Gender The psychological condition of being feminine or masculine as defined by the society in which one lives.

Gender identity Personal sense or awareness of being masculine or feminine, a male or a female.

Gender roles Expression of maleness or femaleness in everyday life.

Gender-role stereotypes Generalizations concerning how males and females should express themselves and the characteristics each possesses.

Genderlect The "dialect," or individual speech pattern and conversational style, of each gender.

General adaptation syndrome (GAS) The pattern followed in the physiological response to stress, consisting of the alarm, resistance, and exhaustion phases.

Generalized anxiety disorder (GAD) A constant sense of worry that may cause restlessness, difficulty in concentrating, and tension.

Generic drugs Drugs marketed by chemical name rather than brand name.

Genital herpes STI caused by the herpes simplex virus.

Genital warts Warts that appear in the genital area or the anus; caused by the human papilloma viruses (HPVs).

German measles (rubella) A milder form of measles that causes a rash and mild fever in children and may cause damage to a fetus or a newborn baby.

Gerontology The study of individual and collective aging processes.

Girth and circumference measures A method of assessing body fat that employs a formula based on girth measurements of various body sites.

Glaucoma Elevation of pressure within the eyeball, leading to hardening of the eyeball, impaired vision, and possible blindness.

Glycogen The polysaccharide form in which glucose is stored in the liver.

Gonadotropin-releasing hormone (GnRH) Hormone that signals the pituitary gland to release gonadotropins.

Gonads The reproductive organs in a male (testes) or female (ovaries).

Gonorrhea Second most common STD in the United States; if untreated, may cause sterility.

Graded exercise test A test of aerobic capacity administered by a physician, exercise physiologist, or other trained person; two common forms are the treadmill running test and the stationary bike test.

GRAE list A list of drugs generally recognized as effective, which work for their intended purpose when used properly.

GRAS list A list of drugs generally recognized as safe, which seldom cause side effects when used properly.

Greenhouse gases Gases that contribute to global warming by trapping heat near the earth's surface.

Grief The state of mental distress that occurs in reaction to significant loss, including one's own impending death, the death of a loved one, or a quasi-death experience.

Grief work The process of accepting the reality of a person's death and coping with memories of the deceased.

Group practice A group of physicians who combine resources, sharing offices, equipment, and staff costs to render care to patients.

Habit A repeated behavior in which the repetition may be unconscious.

Hallucination An image (auditory or visual) that is perceived but is not real.

Hallucinogens Substances capable of creating auditory or visual hallucinations.

Hangover The physiological reaction to excessive drinking, including symptoms such as headache, upset stomach, anxiety, depression, diarrhea, and thirst.

Hashish The sticky resin of the cannabis plant, which is high in THC.

Hay fever A chronic respiratory disorder that is most prevalent when ragweed and flowers bloom.

Hazardous waste Solid waste that, due to its toxic properties, poses a hazard to humans or to the environment.

Health Dynamic, ever-changing process of achieving individual potential in the physical, social, emotional, mental, spiritual, and environmental dimensions.

Health Belief Model (HBM) Model for explaining how beliefs may influence behaviors.

Health promotion Combined educational, organizational, policy, financial, and environmental supports to help people reduce negative health behaviors and promote positive change.

Heart attack A blockage of normal blood supply to an area in the heart.

Heat cramps Muscle cramps that occur during or following exercise in warm or hot weather.

Heat exhaustion A heat stress illness caused by significant dehydration resulting from exercise in warm or hot conditions; frequent precursor to heatstroke.

Heat stroke A deadly heat stress illness resulting from dehydration and overexertion in warm or hot conditions; can cause body core temperature to rise from normal to 105°F to 110°F in just a few minutes.

Hemochromatosis Iron toxicity due to excess consumption.

Hepatitis A virally caused disease in which the liver becomes inflamed, producing symptoms such as fever, headache, and jaundice.

Herbal preparations Substances of plant origin that are believed to have medicinal properties.

Heroin An illegally manufactured derivative of morphine, usually injected into the bloodstream.

Heterosexual Experiencing primary attraction to and preference for sexual activity with people of the other sex.

High-density lipoproteins (HDLs) Compounds that facilitate the transport of cholesterol in the blood to the liver for metabolism and elimination from the body.

Histamines Chemical substances that dilate blood vessels, increase mucous secretions, and produce other symptoms of allergies.

Holographic will A will written in the testator's own handwriting and unwitnessed.

Homeopathy Unconventional Western system of medicine based on the principle that "like cures like."

Homeostasis A balanced physical state in which all the body's systems function smoothly.

Homicide Death that results from intent to injure or kill.

Homophobia Irrational hatred or fear of homosexuals or homosexuality.

Homosexual Experiencing primary attraction to and preference for sexual activity with people of the same sex.

Hope Belief that establishes confidence and courage in facing the future.

Hormone replacement therapy (HRT) Use of synthetic or animal estrogens and progesterone to compensate for decreases in hormones in a woman's body, particularly in postmenopausal women.

Hospice A concept of care for terminally ill patients designed to maximize quality of life.

Human chorionic gonadotropin (HCG) Hormone detectable in blood or urine samples indicating increased levels of estrogen and progesterone secretion if fertilization has taken place.

Human immunodeficiency virus (HIV) The slow-acting virus that causes AIDS.

Human papilloma viruses (HPVs) A small group of viruses that cause genital warts.

Hunger The feeling associated with the physiological need to eat.

Hydrocarbons Chemical compounds that contain carbon and hydrogen.

Hydrostatic weighing techniques Methods of determining body fat by measuring the amount of water displaced when a person is completely submerged.

Hymen Thin tissue covering the vaginal opening.

Hyperglycemia Elevated blood sugar levels.

Hyperlipidemia Elevated levels of lipds in the blood.

Hyperplasia A condition characterized by an excessive number of fat cells.

Hypertension Sustained elevated blood pressure.

Hypertrophy Increased size (girth) of a muscle.

Hypervitaminosis A toxic condition caused by overuse of vitamin supplements.

Hypnosis A process that allows people to become unusually responsive to suggestion.

Hypothalamus A section of the brain that controls the sympathetic nervous system and directs the stress response.

Hypothalamus An area of the brain located near the pituitary gland. The hypothalamus works in conjunction with the pituitary gland to control reproductive functions.

Hypothermia Potentially fatal condition caused by abnormally low body core temperature.

Hysterectomy Surgical removal of the uterus, ovaries, and/or other reproductive organs; done either vaginally or abdominally.

Hysterotomy The surgical removal of the fetus from the uterus.

"I" messages Messages in which a person takes responsibility for communicating his or her own feelings, thoughts, and beliefs by using statements that begin with "I," not "you."

Ice A potent, inexpensive stimulant that has long-lasting effects.

Idiopathic Of unknown cause.

Illicit (illegal) drugs Drugs whose use, possession, cultivation, manufacture, and/or sale are against the law because they are generally recognized as harmful.

Imagined rehearsal Practicing, through mental imagery, to become better able to perform an event in actuality.

Immunological competence/Immunocompetency Ability of the immune system to defend the body from pathogens.

Immunotherapy A process that stimulates the body's own immune system to combat cancer cells.

In vitro fertilization Fertilization of an egg in a nutrient medium and subsequent transfer back to the mother's body.

Incidence   The number of new cases.

Incomplete proteins   Proteins that are lacking in one or more of the essential amino acids.

Incubation period   The time between exposure to a disease and the appearance of the symptoms.

Induction abortion   A type of abortion in which chemicals are injected into the uterus through the uterine wall; labor begins and the woman delivers a dead fetus.

Infertility   Difficulties in conceiving.

Influenza   A common viral disease of the respiratory tract.

Inhalants   Products that are sniffed or inhaled in order to produce highs.

Inhalation   The introduction of drugs through the nostrils.

Inhibited sexual desire (ISD)   Lack of sexual appetite or simply a lack of interest and pleasure in sexual activity.

Inhibition   A type of interaction in which the effects of one drug are eliminated or reduced by the presence of another drug at the receptor site.

Injection   The introduction of drugs into the body via a hypodermic needle.

Insomnia   Difficulty in falling asleep or staying asleep.

Insulin   A hormone produced by the pancreas; required by the body for the metabolism of carbohydrates.

Intact dilation and extraction (D & X)   A late-term abortion procedure in which the body of the fetus is extracted up to the head and then the contents of the cranium are aspirated.

Intentional injuries   Injuries done on purpose with intent to harm.

Interconnectedness   A web of connections, including our relationship to ourselves, to others, and to a larger meaning or purpose in life.

Interferon   A protein substance produced by the body that aids the immune system by protecting healthy cells.

Internal female genitals   The vagina, uterus, fallopian tubes, and ovaries.

Internal male genitals   The testes, epididymides, vasa deferentia, ejaculatory ducts, urethra, and accessory glands.

Internet addiction   Compulsive use of computer activities such as fantasy games, online shopping, and chatrooms.

Intersexuality   Not exhibiting exclusively female or male primary and secondary sex characteristics.

Interspecies transmission   Transmission of disease from humans to animals or from animals to humans.

Intervention   A planned process of confronting an addict, carried out by significant others.

Intestate   Not having made a will.

Intimate relationships   Relationships with family members, friends, and romantic partners, characterized by closeness and understanding.

Intolerance   A type of interaction in which two or more drugs produce extremely uncomfortable symptoms.

Intracytoplasmic sperm injection (ICSI)   Fertilization accomplished by injecting a sperm cell directly into an egg.

Intramuscular injection   The introduction of drugs into muscles.

Intrauterine device (IUD)   A T-shaped device that is implanted in the uterus to prevent pregnancy.

Intravenous injection   The introduction of drugs directly into a vein.

Inunction   The introduction of drugs through the skin.

Ionizing radiation   Radiation produced by photons having high enough energy to ionize atoms.

Irritable bowel syndrome (IBS)   Nausea, pain, gas, or diarrhea caused by certain foods or stress.

Ischemia   Reduced oxygen supply to the heart.

Isometric muscle action   Force produced without any resulting joint movement.

Jealousy   An aversive reaction evoked by a real or imagined relationship involving a person's partner and a third person.

Ketosis   A condition in which the body adapts to prolonged fasting or carbohydrate deprivation by converting body fat to ketones, which can be used as fuel for some brain activity.

Klinefelter's syndrome   A chromosome defect that causes abnormal sexual development.

Labia majora   "Outer lips" or folds of tissue covering the female sexual organs.

Labia minora   "Inner lips" or folds of tissue just inside the labia majora.

Lactose intolerance   The inability to produce lactase, an enzyme needed to convert milk sugar into glucose.

Laxatives   Medications used to soften stool and relieve constipation.

Leach   To dissolve and filter through soil.

Leachate   A liquid consisting of soluble chemicals that come from garbage and industrial waste that seeps into the water supply from landfills and dumps.

Lead   A metal found in the exhaust of motor vehicles powered by fuel containing lead and in emissions from lead smelters and processing plants.

Learned behavioral tolerance   The ability of heavy drinkers to modify behavior so that they appear to be sober even when they have high BAC levels.

Learned helplessness   Pattern of responding to situations by giving up because of repeated failure in the past.

Leukoplakia   A condition characterized by leathery white patches inside the mouth produced by contact with irritants in tobacco juice.

Leveling   The communication of a clear, simple, and honest message.

Loss of control   Inability to predict reliably whether a particular instance of involvement with the addictive object or behavior will be healthy or damaging.

Love   Acceptance, affirmation, and respect for the self and others.

Low sperm count   A sperm count below 60 million sperm per milliliter of semen; the leading cause of infertility in men.

Low-density lipoproteins (LDLs) Compounds that facilitate the transport of cholesterol in the blood to the body's cells.

Lunelle A monthly injection of estrogen and progestin that prevents ovulation and fertilization.

Lupus A disease in which the immune system attacks the body, producing antibodies that destroy or injure organs such as the kidneys, brain, and heart.

Luteinizing hormone (LH) Hormone that signals the ovaries to release an egg and to begin producing progesterone.

Lysergic acid diethylamide (LSD) Psychedelic drug causing sensory disruptions; also called acid.

Macrominerals Minerals that the body needs in fairly large amounts.

Magnetic resonance imaging (MRI) A device that uses magnetic fields, radio waves, and computers to generate an image of internal tissues of the body for diagnostic purposes without the use of radiation.

Mainstream smoke Smoke that is drawn through tobacco while inhaling.

Major depressive disorder Severe depression that entails chronic mood disorder, physical effects such as sleep disturbance and exhaustion, and mental effects such as the inability to concentrate.

Malignant Very dangerous or harmful; refers to a cancerous tumor.

Malignant melanoma A virulent cancer of the melanin (pigment-producing portion) of the skin.

Managed care Cost-control procedures used by health insurers to coordinate treatment.

Marijuana Chopped leaves and flowers of the Cannabis indica or Cannabis sativa plant (hemp); a psychoactive stimulant that intensifies reactions to environmental stimuli.

Masturbation Self-stimulation of genitals.

Measles A viral disease that produces symptoms including an itchy rash and a high fever.

Medicaid Federal-state health insurance program for the poor.

Medical Model A model in which health status was focused primarily on the individual and a biological or diseased organ perspective.

Medicare Federal health insurance program for the elderly and the permanently disabled.

Meditation A relaxation technique that involves deep breathing and concentration.

Meltdown An accident that results when the temperature in the core of a nuclear reactor increases enough to melt the nuclear fuel and the containment vessel housing it.

Menarche The first menstrual period.

Menopause The permanent cessation of menstruation.

Mental health The "thinking" part of psychosocial health; includes your values, attitudes, and beliefs.

Mescaline A hallucinogenic drug derived from the peyote cactus.

Metastasis Process by which cancer spreads from one area to different areas of the body.

Methadone maintenance A treatment for people addicted to opiates that substitutes methadone, a synthetic narcotic, for the opiate of addiction.

Methamphetamine A powerfully addictive drug that strongly activates certain areas of the brain and affects the central nervous system.

Middle-old People age 75 to 84.

Midwives Experienced practitioners who assist with pregnancy and delivery.

Mifepristone A steroid hormone that induces abortion by blocking the action of progesterone.

Migraine A condition characterized by localized headaches that possibly result from alternating dilation and constriction of blood vessels.

Mindfulness Awareness and acceptance of the reality of the present moment.

Minerals Inorganic, indestructible elements that aid physiological processes.

Miscarriage Loss of the fetus before it is viable; also called spontaneous abortion.

Modeling Learning specific behaviors by watching others perform them.

Monogamy Exclusive sexual involvement with one partner.

Monosaccharide A simple sugar that contains only one molecule of sugar.

Mons pubis Fatty tissue covering the pubic bone in females; in physically mature women, the mons is covered with coarse hair.

Morbidity Illness rate.

Morphine A derivative of opium; sometimes used by medical practitioners to relieve pain.

Mortality Death rate.

Mourning The culturally prescribed behavior patterns for the expression of grief.

Multifactorial disease Disease caused by interactions of several factors.

Multiple sclerosis (MS) A degenerative neurological disease in which myelin, an insulator of nerves, breaks down.

Municipal solid waste Solid wastes such as durable goods, nondurable goods, containers and packaging, food wastes, yard wastes, and miscellaneous wastes from residential, commercial, institutional, and industrial sources.

Muscle dysmorphia Sometimes referred to as "bigarexia," a pathological preoccupation with being larger and more muscular, which can lead to exercise addiction.

Muscular endurance A muscle's ability to exert force repeatedly without fatiguing.

Muscular strength The amount of force that a muscle is capable of exerting.

Mutant cells Cells that differ in form, quality, or function from normal cells.

Myocardial infarction (MI) Heart attack.

Narcotics Drugs that induce sleep and relieve pain; primarily the opiates.

Natural immunity Immunity passed to a fetus by its mother.

Naturopathy System of medicine that attempts to restore natural processes of the body and promote healing through natural means.

Negative consequences Physical damage, legal trouble, financial ruin, academic failure, family dissolution, and other severe problems associated with addiction.

Neoplasm A new growth of tissue that serves no physiological function and results from uncontrolled, abnormal cellular development.

Neurotransmitters Biochemical messengers that exert influence at specific receptor sites on nerve cells.

Nicotine The stimulant chemical in tobacco products.

Nicotine poisoning Symptoms often experienced by beginning smokers, including dizziness, diarrhea, lightheadedness, rapid and erratic pulse, clammy skin, nausea, and vomiting.

Nicotine withdrawal Symptoms, including nausea, headaches, and irritability, suffered by smokers who cease using tobacco.

Nitrogen dioxide An amber-colored gas found in smog; can cause eye and respiratory irritations.

Nitrous oxide The chemical name for "laughing gas," a substance properly used for surgical or dental anesthesia.

Nonassertive communicators Individuals who tend to be shy and inhibited in their communication with others.

Nonpoint source pollutants Pollutants that run off or seep into waterways from broad areas of land.

Nonprofit (voluntary) hospitals Hospitals run by religious or other humanitarian groups that reinvest their earnings in the hospital to improve health care.

Nonsurgical embryo transfer In vitro fertilization of a donor egg by the male partner's (or donor's) sperm and subsequent transfer to the female partner's or another woman's uterus.

Nonverbal communication All unwritten and unspoken messages, both intentional and unintentional.

Norplant A long-lasting contraceptive that consists of six silicon capsules surgically inserted under the skin in a woman's upper arm.

Nuclear family Parents (usually married, but not necessarily) and their offspring

Nurse Health practitioner who provides many services for patients and who may work in a variety of settings.

Nurturing through avoidance Repeatedly seeking the illusion of relief to avoid unpleasant feelings or situations, a maladaptive way of taking care of emotional needs.

Nutraceuticals Term often used interchangeably with functional foods; refers to the combined nutritional and pharmaceutical benefit derived through use of foods or food supplements.

Nutrients The constituents of food that sustain us physiologically: proteins, carbohydrates, fats, vitamins, minerals, and water.

Nutrition The science that investigates the relationship between physiological function and the essential elements of foods eaten.

NuvaRing A soft, flexible ring inserted into the vagina that releases hormones, preventing pregnancy.

Obesity A weight disorder generally defined as an accumulation of fat beyond that considered normal for a person based on age, sex, and body type.

Obsession Excessive preoccupation with an addictive object or behavior.

Old-old People age 85 and over.

Oncogenes Suspected cancer-causing genes present on chromosomes.

Oncologists Physicians who specialize in the treatment of malignancies.

One repetition maximum (1 RM) The amount of weight/resistance that can be lifted or moved once, but not twice; a common measure of strength.

Open relationship A relationship in which partners agree that sexual involvement can occur outside the relationship.

Ophthalmologist Physician who specializes in the medical and surgical care of the eyes, including prescriptions for glasses.

Opium The parent drug of the opiates; made from the seedpod resin of the opium poppy.

Optometrist Eye specialist whose practice is limited to prescribing and fitting lenses.

Oral contraceptives Pills taken daily for three weeks of the menstrual cycle that prevent ovulation by regulating hormones.

Oral ingestion Intake of drugs through the mouth.

Oral surgeon Dentist who performs surgical procedures to correct problems of the mouth, jaw, and face.

Organically grown Foods that are grown without use of pesticides or chemicals.

Ortho Evra A patch worn for three weeks at a time that releases hormones similar to those in oral contraceptives.

Orthodontist Dentist who specializes in the alignment of teeth.

Osteoarthritis A progressive deterioration of bones and joints that has been associated with the "wear and tear" theory of aging.

Osteopath General practitioner who receives training similar to a medical doctor's but with an emphasis on the skeletal and muscular systems, often using spinal manipulation as part of treatment.

Osteoporosis A degenerative disease characterized by low bone mass, porous bones, and deterioration of bone tissue, which increase risk of fracture.

Outpatient (ambulatory) care Treatment that does not involve an overnight stay in a hospital.

Ovarian follicles (egg sacs) Areas within the ovary in which individual eggs develop.

Ovaries Almond-size organs that house developing eggs and produce hormones.

Overload A condition in which a person feels overly pressured by demands.

Over-the-counter (OTC) drugs Medications that can be purchased without a physician's prescription.

Overuse injuries Injuries that result from the cumulative effects of day-after-day stresses placed on tendons, muscles, and joints.

Overweight Increased body weight in relation to height.

Ovulation The point of the menstrual cycle at which a mature egg ruptures through the ovarian wall.

Ozone A gas formed when nitrogen dioxide interacts with hydrogen chloride.

Pairings Paired associations (e.g., coffee and a cigarette) that trigger cravings.

Pandemics Global epidemics of diseases.

Panic disorder Severe anxiety disorder in which a particular situation, often for unknown reasons, causes terror and panic attacks.

Pap test A procedure in which cells taken from the cervical region are examined for abnormal cellular activity.

Parasitic worms The largest of the pathogens, most of which are more a nuisance than a threat.

Parasympathetic nervous system Part of the autonomic nervous system responsible for slowing systems stimulated by the stress response.

Parkinson's disease A chronic, progressive neurological condition that causes tremors and other symptoms.

Particulates Nongaseous air pollutants.

Passive euthanasia The intentional withholding of treatment that would prolong life.

Passive immunity Antibodies formed in another person or animal, then given to someone with a weakened immune system.

Pathogen A disease-causing agent.

Pelvic inflammatory disease (PID) Term used to describe various infections of the female reproductive tract; results in inflammation and other symptoms.

Penis Male sexual organ that releases sperm into the vagina.

Peptic ulcer Damage to the stomach or intestinal lining, usually caused by digestive juices.

Perception The process of filtering and interpreting information gathered through the senses.

Perineum The area between the vulva and the anus.

Periodontal diseases Diseases of the tissue around the teeth.

Personal control Belief that one's own internal resources can control a situation.

Pesticides Chemicals that kill pests.

Peyote A cactus with small "buttons" that, when ingested, produce hallucinogenic effects.

Phencyclidine (PCP) A deliriant commonly called "angel dust."

Phobia A deep and persistent fear of a specific object, activity, or situation that results in a compelling desire to avoid the source of the fear.

Photochemical smog The brownish yellow haze resulting from the combination of hydrocarbons and nitrogen oxides.

Physical fitness The ability to perform regular moderate-to-rigorous physical activity without great fatigue.

Physician assistant A midlevel practitioner trained to handle most standard cases of care.

Phytomedicines Another name for medicinal herbs, many of which are sold over the counter in Europe.

Pica Iron deficiency disease characterized by craving for certain foods and substances.

Pilates Exercise programs that combine stretching with movement against resistance, aided by devices such as tension springs and heavy bands.

Pinch test A method of determining body fat whereby a fold of skin just behind the triceps is pinched between the thumb and index finger to determine the relative amount of fat.

Pituitary gland The endocrine gland located deep within the brain; controls hormonal release and reproductive functions.

Placebo effect An apparent cure or improved state of health brought about by a substance or product that has no medicinal value.

Placenta The network of blood vessels, connected to the umbilical cord, that carries nutrients to the developing infant and carries wastes away.

Plaque Cholesterol buildup on the inner walls of arteries, causing a narrowing of the channel through which blood flows; a major cause of atherosclerosis.

Plateau That point in a weight-loss program at which the dieter finds it difficult to lose more weight.

Platelet adhesiveness Stickiness of red blood cells associated with blood clots.

Pneumonia Bacterially caused disease of the lungs.

Point source pollutants Pollutants that enter waterways at a specific point.

Polychlorinated biphenyls (PCBs) Toxic chemicals that were once used as insulating materials in high-voltage electrical equipment.

Polydrug use The use of multiple medications or illicit drugs simultaneously.

Polysaccharide A complex carbohydrate formed by the combination of long chains of saccharides.

Positive reinforcement Presenting something positive following a behavior that is being reinforced.

Positron emission tomography (PET scan) Method for measuring heart activity by injecting a patient with a radioactive tracer that is scanned electronically to produce a three-dimensional image of the heart and arteries.

Postpartum depression The experience of energy depletion, anxiety, mood swings, and depression that women may feel during the postpartum period.

Power The ability to make and implement decisions.

Prader-Willi syndrome A disorder characterized by mental retardation and obesity.

Preconception care Medical care received prior to becoming pregnant that helps a woman assess and address potential maternal health.

Preeclampsia A complication in pregnancy characterized by high blood pressure, protein in the urine, and edema.

Prejudice   Negative attitudes and beliefs about an entire group of people that is typically based on unfavorable and often bigoted/biased ideas about the group.

Premature ejaculation   Ejaculation that occurs prior to or almost immediately following penile penetration of the vagina.

Premenstrual dysphoric disorder (PMDD)   Collective name for a group of negative symptoms similar to but more severe than PMS, including severe mood disturbances.

Premenstrual syndrome (PMS)   Comprises the mood changes and physical symptoms that occur in some women during one or two weeks prior to menstruation.

Prescription drugs   Medications that can be obtained only with the written prescription of a licensed physician.

Prevalence   The number of existing cases.

Primary aggression   Goal-directed, hostile self-assertion, destructive in character.

Primary care practitioner   A medical practitioner who treats routine ailments, advises on preventive care, gives general medical advice, and makes appropriate referrals when necessary.

Primary prevention   Actions designed to stop problems before they start.

Prions   One of the newest, more frightening pathogens to infect humans and animals in recent years; a self-replicating protein-based agent that systematically destroys brain cells.

Process addictions   Behaviors such as money addictions, work addictions, exercise addictions, and sex addictions that are known to be addictive because they are mood-altering.

Progesterone   Hormone secreted by the ovaries; helps keep the endometrium developing in order to nourish a fertilized egg; also helps maintain pregnancy.

Proof   A measure of the percentage of alcohol in a beverage.

Proprioceptive neuromuscular facilitation (PNF) stretching   Techniques that involve the skillful use of alternating muscle contractions and static stretching in the same muscle.

Prostaglandin inhibitors   Drugs that inhibit the production and release of prostaglandins associated with arthritis or menstrual pain.

Prostate gland   Gland that secretes nutrients and neutralizing fluids into the semen.

Prostate-specific antigen (PSA)   An antigen found in prostate cancer patients.

Proteins   The essential constituents of nearly all body cells; necessary for the development and repair of bone, muscle, skin, and blood; the key elements of antibodies, enzymes, and hormones.

Protooncogenes   Genes that can become oncogenes under certain conditions.

Protozoa   Microscopic, single-celled organisms.

Psilocybin   The active chemical found in psilocybe mushrooms; it produces hallucinations.

Psychedelics   Drugs that distort the processing of sensory information in the brain.

Psychiatric nurse specialist   A registered nurse specializing in psychiatric practice.

Psychiatrist   A licensed physician who specializes in treating mental and emotional disorders.

Psychoactive drugs   Drugs that have the potential to alter mood or behavior.

Psychoanalyst   A psychiatrist or psychologist having special training in psychoanalysis.

Psychoeducation   The teaching of crucial psychological skills, giving people knowledge so they can help themselves.

Psychological hardiness   A personality trait characterized by control, commitment, and challenge.

Psychologist   A person with a Ph.D. degree and training in psychology.

Psychoneuroimmunology (PNI)   Science of the interaction between the mind and the immune system.

Psychosocial health   The mental, emotional, social, and spiritual dimensions of health.

Puberty   The maturation of the female or male reproduction system.

Pubic lice   Parasites that can inhabit various body areas, especially the genitals; also called "crabs."

Qi   Element of traditional Oriental medicine that refers to the vital energy force that courses through the body. When qi is in balance, health is restored.

Quasi-death experience   A loss or experience that resembles death, in that it involves separation, termination, significant loss, a change of personal identity, and grief.

Rabies   A viral disease of the central nervous system often transmitted through animal bites.

Radiation absorbed doses (rads)   Units that measure exposure to radioactivity.

Radiotherapy   The use of radiation to kill cancerous cells.

Radon   A naturally occurring radioactive gas resulting from the decay of certain radioactive elements.

Rape   Sexual penetration without the victim's consent.

Rational suicide   The decision to kill oneself rather than endure constant pain and slow decay.

Raynaud's syndrome   A disease in which exposure to cold temperatures produces exaggerated constriction of the small arteries in the extremities, causing fingers and toes to go numb, turn white, and then turn deep purple.

Reactive aggression   Emotional reaction brought about by frustrating life experiences.

Rebound effects   Severe withdrawal effects experienced by users of stimulants, including depression, nausea, and violent behavior.

Receptor sites   Specialized cells to which drugs can attach themselves.

Recommended Dietary Allowances (RDAs)   The average daily intakes of energy and nutrients considered adequate to meet the needs of most healthy people in the United States under usual conditions.

Recreational drugs   Legal drugs that contain chemicals that help people relax or socialize.

Reference Daily Intake (RDIs)   Recommended amounts of 19 vitamins and minerals, also know as micronutrients..

Referred pain   Pain that is present at one point, but the source of pain is elsewhere.

Relapse   The tendency to return to the addictive behavior after a period of abstinence.

Relative risk   A measure of the strength of the relationship between risk factors and the condition being studied, such as a particular cancer.

Repetitive stress injury (RSI)   An injury to nerves, soft tissue, or joints due to the physical stress of repeated motions.

Resistance exercise program   A regular program of exercises designed to improve muscular strength and endurance in the major muscle groups.

Respite care   The care provided by substitute caregivers to relieve the principal caregiver from his or her continuous responsibility.

Resting metabolic rate (RMR)   The energy expenditure of the body under BMR conditions plus other daily sedentary activities.

Reticular formation   An area in the brain stem that is responsible for relaying messages to other areas in the brain.

Rh factor   A blood protein related to the production of antibodies. If an Rh-negative mother is pregnant with an Rh-positive fetus, the mother will manufacture antibodies that can kill the fetus, causing miscarriage.

Rheumatic heart disease   A heart disease caused by untreated streptococcal infection of the throat.

Rheumatoid arthritis   A serious inflammatory joint disease.

RICE   Acronym for the standard first-aid treatment for virtually all traumatic and overuse injuries: rest, ice, compression, and elevation.

Rickettsia   A small form of bacteria that live inside other living cells.

Risk behaviors   Behaviors that increase susceptibility to negative health outcomes.

Rohypnol ("roofies," "rope," "forget pill")   A drug that is sometimes used in combination with alcohol to facilitate date rape by making a woman unaware of what is happening to her.

Route of administration   The manner in which a drug is taken into the body.

Saliva   Fluid secreted by the salivary glands; enzymes in the fluid aid in the breakdown of certain foods for digestion.

Sarcopenia   Age-related loss of muscle mass.

Satiety   The feeling of fullness or satisfaction at the end of a meal.

Saturated fats   Fats that are unable to hold any more hydrogen in their chemical structure; derived mostly from animal sources; solid at room temperature.

Schizophrenia   A mental illness with biological origins that is characterized by irrational behavior, severe alterations of the senses (hallucinations), and, often, an inability to function in society.

Scleroderma   A disease in which fibrous growth of connective tissue underlying the skin and body organs hardens and makes movement difficult.

Scrotum   Sac of tissue that encloses the testes.

Seasonal affective disorder (SAD)   A type of depression that occurs in the winter months, when sunlight levels are low.

Secondary hypertension   Hypertension caused by specific factors, such as kidney disease, obesity, or tumors of the adrenal glands.

Secondary prevention (intervention)   Intervention early in the development of a health problem.

Secondary sex characteristics   Characteristics associated with gender but not directly related to reproduction, such as vocal pitch, degree of body hair, and location of fat deposits.

Sedatives   Central nervous system depressants that induce sleep and relieve anxiety.

Self-disclosure   The process of revealing one's inner thoughts, feelings, and beliefs to another person.

Self-efficacy   Belief in one's own ability to perform a task successfully.

Self-esteem   Sense of self-respect or self-confidence.

Self-nurturance   Developing individual potential through a balanced and realistic appreciation of self-worth and ability.

Semen   Fluid containing sperm and nutrient fluids that increase sperm viability and neutralize vaginal acid.

Seminal vesicles   Storage areas for sperm where nutrient fluids are added to them.

Senility   A term associated with the loss of memory and judgment and orientation problems occurring in a small percentage of the elderly.

Serial monogamy   A series of monogamous sexual relationships.

Setpoint theory   A theory of obesity causation that suggests that fat storage is determined by a thermostatic mechanism in the body that acts to maintain a specific amount of body fat.

Sexual abuse of children   Sexually suggestive conversations; inappropriate kissing; touching; petting; oral, anal, or vaginal intercourse; and/or other kinds of sexual interaction between a child and an adult or older child.

Sexual addiction   Compulsive involvement in sexual activity.

Sexual assault   Any act in which one person is sexually intimate with another person without that other person's consent.

Sexual aversion disorder   Type of desire dysfunction characterized by sexual phobias and anxiety about sexual contact.

Sexual dysfunction   Problems associated with achieving sexual satisfaction.

Sexual fantasies   Sexually arousing thoughts and dreams.

Sexual harassment   Any form of unwanted sexual attention.

Sexual identity   Recognition of oneself as a sexual being; a composite of biological sex, gender identity, gender roles, and sexual orientation.

Sexual orientation   A person's enduring emotional, romantic, sexual, or affectionate attraction to other persons.

Sexual performance anxiety   A condition of sexual difficulties caused by anticipating some sort of problem with the sex act.

Sexually transmitted infections (STIs)   Infectious diseases transmitted via some form of intimate, usually sexual, contact.

Shaping   Using a series of small steps to get to a particular goal gradually.

Sick building syndrome (SBS)   Problem that exists when 80 percent of a building's occupants report maladies that tend to lessen or vanish when they leave the building.

Sickle-cell anemia   Genetic disease commonly found among African Americans; results in organ damage and premature death.

Sidestream smoke   The cigarette, pipe, or cigar smoke breathed by nonsmokers; also called *secondhand smoke.*

Simple rape   Rape by one person known to the victim that does not involve a physical beating or use of a weapon.

Simple sugars   Major types of carbohydrate, which provide short-term energy.

Sinoatrial node (SA node)   Node serving as a form of natural pacemaker for the heart.

Situational inducement   Attempt to influence a behavior through situations and occasions that are structured to exert control over that behavior.

Skinfold caliper test   A method of determining body fat whereby folds of skin and fat at various points on the body are grasped between thumb and forefinger and measured with calipers.

Sleep apnea   Disorder in which a person has numerous episodes of breathing stoppage during a normal night's sleep.

Slow-acting viruses   Viruses having long incubation periods and causing slowly progressive symptoms.

Small intestine   Muscular, coiled digestive organ; consists of the duodenum, jejunum, and ileum.

Snuff   A powdered form of tobacco that is sniffed and absorbed through the mucous membranes in the nose or placed inside the cheek and sucked.

Social bonds   Degree and nature of interpersonal contacts.

Social death   An irreversible situation in which a person is not treated like an active member of society.

Social learning theory   Theory that people learn behaviors by watching role models—parents, caregivers, and significant others.

Social phobia   A phobia characterized by fear and avoidance of social situations.

Social physique anxiety (SPA)   A desire to look good that has a destructive effect on a person's ability to function effectively socially.

Social supports   Structural and functional aspects of social interactions.

Social worker   A person with an M.S.W. degree and clinical training.

Socialization   Process by which a society communicates behavioral expectations to its individual members.

Soft-tissue roentgenogram   A technique of body fat assessment in which radioactive substances are used to determine relative fat.

Solo practitioner   Physician who renders care to patients independently of other practitioners.

Spermatogenesis   The development of sperm.

Spermicides   Substances designed to kill sperm.

Spirituality   A form of well-being in which a person acknowledges the need for having, relating, being, and transcendence in the quest for meaning and purpose in life.

Spontaneous remission   The disappearance of symptoms without any apparent cause or treatment.

Staphylococci   Round, gram-positive bacteria, usually found in clusters.

Static stretching   Techniques that gradually lengthen a muscle to an elongated position (to the point of discomfort) and hold that position for 10 to 30 seconds.

Sterilization   Permanent fertility control achieved through surgical procedures.

Stillbirth   The birth of a dead baby.

Stomach   Large muscular organ that temporarily stores, mixes, and digests foods.

Strain   The wear and tear sustained by the body and mind in adjusting to or resisting a stressor.

Streptococci   Round bacteria, usually found in chain formation.

Stress   Mental and physical responses to change.

Stress inoculation   Newer stress management technique in which a person consciously tries to prepare ahead of time for potential stressors.

Stressor   A physical, social, or psychological event or condition that requires an adjustment.

Stroke   A condition occurring when the brain is damaged by disrupted blood supply.

Subcutaneous injection   The introduction of drugs into the layer of fat directly beneath the skin.

Subjective well-being (SWB)   Feeling characterized by satisfaction with present life, relative presence of positive emotions, and relative absence of negative emotions.

Sudden cardiac death   Death that occurs as a result of sudden, abrupt loss of heart function.

Sudden infant death syndrome (SIDS)   The sudden death of an infant under one year of age for no apparent reason.

Sulfur dioxide   A yellowish brown gaseous by-product of the burning of fossil fuels.

Superfund   Fund established under the Comprehensive Environmental Response Compensation and Liability Act to be used for cleaning up toxic waste dumps.

Suppositories   Mixtures of drugs and a waxy medium designed to melt at body temperature that are inserted into the anus or vagina.

Sympathetic nervous system   Branch of the autonomic nervous system responsible for stress arousal.

Sympathomimetics   Drugs found in appetite suppressants that affect the sympathetic nervous system.

Synergism   An interaction of two or more drugs that produces more profound effects than would be expected if the drugs were taken separately.

Synesthesia   A (usually) drug-created effect in which sensory messages are incorrectly assigned—for example, hearing a taste or smelling a sound.

Syphilis   One of the most widespread STDs; characterized by distinct phases and potentially serious results.

Systolic blood pressure   The upper number in the fraction that measures blood pressure, indicating pressure on the walls of the arteries when the heart contracts.

Tai chi   An ancient Chinese form of exercise widely practiced in the West today that promotes balance, coordination, stretching, and meditation.

Tar   A thick, brownish substance condensed from particulate matter in smoked tobacco.

Target heart rate   Calculated as a percentage of maximum heart rate (220 minus age); heart rate (pulse) is taken during aerobic exercise to check if exercise intensity is at the desired level (e.g., 70 percent of maximum heart rate).

Temperature inversion   A weather condition occurring when a layer of cool air is trapped under a layer of warmer air.

Teratogenic   Causing birth defects; may refer to drugs, environmental chemicals, x-rays, or diseases.

Terrorism   The use of unlawful force or violence against persons or property to intimidate or coerce a government, the civilian population, or any segment thereof, in furtherance of political or social objectives.

Tertiary prevention   Treatment and/or rehabilitation efforts.

Testator   A person who leaves a will or testament at death.

Testes   Two organs, located in the scrotum, that manufacture sperm and produce hormones.

Testosterone   The male sex hormone manufactured in the testes.

Tetrahydrocannabinol (THC)   The chemical name for the active ingredient in marijuana.

Thanatology   The study of death and dying.

Theory of Reasoned Action   Model for explaining the importance of our intentions in determining behaviors.

Thrombolysis   Injection of an agent to dissolve clots and restore some blood flow, thereby reducing the amount of tissue that dies from ischemia.

Thrombus   Blood clot.

Thyroid gland   A two-lobed endocrine gland located in the throat region that produces a hormone that regulates metabolism.

Tinctures   Herbal extracts usually combined with grain alcohol to prevent spoilage.

Tolerable Upper Intake Level (UL)   The highest amount of a nutrient that an individual can safely consume every day without risking adverse health effects.

Tolerance   Phenomenon in which progressively larger doses of a drug or more intense involvement in a behavior is needed to produce the desired effects.

Total body electrical conductivity (TOBEC)   Technique using an electromagnetic force field to assess relative body fat.

Toxic shock syndrome (TSS)   A potentially life-threatening disease that occurs when specific bacterial toxins are allowed to multiply unchecked in wounds or through improper use of tampons or diaphragms.

Toxins   Poisonous substances produced by certain microorganisms that cause various diseases.

Toxoplasmosis   A disease caused by an organism found in cat feces that, when contracted by a pregnant woman, may result in stillbirth or an infant with mental retardation or birth defects.

Trace minerals   Minerals that the body needs in only very small amounts.

Traditional Oriental medicine (TOM)   Comprehensive system of diagnosis and treatment in which dietary change, touch, massage, medicinal teas, and other herbal medicines are used extensively.

Tranquilizers   Central nervous system depressants that relax the body and calm anxiety.

Trans-fatty acids   Fatty acids that are produced when polyunsaturated oils are hydrogenated to make them more solid.

Transgendered   Refusing to follow the sexual and gender scripts prescribed based on biology and resisting the division of gender into two distinct categories.

Transient ischemic attacks (TIAs)   Brief interruptions of the blood supply to the brain that cause only temporary impairment; often an indicator of impending major stroke.

Transition   The process during which the cervix becomes nearly fully dilated and the head of the fetus begins to move into the birth canal.

Transsexual   Experiencing the feeling the body one is born into is the wrong sex.

Traumatic injuries   Injuries that are accidental in nature, which occur suddenly and violently (e.g., fractured bones, ruptured tendons, and sprained ligaments).

Trichomoniasis   Protozoan infection characterized by foamy, yellowish discharge and unpleasant odor.

Triglycerides   The most common form of fat in the body; excess calories are converted into triglycerides and stored as body fat.

Trimester   A three-month segment of pregnancy; used to describe specific developmental changes that occur in the embryo or fetus.

Trust   The degree of confidence felt in a relationship.

Tubal ligation   Sterilization of the female that involves the cutting and tying off or cauterizing of the fallopian tubes.

Tuberculosis (TB)   A disease caused by bacterial infiltration of the respiratory system.

Tumor   A neoplasmic mass that grows more rapidly than surrounding tissue.

Ulcerative colitis   An inflammatory disorder that affects the mucous membranes of the large intestine, producing bloody diarrhea.

Unintentional injuries   Injuries done without intent to harm.

Unsaturated fats   Fats that do have room for more hydrogen in their chemical structure; derived mostly from plants; liquid at room temperature.

Urethral opening   The opening through which urine is expelled.

Urinary incontinence   The inability to control urination.

U.S. Recommended Daily Allowance (USRDA)   Dietary guidelines developed by the Food and Drug Administration (FDA) and the United States Department of Agriculture.

Uterus (womb)   Hollow, pear-shaped muscular organ whose function is to contain the developing fetus.

Vaccination   Inoculation with killed or weakened pathogens or similar, less dangerous antigens in order to prevent or lessen the effects of some disease.

Vacuum aspiration   The use of gentle suction to remove fetal tissue from the uterus.

Vagina   The passage in females leading from the vulva to the uterus.

Vaginal intercourse   The insertion of the penis into the vagina.

Vaginismus   A state in which the vaginal muscles contract so forcefully that penetration cannot be accomplished.

Vaginitis   Set of symptoms characterized by vaginal itching, swelling, and burning.

Validating   Letting your partner know that although you may not agree with his or her point of view, you still respect the fact that he or she thinks or feels that way.

Variant sexual behavior   A sexual behavior that is not engaged in by most people.

Vas deferens   A tube that transports sperm toward the penis.

Vasectomy   Sterilization of the male that involves the cutting and tying off of both vasa deferentia.

Vasocongestion   The engorgement of the genital organs with blood.

Vegetarian   A term with a variety of meanings: Vegans avoid all foods of animal origin; lacto-vegetarians avoid flesh foods but eat dairy products; ovo-vegetarians avoid flesh foods but eat eggs; lacto-ovo-vegetarians avoid flesh foods but eat both dairy products and eggs; pesco-vegetarians avoid meat but eat fish, dairy products, and eggs; semivegetarians eat chicken, fish, dairy products, and eggs.

Veins   Vessels that carry blood back to the heart from other regions of the body.

Venereal warts   Warts that appear in the genital area or the anus; caused by the human papillomaviruses (HPVs).

Ventricles   The two lower chambers of the heart, which pump blood through the blood vessels.

Very low calorie diets (VLCDs)   Diets with a caloric value of 400 to 700 calories.

Violence   A set of behaviors that produce injuries, as well as the outcomes of these behaviors (the injuries themselves).

Virulent   Strong enough to overcome host resistance and cause disease.

Viruses   Minute parasitic microbes that live inside another cell.

Vitamins   Essential organic compounds that promote growth and reproduction and help maintain life and health.

Vulva   The female's external genitalia.

Wake or **viewing**   Displaying of the deceased to formalize last respects and increase social support of the bereaved.

Wellness   The achievement of the highest level of health possible in each of several dimensions.

Western blot   A test more accurate than the ELISA to confirm presence of HIV antibodies.

Withdrawal   A method of contraception that involves withdrawing the penis from the vagina before ejaculation. Also called *coitus interruptus*.

Withdrawal   A series of temporary physical and biopsychosocial symptoms that occur when the addict abruptly abstains from an addictive chemical or behavior.

Women's Health Initiative (WHI)   National study of postmenopausal women, in conjunction with the NIH mandate for equal research priorities for women's health issues.

Work addiction   The compulsive use of work and the work persona to fulfill needs for intimacy, power, and success.

Xanthines   The chemical family of stimulants to which caffeine belongs.

Yoga   A variety of Indian traditions geared toward self-discipline and the realization of unity; includes forms of exercise widely practiced in the West today that promote balance, coordination, flexibility, and meditation.

Young-old   People age 65 to 74.

Yo-yo diets   Cycles in which people repeatedly gain weight, then starve themselves to lose weight. This lowers their BMR, which makes regaining weight even more likely.

References

Chapter 1

1. Rossouw, J. and Writing Group for the Women's Health Initiative Investigators. Risks and Benefits of Estrogen Plus Progestin in Health of Postmenopausal Women. *Journal of the American Medical Association,* July 17, 2002, Vol 288, No. 3.
2. World Health Organization, "Constitution of the World Health Organization," *Chronicles of the World Health Organization* (Geneva, Switzerland, 1947).
3. R.Dubos, *So Human the Animal* (New York: Scribners, 1968), 15.
4. Department of Health and Human Services, *Healthy People 2000: National Health Promotion and Disease Prevention Objectives for the Year 2000* (Washington, DC: Government Printing Office, 1990).
5. National Center for Health Statistics, "About Healthy People 2010," 2002. http://www.health.gov/healthypeople/About/hpfact.htm.
6. Centers for Disease Control and Prevention, *Best Practices for Comprehensive Tobacco Control Programs—August 1999.* (Atlanta, GA: U.S. Department of Health and Human Services, Centers for Disease Control and Prevention, National Center for Chronic Disease Prevention and Health Promotion, Office on Smoking and Health, August 1999). Reprinted, with corrections.
7. R. Donatelle and S. Prows, *The Use of Financial Incentives and Social Support to Motivate Smoking Cessation Among High-Risk Pregnant Smokers,* technical report submitted to R.W. Johnson, Smoke-Free Families Office, Birmingham, AL.
8. Adapted from "Ten Great Public Health Achievements—United States, 1900–1999," *MMWR Weekly,* 48 (12) (April 1999): 241–243 (see website: http://www.cdc.gov/epo/mmwr/preview/mmwhtml/00056796.htm).
9. L. Strohl, "A Special Health Report: A look at the Future of Medicine," *USA Weekend* (October 1–3, 1999): 6–9.
10. Institute of Medicine, Board on International Health, *America's Vital Interest in Global Health: Protecting our People, Enhancing our Economy, and Advancing our International Interests.* (National Academy Press, Washington, DC 2002) (see http://www.stills.nap.edu/readingroom/books/avi/index.html).
11. Ibid.
12. L. Miller, "Medical Schools Put Women in Curricula," *The Wall Street Journal* (May 24, 1994): B1,B7.
13. F. Austin, "Women in Focus," *Shape* (September 1994): 46–47.
14. C. Tavris, *The Mismeasure of Woman* (New York: Touchstone, 1992), 99.
15. Ibid.
16. National Heart, Blood, and Lung Institute, "Facts about the Women's Health Initiative" (see http://www.nhlbi.nih.gov).
17. Ibid., Chapter 4.
18. Ibid., Chapter 8
19. M. DiMatteo, *The Psychology of Health, Illness, and Medical Care: An Individual Perspective* (Pacific Grove, CA: Brooks/Cole, 1994), 101–103.
20. E.P. Sarafino, *Health Psychology* (New York: Wiley, 1990), 189–191.
21. G.D. Bishop, *Health Psychology* (Boston: Allyn & Bacon, 1994), 84–86.
22. K. Glanz, F. Lewis, and B. Rimer, *Health Behavior and Health Education* (San Francisco: Jossey Bass, 2003), Chapters 8 and 9.
23. Ibid.
24. R. Donatelle, S. Prows, D. Champeau, and D. Hudson, "Randomized Controlled Trial Using Social Support and Financial Incentives for High-Risk Pregnant Smokers: Significant Other Supporter (SOS) Program," *Tobacco Control 9* Suppl. III (2000): iii, 67–69; S. Higgins et al., "Participation of Significant Others in Outpatient Behavioral Treatment Predicts Greater Cocaine Abstinence," *American Journal of Drug and Alcohol Abuse* (1994): 2047.
25. A. Ellis and M. Benard, *Clinical Application of Rational Emotive Therapy* (New York: Plenum, 1985).
26. P. Watson and R. Tharp, *Self-Directed Behavior: Self-Modification for Personal Adjustment* (Pacific Grove, CA: Brooks/Cole, 1993), 13.

Chapter 2

1. Steven Hyman and G. Fischbach. Mental Health: A Report of the Surgeon General NIH, NIMH http://www.surgeongeneral.gov/Library/mental health/chapter2/sec1.html 2002.
2. R. Lazarus, *Emotion and Adaptation* (New York: Oxford Press, 1991).
3. Catherine Heaney and Barbara A. Israel. Social Networks and Social Support. In Karen Glanz, et al. *Health Behavior and Health Education: Theory, Research and Practice,* 3E. 2002. (Jossey Bass Publishing, San Francisco.), 185-210.
4. MEP Seligman and D.M.Isaacowitz (2002). Learned Helplessness. In the *Encyclopedia of Stress.* San Diego: Academic Press.
5. J.R. Grant, Editor. *Journal of Humanistic Psychology:* Special Issue on Positive Psychology. Vol. 4, No. 1, 2001.
6. Steve Proffitt, "Pursuing Happiness with a Positive Outlook, not a Pill," *Los Angeles Times,* January 24, 1999, (see http://www.apa.org/releases/pursuing.html); "'Learned Optimism' Yields Health Benefits," APA HelpCenter: Mind/Body Connection, American Psychological Association, (see http://helping.apa.org).
7. M. Seligman. *Learned Optimism* (New York: Knopf, 1990).
8. James H. Martin. Motivation Processes and Performance: The Role of Global and Facet Personality. Doctoral Dissertation. University of North Carolina at Chapel Hill. 2002.
9. American Sleep Apnea Association. Washington, DC. http://www.sleepapnea.org 2002.
10. National Institutes of Health: National Center on Sleep Disorder Research, NHLBI. 2002. http://www.nhlbisupport.com/Sleep/research-a.html.
11. Ibid. 2002.
12. S. Hawks, M. Hull, R. Thalman, and P. Richins, "Review of Spiritual Health: Definition, Role, and Intervention Strategies in Health Promotion," *American Journal of Health Promotion* 9 (5) (1995): 371–378.
13. A. Scandurra, "Everyday Spirituality: A Core Unit in Health Education and Lifetime Wellness," *Journal of Health Education* 30 (2) (1999): 104–109.
14. Ibid., 106
15. L. Chapman, "Developing a Useful Perspective on Spiritual Health: Love, Joy, Peace and Fulfillment," *American Journal of Health Promotion* 2 (1987): 121–127.
16. Ibid., 122
17. Ibid., 124
18. R. Sloan, E. Bagiella, and T. Powell, "Religion, Spirituality, and Medicine," *The Lancet* 353-9153 (1999): 664–672.

19. D. Elkins, *Beyond Religion—A Personal Program for Building a Spiritual Life Outside the Walls of Traditional Religion* (Wheaton, IL: Quest Books, 1998).
20. Ibid.
21. Ibid.
22. D.Elkins, "Spirituality: It's What's Missing in Mental Health," *Psychology Today* (September/October, 1999), 48.
23. D.G. Myers and E. Diener, "Who Is Happy?" *Psychological Science* 6 (1995): 10–19.
24. Ibid.
25. Ibid.
26. Barbara L. Fredrickson, "Cultivating Positive Emotions to Optimize Health and Well-Being," American Psychological Association: *Prevention & Treatment*, 3, Article 0001a, posted March 7, 2000.
27. P. Doskoch, "Happily Ever Laughter," *Psychology Today* 29 (1996): 32–34.
28. Fredrickson, op. cit.
29. B. Siegel, *Love, Medicine, and Miracles* (New York: HarperCollins, 1988).
30. Fredrickson, op. cit.
31. D. Grady, "Think Right, Stay Well" *American Health* xi (1992): 50–54.
32. L. Temoshock, *The Type C Connection* (New York: Random House, 1989).
33. L. Cool, "Is Mental Illness Catching?" *American Health For Women* 16 (1997) 72–74.
34. L.A. Lefton, *Psychology* 7th ed. (Boston: Allyn and Bacon, 2000).
35. R. Hirshchfeld et al., "The National Depressive and Manic Depressive Association Consensus Statement on the Undertreatment of Depression," *Journal of the American Medical Association* 277 (4) (1997): 333–340.
36. Lefton, op. cit., 540.
37. National Institute for Mental Health (2000) (see http://www.nimh.nih.gov/); Lefton, op. cit., 541.
38. I. Levav, R. Kohn, J. Golding, and M. Weissman, "Vulnerability of Jews to Affective Disorders" *American Journal of Psychiatry* 154 (1997): 941–947.
39. S. Wood and E. Wood, *The World of Psychology* (Boston: Allyn and Bacon, 1999), 513.
40. S. Banks and R. Kerns, "Explaining High Rates of Depression in Chronic Pain: A Diathesis–Stress Framework," *Psychological Bulletin* 119 (1996): 995–110.
41. Lefton, op. cit., 543.
42. Adapted by permission of the author from Kathryn Rose Gertz, "Mood Probe: Pinpointing the Crucial Differences between Emotional Lows and the Gridlock of Depression," *Self* (November 1990): 165–168, 204.
43. R. G. Gladstone and L. Koenig, " Sex Differences in Depression Across the High School to College Transition," *Journal of Youth and Adolescence* 23 (1994): 643–669.
44. S. Scott, "Biology and Mental Health: Why Do Women Suffer More Depression and Anxiety?" *Maclean's* (Journal 12, 1998): 62–64.
45. L. Rabasca, "Psychotherapy May Be as Useful as Drugs in Treating Depression, Study Suggests," American Psychological Association: *The APA Monitor Online*, 30 (8) (September 1999).
46. NIMH, op. cit.
47. Ibid., 13.
48. "Anxiety Disorders," *USA Weekend* (October 12, 2000): 12.
49. Zimbardo et al., op. cit., 505.
50. Ibid, 506.
51. G. Wilson, P. Nathan, K. O'Leary, and L. Clark, *Abnormal Psychology* (Boston: Allyn and Bacon, 1996), 147.
52. Ibid., 147.
53. R. Saltus, "The PMS Debate," *Boston Globe Magazine* (July 25, 1999): 8–9.
54. U.S. Health Centers for Disease Control and Prevention (2000) (see http://www.cdc.gov).
55. K. Kendler and C. Gardner, "Boundaries of Major Depression: An Evaluation of DSM-IV Criteria," *American Journal of Psychiatry* 155 (1998): 172–176.
56. Ibid., 542.
57. "How to Choose a Therapist," *CBS This Morning* (July 24–26, 1996); D. Meyers, "Chapter 16: Therapy," in *Psychology* (New York: Worth, 2001), 537–572; J.W. Kalat, "Treatment of Psychologically Troubled People," in *Introduction to Psychology*, 4th ed. (Pacific Grove, CA: Brooks/Cole, 1996), 648–678.

Chapter 3

1. Sue Shellenbarger, "Learning How to Work with the Good Stress, Live without the Bad," *The Wall Street Journal*, July 25, 2001, B1.
2. H. Selye, *Stress Without Distress* (New York: Lippincott, 1974), 28–29.
3. Kenny, Diana, F. J. McGuigan and J. Sheppard (Eds). *Stress and Health Research and Clinical Applications* (New York: Gordon and Breach Pub., 2000).
4. H. Anismam and Z. Merali "Cytokines, Stress and Depressive Illness." *Brain, Behavior, and Immunity*. Vol 16. No 5 (2002): 513–524.
5. M. D. Jeremko, "Stress Inoculation Training: A Generic Approach for the Prevention of Stress-Related Disorders," *The Personal and Guidance Journal* 62 (1984): 544–550; H. S. Friedman, and S. Booth-Kewley, "The Disease-Prone Personality: A Meta-analytic View of the Construct." *American Psychologist* 42 (1987): 539–555.
6. G. E. Vaillant, *Adaptation to Life* (Boston: Little, Brown, 1977).
7. S. A. Lyness, "Predictions of Differences Between Type A and B Individuals in Heart Rate and Blood Pressure Reactivity,"*Psychological Bulletin* 114 (1993): 266–295: J. C. Barefoot and M. Schroll, "Symptoms of Depression, Acute Myocardial Infarction, and Total Mortality in a Community Sample, 1976–1980." *Circulation* 93 (1996); Schiraldi, G. T. Spalding, and C. Holford, "Expanding Health Educators' Roles to Meet Critical Needs in Stress Management and Mental Health," *Journal of Health Education* (1998):70.
8. R. Glaser, B. Rabin, M. Chesney, S. Cohen, and B. Natelson, "Updates Linking Evidence and Experience: Stress-Induced Immunomodulation," *Journal of the American Medical Association* 281 (24) (1999):2268–2270.
9. B. Rabin, *Stress, Immune Function, and Health: The Connection* (New York: Wiley-Liss, 1999).
10. D. Padgett, J. Sheridan, J. Dome, G. Berntson, J. Candelora, and R. Glaser, "Social Stress and the Reactivation of Latent Herpes Simplex Virus-Type 1," *Proceedings of the National Academy of Sciences, USA* 9 (1998): 7231–7235.
11. J Kiecolt-Glaser, R. Glaser, S. Gravenstein, W. Malarkey, and J. Sheridan, "Chronic Stress Alters the Immune Response to Influenza Virus Vaccines in Older Adults," *Proceedings of the National Academy of Sciences, USA* 93 (1996): 3043–3047.
12. S. Cohen, E. Frank, W. Doyle, D. Skoner, B. Rabin, and J. Gwaltney, "Types of Stressors That Increase Susceptibility to the Common Cold in Adults." *Health Psychology* 17 (1998): 214–223.
13. S. Cohen, W. Doyle, D. Skoner, B. Rabin, and J. Gwaltney, "Social Ties and Susceptibility to the Common Cold," *Journal of the American Medical Association* 277 (1997): 1940–1944.
14. N. Cherney et al. "Positive Thinking Does Not Improve Health." 2002. Report: Meeting of the European Society of Medical Oncology. http://www.esmo.org.
15. Schiraldi et al., op. cit., 69.
16. T. Holmes and R. Rahe, "The Social Readjustment Rating Scale," *Journal of Psychosocial Research* (1967): 213–217.
17. Ibid., 214.
18. R. Lazarus, "The Trivialization of Distress," in *Preventing Health Risk Behaviors and Promoting Coping with Illness*, ed. J. Rosen and L. Solomon (Hanover, NH: University Press of New England, 1985), 279–298.
19. L. Lefton, *Psychology* (Boston: Allyn and Bacon, 1994), 471.
20. M. Kenny and K. Rice, "Attachment to Parents and Adjustment in College Students: Current Status, Applications, and Future Considerations," *Counseling-Psychologist* 23 (1995): 433–456.

21. Kevin Nadal, "Ethnic Minority Students' Stressors: Their Impact on Campus Climate Perceptions and Academic Achievement," R. E. McNair Fellowship paper. http://members.tripod.com/~knall/minoritystress.html

22. Ibid.

23. R. C. Kessler, K. S. Kendler, A. C. Health, M. C. Neale, and L. J. Eaves, "Social Support, Depressed Mood, and Adjustment to Stress: A Genetic Epidemiological Investigation," *Journal of Personality and Social Psychology* 62 (1992): 257–272.

24. M. Friedman and R. H. Rosenman, *Type A Behavior and Your Heart* (New York: Knopf, 1974).

25. R. Ragland and R. Brand, "Distrust, Rage May be Toxic Cores That Put Type A Person at Risk," *Journal of American Medical Association* 261 (1989): 813, 814.

26. P. L. Rice, *Stress and Health* (Belmont, CA: Wadsworth Publishing, 1998), 378.

27. Kivimaki, M. et al. "Job Stress and Negative Health Effects," *British Medical Journal.* 325 (2002): 857–860.

28. L. Towbes and L. Cohen, "Chronic Stress in the Lives of College Students: Scale Development and Prospective Prediction of Distress," *Journal of Youth and Adolescence* 25 (1996): 206–217.

29. C. Crandell, J. Preisler, and J. Ausspring, "Measuring Life Event Stress in the Lives of College Students: The Undergraduate Stress Questionnaire (USQ)," *Journal of Behavioral Medicine* 15 (1992): 627–642.

30. "Hearts and Minds," *Harvard Mental Health Letter* 14 (1991): 1–4.

Chapter 4

1. D. Zucchio, "Todays's Violent Crime Is an Old Story with a New Twist," *San Jose Mercury News* (November 21, 1994), transmitted via America Online.

2. Bureau of Justice Statistics, "Expenditures and Employment Report: 1997" (Washington, DC: U.S. Department of Justice, 1998) (see http://www.ojp.usdoj.gov/bjs/).

3. Bureau of Justice Statistics, 2002 (see http://www.ojp.usdoj.gov/bjs).

4. Ibid.

5. U.S. Center for Health Statistics, "Health, United States, 2001" (Atlanta, GA: Centers for Disease Control and Prevention, 2001).

6. M. Leeds, Violence Prevention Conference (1996), Linnfield Community College, McMinnville, OR.

7. Ibid.

8. Ibid.

9. L. Lamberg, "Prediction of Violence Both Art And Science," *Journal of the American Medical Association* 275 (1996): 1713.

10. Leeds, op. cit.

11. Ibid.

12. Ibid.

13. F. Rivera, B. Mueller, G. Somas, Mendosa, and C. N. Rushfork, "Alcohol and Illicit Drugs and the Risk of Violent Death in the Home," *Journal of the American Medical Association* 278 (1997): 569–572.

14. "Substance Abuse: A Significant Characteristic in Domestic Violence Assailants," *Brown University Digest of Addiction Theory and Application* 16: 1–3.

15. M. Swartz, J. Swanson, et al., "Violence and Severe Mental Illness: The Effects of Substance Abuse and Non-Adherence to Medication," *American Journal of Psychiatry* 155 (1998): 226.

16. Rivera et al., op. cit., 571.

17. U.S. Center for Health Statistics, "Health, United States, 2000" (Atlanta, GA: Centers for Disease Control and Prevention, 2000).

18. U.S. Center for Health Statistics, "Health: United States, 2001. Highlights: Health Status and Determinants—Disparities in Mortality" (Atlanta, GA: Centers for Disease Control and Prevention, 2001): 6.

19. U.S. Center for Health Statistics, "Health, United States, 2000."

20. Ibid., 44.

21. Ibid., 46.

22. R. Lacyo, "Still Under the Gun?" *Time* (July 6, 1998): 32–56.

23. FBI, "Hate Crime Statistics Report, 1999" (2000) (see http://www.fbi.gov/ucr/99hate.pdf).

24. R. Fenske and L. Gordon, "Reducing Racial and Ethnic Hate Crimes on Campus: The Need for Community," in *Violence on Campus: Defining the Problems, Strategies for Action,* ed. A. Hoffman et al. (Gaithersburg, MD: Aspen, 1998).

25. Ibid.

26. Ibid.

27. Bureau of Justice Statistics, "2001 National Crime Victimization Survey" (Washington, DC: U.S. Department of Justice, 2002).

28. National Center for Domestic Violence and Abuse. Fact Sheet (2000).

29. J. Barley et al., "Risk Factors for Violent Death in the Home," *Archives of Internal Medicine* 157 (1997): 786.

30. D. Brookkoff, K. Obrien, C. Cook, T. Thompson, and C. Williams, "Characteristics of Participants in Domestic Violence: Assessment at the Scene of Domestic Violence," *Journal of the American Medical Association* 277 (1997): 1369.

31. "Injury and Domestic Violence Prevention," *Nurse Practitioner* 22 (1997): 122.

32. F. Trevino, S. Walker, and G. Ramirez, "Violent Crime in American Society," in *Violence on Campus: Defining the Problems, Strategies for Action,* ed. A. Hoffman et al. (Gaithersburg, MD: Aspen, 1998); Federal Bureau of Investigation, *Uniform Crime Report* (Washington, DC: U.S. Department of Justice, 1997).

33. A. Joerger and L. McClellan, "Why Men Batter: Why Women Stay," *Community Safety Quarterly* 5 (1992): 22–23.

34. N. West, "Crimes Against Women," *Community Safety Quarterly* 5 (1992): 3.

35. M. A. Straus and R. Gelles, eds., *Physical Violence in American Families: Risk Factors and Adaptions to Violence in 8,145 Families* (New Brunswick, NJ: Transaction, 1993), 101–201.

36. H. Pan, P. Neidig, and K. O'Leary, "Physical Aggression in Early Marriage: Pre-relationship and Relationship Effects," *Journal of Consulting and Clinical Psychology.*

37. G. T. Wilson, P. Nathan, K. D. O'Leary, and L. A. Clark, *Abnormal Psychology* (Boston: Allyn & Bacon, 1996).

38. Ibid.

39. Ibid.

40. E. Newberger, "Child Sexual Abuse," in *Violence in America: A Public Health Approach,* ed. M. Rosenberg and M. Fenley (New York: Oxford University Press, 1991), 85.

41. M. Whittaker, "The Continuum of Violence Against Women: Psychological and Physical Consequences," *Journal of American College Health* 40 (1992): 155.

42. D. Finkelhor, "Child Sexual Abuse," in *Violence in America: A Public Health Approach,* ed. M. Rosenberg and M. Fenley (New York: Oxford University Press, 1991), 25.

43. N. West, "Children: The Invisible Victims of Domestic Violence," *Community Safety Quarterly* 5 (1992): 20.

44. Whittaker, op. cit., 152.

45. K. Hunnicutt, "Women and Violence on Campus," in *Violence on Campus: Defining the Problems, Strategies for Action,* ed. A. Hoffman et al. (Gaithersburg, MD: Aspen, 1998), 150.

46. Ibid., 149.

47. A. Berkowitz, "College Men as Perpetrators of Acquaintance Rape and Sexual Assualt: A Review of Recent Literature," *Journal of American College Health* 40 (1992): 175.

48. J. Lenssen, "Update on Violence Statistics for Young Adults," Violence Prevention Summer Institute (2000), Corvallis, OR.

49. Bureau of Justice Statistics, "2001 National Crime Victimization Survey."

50. Ibid.

51. A. Hoffman, J. Schuh, and R. Fenske, *Violence on Campus* (Gaithersburg, MD: Aspen, 1998), 149–168.

52. D. Benson, C. Charlton, and F. Goohart, "Acquaintance Rape on Campus: A Literature Review," *Journal of American College Health* (1992): 157.

53. Wilson et al., op. cit.

54. Raquel Kennedy Bergen, *Violence Against Women Online Resources,* University of Minnesota, 2002 (see http://www.vaw.umn.edu/Vawnet/mrape.htm).

55. Ibid.

56. Benson et al., op. cit., 158.

57. M. W. Leidig, "The Continuum of Violence Against Women: Psychological and Physical Consequences," *Journal of American College Health* 40 (1992): 151. Reprinted with permission of the Helen Dwight Reid Education Foundation. Published by Heldref Publications, 1319 Eighteenth Street NW, Washington, DC 20036-1802. Copyright © 1992.

58. Berkowitz, op. cit., 177.

59. Ibid., 175.

60. Whittaker, op. cit., 153–154.

61. Berkowitz, op. cit., 718.

62. Ibid., 175.

63. Ibid., 176.

64. Hoffman et al., op. cit., 1–40.

65. Ibid., 175.

66. Ibid., 183.

67. J. Baier, M. Rosenzweig, and E. Shipple, "Patterns of Sexual Behavior, Coercion, and Victimization of University Students," *Journal of College Student Development* 32 (1991): 178.

68. M. Koss, "Rape: Scope, Impact, Interventions, and Public Policy Responses," *American Psychologist* 48 (1993): 1062–1069.

69. Hoffman et al., op. cit., 242.

70. E. Dersinger, C. Cychosz, and L. Jaeger, "Strategies for Dealing with Campus Violence," in *Violence on Campus: Defining the Problems, Strategies for Action,* ed. A. Hoffman et al. (Gaithersburg, MD: Aspen, 1998).

71. American Association of University Professors *Hostile Hallways, The AAUW Survey on Sexual Harrassment in America's Schools,* 1996; Hunnicutt, op. cit., 160.

72. Ibid., 161.

73. Ibid., 162.

74. A. Matthews, "Campus Crime 101," *Eugene Register Guard* (March 1993): 4B.

75. Dersinger et al., op. cit., 248.

76. B. Moyers, "What Can We Do About Violence?" Public Broadcasting Service, January 1995.

77. U.S. Center for Health Statistics, "Health, United States, 2001. U.S. Department of Labor, Bureau of Labor Statistics, Census of Fatal Occupational Injuries."

78. "National Census of Fatal Occupational Injuries, 1999." Bureau of Labor Statistics, U.S. Dept of Labor.

Chapter 5

1. G.Goenthals, S. Worchel, and L. Heatherington, *Pathways to Personal Growth: Adjustments in Today's World* (Boston: Allyn & Bacon, 1999), 480.

2. "Nurture Relationships: A Healthy Investment," MayoClinic.com, 2002, Mayo Foundation for Medical Education and Research (MFMER) (see http://www.mayohealth.org/home).

3. S.L. Michaud and R. M. Warner, "Gender Differences in Self-Reported Response in Troubles Talk," *Sex Roles: A Journal of Research* 37 (1997): 527–541; D.J. Canary and M.J. Cody, *Interpersonal Communication* (New York: St. Martin's, 1994), 33.

4. Dean M. Busby, and Vicki L. Loyer-Carlson, *Pathways to Marriage with RELATE Online Relationship Inventory: Premarital and Early Marital Relationships.* (Boston: Allyn & Bacon/Longman, 2003).

5. K. Galvin and P. Cooper, *Making Connections* (Los Angeles: Roxbury Press, 2000), 4.

6. Ibid., 6.

7. R. Adler and G. Rodman, "Perceiving the Self," in *Making Connections,* ed. K. Galvin and P. Cooper (Los Angeles: Roxbury Press, 2000), 23.

8. J. Caputo, H.C. Hazel, and C. McMahon, *Interpersonal Communication* (Boston: Allyn & Bacon, 1994), 224.

9. Ibid., 100.

10. Larry A. Nadig, (2002), "Effective Listening" (see http://www.drnadig.com/listening.htm).

11. Ibid.

12. Ibid.

13. M.E. Guffy, *Business Communication: Process and Products* (Belmont, CA: Wadsworth, 1994), 38.

14. Ibid., 38.

15. L.A. Nadig (2002), "How to Express Difficult Feelings" (see http://www.drnadig.com/feelings.htm).

16. M.Beard, *Interpersonal Relationships* (Dubuque, IA:Kendall/Hunt, 1989); N. Coupland, H. Giles, and W. Wieman, *Miscommunication and Problematic Talk* (London: Sage, 1991).

17. L.A. Nadig. (2002) "Relationship Conflict: Healthy or Unhealthy" (see http://www.drnadig.com.conflict.htm).

18. S.S. Brehm, *Intimate Relationships* (New York: McGraw-Hill, 1992), 4–5.

19. L. Lefton, *Psychology* (Boston: Allyn & Bacon, 2000) 480.

20. Ibid., 481.

21. C. Weiskopf, "Real Friends," *Current Health* 24 (1998): 16–18.

22. J. Turner and L. Rubinson, *Contemporary Human Sexuality* (Englewood Cliffs, NJ: Prentice Hall, 1993), 457.

23. D. McAdams, *Intimacy: The Need to Be Close* (New York: Doubleday, 1989), 87–91.

24. Turner and Rubinson, op. cit., 457.

25. G. Levinger, "Can We Picture Love?" in *The Psychology of Love,* ed. R. J. Sternberg and M. Barnes (New Haven: Yale University Press, 1988), 139–159.

26. E. Hatfield "Passionate and Compassionate Love" in *The Psychology of Loves,* ed. R. J. Sternberg and M. Barnes (New Haven: Yale University Press, 1988), 191–217.

27. R. A. Baron and D. Byrne, *Social Psychology* (Boston: Allyn & Bacon, 1997), 290–295.

28. E. Hatfield and G. W. Walster, *A New Look at Love* (Reading, MA: Addison Wesley, 1981).

29. A. Toufexis and P. Gray, "What Is Love? The Right Chemistry," *Time* (1993), 47–52.

30. Ibid., 51.

31. Ibid., 49.

32. H. Fisher, *Anatomy of Love: The Natural History of Monogamy, Adultery, and Divorce* (New York: Norton, 1993).

33. E. Hatfield, *Love, Sex, and Intimacy: Their Psychology, Biology, and History* (Reading, MA: Addison Wesley, 1993).

34. D. Tannen, *You Just Don't Understand: Women and Men in Conversation* (New York: William Morrow, 1990).

35. Michaud and Warner, op.cit., 528; Kay Pasley, Jennifer Kerpelman, and Doug Guilbert, "Gender Conflict; Identity Disruption and Marital Instability. Expanding Gottman's Model," *Journal of Social and Personal Relationships.* 18 (1) (2001): 1107–1114; Linda C. Gallo and Timothy W. Smith, "Attachment Style in Marriage: Adjustments and Responses to Interaction," *Journal of Social and Personal Relationships* 18 (2) (2001): J. Manusov and J. Harvey, eds., *Attribution, Communication Behavior, and Close Relationships* (New York: Cambridge University Press, 2001).

36. M. McGill, *The McGill Report on Male Intimacy* (New York: Holt, Rinehart and Winston, 1985), 87–88.

37. C. Gilligan, *In a Different Voice: Psychological Theory and Women's Development* (Cambridge, MA: Harvard University Press, 1982).

38. Caputo et al., op. cit., 302.

39. Ibid.

40. C. Morris, *Understanding Psychology* (Englewood Cliffs, NJ: Prentice Hall, 1993).

41. Ibid.

42. M. Brenton, *Sex Talk* (New York: Stein and Day, 1972); J. Gottman, C. Notarius, and H. Markman, *A Couple's Guide to Communication* (Champaign, IL: Research Press, 1976).

43. McGill, op. cit., 87–88.

44. M. Klausner and B. Hasselbring, *Aching for Love: The Sexual Drama of the Adult Child* (New York: Harper and Row, 1990).

45. Brehm, op. cit., 263.

46. B. Strong, C. DeVault, and B. Sayad, *Human Sexuality* (Mountain View, CA: Mayfield Publishing, 1999), 219.

47. Bureau of the Census, U.S. Department of Commerce, "U.S. Median Age at First Marriage 2001," *World Almanac Book of Facts,* 876.

48. Abraham Greeff and H.L. Malherbe, "Intimacy and Marital Satisfaction in Spouses," *Journal of Sex and Marital Therapy* 27 (93) (May–June 2001) Special Issue: 247–257; "Is Your Love Life Making You Sick?" *Ebony* 56 (9) (July 2001): 38–41; Linda Waite and Maggie Gallagher, *The Case for Marriage: Why Married People are Healthier, Happier, and Better off Financially* (New York: Doubleday, 2000).

49. Michael Young, George Denny, Tamara Young, and Raffy Tuquis, "Sexual Satisfaction among Married Women," *American Journal of Health Studies* 16 (2) (2000): 73–78.

50. Ronald Alsop, "As Same-Sex Households Grow More Mainstream, Businesses Take Note," *The Wall Street Journal,* August 8, 2001, B1, B4.

51. Ibid.

52. Ibid.

53. Ibid.

54. Centers for Disease Control, "National Vital Statistics Report." 49 (6) (August 2001).

55. National Center for Health Statistics and U.S. Census Bureau (2001) (see http://wwwcdc.gov/nchs/fastats/divorce.htm).

Chapter 6

1. The National College Health Assessment (Baltimore, MD. American College Health Association (ACHA), 2000).

2. S. Shaw, and J. Lee, "Learning Gender in a Diverse Society," *Women's Voices, Feminist Visions: Classic and Contemporary Readings* (Mountain View, CA: Mayfield Publishing, 2001).

3. American Psychological Association (see http://www.apa.org/monitor/oct97/conversion.html/).

4. D. J. Bem, "Exotic Becomes Erotic: A Developmental Theory of Sexual Orientation," *Psychological Review* 103 (2) (1996): 320–335; J. P. DeCecco and D. A. Parker, "The Biology of Homosexuality: Sexual Orientation or Sexual Preference?" *Journal of Homosexuality* 28 (1995): 1–28; G. Haumann, "Homosexuality, Biology, and Ideology," *Journal of Homosexuality* 28 (1) (1995): 57–77; S. LeVay, *Queer Science: The Use and Abuse of Research into Homosexuality* (Cambridge, MA: MIT Press, 1996).

5. G. M. Herek, J. Roy Gillis, and J. C. Cogan, "Psychological Sequelae of Hate-Crime Victimization Among Lesbian, Gay and Bisexual Adults," *Journal of Consulting and Clinical Psychology* 67 (6) (1999): 945–951.

6. A. H. Slyper, "Childhood Obesity, Adipose Tissue Distribution, and the Pediatric Practitioner," *Pediatrics* 102 (1998): 4.

7. J. Endicott et al., "Is Premenstrual Dysphoric Disorder a Distinct Clinical Entity?" *Journal of Women's Health and Gender-Based Medicine* 8 (1999): 663–679; F. R. Jelovesk, "Premenstrual Syndrome (PMS) vs. Premenstrual Dysphoric Disorder (PMDD)," *Women's Diagnostic Cyber* (2000) (see www.wdxcyber.com/nmood06.htm)

8. Writing Group for the Women's Health Initiative Investigators, "Risk and Benefits of Estrogen Plus Progestin in Healthy Postmenopausal Women: Principal Results from the Women's Health Initiative Randomized Controlled Trial," *Journal of the American Medical Association* 288 (3): (2002) 321–333.

9. W. H. Masters and V. Johnson, *Human Sexual Response* (Boston: Little, Brown, 1966).

10. G. F. Kelly, "Sexual Individuality and Sexual Values," in *Sexuality Today: The Human Perspective* (Dubuque, IA: McGraw-Hill, 1998), 203–206.

11. Ibid.

12. R. T. Michael, J. H. Gagnon, E. O. Laumann, and G. Kolata, *Sex in America: A Definitive Survey* (Boston: Little, Brown, 1994).

13. Ibid.

14. J. G. Beck, "Hypoactive Sexual Desire Disorder: An Overview," *Journal of Consulting and Clinical Psychology* 36 (6) (1995): 919–927.

15. B. Handy, "The Potency Pill," *Time* (May 4, 1998): 50–57.

16. Arnot Ogden Medical Center, "Frequently Asked Questions" (1998) (see http://www.aomc.org/HOD2/general/ViagraFAQ.html).

17. Men's Health Network, "Erectile Dysfunction Focus" (see www.healthology.com/focus_index.asp).

18. S. A. Lyman, C. Hughes-McLain, and G. Thompson, " 'Date-Rape Drugs': A Growing Concern," *Journal of Health Education* 29 (5) (1998): 271–274.

Chapter 7

1. Centers for Disease Control, *Contraceptive Options: Increasing Your Awareness* (Washington, DC: NAACOG, 1990).

2. University of Southern California School of Medicine, "Noncontraceptive Health Benefits," *Dialogues in Contraception* 3 (1990): 2.

3. National Center for Health Statistics, "Fertility, Family Planning, and Women's Health," 23 (1997): 7.

4. "FDA Approves Emergency Contraceptive Kit," College Health Report 1 (1998): 8.

5. Boston Women's Health Collective, *Our Bodies Ourselves for the New Century: A Book by Women and for Women* (New York: Simon and Schuster, 1998).

6. P. Gober, "The Role of Access in Explaining State Abortion Rates," *Social Science and Medicine* 44 (1997): 7.

7. Allan Guttmacher Institute, "Facts in Brief: Induced Abortion" (2000) (see www.agi-usa.org).

8. J. Gans Epner, H. Jonas, and D. Seckinger, "Late Term Abortion," *Journal of the American Medical Association* 280 (1998): 726.

9. Ibid., 728.

10. K. Schmidt, "The Dark Legacy of Fatherhood," *U.S. News and World Report* (December 14, 1992): 94–95.

11. U.S. Department of Agriculture, Center for Nutrition Policy and Promotion, "Expenditure on Children by Families, 2001 Annual Report" (see www.usda.gov/cnpp/Crc/crc2001.pdf).

12. Babycenter, "Family Finances: Life with a Baby" (2002) (see www.babycenter.com).

13. U.S. Department of Health and Human Services, *The Health Benefits of Smoking Cessation: A Report of the Surgeon General* (Washington, DC: Government Printing Office, 1990).

14. H. Klonoff-Cohen et al., "The Effects of Passive Smoking and Tobacco Exposure Through Breast Milk on Sudden Infant Death Syndrome," *Journal of the American Medical Association* 273 (1995): 795–798.

15. Centers for Disease Control and Prevention, "Cigarette Smoking among Pregnant Women," *Women and Smoking: A Report of the Surgeon General* (2001) (see CDC.gov/tobacco).

16. American College of Obstetricians and Gynecologists, "Nutrition During Pregnancy," *Patient Education Pamphlet* (AP001), March 1996.

17. National Down Syndrome Society (1998): (see http://www.ndss.org/).

18. Eleena de Lisser, "Breast-Feeding Boosts Adult IQ, Research Suggests," *The Wall Street Journal,* May 8, 2002, D2.

19. M. Avery, L. Duckett, J. Dodgson, K. Savik, and S. Henly, "Factors Associated with Very Early Weaning Among Primiparas Intending to Breastfeed," *Maternal and Child Health Journal* 2 (1998): 167–179.

20. Centers for Disease Control and Prevention. Cesarean Births in the United States. 2002. http://www.cdc.gov.

21. Centers for Disease Control and Prevention. Pelvic Inflammatory Disease. 2002. http://www.cdc.gov.

22. Ibid.

Chapter 8

1. Oregon Dairy Council, Nutrition Education Services, "Quotable Nutrition: It's All About You," news press release, 1998.

2. American Dietetic Association, "Nutrition and You Survey" (2002) (see http://www.eatright.org/pr/2002/052002a.html).

3. J. Beary and R. Donatelle, unpublished doctoral dissertation, 1994, Oregon State University.

4. C. Georgiou et al., "Among Young Adults, College Students and Graduates Practiced More Healthful Habits and Made More Healthful

Food Choices Than Did Non-Students," *Journal of the American Dietetic Association* 97 (1997): 754–762.

5. American Institute of Cancer Research, "Food, Nutrition and the Prevention of Cancer: A Global Perspective," (Washington, DC:1997).

6. Centers for Disease Control. Health, United States, 2002. Overview of Obesity in the United States. http://www.cdc.gov.

7. E. Whitney and S. Rolfes, *Understanding Nutrition,* 8th ed. (Belmont, CA: Wadsworth, 1999), 3–4.

8. David Ludwig, "Obesity: A New Dietary Treatment for a Major Public Health Threat," paper presented at the Linus Pauling Institute International Conference on Diet and Optimum Health (Portland, OR: May 2001).

9. National Center for Health Statistics, *Prevalence of Overweight and Obesity Among Adults: United States* (1999) (see http://www.cdc.gov/nchs/products/pubs/pubd/hestats/obese/obse99/htm).

10. Office of the Surgeon General, "Call to Action to Prevent and Decrease Overweight and Obesity: The Health Consequences of Obesity" (2001) (see http://www.surgeongeneral.gov/topics/obesity).

11. Ludwig, op. cit.

12. American Dietetic Association, "American Dietetic Association Survey Shows Americans Can Use Some Help in Sizing Up Their Meals" (May 20, 2002) (see http://www.eatright.org/pr/2002/052002b.html).

13. "Proteins," *Harvard Women's Health Watch,* 5 (1998):4.

14. Ibid., 4.

15. J.W. White and M. Wolraich, "Effect of Sugar on Behavior or Cognition in Children: A Meta-Analysis," *Journal of the American Medical Association* 274 (1995): 1617–1621.

16. "Do Potato Chips Cause Cancer? Don't Panic Yet, Say Experts," *Environmental Nutrition* 25 (6) (June 2002.): 3.

17. Center for Science in the Public Interest, "New Tests Confirm Acrylamide in American Foods—Snack Chips and French Fries Show Highest Levels of Known Carcinogens" (see http://www.cspinet.org/new/200206251.html).

18. *Food, Nutrition, and the Prevention of Cancer: A Global Perspective* (World Cancer Research Fund and the American Institute for Cancer Research, 1997); C. Fuchs et al., "Dietary Fiber and the Risk of Colorectal Cancer and Adenoma in Women," *New England Journal of Medicine* 340 (1999): 169–176.

19. Ibid., 170.

20. C. Fuchs, et al., op. cit.

21. L. K. Mahan and S. Escott-Stump, *Krause's Food, Nutrition, and Diet Therapy* (Philadelphia: Saunders, 2000), 578 + .

22. American Dietetic Association, "Position Statement: Diabetic Care," (22 suppl.) 1:542, 1999.

23. R. Mensink and M. Katan, "Effect of Dietary Trans-Fatty Acids on High-Density and Low-Density Lipoprotein and Cholesterol Levels in Healthy Subject," *New England Journal of Medicine* (August 16, 1990).

24. G. Ruoff, "Reducing Fat Intake with Fat Substitutes," *American Family Physician* 43 (1991): 1235–1242.

25. *Food, Nutrition and the Prevention of Cancer,* op. cit., 532.

26. W. Willet and A. Ascherio, "Health Effects of Trans-Fatty Acids," *American Journal of Clinical Nutrition* 66 (1997): 1006S–1010S.

27. Whitney and Rolfes, op. cit., 144.

28. American Heart Association, Nutrition Advisory Committee, News Release, on trans-fatty acids, May 13, 1994.

29. Willet and Ascherio, op. cit.

30. Whitney and Rolfes, op. cit., 144.

31. Elizabeth M. Ward., R.D., "Balancing Essential Dietary Fats: When More Might Be Better," *Environmental Nutrition* 24 (12) (2002): 1–6.

32. Ibid.

33. "MUFAs and PUFAs," *Food and Fitness Advisor* (9) (September 2002): 7:6.

34. Ibid.

35. J. Midgley, A. Matthew, C. Greenwood, and A. Logan, "Effects of Reduced Dietary Sodium on Blood Pressure: A Meta-Analysis of Randomized Controlled Trials," *Journal of the American Medical Association* 275 (1996): 1590–1598.

36. Whitney and Rolfes, op. cit., 412.

37. A.C. Looker et al., "Prevalence of Iron Deficiency in the United States, *Journal of the American Medical Association* 277 (1997): 973–976; "Recommendations to Prevent and Control Iron Deficiency in the United States," *Morbidity and Mortality Weekly Report* 47 (1998 supplement).

38. G.T. Sempos, A.C. Looker, and R.E. Gillum, "Iron and Heart Disease: the Epidemiological Data," *Nutrition Reviews* 54 (1996): 73–84.

39. Whitney and Rolfes, op. cit., 412.

40. "Food as Medicine," *Harvard Women's Health Watch* 5 (1998): 4–5.

41. J. Blumber, "Changing Vitamin Requirements"; Lawrence Kolonel, "Overview of Diet and Cancer Epidemiology"; Michael Gould, "The Anticancer Effects of Plant Monoterpenes"; John Potter, "Diet and Colorectal Cancer." Papers Presented at the Linus Pauling Institute International Conference on Diet and Optimum Health (Portland, OR: May 2001).

42. "Food as Medicine," op. cit., 5.

43. Melinda Manor and Janice Thompson, *Sport Nutrition for Health and Performance* (Champaign, IL: Human Kinetics Publishing, 2000), 278–283.

44. Ibid., 283.

45. E. Giovanucci, et al., "Intake of Carotenoids and Retinol in Relation to Risk of Prostate Cancer, *"Journal of the National Cancer Institute."* 87 (1995): 1767.

46. "Kale, Collards and Spinach Beat Carrots for Protecting Aging Eyes," *Environmental Nutrition* 24 (4) (2001): 1+ .

47. Ibid.

48. Jean Carper, R.D., "Eat Smart," *USA Weekend.* May 3–5, 2002, p. 6.

49. J. Smythies, *Every Person's Guide to Antioxidants* (Newark, NJ: Rutgers University Press, 1998).

50. Ibid.

51. B. Frie, OSU Linus Pauling Institute Seminar Series (2000).

52. Ibid.

53. Malinow, op. cit.

54. Rene Malinow, "Homocysteine, Folic Acid and CVD". Paper presented at the Linus Pauling Institute International Conference on Diet and Optimum Health (Portland, OR: May 2001).

55. Ibid.

56. N. T. Crane, V. S. Hubbard, and C. J. Lewis, "National Nutrition Objectives and Dietary Guidelines for Americans," *Nutrition Today* 33 (1998): 186–188.

57. Ibid.

58. Mahan and Escott-Stump, op. cit., 343–345.

59. Steffen Loft, "Diet, Oxidative DNA Damage and Cancer". Lawrence Kolonel, "Overview of Diet and Cancer Epidemiology." Papers presented at the Linus Pauling Institute International Conference on Diet and Optimum Health (Portland, OR: May 2001).

60. K. M. Fairfield and R. H. Fletcher, "Vitamins for Chronic Disease Prevention in Adults: Scientific Review," *JAMA* 2001, 287 (23): 3116–3126.

61. David Bender, "Daily Doses of Multivitamin Tablets," editorial in the *British Medical Journal* 325 174 (July 27): 173–174.

62. Centers for Disease Control and Prevention, Center for Infection Diseases. Food Borne Illnesses. http://www.cdc.gov. 2002.

63. Ibid.

64. Ibid.

65. Ibid.

66. Ibid.

67. Luanne Hughes, "Don't Let Unexpected Visitors 'Spoil' Summer Meals," *Environmental Nutrition* 25 (6) (June 2002): 2.

68. P. Morris, Y. Motarjemi, and F. Kaferstein, "Emerging Food-Borne Diseases," *World Health* 50 (1997): 16–22. Also see CDC website indicated in this chapter.

69. "Special Report: Irradiation Plants Geared to 'Zap' Meat and Poultry—Is it Safe?" *Tufts University Health and Nutrition Letter* 18 (1) (2000): 4–7.

70. Ibid., 5.
71. National Institute of Allergy and Infectious Diseases, NIH, "Fact Sheet: Food Allergy and Intolerances" (August 2002) (see http://www.niaid.gov/factsheets/food.htm).
72. Ibid.
73. Ibid.

Chapter 9

1. Centers for Disease Control, "Nutrition: Overweight and Obesity Trends: 1985–2000" (see http://www.cdc.gov/nccdphp/dnpa/obesity/trend/maps/index.htm), 2002.
2. A. H. Mokdad, B. A. Bowman, E. S. Ford, F. Vinicor, J. S. Marks, and J. P. Koplan, "Prevalence of Obesity in America," *Journal of the American Medical Association*, 286 (10) (2001): 1195–1200.
3. Centers for Disease Control and Prevention, National Center for Chronic Disease Prevention and Health Promotion, "Nutrition: Defining Overweight and Obesity" (see http://www.cdc.gov/nccdphp/dnpa/obesity/defining.htm). September 2002.
4. J. P. Boyle, A. A. Honeycutt, N. Venkat, T. J. Hoerger, L. S. Geiss, H. Chen, T. J. Thompson, *Diabetes Care* 24 (11) (2001): 1936–1940.
5. G. Cowley, "Generation XXL," *Newsweek* (July 3, 2000): 40–46.
6. Ibid., 42.
7. Centers for Disease Control and Prevention, National Center for Chronic Disease Prevention and Health Promotion, op cit.
8. Ibid.
9. National Center for Health Statistics (see www.cdc.gov/nchs/products/pubs/pubd/hestats/obese/obse99.htm).
10. Ibid.
11. Ibid.
12. Ibid.
13. R. Ross, "Atherosclerosis—An Inflammatory Disease," *New England Journal of Medicine* 340 (1999): 115–126.
14. ADA Position adopted by the House of Delegates, October 20, 1996. ADA headquarters at 800-877-1600, ext. 4896.
15. Centers for Disease Control and Prevention, National Center for Chronic Disease Prevention and Health Promotion, op. cit.
16. S. Cummings, K. Goodrick, and J. Foreyt, "Position of the American Dietetic Association: Weight Management 97" (1997): 71–75.
17. J. G. Meisler and S. St. Jeor, "Summary and Recommendations from the American Health Foundation's Expert Panel on Healthy Weight," *American Journal of Clinical Nutrition* 63 (1996): 474S–477S.
18. Cummings et al., op. cit., 72.
19. U.S. Department of Health and Human Services, "The Surgeon General's Call to Action to Prevent and Decrease Overweight and Obesity" (2001) (see http://www.surgeongeneral.gov/topics/obesity/).
20. A. Forman, "The Threat of Insulin Resistance to Your Heart," *Environmental Nutrition* 23 (8) (2000): 4–6.
21. American Heart Association web site, "2001 Heart and Stroke Statistical Update," 11.
22. Ibid., 13.
23. Ibid., 19.
24. Ibid., 20.
25. Ibid., 19–20.
26. Ibid., 14.
27. "Special Report: Weight Control," from *Women's HealthSource* (Mayo Clinic, 1997), 3.
28. A. Stunkard et al., "The Body Mass Index of Twins Who Have Been Raised Apart," *New England Journal of Medicine* 322 (1990): 1477–1482.
29. C. Bouchard et al., "The Response to Long-Term Overfeeding in Identical Twins," *New England Journal of Medicine* 322 (1990): 1483–1487.
30. Ibid.
31. Cummings et al., op. cit., 73.
32. P. Jaret, "The Way to Lose Weight," *Health* (January/February 1995): 52–59.

33. A. Novitt-Morena, "Obesity: What's the Genetic Connection?" *Current Health* 24 (1998): 18–23.
34. "Genes and Appetite," *Harvard Women's Health Watch*, January 1996; L. Tartaglia et al., "Identification and Expression Cloning of a Leptin Receptor," *Cell* 83 (1995): 1263–1271.
35. "Special Report: Weight Control," op. cit.
36. M. Turton, D. O'Shea, I. Gunn, et al., "A Role of Glucagon-like Peptide 1 in the Central Regulation of Feeding," *Nature* 379 (1996): 69–72.
37. F. Katch and W. McArdle, *Introduction to Nutrition, Exercise, and Health*, 4th ed. (Philadelphia: Lea and Febiger, 1992), 53.
38. "Special Report: Weight Control," op. cit., 4.
39. P. Elmer-Dewitt, "Fat Times" *Time* (January 16, 1995): 60.
40. Cowley, op. cit., 43.
41. S. Lichman et al., "Discrepancy Between Self-Reported and Actual Caloric Intake and Exercise in Obese Subjects," *New England Journal of Medicine* 327 (1992): 1894–1897.
42. K. Brownell, "Comments on the Latest Study on Yo-Yo Diets by Steven Blair of the Institute for Aerobics Research" (paper originally presented in 1993, newer report in paper presented at Oregon State University by Steven Blair, Fall, 1998).
43. National Center for Health Statistics, "Prevalence of Sedentary Leisure-Time Behavior Among Adults in the United States," December 2000 (see http://www.cdc.gov/nchs/products/pubs/pubd/hestats/3and4/sedentary.htm).
44. Ibid.
45. Ibid.
46. "Special Report: Weight Control," op. cit., 4.
47. N. Diehl, C. Johnson, and R. Rogers, "Social Physique Anxiety and Disordered Eating: What's the Connection?" *Addictive Behaviors* 23 (1998): 1–16.
48. "Special Report: Weight Control," op. cit., 4.
49. G. K. Goodrick and J. P. Foreyt, "Why Treatments for Obesity Don't Last," *Journal of the American Dietetic Association* 91 (1991): 1243–1247.
50. C. F. Telch and W. S. Agras, "The Effects of Very Low Caloric Diet on Binge Eating," *Behavior Therapy* 24 (1993): 177–193.
51. *USA Today Weekend* (July 14–16, 2000): 6.
52. R. L. Atkinson, "Use of Drugs in the Treatment of Obesity," *Annual Review of Nutrition* 17 (1997): 383–403, as reported in Eleanor Whitney and S. R. Rolfes, *Understanding Nutrition* 9th ed. (Belmont, CA: Wadsworth, 2002), 278.
53. "Fen-Phen Legal Resources," (2002) (see http://www.fen-phen-legal-resources.com).
54. Food and Drug Administration, "FDA Approves Orlistat for Obesity" (1999) (see http://www.fda.gov/bbs/topics/ANSWERS/ANS00951.html).
55. Eleanor Whitney and S. R. Rolfes, *Understanding Nutrition*, 9th ed. (Belmont, CA: Wadsworth, 2002), 279.
56. Ibid.

Chapter 10

1. National Center for Chronic Disease Prevention and Health Promotion, "Physical Activity and Health: A Report of the Surgeon General" (2002) (see http://www.cdc.gov/nccdphp/sgr/mm.htm); National Center for Chronic Disease Prevention and Health Promotion, "The Surgeon General's Call to Action to Prevent and Decrease Overweight and Obesity" (2002) (see http://www.cdc.gov).
2. Centers for Disease Control and Prevention, "Physical Activity and Health: The Link between Physical Activity and Morbidity and Mortality." (see http://www.cdc.gov/nccdphp/sgr/mm.htm).
3. American College of Sports Medicine, "ACSM Position Stand on the Recommended Quantity and Quality of Exercise for Developing and Maintaining Cardiorespiratory and Muscular Fitness, and Flexibility in Adults," *Medicine and Science in Sports and Exercise* 30 (1998): 975–991.
4. C. J. Caspersen, K. E. Powell, and G. M. Christianson, "Physical Activity, Exercise, and Physical Fitness: Definitions and Distinctions

for Health-Related Research," *Public Health Report* 100 (1985): 126–131.

5. L. Bernstein et al., "Adolescent Exercise Reduces Risk of Breast Cancer in Younger Women," *Journal of the National Cancer Institute,* September 1994.

6. U.S. Department of Health and Human Services, *Physical Activity and Health: A Report of the Surgeon General,* op. cit.

7. R. Gates, "Fitness Is Changing the World: For Women," *IDEA Today* (July–August 1992): 58.

8. Ibid.

9. C. B. Corbin and R. Lindsey, *Concepts in Physical Education with Laboratories,* 8th ed. (Dubuque, IA: Times Mirror, 1994).

10. U.S. Department of Health and Human Services, *Physical Activity and Health: A Report of the Surgeon General,* op cit.

11. A. Lubell, "Can Exercise Help Treat Hypertension in Black Americans?" *The Physician and Sportsmedicine* 16 (September 1988): 165–168.

12. V. H. Heyward, *Advanced Fitness Assessment and Exercise Prescription,* 2nd ed. (Champaign, IL: Human Kinetics Publishers, 1991).

13. W. L. Haskell et al., "Cardiovascular Benefits and Assessment of Physical Activity and Physical Fitness in Adults," *Medicine and Science in Sports and Exercise* 24 (6) Supplement (1992): S201–S220.

14. C. Christmas, "Fitness for Reducing Osteoporosis," *The Physician and Sportsmedicine* 28 (October 2000): 33–34.

15. National Institute of Health Osteoporosis and Related Bone Disease National Resource Center, "Fast Facts on Osteoporosis" (December 2001).

16. C. M. Snow, J. M. Shaw, and C. C. Matkin, "Physical Activity and Risk for Osteoporosis," in *Osteoporosis,* eds. R. Marcus, D. Feldman, and J. Kelsey (San Diego: Academic Press, 1996), 511–528.

17. Christine Snow, and Toby Hayes, Guest Lecture, "Bone Health" in Modern Maladies Class Oregon State University, 2001.

18. W. McArdle, F. Katch, and V. Katch, *Exercise Physiology, Fifth Edition* (Philadelphia: Lippincott, Williams and Wilkins, 2001), 60–65.

19. American College of Sports Medicine, *ACSM's Guidelines for Exercise Testing and Prescription,* 6th ed. (Baltimore: Lippincott, Williams and Wilkins, 2000).

20. R. Ross, J. A. Freeman, and I. Janssen, "Exercise Alone Is an Effective Strategy for Reducing Obesity and Related Comorbidities," *Exercise and Sport Sciences Reviews* 28 (4) (2000): 165–170.

21. Ibid.

22. National Institutes of Health, "Consensus Development Conference Statement on Diet and Exercise in Non-Insulin-Dependent Diabetes Mellitus," *Diabetes Care* 10 (1987): 639–644.

23. S. P. Helmrich, D. R. Ragland, and R. S. Paffenbarger, Jr., "Prevention of Non-Insulin-Dependent Diabetes Mellitus with Physical Activity," *Medicine and Science in Sports and Exercise* 26 (1994): 824–830.

24. S. N. Blair et al., "Physical Fitness and All-Cause Mortality: A Prospective Study of Healthy Men and Women," *Journal of the American Medical Association* 262 (1989): 2395–2401.

25. E. R. Eichner, "Infection, Immunity, and Exercise: What to Tell Patients?" *The Physician and Sportsmedicine* 21 (January 1993): 125–135.

26. W. A. Primos, Jr., "Sports and Exercise During Acute Illness: Recommending the Right Course for Patients," *The Physician and Sportsmedicine* 24 (January 1996): 44–53.

27. D. C. Nieman et al., "Infectious Episodes in Runners Before and After the Los Angeles Marathon," *Journal of Sports Medicine and Physical Fitness* 30 (1990): 316–328.

28. Eichner, op. cit.

29. Ibid.

30. R. Gates, "Fitness Is Changing the World: For Women," op. cit.

31. E. T. Howley and D. B. Franks, *Health Fitness Instructor's Handbook,* 2nd ed. (Champaign, IL: Human Kinetics Books, 1992).

32. U.S. Department of Health and Human Services, *Physical Activity and Health: A Report of the Surgeon General,* op. cit.

33. B. Stamford, "Tracking Your Heart Rate for Fitness," *The Physician and Sportsmedicine* 21 (March 1993): 227–228.

34. U.S. Centers for Disease Control and Prevention and American College of Sports Medicine, "Summary Statement: Workshop on Physical Activity and Public Health," *Sports Medicine Bulletin* 28 (4) (1993): 7.

35. G. A. Klug and J. Lettunich, *Wellness: Exercise and Physical Fitness* (Guilford, CT: Dushkin Publishing Group, 1992).

36. P. D. Wood, "Physical Activity, Diet, and Health: Independent and Interative Effects," *Medicine and Science in Sports and Exercise* 26 (1994): 838–843.

37. American College of Sports Medicine," ACSM Position Stand on the Recommended Quantity and Quality of Exercise for Developing and Maintaining Cardiorespiratory and Muscular Fitness, and Flexibility in Adults," op. cit.

38. Ibid.

39. M. Cyphers, "Flexibility," in *Personal Trainer Manual,* 2nd ed. (San Diego: American Council on Exercise, 1996), 291–308.

40. P. A. Sienna, *One Rep Max: A Guide to Beginning Weight Training* (Indianapolis: Benchmark Press, 1989).

41. H. G. Knuttgen and W. J. Kraemer, "Terminology and Measurement in Exercise Performance," *Journal of Applied Sport Science Research* 1 (1987): 1–10.

42. M. S. Feigenbaum and M. L. Pollock, "Prescription of Resistance Training for Health and Disease," *Medicine and Science in Sports and Exercise* 31 (1999): 38–45.

43. M. L. Pollock and W. J. Evans, "Resistance Training for Health and Disease: Introduction," *Medicine and Science in Sports and Exercise* 31 (1999): 10–11.

44. American College of Sports Medicine, "ACSM Position Stand on the Recommended Quantity and Quality of Exercise for Developing and Maintaining Cardiorespiratory and Muscular Fitness, and Flexibility in Adults," op. cit.

45. C. L. Wells, *Women, Sport, and Performance: A Physiological Perspective,* 2nd ed. (Champaign, IL: Human Kinetics, 1991).

46. American College of Sports Medicine, "ACSM Position Stand on the Recommended Quantity and Quality of Exercise for Developing and Maintaining Cardiorespiratory and Muscular Fitness, and Flexibility in Adults," op. cit.

47. W. C. Whiting and R. F. Zernicke, *Biomechanics of Musculoskeletal Injury* (Champaign, IL: Human Kinetics, 1998).

48. D. M. Brody, "Running Injuries: Prevention and Management," *Clinical Symposia* 39 (1987).

49. J. C. Erie, "Eye Injuries: Prevention, Evaluation, and Treatment," *The Physician and Sportsmedicine* 19 (November 1991): 108–122.

50. R. C. Wasserman and R. V. Buccini, "Helmet Protection from Head Injuries Among Recreational Bicyclists," *American Journal of Sports Medicine* 18 (1990): 96–97.

51. S. M. Simons, "Foot Injuries of the Recreational Athlete," *The Physician and Sportsmedicine* 27: (January 1999): 57–70.

52. J. Andrish and J. A. Work, "How I Manage Shin Splints," *The Physician and Sportsmedicine* 18 (December 1990): 113–114.

53. E. A. Arendt, "Common Musculoskeletal Injuries in Women," *The Physician and Sportsmedicine* 24 (July 1996): 39–48.

54. American Academy of Orthopaedic Surgeons, *Athletic Training and Sports Medicine,* 3rd ed., (Park Ridge, IL: AAOS, 2000).

55. J. J. Mistovich, B. Q. Hafen, and K. J. Karren, *Prehospital Emergency Care,* 6th ed. (Upper Saddle River, NJ: Prentice-Hall, 2000).

56. American College of Sports Medicine, "Position Stand—Heat and Cold Illnesses During Distance Running," *Medicine and Science in Sports and Exercise* 28 (December 1996): i–x.

57. American College of Sports Medicine, "Position Stand—Exercise and Fluid Replacement," *Medicine and Science in Sports and Exercise* 28 (January 1996): i–vii.

58. P. R. Below, P. Mora-Rodriguez, J. Gonzalez-Alonso, and F. F. Coyle, "Fluid and Carbohydrate Ingestion Independently Improve Performance During 1 Hr. of Intense Exercise," *Medicine and Science in Sports and Exercise* 27 (1995): 200–210.

59. D. J. Casa et al., "National Athletic Trainers' Association Position Statement: Fluid Replacement for Athletes," *Journal of Athletic Training* 35 (2) (2000): 212–224.

60. J. S. Thornton, "Hypothermia Shouldn't Freeze Out Cold-Weather Athletes," *The Physician and Sportsmedicine* 18 (January 1990): 109–113.

61. American College of Sports Medicine, "Position Stand: Heat and Cold Illnesses During Distance Running," op. cit.

62. Nancy Clark, "Muscle Cramps: Do They Cramp Your Style?" *Newsletter of the American College of Sports Medicine* (Summer 2001), 7.

63. Ibid.

64. Ibid.

65. Ibid.

Chapter 11

1. H. F. Doweiko, *Concepts of Chemical Dependency* (Pacific Grove, CA: Brooks/Cole, 1993), 9.

2. C. Nakken, *The Addictive Personality* (Center City, MN: Hazelden, 1996), 24.

3. K. Blum and J. E. Payne, *Alcohol and the Addictive Brain* (New York: The Free Press, 1991), 186.

4. S. Peele, *Diseasing of America: How We Allowed Recovery Zealots and the Treatment Industry to Convince Us We Are Out of Control* (Lexington, MA: Lexington Books, 1995), 61.

5. V. Fox, *Addiction, Change, and Choice: The New View of Alcoholism* (Tucson, AZ: See Sharp Press, 1998), 11.

6. G. Hansen and P. Venturelli, *Drugs and Society,* 5th ed. (Boston: Jones and Bartlett, 1998), 47.

7. Ibid., 40.

8. Ibid.

9. L. Kurtz, *Self Help and Support Groups: A Handbook for Practitioners* (Thousand Oaks, CA: Sage, 1997), 12.

10. J. R. Wilson and J. A. Wilson, *Addictionary* (New York: Simon & Schuster, 1992), 166.

11. Nakken, op. cit, 24.

12. D. Gerstein et. al, "Gambling Impact and Behavior Study: Report to the National Gambling Impact Study Commission," April 1999, National Opinion Research Center at the University of Chicago (see http://www.norc.uchicago.edu/new/pdf/gamble.pdf.

13. Ibid., 28.

14. A. Washton and D. Boundy, *Willpower's Not Enough: Recovering from Addictions of Every Kind* (New York: HarperCollins, 1990), 14.

15. Performance Resource Press, "Health Sentry Newsletter" 15 (1) (2002) (see http://www.prponline.net).

16. B. Yoder, *The Resource Recovery Book* (New York: Simon & Schuster, 1992), 259.

17. R. Olivardia, H. Pope, and J. Hudson, "Muscle Dysmorphia in Male Weightlifters: A Case-Control Study," *American Journal of Psychiatry* 157 (2000): 1291–1296.

18. M. Maine, *Body Wars: Making Peace with Women's Bodies* (Carlsbad, CA: Gurze, 2000), 282.

19. K. Young, M. Pistner, J. O'Mara, and J. Buchanan, "Cyber-Disorders: The Mental Health Concern for the New Millennium," paper presented at 107th APA convention, August 20, 1999 (see http://www.netaddiction.com/articles/cyberdisorders.htm).

20. K. Young, "Net Compulsions: The Latest Trends in the Area of Internet Addiction," 1999 (see http://www.netaddiction.com/net_compulsions.htm).

21. Ibid.

22. Nakken, op. cit., 16.

23. Wilson and Wilson, op. cit., 167.

24. National Institute on Alcohol Abuse and Alcoholism, Alcohol Alert Number 36, *Patient-Treatment Matching,* April 1997.

Chapter 12

1. L. D. Johnson, P. M. O'Malley, and J. G. Bachman, *The Monitoring the Future Study, 1975–2001,* vol. 2 (Rockville, MD: NIDA, 2002), 204.

2. A. Cohen, "Battle of the Binge," *Time* (September 8, 1997).

3. H. Wechsler et al., "Trends in College Binge Drinking during a Period of Increased Prevention Efforts: Findings from Four Harvard School of Public Health College Study Surveys: 1993–2001," *Journal of American College Health* 50 (5) (2002): 207.

4. Johnson et al., op. cit., 45.

5. Wechsler et al., op. cit.

6. H. Wechsler et al., "College Binge Drinking in the 1990s: A Continuing Problem," *Journal of American College Health* 28 (2000): 202.

7. J. Knight, H. Wechsler, K. Meichun, M. Seibring, E. Weitzman, and M. Schnuckit, "Alcohol Abuse and Dependence among U.S. College Students," *Journal of Studies on Alcohol* 63 (3) (2002): 263–270.

8. National Institute on Alcohol Abuse and Alcoholism, "Surveillance Report #55. Apparent Per Capita Alcohol Consumption: National, State, and Regional Trends, 1977–98," December 2000.

9. T. Katsouyanni et al., "Ethanol and Breast Cancer: An Association That May Be Both Confounded and Causal," *International Journal of Cancer* 58 (3) (1994): 356–361.

10. C. Ikonomidou et al., "Ethanol-Induced Apoptotic Neurodegeneration and the Fetal Alcohol Syndrome," *Science* 287 (2000): 1056–1060.

11. National Organization on Fetal Alcohol Syndrome (see http://www.nofas.org).

12. National Highway Traffic Safety Administration, "Traffic Safety Facts," 2000, 2001.

13. H. Wechsler et al., "Changes in Binge Drinking and Related Problems among American College Students Between 1993 and 1997," *Journal of American College Health* 47 (2) (1998): 57–68.

14. National Highway Traffic Safety Administration, "Traffic Safety Facts" 1996, Alcohol, Washington, DC: National Center for Statistics and Analysis, 1997.

15. National Highway Traffic Safety Administration, "Traffic Safety Facts," 2000, 2001.

16. Ibid.

17 Insurance Institute for Highway Safety, "Fatality Facts: Alcohol," October 2000.

18. F. K. Goodwin and E. M. Gause, "Alcohol, Drug Abuse, and Mental Health Administration," *Prevention Pipeline* 3 (1990): 19.

19. Marc A. Shockit, "New Findings on Genetics of Alcoholism," *Journal of American Medical Association* 281 (20) (1999): 1075–1976.

20. W. S. Slutske et al., "The Heritability of Alcoholism Symptoms: Indicators of Environmental Influence in Alcohol Dependent Individuals—Revisited," *Alcoholism and Experimental Research* 23(5) (1999): 759.

21. "Adult Children of Alcoholics" *Alcohol Issues and Solutions* 6 (2) (2000): 6.

22. B. F. Grant, "Estimates of U.S. Children Exposed to Alcohol Abuse and Dependence in the Family," *American Journal of Public Health* 90 (1) (2000).

23. U.S. Department of Health and Human Services, *Ninth Special Report to the U.S. Congress on Alcohol and Health* (1997): 261.

24. E. Gomberg, "Women and Alcohol: Issues for Prevention Research," *National Institute on Alcohol Abuse and Alcohol Research Monograph* 32 (1996): 185–214.

25. Ibid.

Chapter 13

1. J. M. McGinnis and W. H. Foege, "Actual Causes of Death in the United States," *Journal of the American Medical Association* 270 (1993): 2207–2212.

2. American Lung Association, Best Practices and Program Services, Epidemiology and Statistics Unit, June 2002.

3. Centers for Disease Control and Prevention, "Trends in Cigarette Smoking Among High School Students—United States, 1991–2001," *Morbidity and Mortality Weekly* 51 (19): 409–412.

4. Centers for Disease Control and Prevention, "Annual Smoking-Attributable Mortality, Years of Potential Life Lost, and Economic Costs—United States," Vol. 51 (14).

5. N. Rigotti, J. Lee, and H. Wechsler, "U.S. College Students' Use of Tobacco Products," *Journal of the American Medical Association* 284 (2000): 699–705.

6. Everett et al., "Smoking Initiation and Smoking Patterns Among U.S. College Students," *Journal of American College Health* 48 (1999): 55.
7. American Cancer Society, Tobacco Information: Cigar Smoking and Cancer, 1998.
8. American Lung Association, "Trends in Cigarette Smoking," March 1999.
9. S. Hansen, The University of Iowa Student Health Service Website, downloaded August 21, 2000.
10. National Institutes of Health, *Smokeless Tobacco or Health,* Monograph 2 (May 1993): 3.
11. Oral Cancer Foundation, 2002, (see http://www.oralcancer.org).
12. National Institute on Drug Abuse Research Report Series, "Nicotine Addiction," U.S. Department of Health and Human Services, NIDA Publication No. 98-4342, 1998.
13. National Institute on Drug Abuse, "Evidence Builds that Genes Influence Cigarette Smoking." NIDA Notes, U.S. Department of Health and Human Services, NIDA Publication 00-3478, 2000.
14. American Cancer Society, "Cancer Facts and Figures" (2000), 18.
15. American Cancer Society, op. cit.
16. "Study Links Smoking to Pancreatic Cancer," *Science News* (October 22, 1994): 261.
17. WHO Collaborative Study of Cardiovascular Disease and Steroid Hormone Contraception, "Acute Myocardial Infarction and Combined Oral Contraceptives: Results of an International Multicentre Case-Control Study," *Lancet* (April 26, 1997): 1202–1209.
18. American Cancer Society, op. cit.
19. NIDA Notes, "Nicotine Conference Highlights Research Accomplishments and Challenges" (September/October 1995): 11–12.
20. American Lung Association Website, "Secondhand Smoke" (see http://ala.org).
21. K. Steenland, "Passive Smoking and the Risk of Heart Disease," *Journal of the American Medical Association* 267 (1992): 94–99.
22. P. Hilts, "Wide Peril is Seen in Passive Smoking," *New York Times* (May 9, 1990): A25.
23. American Lung Association Website, op. cit.
24. D. Mannino, "Children Exposed to ETS Miss More School," *Tobacco Control* (May 1996).
25. The State Tobacco Information Center at http://stic.neu.edu. National Association of Attorneys General, "Multistate Settlement with Tobacco Industry." Downloaded August 23, 2000.
26. "Nicotine Patches Seen to Help Smokers Quit," *Boston Globe* (June 23, 1994): 3.
27. "Grounds for Breaking the Coffee Habit," *Tufts University Diet and Nutrition Newsletter* 7 (1990): 4.
28. "Fetal Loss Associated with Caffeine," *Fact and Comparisons Drug Newsletter* 13 (March 1994): 39.

Chapter 14

1. U.S. Department of Health and Human Services, "National Household Survey on Drug Abuse Main Findings 2001" (2002).
2. Ibid.
3. National Institute on Drug Abuse, "National Survey Results on Drug Use, 1975–2001: College Students and Adults," *Monitoring the Future* (2002).
4. Ibid.
5. M. Fisherman and C. Johanson, "Cocaine," in *Pharmacological Aspects of Drug Dependence: Towards an Integrated Neurobehavior Approach (Handbook of Experimental Pharmacology),* ed. C. Schuster and M. Kuhar (Hamburg: Springer Verlag, 1996), 159–195.
6. Ibid.
7. National Institute on Drug Abuse, *Capsules* (1996).
8. H. C. Ashton, "Pharmacology and Effects of Cannabis: A Brief Review," *British Journal of Psychiatry* 178 (2001): 101–106.
9. American Academy of Ophthalmology, Medical Library, "The Use of Marijuana in the Treatment of Glaucoma" (see http://www.medem.com.2002).
10. R. Mathias, "Marijuana Impairs Driving-Related Skills and Workplace Performance," *NIDA Notes 11* (1) (January/February 1996): 6.

11. National Institute on Drug Abuse, "Heroin, 0–12," *Infofax* (1998): 1.
12. National Institute on Drug Abuse, "National Survey Results on Drug Use, 1975–2001," op. cit.
13. National Institute on Drug Abuse, "NIDA Launches Initiative to Combat Club Drugs," *NIDA Notes* 14 (2) (2000).
14. National Institute on Drug Abuse, "Anabolic Steroid Abuse," *NIDA Research Report Series* (2000).
15. Office of National Drug Control Strategy, "2002 National Drug Control Strategy" (see http://www.whitehousedrugpolicy.gov. 2002).
16. Ibid.
17. National Institute on Drug Abuse, "Worker Drug Use and Workplace Policies and Programs: Results from the 1994 and 1997 National Household Survey on Drug Abuse" (1999).
18. Ibid.

Chapter 15

1. American Heart Association, "2002 Heart and Stroke Statistical Update" (Dallas, TX: American Heart Association, 2002).
2. Ibid.
3. Ibid.
4. Ibid.
5. Ibid.
6. Centers for Disease Control, *Mortality and Morbidity Weekly Report* 49, (55-2), March 24, 2000.
7. American Heart Association, "2002 Heart and Stroke Statistical Update" (see http://www.americanheart.org).
8. Ibid.
9. American Heart Association, "2001 Heart and Stroke Statistical Update."
10. Ibid.
11. American Heart Association, "2002 Heart and Stroke Facts," 18.
12. W. McArdle, , F. Katch, and V. Katch, *Exercise Physiology* 5th ed. (Philadelphia: Lippincott, Williams and Wilkins, 2001), 896.
13. Debra Krummel, "Nutrition in Cardiovascular Disease," in L. K. Mahan, and S. Escott-Stump, *Krause's Food, Nutrition, and Diet Therapy.* (New York: W. B. Saunders 2000).
14. C. Napoli, E. P. D'Armiento, F. P. Mancini, et. al., "Fatty Streak Formation Occurs in Human Fetal Aortas and Is Greatly Enhanced by Maternal Hypercholesterolemia: Intimal Accumulation of Low-Density Lipoprotein and Its Oxidative Precede Monocyte Recruitment into Early Atherosclerotic Lesions," *Journal of Clinical Investigation* 100 (1997): 2680–2690.
15. J. L. Breslow, "Cardiovascular Disease Burden Increases, NIH Funding Decreases," *Nature Medicine* 3 (1997): 6000–6009.
16. R. Ross, "Atherosclerosis—An Inflammatory Disease," *New England Journal of Medicine* 340 (1999): 115.
17. J. Danesh, R. Collins, and R. Peto, "Chronic Infections and Coronary Heart Disease: Is There a Link?" *Lancet* 350 (1997): 430–436.
18. E. Braunwald, "Cardiovascular Medicine at the Turn of the Millennium: Triumphs, Concerns, and Opportunities," *New England Journal of Medicine* 337 (1997): 1360–1369.
19. Ross, op cit., 122.
20. A. Forman, "The Threat of Insulin Resistance to Your Heart," *Environmental Nutrition* 23 (8) (2000): 4–6.
21. American Heart Association, "2001 Heart and Stroke Statistical Update," 11.
22. Ibid., 13.
23. American Heart Association, "2002 Heart and Stroke Statistical Update," 19.
24. Ibid.
25. Ibid., 20.
26. Ibid.
27. American Heart Association, "2002 Heart and Stroke Facts," 16.
28. Ibid.
29. Ibid., 17.
30. American Heart Association, "2002 Heart and Stroke Statistical Update."

31. American Heart Association, "2001 Heart and Stroke Statistical Update."
32. Ibid., 24.
33. Ibid.
34. National Heart, Lung, and Blood Institute: "Third Report of the National Cholesterol Education Program (NCEP) Expert Panel on Detection, Evaluation, and Treatment of High Cholesterol in Adults" (Adult Treatment Panel III), May 2001 (see http://www.nhlbi.nih.gov).
35. Ibid.
36. American Heart Association, "2001 Heart and Stroke Statistical Update."
37. National Heart, Lung, and Blood Institute, op. cit.
38. Ibid.
39. Ibid.
40. Ibid., 15; Center for Science in the Public Interest, Nutrition Action Health Letter 22 (1995): 4.
41. U.S. Department of Health and Human Services, Surgeon General's Report on Physical Activity (1996); American Heart Association, "2001 Heart and Stroke Statistical Update," 11.
42. American Heart Association, "2001 Heart and Stroke Statistical Update."
43. Ibid.
44. National Heart, Lung, and Blood Institute, "Understanding High Blood Pressure," 2002 (see http://www.nhlbi.nih.gov/hbp/hbp/intro.htm).
45. Ross, op. cit., 117.
46. R. Eliot, "Changing Behavior: A New Comprehensive and Quantitative Approach" (keynote address at the annual meeting of the American College of Cardiology on stress and the heart, Jackson Hole, Wyoming, July 3, 1987).
47. American Heart Association, "2001 Heart and Stroke Facts," 2.
48. A. G. Boston et al., "Elevated Plasma Lipoprotein(a) and Coronary Heart Disease in Men Aged 55 Years and Younger: A Prospective Study," Journal of the American Medical Association 276 (1996): 555–558.
49. Ibid., 555.
50. Ibid., 556.
51. National Heart, Lung and Blood Institute, "Heart Memo: The Cardiovascular Health of Women" (1995): 5.
52. Ibid., 5.
53. American Heart Association, "2001 Heart and Stroke Facts," 25.
54. J. E. Willard, R. A. Lange, and D. L. Hillis, "The Use of Aspirin in Ischemic Heart Disease," New England Journal of Medicine 327 (1992): 175–179.
55. Agency for Health Care Policy and Research, "Cardiac Rehabilitation: Exercise, Training, Education, Counseling, and Behavioral Interventions," Publication #96-0672 (1996).

Chapter 16

1. American Cancer Society, Cancer Facts and Figures, 2003 (Atlanta: American Cancer Society, 2003), 4 (see www.cancer.org).
2. Ibid.
3. Ibid., 28.
4. Ibid., 29.
5. Ibid., 3.
6. Julian Peto, "Cancer Epidemiology in the Last Century and Next Decade," Nature 411 (2001): 390–395.
7. L. Remennick, "The Cancer Problem in the Context of Modernity, Sociology, Democracy and Politics," Current Sociology 46 (1998): 144.
8. M. Osborne, P. Boyle, and M. Lipkin, "Cancer Prevention," The Lancet 349 (1997): 1–8 (special oncology supplement).
9. Ibid.
10. American Cancer Society, op. cit.
11. Osborne et al., op. cit.
12. Ibid., 2; Peto, op. cit.
13. Peto, op. cit.
14. American Cancer Society, op. cit., 11.
15. Ibid.
16. Ibid.
17. Ibid.
18. Ibid., 10.
19. Ibid.
20. Ibid., 10.
21. Ibid.
22. Ibid.
23. Ibid.; Peto, op. cit.
24. Peto, op. cit.
25. A. Bergstrom, P. Pisani, V. Tenet, A. Wolk, and O. Adamis, "Overweight as an Avoidable Cause of Cancer in Europe," International Journal of Cancer 91 (2001): 421–430.
26. American Cancer Society, op. cit., 9.
27. Ibid., 20.
28. Ibid., 21.
29. P. A. Janne, and R. J. Mayer, "Chemoprevention of Colorectal Cancer," New England Journal of Medicine 342 (2000): 1960–1968; Writing Group—WHI, "Risks and Benefits of Estrogen Plus Progesterone on the Health of Postmenopausal Women," Journal of the American Medical Association, 288 (3) (July 17, 2002).
30. American Cancer Society, op. cit., 20.
31. L. Seeff, et al., "Screening for Colorectal Cancer in the U.S.," Journal of Family Practice 51 (2002): 761–766.
32. American Cancer Society, op. cit., 21.
33. Ibid., 22.
34. Ibid., 23.
35. Ibid., 10.
36. Ibid.
37. Ibid., 15.
38. Ibid., 15.
39. University of Wisconsin Health Service, "Sunburn: Prevention/Treatment" (2002) (see http://www.uhs.wisc.edu/ex/selfcare/resource/sunburn.php).
40. American Cancer Society, op. cit., 15.
41. University of Wisconsin Health Service, op. cit.
42. American Cancer Society, op. cit., 15.
43. University of Wisconsin Health Service, op. cit.
44. Ibid.
45. American Academy of Dermatology (2002) (see www.aad.org).
46. American Cancer Society, op. cit.
47. Ibid.
48. Ibid., 13.
49. National Ovarian Cancer Coalition (2002) (see www.ovarian.org).
50. American Cancer Society, op. cit.
51. A. Harvey, M. J. Risch, L. D. Marrett, and G. R. Howe, "Dietary Fat Intake and Risk of Epithelial Ovarian Cancer," Journal of the National Cancer Institute 86 (1994): 21.
52. American Cancer Society, op. cit., 14.
53. Ibid., 16.
54. Ibid.
55. Ibid.
56. Ibid.
57. Ibid., 14.
58. Ibid.
59. Ibid.
60. Ibid., 11.
61. Ibid.

Chapter 17

1. K. Nelson, C. Williams, and N. Graham, Infectious Disease Epidemiology: Theory and Practice (Gaithersburg, MD: Aspen, 2001), 17–39.
2. "Group B Streptococcal Infections," Respiratory Disease Branch, Division of Bacterial and Mycotic Diseases, National Center for Infectious Diseases, Centers for Disease Control and Prevention (CDC), 2000 (see http://www.cdc.gov/ncidod/diseases/bacter/strep_b.htm).

3. Ibid.
4. "Preventing Emerging Infectious Diseases: A Strategy for the 21st Century," U.S. Department of Health and Human Services (Atlanta, GA: CDC, 1998).
5. A. Evans and P. Brachman, *Bacterial Infections of Humans: Epidemiology and Control.* 3rd ed. (New York: Plenum, 1998).
6. Centers for Disease Control and Prevention, National Center for HIV, STD, and TB Prevention, "Reported TB in the U.S.—2001," 2001 (see http://www.cdc.gov/nchstp/tb/surv/surv2001/default.htm).
7. Ibid.
8. Ibid.
9. Nelson et al., op. cit., 411.
10. Global Tuberculosis Program, "Tuberculosis Fact sheet No. 104" (see http://wwwwho.int/inffs/en/fact104.html; accessed January 2000).
11. Ibid.
12. Ibid.
13. Centers for Disease Control and Prevention, National Center for HIV, STD, and TB Prevention, op. cit.
14. Global Tuberculosis Program, op. cit.
15. Centers for Disease Control and Prevention, National Center for Infectious Disease, Division of Viral and Rickettsial Diseases, 2002 (see http://www.cdc.gov/ncidod/dvrd/branch/vrzb.htm).
16. A. Evans and R. Kaslow, *Viral Infections in Humans: Epidemiology and Control,* 4th ed. (New York: Plenum, 1997), 6–11.
17. Centers for Disease Control and Prevention, National Center for Infectious Diseases, "Viral Hepatitis A Fact Sheet," 2002 (see http://www.cdc.gov/ncidod/diseases/hepatitis/a/fact.htm).
18. National Institutes of Health, "Promote Prevention: Hepatitis—Education and Information for Patients and Professionals" (National Digestive Diseases Information Clearinghouse, 2000) (see http://www.niddk.nih.gov/health/digest/digest.htm).
19. Centers for Disease Control and Prevention: National Center for Infectious Diseases: "Viral Hepatitis B Fact Sheet," 2002. (see http://www.cdc.gov/ncidod/diseases/hepatitis/b/fact.htm).
20. Ibid.
21. Ibid.
22. Centers for Disease Control and Prevention, National Center for Infectious Diseases, "Viral Hepatitis C Fact Sheet," 2002 (see http://www.cdc.gov/ncidod/diseases/hepatitis/c/fact.htm).
23. Ibid.
24. Nelson et al., op. cit., 17–39.
25. Centers for Disease Control and Prevention, National Center for Infectious Diseases, "BSE and CJD Information and Resources," 2002 (see http://www.cdc.gov/ncidod/diseases/cjd/cjd.htm).
26. Ibid.
27. Nelson et al., op. cit., 315–318.
28. Ibid.
29. Centers for Disease Control, Special Pathogens Branch, "Diseases—Ebola Hemorrhagic Fever," 2002 (see http://www.cdc.gov/ncidod/dvrd/spb/mnpages/dispages/ebola.htm).
30. Ibid.
31. Nelson, et al., op. cit., 325.
32. R. Fenner, *The History of Smallpox and Its Spread Around the World* (Geneva, Switzerland: World Health Organization, 1988).
33. T. J. Torok, R. V. Tauxe, and R. P. Wise, "A Large Community Outbreak of Salmonellosis Carried by Intentional Contamination of Restaurant Salad Bars," *Journal of the American Medical Association* 279 (1997): 389–395.
34. Centers for Disease Control, National Prevention Information Network, "STD Prevention," 2002 (see http://www.cdcnpin.org/std/start.htm).
35. K. Painter, "STI Rate Higher Than Previously Believed," *USA Today* (December 3, 1998): D1 (taken from CDC December 1998 report).
36. "Chlamydia Fact Sheet," National Institute of Allergy and Infectious Diseases, National Institutes of Health, November 2000 (see http://www.niaid.nih.gov).
37. "Pelvic Inflammatory Disease," National Institute of Allergy and Infectious Diseases, National Institutes of Health, November 2000 (see http://www.niaid.nih.gov).
38. "PID: Guidelines for Prevention, Detection, and Management," *Clinical Courier* 10 (1992): 1–5.
39. "Gonorrhea Fact Sheet," National Institute of Allergy and Infectious Diseases, National Institutes of Health, October 2000 (see http://www.niaid.nih.gov).
40. Ibid.
41. Evans and Brachman, op. cit., 285.
42. "Genital Herpes Fact Sheet," National Institute of Allergy and Infectious Diseases, National Institutes of Health, March 2000 (see http://www.niaid.nih.gov).
43. Ibid.
44. G. Stine, *AIDS Update 2000* (Upper Saddle River, NJ: Prentice Hall, 2000), 349.
45. Centers for Disease Control, National Center for HIV, STD, and TB Prevention, Division of HIV/AIDS Prevention, "Basic Statistics: HIV/AIDS Surveillance Report," December 2001—year-end edition, vol. 13, no 2 (see http://www.cdc.gov/hiv/stats.htm).
46. National Institutes of Health, National Institute of Allergy and Infectious Disease. HIV Infection in Women—Fact Sheet. December, 2002. http://www.niaid.nih.gov/factsheets/womenhiv.htm.
47. Ibid., 243–349; Society for the Advancement of Women's Health Research, "Some Ailments Found Guilty of Sex Bias," *New York Times* (November 11, 1998): D12; B. M. Branson, "Home Sample Collection Tests for HIV Infection," *Journal of the American Medical Association* 280 (1998): 1699–1701.
48. Centers for Disease Control, "Revised Recommendations for HIV Screening of Pregnant Women," MMWR, November 9, 2001 (50)(RR19): 59–86 (see http://www.cdc.gov/mmwr/review).
49. Centers for Disease Control, National Center for HIV, STD, and TB Prevention, Division of HIV/AIDS Prevention, January 2002 (see http://www.cdc.gov/pubs/facts.htm).
50. F. Cox, *The AIDS Booklet,* 6th ed. (Boston: McGraw-Hill Higher Education, 2000), 27–30.
51. Richard Conviser, "Changing Care Costs for HIV/AIDS," Office of Science and Epidemiology, HIV/AIDS Bureau, HRSA, DHHS, 2002 (see http://hab.hrsa.gov/reports/changingcost/sld001.htm).

Chapter 18

1. R. Brownson, P. Remington, and J. Davis, eds., *Chronic Disease Epidemiology and Control* (Washington, DC: American Public Health Association, 1998), 379–382.
2. Asthma and Allergy Foundation of America, "Asthma Facts and Figures," 2002. (see http://www.aafa.org/temp/display2.cfm?id = 2).
3. Ibid.
4. Brownson et al., op. cit., 389.
5. American Lung Association, accessed January 2001 (see http://www.lungusa.org).
6. Brownson et al., op. cit., 401.
7. Ibid., 516.
8. J. Adler and A. Rogers, "The New War Against Migraines," *Newsweek* (January 11, 1999): 46–55.
9. Ibid., 48.
10. Ibid., 49.
11. J. Allen, "Oh, My Aching Head" *Life* (1994): 66–76.
12. Ibid., 72.
13. Adler and Rogers, op. cit., 52.
14. E. Mignot, T. Yount, L. Ling, and M. Patta, "Reduction of REM Sleep Latency Associatied with HLA-DQB1*0602 in Normal Adults," *The Lancet* 351 (1998): 729.
15. G. Cowley, "The New War on Parkinson's," *Newsweek* (May 22, 2000): 52–58; Mayo Clinic website accessed January 2001 (see http://www.mayo.edu/fpd/2_new/article.htm).
16. Ibid.

17. R. Schapiro, International MS Support Foundation, 2001 (see http://www.msnews.org/fair2.shtml).
18. Jeffrey Koplan, "Diabetes Is a Growing Public Health Concern," 2002 (see http://www.cdc.gov/diabetes/pubs/glance.htm).
19. J. Adler and C. Kalb, "An American Epidemic: Diabetes," *Newsweek*, (September 4, 2000): 40–48; Centers for Disease Control and Prevention, accessed January 2001 (see http://cdc.gov).
20. Koplan, op. cit.
21. Ibid.
22. Brownson et. al., op. cit., 424.
23. Koplan, op. cit.
24. Ibid.
25. Adler and Kalb, op. cit., 424.
26. Koplan, J. op. cit.
27. P. Lustman and A. Keegan, "Depression," *Diabetes Forecast* 51 (1998): 56–64.
28. Koplan,. op. cit.
29. Brownson et al., op. cit., 424.
30. Arthritis Foundation, "Disease Center," 2002 (see http://www.arthritis.org/conditions/DiseaseCenter/oa.asp).
31. Ibid.
32. Ibid.
33. Ibid.
34. Ibid.
35. Brownson et al., op. cit.
36. "Is the Prevalence of Back Pain Rising?" *The Back Letter*, 2002. Volume 17, No. 11. Philadelphia: Lippincott, Williams and Wilkins.
37. N. Hadler and T. Carey, "Low Back Pain: An Intermittent Predicament in Life," *Annals of the Rheumatic Diseases* 57 (1998): 1–3.
38. K. Nelson, C. Williams, and N. Graham, *Infectious Disease Epidemiology* (Gaithersburg, MD: Aspen, 2001), 348–349.

Chapter 19

1. J. Kavenaugh, *Adult Development and Aging* (Pacific Grove, CA: BrooksCole/ITP, 1996), 45.
2. W. Madar, "Life Stories as Well as Theory Needed to Understand Aging," *Center for the Humanities Newsletter* (Consortium of Humanities Centers and Institutes, Oregon State University, Spring 2000), 8.
3. Department of Health and Human Services, Administration on Aging, *A Profile of Older Americans: 2001*, January 2002. (see http://www.aoa.gov/aoa/stats/profile/2001/hightlights.html)
4. Ibid.
5. Ibid.
6. Ibid.
7. Ibid.
8. U.S. Senate Special Committee on Aging. (2002). Aging Committee: Hearing finding summary. (Report to Congress). Washington, DC: U.S. Government Printing Office.
9. Alliance for Health Reform. 2002 (see: http://www.allhealth.org/sourcebook/2002.)
10. National Institutes of Health, Osteoporosis and Related Bone Diseases National Resource Center (December 2002) (see http://www.osteo.org/osteo.html).
11. National Kidney and Urologic Diseases Information Clearinghouse. 2002 (see http://www.Niddk.Nih.gov/health/uralog/pubs/uiwomen.html).
12. Ibid., 137–138.
13. National Council on Aging, press release, "Half of Older Americans Report They Are Sexually Active, 4 in 10 Want More Sex, Says New Survey" (September 28, 1998) (see http://ncoa.org/news/archives/sexsurvey.htm).
14. Alzheimer's Association, "Understanding Alzheimers: Statistics and Prevalence" (Chicago, IL: The Alzheimer's Association, 2002).
15. Alzheimer's Association, "Fact Sheet: Cholinesterase Inhibitors" (2002). (see http://www.alz.org/ResourceCenter/ByTopic/cholinesterase.htm).

Chapter 20

1. *Oxford English Dictionary* (Oxford, UK: Oxford University Press, 1969), 72, 334, 735.
2. President's Commission for the Study of Ethical Problems in Medicine and Biomedical and Behavioral Research, *Deciding to Forgo Life-Sustaining Treatment* (New York: Concern for Dying, 1983), 9.
3. Ad Hoc Committee of the Harvard Medical School to Examine the Definition of Brain Death, "A Definition of Irreversible Coma," *Journal of the American Medical Association* 205 (1968): 377.
4. L. R. Aiken, *Dying, Death, and Bereavement*, 3rd ed. (Boston: Allyn & Bacon, 1994), 4.
5. *Civilization*, 6 (6) (2000): 30, 33–34.
6. E. Kübler-Ross, *On Death and Dying* (New York: Macmillan, 1969), 113.
7. R. J. Kastenbaum, *Death, Society, and Human Experience*, 6th ed. (Boston: Allyn & Bacon, 1998), 95.
8. Ibid., 336–337.
9. K. J. Doka (ed.), *Disenfranchised Grief: Recognizing Hidden Sorrow* (Lexington, MA: Lexington Books, 1989).
10. J. B. Kamerman, *Death in the Midst of Life* (Englewood Cliffs, NJ: Prentice Hall, 1988), 126.
11. J. W. Worden, *Children and Grief: When a Parent Dies* (New York: Guilford Press, 1996).
12. The term *quasi-death experience* was coined by J. B. Kamerman, op. cit., 71.
13. C. M. Parkes, *Bereavement* (New York: International Universities Press, 1972), 6.
14. "Last Rights: Why a 'Living Will' Is Not Enough," *Consumer Reports on Health* (September 1993): 5, 9.
15. J. G. Bachman, K. H. Alcser, D. J. Doukas, R. L. Lichenstein, A. D. Corning, and H. Brody, "Attitudes of Michigan Physicians and the Public Toward Legalizing Physician-Assisted Suicide and Voluntary Euthanasia," *New England Journal of Medicine* 334 (1996): 303.
16. M. A. Lee, H. D. Nelson, V. P. Tilden, L. Ganzini, T. A. Schmidt, and S. W. Tolle, "Legalizing Assisted Suicide: Views of Physicians in Oregon," *New England Journal of Medicine* 334 (1996): 310–315.

Chapter 21

1. M. Renner, "Economic Features," *Vital Signs 1997: The Environmental Trends that Are Shaping our Future* (New York: W. W. Norton & Co., 1997).
2. R. Caplan, *Our Earth, Ourselves* (New York: Bantam, 1990), 247.
3. United Nations, *Global Population Policy Database* (New York: UN Population Division, 1995); *The World Gazetter*, October 4, 2002 (see http://www.worldgazetteer.com/home.htm).
4. J. Abramovitz and S. Dunn, "Record Year for Weather-Related Disasters," in *Vital Signs Brief 98-5* (Washington, DC: Worldwatch Institute, 1998).
5. L. R. Brown, M. Renner, and C. Flavin, *Vital Signs 1998: The Environmental Trends That Are Shaping Our Future* (New York: W. W. Norton & Co., 1998).
6. Ibid.
7. L. Gordon, "Environmental Health and Protection. Century 21 Challenges," *Journal of Environmental Health* 57 (1995): 28–34.
8. L. R. Brown, G. Gardner, and B. Halweil, *Beyond Malthus: Sixteen Dimensions of the Population Problem* (Washington, DC: Worldwatch Institute, 1998).
9. Ibid.
10. J. Schwartz, "Health Effects of Particulate Air Pollution," *The Center for Environmental Health Newsletter* 7 (1998) (University of Connecticut, College of Agriculture & Natural Resources).
11. National Center for Environmental Health, *Screening Young Children for Lead Poisoning: Guidance for State and Local Public Health Officials*. (Atlanta: Centers for Disease Control and Prevention, U.S. Public Health Service, 1997).

12. L. Brown, "A New Era Unfolds," in *State of the World, 1993,* Lester Brown, ed. (New York: W. W. Norton Co., 1993), 107.
13. Environmental Protection Agency, "The Inside Story: A Guide to Indoor Air Quality," EPA Document #402-K-93-007, January 2002 (see http://epa.gov/iaq/pubs/insidest.html).
14. Ibid.
15. Ibid.
16. K. E. Warner, D. Mendez, and P. N. Courant, "Toward a More Realistic Appraisal of the Lung Cancer Risk from Radon," *American Journal of Public Health* 86 (1996): 1222–1227.
17. Environmental Protection Agency, op. cit.
18. B. Condor, "Alternative Watch: Clearing the Air in Classrooms," *Chicago Tribune,* 2000.
19. N. Carpenter, " 'Sick' Buildings Can Be Root of Work-Related Maladies," *Boston Business Journal* 20 (2000): 36–37.
20. U.S. Environmental Protection Agency, *Questions and Answers on Ozone Depletion* (Washington, DC: Stratospheric Protection Division, 1998).
21. Environmental Protection Agency. "Global Warming-Climate" 2002. (see http://yosemite.epa.gov/oar/globalwarming.nsf/content/climate.html).
22. Ibid.
23. Ibid.
24. J. Abramovitz, *Taking a Stand: Cultivating a New Relationship with the World's Forests* (Washington, DC: Worldwatch Institute, 1998).
25. American Water Works Association, "Drop by Drop: A Guide to Starting a Water Conservation Program," 2002 (see http://www.awwa.org/community).
26. U.S. Environmental Protection Agency, *Water on Tap: A Consumer's Guide to the Nation's Drinking Water* (Washington, DC: Safe Drinking Water Information System, 1997).
27. Monroe Morgan. *Environmental Health* (Belmont, CA: Wadsworth Publishing, 2003), 73.
28. Environmental Protection Agency, *Water on Tap,* op. cit.
29. Ibid.
30. Ibid.
31. Brown et al., op. cit.
32. A. Hoyer, "Organochlorine Exposure and Risk of Breast Cancer," *Lancet* 352 (1998): 1816–1831.
33. B. L. Johnson and C. T. DeRosa, "The Toxicologic Hazard of Superfund Hazardous Waste Sites," *Environmental Health* 12 (1997): 235–251.
34. Ibid., 243.
35. U.S. Environmental Protection Agency, *Meeting the Environmental Challenge: EPA's Review of Progress and New Directions in Environmental Protection* (EPA Publication No. 21K-2001, 1990), 4.
36. Ibid.
37. Environmental News Network (see http://www.enn.com).

Chapter 22

1. L. C. Baker and L. S. Baker, "Excess Cost of Emergency Department Visits for Nonurgent Care," *Health Affairs* (winter 1994): 162–180.
2. Hospital Health Network, "Emergency Care: The Number of Visits to U.S. Hospital Emergency Departments Has Declined," *Hospital Health Network* 70 (1966): 14.
3. R. M. Williams, "The Costs of Visits to Emergency Departments," *New England Journal of Medicine* 334 (1996): 642–646.
4. J. Schmittdiel, J. V. Selby, K. Grumbach, and C. P. Quesenberry, "Choice of a Personal Physician and Patient Satisfaction in a Health Maintenance Organization," *Journal of the American Medical Association* 278 (1997): 1596–1599.
5. Charnicia Huggins, "Poll Shows Most Americans Trust Their Doctors," *Medline Plus Health Information,* 2002 (see http://www.nlm.nih.gov/medlineplus/news/fullstory_10844.html).
6. J. Schuster, "Insomnia: Understanding Its Pharmacological Treatment Options," *Pharmacy Times* 62 (1996): 67–76.

7. Food and Drug Administration, "Phenylpropanolamine (PPA) Information Page," 2002 (see http://www.fda.gov/cder/drug/infopage/ppa/default.htm).
8. G. Annas, *The Rights of Patients: The Basic ACLU Guide to Patient Rights,* 2nd ed. (Chicago: Southern Illinois University Press, 1989), 105.
9. Pennsylvania Medicine, "Use of Non-Physician Practitioners," *Pennsylvania Medicine* 101 (1998): 17–19.
10. C. Hafner-Eaton, "Patterns of Hospital and Physician Utilization Among the Uninsured," *Journal of Health Care for the Poor and Unserserved* 5 (1994): 297–315.
11. National Center for Chronic Disease Prevention and Health Promotion, "Chronic Disease Overview," 2002 (see http://www.cdc.gov/nccdphp/overview.htm).
12. Ibid.
13. National Academy of Sciences, *The Future of the Public's Health in the 21st Century,* 2003, 2.
14. Centers for Disease Control and Prevention, *Morbidity and Mortality Weekly Report* 49 (2000): 1–39.
15. *Medical Group Practice Digest: Managed Care Digest Series 1998* (Kansas City: Hoechst Marion Roussel, Inc., 1998).
16. Ibid.
17. Ibid.
18. Ibid.
19. Ibid.
20. Steffie Woolhandler and David Himmelstein, "Paying for National Health Insurance and Not Getting It," 2002, *Health Affairs* 21(4): 90.

Chapter 23

1. "Health for Life: Inside the Science of Alternative Medicine," *Newsweek* (December 2, 2002): 45–70.
2. Ibid.
3. E. Eisenberg et al. "Trends in Alternative Medicine Use in the United States, 1990–97: Results of a Follow-up National Study," *Journal of the American Medical Association* 280 (1998): 1569–1579.
4. National Center for Complementary and Alternative Medicine, "What Is Complementary and Alternative Medicine (CAM)?" 2002 (see http://nccam.nih.gov/health.whatiscam).
5. L. C. Paramore, "Use of Alternative Therapies," *Journal of Pain and Symptom Management* 13 (1997): 83–89; Landmark Healthcare, *The Landmark Report on Public Perceptions of Alternative Care* (Sacramento, CA: Landmark Healthcare, 1998).
6. National Center for Complementary and Alternative Medicine, op. cit.
7. D. M. Eisenberg, R. C. Kessler, C. Foster, et al., "Unconventional Medicine in the United States," *New England Journal of Medicine* 328 (1993): 246–252.
8. "Health for Life," *Newsweek,* op. cit.
9. Eisenberg, op. cit., 247: Eisenberg et al., op. cit., 1570.
10. A. Weil, *Spontaneous Healing* (New York: Fawcett Columbine, 1995), 233.
11. National Center for Complementary and Alternative Medicine, op. cit.
12. N. Rasmussen and J. Morgall, "The Use of Alternative Treatments in the Danish Adult Population," *Complementary Medicine Research* 4 (1990): 16–22; A. MacLennan, D. Wilson, and A. Taylor, "Prevalence and Cost of Alternative Medicine in Australia," *The Lancet* 347 (1996): 569–573; P. Fisher and A. Ward, "Complementary Medicine in Europe," *British Medical Journal* 309 (1994): 107–111; W. Miller, "Use of Alternative Health Care Practitioners by Canadians, *Canadian Journal of Public Health* 88 (1997): 154–158.
13. M. Angell and J. P. Kassirer, "Alternative Medicine—The Risks of Untested and Unregulated Remedies," *New England Journal of Medicine* 339 (1998): 839–841.
14. National Center for Complementary and Alternative Medicine, op. cit.
15. Ibid.
16. Ibid.

17. Ibid.
18. Ibid.
19. J. Greenwald, "Herbal Healing," *Time* (November 23, 1998): 63–65.
20. Weil, op. cit., 205.
21. Food and Drug Administration, Center for Food Safety and Applied Nutrition, "Consumer Advisory," 2002 (see http://www.cfsan.fda.gov/~dms/ds-ltr29.html).
22. Ibid., 241.
23. J. Kleignene and P. Knipschild, "Ginkgo Biloba," *The Lancet* 340 (1992): 1136–1139.
24. M. Murray, "Ginkgo Biloba Extract and Ginkgo Phytosome," Ask the Doctor, Vital Communication, 1998.
25. P. L. LeBars et al., "A Placebo-Controlled, Double Blind, Randomized Trial of an Extract of Ginkgo Biloba for Dementia," *Journal of the American Medical Association* 278 (1997): 1327–1332.
26. "The Pill That Helps You Think?" *Tufts University Health and Nutrition Letter* 15 (1997): 8–10.
27. "St. John's Wort," Nature's Life Brochure, 1998.
28. H. Schultz, "St. John's Wort for Depression," *British Medical Journal* 7052 (1996): 313–319.
29. K. D. Hansgen et al., "Multicenter Double Blind Study Examining the Anti-Depressant Effectiveness of the Hypericum Extract L1160," *Journal of Psychiatric Neurology,* Supplement 1 (October 7, 1994): x15–18; H. Schultz et al., "Effects of Hypericum Extract on the Sleep EEG in Older Volunteers," *American Journal of Geriatric Psychiatry,* Supplement 1 (1994): x65–68.
30. Schultz et al., op. cit., 66.
31. Ibid.
32. H. Martin, "St. John's Wort vs. Tricyclic Antidepressants," *American Journal of Naturopathic Medicine* 2 (1995): 42.
33. Schultz, op. cit., 66.
34. R. J. Davidson et al., "Effect of SJW in Major Depressive Disorder: A Randomized, Controlled Trial," *Journal of the American Medical Association* 287 (2002): 1807–1814.
35. J. Blair, "Echinacea—New Wonder Drug? *Archives of Family Medicine* (November 24, 1998): 1332–1339.
36. S. Momiyama, "Green Tea as Protection from Heart Attack," *American Journal of Cardiology* (2002), 909:1150–1153.
37. D. Ahrendt, "Ergogenic Aids: Counseling the Athlete," *American Family Physician* (2002), 63:913–922. (See http://www.aafp.org/afp/2001/0301/913.htm)
38. Ibid., 220.
39. E. Ernst, "The Risk-Benefit Profiles of Commonly used Herbal Therapies: Ginkgo, St. John's Wort, Ginseng, Echinacea, Saw Palmetto and Kava," *Annals of Internal Medicine* (January 1, 2002): Vol. 136, No. 1, 42–53.
40. Ibid., 45.
41. D. Ahrendt, 2001: 917.
42. Ibid., 915.
43. Agency for Healthcare Research and Quality, "S-Adenosyl-L Methionine for Treatment of Depression, Osteoarthritis, and Liver Disease," *Evidence Report/Technology Assessment: Number 64"* (August 2002). (See http://www.ahrq.gov/clinic/epcsums/samesum.htm).
44. Ibid.
45. Ibid.
46. S. Dixon, "Food for Thought: Prebiotic and Probiotics: What Are They and Why Should You Eat Them?" University of Michigan Comprehensive Cancer Center (January 15, 2003). (See http://www.cancer.med.umich.edu/newspro09spr02.htm).
47. D. Wilson, "Health Food Masquerade," *Corvallis Gazette Times* (August 11, 1999), C-4.
48. American Botanical Council. "Commission E." January, 2003. (See http://www.herbab/ram.org/default.asp?c = comm_e_catalog).
49. Ibid.
50. M. Angell and J. P. Kassirer, op. cit., 839–841; "CAM Centers of Research; Overview of the Specialty Centers," National Center for Complementary and Alternative Medicine (2002) (See http.//nccam nih.gov/nccam/research/centers.html).
51. "Health for Life," *Newsweek,* op. cit., 53.

Index

Disaccharides, 228
Discrimination, 102
    violence and, 98
Disease. *See also* Infectious diseases;
        Noninfectious conditions
    Category A, B, and C, 106
    disparities in trends in, 514
    emergent/resurgent, 486
    environment and, 8
    genetic propensity to, 30
    infectious disease control and, 17, 18
    prevention of, 16–17
    research funds allocation for, 531
    self-esteem and, 79
Disenfranchised grief, 526
Dissociation, in PTSD, 80
Distillation, 346
Distress, 68
    background, 77
Disulfiram (Antabuse), 360
Diuretic, 243, 611
    alcohol as, 349–350
Diverticulosis, 527–528
    fiber and, 231
Divorce
    statistics on, 146–147
    studies of, 142
    world rates of, 147
DNA. *See* Deoxyribonucleic acid (DNA)
Doctors. *See* Physicians
Documenting, in communication within
        couples, 137
Domestic violence, 107–109
Downshifting, 82–83
Down syndrome, 194, 198
DRGs. *See* Diagnosis related groups (DRGs)
DRI. *See* Dietary Reference Intake (DRI)
Drinking. *See* Alcohol; Alcohol abuse
        (alcoholism); Binge drinking
Drinking water, fluoridated, 17
Driving
    alcohol and, 344, 352–353
    marijuana and, 401
    risk management, 653
Drug abuse, 392. *See also* Drugs
    recognizing, 395
    by women, 397
Drug addiction, impact of, 334
Drug Free America Act (1986), 394
Drug misuse, 392. *See also* Drugs
Drug-resistant bacteria, 607
Drugs, 17. *See also* Alcohol; Over-the-counter
        (OTC) drugs; Prescription drugs; Tobacco
    addiction across cultures, 393
    alcohol interactions with, 350
    amphetamines and, 398–399
    antidepressant, 54
    antidrug strategies, 410–411
    caffeine as, 382–383
    categories of, 390–391
    cocaine as, 325, 393, 394–398
    communication barriers and, 139
    controlled substances, 394–409
    culture and, 325
    hallucinogens (psychedelics) as, 404–406
    HIV/AIDS from injections of, 505
    illegal drug use in United States, 409–411
    illicit, 390–411

inhalants as, 406, 407–409
marijuana as, 325, 399–401
metabolizing of, 390
multiple addictions and, 334
opiates as, 393, 401–403
during pregnancy, 195–196
prevalence of use, 393
protecting illicit users of, 408
risk of dependence, 394
routes of administration, 391–392
schedules of, 394, 396
sex and, 171
use of, 392
users of, 393–394
violence and, 98
in workplace, 410
worldwide access to, 18
Drug testing, in workplace, 410
Drug treatment, for weight loss, 285–288
DRVs. *See* Daily Reference Values (DRVs)
Dry-cleaning chemicals, 585
DSA. *See* Digital cardiac angiography
        (DCA, DSA)
DSM-IV, 59
DTs. *See* Delirium tremens (DTs)
Dual-career family, 144
Dubos, René, 8, 9
Duodenum, 224
    peptic ulcer and, 528
DV. *See* Daily Values (DV)
Dyathanasia, 568
Dying. *See also* Death
    defined, 558
    hospice care for, 568–570
    Kübler-Ross's stages of, 560, 561
    process of, 560–565
    right to die and, 566
    supporting dying person, 570
Dysfunction, sexual, 168–172, 376
Dysfunctional families, 44
    alcoholism and, 356–357
    communication barriers and, 139
Dysmenorrhea, 161
Dyspareunia, 170
Dyspnea, 514

E

Eades, Mary and Michael, 287
Eating. *See also* Diet; Nutrition
    aging and, 551
    assessing behaviors, 214–215
    behavior triggers for, 284
    changing habits of, 283–284
    digestive process and, 221–224
    health and, 218–224
    improving, 250–253
    psychosocial factors in, 278
    self-assessment of, 216–218
Eating disorders
    anorexia nervosa, 288, 289, 290
    binge eating disorder (BED), 289–290
    bulimia nervosa, 289, 290
    physical activity and, 299
    treatment for, 290
Eating Well for Optimum Health (Weil), 287
Ebola hemorrhagic fever (Ebola HF), 487
Eccentric muscle action, 308, 309
ECG. *See* Electrocardiogram (ECG)

Echinacea, 640
Eclampsia, 204
E. coli bacteria, 254, 474, 487, 489
    antibiotics and, 607
Ecological (Public Health) Model, 7, 8
Economies of scale, health care
        costs and, 620
ECPs. *See* Emergency contraceptive pills (ECPs)
Ecstasy (MDMA), 406, 407
    PMA and, 408
    water intoxication and, 226
ECT. *See* Electroconvulsive therapy (ECT)
Ectopic pregnancy, 205
Ecuador, pollution of rain forests in, 593
Edamamé, 228
Editing, in communication within couples, 137
Education
    as antidrug strategy, 410–411
    health risks and, 30
    zero population growth and, 579
Egg, fertilization of, 154, 197
Egg sacs, 160
Ejaculation, 162
    premature, 169–170
Elderly. *See* Aging; Older adults
Electrical shock, emergency treatment for,
        657–658
Electric and magnetic fields (EMFs), 594
Electrocardiogram (ECG), 436
Electroconvulsive therapy (ECT), 54
Electromagnetic fields, in bioelectromagnetic
        therapy, 636
Eliot, Robert S., 85, 431
ELISA test, 507
Embalming, 571
Embolism, 427
Embolus, 422, 423, 426
Embryo, 198, 199
    abortion and, 190
    adoption programs, 208
    freezing of, 208
    transfer of, 207
Emergency care, 655–660
    for heart attack, 425
Emergency contraception
    effectiveness of, 178
    pills (ECPs) for, 186
Emergency minipills, 186
Emerging diseases, 486–491
EMFs. *See* Electric and magnetic fields (EMFs)
Emotion(s), 41–42
    over abortion, 192
    eating and, 215, 264, 278
    managing responses and, 83
    negative, 89
    positive, 51
    in pregnancy process, 199
Emotional attachment, 131, 132
Emotional availability, 131, 132
Emotional component of love, 134
Emotional health, 9, 41–42
    for pregnancy, 193–194
Empathy, listening and, 127
Emphysema, 516, 517
    smoking and, 376, 377
EMR. *See* Exercise metabolic rate (EMR)
Enablers, 334, 335
Enabling factors, in change, 25

Endemic disease, colds as, 478
Endocrine glands, weight loss and, 278
Endocrine system, menstruation and, 159
Endogenous microorganisms, 472
Endometrial (uterine) cancer, 456, 462
    early detection of, 456
    obesity and, 447
Endometriosis, 206, 520, 521–522
    environmental influences on, 590
Endometrium, 159
Endorphins
    addiction and, 326
    in love, 134
    opium addiction and, 403
Endothelium, 422
Endurance, muscular, 306–309
Energy healing, 635
    therapies in, 636–637
Energy/vigor, physical activity and, 299
Enjoyment, in friendships, 133
Enkephalin, addiction and, 326
Enterococcus, antibiotics and, 607
Environment
    addiction and, 327–328
    anxiety disorders and, 58
    cancer risks and, 450
    disease and, 8
    health risks and, 30
    infectious diseases and, 473
    obesity and, 274–275
    psychosocial health and, 44
Environmental health, 9
    air pollution and, 378, 580–587
    environmental racism and, 593
    land pollution and, 590–593
    noise pollution and, 590
    overpopulation and, 578–579
    radiation and, 594–597
    speaking out about, 596
    water pollution and, 587–590
Environmental Protection Agency (EPA), 581
    hazardous waste management by, 592–593
    on secondhand tobacco smoke, 378
    water quality and, 587
Environmental stress, 77
Environmental (passive) tobacco smoke
    (ETS), 378, 450–451, 453
Enzymes, 482
    in digestion, 221
EPA. See Environmental Protection
    Agency (EPA)
Ephedra, 644
Epidemics, 6, 472
Epidermis, 475
Epididymis, 162
Epilepsy, 518, 519–520
Epinephrine, 68, 70
Episiotomy, 202
Epstein-Barr virus
    cancer and, 451
    infectious mononucleosis and, 477
Equipment, exercise, 318
Erectile dysfunction, 169
Ergogenic aids, 641
Ergogenic drug, 408, 409
Ergot, for migraines, 519
Erickson v. Bartell Drug Co., 183
Erikson, Erik, 544

Erogenous zones, 166, 167
ERT. See Estrogen replacement therapy (ERT)
Escherichia coli O157:H7. See E. coli bacteria
Esophagus, 221
    cancer of, 246
Essential amino acids, 226
Essential hypertension, 431
Estrogen, 160
    Alzheimer's disease and, 549
    breast cancer risk and, 450
    heart disease and, 433–435
    menopause and, 161–162
    in oral contraceptives, 181
    osteoporosis and, 240
    tamoxifen and, 464
Estrogen Replacement and Atherosclerosis
    (ERA) Trial (2000), 434
Estrogen replacement therapy (ERT), 166. See
    also Hormone replacement therapy (HRT)
Ethical issues
    in health care for elderly, 543
    Philip Morris's charitable work as, 368
    students' right to privacy and, 344
Ethnicity, 5. See also Race; specific groups
    cardiovascular disease and, 432
    diabetes and, 523
    leading causes of death and, 514
    osteoporosis and, 546
    tuberculosis and, 476
    and women's marriage success, 146
Ethnoviolence, 102
Ethyl alcohol (ethanol), 346
ETS. See Environmental (passive) tobacco
    smoke (ETS)
Europe
    drug addiction in, 325, 393
    HIV/AIDS in, 502, 503
European Athletics Championships, sex
    testing at, 157
Eustress, 68
Euthanasia, 568
Every Person's Guide to Antioxidants
    (Smythies), 244
Excitement/arousal phase, of sexual
    response, 165
Exclusiveness, of love relationships, 133
Exelon, 549
Exercise. See also Aerobic exercise;
    Physical activity
    addiction to, 331
    aging and, 546, 552
    benefits of, 311
    cardiovascular disease and, 430
    in cold, 315
    duration of, 303
    equipment for, 312
    for flexibility and strength, 304–306
    frequency of, 301
    in heat, 313–315
    intensity of, 301–302
    as obsession, 300
    for osteoporosis prevention, 546
    during pregnancy, 195, 196
    resistance, 307–308
    starting program of, 304, 317
    stress management through, 85
    tips for buying products and services, 318
    weight and, 280, 283

Exercise-induced asthma, 517
Exercise metabolic rate (EMR), 283
Exercise training, 296
Exhaustion phase, of general adaptation
    syndrome, 70–71
Exhibitionism, 168
Exogenous microorganisms, 472
Expectations, realistic, 46
Expectorants, 610
Expulsion stage, of labor, 201–202
External bleeding, 657
External female genitals, 157–158
External locus of control, 79
External male genitals, 162
Extrinsic (slow onset) asthma, 516, 517
Eye(s)
    aging and, 545–547
    disease from diabetes, 526
    foods and, 241
    injuries during exercise, 312

F

Facial expression, of men vs. women, 138
Factor VII, 427
FAE. See Fetal alcohol effects (FAE)
Faith, 49, 50
    in relationships, 149
    stress management and, 89
Fallopian tubes, 159
Fallout, from Chernobyl disaster, 596–597
False-negative results, in HIV tests, 507
False-positive results, in HIV tests, 507
Family, 132. See also Commitment;
    Marriage; Relationships
    alcoholism and, 354–355, 356–357
    of Alzheimer's patient, 549
    as change agent, 26–27
    children and, 144
    dysfunctional, 139
    impact of addiction on, 334
    osteoporosis and, 546
    psychosocial health and, 44
    smoking and, 377
    in twenty-first century, 145
Family/couples therapy, 62
Family of origin, 132
Family planning, 17. See also
    Contraception
    information about, 579
Family practitioner, 195, 616
Family therapy, for alcohol abuse, 359
FAMs. See Fertility awareness methods
FAS. See Fetal alcohol syndrome (FAS)
Fascination, in love relationships, 133
Fast foods, 224, 250–251
Fasting, 285
Fat (body), 270
    assessing levels of, 270–274
    BMI and, 269, 270–272
    measures of, 272–274
    waist circumference and, 272
    waist-to-hip ratio and, 272
Fat (dietary), 218, 231–233, 234
    limiting, 220
    needs for, 233
    reducing, 232, 427
    saturated, 232, 429
    unsaturated, 232

Hydrostatic weighing techniques, 272, 273
Hydrotherapy, 635
Hymen, 159
Hyperactivity, sugar and, 229
Hyperglycemia, 523
Hyperlipidemia, 422
Hyperplasia, 276, 277
Hypertension, 431
    diet and, 241
    physical fitness and, 297–298
    stress and, 71
Hypertrophy, 276, 277, 308
Hypervitaminosis, 235
Hypnosis, 635, 637
    for stress management, 87
Hypothalamus, 70
Hypothermia, 315
    emergency treatment for, 659
Hysterectomy, 185, 520, 521–522

I

IBS. See Irritable bowel syndrome (IBS)
Ibuprofen, 609
Ice (methamphetamine), 399
ICSI. See Intracytoplasmic sperm
    injection (ICSI)
Idiopathic disorders, 514
Ileum, 224
Illicit (illegal) drugs, 390–411. See also
    Addiction; Drugs; specific drugs
Illness. See also specific conditions
    food-borne, 253, 254
    mind-body connection and, 49–52
Imagined rehearsal, for change, 27
"I" messages, 128–129
Imitrex, 519
Immune deficiency syndrome, 484
Immune system, 482–483
    aging and, 544
    autoimmune diseases and, 590
    bolstering, 483
    cancer risk and, 450
    laughter and, 51
    stress and, 71, 79
    Type C personality and, 52
Immunity
    acquired vs. natural, 485
    active and passive, 485–486
    physical activity and, 299
    spirituality and, 50
    vaccines and, 484–485
Immunization, childhood schedule of, 485
Immunocompetence, 71
Immunotherapy, 464
IMPACT (Initiatives to Mobilize for the
    Prevention and Control of Tobacco Use),
    379
Implants, for contraception, 177
Impotence, 169
Imprinting, in love, 134
Incidence, 17
Incomes, dual, 144
Incomplete proteins, 226
Incontinence, 545
Incubation periods, for viruses, 478
Independence, developmental tasks and, 45
Independent practice association (IPA), of
    HMO, 623

India
    drug addiction in, 393
    gutka (smokeless tobacco) in, 373
    heroin addiction in, 325
    overpopulation in, 578
Indians. See Native Americans
Indirect contact, disease spread by, 474
Individual biological therapies, 638
Individuality, weight and, 281
Individual therapy, for alcohol abuse, 359
Indoor air pollution, 583–585
    health effects of, 584
Induction abortions, 192
Industrialization, population and, 579
Infant, death of, 564
Infant care, 17
Infectious diseases
    antibiotic treatment of, 607
    control of, 17
    resistance to, 72
    risk assessment for, 472–473
    risk factors one can control, 473
    risk factors one can't control, 472–473
    sexually-transmitted, 491–509
    stress and, 72
    treatment of, 18
Infectious mononucleosis, 478–479
Infertility, 206–209
    pill and, 182
    treatment of, 206–207
Influenza, 18, 478
    cold and, 479
    diabetes and, 526
    pandemic, 472
Information
    about health care professionals, 605
    on health care quality, 619
    about health issues, 30–31
    trusting, 7
    from Web, 604, 631
Informed consent, 616
Inhalants, 406, 407–409
    risk of dependence on, 394
Inhalation, of drugs, 392
Inhibition, among drugs, 613
Injections
    contraceptive, 177
    of drugs, 391
    HIV/AIDS and, 505
Injuries. See also specific injuries
    as cause of death, 3
    fitness, 310–316
    intentional, 96, 99–115
    preventing, 653–654
    unintentional, 96, 118–119
Inner critic, 46
Insect vector, for rickettsia, 477
Insoluble fiber, 230
Insomnia, 47
Institute for Aerobics Research, on
    exercise, 299
Institute of Social and Economic Research
    (Cornell University), harassment
    study at, 115
Insulin, 523, 524–525
Insurance. See also Health insurance
    help from, 645
Intact dilation and extraction (D&X), 192

Intellectual health, 9
Intelligence, aging and, 547
Intentional injuries, 96
    campus crime and, 114–115
    domestic violence and, 107–109
    gratuitous violence and, 99–100
    sexual victimization and, 109–114
    terrorism and, 105, 106
Interconnectedness, through spirituality, 48
Intercountry adoption, 209
Intercourse
    anal, 168
    vaginal, 168
Interdependence, behavioral, 132
Interferon, 478
    laughter and, 51
Internal bleeding, 657
Internal female genitals, 159
Internal locus of control, 79
Internal male genitals, 162–165
Internal mammary artery, 437
International Olympic Committee, sex
    testing and, 157
International Planned Parenthood Federation,
    579. See also Planned Parenthood
Internet
    hoaxes and rumors on, 7
    medical resources on, 604, 631
Internet addiction, 331, 332–333
Internist, 616
Interpersonal therapy, for depression, 54
Interrupting, listening and, 128
Intersexuality, 154, 156
Interspecies transmission of disease, 474
Intervention, 16
    for addiction, 335
    for alcohol abuse, 357–359
Interstate, 573
Intestine, small, 224
Intimacy, 132. See also Love
    in healthy relationships, 149
    in love, 134
    overcoming barriers to, 138–140
Intimate relationships, 131–138
Intolerance
    among drugs, 613
    sources of, 102
Intracytoplasmic sperm injection (ICSI), 207
Intramuscular injection, of drugs, 392
Intrauterine device (IUD), 178, 186
Intravenous injection of drugs, 391
    of cocaine, 394–395
Intrinsic asthma, 516
Intuition, stress management and, 91
Inunction, of drugs, 392
Inversion, temperature, 582
In vitro fertilization, 207
Iodine, 238–239
Ionizing radiation (IR), 594
    cancer risk and, 450
Ireland, drug addiction in, 325, 393
Iron, 234, 238–239, 240
Iron-deficiency anemia, 240
Ironman triathlons, 316
Irradiation, of food, 255
Irritable bowel syndrome (IBS), 527
Ischemia, 422, 423–424
ISD (inhibited sexual desire), 169

Staff model, of HMO, 623
"Stage theory," of Kübler-Ross, 561
Staphylococcal infections, 254, 475
    antibiotics and, 607
    staphylococcus aureus, 488
Starch, 228–229
States
    CVD death rates by, 417
    medical marijuana laws in, 400–401
    smoking controls in, 379
Static stretching, 304–305
Statins, 429
Stereotypes, of gender roles, 43
Sterilization, 185
    effectiveness of, 178
Sternberg, Robert, on love, 134
Steroids, 409, 641–642
    anabolic, 408, 409
Steward, H. Leighton, 287
Stewart, Felicia, 492
Stillbirth, 205
Stimulants, 394–399
    amphetamines as, 398
    cocaine as, 394–398
    methamphetamines as, 398–399
    OTC, 611
STIs. See Sexually transmitted infections (STIs)
Stomach, 221
Strain, 68
Strength
    benefits of training, 309
    development principles, 307–308
    exercises for, 304–306
    muscular, 306–309
    overload principle and, 308
Streptococcal infections, 475, 488
    antibiotics and, 607
    flesh-eating, 491
    rheumatic heart disease and, 426
Stress. See also Exercise
    body's response to, 68–69
    buffers for, 87–88
    cancer risk and, 450
    changing responses to, 81–82
    cognitive stress system and, 77–79
    college students and, 80–81
    CVD and, 71, 72
    defined, 68
    downshifting and, 82–83
    emotional response management and, 83
    environmental, 77–79
    general adaptation syndrome and, 69–71
    health effects of, 71–73
    immune system and, 71, 79, 483
    "isms" and, 77
    managing, 67–91, 431
    mental action for controlling, 84–85
    mind and, 72–73
    negative emotions and, 89
    persistent symptoms in PTSD, 80
    personality types and, 79
    physical activity and, 85, 299–300
    psychosocial sources of, 73–77
    St. John's Wort and, 86
    self-assessment of, 74–76
    self-imposed, 77–79
    spirituality and, 50
    support groups for, 87–88

    technostress, 78
    time management and, 85–86
Stress inoculation, 82
Stressors, 68. See also Alcohol
    assessing, 81
    chronic, for college students, 73
Stretching
    aging and, 552
    designing own program for, 306
    exercises for, 304–305
    for flexibility, 307
Stroke, 426–427
    advances against, 438
    deaths from, 17
    smoking and, 376
    warning signs of, 426–427
Student health insurance, contraceptives
    covered by, 183
Subcutaneous injection, of drugs, 392
Subjective well-being (SWB), 50
Substance abuse. See also Alcohol abuse
    (alcoholism); Drug abuse
    violence and, 98
Sucrose, 228
Sudden cardiac death, 416, 417
Sudden infant death syndrome (SIDS),
    205–206
    smoking and, 377
Sudden sniffing death (SSD) syndrome, 408
Sugar
    athletic performance and, 229
    in diet, 228
    hyperactivity and, 229
    intake of, 218
    use of, 220
Sugar Busters (Steward, Bethea, Andrews,
    and Balart), 287
Sugar metabolism, abnormal, 525
Suicide, 59–60
    as cause of death, 3
    drinking and, 343
    preventing, 60
    rates among diverse populations, 59
    rational, 566–568
    warning signs of, 60
Suits, malpractice, 620, 621
Sulfites, as food additive, 256
Sulfur dioxide, 580
Summers, Gemma, 43
Sun, skin cancer and, 459–461
Sunflower, 643
Sunscreens, 460
Sunstroke. See Heat stroke
Superficial adaptation energy stores, 70–71
Superfund, 592
Super-sized meals, 264
Supplements. See Vitamin(s)
Support groups, 45–46
    for stress management, 87–88
Suppositories
    as contraceptives, 180
    for drug administration, 392
"Supressor T's," 483–484
Surgeon General, Healthy People 2000
    and, 9
Surgery
    for contraception, 185
    for weight loss, 288

Surrogate motherhood, 144, 208
Survival rates, for cancer, 466
Susceptibility, to infectious diseases, 472
SWB. See Subjective well-being (SWB)
Sweden, amphetamine use in, 325
Swimming, safety and, 654
Sympathetic nervous system, 70
Sympathomimetic ingredient, 611
Sympathy, listening and, 127
Syndrome X: Overcoming the Silent Killer That
    Can Give You a Heart Attack (Reaven), 423
Synergism, 612
Synesthesia, 404
Syphilis, 496–497
Systemic lupus erythematosus (SLE),
    484, 530
Systolic blood pressure, 297, 431

T

Tai chi, 305, 637
Tamoxifen, 464
Tan, Stanley, 51
Tannen, Deborah, 135, 138
Taoism, tai chi and, 306
Tar, in cigarette smoke, 370
Target heart rate, 301–303
Tattooing, health risks from, 506
Tavris, Carol, 20
Taxol, 464
TB. See Tuberculosis
T-cell lymphotropic virus type III
    (HTLV-III), 501
T-cells, stress and, 72
Tea, 644
    green, 640, 643
    white, 234
Technology
    car safety, 653
    medical care costs and, 619
Technostress, 78
Teeth, smoking and, 377
Teff (grain), 223
Temoshok, Lydia, 52
Tempeh, 228
Temperature inversion, 582
Tension headaches, 518, 519
Tension principle, for strength development,
    307–308
Teratogenic effects, 195
Termination stage, of change, 24
Terrorism, 97. See also September 11, 2001
    bioterrorism and, 106, 491
    defined, 105
    fears after, 97
    increased risks of, 105–106
    Oklahoma City bombing and PTSD, 80
    post-traumatic stress after, 79, 80
    as result of hatred, 103
    violence after, 95, 100
Tertiary prevention, 16
Testator, 573
Testes, 154, 162
Testicular cancer, 461
Testosterone, 162
    as male contraceptive, 177
Test-taking anxiety, 82
Tetanus, from body piercing and tattooing, 506
Tetrachloroethylene, 589

Tetrahydrocannabinol (THC), 399
Thai food, 224
Thallium test, 436
Thanatology, 561
THC. *See* Tetrahydrocannabinol (THC)
Theobromine, 382
Theophylline, 382
Theory of Reasoned Action, 26
Therapeutic touch, 636
Therapist, choosing, 62–63
Therapy
  for alcohol abuse, 359
  process of, 63
  rational-emotive, 28
  for sexual dysfunction, 170–171
Thiamin, 236–237
Thinking. *See also* Mental health
  alcohol impairment and, 343
Third Report on Detection, Evaluation, and Treatment of Cholesterol National Guidelines, 427
Third trimester of pregnancy
  emotions during, 200
  fetal development during, 199
Third world, population growth in, 578
Thomas, Clarence, sexual harassment charges against, 113
Thoreau, Henry David, 83, 90
Three Mile Island, 596
Thrombolysis, 438
Thrombus, 426, 427
Thyroid gland
  Graves' disease and, 532
  weight loss and, 278
TIAs. *See* Transient eschemic attacks (TIAs)
Tibetan medicine, 634
Time, for self, 46
Time management, stress management and, 85–86
Tinctures, 638
Title VII, of Civil Rights Act (1964), 183
T-lymphocytes, 483
Tobacco, 366–382. *See also* Smoking
  addiction to, 374
  advertising of, 367–368
  cancer and, 447
  as cardiovascular disease risk, 427
  deaths from, 19
  environmental tobacco smoke and, 378
  as health hazard, 17
  health-related costs of, 368
  industry, 378–379
  nicotine and, 369, 370
  politics and, 378–379
  products made from, 370–373
  smokeless, 372–373
  social issues and, 366–368
Tobacco smoke, air pollution from, 378, 584
TOBEC. *See* Total body electrical conductivity (TOBEC)
Tofu, 228
Token economy system, as reinforcement, 28
Tolerable upper intake level (UL), 246
Tolerance, of drugs, 326
Toluene, 584

TOM. *See* Traditional Oriental Medicine (TOM)
Tomato-based foods, 241
Total body electrical conductivity (TOBEC), 272, 273–274
Touching, erotic, 167
Toxic shock syndrome (TSS), 161, 180–181, 475
Toxins, 475
Toxoplasmosis, 196, 254
Trace minerals, 235
Traditional medicine. *See* Allopathic medicine
Traditional Oriental medicine (TOM), 633–634
Trager work, 637
Tranquilizers, 608
  Rohypnol as, 407
Transcendence, need for, 49
Trans-fatty acids, 232–234
Transgendered people, 155
Transient eschemic attacks (TIAs), 426
Transition stage, of labor, 201
Transsexual, 155
Transvestism, 168
Trash, disposal of, 592
Traumatic injuries, 310, 311
Trazodone (Desyrel), 55
Treatment. *See* specific conditions and treatments
Tremors, in Parkinson's disease, 521
Trial Lawyers for Public Justice, 183
Trial separations, 146
"Triangular Theory of Love, The" (Sternberg), 134
Trichlorethylene (TCE), 584, 589
Trichomoniasis, 498–499
Tricuspid valve, 418
Tricyclics, 54, 55, 608
Trigeminus nerve, 519
Triglycerides, 231, 428
Trimesters of pregnancy, 198, 199
Trips, LSD and, 405
Triptans, for migraines, 519
Triticale (grain), 223
Tropical diseases, 482
Tropical rain forests, deforestation of, 586
Trust, in relationships, 133, 148, 149
TSS. *See* Toxic shock syndrome (TSS)
Tubal ligation, 185
Tuberculosis, 476, 488
  antibiotics and, 607
Tumor, 444
Turner, Jeffrey, 133
Turner's Syndrome, 156
Twain, Mark, 23
12-step abstinence-based treatment, 336, 337
Twin studies, body type and, 276
Two-person standard, for sexual behavior, 166
Type 1 alcoholics, 354
Type 1 diabetes, 523
  race, ethnicity, and, 514
Type 2 alcoholics, 354
Type A personality, 79
Type B personality, 79
Type C personality (illness-related), 52
  cancer risk and, 450

Type C personality (stress-related), 79
Typical use failure rate, for contraceptive methods, 176

U

Ulcerative colitis, 527
Ulcers, 528
Ultrasound, during pregnancy, 199
Ultraviolet rays, skin cancer and, 459
Underage students, drinking by, 343
Undergraduates, drinking by, 342
Underinsurance, 621
Understanding, in friendships, 133
Unemployment, violence and, 97
Uniform Determination of Death Act (1981), 558
Uniform donor cards, 573–574
Unintentional injuries, 96, 118–119
  as cause of death, 3
United Nations, on world population, 578
United States
  CAM in, 632
  divorce rates in, 147
  environmental racism in, 593
  illegal drug use in, 409–411
  leading causes of death in, 514
  national health care insurance and, 624
  population 65 and over, 541
  violence in, 96–98
United States Department of Agriculture (USDA)
  dietary guidelines of, 221
  Food Guide Pyramid of, 218–220
  organic foods certified by, 257
U.S. Dietary Guidelines, 234
  on weight gain, 272
U.S. Recommended Daily Allowances (USRDA), 247
Unsaturated fats, 232
"Uppers," 398
Urban areas, population growth in, 578
Urethra, 162
Urethral opening, 159
Urinary incontinence, 545
Urinary tract, aging and, 545
USDA. *See* United States Department of Agriculture (USDA)
USRDA. *See* U.S. Recommended Daily Allowances (USRDA)
Utah, Healthy Aging program in, 540–541
Uterine cancer. *See* Endometrial (uterine) cancer
Uterine fibroids, 522
Uterus, 159
UTIs. *See* General urinary tract infections (UTIs)

V

Vaccinations, 17, 485
Vaccines
  cancer-fighting, 465
  contraceptive, 177
  for flu, 478
  for hepatitis B, 480
  immunity and, 484–485
Vacuum aspiration, 191
Vagina, 159
  spermicides and, 180

Credits

Chapter Opening Art

CHAPTER 1, **p. 2:** Paul Klee, *Color Shapes*. Reproduced with permission from the Artist Rights Society, N.Y., Superstock. CHAPTER 2, **p. 36:** Bob Commander, Stock Illustration Source, Inc. CHAPTER 3, **p. 66:** *Racer, Diana Ong*, Superstock. CHAPTER 4, **p. 94:** Noma, The Stock Illustration Source, Inc. CHAPTER 5, **p. 122:** *Rainy Day Crowd,* Diana Ong, Superstock. CHAPTER 6, **p. 152:** Jose Ortega, The Stock Illustration Source, Inc. CHAPTER 7, **p. 174:** Russell Thurston/Getty Images. CHAPTER 8, **p. 212:** *Woman with Fruit,* Louise Williams, Superstock. CHAPTER 9, **p. 260:** Michael Shumate/Getty Images. CHAPTER 10, **p. 294:** *The Runners,* Robert Delaunay, Superstock. CHAPTER 11, **p. 322:** Patria B. Alejandro, *Xul Solar,* Superstock. CHAPTER 12, **p. 340:** *Integration,* Diana Ong, Superstock. CHAPTER 13, **p. 364:** Stephanie Dalton Cowan/Getty Images. CHAPTER 14, **p. 388:** *Wet Paint on Canvas,* Diana Ong, Superstock. CHAPTER 15, **p. 414:** Gayle Ray/Superstock. CHAPTER 16, **p. 442:** Timothy John, The Stock Illustration Source, Inc. CHAPTER 17, **p. 470:** Mick Wiggens, Jacquilee Dedelle, Inc. CHAPTER 18, **p. 512:** Bruno Budrovic, The Stock Illustration Source, Inc. CHAPTER 19, **p. 536:** Dave Cutler/ Images.com, Inc. CHAPTER 20, **p. 556:** Harold Stevenson/Chisolm Gallery, West Palm Beach, Florida/Superstock. CHAPTER 21, **p. 576:** John S. Dykes, The Stock Illustration Source, Inc. CHAPTER 22, **p. 600:** Timothy John, The Stock Illustration Source, Inc. CHAPTER 23, **p. 628:** Stephanie Dalton Cowan/Getty Images.

Photo Credits

CHAPTER 1, **p. 6:** Digital Stock/CORBIS; **p. 16:** Bob Daemmrich/Stock Boston; **p. 26:** Tom Prettyman/PhotoEdit. CHAPTER 2, **p. 42:** Kent Meireis/The Image Works; **p. 47:** Topham/Picturepoint/The Image Works; **p. 54:** Jonathan Nourok/PhotoEdit; **p. 61:** Penny Tweedie/Stone. CHAPTER 3, **p. 68:** Mike Greenlar/The Image Works; **p. 71:** Bob Daemmrich/The Image Works; **p. 81:** Bob Daemmrich/The Image Works; **p. 90:** David Weintraub/Stock Boston. CHAPTER 4, **p. 100:** Zed Nelson-IPG/Matrix; **p. 103:** Rudi Von Briel/PhotoEdit; **p. 108:** Bill Aron/PhotoEdit; **p. 114:** AP/Wide World Photos. CHAPTER 5, **p. 126:** David Young-Wolff/PhotoEdit; **p. 131:** Jeff Greenberg/Stock Boston; **p. 140:** Owen Franken/CORBIS; **p. 144:** Ellen Senisi/The Image Works. CHAPTER 6, **p. 154:** John Curtis/Offshoot Stock; **p. 157:** Joel Gordon; **p. 168:** Frank Siteman/PhotoEdit; **p. 171:** Bill Stanton/Rainbow. CHAPTER 7, **p. 176:** Charles Thatcher/Getty Images; **p. 184:** Joel Gordon; **p. 196:** Michael Newman/PhotoEdit; **p. 198a:** Claude Edelman/Photo Researchers; **p. 198b:** Petit Format-Nestle/Photo Researchers; **p. 198c:** Petit Format-Nestle/Photo Researchers; **p. 203:** Myrleen Ferguson Cate/PhotoEdit. CHAPTER 8, **p. 215:** Steven Rubin/The Image Works; **p. 246:** Novastock/Rainbow; **p. 252:** Bill Aron/PhotoEdit. CHAPTER 9, **p. 263:** Reuters/Fred Prouser/Archive Photos; **p. 273:** David Young-Wolff/PhotoEdit; **p. 274:** Bob Daemmrich/The Image Works. CHAPTER 10, **p. 298:** Topham/The Image Works; **p. 306:** Jim Craigmuyle/CORBIS; **p. 313:** Bob Daemmrich/The Image Works; **p. 316:** Bob Mahoney/The Image Works. CHAPTER 11, **p. 324:** Bonnie Kamin/PhotoEdit; **p. 329:** Mary Kate Denny/PhotoEdit; **p. 331:** Peter Cade/Stone; **p. 335:** Jon Bradley/Stone. CHAPTER 12, **p. 342:** AP/Wide World Photos; **p. 352:** Yva Momatiuk & John Eastcott/Stock Boston; **p. 356:** Richard Hutchings/ Photo Researchers; **p. 359:** AP/Wide World Photos. CHAPTER 13, **p. 368:** Bob Daemmrich/Stock Boston; **p. 371:** David Young-Wolff/PhotoEdit;

p. 372: Courtesy of Romano & Associates Inc./Oral Health America; **p. 379:** Mark C. Burnett/Stock Boston. CHAPTER 14, **p. 397:** Michael Newman/PhotoEdit; **p. 401:** AP/Wide World Photos; **p. 405:** Courtesy of NIDA; **p. 406:** Luc Beziat/Getty Images. CHAPTER 15, **p. 423:** Mike Fiala/CORBIS; **p. 426:** Michal Heron/CORBIS; **p. 433:** Larry Mulvehill/ The Image Works; **p. 437:** Bruce Ayres/Stone. CHAPTER 16, **p. 454:** Charles Gupton/Stock Boston; **p. 458:** Christopher Brown/Stock Boston; **p. 459 left:** James Stevenson/SPL/Photo Researchers, Inc; **p. 459 middle** and **right:** Dr. P. Marazzi/SPL/Photo Researchers, Inc; **p. 465:** Bill Greenblatt/ Newsamakers/ Liaison Agency. CHAPTER 17, **p. 474:** Rudi Von Briel/ PhotoEdit; **p. 484:** Richard Hutchings/PhotoEdit; **p. 496:** SPL/Photo Researchers, Inc; **p. 497:** Dr. P. Marazzi/SPL/Photo Researchers, Inc; **p. 499:** Steven J. Nussenblatt/Custom Medical Stock Photo; **p. 500:** Dan McCoy/Rainbow; **p. 501:** A Ramy/Stock Boston. CHAPTER 18, **p. 516:** John Millar/Stone; **p. 519:** Elena Dorfman/Offshoot Stock; **p. 523:** Donna Day/Getty Images; **p. 528:** Bonnie Kamin; **p. 533:** Spencer Grant/ PhotoEdit CHAPTER 19, **p. 538:** Dan Bosler/Stone; **p. 540 left:** Fred Prouser/CORBIS; **p. 540 middle:** AP/Wide World Photos; **p. 540 right:** AP Photo/Eric Risberg; **p. 544:** Yva Momatiuk & John Eastcott/Stock Boston; **p. 550:** Mark E. Gibson/Rainbow. CHAPTER 20, **p. 562:** Arvind Garg/Photo Researchers; **p. 564:** Mark Reinstein/The Image Works; **p. 566:** Mark Richards/PhotoEdit; **p. 571:** Ben Edwards/Stone. CHAPTER 21, **p. 578:** AP/Wide World Photos; **p. 582:** Will and Deni McIntyre/Photo Researchers; **p. 591:** Seth Resnick/Stock Boston; **p. 592:** Bonnie Kamin/ Photo Edit. CHAPTER 22, **p. 605:** Alain Dex/Publiphoto/Photo Researchers; **p. 617:** Spencer Grant/PhotoEdit; **p. 619:** Larry Mulvehill/The Image Works. CHAPTER 23, **p. 636:** Ron Sutherland/SPL/Photo Researchers; **p. 637:** Rich Frishman/Stone; **p. 638:** Michael Newman/PhotoEdit.

Additional Text and Figure Credits

Page 7: Reality Check: Consumer Beware: Hoaxes, Rumors, and Other Perils of the Internet. Copyright © 2001 Dow Jones and Company, Inc. Reproduced with permission by Dow Jones & Co., Inc. in the format Textbook via Copyright Clearance Center. **Page 102:** Reality Check: Superpredators: A New Generation of Violent Adults? Reprinted by permission of the publisher. **Page 158:** Figure 6.1. Reprinted by permission of the publisher. **Page 160:** Figure 6.3. Reprinted by permission of the publisher. **Page 170:** Figure 6.6. Reprinted by permission of the publisher. **Page 179:** Assess Yourself: Contraceptive Comfort and Confidence Scale. Reprinted by permission. **Page 182:** Figure 7.4. Reprinted by permission. **Page 183:** Health Ethics: Conflict and Controversy: Should Prescription Contraceptives Be Covered by Student Health Insurance? Reprinted with permission. **Page 200:** Table 7.4. Reprinted by permission of Lamaze Publishing Company. **Pages 217-218:** Assess Yourself: What's Your EQ (Eating Quotient)? Reproduced with permission of Center for Science in the Public Interest in the format Textbook via Copyright Clearance Center. **Page 220:** Figure 8.2. Adapted with the permission of Simon & Schuster Source, a Division of Simon & Schuster Adult Publishing Group, from *Eat, Drink, and Be Healthy:* The Harvard Medical School Guide to Healthy Eating. Copyright © 2001 by the President and Fellows of Harvard College. **Page 228:** Skills for Behavior Change: A Consumer's Guide to Soy. From "EN Presents a Buyer's Guide to Selected Soy Foods," by Julie Walsh from *Environmental Nutrition,* May 2002, Vol. 25, #5. Reprinted with permission from *Environmental Nutrition,* 52 Riverside

Behavior Change Contract

Complete the Assess Yourself questionnaire and read the Skills for Behavior Change box describing the stages of change (both in Chapter 1). After reviewing your results and considering the various factors that influence your decisions, choose a health behavior that you would like to change, starting this quarter or semester (see other side for a sample filled-in contract). Sign the contract at the bottom to affirm your commitment to making a healthy change and ask a friend to witness it.

My behavior change will be:

_____

My long-term goal for this behavior change is:

_____

These are three obstacles to change (things that I am currently doing or situations that contribute to this behavior or make it harder to change):

1. _____

2. _____

3. _____

The strategies I will use to overcome these obstacles are:

1. _____

2. _____

3. _____

Resources I will use to help me change this behavior include:

a friend/partner/relative: _____

a school-based resource: _____

a community-based resource: _____

a book or reputable website: _____

In order to make my goal more attainable, I have devised these short-term goals:

short-term goal	target date	reward
short-term goal	target date	reward
short-term goal	target date	reward

When I make the long-term behavior change described above, my reward will be:

_____ target date: _____

I intend to make the behavior change described above. I will use the strategies and rewards to achieve the goals that will contribute to a healthy behavior change.

Signed: _____   Witness: _____

Behavior Change Contract

Complete the Assess Yourself questionnaire and read the Skills for Behavior Change box describing the stages of change (both in Chapter 1). After reviewing your results and considering the various factors that influence your decisions, choose a health behavior that you would like to change, starting this quarter or semester (see other side for a sample filled-in contract). Sign the contract at the bottom to affirm your commitment to making a healthy change and ask a friend to witness it.

My behavior change will be:

To snack less on junk food and more on healthy foods

My long-term goal for this behavior change is:

Eat junk food snacks no more than once a week

These are three obstacles to change (things that I am currently doing or situations that contribute to this behavior or make it harder to change):

1. The grocery store is closed by the time I come home from school

2. I get hungry between classes and the vending machines only carry candy bars

3. It's easier to order pizza or other snacks than to make a snack at home

The strategies I will use to overcome these obstacles are:

1. I'll leave early for school once a week so I can stock up on healthy snacks in the morning

2. I'll bring a piece of fruit or other healthy snack to eat between classes

3. I'll learn some easy recipes for snacks to make at home

Resources I will use to help me change this behavior include:

a friend/partner/relative: my roommates: I'll ask them to buy healthier snacks instead of chips when they do the shopping

a school-based resource: the dining hall: I'll ask the manager to provide healthy foods we can take to eat between classes

a community-based resource: the library: I'll check out some cookbooks to find easy snack ideas

a book or reputable website: the USDA nutrient database at www.nal.usda.gov/fnic: I'll use this site to make sure the foods I select are healthy choices

In order to make my goal more attainable, I have devised these short-term goals:

Eat a healthy snack 3 times per week	September 15	new CD
short-term goal	target date	reward
Learn to make a healthy snack	October 15	Concert ticket
short-term goal	target date	reward
Eat a healthy snack 5 times per week	November 15	New shoes
short-term goal	target date	reward

When I make the long-term behavior change described above, my reward will be:

Ski lift tickets for winter break   target date: December 15

I intend to make the behavior change described above. I will use the strategies and rewards to achieve the goals that will contribute to a healthy behavior change.

Signed: Elizabeth King   Witness: Susan Bauer

Lifelong Behavior Change Contract

Behavior change is a process that continues for a lifetime. The strategies that you begin to follow now can contribute to healthy benefits far into the future. Choose a change that will have long-term positive effects, then complete the contract and put your intentions into action (see other side for a sample filled-in contract). Sign the contract at the bottom to affirm your commitment to making a healthy change and ask a friend to witness it.

My behavior change will be:

_____

My long-term goal for this behavior change is:

_____

These are three obstacles to change (things that I am currently doing or situations that contribute to this behavior or make it harder to change):

1. _____

2. _____

3. _____

The strategies I will use to overcome these obstacles are:

1. _____

2. _____

3. _____

Resources I will use to help me change this behavior include:

a friend/partner/relative: _____

a school-based resource: _____

a community-based resource: _____

a book or reputable website: _____

In order to make my goal more attainable, I have devised these short-term goals:

short-term goal	target date	reward
short-term goal	target date	reward
short-term goal	target date	reward

When I make the long-term behavior change described above, my reward will be:

_____ target date: _____

I intend to make the behavior change described above. I will use the strategies and rewards to achieve the goals that will contribute to a healthy behavior change.

Signed: _____   Witness: _____

Lifelong Behavior Change Contract

Behavior change is a process that continues for a lifetime. The strategies that you begin to follow now can contribute to healthy benefits far into the future. Choose a change that will have long-term positive effects, then complete the contract and put your intentions into action (see other side for a sample filled-in contract). Sign the contract at the bottom to affirm your commitment to making a healthy change and ask a friend to witness it.

My behavior change will be:

To incorporate exercise into my daily life

My long-term goal for this behavior change is:

To maintain a healthy weight and feel fit

These are three obstacles to change (things that I am currently doing or situations that contribute to this behavior or make it harder to change):

1. _I get bored doing the same exercise all of the time_

2. _I find myself watching TV I don't even enjoy and then not having time to exercise_

3. _I'm afraid I'll injure myself doing new activities_

The strategies I will use to overcome these obstacles are:

1. _I'll learn several activities so that I have variety in my exercise program_

2. _I'll give myself a set number of "TV hours" and use the extra time for exercise_

3. _I'll get a complete check-up with my physician before I start a new exercise program_

Resources I will use to help me change this behavior include:

a friend/partner/relative: _I'll ask friends to exercise with me so I stay motivated and don't get bored_

a school-based resource: _I'll find out what types of activities are offered by the PE department_

a community-based resource: _I'll join a local club that does the activity I enjoy most_

a book or reputable website: _I'll track my progress in the Fitness section of my Log Book and Wellness Journal_

In order to make my goal more attainable, I have devised these short-term goals:

Walk to school three times a week	_3 months from today_	_dinner out at my favorite restaurant_
short-term goal	target date	reward
Learn a new activity to add to my exercise program	_6 months from today_	_new outfit_
short-term goal	target date	reward
Participate in the local 10k walk/run	_1 year from today_	_weekend vacation_
short-term goal	target date	reward

When I make the long-term behavior change described above, my reward will be:

vacation trip   target date: _2 years from now_

I intend to make the behavior change described above. I will use the strategies and rewards to achieve the goals that will contribute to a healthy behavior change.

Signed: _Barry Snow_   Witness: _Rob Santiago_